Therapy for
Diabetes
Mellitus
and Related Disorders

SIXTH EDITION

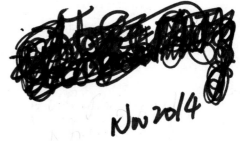

Nov 2014

Edited by
Guillermo E. Umpierrez, MD, CDE

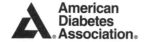

American
Diabetes
Association.

Director, Book Publishing, Abe Ogden; *Managing Editor*, Greg Guthrie; *Acquisitions Editor*, Victor Van Beuren; *Production Manager*, Melissa Sprott; *Cover Design*, Design Literate, LLC; *Printer*, Marquis Imprimeur.

Printed in Canada
1 3 5 7 9 10 8 6 4 2

The suggestions and information contained in this publication are generally consistent with the *Clinical Practice Recommendations* and other policies of the American Diabetes Association, but they do not represent the policy or position of the Association or any of its boards or committees. Reasonable steps have been taken to ensure the accuracy of the information presented. However, the American Diabetes Association cannot ensure the safety or efficacy of any product or service described in this publication. Individuals are advised to consult a physician or other appropriate health care professional before undertaking any diet or exercise program or taking any medication referred to in this publication. Professionals must use and apply their own professional judgment, experience, and training and should not rely solely on the information contained in this publication before prescribing any diet, exercise, or medication. The American Diabetes Association—its officers, directors, employees, volunteers, and members—assumes no responsibility or liability for personal or other injury, loss, or damage that may result from the suggestions or information in this publication.

♾ The paper in this publication meets the requirements of the ANSI Standard Z39.48-1992 (permanence of paper).

ADA titles may be purchased for business or promotional use or for special sales. To purchase more than 50 copies of this book at a discount, or for custom editions of this book with your logo, contact the American Diabetes Association at the address below or at booksales@diabetes.org.

American Diabetes Association
1701 North Beauregard Street
Alexandria, Virginia 22311

DOI: 10.2337/9781580405096

Library of Congress Cataloging-in-Publication Data
Therapy for diabetes mellitus and related disorders. -- 6th edition / [edited by] Guillermo Umpierrez.
　p. ; cm.
　Includes bibliographical references and index.
　ISBN 978-1-58040-509-6 (alk. paper)
　I. Umpierrez, Guillermo E., editor of compilation. II. American Diabetes Association, issuing body.
　[DNLM: 1. Diabetes Mellitus--therapy. 2. Diabetes Complications. WK 815]
　RC660
　616.4'6206--dc23
                    2013042342

Handwritten notes (margin annotations):

ketonemia?
oxidative stress 222 (nutrition excess)
lipohypertrophy
paresthesia
alleviating 缓解
acanthosis Nigricans
polypepsia, polyuria, glycosuria 158
manual dexterity
paronychia
Inflammatory marker - TNF-α, CRP
liver - ↑ fasting glycemic
muscle ↑ postprandial
tenable hypothesis 170
RR
insulin 179
glucagon 423 (primary)

Contents

Preface   ix
List of Contributors   xi

PART I: DIAGNOSIS AND CLASSIFICATION

1. **Diagnosis**   1
   Silvio E. Inzucchi, MD

2. **Classification of Diabetes**   13
   M. Sue Kirkman, MD, and Guillermo E. Umpierrez, MD, CDE

3. **Role of Diabetes Education in Patient Management**   21
   Martha M. Funnell, MS, RN, CDE; Gretchen A. Piatt, MPH, PhD;
   and Robert M. Anderson, EdD

4. **Glucose Monitoring**   28
   Robert A. Vigersky, MD

5. **Medical Nutrition Therapy**   51
   Anne Daly, MS, RDN, BC-ADM, CDE, and Margaret A. Powers,
   PhD, RD, CDE

6. **Exercise**   65
   Judith G. Regensteiner, PhD; Timothy A. Bauer, PhD; and Edward S.
   Horton, MD

7. **Epidemiology of Type 1 and Type 2 Diabetes**   77
   Edward W. Gregg, PhD; Giuseppina Imperatore, MD, PhD; and K.M.
   Venkat Narayan, MD

PART II: TYPE 1 DIABETES

8. **Type 1 Diabetes: Pathogenesis and Natural History**   97
   Guillermo E. Umpierrez, MD, CDE; Francisco Pasquel, MD; and
   Isabel Errazuriz, MD

9. **Assessment and Treatment of Patients with Type 1 Diabetes**   105
   Anne Peters, MD, and Lori Laffel, MD, MPH

paronychia 112

10. **Preservation and Prevention Strategies for Type 1 Diabetes** 116
Jay S. Skyler, MD, MACP

11. **Insulin Pump Therapy: Artificial Pancreas** 128
Jennifer L. Sherr, MD, and William V. Tamborlane, MD

12. **Psychosocial and Family Issues in Children with Type 1 Diabetes** 134
Barbara J. Anderson, PhD, and David D. Schwartz, PhD, ABPP

PART III: DIABETES AND PREGNANCY

13. **Gestational Diabetes Mellitus: Diagnostic Criteria and Epidemiology** 156
Shubhada Jagasia, MD, MMHC *diagnos algorin 160 . liver fasting. insula postprandl* (157)

14. **Gestational Diabetes Mellitus: Management** 168
David A. Sacks, MD

15. **Management of Pregnant Women with Type 1 and Type 2 Diabetes** 197
Elisabeth R. Mathiesen, MD, DMSc; Lene Ringholm, MD, PhD; and
Peter Damm, MD, DMSc

PART IV: TYPE 2 DIABETES

16. **Type 2 Diabetes: Pathogenesis and Natural History** 212
Jack L. Leahy, MD

17. **Obesity and Type 2 Diabetes** 239
Catherine M. Champagne, PhD, RDN, LDN; Frank L. Greenway,
MD; and William T. Cefalu, MD

18. **Obesity and Type 2 Diabetes in Children** 263
Michelle Y. Rivera-Vega, MD; Ingrid Libman, MD, PhD; and Silva
Arslanian, MD

19. **Psychosocial Issues Related to Type 2 Diabetes** 284
Deborah Young-Hyman, PhD

PART V: THERAPEUTICS OF TYPE 2 DIABETES

20. **Prevention Strategies for Type 2 Diabetes** 314
Asqual Getaneh, MD, MPH, and Vanita R. Aroda, MD

21. **Metformin** 341
Clifford J. Bailey, PhD

22. **Insulin Secretagogues: Sulfonylureas and Glinides** 359
Giulio R. Romeo, MD; Martin J. Abrahamson, MD; and Allison B.
Goldfine, MD

23. **Future Use of Thiazolidinediones in Type 2 Diabetes: Practical Lessons** 377
    Kwame Osei, MD, FACE, FACP, and Trudy Gaillard, PhD, RN, CDE

24. **Dipeptidyl-Peptidase 4 Inhibitors** 387
    Pablo Aschner, MD, MSc

25. **Glucagon-Like Peptide-1 Receptor Agonist Therapy for Type 2 Diabetes** 401
    Dima L. Diab, MD, and David A. D'Alessio, MD

26. **α-Glucosidase Inhibitors** 416
    Josée Leroux-Stewart, MD; Rémi Rabasa-Lhoret, MD, PhD; and Jean-Louis Chiasson, MD

27. **Cycloset: A Sympatholytic, D2-Dopamine Agonist for the Treatment of Type 2 Diabetes** 435
    Ralph A. DeFronzo, MD

28. **Sodium-Glucose Cotransporter-2 Inhibitors and Type 2 Diabetes** 445
    Muhammad A. Abdul-Ghani, MD, PhD; Luke Norton, PhD; and Ralph A. DeFronzo, MD

29. **Insulin Therapy in Type 2 Diabetes** 461
    Darin E. Olson, MD, PhD; Mary Rhee, MD, MS; and Lawrence S. Phillips, MD

30. **Current and New Long-Acting Insulin Analogs in Development: The Quest for a Better Basal Insulin** 480
    David R. Owens, CBE, MD, FRCP, and Julio Rosenstock, MD

31. **Combination Therapy in Type 2 Diabetes** 508
    Matthew C. Riddle, MD, and Kevin C.J. Yuen, MD, FRCP (UK)

32. **Role of Bariatric Surgery in the Treatment of Type 2 Diabetes** 522
    Steven K. Malin, PhD, and Sangeeta R. Kashyap, MD

33. **Diabetes in the Elderly** 544
    Medha N. Munshi, MD

PART VI: DIABETES IN THE HOSPITAL SETTING

34. **Diabetes in Intensive Care Units and Non-ICU Settings** 559
    Kara Hawkins, MD; Amy C. Donihi, PharmD, BCPS; and Mary T. Korytkowski, MD

35. **Perioperative Hyperglycemia Management** 582
    Dawn Smiley, MD, MSCR

36. **Post-Transplant Diabetes: Diagnosis, Consequences, and Management**   607
    Brian Boerner, MD; Vijay Shivaswamy, MD; and Jennifer Larsen, MD

PART VII: DIABETES COMPLICATIONS

37. **Diabetic Ketoacidosis and Hyperglycemic Hyperosmolar State in Adults**   621
    Guillermo E. Umpierrez, MD, CDE, and Carlos E. Mendez, MD, FACP

38. **Diabetic Ketoacidosis in Infants, Children, and Adolescents**   641
    Joseph I. Wolfsdorf, MB, BCh

39. **Glycemic Control and Chronic Diabetes Complications**   668
    Samuel Dagogo-Jack, MD

40. **Hypoglycemia in Diabetes**   696
    Anthony L. McCall, MD, PhD, FACP

41. **Ocular Complications**   729
    Paolo S. Silva, MD; Jerry D. Cavallerano, OD, PhD; Lloyd M. Aiello, MD; and Lloyd Paul Aiello, MD, PhD

42. **Management of Diabetic Retinopathy**   748
    Maxwell S. Stem, MD; Thomas W. Gardner, MD, MS; and Grant M. Comer, MD, MS

43. **Chronic Kidney Disease Complicating Diabetes**   760
    Mary C. Mallappallil, MD, and Eli A. Friedman, MD, MACP, FRCP

44. **Peripheral Neuropathy in Diabetes**   793
    Rodica Pop-Busui, MD, PhD; James W. Albers, MD, PhD; and Eva L. Feldman, MD, PhD

45. **Autonomic Neuropathy in Diabetes**   834
    Rodica Pop-Busui, MD, PhD, and Martin Stevens, MD

46. **The Diabetic Foot**   864
    Andrew J.M. Boulton, MD, DSc (Hon), FACP, FRCP

47. **Macrovascular Complications and Coronary Artery Disease: Primary and Secondary Prevention in Patients with Diabetes**   876
    Tina K. Thethi, MD, MPH, FACE, and Vivian Fonseca, MD

48. **Peripheral Arterial Disease: Diagnosis and Management**   898
    Enrico Cagliero, MD

49. Dyslipidemia in Diabetes: Epidemiology, Complications, and Management   **908**
Craig Williams, PharmD, FNLA, BCPS, and Steven Haffner, MD

50. Hypertension in Diabetes   **921**
Jorge Calles-Escandón, MD; Thomas A. Murphy, MD; Georges Saab, MD; and Tariq Khan, MD

51. Infections and Diabetes   **941**
Rajeev Sharma, MBBS, MD; Michael Augenbraun, MD, FACP, FIDSA; and Mary Ann Banerji, MD, FACP

52. Skin and Subcutaneous Tissues   **952**
Jean L. Bolognia, MD, and Irwin M. Braverman, MD

53. Hypogonadotropic Hypogonadism in Type 2 Diabetes   **966**
Paresh Dandona, MBBS, DPhil, FRCP, FACP, FACC, FACE; Ajay Chaudhuri, MBBS, MRCP (UK); and Sandeep Dhindsa, MBBS

54. Clinical Implications of Nonalcoholic Fatty Liver Disease in Type 2 Diabetes   **994**
Maryann Maximos, DO; Fernando Bril, MD; and Kenneth Cusi, MD, FACP, FACE

55. Diabetes and Cancer   **1018**
Daniel J. Rubin, MD, MSc, and Ajay D. Rao, MD, MMSc

Index   **1045**

Preface

Diabetes has reached epidemic proportions in the U.S. and throughout the world. The World Health Organization estimates that 347 million people worldwide have diabetes and that by 2030, this number will rise to 552 million. There are many more individuals who are at risk for diabetes. Data from the population-based U.S. National Health and Nutrition Examination Survey indicate that 35% of U.S. adults, representing an estimated 79 million individuals, have prediabetes. In those over age 65 years, this proportion approaches 50%. Diabetes is projected to be one of the five leading causes of death in high-income countries by 2030 and one of the ten leading causes of death worldwide, emphasizing its worldwide public health importance in the 21st century.

The overall burden of diabetes can be calculated not only by its health impact on individuals but also by the cost to the health care system. Diabetes is the leading cause of end-stage renal disease, adult blindness, and nontraumatic lower-limb amputation. It is a major cause of cardiovascular morbidity and mortality and the seventh leading cause of death in the U.S. The average cost of caring for a person with diabetes is greater than twice that for age-matched peers in our health care system. The estimated cost of diabetes in the U.S. in 2012 was $245 billion, of which $176 billion (72%) represented direct medical costs related to diabetes. This number is expected to climb to $336 billion by 2034. Much of the disability and costs associated with diabetes are related to the care of acute and chronic complications. The major tasks of the health care establishment today are to implement strategies to prevent the development of diabetes in at-risk populations and to implement therapies that prevent or minimize complications.

Since the publication of the first edition of this reference book (affectionately known as the "Green Book") in 1971, remarkable advances in both the diagnosis and management of diabetes and its complications have occurred. In 2009, the American Diabetes Association adopted new recommendations for the diagnosis of diabetes and individuals at risk (prediabetes) to better reflect the impact of hyperglycemia on complication risk. Data from observational and prospective clinical trials have shown that targeting the multiple metabolic factors associated with diabetes reduces risk for complications and improves health-related quality of life. This approach includes not only controlling HbA_{1c}, but also blood pressure and lipid levels.

Improved glycemic control clearly results in improvement in microvascular complications in patients with type 1 and type 2 diabetes. In addition, we have learned that early attention to glucose has a "legacy effect," with observed reductions in cardiovascular events and mortality that persist for more than 10 years following implementation of intensive goal-directed interventions. Despite this evidence, wide variations in the care of people with diabetes persist. A significant number of patients do not achieve and maintain treatment targets, contributing to the absence of any significant reductions in the incidence of acute and chronic diabetes-related metabolic complications. These can be attributed in part to lack of access to high-quality health care to certain segments of the population, inadequate dissemination of practice guidelines to health care providers, and the challenges faced by patients in following clinician recommendations.

In this sixth edition, we have been fortunate to gather a group of distinguished clinicians and scientists to provide up-to-date information on the diagnosis, pathophysiology, and management of type 1 and type 2 diabetes and their complications. The book is divided into seven parts; each is subdivided into individual chapters, for a total of 55 contributions by the experts in each field. The first part covers the new diagnostic criteria, classification and epidemiology of type 1 and type 2 diabetes, as well as current information regarding diabetes self-management education, glucose monitoring, exercise, and medical nutrition therapy. The following three parts discuss new advances in the pathogenesis, prevention strategies, psychosocial issues, and treatment of type 1 diabetes, gestational diabetes, and type 2 diabetes. Part five presents detailed information regarding the expanding therapeutic options for management of patients with type 2 diabetes. Part six covers the management of inpatient hyperglycemia and diabetes in patients in critical and noncritical care settings. The final part includes 19 chapters on management and prevention of diabetes-related complications and comorbidities. Each chapter is written as a focused review to provide up-to-date information to guide health care providers and administrators in their efforts to improve the lives of all people affected by diabetes.

I am grateful to American Diabetes Association for the invitation to serve as Editor-in-Chief on this new edition of *Therapy for Diabetes Mellitus and Related Disorders*. I would like to thank all of our authors for their cooperation and excellent contributions in their respective areas of expertise. Finally, the American Diabetes Association staff deserves special recognition for their editorial support.

Guillermo Umpierrez
March 2014

List of Contributors

VOLUME EDITOR
Guillermo E. Umpierrez, MD, CDE
Professor of Medicine
Director, Grady Hospital Research Unit
Emory University
Atlanta, GA

Section Head, Diabetes & Endocrinology
Grady Health System
Atlanta, GA

CONTRIBUTORS

Muhammad A. Abdul-Ghani, MD, PhD
Associate Professor
Department of Medicine
University of Texas Health Science Center
   at San Antonio
San Antonio, TX

Martin J. Abrahamson, MD
Senior Vice President for Medical Affairs
Joslin Diabetes Center
Boston, MA

Associate Professor of Medicine
Harvard Medical School
Boston, MA

Lloyd M. Aiello, MD
Founding Director
Beetham Eye Institute
Boston, MA
Clinical Professor of Ophthalmology
Harvard Medical School
Boston, MA

Lloyd Paul Aiello, MD, PhD
Director
Beetham Eye Institute
Joslin Diabetes Center
Boston, MA

Head
Section of Eye Research
Joslin Diabetes Center
Boston, MA

Professor of Ophthalmology
Harvard Medical School
Boston, MA

James W. Albers, MD, PhD
Department of Neurology
University of Michigan
Ann Arbor, MI

Barbara J. Anderson, PhD
Professor of Pediatrics
Associate Head, Psychology Section
Pediatrics
Baylor College of Medicine
Houston, TX

Robert M. Anderson, EdD
Professor Emeritus
Department of Medical Education
University of Michigan Medical School
Ann Arbor, MI

Vanita R. Aroda, MD
Physician Investigator
MedStar Health Research Institute
Hyattsville, MD

Assistant Professor of Medicine
Georgetown University School of
  Medicine
Washington, DC

Silva Arslanian, MD
Richard L. Day Endowed Professor of
  Pediatrics
Division of Pediatric Endocrinology,
  Metabolism and Diabetes Mellitus
University of Pittsburgh Department of
  Pediatrics
Pittsburgh, PA

Division of Weight Management
Children's Hospital of University of
  Pittsburgh Medical Center
Pittsburgh, PA

Pablo Aschner, MD, MSc
Professor of Endocrinology
Javeriana University and San Ignacio
  University Hospital
Bogotá, Colombia

Michael Augenbraun, MD, FACP, FIDSA
Professor of Medicine
State University of New York, Downstate
  College of Medicine
Brooklyn, NY

Professor of Epidemiology
State University of New York, Downstate
  School of Public Health
Brooklyn, NY

Director, Division of Infectious Diseases
State University of New York, Downstate
  Medical Center
Brooklyn, NY

Clifford J. Bailey, PhD
Professor of Clinical Science
Life and Health Science
Aston University
Birmingham, UK

Mary Ann Banerji, MD, FACP
Professor of Medicine
Director, Diabetes Treatment Center
State University of New York, Downstate
  Medical Center
Brooklyn, NY

Timothy A. Bauer, PhD
Adjunct Assistant Professor
Department of Medicine
University of Colorado, Denver
Aurora, CO

Brian Boerner, MD
Assistant Professor
Division of Diabetes, Endocrinology, and
  Metabolism
Department of Internal Medicine
University of Nebraska Medical Center
Omaha, NE

Jean L. Bolognia, MD
Professor
Department of Dermatology
Yale Medical School
New Haven, CT

Andrew J.M. Boulton, MD, DSc (Hon), FACP, FRCP
President
European Association for the Study of
  Diabetes
Düsseldorf, Germany

Professor of Medicine
University of Manchester
Machester, UK

Visiting Professor
University of Miami
Miami, FL

Consultant Physician
Manchester Royal Infirmary
Manchester, UK

Irwin M. Braverman, MD
Professor
Department of Dermatology
Yale Medical School
New Haven, CT

Fernando Bril, MD
Postdoctoral Associate
Division of Endocrinology, Diabetes, and
Metabolism
Department of Medicine
University of Florida
Gainesville, FL

Enrico Cagliero, MD
Associate Professor of Medicine
Harvard Medical School
Boston, MA

Jorge Calles-Escandón, MD
Professor of Internal Medicine and Director
Division of Endocrinology
MetroHealth Regional and Case Western
Reserve University
Cleveland, OH

Jerry D. Cavallerano, OD, PhD
Staff Optometrist and Assistant to the
Director
Beetham Eye Institute
Joslin Diabetes Center
Boston, MA

Associate Professor of Ophthalmology
Harvard Medical School
Boston, MA

William T. Cefalu, MD
Douglas L. Manship, Sr., Professor of
Diabetes
Executive Director
Pennington Biomedical Research Center
Louisiana State University System
Baton Rouge, LA

**Catherine M. Champagne, PhD, RDN,
LDN**
Professor and Chief
Nutritional Epidemiology/Dietary
Assessment & Nutrition Counseling
Pennington Biomedical Research Center
Louisiana State University System
Baton Rouge, LA

Ajay Chaudhuri, MBBS, MRCP (UK)
Associate Professor of Medicine
Program Director, Endocrinology
State University of New York at Buffalo
Buffalo, NY

Jean-Louis Chiasson, MD
Professor, Research Unit Director
Medicine Department
Centre de recherche du Centre Hospitalier
de l'Université de Montréal
(CR-CHUM)
Université de Montréal
Montreal, Québec, Canada

Grant M. Comer, MD, MS
Assistant Professor, Ophthalmology and
Visual Sciences
Edward T. and Ellen K. Dryer Career
Development Professor in
Ophthalmology and Visual Sciences
Department of Ophthalmology and Visual
Sciences
University of Michigan, W. K. Kellogg Eye
Center
Ann Arbor, MI

Kenneth Cusi, MD, FACP, FACE
Professor of Medicine
Chief, Endocrinology, Diabetes and
Metabolism Division
University of Florida
Gainesville, FL

Samuel Dagogo-Jack, MD
Department of Medicine
Division of Endocrinology, Diabetes &
Metabolism
University of Tennessee Health Science
Center
Memphis, TN

David A. D'Alessio, MD
Director, Division of Endocrinology
Professor, Department of Medicine
University of Cincinnati
Cincinnati, OH

Anne Daly, MS, RDN, BC-ADM, CDE
Director of Nutrition & Diabetes Education
HSHS Medical Group
Springfield Diabetes & Endocrine Center
Springfield, IL

Peter Damm, MD, DMSc
Professor, Specialist in Obstetrics and
  Gynecology
Center for Pregnant Women with Diabetes
Department of Obstetrics
Rigshospitalet, University of Copenhagen
Copenhagen, Denmark

**Paresh Dandona, MBBS, DPhil, FRCP,
  FACP, FACC, FACE**
Founder, Diabetes-Endocrinology Center of
  WNY
Chief of the Division of Endocrinology
State University of New York at Buffalo
Buffalo, NY

SUNY Distinguished Professor of Medicine
State University of New York at Buffalo
Buffalo, NY

Ralph A. DeFronzo, MD
Professor of Medicine
Chief, Diabetes Division
Department of Medicine
University of Texas Health Science Center
  at San Antonio
San Antonio, TX

Sandeep Dhindsa, MBBS
Associate Professor of Medicine
Fellowship Program Director
Division of Endocrinology and Metabolism
Texas Tech University Health Sciences
  Center
Odessa, TX

Dima L. Diab, MD
Assistant Professor of Clinical Medicine
Associate Program Director
Director, UC Bone Health and
  Osteoporosis Center
Division of Endocrinology, Diabetes and
  Metabolism
University of Cincinnati College of
  Medicine
Cincinnati, OH

Amy C. Donihi, PharmD, BCPS
Associate Professor
Department of Pharmacy and Therapeutics
University of Pittsburgh School of
  Pharmacy
Pittsburgh, PA

Isabel Errazuriz, MD
Postdoctoral Fellow
Division of Endocrinology
Emory University
Atlanta, GA

Eva L. Feldman, MD, PhD
Department of Neurology
University of Michigan
Ann Arbor, MI

Vivian Fonseca, MD
Professor of Medicine and Pharmacology
Tullis Tulane Alumni Chair in Diabetes
Chief, Section of Endocrinology
Tulane University Health Sciences Center
New Orleans, LA

Professor of Medicine
Chief, Section of Endocrinology
Southeast Louisiana Veterans Health Care
  System
New Orleans, LA

Eli A. Friedman, MD, MACP, FRCP
Distinguished Teaching Professor
Department of Medicine
State University of New York
Downstate Medical Center
Brooklyn, NY

Martha M. Funnell, MS, RN, CDE
Associate Research Scientist
Department of Medical Education
University of Michigan Medical School
Ann Arbor, MI

Trudy Gaillard, PhD, RN, CDE
Research Assistant Professor of Medicine
Department of Internal Medicine
Division of Endocrinology, Diabetes and
  Metabolism
The Ohio State University Wexner Medical
  Center
Columbus, OH

Thomas W. Gardner, MD, MS
Associate Chair for Research
Professor, Ophthalmology and Visual
Sciences
Professor, Molecular & Integrative
Physiology
Department of Ophthalmology and Visual
Sciences
University of Michigan, W. K. Kellogg Eye
Center
Ann Arbor, MI

Asqual Getaneh, MD, MPH
Research Physician
MedStar Health Research Institute
Hyattsville, MD

Allison B. Goldfine, MD
Section Head of Clinical Research
Joslin Diabetes Center
Boston, MA

Associate Professor
Harvard Medical School
Boston, MA

Frank L. Greenway, MD
Professor and Head of Outpatient Research
Clinic
Department of Clinical Trials
Pennington Biomedical Research Center
Louisiana State University System
Baton Rouge, LA

Edward W. Gregg, PhD
Chief, Epidemiology and Statistics Branch
Division of Diabetes Translation
National Center for Chronic Disease
Prevention and Health Promotion
Centers for Disease Control and Prevention
Atlanta, GA

Steven Haffner, MD
Professor
Department of Medicine
University of Texas Health Science Center
San Antonio, TX

Kara Hawkins, MD
Staff Endocrinologist
Department of Medicine
Martha Jefferson Medical and Surgical
Associates
Charlottesville, VA

Edward S. Horton, MD
Professor of Medicine, Senior Investigator
Joslin Diabetes Center
Harvard Medical School
Boston, MA

Giuseppina Imperatore, MD, PhD
Leader, Epidemiology Section
Division of Diabetes Translation
National Center for Chronic Disease
Prevention and Health Promotion
Centers for Disease Control and Prevention
Atlanta, GA

Silvio E. Inzucchi, MD
Professor of Medicine
Clinical Chief
Section of Endocrinology
Yale University School of Medicine
New Haven, CT

Director, Yale Diabetes Center
Yale-New Haven Hospital
New Haven, CT

Shubhada Jagasia, MD, MMHC
Associate Professor of Medicine
Associate Director, Clinical Affairs
Division of Endocrinology, Diabetes and
Metabolism
Vanderbilt University Medical Center
Nashville, TN

Sangeeta R. Kashyap, MD
Associate Professor of Medicine
Lerner College of Medicine
Department of Endocrinology, Diabetes and
Metabolism
Cleveland Clinic
Cleveland, OH

Tariq Khan, MD
Assistant Professor of Internal Medicine
Division of Endocrinology
MetroHealth Regional and Case Western
Reserve University
Cleveland, OH

M. Sue Kirkman, MD
Professor
Department of Medicine
University of North Carolina
Chapel Hill, NC

Mary T. Korytkowski, MD
Interim Chief, Division of Endocrinology
Professor
Department of Medicine
University of Pittsburgh
Pittsburgh, PA

Lori Laffel, MD, MPH
Chief, Pediatric, Adolescent and Young
  Adult Section
Joslin Diabetes Center
Boston, MA

Senior Investigator, Genetics and
  Epidemiology Section
Joslin Diabetes Center
Boston, MA

Associate Professor of Pediatrics
Harvard Medical School
Boston, MA

Jennifer Larsen, MD
Louise and Morton Degen Professor
Division of Diabetes, Endocrinology, and
  Metabolism
Department of Internal Medicine
University of Nebraska Medical Center
Omaha, NE

Jack L. Leahy, MD
Chief
Division of Endocrinology, Diabetes and
  Metabolism
University of Vermont
Colchester, VT

Josée Leroux-Stewart, MD
Resident in Endocrinology
Department of Medicine, Division of
  Endocrinology
Centre Hospitalier de l'Université de
  Montréal
Montréal, Québec
Canada

Ingrid Libman, MD, PhD
Assistant Professor
Division of Pediatric Endocrinology,
  Metabolism and Diabetes Mellitus
University of Pittsburgh Department of
  Pediatrics
Pittsburgh, PA

Division of Weight Management
Children's Hospital of University of
  Pittsburgh Medical Center
Pittsburgh, PA

Steven K. Malin, PhD
Postdoctoral Research Fellow
Department of Pathobiology
Lerner Research Institute
Cleveland Clinic
Cleveland, OH

Mary C. Mallappallil, MD
Assistant Professor of Medicine
Continuing Medical Education Director
Division of Nephrology
State University of New York at Downstate
  Medical Center
Brooklyn, NY

Elisabeth R. Mathiesen, MD, DMSc
Professor, Specialist in Endocrinology
Center for Pregnant Women with Diabetes
Department of Endocrinology
Rigshospitalet, University of Copenhagen
Copenhagen, Denmark

Maryann Maximos, DO
Fellow
Division of Gastroenterology, Hepatology,
  and Nutrition
Department of Pediatrics
University of Florida
Gainesville, FL

Anthony L. McCall, MD, PhD, FACP
James M. Moss Professor of Diabetes
Department of Medicine
Division of Endocrinology & Metabolism
University of Virginia School of Medicine
Charlottesville, VA

Carlos E. Mendez, MD, FACP
Director, Diabetes Management Program
Samuel Stratton VA Medical Center
Albany, NY

Assistant Professor, Department of Medicine
Albany Medical College
Albany, NY

Medha N. Munshi, MD
Director
Joslin Geriatric Diabetes Clinic
Department of Medicine, Division of
    Geriatrics
Beth Israel Deaconess Medical Center
Harvard Medical School
Boston, MA

Thomas A. Murphy, MD
Associate Professor of Internal Medicine
Division of Endocrinology
MetroHealth Regional and Case Western
    Reserve University
Cleveland, OH

Luke Norton, PhD
Assistant Professor
Department of Medicine
University of Texas Health Science Center
    at San Antonio
San Antonio, TX

Darin E. Olson, MD, PhD
Assistant Professor of Medicine
Division of Endocrinology, Metabolism and
    Lipids
Emory University School of Medicine
Atlanta, GA

Kwame Osei, MD, FACE, FACP
Professor Emeritus of Medicine and
    Exercise Physiology
Director, Diabetes Research Center
Division of Endocrinology, Diabetes and
    Metabolism
The Ohio State University Wexner Medical
    Center
Columbus, OH

David R. Owens, CBE, MD, FRCP
Professor of Diabetes
Institute of Life Sciences College of
    Medicine
Swansea University
Wales, UK

Francisco Pasquel, MD
Assistant Professor of Medicine
Division of Endocrinology
Emory University
Atlanta, GA

Anne Peters, MD
Professor
Keck School of Medicine of USC
Division of Endocrinology
University of Southern California
Los Angeles, CA

Lawrence S. Phillips, MD
Professor of Medicine
Atlanta VA Medical Center
Atlanta, GA

Division of Endocrinology
Department of Medicine
Emory University School of Medicine
Atlanta, GA

Gretchen A. Piatt, MPH, PhD
Assistant Professor
Department of Medical Education
University of Michigan Medical School
Ann Arbor, MI

Rodica Pop-Busui, MD, PhD
Associate Professor of Internal Medicine
Metabolism, Endocrinology and Diabetes
University of Michigan
Ann Arbor, MI

Margaret A. Powers, PhD, RD, CDE
Research Scientist
International Diabetes Center at Park
    Nicollet
Minneapolis, MN

Rémi Rabasa-Lhoret, MD, PhD
Associate Professor, Research Unit Director
Nutrition Department
Institut de Recherches Cliniques de
    Montréal (IRCM)
Université de Montréal
Montreal, Québec, Canada

Ajay D. Rao, MD, MMSc
Assistant Professor of Medicine
Section of Endocrinology, Diabetes and
    Metabolism
Temple University School of Medicine
Philadelphia, PA

Judith G. Regensteiner, PhD
Professor of Medicine
Director, Center for Women's Health
    Research
Judith and Joseph Wagner Chair of
    Women's Health Research
Department of Medicine
University of Colorado School of Medicine
Aurora, CO

Mary Rhee, MD, MS
Assistant Professor
Department of Medicine
Division of Endocrinology, Metabolism and
    Lipids
Emory University School of Medicine
Atlanta, GA

Matthew C. Riddle, MD
Professor
Division of Endocrinology, Diabetes, &
    Clinical Nutrition
Department of Medicine
Oregon Health & Science University
Portland, OR

Lene Ringholm, MD, PhD
Specialist in Endocrinology
Center for Pregnant Women with Diabetes
Department of Endocrinology
Rigshospitalet, University of Copenhagen
Copenhagen, Denmark

Michelle Y. Rivera-Vega, MD
Pediatric Endocrinology Fellow
Division of Pediatric Endocrinology,
    Metabolism and Diabetes Mellitus
University of Pittsburgh Department of
    Pediatrics
Pittsburgh, PA

Division of Weight Management
Children's Hospital of University of
    Pittsburgh Medical Center
Pittsburgh, PA

Giulio R. Romeo, MD
Clinical Fellow
Joslin Diabetes Center
Boston, MA

Division of Endocrinology, Diabetes and
    Metabolism
Beth Israel Deaconess Medical Center
Harvard Medical School
Boston, MA

Julio Rosenstock, MD
Director
Dallas Diabetes and Endocrine Center at
    Medical City
Dallas, TX

Clinical Professor of Medicine
University of Texas Southwestern Medical
    Center
Dallas, TX

Daniel J. Rubin, MD, MSc
Assistant Professor of Medicine
Section of Endocrinology, Diabetes and
    Metabolism
Temple University School of Medicine
Philadelphia, PA

Georges Saab, MD
Assistant Professor of Internal Medicine
Division of Nephrology
MetroHealth Regional and Case Western
    Reserve University
Cleveland, OH

David A. Sacks, MD
Associate Investigator
Department of Research and Evaluation
Kaiser Permanente Southern California
Pasadena, CA

Clinical Professor
Department of Obstetrics and Gynecology
Keck School of Medicine
University of Southern California
Los Angeles, CA

David D. Schwartz, PhD, ABPP
Assistant Professor of Pediatrics
Department of Pediatrics
Baylor College of Medicine
Houston, TX

Rajeev Sharma, MBBS, MD
Clinical Fellow
Division of Endocrinology
State University of New York, Downstate
    Medical Center
Brooklyn, NY

Jennifer L. Sherr, MD
Assistant Professor of Pediatrics
Department of Pediatrics
Yale School of Medicine
New Haven, CT

Vijay Shivaswamy, MD
Associate Professor
Division of Diabetes, Endocrinology, and
    Metabolism
Department of Internal Medicine
University of Nebraska Medical Center
Omaha, NE

Paolo S. Silva, MD
Staff Ophthalmologist and Assistant Chief
    of Telemedicine
Beetham Eye Institute
Joslin Diabetes Center
Boston, MA

Instructor in Ophthalmology
Harvard Medical School
Boston, MA

Jay S. Skyler, MD, MACP
Professor
Division of Endocrinology, Diabetes, &
    Metabolism
University of Miami Miller School of
    Medicine

Deputy Director—Diabetes Research
    Institute
University of Miami Miller School of
    Medicine
Miami, FL

Dawn Smiley, MD, MSCR
Associate Professor of Medicine
Division of Endocrinology, Metabolism and
    Lipids
Emory University School of Medicine
Atlanta, GA

Maxwell S. Stem, MD
Resident Physician
Department of Ophthalmology and Visual
    Sciences
University of Michigan, W. K. Kellogg Eye
    Center
Ann Arbor, MI

Martin Stevens, MD
School of Clinical and Experimental
    Medicine
University of Birmingham
Heart of England NHS Foundation Trust
Birmingham, UK

William V. Tamborlane, MD
Professor of Pediatrics
Department of Pediatrics
Yale School of Medicine
New Haven, CT

Tina K. Thethi, MD, MPH, FACE
Assistant Professor of Medicine
Section of Endocrinology
Tulane University Health Sciences Center
New Orleans, LA

Assistant Professor of Medicine
Section of Endocrinology
Southeast Louisiana Veterans Health Care
    System
New Orleans, LA

K.M. Venkat Narayan, MD
Director, Emory Global Diabetes Research
   Center
Ruth and O.C. Hubert Chair in Global
   Health
Professor of Epidemiology and Medicine
Emory University
Atlanta, GA

Robert A. Vigersky, MD
Director, Diabetes Institute
Endocrinology, Diabetes and Metabolism
   Service
Walter Reed National Military Medical
   Center
Bethesda, MD

Craig Williams, PharmD, FNLA, BCPS
Professor of Pharmacy Practice
Department of Pharmacy Practice
OSU/OHSU College of Pharmacy
Portland, OR

Joseph I. Wolfsdorf, MB, BCh
Clinical Director and Associate Chief
Division of Endocrinology
Department of Medicine
Boston Children's Hospital
Boston, MA

Deborah Young-Hyman, PhD
Health Scientist Administrator
Office of Behavioral and Social Sciences
   Research
Office of the Director, NIH
Bethesda, MD

Kevin C.J. Yuen, MD, FRCP (UK)
Associate Professor
Division of Endocrinology, Diabetes, &
   Clinical Nutrition
Department of Medicine
Oregon Health & Science University
Portland, OR

Chapter 1

Diagnosis

Silvio E. Inzucchi, MD

INTRODUCTION

D iabetes is a chronic multisystem disease of complex and variable pathogenesis, associated with multiple long-term complications, predominately involving the vasculature. Its diagnosis is based on the documentation of hyperglycemia, either through the direct measurement of plasma glucose concentrations or elevations in glycated hemoglobin, a stable measure of long-term systemic glucose concentrations. In some circumstances, symptoms of hyperglycemia also may be used for diagnostic purposes, in conjunction with direct measurement of plasma glucose.

Type 1 diabetes (T1D) occurs from autoimmune destruction of pancreatic β-cells, which are responsible for the secretion of insulin. This typically is encountered in children, teens, and young adults, but the diagnosis of T1D may be made at any age. Because circulating glucose concentrations usually are elevated markedly in this condition, the diagnosis is straightforward. Indeed, the presentation may be fulminant, accompanied by metabolic decompensation (i.e., diabetic ketoacidosis.) In contradistinction, type 2 diabetes (T2D) evolves over many years and has a lengthy asymptomatic period. Its identification therefore is more challenging and relies predominately on the clinical laboratory. This condition is preceded by years of mildly elevated glucose levels that are above the normal range but not high enough to indicate diabetes. This period often is referred to as *prediabetes*, encompassing stages referred to as "impaired fasting glucose" or "impaired glucose tolerance," each having specific diagnostic criteria. Admittedly, glycemia in the development of T2D is a continuum and the cut points used for its diagnosis remain somewhat arbitrary. Gestational diabetes mellitus (GDM) is a distinct condition that is related to T2D and presents during pregnancy; its identification is discussed in chapter 13.

DIAGNOSIS AND SCREENING FOR DIABETES

The American Diabetes Association (ADA) recommends the periodic screening of individuals at risk for T2D. Criteria for whom to screen and when are listed in Table 1.1.[1] Before 1997, the diagnosis of diabetes had been defined by the ADA as a fasting plasma glucose (FPG) ≥140 mg/dl (7.8 mmol/l) or a 2-hour PG during a 75-gram oral glucose tolerance test (OGTT) of ≥200 mg/dl (11.1 mmol/l). These criteria were based on recommendations of a widely cited consensus document

DOI: 10.2337/9781580405096.01

A1C

7

FPG

126

from the National Diabetes Data Group.[2] The cut points were selected because they identified a group of individuals who were subsequently at risk for developing symptoms of uncontrolled hyperglycemia. Two decades later, the Expert Committee on the Diagnosis and Classification of Diabetes[3] recommended that the criteria be changed to better reflect the impact of hyperglycemia on complication risk. They advised that the diagnostic threshold for FPG be lowered to 126 mg/dl (7.0 mmol/l), since this was the range at which the risk of diabetic retinopathy appeared to initiate. The ADA endorsed this recommendation and has used this arguably more biologically relevant diagnostic criterion ever since. (The OGTT threshold remained unchanged [≥200 mg/dl (11.1 mmol/l) at 2 hours].) Although the OGTT is known to be a more sensitive test, its reproducibility is lower than that of FPG. It is also more inconvenient, cumbersome, and expensive; outside of the research setting, and screening for GDM, it is not widely used in the United States. As a result, the FPG has remained the favored test in the U.S., although the OGTT still is considered the gold standard in many parts of the world.[4]

Glycated hemoglobin (or hemoglobin A1C) is used in clinical diabetes care and research studies as a simple method to evaluate the quality of blood glucose control over the previous 2–3 months. The test measures the result of nonenzymatic glycation of the most prevalent protein in blood, namely hemoglobin. Lack of global standardization prevented its use for diagnostic purposes for many years. However, the International Federation of Clinical Chemistry in conjunction with the National Glycohemoglobin Standardization Program established an international reference method and A1C reference standard, the latter based on the assay

Table 1.1 Recommendations of the ADA for Screening Asymptomatic Individuals for Diabetes

1. Screen beginning at age 45 years at least every 3 years.
2. Screen at any age and more frequently if overweight (BMI ≥25 kg/m²) and at least one additional risk factor:
   - Family history of diabetes (first-degree relative)
   - High-risk race or ethnicity (African Americans, Hispanic Americans, Native Americans, Asian Americans, Pacific Islanders)
   - A1C ≥5.7%, IFG, or IGT on prior testing
   - History of gestational diabetes or delivery of a baby weighing >9 pounds
   - Women with polycystic ovary syndrome
   - Hypertension (≥140/90 mmHg or therapy for hypertension)
   - HDL cholesterol <35 mg/dl (0.90 mmol/l) or a triglyceride level >250 mg/dl (2.82 mmol/l)
   - History of cardiovascular disease
   - Physical inactivity
   - Other clinical conditions associated with insulin resistance (severe obesity, acanthosis nigricans)

Note: ADA = American Diabetes Association; BMI = body mass index; A1C = hemoglobin A1C; IFG = impaired fasting glucose; IGT = impaired glucose tolerance; HDL = high-density lipoprotein.

Source: Adapted from American Diabetes Association. Standards of medical care in diabetes-2014. *Diabetes Care* 2014;37(Suppl1):S14.

used in two large clinical trials (Diabetes Control and Complications Trial and U.K. Prospective Diabetes Study) that validated its relationship to clinical outcomes in both T1D and T2D, respectively.[5] In response to these improvements, the International Expert Committee, in 2009, recommended that the A1C be used for screening and diagnosis purposes, with a cut point of ≥6.5%. The committee actually felt that A1C should become the *preferred* test for the diagnosis of diabetes. This recommendation was based on the clear demonstration from several large observational studies that the threshold of 6.5% correlated as well with retinopathy risk as did the glucose-based measures (FPG, OGTT). In addition, there were several recognized advantages to A1C versus fasting glucose, including global standardization, the lack of requirement for fasting by the patient, its reflection of long-term glycemia without any perturbations from acute illness, and physical sample stability (see Table 1.2).[6] While endorsing the committee's recommendation for use of A1C for diagnosis, the ADA did not adopt its status as the preferred test, acknowledging ongoing uncertainties about A1C testing (see Table 1.3) and the lack of availability in certain parts of the world. Accordingly, as of 2010, the ADA recommends that *either* FPG, OGTT, *or* A1C can be used for screening and diagnostic purposes (see Table 1.3), with the choice left to the clinician, depending on patient and visit circumstances.[7] Per these guidelines, the diagnosis of diabetes is confirmed when two abnormal results of the same test on separate days (e.g., A1C 6.7 and 6.8% or FPG 128 and 131 mg/dl [7.1 and 7.3 mmol/l]) or an abnormal result of two separate tests on the same (or a different) day (e.g., A1C 6.7% and FPG 128 mg/dl [7.1 mmol/l]).[1,7]

In spite of its advantages, A1C testing has several drawbacks,[8] including falsely high or falsely low values in some assays in certain hemoglobinopathies (e.g., thalassemia) and in any hematological condition characterized by *increased* red blood cell turnover (e.g., hemolytic anemias; see Table 1.2). Lower values than would be anticipated by ambient glucose levels also are seen in patients with chronic kidney disease (CKD), especially those on erythropoietin analog therapy for CKD-associated anemia. In contrast, iron deficiency and other states characterized by *decreased* red cell turnover may result in falsely elevated A1C levels. Moreover, inconsistencies in measured A1C levels between various ethnic and racial groups suggest some influence of genetic factors on intracellular glycation.[9] A *glycation gap* has been described by several groups as the phenomenon of significantly different A1C levels in patients with similar ambient glycemia.[10,11] Because the glycation reaction is nonenzymatic and should be relatively consistent from individual to individual exposed to similar glucose concentrations, the gap may stem from differential access of glucose to the intracellular compartment or from variations in red cell life span. These caveats must be considered when interpreting A1C levels for diagnosing (and also for managing) diabetes.

On the basis of these disadvantages, since the International Expert Committee and ADA recommendations were released, several investigative groups have called into question the appropriateness of A1C testing for diagnosis.[12–17] Several studies have compared the diagnostic accuracy of A1C to traditional glucose based criteria. Most have demonstrated that A1C testing identifies *fewer* patients with diabetes than either FPG or OGTT. In addition, most studies have revealed significant discrepancies among these various measures with regard to which individuals are

Table 1.2 Advantages and Disadvantages of Three Screening Tests for Diabetes

Testing Method	Advantages	Disadvantages
FPG	■ Extensive experience	■ Fasting required
	■ Widespread availability	■ Reflects glycemic status only at moment of sampling
	■ Low cost	■ Significant biological variability
		■ Potential effects of acute illness
		■ Less tightly linked to chronic complications
		■ Lower sample stability (in collection/transport vessel)
		■ Results influenced by sample source (blood plasma, serum)
		■ Glucose assay not globally standardized
OGTT	■ Most sensitive test	■ Fasting and patient preparation required
	■ Earliest marker of glucose dysregulation	■ Significant biological variability
		■ Poor reproducibility from test to test
		■ Less tightly linked to chronic complications
		■ Lower sample stability
		■ Time-consuming
		■ Inconvenient
		■ Higher cost
		■ Glucose assay not globally standardized
A1C	■ Fasting not required	■ Unreliable in certain hemoglobinopathies
	■ Low biological variability	■ Unreliable in certain anemias (high or low RBC turnover)
	■ Marker of long-term glycemia	■ Unreliable in the recently transfused
	■ Stable during acute illness	■ Falsely low in advanced renal disease
	■ Greater sample stability	■ Racial and ethnic differences
	■ Globally standardized	■ Glycation gap
	■ Tightly linked to chronic complications	■ Higher cost
		■ Not globally available

Note: FPG = fasting plasma glucose; OGTT = oral glucose tolerance test; A1C = hemoglobin A1C; RBC = red blood cell.

Source: Adapted from Sacks DB. A1C versus glucose testing: a comparison. *Diabetes Care* 2011;34:518.

Table 1.3 Major Diagnostic Criteria for Diabetes and Prediabetes/At-Risk States from ADA and WHO

	American Diabetes Association[17]		World Health Organization[11,18]	
	Diabetes	Prediabetes	Diabetes	Impaired Glucose Regulation
Fasting plasma* glucose†	>126 mg/dl (7.0 mmol/l)	100–125 mg/dl (5.6–6.9 mmol/l) [IFG]	>126 mg/dl (7.0 mmol/l)	110–125 mg/dl (6.1–6.9 mmol/l) [IFG]
2-hour plasma glucose† (during 75-gram OGTT)	>200 mg/dl (11.1 mmol/l)	140–199 mg/dl (7.8–11.0 mmol/l) [IGT]	>200 mg/dl (11.1 mmol/l)	140–199 mg/dl (7.8–11.0 mmol/l) [IGT]
Casual (or random) plasma glucose (if obtained in a patient with classic symptoms of hyperglycemia)	>200 mg/dl (11.1 mmol/l)	140–199 mg/dl (7.8–11.0 mmol/l) [IGT]	>200 mg/dl (11.1 mmol/l)	140–199 mg/dl (7.8–11.0 mmol/l) [IGT]
Hemoglobin A1C†	>6.5%	5.7–6.4%	>6.5%	—

Note: ADA = American Diabetes Association; WHO = World Health Organization; IFG = impaired fasting glucose; OGTT = oral glucose tolerance test; IGT = impaired glucose tolerance; PG = plasma glucose.

*All plasma glucoses denoted on this table are from venous sampling.

†All tests (except for casual PG in a symptomatic patient) should be repeated and confirmed on a separate day. (ADA allows for A1C to be paired with FPG on same day—if both are in the diabetic range, the diagnosis is confirmed.)

Source: Adapted from American Diabetes Association. Standards of medical care in diabetes-2013. *Diabetes Care* 2013;36(Suppl.1):S13.

identified with diabetes. As in prior comparison between FPG and OGTT, when both FPG and A1C are tested, three separate patient groups are identified:

- Those who are diagnosed with diabetes using either measure (i.e., have *both* FPG ≥126 mg/dl and A1C ≥6.5%)
- Those with an abnormal FPG only (i.e., FPG ≥126 mg/dl but with A1C <6.5%)
- Those with abnormal A1C only (i.e., with A1C ≥6.5% but with FPG <126 mg/dl)

The lack of overlap in individuals identified by these now commonly used measures is somewhat disconcerting and the implications of being diagnosed by one but not the other are not entirely clear. It is interesting to note that such discordance between FPG and OGTT has not been a well-recognized clinical problem in the U.S. because of the uncommon use of the latter for diagnosis. Given the ease with which FPG and A1C are measured, however, and the fact that both tests frequently are encountered in clinical practice, practitioners now confront discordant data sets. Lack of agreement between tests may stem from inherent measurement variability, from change in glycemic status over time, or from the fact that FPG and A1C (as well as post-OGTT challenge glucose) actually assess different physiological processes. Admittedly, in most circumstances when the tests are discordant, the values are near the margins of the abnormal thresholds, and these differences therefore are less relevant clinically.

Several investigators have reported that a greater proportion of African Americans make up the A1C-only group, and others have found an A1C level in African Americans 0.2–0.4% higher than in other racial groups.[9,15,16] It is not known whether this pattern results from higher postprandial glucose levels in this group or fundamental (i.e., genetically determined) differences in glycation rates or red cell turnover. With increasing use of A1C testing for diagnosis, these differences between groups are important to recognize. Some have proposed race-based A1C cut points for this purpose, although this may be difficult to implement.[18]

The main concern with each of these studies is their definition of the glucose-based tests as gold standards. Because FPG, 2-hour PG, and A1C *each* correlate *equally* well with the risk of retinal microvascular complications, it remains arguable which measure is truly best. To determine this would require a large, long-term, prospective study, which currently is not available. A1C actually may yield a closer relationship to complications because one theory as to the development of microvascular disease is the glycation of cellular proteins. It may be proposed logically that A1C is the optimal diagnostic test because it may directly reflect an individual's susceptibility to the pernicious effects of hyperglycemia. Preliminary data would suggest that those identified as having diabetes by A1C (which represents and integrates both fasting and postprandial glucose over many weeks), might be better predictor of cardiovascular complications, but these data require confirmation.[19] Clearly, more research is needed to better characterize those individuals whose glycemic status is categorized differently by the available tests (i.e., FPG, OGTT, and A1C).

The ADA currently recommends that when two tests are available (e.g., FPG and A1C) and their results are discordant (e.g., FPG 130 mg/dl but A1C 6.3% or FPG 124 mg/dl but A1C 6.7%), clinicians should default to the most abnormal test (if it is repeated and confirmed). Repeat testing should be performed as soon as is feasible.[7]

IDENTIFYING AT-RISK STATES

As β-cell function begins to decline and is no longer able to maintain normal glucose concentrations in the face of insulin resistance, T2D is preceded by an asymptomatic state of mild but usually progressive hyperglycemia. The only recognized at-risk category for T2D before 1997 was referred to as impaired glucose

IGT
IFG

sael 48 g

tolerance (or IGT). It was identified during a 75-gram OGTT when the 2-hour PG fell between 140 and 199 mg/dl (7.8 and 11.1 mmol/l). When the diabetes diagnostic criteria were revised in 1997, there was a need to develop an analogous criterion for an equally impaired and at-risk level based on FPG. Thus, the category of impaired fasting glucose (or IFG) emerged, defined by a fasting glucose substantially above (>110 mg/dl [6.1 mmol/l]) the normal range of 70–99 mg/dl (3.9–5.5 mmol/l) but lower than the diagnostic threshold for diabetes itself (126 mg/dl [7.0 mmol/l]). In 2003, with the intent to approximate the proportion of the population who might be identified at risk by either OGTT or FPG, the Expert Committee recommended reducing the lower bounds of this diagnostic category to 100 mg/dl (5.6 mmol/l).[29] This recommendation was incorporated by the ADA, although the World Health Organization, which had agreed with the revised criteria of 1997, continues to use the 110 mg/dl (6.1 mmol/l) threshold to define IFG (see Table 1.3).

Both these categories sometimes are referred to as prediabetes, denoting their underlying purpose, that is, to identify those at risk for future T2D. Longitudinal studies show that people with either IGT or IFG proceed, without intervention, to develop diabetes at a rate of ~5–10% per year, with those at the higher ends of the glycemic ranges at the greatest risk. Notably, as with the diagnosis of diabetes using different measures, some individuals are identified as having IFG but not IGT, and vice versa, and some individuals fall into both abnormal categories. The last group appears to include individuals who are at the highest risk for developing diabetes. The risk in those with isolated IFG (i.e., without IGT) and isolated IGT (i.e., without IFG) is similar in most analyses.[21] Because the proportion of patients with IGT tends to be greater than IFG in most populations (particularly in women), the former category represents a proportionately greater number of people at risk. Although both prediabetic states carry with them an increased risk of mortality, particularly cardiovascular mortality, IGT has been demonstrated to be a more robust marker for this specific adverse outcome, perhaps because it is more tightly aligned to insulin resistance, which independently has been associated with incident cardiovascular disease.[21]

The 2009 International Expert Committee report on using A1C for diabetes diagnosis underscored the continuum of risk for diabetes with each glycemic measure.[6] Accordingly, the committee elected to actually not identify an equivalent intermediate glycemic category for A1C as it already had been defined for both FPG and OGTT. It did note, however, that people with levels above the laboratory normal range but below the diagnostic cut point for diabetes (i.e., 6.0 to <6.5%) were at very high risk of developing diabetes—more than 10 times that of individuals with lower levels.

In considering these recommendations, the ADA observed that this high (but not quite diabetic) A1C range did not adequately identify a large enough number of individuals who would be categorized as having IFG or IGT by the prevailing conventional criteria. In fact, several prospective studies have demonstrated that the relative incidence of diabetes in those with A1C levels in the range of 5.5 to 6.0% is substantially increased as well, with relative risks three to eight times that of the general U.S. population—a risk not dissimilar to individuals with more mild degrees of IFG or IGT. Data from the National Health and Nutrition Examination Survey (NHANES) indicate that the A1C value that most accurately identifies people known to have IFG or IGT actually falls somewhere between 5.5 and 6.0%.[22] In addition, in the Diabetes Prevention Program (DPP), the clinical trial that confirmed the value of identifying and treating patients with prediabetes, the mean baseline A1C was 5.9 ± 0.5%.[23] This finding indicates that preventive interventions are effective in those with A1C levels both <5.9 and >5.9%. When it revised its criteria to incorporate use of A1C in 2010, the ADA felt that any cut point for prediabetes needed to balance failing to identify those who are destined to develop diabetes with the costs of resource expenditures on falsely identifying individuals who will not. Receiver operating curve analyses of nationally representative U.S. data (NHANES 1999–2006) indicate that an A1C value of 5.7% has modest sensitivity (39–45%) but high specificity (81–91%) to identify cases of IFG (FPG >100 mg/dl [5.6 mmol/l]) or IGT (R.T. Ackerman, personal communication). Another study suggested than an A1C of 5.7% is associated with similar diabetes risk to the high-risk participants in the DPP.[24] After some deliberation, the ADA decided that a reasonable A1C range to identify individuals at risk for diabetes (i.e., prediabetes) would be 5.7 to 6.4%.[7] As with other glycemic measures, however, those with the A1C levels closest to the diabetic threshold are at the highest risk. Accordingly, prevention interventions and follow-up should be most aggressive for those with A1C >6.0%. Other risk factors, including obesity and family history, should be incorporated into this risk assessment as well. Subsequent economic analysis involving nondiabetic patients in the NHANES has suggested that interventions prompted by the ADA's A1C range for prediabetes would be cost-effective.[25]

Discordant results also may be obtained in the evaluation of prediabetes when two different measures are available. In a recent NHANES analysis, the crude prevalence of prediabetes in U.S. adults >18 years of age was found to be 14.2% for A1C 5.7–6.4%, 26.2% for IFG (≥100 mg/dl [5.6 mmol/l]), and 13.7% for IGT. Not unexpectedly, there was considerable discordance between the various definitions of prediabetes. Among those with IGT, 58.2% had IFG and 32.3% had an A1C between 5.7 and 6.4%; 67.1% had the combination of either IFG or A1C 5.7–6.4%.[26] It remains unknown whether prediabetes by FPG but not by A1C (or vice versa) identifies a group at lower (or higher) risk for developing diabetes. Preliminary data suggest that using both tests (i.e., A1C and FPG) to reveal at-risk states may increase the diagnostic yield substantially versus one or the other test. Similar reports concerning the suboptimal performance of A1C to identify at-risk individuals (if compared with glucose-based testing as the gold standard) also have emerged.[16,27,28] Here, the challenges versus FPG (and OGTT) are accentuated by the larger number of individuals who make up these mildly abnormal metabolic states and the inherent imprecision of distinguishing a normal from a mildly increased glycemia. The ADA does not prefer any single test in the evaluation of prediabetes and has no recommendations as to which test may be favored for patient categorization when the results are discordant. Because diabetes risk as determined by any measure is actually on a gradual continuum, any differences between testing results are likely to be less clinically relevant.

A proposed algorithm for diabetes screening is presented in Figure 1.1.

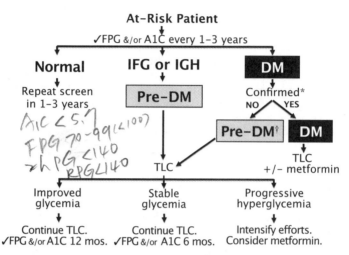

Figure 1.1—Suggested algorithm for diabetes screening.

From: Inzucchi SE. Clinical practice. Diagnosis of diabetes. *N Engl J Med* 2012;367(6):548. Reprinted with permission.

CONCLUSION

Patients with risk factors for diabetes should be screened periodically for diabetes. Three screening tests are now endorsed by the ADA. Which test to use is dependent on several factors, including convenience, availability, cost, and specific patient characteristics that might invalidate a certain measure. Abnormal values generally should be repeated and confirmed on a different day, unless two abnormal tests (e.g., FPG and A1C) already are available from the same day. In certain high-risk individuals, combined A1C and FPG testing is an option. Patients identified as having diabetes should be treated following recent guidelines.[29] Patients with levels above the normal but still not in diagnostic range are at risk for developing progressive hyperglycemia. Recommendations for these individuals to prevent future diabetes mainly include lifestyle changes.[30]

When testing results are discordant, diabetes diagnosis should default to the most abnormal test, if it is repeated and confirmed. In these circumstances, the nondiagnostic test usually hovers near the abnormal range, adding confidence in assigning the diagnosis of diabetes. When test results are widely disparate, however (e.g., FPG 128 mg/dl [7.1 mmmol/l] but A1C 5.3% or A1C 6.9% but FPG 83 mg/dl [4.6 mmol/l]), one of the measures may be misleading or unreliable. This may result from the effects of acute illness on glycemia or, potentially, an aberrant glycation pattern in a specific patient. In such a circumstance, repeat testing is mandatory before diagnostic assignment. Consideration should be given to conducting an OGTT to better clarify the patient's actual status. Recommendations have not addressed the implications of discordant values for prediabetes, although it is reasonable to recommend simple, healthy lifestyle changes in any patient with any test in this range, unless it is clearly an outlier. Evaluation of patients at risk also should incorporate a global risk factor assessment for both diabetes and cardiovascular disease. Importantly, screening for and counseling about the risk of diabetes always should be in the realistic context of the patient's comorbidities, life expectancy, personal capacity to engage in lifestyle change, and overall health goals.

REFERENCES

1. American Diabetes Association. Standards of medical care in diabetes-2014. *Diabetes Care* 2014;37(Suppl 1):S14–S80.

2. National Diabetes Data Group. Classification and diagnosis of diabetes mellitus and other categories of glucose intolerance. *Diabetes* 1979;28:1039–1057.

3. Report of the Expert Committee on the Diagnosis and Classification of Diabetes Mellitus. *Diabetes Care* 1997;20:1183–1197.

4. Alberti KGMM, Zimmet PZ for the WHO Consultation. Definition, diagnosis and classification of diabetes mellitus and its complications. Part 1: Diagnosis and classification of diabetes mellitus. Provisional report of a WHO Consultation. *Diabet Med* 1998;15:539–553.

5. Hanas R, John G; International HBA1c Consensus Committee. 2010 consensus statement on the worldwide standardization of the hemoglobin A1C measurement. *Diabetes Care* 2010;33:1903–1904.

6. International Expert Committee. International Expert Committee report on the role of the A1C assay in the diagnosis of diabetes. *Diabetes Care* 2009;32:1327–1334.

7. American Diabetes Association. Diagnosis and classification of diabetes mellitus. *Diabetes Care* 2013;36(Suppl 1):S67–S74.

8. Sacks DB. A1C versus glucose testing: a comparison. *Diabetes Care* 2011;34:518–523.

9. Ziemer DC, Kolm P, Weintraub WS, Vaccarino V, Rhee MK, Twombly JG, Narayan KM, Koch DD, Phillips LS. Glucose-independent, black-white differences in hemoglobin A1c levels: a cross-sectional analysis of 2 studies. *Ann Intern Med* 2010;152:770–777.

10. Khera PK, Joiner CH, Carruthers A, Lindsell CJ, Smith EP, Franco RS, Holmes YR, Cohen RM. Evidence for interindividual heterogeneity in the glucose gradient across the human red blood cell membrane and its relationship to hemoglobin glycation. *Diabetes* 2008;57:2445–2452.

11. Nayak AU, Holland MR, Macdonald DR, Nevill A, Singh BM. Evidence for consistency of the glycation gap in diabetes. *Diabetes Care* 2011;34:1712–1716.

12. Kramer CK, Araneta MR, Barrett-Connor E. A1C and diabetes diagnosis: the Rancho Bernardo Study. *Diabetes Care* 2010;33:101–103.

13. Jørgensen ME, Bjerregaard P, Borch-Johnsen K, Witte D. New diagnostic criteria for diabetes: is the change from glucose to HbA1c possible in all populations? *J Clin Endocrinol Metab* 2010;95:E333–E336.

14. Olson DE, Rhee MK, Herrick K, Ziemer DC, Twombly JG, Phillips LS. Screening for diabetes and pre-diabetes with proposed A1C-based diagnostic criteria. *Diabetes Care* 2010;33:2184–2189.

15. Carson AP, Reynolds K, Fonseca VA, Muntner P. Comparison of A1C and fasting glucose criteria to diagnose diabetes among U.S. adults. *Diabetes Care* 2010;33:95–97.

16. Lipska KJ, De Rekeneire N, Van Ness PH, Johnson KC, Kanaya A, Koster A, Strotmeyer ES, Goodpaster BH, Harris T, Gill TM, Inzucchi SE. Identifying dysglycemic states in older adults: implications of the emerging use of hemoglobin A1c. *J Clin Endocrinol Metab* 2010;95:5289–5295.

17. Malkani S, Mordes JP. Implications of using hemoglobin A1C for diagnosing diabetes mellitus. *Am J Med* 2011;124:395–401.

18. James C, Bullard KM, Rolka DB, Geiss LS, Williams DE, Cowie CC, Albright A, Gregg EW. Implications of alternative definitions of prediabetes for prevalence in U.S. adults. *Diabetes Care* 2011;34:387–391.

19. Selvin E, Steffes MW, Zhu H, Matsushita K, Wagenknecht L, Pankow J, Coresh J, Brancati FL. Glycated hemoglobin, diabetes, and cardiovascular risk in nondiabetic adults. *N Engl J Med* 2010;362:800–811.

20. Expert Committee on the Diagnosis and Classification of Diabetes Mellitus. Follow-up report on the diagnosis of diabetes mellitus. *Diabetes Care* 2003;26:3160–3167.

21. Unwin N, Shaw J, Zimmet P, Alberti KG. Impaired glucose tolerance and impaired fasting glycaemia: the current status on definition and intervention. *Diabet Med* 2002;19:708–723.

22. Zhang X, Gregg EW, Williamson DF, Barker LE, Thomas W, Bullard KM, Imperatore G, Williams DE, Albright AL. A1C level and future risk of diabetes: a systematic review. *Diabetes Care* 2010;33:1665–1673.

23. Diabetes Prevention Program Research Group. Reduction in the incidence of type 2 diabetes with lifestyle intervention or metformin. *N Engl J Med* 2002;346:393–403.

24. Ackermann RT, Cheng YJ, Williamson DF, Gregg EW. Identifying adults at high risk for diabetes and cardiovascular disease using hemoglobin A1c: National Health and Nutrition Examination Survey 2005-2006. *Am J Prev Med* 2011;40:11–17.

25. Zhuo X, Zhang P, Selvin E, Hoerger TJ, Ackermann RT, Li R, Bullard KM, Gregg EW. Alternative HbA1c cutoffs to identify high-risk adults for diabetes prevention: a cost-effectiveness perspective. *Am J Prev Med* 2012;42:374–381.

26. James C, Bullard KM, Rolka DB, Geiss LS, Williams DE, Cowie CC, Albright A, Gregg EW. Implications of alternative definitions of prediabetes for prevalence in U.S. adults. *Diabetes Care* 2011;34:387–391.

27. Mann DM, Carson AP, Shimbo D, Fonseca V, Fox CS, Muntner P. Impact of A1C screening criterion on the diagnosis of pre-diabetes among U.S. adults. *Diabetes Care* 2010;33:2190–2195.

28. Lorenzo C, Wagenknecht LE, Hanley AJ, Rewers MJ, Karter AJ, Haffner SM. A1C between 5.7 and 6.4% as a marker for identifying pre-diabetes, insulin sensitivity and secretion, and cardiovascular risk factors: the Insulin Resistance Atherosclerosis Study (IRAS). *Diabetes Care* 2010;33:2104–2109.

29. Inzucchi SE, Bergenstal RM, Buse JB, Diamant M, Ferrannini E, Nauck M, Peters AL, Tsapas A, Wender R, Matthews DR. Management of hyperglycemia in type 2 diabetes: a patient-centered approach. Position Statement of the American Diabetes Association (ADA) and the European Association for the Study of Diabetes (EASD). *Diabetes Care* 2012;35(6):1364–1379.

30. Nathan DM, Davidson MB, DeFronzo RA, Heine RJ, Henry RR, Pratley R, Zinman B; American Diabetes Association. Impaired fasting glucose and impaired glucose tolerance: implications for care. *Diabetes Care* 2007;30:753–759.

31. Inzucchi SE. Clinical practice. Diagnosis of diabetes. *N Engl J Med* 2012;36:542–550.

Chapter 2

Classification of Diabetes

M. Sue Kirkman, MD
Guillermo E. Umpierrez, MD, CDE

Diabetes mellitus includes a group of metabolic diseases leading to hypergly-cemia, the *sine qua non* of the disorder. The name emphasizes the patho-logic signs and symptoms of advanced hyperglycemia: diabetes, from the Ancient Greek word for a passer-through or siphon, eloquently describes polydip-sia and polyuria; mellitus, Latin for honey-sweet, was added in the 1600s to con-note that the urine from people with diabetes tasted sweet. The primary metabolic disorders of diabetes stem from deficient or abnormal secretion of insulin or impairment in the hormone's action.

The majority of prevalent cases of diabetes fall into two major classes: type 1 diabetes (T1D) and type 2 diabetes (T2D), which have distinct pathophysiologies. Gestational diabetes, which might be considered a *forme fruste* of T2D, occurs during the insulin-resistant phase of later pregnancy in predisposed women. Myr-iad other types of diabetes have been identified, including monogenic forms, cys-tic-fibrosis–related diabetes (CFRD), diabetes due to pancreatic damage or resection, and drug-induced diabetes. Classifying an individual patient's type of diabetes is not always straightforward, as will be discussed, and there is likely more overlap and ambiguity among the types than classically has been taught.

TYPE 1 DIABETES

T1D is characterized by progressive destruction of the insulin-producing β-cells of the pancreatic islets, leading to severe insulin deficiency or absence. In its clas-sic form (type 1A diabetes), the β-cell destruction is autoimmune in nature. More rarely, patients may develop severe insulin deficiency without evidence of autoim-munity (type 1B diabetes). T1D accounts for ~5% of cases of diagnosed diabetes in the U.S. It is more common in Caucasians than in other ethnic groups and has equal incidence between sexes. Its onset occurs most often during childhood or adolescence, but the disease can occur at any age; incidence in adulthood accounts for a significant, but not precisely known, proportion of new cases of T1D. This fact plus the reality in most of the world that children with T1D grow into adult-hood means that most people with T1D are adults.

The pathophysiology of type 1A diabetes involves a complex and as yet incom-pletely understood interplay between genetic risk and environmental triggers to autoimmunity. Although 90% of cases occur in the absence of family history, rela-tives of those with T1D are at substantially higher risk of developing the disease

DOI: 10.2337/9781580405096.02

antibody:

Factor	OR	p
GAD +	1.32	0.69
ICA +	1.14	0.848
IAA +	4.93	0.017

antigen:

HLA - DR3

HLA - DR4

than those in the general population. The strongest genetic determinants are those in the human leukocyte antigen (HLA) complex on chromosome 6; specifically, two HLA class II haplotypes (DR3 and DR4, DQA0302/501 and DQB0301/0201). More than 90% of children with T1D carry one or both haplotypes. At least one of the high-risk DR haplotypes, however, is found in ~20% of the Caucasian population, and <5% of population with one or both haplotypes develops T1D. Protective haplotypes also have been discovered, particularly the DR haplotype DQB1*0602 gene, which is found in <1% of those with T1D but in 20% of the Caucasian population without diabetes. Weaker genetic associations include the protein tyrosine phosphatase gene PTPN22 on chromosome 1 and the insulin gene on chromosome 11. Genetic predisposition alone is clearly not sufficient to lead to T1D. The concordance rate in identical twins is only 50–65%, and the age of onset between twins can vary by decades, suggesting that one or more environmental factors must combine with genetic risk to trigger the disease.

Autoimmunity is a central feature of the pathogenesis of T1D. Antibodies to islet cells or specific islet antigens are found in most patients before and at the time of diagnosis, while in relatives of index cases, islet antibodies are strong predictors of future development of the disease. Validated antibodies include those to islet cells (ICA), glutamic acid decarboxylase (GAD), tyrosine phosphatase (IA-2), insulin (IAA), or the zinc transporter (ZnT8). It is clear, however, that the antibodies themselves are not pathologic and that cellular immunity is the cause of islet destruction. Histologic examination of pancreatic specimens from people with T1D demonstrates infiltration of lymphocytes (insulitis) with the absence of β-cells and distorted islet architecture. This seems to be the result of activation of CD8 T-cells with specificity for β-cell destruction. β-Cell death results in the release of intracellular antigens accessed by CD4 T-cells and mature B-lymphocytes, with the latter producing the islet-specific antibodies as a result of exposure to autoantigens.

Potential environmental triggers to islet autoimmunity in those with genetic risk have been studied widely, but as yet no clear candidate has been found. Proposed triggers include infections, early introduction of specific dietary components (cow's milk, gluten), vitamin D deficiency, nitrosamine compounds, vaccines, and many others. Conflicting evidence has been found for most. The increased incidence of T1D along with that of asthma and allergies has led to the "hygiene hypothesis," which suggests that reduced exposure to infectious agents early in life may shift immune pathways toward autoimmunity or allergy.

Classifying a patient with newly diagnosed diabetes as having T1D is sometimes, but not always, straightforward. A classic presentation would be a lean child presenting with a few days or weeks of hyperglycemic symptoms that then progress to diabetic ketoacidosis (DKA). The disease can present at any age, however, and many adults have a more indolent presentation. Some adults have mild hyperglycemia that may respond to oral agents for months or even several years before progressing to absolute insulin deficiency requiring replacement, a condition referred to as latent autoimmune diabetes of adults (LADA). The epidemic of overweight and obesity in the industrial world has not spared those at risk for T1D, so new-onset T1D in an overweight child or adult can be confused with T2D. Finally, as will be discussed, ketoacidosis (even unprovoked) can occur in patients who otherwise phenotypically have T2D. Autoantibody testing may be helpful when the type of diabetes is unclear; patients with one or more islet-directed antibodies are likely to have T1D.

TYPE 2 DIABETES

T2D is the most prevalent form of diabetes, accounting for ~90–95% of all cases. It is a heterogeneous disease characterized by peripheral insulin resistance, impaired regulation of hepatic glucose production, and declining b-cell function, eventually leading to b-cell failure. Insulin resistance is present in people predisposed to T2D before the onset of hyperglycemia, which may suggest that insulin resistance is the primary abnormality that is responsible for the development of diabetes. Defective β-cell function is also present before the onset of T2D in subjects with prediabetes and impaired glucose tolerance (IGT), and in first-degree relatives of people with diabetes who have normal plasma glucose concentrations. Therefore, although there is still controversy on the primary defect in T2D, both defects are present in essentially all subjects with the disorder, often from an early preclinical stage.

T2D is caused by complex interactions between adverse environmental and genetic factors. Several risk factors include common, easily measurable phenotypic features such as overweight and obesity, hypertension, elevated triglyceride levels, and a sedentary lifestyle. The prevalence of T2D increases with age; however, the prevalence in children is rising. Between 8 and 45% of children with newly diagnosed diabetes have T2D, in particular in minority adolescent populations compared with non-Hispanic whites. Most patients with this form of diabetes are obese, and obesity itself causes some degree of insulin resistance. Patients who are not obese by traditional weight criteria may have an increased percentage of body fat distributed predominantly in the abdominal region; this phenomenon is common in many Asian populations. T2D prevalence is higher in non-Caucasian populations. It is estimated that African Americans and Hispanic Americans are 1.5–1.7 and 2 times more likely to have diabetes, respectively, compared with non-Hispanic whites.

Epidemiological, observational, and experimental evidence suggests the role of genes in development of T2D, including ethnic variation in prevalence, a concordance rate of 60–90% in identical twins, and strong familial aggregation. Multiple genes that are associated with the risk of developing diabetes or the risk of diabetes complications have been identified by candidate gene analysis and genome-wide scanning. With the exception of specific monogenic forms of the disease that might result from defects largely confined to the pathways that regulate insulin action in muscle, liver, and fat or defects in insulin secretory function in the pancreatic β-cell, there is an emerging consensus that the common forms of T2D are polygenic in nature and are caused by a combination of insulin resistance, abnormal insulin secretion, and other factors. Whole genome scans have identified numerous regions on many different chromosomes that are linked to diabetes. The contribution to disease risk by any one of these genetic factors is small (typically <1.5-fold increased risk) and is less strong than environmental factors.

The clinical presentation of T2D is heterogeneous, with a wide range in age at onset, severity of associated hyperglycemia, and degree of obesity. Frequently, this form of diabetes goes undiagnosed for many years because the hyperglycemia develops gradually and at earlier stages often is not severe enough for the patient to notice any of the classic symptoms of diabetes. On the other hand, some patients present with severe hyperglycemia, even with DKA. DKA is rare in patients with established T2D; when seen, it usually arises in association with the stress, trauma, or another illness such as infection. In recent years, however, it has been well described that some children and adult subjects with T2D can debut with DKA without precipitating cause.[1-3] At presentation, they have markedly impaired insulin secretion and insulin action.[3,4] Intensified diabetes management results in significant improvement in β-cell function and insulin sensitivity sufficient to allow discontinuation of insulin therapy within a few months of follow-up.[5,6] This clinical presentation has been reported primarily in Africans and African Americans, but also in other ethnic groups, and has been referred to in the literature as idiopathic T1D (type 1B), atypical diabetes mellitus, type 1.5 diabetes, and more recently as ketosis-prone T2D. Despite their presentation in DKA, the majority of these patients appear to have T2D, given the presence of obesity, a strong family history of diabetes, measurable insulin secretion, and a low prevalence of autoimmune markers of β-cell destruction.

Patients with T2D often can be managed effectively with lifestyle modifications or oral hypoglycemic agents. At least initially, and for many people throughout their lifetime, these individuals do not need insulin treatment to survive. The progressive nature of β-cell failure that characterizes the disease means that many patients eventually will require insulin replacement therapy to manage hyperglycemia.

GESTATIONAL DIABETES

For many years, gestational diabetes mellitus (GDM) was defined as any degree of glucose intolerance with onset or first recognition during pregnancy.[1] Although most cases resolved with delivery, the definition applied whether or not the condition persisted after pregnancy and did not exclude the possibility that unrecognized T2D or other forms of diabetes may have antedated or begun concomitantly with the pregnancy. This definition facilitated a uniform strategy for detection and classification of GDM, but its limitations were recognized for many years. As the ongoing epidemic of obesity and diabetes has led to more T2D in women of childbearing age, the number of pregnant women with previously undiagnosed T2D has increased.

After deliberations in 2008–2009, the International Association of Diabetes and Pregnancy Study Groups (IADPSG) recommended that high-risk women found to have diabetes at their initial prenatal visit, using standard criteria, receive a diagnosis of overt, not gestational, diabetes, and that GDM be used to describe hyperglycemia that develops during midpregnancy. The American Diabetes Association (ADA) subsequently promulgated this same recommendation. Approximately 7% of all pregnancies (ranging from 1 to 14%, depending on the population studied and the diagnostic tests employed) are complicated by GDM, resulting in >200,000 cases annually in the U.S.

Pregnancy normally is marked by progressive, significant insulin resistance that begins after ~20 weeks of gestation. The insulin resistance is primarily

Stomach growling

thought to be due to anti-insulin hormones secreted by the placenta, as it resolves rapidly after delivery. In normal women, pancreatic β-cells increase secretion of insulin to compensate for this insulin resistance, preserving normoglycemia. Elegant studies of women who develop GDM have shown that most have chronic insulin resistance that predates (and continues after) pregnancy. These women are able to increase insulin secretion in response to the additional acquired insulin resistance of pregnancy, but along an insulin sensitivity–secretion curve that is ~50% lower than in pregnant women without GDM.

A history of GDM is a strong risk factor for later development of T2D, with roughly a 50% risk by 10 years after the index pregnancy and long-term risk as high as 70%. Risk factors for GDM overlap with those for T2D (obesity, older age, non-Caucasian ethnicity), and progressive β-cell function has been found in Hispanic women who develop hyperglycemia after a GDM pregnancy. Taken together, these data suggest that GDM could be considered incipient T2D that temporarily was unmasked during the metabolic stress of pregnancy.

How to diagnose GDM (and therefore classify a woman as having this form of diabetes) is controversial. Five decades ago, the first diagnostic criteria were developed to identify women at high risk of later development of T2D. With the recognition that GDM was associated with adverse maternal, fetal, and neonatal outcomes, screening and diagnosis evolved to identify high-risk pregnancies. There was no worldwide consensus on the means of testing or glycemic cut points. The multinational Hyperglycemia and Adverse Pregnancy Outcomes (HAPO) study demonstrated a linear relationship between multiple pregnancy outcomes and the fasting, 1-hour, and 2-hour glucose values during a 75-gram oral glucose tolerance test (OGTT) performed at 24–28 weeks of gestation. The lack of any clear cut points above which rates of adverse outcomes accelerated markedly meant that a dichotomous GDM diagnosis was somewhat arbitrary.

A working group assembled by the IADPSG looked closely at the HAPO data and proposed that GDM be diagnosed when any one of the three OGTT values was above the point at which rates of adverse perinatal outcomes (particularly macrosomia and neonatal adiposity) were 1.75 times higher than adverse outcome rates at the mean glucose values for women in the HAPO study. Use of the IADPSG criteria subsequently was adopted by a number of countries. The IADPSG criteria, however, would identify significantly more pregnancies as being affected by GDM, and there is ongoing controversy as to whether treatment of mild hyperglycemia in pregnancy significantly reduces major adverse outcomes. Many countries have not changed from prior criteria, and in the U.S. both the American College of Obstetrics and Gynecology and a National Institutes of Health consensus panel recommended continuing with older diagnostic criteria. The ADA, citing the uncertainty in the field, currently recommends that either the IADPSG or prior methods and criteria be used for GDM screening and diagnosis.

OTHER TYPES OF DIABETES

The "other" category includes many disorders associated with hyperglycemia, although most are rare. A summary of several broad classes follows.

MONOGENIC DIABETES

Genetic Defects of the β-Cell   *chromosome 12*

Several forms of diabetes are associated with monogenetic defects in β-cell function. These forms of diabetes are inherited in an autosomal dominant fashion, usually are characterized by onset of hyperglycemia at an early age (generally <25 years old), and therefore are referred to as maturity-onset diabetes of the young (MODY). Abnormalities at six genetic loci on different chromosomes have been identified to date. The most common form is associated with mutations on chromosome 12 in a hepatic transcription factor referred to as hepatocyte nuclear factor (HNF)-1α. A second form is associated with mutations in the glucokinase gene on chromosome 7p and results in a defective glucokinase molecule, the "glucose sensor" for the β-cell. Less common forms result from mutations in other transcription factors, including HNF-4α, HNF-1β, insulin promoter factor (IPF)-1, and NeuroD1.

Most children with diabetes diagnosed in the first 6 months of life have monogenic diabetes and do not have autoimmune T1D. This so-called neonatal diabetes can be either transient or permanent. The most common genetic defect causing transient disease is a defect on ZAC/HYAMI imprinting, whereas permanent neonatal diabetes is most commonly a defect in the gene encoding the Kir6.2 subunit of the β-cell K_{ATP} channel. Diagnosing the latter has implications, as such children can be well managed with sulfonylureas.

Genetic Defects in Insulin Action

Uncommonly, diabetes results from genetically determined abnormalities of insulin action. The metabolic abnormalities associated with mutations of the insulin receptor may range from hyperinsulinemia and modest hyperglycemia to severe diabetes. Some individuals with these mutations have acanthosis nigricans, and women may have virilization and cystic ovaries. Leprechaunism and the Rabson-Mendenhall syndrome are two pediatric syndromes with mutations in the insulin receptor gene that cause extreme insulin resistance. The former has characteristic facial features and is usually fatal in infancy, while the latter is associated with abnormalities of teeth and nails and pineal gland hyperplasia. Alterations in the structure and function of the insulin receptor cannot be demonstrated in patients with insulin-resistant lipoatrophic diabetes, implying that defects must reside in postreceptor signal transduction pathways.

Diseases of the Exocrine Pancreas   *胰腺 癌 cancer trauma*

Any process that diffusely injures the pancreas can cause diabetes. Acquired processes include pancreatitis, trauma, infection, pancreatectomy, and pancreatic carcinoma. With the exception of the last example, common wisdom is that damage to the pancreas must be extensive for diabetes to occur. Adenocarcinomas involving only a small portion of the pancreas have been associated with diabetes, implying mechanisms beyond just reduction in β-cell mass. Genetic defects such as cystic fibrosis and hemochromatosis also can damage β-cells and impair insulin secretion. CFRD is common in teens and adults with cystic fibrosis. It shares

cystic fibrosis related disease

phenotypic features with both T1D and T2D, with both β-cell dysfunction or loss and insulin resistance, perhaps related to chronic inflammation.

Endocrinopathies

Excess amounts of these insulin-antagonizing hormones (e.g., acromegaly, Cushing's syndrome, glucagonoma, pheochromocytoma) can cause diabetes. This generally occurs in individuals with preexisting defects in insulin secretion, and hyperglycemia typically resolves when the hormone excess is resolved. Somatostatinomas and aldosteronoma-induced hypokalemia can cause diabetes, at least in part, by inhibiting insulin secretion. Hyperglycemia generally resolves after successful removal of the tumor.

Drug- or Chemical-Induced Diabetes

Rarely encountered toxins such as the rat poison Vacor and administration of intravenous pentamidine can permanently destroy β-cells. High-dose thiazide diuretics are associated with the development of T2D, perhaps due to hypokalemia, but lower doses used in current practice generally do not. In clinical practice, common causes of drug-induced hyperglycemia include glucocorticoids, nicotinic acid, and atypical antipsychotics. Patients who develop hyperglycemia on these drugs often have risk factors for T2D. Like GDM, this may represent unmasking of latent T2D. Patients receiving α-interferon can develop autoimmune diseases of the thyroid and other organs, including severely insulin-deficient diabetes associated with islet cell antibodies. The use of statins has been associated with development of T2D, especially in those with underlying prediabetes, through unknown mechanisms.

Uncommon Forms of Immune-Mediated Diabetes

The stiff-man syndrome is an autoimmune disorder of the central nervous system characterized by stiffness of the axial muscles with painful spasms. Patients usually have high titers of the glutamic acid decarboxylase (GAD) autoantibodies, and approximately one-third will develop diabetes. Anti-insulin receptor antibodies, occasionally found in patients with lupus or other autoimmune diseases, can cause diabetes by binding to the insulin receptor, blocking the binding of insulin to its receptor in target tissues. In some cases, however, these antibodies can act as an insulin agonist and cause hypoglycemia.

Other Genetic Syndromes Sometimes Associated with Diabetes

Genetic syndromes that are accompanied by an increased incidence of diabetes include the chromosomal abnormalities Down syndrome, Klinefelter syndrome, and Turner syndrome. Wolfram syndrome is an autosomal recessive disorder characterized by insulin-deficient diabetes, absence of β-cells at autopsy, diabetes insipidus, hypogonadism, optic atrophy, and neural deafness.

CONCLUSION

Although there are numerous causes of diabetes, the majority of cases are either T1D or T2D. Nevertheless, the varying clinical onset of even the common types of diabetes means that classification is not always straightforward. Features that might prompt consideration of alternative classification of a patient include atypical features in the age of onset, family history, body weight, or response to conventional therapies for the presumed type of diabetes.

REFERENCES

1. American Diabetes Association. Diagnosis and classification of diabetes mellitus. *Diabetes Care* 2014;37(Suppl 1):S81–S90.

2. Centers for Disease Control and Prevention. *National Diabetes Fact Sheet: National Estimates and General Information on Diabetes and Prediabetes in the United States, 2011.* Atlanta, GA, U.S. Department of Health and Human Services, Centers for Disease Control and Prevention, 2011.

3. Haller MJ. Type 1 diabetes in the 21st century: a review of the landscape. In *Type 1 Diabetes Sourcebook.* Peters A, Laffel L., Eds. Alexandria, VA, American Diabetes Association, 2013.

4. Umpierrez GE, Smiley D, Kitabchi AE. Narrative review: ketosis-prone type 2 diabetes mellitus. *Ann Intern Med* 2006;144(5):350–357.

5. Buchanan TA, Xiang AH. Gestational diabetes mellitus. *J Clin Invest* 2005;115:485–491.

6. American College of Obstetrics and Gynecology, Committee on Obstetric Practice. ACOG Committee Opinion No. 435: postpartum screening for abnormal glucose tolerance in women who had gestational diabetes mellitus. *Obstet Gynecol* 2009;113:1419–1421.

Chapter 3

Role of Diabetes Education in Patient Management

Martha M. Funnell, MS, RN, CDE
Gretchen A. Piatt, MPH, PhD
Robert M. Anderson, EdD

R ecent advances in knowledge, therapies, and technology have greatly
enhanced our ability to effectively care for patients with diabetes. In spite of
these advances, people with diabetes still experience less-than-optimal
blood glucose, blood pressure, and cholesterol levels as well as acute and long-term
complications. Health care professionals often are frustrated by their patients'
inability to make changes in their behavior, and people with diabetes sometimes
feel that they are "just a blood sugar number" to their providers. Clearly, there is a
gap between the promise and the reality of diabetes care. One of the keys to closing
the gap is effective self-management.

DIABETES SELF-MANAGEMENT

Diabetes self-management refers to all of the activities in which patients engage
to care for their illness; promote health; augment physical, social, and emotional
resources; and prevent long- and short-term effects from diabetes. Patient education is the essential first step in becoming an effective self-manager. Traditional
views of diabetes self-management education (DSME) were based on information
transfer with the goal of compliance or adherence. On the basis of the current
evidence, DSME has evolved to recognize the right and responsibility of patients
to make decisions and set self-selected goals that make sense within the context of
their lives. There is also increasing recognition of the need to address psychosocial
issues, such as diabetes-related distress and depression, as a component of DSME
because of their prevalence, impact on glycemic outcomes, and self-management
behaviors. Therefore, the current goals of DSME are to help patients make
informed decisions and then to evaluate the costs and benefits of those choices in
order to cope with the self-management demands of a complex chronic illness
such as diabetes.

Although patients need a comprehensive understanding of diabetes, its effect
on their lives, and how to change behavior, it is unreasonable to think that a one-
time educational intervention is adequate to manage diabetes for a lifetime. Diabetes self-management support (DSMS) is the ongoing assistance that patients
need from health care professionals, the community, family and friends, and other
relevant organizations to make and sustain behavioral changes and cope with diabetes. DSMS incorporates the provision of the needed emotional, behavioral,
clinical, psychosocial, and tangible resources to enable patients to manage their

DOI: 10.2337/9781580405096.03

illness effectively. Strategies for providing ongoing self-management support include the following:

- Assess patient self-management knowledge, behaviors, confidence, coping skills, and barriers.
- Incorporate effective interventions and ongoing support from family, peers, and professionals.
- Incorporate strategies including effective communication to help patients cope with the distress that often results from the many physical, self-management, and emotional demands of living with diabetes.
- Ensure collaborative care planning and problem solving with a team of health care professionals.
- Redesign practice patterns and health care systems to be better able to provide continuing education and support for patients over a lifetime of a chronic illness.

DIABETES SELF-MANAGEMENT EDUCATION AND SUPPORT

Because of the growing body of evidence about the importance of ongoing self-management support following DSME, the title of the national standards was changed in the most recent revision to the National Standards for Diabetes Self-Management Education and Support (DSME/S). These standards were developed by key diabetes organizations based on a review of the evidence.

Recent reviews and meta-analysis indicate that DSME/S is effective for improving metabolic outcomes, enhancing quality of life and healthy coping, increasing use of primary and preventive services, and reducing diabetes-related costs, at least in the short term. More time spent with the educator increases the effect. In addition, DSME/S interventions that integrate the physiological, behavioral, and psychosocial aspects of diabetes are more effective than programs that focus strictly on knowledge.

DSME is primarily available through outpatient group programs often offered by hospitals or community-based organizations. Programs that achieve American Diabetes Association (ADA) Recognition or American Association of Diabetes Educators Accreditation by meeting standards for process, structure, and outcomes are eligible to bill for education services and receive reimbursement from the Centers for Medicare and Medicaid Services and other payers. Both ADA Recognition and AADE Accreditation certify that the program both meets quality standards and can be reimbursed for services.

PROVISION OF DIABETES SELF-MANAGEMENT EDUCATION AND SUPPORT

Essential content areas have been defined in the National Standards for DSME/S (Table 3.1). These content areas were written in behavioral terms to maximize creativity on the part of the educator and to allow programs to match instruction and methodology to the culture, literacy, and other needs of their target populations. The particular content areas provided to an individual patient are based on an assessment of needs, personal priorities, learning style, cultural influences, health literacy, and coping style. Evaluation of the effectiveness of DSME/S is based on patient achievement of self-selected behavior change goals, metabolic measures, and psychosocial and other outcomes.

Table 3.1 Recommended DSME/S Content Areas   obesity.

- Describing the diabetes disease process and treatment options   weight loss
- Incorporating nutritional management into lifestyle
- Incorporating physical activity into lifestyle   ordering strips
- Using medications safely and for maximum therapeutic effectiveness
- Monitoring blood glucose and other parameters and interpreting and using the results for self-management decision making
- Preventing, detecting, and treating acute complications
- Preventing, detecting, and treating chronic complications
- Developing personal strategies to address psychosocial issues and concerns

Any health care professional who provides diabetes education is a diabetes educator. A certified diabetes educator is a health care professional who has specialized knowledge and practical experience in diabetes education and who has passed an examination developed by the National Certification Board for Diabetes Education. Board-Certified–Advanced Diabetes Managers are advanced practice nurses, dietitians, or pharmacists who have passed an examination administered jointly by the American Nurses Credentialing Center and the American Association of Diabetes Educators.   N CBDE

ROLE OF THE PROVIDER IN DIABETES SELF-MANAGEMENT EDUCATION AND SUPPORT

Models of chronic illness care, including the chronic care model, were designed to address the epidemic of chronic diseases and aid in their management. The chronic care model includes six elements (health systems, community resources and policies, self-management support, delivery system design, decision support, and clinical information systems) that when implemented successfully result in more actively involved patients working in partnership with a proactive practice team. Thus, effective diabetes management occurs at the individual, practice, and system levels. Although it is unrealistic to expect providers to provide comprehensive DSME in the context of a busy practice, they do have an essential role to play in providing DSME and DSMS.

Starting at the time of diagnosis, providers need to provide key messages about diabetes, its treatment and the value of DSME and DSMS. Key messages for patients and their family members include the following:

- All types of diabetes need to be taken seriously.

OSA is a self-managent disease

- Diabetes is a self-managed disease, which means that your day-to-day care is in your hands. DSME/S can help you make informed and wise decisions as you go through each day, teach you how to cope with diabetes, and make changes in your health behaviors.
- The decisions you make each day will have a major impact on your future health and quality of life. It is a big responsibility and a lot of work, but it is worth the effort. The long-term complications of diabetes are not inevitable.
- It is common to have a strong feelings about having and living with diabetes. A collaborative partnership between you, your family, and your health care team is essential to provide you with the ongoing support and strategies you need to live a long and healthy life.

Because of the increasing emphasis on shared decision making and patient engagement, it is also useful to discuss the roles of the patient and the provider in diabetes care. Because chronic illness care differs from acute care, many patients will not have experienced working in a collaborative partnership with their health care team. It is important to stress that the person with diabetes is the primary decision maker and is responsible for the daily care of diabetes. It takes the provider's knowledge about diabetes combined with the expertise of the patients about their own goals and priorities to create a truly workable care plan. A plan that is not working is not a negative reflection on either the patient or the provider but simply needs to be revised using what was learned from that experience.

Providers also need to stress the importance of DSME/S for successful self-management and shared decision making and actively offer referral to approved DSME/S programs and registered dietitians. Patients value physician opinions and recommendations. Providers need to let patients know that DSME/S is a wise investment in their future health and will provide the knowledge they need to make informed decisions as they care for themselves each day.

Providers can acknowledge how difficult it is to live with diabetes and provide reinforcement for the education that has been provided based on feedback from the patient and the DSME/S program. Although most practices cannot offer comprehensive DSME/S, practitioners can take advantage of teachable moments that present during any patient encounter. For example, pointing out at-risk areas during a foot examination or making the link between heart disease and diabetes when reviewing lab results are powerful education moments. Specific strategies that can be used with individual patients are listed in Table 3.2.

Physicians can not only ensure that individual patients receive DSME but also can design their practices to facilitate ongoing self-management support. Including a diabetes educator into the practice or models, such as patient-centered medical homes that incorporate team members designated and trained to provide ongoing care management, are consistent with recent recommendations for both DSME/S and for improving chronic care delivery.

Although DSME and DSMS work best when provided by a team of health care professionals, the team does not need to work in the same setting or in traditional roles. Better use of technology allows "virtual" teams to work and communicate effectively with each other and with patients. Table 3.3 lists strategies shown to be effective in facilitating self-management education and ongoing support in a variety of practice settings.

Table 3.2 Effective Provider-Based Strategies for Self-Management Support

- Stress the importance of taking diabetes seriously.
- Stress the importance of both DSME and ongoing DSMS.
- Stress the importance of the patient's role in self-management
- Reinforce education provided in the DSME program.
- Begin each visit by asking the patient to identify their concerns, questions, and progress toward metabolic and self-determined behavioral goals.
- Assess and address patient-identified fears and concerns.
- Ask for the patient's opinions about home blood glucose monitoring results and other laboratory and outcome measures.
- Review and revise the diabetes care plan as needed based on both the patient and provider assessment of its effectiveness.
- Provide ongoing information about the costs and benefits of therapeutic and behavioral options to promote shared decision making.
- Take advantage of teachable moments that occur during each visit.
- Ask patients to "teach back" what you have discussed at the end of each visit.
- Ask patients to identify one thing they will do differently to manage their diabetes before the next visit.
- Establish a partnership with patients and their families to develop collaborative goals.
- Provide information about behavior change and problem-solving strategies to assist patients to overcome barriers to self-management.
- Support and facilitate patients' efforts in their role as the primary decision maker in their self-management.
- Encourage the use of self-management experiments, such as monitoring blood glucose before and after exercise or before and 2 hours after a meal to help patients understand the metabolic consequences of their choices.
- Abandon traditional dysfunctional models of care (e.g., adherence and compliance; provider-centered care).

Source: Adapted from Funnell MM, Anderson RM: Patient empowerment. In: *Psychology in Diabetes Care*, 2nd edition. FJ Snoek and TC Skinner, eds. West Sussex, U.K., John Wiley & Sons, 95–108, 2005.

Table 3.3 Effective Practice-Based Strategies for Self-Management Support

- Use continuous quality improvement to develop, implement, maintain, and enhance DSME/S and improve practice.
- Create a patient-centered model of care.
- Incorporate care management into your practice to provide DSME/S.
- Link patient self-management support with provider support (e.g., use of the electronic medical record [EMR], patient flow, logistics).
- Supplement self-management support with information technology.
- Create a team with other health care professionals in your system or area with additional experience or training in the educational, behavioral, psychosocial, or clinical aspects of diabetes care.
- Incorporate a diabetes educator into your practice. Evidence demonstrates that this can improve clinical and behavioral outcomes and is cost-effective.
- Assist patients to establish a self-selected behavioral goal that is incorporated into the EMR and can be reinforced by all team members.
- Create a patient-centered environment that incorporates self-management support from all practice personnel and is integrated into the flow of the visit.

CONCLUSION

All types of diabetes are serious and can result in acute and long-term complications that diminish both the quality and length of patients' lives. Patients make multiple decisions each day that directly affect their health outcomes, and they experience the consequences of their daily choices and self-care efforts. The key to closing the gap between the promise and reality of diabetes care is through the development of collaborative relationships and patient-centered practices that support patients' self-management efforts. Effective DSME/S recognizes the patient's role as a collaborator, decision maker, and expert on his or her own life and provides ongoing self-management support. DSME/S can help relieve the burden of diabetes care on your practice by helping patients to become informed, active participants in their own care. Staff members of a Recognized DSME program can become a valuable resource for you, your patients, and your staff. You can find an ADA Recognized DSME/S program in your area at www.diabetes.org. You can find a diabetes educator in your area at www.aadenet.org.

BIBLIOGRAPHY

Anderson RM, Patrias R. Getting out ahead: The Diabetes Concerns Assessment Form. *Clinical Diabetes* 2007;25:141–143.

Bodenheimer T, MacGregor K, Sharifi C. *Helping Patients Manage Their Chronic Conditions.* Oakland, CA, California Healthcare Foundation, 2005.

Duncan I, Birkmeyer C, Coughlin S, Li QE, Sherr D, Boren S. Assessing the value of diabetes education. *Diabetes Educ* 2009;35:752–760.

Funnell MM, Anderson RM. Patient empowerment. In *Psychology in Diabetes Care.* 2nd edition. FJ Snoek, TC Skinner, Eds. West Sussex, U.K., John Wiley & Sons, 2005, p. 95–108.

Funnell MM, Tang TS, Anderson RM. From DSME to DSMS: developing empowerment based self-management support. *Diabetes Spectrum* 2007;20:221–226.

Haas L, Maryniuk M, Beck J, Cox CE, et al. National Standards for Diabetes Self-Management Education and Support. *Diabetes Care* 2013;36(Suppl 1):S100–S108.

Marrero DG, Ard J, Delamater AM, Peragallo-Dittko V, Mayer-Davis EJ, Nwankwo R, Fisher EB. Twenty-first century behavioral medicine: a context for empowering clinicians and patients with diabetes: a consensus report. *Diabetes Care* 2013;36:463–470.

Peyrot, M, Rubin RR, Lauritzen T, Snoek FJ, Matthews DR, Skovlund SE. Psychosocial problems and barriers to improved diabetes management: results of the Cross-National Diabetes Attitudes, Wishes and Needs (DAWN) Study. *Diabet Med* 2005;22:1379–1385.

Piatt G, Orchard T, Emerson S, et al. Translating the chronic care model into the community: results from a randomized controlled trial of a multifaceted diabetes care intervention. *Diabetes Care* 2006;29:811–817.

Piatt GA, Seidel MC, Powell TO, Zgibor JC. Comparative effectiveness of lifestyle intervention efforts in the community: results of the Rethinking, Eating and ACTivity (REACT) study. *Diabetes Care* 2013;36:202–209.

Shojania KG, Ranji SR, McDonald KM, et al. Effects of quality improvement strategies for type 2 diabetes on glycemic control: a meta-regression analysis. *JAMA* 2007;296:427–440.

Stellefson M, Dipnarine K, Stopka C. The chronic care model and diabetes management in US primary care settings: a systematic review. *Prev Chronic Dis* 2013;10:120180.

Tricco AC, Ivers NM, Grimshaw JM, et al. Effectiveness of quality improvement strategies on the management of diabetes: a systematic review and meta-analysis. *Lancet* 2012;379:2252–2261.

ACKNOWLEDGMENT

The authors were supported in part by the Michigan Center for Diabetes Translational Research (MCDTR) Intervention and Technology Core, Grant Number P30DK092926 (MCDTR) from the National Institute of Diabetes and Digestive and Kidney Diseases.

Chapter 4

Glucose Monitoring

ROBERT A. VIGERSKY, MD

INTRODUCTION

In the decades following the publication of the landmark Diabetes Control and Complications Trial and the U.K. Prospective Diabetes Study—both showing a reduction in diabetes complications with improved glycemic control as measured by A1C—there has been a progressive improvement in the overall health of patients with diabetes.[1-3] Arguably, glucose monitoring has been one of the key developments, along with improved pharmacotherapy, in permitting patients with diabetes to achieve the glycemic control necessary to prevent or reduce the microvascular and macrovascular complications that have been long associated with the disease. In this same time frame, there has been a progressive improvement in the technology for glucose monitoring with more accurate and faster meters requiring less blood for self-monitoring of blood glucose (SMBG) and an evolution from an era of single blood glucose measurement by capillary blood test to continuous glucose monitoring (CGM). CGM has emerged as an important tool not only for retrospective analysis of glycemic patterns but also for real-time tracking and trending. The most recent application of CGM is its use as one of the components of a semi-closed-loop "artificial pancreas," which preemptively suspends insulin delivery when the glucose approaches a preset threshold.[4] These developments essentially have relegated urine testing to only measurement of ketones. Furthermore, one of the newly U.S. Food and Drug Administration (FDA)–approved classes of medications, the sodium-glucose cotransporter-2 inhibitors, makes urine glucose testing obsolete and inaccurate because the mechanism of action of these agents increases urine glucose.[5] This chapter will review the technology of SMBG and CGM and their use in patients with both type 1 diabetes (T1D) and type 2 diabetes (T2D).

BLOOD GLUCOSE METERS

TECHNOLOGY

One of the most important technological advances in diabetes care—both for patient home use and for hospital use—has been the development and deployment of increasingly accurate, faster, and portable glucose meters requiring minimal amounts of blood. This began >50 years ago when the dry-reagent test strips

 DOI: 10.2337/9781580405096.04

used for urine glucose testing were adapted for use with blood.[6,7] The chemistry in these and many subsequent methods of glucose monitoring generally has relied on the enzyme glucose oxidase reacting with glucose, which in the presence of oxygen, results in the formation of gluconic acid and hydrogen peroxide (H_2O_2). A major advance in glucose measurement technology occurred in 1987 when a biosensor system was developed employing artificial electron acceptors (i.e., electron mediators or redox dyes) instead of oxygen.[8] The resultant current was read amperometrically, permitting the development of smaller and more accurate meters that could be used at home.

Other enzymes such as glucose dehydrogenase (GDH) have been used as the basis of glucose-monitoring technology. They have an advantage over glucose oxidase in that they are not dependent on oxygen, and therefore results are not affected by oxygen tension that may vary considerably in hospitalized patients in critical care settings. On the other hand, the GDH-based technology, particularly GDH pyrroloquinolinequinone (GDH-PQQ) has the disadvantage of having significant cross-reactivity with other clinically important compounds, such as the maltose-containing icodextrin, which is present in peritoneal dialysis fluids and intravenous immunoglobulin (IVIG) and also contains maltose. The use of GDH-PQQ-based meters has led to severe hypoglycemia and death when used in patients receiving those compounds because of falsely elevated glucose readings, resulting in inappropriate insulin doses.[9] As a result, the use of GDH-PQQ has been abandoned. Bioengineering this enzyme, however, may allow its non–oxygen-dependency advantage to be utilized in the future. Thus, the next generation of glucose sensors may use direct electron transfer technology using "designer" fungus- or bacterial-derived GDHs that contain flavin adenine dinucleotide (FAD) as the catalytic cofactor and cytochrome-c as the electron transfer subunit to provide a glucose-specific assay.[10,11]

Other enhancements to the basic glucose monitoring technology that have promoted its utilization include alternate site testing, no coding systems, and memory enhancement features that allow display of summary statistics like 7, 14, and 30 days mean glucose and the ability to mark events like meals and exercise. Some meters contain decision support algorithms that can provide advice to patients such as when to do ketone testing or have a snack. The ability to download meter data to desktop software or to a website provides useful features, such as detailed statistics and graphic display of glycemic patterns.

Alternate site testing, which is less painful than finger-sticks because there are fewer pain receptors in the forearm or palms than the fingertips, has been embraced eagerly by some patients. There is, however, no clear evidence that it enhances adherence to testing[12-14] or that it improves glycemic control.[13] A drawback of alternate site testing is that it may be inaccurate in times of fluctuating blood glucose levels. Thus, alternate sites are not recommended immediately after insulin administration, within 1–2 hours after ingestion of food or initiation of exercise, or when feeling hypoglycemic.[15,16] Furthermore, these alternate sites should never be used to calibrate a CGM.

"No coding" systems have been developed by several glucose meter manufacturers, and these systems appear to be as accurate as those that require patient coding with each new batch of strips.[17] Most meters on the market today are "no code" meters. In fact, these strips are still coded, but the manufacturer has incorporated the technology into the strip itself. Abolishing the coding by the patient eliminates the possibility of miscoding, which has been estimated to occur up to 25% of the time,[18] resulting in potential insulin dosing errors of up to 5 units 50% of the time. It also eliminates a barrier to glucose monitoring because there is one less step to remember when opening a new batch of strips.

Software for uploading glucose information has become available with most meter brands. Unfortunately, each brand uses its own proprietary software, which is generally incompatible with those of other manufacturers, precluding the integration of data from different brands of meters if a patient is using more than one brand. It also requires that diabetes care providers have the software for all meter brands that are being used by their patients as well as multiple cables and infrared, Bluetooth, or radio frequency data transfer devices to upload the data. Evidence suggests that use of such software significantly improves glycemic control compared with the use of logbooks alone.[19,20] A number of strategies to circumvent these barriers to efficiently obtaining the meter data have been devised, including the use of flash memory drives plugged into universal serial bus (USB) ports.[21] Meters also have incorporated a pen-drive USB system, such as the Bayer Contour USB meter. Emerging web-based software ultimately will make it seamless to upload glucose data to a secure cloud-based platform from any device using open-source code and open-reference designs.

Software for analyzing glucose data permits its presentation statistically or graphically. Such displays may provide valuable information about patterns of glycemia not readily obvious on handwritten logbooks.[22] Using such tools also reduces the likelihood of patient recording errors. The ability to collect and upload glucose data has led to a panoply of mobile applications and has focused a number of studies investigating web-based diabetes management.[23-26] The wireless transfer of data from the meter to the web-based application, however, is present only in a limited number of devices.[25] Recent advances include the integration of a meter and phone into one device (iBGStar®, a plug-in to the iPhone 4 but not iPhone 5) and the Telcare® blood glucose device—a 3G wireless glucose meter connecting directly to a data organizer via an online portal. Such systems permit the sharing of data with a patient's health care provider, family, or other self-authorized person. Extension of this concept to using a mobile phone that links the SMBG (along with other self-care information) with a web-based automated mobile coaching system has shown promising results in patients with T2D.[27]

ACCURACY OF GLUCOSE METERS

The analytic accuracy of a glucose meter is measured by how closely it provides true readings as determined by a laboratory-quality instrument such as the Yellow Springs Instrument (YSI) 2300. A meter's precision is measured by its reproducibility. Bias is the tendency for all readings to favor higher or lower than actual values but to the same degree. To have a meter that is clinically useful, it has to be accurate, precise, and without significant bias (Figure 4.1). A meter's ability to achieve these requirements can be described statistically. Laboratory-quality instruments should be within 20% (for a blood glucose ≥60 mg/dl) or 12 mg/dl (for a blood glucose <60 mg/dl) of true glucose, whichever is greater, as mandated by the Clinical Laboratory Improvement Amendments.

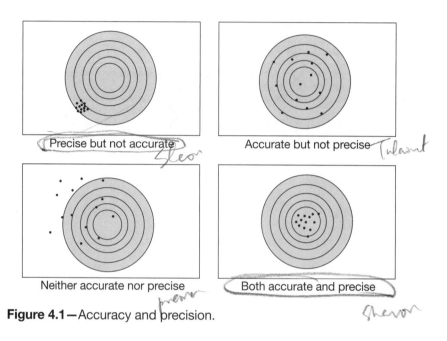

Precise but not accurate

Accurate but not precise

Neither accurate nor precise

Both accurate and precise

Figure 4.1—Accuracy and precision.

The International Organization for Standardization (ISO) recently updated its standards for the point accuracy of glucose meters used in the home, and the Clinical Laboratory Standards Institute established standards for meters that are used in professional health care settings (such as physicians' offices and acute and chronic care facilities).

The FDA has new draft guidance for meter accuracy that differentiates between the meters for home use and those that are for use in professional health care settings (Table 4.1).[28,29] Patient safety is the main reason that professional health care settings have more stringent criteria, because these patients may be frail or critically ill and are "more likely to present physiological and pathological factors that could interfere with glucose measurements as compared to the lay population."[29] Stricter standards were driven by computer modeling studies, which have demonstrated that as the accuracy deteriorates there is a significant increase in the likelihood that either the wrong insulin dose will be given or hypoglycemia will not be recognized and treated. For example, there is a 6–20% likelihood of making significant errors of insulin dosing if the total analytic error is 20% versus 0.2% likelihood when the error is 10%.[30] Because professional-use meters likely will be used on multiple patients, the FDA's draft guidance also requires that they be designed to withstand rigorous disinfecting measures to prevent the spread of blood-borne pathogens. Transmission of hepatitis B and C through the use of the same meter on multiple patients prompted the FDA to issue guidelines about such use.[31]

Table 4.1 Standards for Analytic Accuracy of Blood Glucose Meters

Glucose level	ISO 15197:2013	CLSI POCT 12-A3	FDA for prescription meters*	FDA for nonprescription meters*
>70 mg/dl			99% within ±10% and 0% exceed ±20%	95% within ±15% and 99% within ±20%
>75 mg/dl		98% within ±20%		
>100 mg/dl	95% within ±15% 99% within Zones A+B of Error Grid	95% within ±12.5%		
<70 mg/dl			99% within ±7 mg/dl and 0% within ±15 mg/dl	95% within ±15% and 99% within ±20%**
<75 mg/dl		98% within ±15 mg/dl		
<100 mg/dl	95% within ±15 mg/dl	95% within ±12 mg/dl		

Note: ISO = International Organization for Standardization; CLSI POCT = Clinical and Laboratory Standards Institute Point-of-Care Testing; FDA = U.S. Food and Drug Administration.

*Draft Guidance as of January 7, 2014.

**For those meters unable to reliably measure within 15% at very low glucose concentrations, the lower end of the claimed accuracy must be raised to the point at which the criteria are met.

A number of factors can interfere with the ability of a glucose meter to give a true reading. Some of these are intrinsic to the device or strip, such as the effect of temperature, humidity, altitude, or poor storage; and some are extrinsic, that is, unrelated to the hardware itself. For example, in the hospital setting, substantial errors may be induced by the presence of interfering substances such as maltose (in IVIG) or icodextrin (in peritoneal dialysis) with the use of GDH-PQQ–based strips (see the section on Technology). In glucose oxidase–based strips, oxygen, anemia (causing higher than actual readings), polycythemia (causing lower than actual readings), and the use of ascorbate or acetaminophen may produce significant measurement errors.[32-37] A list of the potential interferents for both over-the-counter (OTC) and point-of-care SMBG devices is shown in Table 4.2.[28,29] The FDA requires that each meter being submitted for approval be tested at a therapeutic level and a toxic concentration of interferents as well as high and low levels of hemoglobin. It behooves the user to carefully review the limitations of the meters being employed in

Table 4.2 Potential Interferents for SMBG Devices

Acetaminophen	Ibuprofen
Ascorbic acid	L-Dopa
Bilirubin	Maltose
Cholesterol	Methyldopa
Creatinine	Salicylate
Dopamine	Sodium
EDTA	Tolbutamide
Galactose	Tolazamide
Gentisic acid	Triglycerides
Glutathione	Uric acid
Hemoglobin	Xylose
Heparin	Sugar alcohols*

Note: EDTA = ethylenediaminetetraacetic acid; SMBG = self-monitoring of blood glucose.

*Including mannitol, sorbitol, xylitol, lactitol, isomalt, maltitol, and hydrogenated starch hydrolysates.

their setting. The site from which the sample is obtained also affects accuracy. For example, capillary samples have been shown to be more accurate than arterial or venous samples in an intensive care unit setting.[38] Other extrinsic errors are "user errors" while miscoding, improper hand washing, and using testing sites damp from topical alcohol.

In addition to analytic accuracy, the concept of clinical accuracy has emerged as an important factor in assessing a meter's performance. A meter has to be accurate enough so that errors in insulin dosing are not made leading to unnecessary and potentially dangerous hypo- or hyperglycemia. Error grids have been used for the past 25 years to help define how clinically accurate a meter is compared with a "gold standard." The Clarke Error Grid (CEG) and the Parkes Consensus Error Grid (PEG) are the most commonly used to date.[39,40] Blood sample data points are displayed on a graph where the y-axis is the new meter and the x-axis is the reference device. The percent of data points falling within grid zones can define the clinical accuracy of the meter (Figure 4.2). Since the CEG and PEG were developed, there have been many advances in medical practice, including the use of analog insulins and more accurate glucose monitors. Therefore, several professional societies and the FDA recently have collaborated to develop a new error grid called the Surveillance Error Grid (SEG)[41] in which four clinical scenarios were presented to 206 diabetes clinicians who scored the clinical impact of various degrees of meter inaccuracy. The resulting error grid uses color gradations, thereby eliminating the hard boundaries that separate the zones in the currently

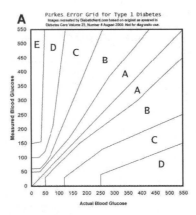

Figure 4.2—Parkes error grid. A meter generating results that fall in Zone A would have no effect on clinical action. Results that fall into the other four zones will have some altered clinical action as follows: Zone B = little or no effect on clinical outcome; Zone C = likely to affect clinical outcome; Zone D = could have significant medical risk; and Zone E = could have dangerous consequences.

used error grids and thus providing more granularity to the understanding of a meter's clinical accuracy.[41]

A new concern about the analytic and clinical accuracy of glucose meters is that a meter that initially meets FDA standards may not do so after introduced into the marketplace. There are many potential reasons for this. For instance, studies performed for FDA approval are done by trained professionals under ideal conditions. This does not take into account the environment that the meters and strips encounter in shipping, storing, and actual use. In addition, once FDA-approved, meter manufacturers may produce and release strip lots whose specifications are too broad. Indeed, many currently available meters do not even meet former ISO (2003) standards and even more of them do not meet the 2013 standards.[42] A program for routine postmarketing surveillance of glucose meters that will identify those meters not meeting the extant FDA standards has been proposed.[43]

CLINICAL USE OF GLUCOSE METERS

The technical improvements in meter performance described previously have permitted SMBG to become one of the essential tools in achieving improved glycemic control in patients with diabetes. Indeed, there is a direct, strongly positive relationship between the frequency of SMBG and glycemic control in those receiving pharmacotherapy.[44–47] Accordingly, for people with T1D treated with multiple-dose insulin or an insulin pump, the American Diabetes Association (ADA) recommends SMBG be performed at least "prior to meals and snacks, occasionally postprandially, at bedtime, prior to exercise, when they suspect low blood glucose, after treating low blood glucose until they are normoglycemic, and prior to critical tasks such as driving."[48] This means that testing may occur eight times per day or more. Although there is little controversy about the use of SMBG in those with T1D and in those patients with T2D on multiple-dose insulin regimens, there is considerable debate about its utility in those patients with T2D using basal insulin, noninsulin injectables such as glucagon-like peptide-1 (GLP-1) agonists, or oral medications. Professional and governmental organizations have provided recommendations for testing in patients with T2D that are more similar than they are different (Table 4.3).

Although professional organizations recommend that patients with T2D who are not using insulin perform SMBG as noted in Table 4.3, its routine use in this

Table 4.3 Recommendations for SMBG in Non–Insulin-Treated Patients with Type 2 Diabetes

Organization and evidence level	Recommendation for SMBG in non–insulin-treated patients with type 2 diabetes
American Diabetes Association (E = Expert opinion)	When prescribed as part of a broader educational context, SMBG results may be helpful to guide treatment decisions or patient self-management for patients using less frequent insulin injections or noninsulin therapies.
American Association of Clinical Endocrinologists (Grade D; Best Evidence Level 4)	Patients not requiring insulin therapy may benefit from SMBG, especially to provide feedback about the effects of their lifestyle and pharmacologic therapy; testing frequency must be personalized.
Veterans Administration/ Department of Defense (Strength of Recommendation = B)	The schedule of SMBG in patients on oral agents (not taking insulin) should be individualized, and continuation justified based on individual clinical outcomes. Consider more frequent SMBG for the following indications: • Initiation of therapy or active adjustment of oral agents • Acute or ongoing illness • Detection and prevention of hypoglycemia when symptoms are suggestive of such, or if there is documented hypoglycemia unawareness • Detection of hyperglycemia when fasting or postprandial blood glucose levels are not consistent with A1C

Note: SMBG = self-monitoring of blood glucose.

Sources: American Diabetes Association. Standards of medical care in diabetes—2014. *Diabetes Care* 2014;36(Suppl 1):S14–S80; Handelsman Y, Mechanick JI, Blonde L, Grunberger G, Bloomgarden ZT, Bray GA, Dagogo-Jack S, Davidson JA, Einhorn D, Ganda O, Garber AJ, Hirsch IB, Horton ES, Ismail-Beigi F, Jellinger PS, Jones KL, Jovanovic L, Lebovitz H, Levy P, Moghissi FS, Orzeck FA, Vinik AI, Wyne KI. American Association of Clinical Endocrinologists Medical Guidelines for Clinical Practice for developing a diabetes mellitus comprehensive care plan. *Endo Pract* 2011;17(Suppl 2):3–53; Veterans Administration/Department of Defense. Clinical practice guideline for the management of diabetes mellitus, version 4.0, August 2010. Available at www.healthquality.va.gov/Diabetes_Mellitus.asp. Accessed November 2013.

population has been questioned. Several meta-analyses have demonstrated only small (but statistically significant) decreases of 0.2–0.4% in A1C with SMBG.[47,49–51] The studies included in these meta-analyses were limited in important ways, however, mitigating the conclusions that otherwise might be drawn from them. The most important limitation is that most of the studies purposely did not instruct patients on how to use SMBG data or how to respond to the results. In addition, health care providers in these studies did not use the SMBG data to titrate medication. Several recent studies have shown more robust effects of SMBG when it was employed in a structured program of paired testing (pre- and postmeals) combined with algorithms addressing the SMBG pattern to assist health care providers.[52–55] The A1C reduction in these studies (–0.5% to –1.4%) approaches or equals the efficacy of several FDA-approved drugs for glycemic management of T2D. In addition, the paired-testing approach increases patient awareness of postprandial glycemic effects of their food choices that lead to salutary lifestyle changes.[56] Other studies have demonstrated that in subjects with T2D SMBG resulted in not only improvement in A1C but also better control of lipids and weight[57,58] and significantly less depression with an improved sense of well-being.[59] Consequently, a recent consensus statement concluded that SMBG should be performed in a structured format in which the data are used to guide treatment.[60]

Despite the growing evidence in favor of SMBG, most patients with T2D do not test as frequently as recommended.[45,61] There are multiple reasons for this ranging from poor literacy and numeracy skills, inability to understand relevance of the result, fear of finger-pricking, and cost. Perhaps one of the most important factors in patients' failing to test at the recommended frequency is that diabetes health care providers do not teach them how to set glucose targets, interpret the results of SMBG, and thereby make changes in food choices and physical activity. Unless the patient sees the value of glucose monitoring and understands the multiple ways SMBG increases personal safety and enables lifestyle choices, there is little motivation to continue a practice that is uncomfortable and expensive. The fact that diabetes health care providers often do not routinely review the data in a timely, efficient, and interactive manner (usually because of the time limits of a typical clinic encounter) further contributes to the problem. Ultimately, the discussion of how to use the glucose results must occur between patient and provider to make this a meaningful practice. Development of software with decision support holds the promise of improving the usefulness of SMBG.

CONTINUOUS GLUCOSE MONITORING

TECHNOLOGY

The first CGM using venous blood was contained in an artificial pancreas system ~40 years ago.[62] Further development of such systems such as the Biostator provided valuable information about subcutaneous insulin dosing in patients with T1D who were considered "brittle."[63,64] Since that time, key technologic advancements have permitted the subcutaneous placement of a glucose sensor, which provides interstitial glucose readings about every 5 minutes. Intravascular CGMs are under development as well. Thus, a new era has emerged in which we can better and more conveniently understand the real-time, real-world effects of diet, exercise, and medication as well as other physiologic processes, such as sleep and stress, on glucose dynamics. Furthermore, CGM has permitted the observation of intraday glycemic variability, which has been proposed to cause oxidative stress,[65] leading to increased micro- and macrovascular complications independent of A1C.[66] Although a cause-and-effect relationship between glycemic variability and adverse effects that are independent of A1C has yet to be proven,[67] a number of tantalizing associations have been demonstrated.[68–72] The future use of CGM in hospital settings should permit the safe achievement of tight glycemic control that may be beneficial in some (e.g., cardiac surgery) but not all patient populations.[48,73–78] Finally, CGM technology is the linchpin in sensor-augmented pumping and in the low–glucose threshold suspend pump,[4] as discussed elsewhere in this book.

Currently available CGMs utilize interstitial fluid glucose to provide real-time glucose values. Glucose sensors are 27–33 gauge (or 0.36–0.23 mm) and are 8.75–13 mm long. The sensor resides in the subcutaneous space for up to 1 week and is connected to a transmitter that relays a signal to either a handheld receiver or directly to an insulin pump where the interstitial glucose level is displayed along with directional information and trends over the previous 1–24 hours. CGMs must be calibrated using a standard glucose meter two to three times a day. Because of the lag time between blood glucose and interstitial glucose, calibration should not be done when there is a high rate of change in glucose such as in the first hour after eating or when a rapid change arrow appears on the display screen.

CGM utilizes much of the same underlying technology that is present in strip-based meters (i.e., glucose oxidase). Devices are using other methodologies, however, such as microdialysis[79] and fluorescence,[80] that permit them to be placed in a central vein, thereby making them suitable for hospital use and ultimately for a fully implantable artificial pancreas. Such devices would circumvent the error risks presented by interfering substances, such as acetaminophen, that otherwise may prevent accurate measurement. Indeed, intravenous acetaminophen's use is increasingly common in critical care settings.[81]

ACCURACY OF CONTINUOUS GLUCOSE MONITORS

There has been considerable improvement in the both analytic and clinical accuracy of CGM sensors over the past decade as determined by a key analytic statistical metric of Mean Absolute Relative Difference (MARD), which is the difference between the reference method (e.g., YSI) and the sensor value in either direction. Most current sensors now have MARDs of 12–18% over the entire range of glucose levels, although newer sensors in development have shown that performance in the 10–11% range is possible.[82] Sensor performance may be better or worse at the extremes of glucose levels depending on the manufacturer. An additional performance metric of CGM is trend accuracy. To this end, continuous error grids have been devised that can demonstrate both point and trend accuracy.[83]

Among the technical challenges of CMG is the fact that the interstitial fluid compartment glucose lags behind serum blood glucose by 10–15 minutes because of the time of diffusion into the subcutaneous space where the CGM electrode resides. In addition, there is additional processing lag time related to the processing delay of the device because displayed result may be a weighted average over several prior measurements. CGM devices also have other problems, including unpredictable loss of sensitivity over the days of use, which may be due to biofouling, "noise" that may occur in the sensor signal for unknown reasons, sensor "dropout," and risks from interfering substances, such as acetaminophen. Nevertheless, the ability to show trends in glucose and to trigger alarms at preset thresholds is a powerful offset to these problems.

CLINICAL USE OF CONTINUOUS GLUCOSE MONITORS

There are currently two clinical applications of CGM technology. One is a diagnostic or "professional" version in which a CGM is worn for 3–7 days in the "masked" mode so that patient is unable to see the results in real time. This "continuous snapshot" is reviewed by the patient's diabetes health care provider for assessment of trends and areas of previously unrecognized hyper- or hypoglycemia. The other application is real-time CGM (RT-CGM), in which the patient uses the device for an indefinite period of time permitting the tracking and trending of glucose. The FDA has approved RT-CGM devices only for this tracking purpose and not for use in dosing insulin—a blood glucose sample must be used to calculate an insulin dose. Indications for each of these forms of CGM are shown in Table 4.4. Studies using both approaches generally have shown positive effects on A1C with a decrease of 0.5% with diagnostic CGM and 0.4% with RT-CGM.[84]

Diagnostic CGM

The first use of modern CGMs was diagnostic, using 3–7 days of "masked" CGM data—that is, the patient is unaware of the readings and there are no alarms for hyper- or hypoglycemia. The sensor is inserted into the patient in the

Table 4.4 Indications for Real-Time Versus Diagnostic Use of Continuous Glucose Monitors

Diagnostic CGM	Real-time CGM
Inconsistency between glucose record diary and A1C	Improving diabetes management in patients with unstable diabetes
Assessing the frequency and severity of hyper- and hypoglycemia	Tracking and trending glucose, thereby enabling patients to intervene and prevent unwanted glucose excursions
Evaluation of the adequacy of timing and frequency of self-monitored blood glucose	Assisting patients with hypoglycemia unawareness, repeated severe hypoglycemic episodes, or undetected hypoglycemia
Enhancing patient education and psychological motivation for optimal diabetes management	Providing parents the ability to monitor their children in real time

Note: CGM = continuous glucose monitoring.

provider's office and the patient is instructed to calibrate the sensor two or more times a day using a blood glucose meter and to maintain a food and activity diary while wearing the device. The diary is an intergral element of the procedure because patients often forget what they ate or what activities might have affected their glucose levels. Upon return of the device to the provider's office, the uploaded data can be analyzed in conjunction with the diary. This leads to a detailed conversation between the patient and provider about the glycemic patterns and events that might be responsible for them, resulting in recommendations for changes in management. Substantial evidence supports the use of diagnostic CGM to detect and treat hypo- and hyperglycemia that was either previously unsuspected or whose frequency and severity was underestimated. The overall results of these studies are that management changes made by the provider as a result of this information reduce the frequency and duration of hypoglycemia and improve overall glycemic control as measured by A1C. A wide variety of patients have been shown to benefit from diagnostic CGM, including those with T1D and T2D,[85,86] including children,[87,88] pregnant women,[89] and elderly patients.[90] The use of diagnostic CGM may have an increasingly important role in older adults because hypoglycemia is common among elderly patients with T2D even in those with A1Cs of ≥9% and those not on insulin.[91] Hypoglycemia is also an increasingly common reason for hospital admissions among Medicare beneficiaries.[92] Diagnostic CGM use may offer additional benefits. For example, reviewing the CGM results with women who have T2D allowed them to independently apply problem-solving skills to identify reasons for the episodes of glycemic excursions (e.g., food intake, physical activity, or stress).[93] Finally, counseling following diagnostic CGM improves physical activity behaviors and leads to weight reduction.[94] Diagnostic CGM is reimbursable by most third-party payers, including Medicare under current procedural terminology codes 95250 and 95251.[95]

Real-Time CGM

The glucose values displayed every 5 minutes by RT-CGM along with the trending information and high- and low-glucose alarms provide important, actionable information for patients who use these devices. Randomized clinical trials in patients with T1D have demonstrated that compared with SMBG, adults with A1Cs >7% have an improvement of A1C with fewer hypoglycemic episodes and that in those beginning with an A1C <7%, there is a reduction in hypoglycemic episodes without a deterioration in A1C.[96-98] Recent meta-analyses confirm these results, that is, RT-CGM is superior to SMBG in improving A1C (by 0.3% on average), although greater effects are seen at higher baseline A1Cs.[99,100] Not surprisingly, RT-CGM's effect was greatest in those using the device for >60% of the time.[100,101] The benefit appears in all age-groups >8 years. In addition, when combined with an insulin pump—so-called sensor-augmented pumping (SAP)—there is a significant improvement in A1C and a reduction of hypoglycemia rates as well as overall glycemic control as measured by A1C compared with those using multiple daily insulin dosing with SMBG.[101] As yet, evidence has not been convincing that RT-CGM is more beneficial than usual care in pregnant women with diabetes.[102]

Hospital use of RT-CGM, whether in the perioperative period or in critical care units, cannot yet be recommended because of concerns with sensor inaccuracy as a result of drug interference, anemia, hypothermia, and hypotension among others.[103] A recent study in the critical care setting, however, suggested that it may be useful despite these drawbacks.[104]

Beneficial results of RT-CGM have been found in those with T2D taking insulin for reasons similar to those with T1D.[105–108] In addition, RT-CGM may be effective both as a "motivational device" and as a tool to refine problem-solving skills not only improving A1C but also promoting weight loss.[94,107] This notion is strengthened by studies in which patients with either T1D or T2D underwent a period of masked CGM followed by unmasking; the unmasking resulted in a markedly improved A1C within 6 days without a change in the prescribed regimen (Figure 4.3).[109,110] Even patients with T2D who are not on prandial insulin may benefit from RT-CGM presumably because it acts as a behavioral modification tool.[111]

RT-CGM use is not without its challenges. Patients develop alarm "fatigue" particularly if the alarms are set too high for hypoglycemia alerting and too low for hyperglycemia alerting, and loss of sensor signal can occur when lying directly on the sensor site.[112] In fact, continuous use of RT-CGM is the exception rather than the rule, particularly in children and adolescents who stop using it for a variety of reasons, including inaccuracy, discomfort, and an additional burden for managing their disease.[113] This, in part, may explain why only 10% of the 26,000 patients with T1D who are registered in the T1D Exchange currently are using RT-CGM.[114] Finally, because clinically relevant decision support tools for both interpreting RT-CGM data and providing actionable advice about the data are not available, reviewing CGM data remains time consuming and largely subjective.

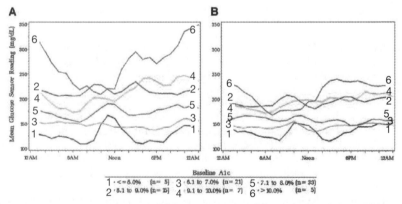

Figure 4.3—Modal day under (a) masked and (b) unmasked conditions, according to baseline A1C. *Source:* From Garg S, Jovanovic L. Relationship of fasting and hourly blood glucose levels to HbA1c values. *Diabetes Care* 2006;29:2644–2649.

CONCLUSION

The foundation and success of current diabetes management for both T1D and T2D are based on the tripod of lifestyle modification (including education), glucose monitoring, and pharmacotherapy. Each leg of the tripod plays an essential yet interactive role in achieving a patient's glycemic goal safely and effectively. By making SMBG more accurate, accessible, and reliable, glucose monitoring has materially advanced our goal of improving dysglycemia and reducing complications over the past decade. Yet, challenges still exist for both patients and diabetes health care providers in making glucose monitoring a seamless part of glycemic management, which ultimately will be solved by improved software and decision-support systems. With improving accuracy, decision-support software, and reduction in costs, it is likely that RT-CGM eventually will supplant SMBG for management of patients using prandial insulin.

REFERENCES

1. Diabetes Control and Complications Trial Research Group. The effect of intensive treatment of diabetes on the development and progression of long-term complications in insulin-dependent diabetes mellitus. *New Engl J Med* 1993;329:977–986.

2. U.K. Prospective Diabetes Study Group. Association of systolic blood pressure with macrovascular and microvascular complications of type 2 diabetes (UKPDS 36): prospective observational study. *BMJ* 2000;321:412–419.

3. Centers for Disease Control and Prevention. Diabetes report card 2012: national and state profile of diabetes and its complications, 2012. Available at www.cdc.gov/diabetes/pubs/reportcard/trends.htm. Accessed November 2013.

4. Bergenstal RM, Klonoff DC, Garg SK, Bode BW, Meredith M, Slover RH, Ahmann AJ, Welsh JB, Lee SW, Kaufman FR; for the ASPIRE In-Home Study Group. Threshold-based insulin pump interruption for reduction of hypoglycemia. *N Eng J Med* 2013;369:224–232.

5. Chao R, Henry RR. SGLT2 inhibition: a novel strategy for diabetes treatment. *Nat Rev Drug Discov* 2010;9:551–559.

6. Free AH, Adams EC, Kercher ML, Free HM, Cook MH. Simple specific test for urine glucose. *Clin Chem* 1957;3:163–167.

7. Kohn J. A rapid method of estimating blood glucose ranges. *Lancet* 1957;273: 119–121.

8. Clarke SF, Foster JR. A history of blood glucose meters and their role in self-monitoring of diabetes mellitus. *Brit J Biomed Sci* 2012;69:83–93.

9. Frias JP, Lim CG, Ellison JM, Montandon CM. A review of adverse events associated with false glucose readings measured by GDH-PQQ–based glu-

cose test strips in the presence of interfering sugars. *Diabetes Care* 2010;33:728–729.

10. Ferri S, Kojima K, Sode K. Review of glucose oxidases and glucose dehydrogenases: a bird's eye view of glucose sensing enzymes. *J Diab Sci Tech* 2011;5:1068–1976.

11. Yamashita Y, Ferri S, Huynh ML, Shimizu H, Yamaoka H, Sode K. Direct electron transfer type disposable sensor strip for glucose sensing employing an engineered FAD glucose dehydrogenase. *Enz Microb Techol* 2013;52:123–128.

12. Bennion N, Christensen NK, McGarraugh G. Alternate site glucose testing: a crossover design. *Diab Technol Ther* 2002;4:25–33.

13. Knapp PE, Showers KM, Phipps JC, Speckman JL, Sternthal E, Freund KM, Ash AS, Apovian CM. Self-monitoring of blood glucose with finger tip versus alternative site sampling: effect on glycemic control in insulin-using patients with type 2 diabetes. *Diab Technol Ther* 2009;11:219–225.

14. Suzuki Y, Atsumi Y, Matusoka K. Alternative site testing increases compliance of SMBG (preliminary study of 3 years cohort trials). *Diab Res Clin Pract* 2003;59:233–234.

15. Bina DM, Anderson RL, Johnson ML, Bergenstal RM, Kendall DM. Clinical impact of prandial state, exercise, and site preparation on the equivalence of alternative-site blood glucose testing. *Diabetes Care* 2003;26:981–985.

16. Jungheim K, Koschinsky T. Glucose monitoring at the arm: risky delays of hypoglycemia and hyperglycemia detection. *Diabetes Care* 2002;25:956–960.

17. Ginsberg B. An analysis: to code or not to code—that is the question. *J Diabetes Sci Technol* 2008;2:819–821.

18. Schrock LE. Miscoding and other user errors: importance of ongoing education for proper blood glucose monitoring procedures. *J Diabetes Sci Technol* 2008;2:563–567.

19. Hirsch IB. Blood glucose monitoring technology: translating data into practice. *Endocrine Pract* 2004;10:67–76.

20. Janssen M, Portalatin M, Wallace J, Zhong W, Parkes JL. Ascensia® WinGLUCOFACTS® professional software improves diabetes health outcomes. *J Diab Sci Technol* 2007;1:47–53.

21. Crowe DJ. Analysis of the evaluation of a new glucose meter with integrated self-management software and USB connectivity. *J Diab Sci Technol* 2011;5:1154–1156.

22. Ginsberg B. Practical use of self-monitoring of blood glucose data. *J Diab Sci Technol* 2013;7:532–541.

23. Arsand E, Froisland DH, Skrovseth SO, Chomutare T, Tatara N, Hartvigsen G, Tufano JT. Mobile health applications to assist patients with diabetes: lessons learned and design implications. *J Diab Sci Technol* 2012;6:1197–1206.

24. Fonda SJ, Kedziora RJ, Vigersky RA, Bursell S-E. Combining iGoogle and personal health records to create a prototype personal health application for diabetes self-management. *Telemed and e-Health J* 2010;16:480–489.

25. Goyal S, Cafazzo JA. Mobile phone healthy apps for diabetes management: current evidence and future developments. *Quart J Med* 2013;106:1067–1069.

26. Harris LT, Tufano J, Le T, Rees C, Lewis GA, Evert AB, Flowers J, Collins C, Hoath J, Hirsch IB, Goldberg HI, Ralston JD. Designing mobile support for glycemic control in patients with diabetes. *J Biomed Inform* 2010;43(5Suppl):S37–S40.

27. Quinn CC, Shardell MD, Terrin ML, Barr EA, Ballew SH, Gruber-Baldini AL. Cluster-randomized trial of a mobile phone personalized behavioral intervention for blood glucose control. *Diabetes Care* 2011;34:1934–1942.

28. U.S. Food and Drug Administration. Self-monitoring blood glucose test systems for over-the-counter use, 2014. Available at www.fda.gov/downloads/MedicalDevices/DeviceRegulationandGuidance/GuidanceDocuments/UCM380327.pdf. Accessed February 2014.

29. U.S. Food and Drug Administration. Blood glucose monitoring test systems for prescription point-of-care use, 2014. Available at www.fda.gov/downloads/MedicalDevices/DeviceRegulationandGuidance/GuidanceDocuments/UCM380325.pdf. Accessed February 2014.

30. Karon BS, Boyd JC, Klee GG. Empiric validation of simulation models for estimating glucose meter performance criteria for moderate levels of glycemic control. *Diab Tech Ther* 2013;15:996–1003.

31. U.S. Food and Drug Administration. Fingerstick devices to obtain blood specimens: initial communication—risk of transmitting bloodborne pathogens. Reusable fingerstick (blood lancing) devices and point of care (POC) blood testing devices (e.g., blood glucose meters, PT/INR anticoagulation meters, cholesterol testing devices), 2010. Available at www.fda.gov/MedicalDevices/Safety/AlertsandNotices/ucm224025.htm. Accessed 2 February 2014.

32. Dungan K, Chapman J, Braithwaite SS, Buse J. Glucose measurement: confounding issues in setting targets for inpatient management. *Diabetes Care* 2007;30:403–409.

33. Lyon ME, Baskin LB, Braakman, Presti S, Dubois J, Shirey T. Interference studies with two hospital-grade and two home-grade glucose meters. *Diab Technol Ther* 2009;11:641–647.

34. Karon BS, Griesmann L, Scott R, Bryant SC, Dubois JA, Shirey TL, Presti S, Santrach PJ. Evaluation of the impact of hematocrit and other interference on the accuracy of hospital-based glucose meters. *Diab Technol Ther* 2008;10:111–120.

35. Tang Z, Du X, Louie RF, Kost GJ. Effects of drugs on glucose measurements with handheld glucose meters and a portable glucose analyzer. *Am J Clin Path* 2000;113:75–86.

36. Tang Z, Louie R, Lee J, Lee D, Miller E, Kost GJ. Oxygen effects on glucose meter measurements with glucose dehydrogenase- and oxidase-based test strips for point-of-care testing. *Crit Care Med* 2001;29:1062–1070.

37. Heinemann L. Quality of glucose measurement with blood glucose meters at the point-of-care: relevance of interfering factors. *Diab Tech Ther* 2010;12:847–857.

38. Karon BS, Gandhi GY, Nuttall GA, Bryant SC, Schaff HV, McMahon MM, Santrach PJ. Accuracy of Roche Accu-Chek Inform whole blood capillary, arterial, and venous glucose values in patients receiving therapy after cardiac surgery. *Am J Clin Path* 2007;127:919–926.

39. Clarke WL, Cox D, Gonder-Frederick LA, Carter W, Pohl SL. Evaluating clinical accuracy of systems for self-monitoring of blood glucose. *Diabetes Care* 1987;10:622–628.

40. Parkes JL, Slatin SL, Pardo S, Ginsberg BH. A new consensus error grid to evaluate the clinical significance of inaccuracies in the measurement of blood glucose. *Diabetes Care* 2000;23:1143–1148.

41. Klonoff DC, Lias C, Vigersky R, Clarke W, Parkes JL Sacks DB Kirkman MS, Kovatchev B; The Error Grid Panel. The Surveillance Error Grid. *J Diab Sci Tech* (in press).

42. Freckmann G, Schmid C, Baumstark A, Pleus S, Link M, Haug C. System accuracy evaluation of 43 blood glucose monitoring systems for self-monitoring of blood glucose according to DIN EN ISO 15197. *J Diab Sci Technol* 2012;6:1060–1075.

43. Klonoff DC, Reyes JS. Do currently available blood glucose monitors meet regulatory standards? 1-day public meeting in Arlington, Virginia. *J Diab Sci Technol* 2013;7:1071–1083.

44. Blonde L, Ginsberg BH, Horne S. Frequency of blood glucose monitoring in relation to glycemic control in patients with type 2 diabetes. *Diabetes Care* 2002;25:245–246.

45. Evans JMM, Newton RW, Ruta DA, MacDonald TM, Stevenson RJ, Morris AD. Frequency of blood glucose monitoring in relation to glycaemic control: observational study with diabetes database. *BMJ* 1999;319:83–86.

46. Karter AJ, Parker MM, Moffet HH, Spence MM, Chan J, Ettner SL, Selby JV. Longitudinal study of new and prevalent use of self-monitoring of blood glucose. *Diabetes Care* 2006;29:1757–1763.

47. Ziegler R, Heidtmann B, Hilgard D, Hofer S, Rosenbauer J, Holl R; for the DPV-Wiss-Initiative. Frequency of SMBG correlates with HbA1c and acute complications in children and adolescents with type 1 diabetes. *Pediatr Diab* 2011;12:11–17.

48. American Diabetes Association. Standards of medical care in diabetes—2013. *Diabetes Care* 2013;37(Suppl 1):S14–S80.

49. Clar C, Barnard K, Cummins E, Royle P, Waugh N; Aberdeen Health Technology Assessment Group. Self-monitoring of blood glucose in type 2 diabetes: systematic review. *Health Technol Assess* 2010;14:1–140.

50. Malanda UL, Welschen LC, Riphagen II, Dekker JM, Nijpels G, Bot SDM. Self-monitoring of blood glucose in patients with type 2 diabetes mellitus who are not using insulin. *Cochrane Database Syst Rev* 2012;1:CD005060.

51. St. John A, Davis WA, Price CP, Davis TM. The value of self-monitoring of blood glucose: a review of recent evidence. *J Diab Comp* 2010;24:129–141.

52. Durán A, Martín P, Runkle I, Pérez N, Abad R, Fernández M, Del Valle L, Sanz MF, Calle-Pascual AL. Benefits of self-monitoring blood glucose in the management of new-onset type 2 diabetes mellitus: the St Carlos Study, a prospective randomized clinic-based interventional study with parallel groups. *J Diabetes* 2010;2:203–211.

53. Franciosi M, Lucisano G, Pellegrini F, Cantarello A, Consoli A, Cucco L, Ghidelli R, Sartore G, Sciangula L, Nicolucci A; on behalf of the ROSES Study Group. ROSES: Role of self-monitoring of blood glucose and intensive education in patients with type 2 diabetes not receiving insulin. A pilot randomized clinical trial. *Diabet Med* 2011;28:789–796.

54. Lalic N, Tankova T, Nourredine M, Parkin C, Schweppe U, Amann-Zalan I. Value and utility of structured self-monitoring of blood glucose in real world clinical practice: findings from a multinational observational study. *Diab Tech Ther* 2012;14:338–343.

55. Polonsky WH, Fisher L, Schikman CH, Hinnen DA, Parkin CG, Jelsovsky Z, Petersen B, Schweitzer M, Wagner RS. Structured self-monitoring of blood glucose significantly reduces A1C levels in poorly controlled, noninsulin-treated type 2 diabetes: results from the Structured Testing Program study. *Diabetes Care* 2011;34:262–267.

56. Bergenstal R, Bode BW, Tamler R, Trence DL, Stenger P, Schachner HC, Fullam J, Pardo S, Kohut T, Fisher WA. Advanced meter features improve postprandial and paired self-monitoring of blood glucose in individuals with diabetes: results of the Actions with the CONTOUR Blood Glucose Meter and Behaviors in Frequent Testers (ACT) study. *Diab Tech Ther* 2012;14:851–857.

57. McAndrew LM, Napolitano MA, Pogach LM, Quigley KS, Shantz KL, Vander Veur SS, Forster GD. The impact of self-monitoring of blood glucose on a behavioral weight loss intervention for patients with type 2 diabetes. *Diabetes Educ* 2013;39:397–405.

58. Zhang DA, Katznelson L, Li M. Postprandial glucose monitoring further improved glycemia, lipids, and weight in persons with type 2 diabetes mellitus who had already reached hemoglobin A1c goal. *J Diabetes Sci Tech* 2012;6:289–293

59. Schwedes U, Siebolds M, Mertes. Meal-related structured self-monitoring of blood glucose: effect on diabetes control in non-insulin-treated type 2 diabetic patients. *Diabetes Care* 2002;25:1928–1932.

60. Klonoff, DC, Blonde, L, Cembrowski, G, Chacra AR, Charpentier, G, Colagiuri, S, Dailey, G, Gabbay, RA, Heinemann, L, Kerr, D, Nicolucci, A, Polonsky, W, Schnell, O, Vigersky, R, Yale, J-F. Consensus report: The current role of self-monitoring of blood glucose in non-insulin-treated type 2 diabetes. *J Diab Sci Tech* 2011;6:1529–1154.

61. Karter AJ, Ackerson LM, Darbinian JA, D'Agostino RB Jr, Ferrara A, Liu J, Selby JV. Self-monitoring of blood glucose levels and glycemic control: the Northern California Kaiser Permanente Diabetes Registry. *Am J Med* 2001;111:1–9.

62. Albisser AM, Leibel BS, Ewart TG, Davidovac Z, Botz CK, Zingg W, Schipper H, Gander R. Clinical control of diabetes by the artificial pancreas. *Diabetes* 1974;23:397–404.

63. Ratzmann KP, Bruns W, Schulz B, Zander E. Use of Biostator in improving insulin therapy in unstable insulin-dependent diabetes. *Diabetes Care* 1982;4:11–17.

64. Mayfield RK, Sullivan FM, Colwell JA, Wohltmann H. Predicting insulin requirements for a portable insulin pump using the Biostator. *Diabetes* 1983;32:908–914.

65. Brownlee M. The pathobiology of diabetic complications: a unifying mechanism. *Diabetes* 2005;54:1615–1625.

66. Brownlee M, Hirsch IB. Glycemic variability: a hemoglobin A1C-independent risk factor for diabetic complications. *JAMA* 2006;295:1707–1708.

67. Siegelaar SE, Holleman F, Hoekstra JBL, DeVries JH. Glucose variability: does it matter? *Endocrine Reviews* 2010;3:171–182.

68. Hermanides J, Vriesendorp TM, Bosman RJ, Zandstra DF, Hoekstra JB, Devries JH. Glucose variability is associated with intensive care unit mortality. *Crit Care Med* 2010;38:838–842.

69. Hu Y, Liu W, Huang R, Zhang X. Postchallenge plasma glucose excursions, carotid intima-media thickness, and risk factors for atherosclerosis in Chinese population with type 2 diabetes. *Atherosclerosis* 2010;210:302–306.

70. Su G, Mi S, Tao H, Li Z, Yang H, Zheng H, Hou Y, Ma C. Association of GV and the presence and severity of coronary artery disease in patients with type 2 diabetes. *Cardiovasc Diabet* 2011;10:19–27.

71. Sun J, Xu Y, Sun S, Sun Y, Wang X. Intermittent high glucose enhances cell proliferation and VEGF expression in retinal endothelial cells: the role of mitochondrial reactive oxygen species. *Mol Cell Biochem* 2010;343:27–35.

72. Temelkova-Kurktschiev TS, Koehler C, Henkel E, Leonhardt W, Fuecker K, Hanefeld M. Postchallenge plasma glucose and glycemic spikes are more

strongly associated with atherosclerosis than fasting glucose or HbA1c level. *Diabetes Care* 2000;23:1830–1834.

73. Qaseem A, Humphrey LL, Chou R, Snow V, Shekelle P. Use of intensive insulin therapy for the management of glycemic control in hospitalized patients: a clinical practice guideline from the American College of Physicians. *Ann Int Med* 2011;154:260–267.

74. Buchleitner AM, Martinez-Alonso M, Hernandez M, Sola I, Mauricio D. Perioperative glycaemic control for diabetic patients undergoing surgery. The Cochrane Collaboration. *Cochrane Database Syst Rev* 2012;1-95. Available at www.thecochranelibrary.com. Accessed November 2013.

75. Desai SP, Henry LL, Holmes SD, Hunt Sl, Martin CT, Hebsur S, Ad N. Strict versus liberal target range for perioperative glucose in patients undergoing coronary artery bypass grafting: a prospective randomized controlled trial *J Thorac Cardiovasc Surg* 2012;143:310–325.

76. Furnary A. Clinical benefits of tight glycaemic control. *Best Pract Res Clin Anaesth* 2009;23:411–420.

77. Sathya B, Davis R, Taveira T, Whitlatch H, Wu W-C. Intensity of peri-operative glycemic control and post-operative outcomes in patients with DM: a meta-analysis. *Diab Res Clin Pract* 2013;102:8–15.

78. Umpierrez GE, Hellman R, Korytkowski MT, Kosiborod M, Maynard GA, Montori VM, Seley JJ, Van Den Berghe G. Management of hyperglycemia in hospitalized patients in non-critical care setting: an Endocrine Society Clinical Practice Guideline. *J Clin Endo Metab* 2012;97:16–38.

79. Schierenbeck, F, Öwall A, Franco-Cereceda A, Liska J. Evaluation of a continuous blood glucose monitoring system using a central venous catheter with an integrated microdialysis function. *Diabetes Technol Ther* 2013;15:26–31.

80. Klonoff DC. Overview of fluorescence glucose sensing: a technology with a bright future. *J Diab Sci Technol* 2012;6:1242–1250.

81. Jones VM. Acetaminophen injection: a review of clinical information. *J Pain Palliat Care Pharmacother* 2011;25:340–349.

82. Zschornack E, Schmid C, Pleus S, Link M, Klotzer H-M, Obermaier K, Schoemaker M, Strasser M, Frisch G, Schmelzeisen-Redeker G, Haug C, Freckmann G. Evaluation of the performance of a novel system for continuous glucose monitoring *J Diab Sci Technol* 2013;7:815–823.

83. Clarke W, Kovatchev B. Statistical tools to analyze continuous glucose monitor data. *Diab Technol Ther* 2009;11:S45–S54.

84 Floyd B, Chandra P, Hall S, Phillips C, Alema-Mensah E, Strayhorn G, Ofili EO, Umpierrez GE. Comparative analysis of the efficacy of continuous glucose monitoring and self-monitoring of blood glucose in type 1 diabetes mellitus. *J Diab Sci Technol* 2012;6:1094–1102.

85. Chico A, Vidal-Rios P, Subira M, Novials A. The continuous glucose monitoring system is useful for detecting unrecognized hypoglycemia in patients with type 1 and type 2 diabetes but is not better than frequent capillary glucose measurements for improving metabolic control. *Diabetes Care* 2003;26:1153–1157.

86. Tanenberg R, Bode B, Lane W, Levetan C, Mestman J, Harmel AP, Tobian J, Gross T, Mastrototaro J. Use of the continuous glucose monitoring system to guide therapy in patients with insulin-treated diabetes: a randomized controlled trial. *Mayo Clin Proc* 2004;79:1521–1526.

87. Boland E, Monsod T, Delucia M, Brandt CA, Fernando S, Tamborlane WV. Limitations of conventional methods of self-monitoring of blood glucose: Lessons learned from 3 days of continuous glucose sensing in pediatric patients with type 1 diabetes. *Diabetes Care* 2001;24:1858–1862.

88. Kaufman FR, Gibson LC, Halvorson M, Carpenter S, Fisher LK, Pitukcheewanont P. A pilot study of the continuous glucose monitoring system: clinical decisions and glycemic control after its use in pediatric type 1 diabetic subjects. *Diabetes Care* 2001;24:2030–2034.

89. Murphy HR, Rayman G, Lewis K, Kelly S, Johal B, Duffield K, Fowler D, Campbell PJ, Temple RC. Effectiveness of continuous glucose monitoring in pregnant women with diabetes: randomized clinical trial. *BMJ* 2008; 337:a1680.

90. Munshi MN, Segal AR, Suhl E, Staum E, Desrochers L, Sternthal A, Giusti J, McCartney R, Lee Y, Bonsignore P, Weinger K. Frequent hypoglycemia among elderly patients with poor glycemic control. *Arch Intern Med* 2011;171:362–364.

91. Lipska KJ, Warton EM, Huang ES, Moffet HH, Inzucchi SE, Krumholz HM, Karter AJ. HbA1c and risk of severe hypoglycemia in type 2 diabetes: the Diabetes and Aging study. *Diabetes Care* 2013;36:3535–3542.

92. Lipska KJ, Want Y, Ross JS, Inzucchi SE, Huang ES, Karter AJ, Minges KE, Dsai MM, Krumholz HM. National trends in hospital admissions for hyperglycemia and hypoglycemia among Medicare beneficiaries, 1999–2010. American Diabetes Association 73rd Scientific Session, Abstract Number 274-OR, June 24, 2013.

93. Fritschi C, Quinn L, Penckofer S, Surkyk PM. Continuous glucose monitoring: the experience of women with type 2 diabetes. *Diabetes Educ* 2010;36:250–257.

94. Allen NA, Fain JA, Braun B, Chipkin SR. Continuous glucose monitoring counseling improves physical activity behaviors of individuals with type 2 diabetes: a randomized clinical trial. *Diab Res Clin Pract* 2008;80:371–379.

95. Blevins TC. Professional continuous glucose monitoring in clinical practice. *J Diab Sci Technol* 2010;4:440–446.

96. Juvenile Diabetes Research Foundation Study Group. Effect of CGM in well-controlled type 1. *Diabetes Care* 2009;32:1378–1383.

97. Deiss D, Bolinder J, Riveline JP, Battelino T, Bosi E, Tubiana-Rufi N, Kerr D, Phillip M. Improved glycemic control in poorly controlled patients with type 1 diabetes using real-time continuous glucose monitoring. *Diabetes Care* 2006;29:2730–2732.

98. O'Connell MA, Donath S, O'Neal DN, Colman PG, Ambler GR, Jones TW, Davis EA, Cameron FJ. Glycaemic impact of patient-led use of sensor-guided pump therapy in type 1 diabetes: a randomized controlled trial. *Diabetolgia* 2009;52:1250–1257.

99. Liebl A, Henrichs HR, Heinemann L, Freckmann G, Biermann E, Thomas A. Continuous glucose monitoring: evidence and consensus statement for clinical use. *J Diab Sci Tech* 2013;7:500–519.

100. Pickup JC, Freeman SC, Sutton AJ. Glycaemic control in type 1 diabetes during real time continuous glucose monitoring compared with self-monitoring of blood glucose: meta-analysis of randomized controlled trials using individual patient data. *BMJ* 2011;343:d3805.

101. Golden SH, Brown T, Yeh H-C, Maruthur N, Ranasinghe P, Berger Z, Suh Y, Wilson LM, Haberl EB, Bass EB. Methods for insulin delivery and glucose monitoring: comparative effectiveness. Agency for Healthcare Research and Quality Comparative Effectiveness Review 2012;57:12-EHC036-EF.

102. Secher AL, Ringholm L, Andersen HU, Damm P, Mathiesen ER. The effect of real-time continuous glucose monitoring in pregnant women with diabetes. *Diabetes Care* 2013;36:1877–1883.

103. Klonoff D. Buckingham B, Christiansen JS, Montori VM, Tamborlane WV, Vigersky RA, Wolpert H. Continuous glucose monitoring: an Endocrine Society clinical practice guideline. *J Clin Endocrinol Metab* 2011;96:2968–2979.

104. Holzinger U, Warszawska J, Kitzberger R, Wewalka M, Miehsler W, Herkner H, Madl C. Real-time continuous glucose monitoring in critically ill patients. *Diabetes Care* 2010;33:467–472. RT- CGM useful in ICU

105. Bailey TS, Zisser HC, Garg SK. Reduction in hemoglobin A1C with real-time continuous glucose monitoring: results from a 12-233k observational study. *Diab Technol Ther* 2007;9:203–210.

106. Garg S, Zisser H, Schwartz S, Bailey T, Kaplan R, Ellis S, Jovanovic L. Improvement in glycemic excursions with a transcutaneous, real-time continuous glucose sensor. *Diabetes Care* 2006;29:44–50.

107. Yoo HJ, An HG, Park SY, Ryu OH, Kim HY, Seo JA, Hong EG, Shin DH, Kim YH, Kim SG, Choi KM, Park IB, Yu JM, Baik SH. Use of a real time continuous glucose monitoring system as a motivational device for poorly controlled type 2 diabetes. *Diab Res Clin Pract* 2008;82:73–79.

108. Zick R, Petersen B, Richter M, Haug C; SAFIR Study Group. Comparison of continuous blood glucose measurement with conventional documentation of hypoglycemia in patients with type 2 diabetes on multiple daily insulin injection therapy. *Diab Technol Ther* 2007;9:483–492.

109. Garg S, Jovanovic L. Relationship of fasting and hourly blood glucose levels to HbA1c values. *Diabetes Care* 2006;29:2644–2649.

110. Rodbard D, Bailey T, Jovanovic L, Zisser H, Kaplan R, Garg SK. Improved quality of glycemic control and reduced glycemic variability with use of continuous glucose monitoring. *Diab Tech Ther* 2009;11:717–723.

111. Vigersky RA, Fonda SJ, Chellappa M, Walker MS, Ehrhardt NM. Short- and long-term effects of real-time continuous glucose monitoring in patients with type 2 diabetes. *Diabetes Care* 2012;35:32–38.

112. Helton KL, Ratner BD, Wisniewski NA. Biomechanics of the sensor-tissue interface-effects of motion, pressure, and design on sensor performance and foreign body response – part II: examples and application. *J Diabetes Sci Technol* 2011;5:647–656.

113. Ramchandani N, Arya S, Ten S, Bhandari S. Real-life utilization of real-time continuous glucose monitoring: the complete picture. *J Diab Sci Technol* 2011;5:860–870.

114. Unitio. T1D Exchange. 2014. Available at https://unitio.org/pages/t1d-exchange/t1d-exchange-data-search. Accessed February 2014.

ACKNOWLEDGMENT

The opinions expressed in this paper reflect the personal views of the authors and not the official views of the United States Army or the Department of Defense.

Chapter 5

Medical Nutrition Therapy

Anne Daly, MS, RDN, BC-ADM, CDE
Margaret A. Powers, PhD, RD, CDE

Medical nutrition therapy (MNT) is an essential component of preventing diabetes, managing existing diabetes, and preventing and slowing diabetes complications. In newly diagnosed people with type 2 diabetes (T2D), A1C levels often decrease 1–2% within 6–12 weeks of initiating MNT. Additionally, MNT is effective in lowering blood pressure, improving lipid profiles, and promoting weight loss. MNT is first-line T2 diabetes therapy, yet as diabetes progresses, medications typically need to be added as an adjunct to MNT. With such a clinically significant treatment tool available, why do so many health care professionals not encourage its full use? Perhaps it is because they are unaware of the effectiveness of MNT. Perhaps some think it is too hard to follow a "diet." Perhaps a referral process for MNT has not been established. Perhaps health care professionals or their patients do not believe that MNT can be reimbursed. This chapter will address these issues so that patients can receive the full benefit of MNT.

OVERVIEW OF MNT

The ultimate goal of diabetes nutrition therapy is for people with diabetes to be comfortable and confident in making daily food choices that contribute to improved metabolic status. This goal is achieved through the development of a personalized food plan that incorporates an individual's favorite foods and typical eating patterns. Nutrition therapy needs to be matched with physiology of the phase of the diabetes disease process (see Figure 5.1). Additionally, counseling and coaching about behavioral strategies particular to the individual support the achievement of short- and long-term goals related to nutrition therapy.

Table 5.1 lists the goals of MNT. Because 75% of deaths in individuals with diabetes are attributed to cardiovascular disease, it is critical that the focus of care be expanded beyond glycemic control. The first goal encompasses the ABCs of diabetes care—managing A1C, blood pressure, and cholesterol. Nutrition therapy is the first-line therapy for managing elevations in each of these areas and heightens the effectiveness of medication when it is necessary. Table 5.2 details the effectiveness of MNT in lowering blood glucose, blood pressure, and cholesterol.

Diabetes medication therapy supports the nutrition therapy and should be prescribed to correspond with eating times and food patterns. The medication should not force an individual to eat at inappropriate or unusual times or to consume excess food to prevent hypoglycemia caused by excess medication. The fact

DOI: 10.2337/9781580405096.05

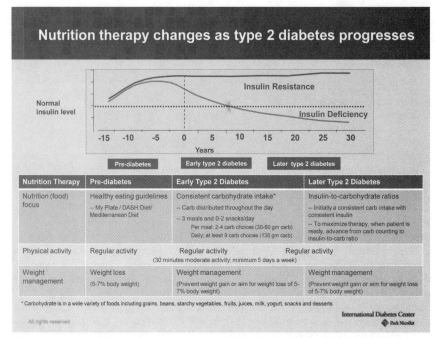

Figure 5.1 — Matching nutrition therapy to disease physiology.

Source: Published with permission of International Diabetes Center, ©2014.

Table 5.1 — Goals of MNT

1. To promote and support healthful eating patterns, emphasizing a variety of nutrient-dense foods in appropriate portion sizes, to improve overall health and specifically to attain the following recommended goals:
   - A1C <7.0
   - Blood pressure <140/80 mmHg
   - Low-density lipoprotein (LDL) cholesterol <100 mg/dl; triglycerides <150 mg/dl; high-density lipoprotein (HDL) cholesterol >40 mg/dl for men; HDL cholesterol >50 mg/dl for women
2. Achieve and maintain body weight goals.
3. Delay and prevent complications of diabetes.
4. Address individual nutrition needs based on personal and cultural preferences, health literacy and numeracy, access to healthful food choices, and willingness and ability to make behavioral changes as well as barriers to change.
5. Maintain the pleasure of eating by providing positive messages about food choices while limiting food choices only when indicated by scientific evidence.
6. Provide the person with diabetes with practical tools for day-to-day meal planning rather than focusing on individual macronutrients, micronutrients, or single foods.

Table 5.2 MNT Effectiveness in Patients with Diabetes

Glycemic control

- ~1% decrease in A1C in newly diagnosed patients with type 1 diabetes (T1D)
- ~2% decrease in A1C in newly diagnosed patients with T2D
- ~1% decrease in A1C with an average 4-year duration of T2D
- 50–100 mg/dl decrease in fasting plasma glucose
- Outcomes will be known by 6 weeks to 3 months

Lipids (intake goal: 7–10% saturated fat, 200–300 mg cholesterol)

- 10–13% decrease in total cholesterol (24–32 mg/dl)
- 12–16% decrease in LDL cholesterol (15–25 mg/dl)
- 8% decrease in triglycerides (15–35 mg/dl)
- Without exercise, HDL cholesterol decreases by 7%; with exercise, no decrease

Hypertension (intake goal: <2,300 mg sodium)

- 5 mmHg decrease in systolic blood pressure and 2 mmHg decrease in diastolic blood pressure in hypertensive patients

that the medication needs of individuals with T2D become more complex as their diabetes progresses is typical and should be expected. Combinations of oral agents or noninsulin injectable medications eventually are needed, with 40–60% of patients requiring insulin. Continuous reliance on MNT alone, or MNT and one diabetes agent, to achieve glycemic control may not be sufficient to achieve desired glycemic control. As medication therapy advances, MNT needs to be evaluated continuously and also may need to advance (see Figure 5.1).

Table 5.3 lists primary nutrition messages that apply to all people with diabetes and would be helpful in achieving the goals of MNT listed previously.

Table 5.3 Primary Nutrition Messages for All People with Diabetes

1. Manage portion sizes to help with meeting carbohydrate prescription, weight loss, and maintenance.
2. Carbohydrate-containing foods and beverages and endogenous insulin production are the greatest determinant of the postmeal blood glucose level; therefore, it is important to know what foods contain carbohydrates—starchy vegetables, whole grains, fruits, milk and milk products, vegetables, and sugar.
3. When choosing carbohydrate-containing foods, choose nutrient-dense, high-fiber foods whenever possible instead of processed foods with added sodium, fat, and sugars. Nutrient-dense foods and beverages provide vitamins, minerals, and other healthful substances with relatively few calories. Calories have not been added to them from solid fats, sugars, or refined starches.
4. Avoid sugar-sweetened beverages, such as soda pop, sweet tea, juices, and punches.
5. Select leaner protein sources and meat alternatives.
6. Limit alcohol intake to one drink/day or less for adult women and two drinks or less for adult men.
7. Add 30 minutes of physical activity each day.

Tables 5.4 and 5.5 outline MNT principles for T1D versus T2D. Table 5.6 summarizes frequently asked questions about diabetes medical nutrition therapy.

Table 5.4 Principles of Nutrition Therapy for T1D and Insulin-Requiring T2D

■ Learn how to count carbohydrates or use another meal planning approach to quantify carbohydrate intake. The objective of using such a meal-planning approach is to "match" mealtime insulin to carbohydrates consumed.
■ If on multiple-daily injection plan or on an insulin pump:
  • Take mealtime insulin before eating.
  • Meals can be consumed at different times, usually within 1 hour of usual time.
  • If physical activity is performed within 1–2 hours of mealtime insulin injection, this dose may need to be lowered to reduce risk of hypoglycemia.
■ If on a premixed insulin plan: *(Combination of Intermediate/Regular)*
  • Insulin doses need to be taken at consistent times every day.
  • Meals need to be consumed at similar times every day.
  • Do not skip meals to reduce risk of hypoglycemia.
  • Physical activity may result in low blood glucose depending on when it is performed. Always carry a source of quick-acting carbohydrates to reduce risk of hypoglycemia. *(Intermediate)*
■ If on a fixed insulin plan:
  • Eat similar amounts of carbohydrate each day to match the set doses of insulin.

Table 5.5 Principles of Nutrition Therapy for T2D

■ Promote overall healthy nutritional food intake and activity.
  • Carbohydrates: Avoid excess intake of carbohydrate foods at any one time of day (aim for consistency in the amount of carbohydrate and timing of intake from day to day); use self–glucose monitoring to evaluate the distribution of carbohydrate.
  • Fat: Limit saturated and trans fatty acids, and cholesterol. For those with elevated total and LDL cholesterol, consuming 1.6–3 grams/day of plant stanols or sterols found in enriched foods can reduce cholesterol levels.
  • Sodium: Follow national recommendations and individual needs.
  • If overweight or obese: Modify calories for weight management, using portion control.
  • Increase physical activity to reach 150 minutes a week or 30 minutes on most days of week.
  • Monitor blood glucose to determine whether adjustments in food and meals will be sufficient to reach blood glucose goals or whether medications need to be added.
■ Add and advance diabetes medication therapy, as needed
  • When secretagogues are used—carbohydrate intake (amount and time consumed) usually needs to be consistent from day to day.

5.6 Frequently Asked Questions About Diabetes Medical Nutrition Therapy

ould provide MNT?

nplexity of nutrition issues requires a coordinated team effort, including the person diabetes or diabetes. To achieve nutrition goals, the American Diabetes Associa-
)A) recommends that an RD, who is knowledgeable and skilled in implementing
principles and recommendations for diabetes, oversee the provision of nutrition
. It is important, however, that all team members, including physicians, nurse prac-
, nurses, and others, be knowledgeable about MNT, support its role in diabetes
d ensure that the patient has access to therapy support.

an ADA diet?

no "one-size-fits-all" food plan that applies to all individuals with diabetes. The
commends that a person with diabetes have an individualized food or meal plan
n assessment, therapy goals, and use of approaches that meet the patient's needs
and abilities. That said, there are certainly principles of a diabetes food plan that are recommended. See Tables 5.2, 5.3, and 5.4.

How can I get my patients to follow the diet I give them?

For people to make lifestyle changes that result in positive clinical outcomes, especially in
the areas of nutrition and physical activity, knowledge, application education, and ongoing
support are required. Handing out booklets and/or educational materials about diet is NOT
a substitute for individualized MNT. ADA states that ideally the individual with diabetes
should be referred to an RD for nutrition therapy at, or soon after, diagnosis and for ongoing follow-up. A dietitian will, in collaboration with the patient, develop an individualized
food or meal plan focused on "to do" behaviors, not a list of dietary restrictions. Also see
Chapter 3 on diabetes education.

What is the medical provider's role in nutrition therapy?

Medical providers play an important role is setting the tone and expectations regarding
nutrition therapy and providing an overview of a diabetes food plan. Setting the patient up
for a positive, successful experience with nutrition therapy contributes greatly to the overall treatment regimen success. Ensure that all patients have access to initial and ongoing
nutrition therapy that is individualized for them. This includes the specific food plan that is
balanced with their diabetes medication as well as the behavioral aspects of implementing
the plan, including purchasing, preparing, and portioning food choices. Setting the expectation that nutrition therapy is a critical component of overall diabetes care and supporting
patient efforts are roles for all medical providers.

So many of my patients need to lose weight, what is the best approach?

Weight loss is typically a helpful but not essential treatment for improving blood glucose
levels. Often weight maintenance is the weight-focused goal. It has been shown that
patients who moderate their carbohydrate intake to achieve glucose goals often lose some
weight.

continued

Table 5.6 Frequently Asked Questions About Diabetes Medical Nutrition Therapy *(continued)*

Sometimes overweight patients have tried many weight-loss programs and approaches and feel frustrated, defeated, and embarrassed about this topic. Sequencing health-related behavior goals based on patient-driven goals may prove to be the best approach. Thus, the first behavior goal may be to walk 10 minutes a day, carry their lunch to work instead of eating out frequently, and have a healthy afternoon snack rather than a high-calorie vending machine choice.

Some of my patients who are obese want to have a normal BMI. What should I do?

- If weight loss is a priority along with glucose control, ensure that they have the education, resources, and support to achieve and maintain the goal.
- Weight loss of 5–7% of current weight is proven effective to reduce health risk for a number of health conditions. Although such weight loss is success, many patients do not define that as success. The health care team can help identify short-term and long-term goals and balance weight management success with other successes such as more healthful food choices, increased activity, reduction of blood pressure, and improved cholesterol levels.

How many visits are necessary for nutrition therapy?

- As with any therapy there is planning, implementation, and ongoing evaluation.
- The planning typically requires two nutrition visits, each ~1 hour long.
- The implementation of the nutrition therapy is the component that, for many, requires additional time. Because nutrition therapy requires lifestyle behavior changes, research reports that frequent contact with individualized goal setting and implementation plans is recommended. This may be as frequent as weekly or monthly for 15–60 minutes. Medicare reimburses for MNT for people with diabetes (3 hours in the first calendar year, 2 hours in subsequent calendar years) and many health plans provide similar or better coverage. For some patients, psychotherapy may be needed to address implementation barriers.
- Evaluation of nutrition therapy effectiveness and any necessary changes is recommended once to twice a year.

I'm confused about sugars, glycemic intake, and the Mediterranean diet. What's best?

- Healthy eating principles are the foundation for any diet (food plan). Guidelines are well described in the Dietary Guidelines for Americans.[1]
- These guidelines limit sugar intake, especially sweetened beverages, promote less processed food and foods higher in fiber (often have a lower glycemic index), suggest eating more fruits and vegetables, and encourage the use of plant-based oils and fats (Mediterranean diet).
- Evidence from many clinical studies has demonstrated that sugars do not increase glycemia more than isocaloric amounts of starch. Therefore, the total amount of carbohydrate eaten is more important than the source of the carbohydrate.
- Glucose monitoring will help guide decisions about food choices and their impact on glucose levels.

DIABETES PREVENTION

Key clinical research, including the Diabetes Prevention Program (DPP), concluded that the incidence of T2D can be decreased by 58% in at-risk individuals who engage in lifestyle-structured intervention programs (Table 5.7). These programs emphasize reduced fat and energy intake, regular physical activity, and frequent participant contact. The intervention is well defined and available online.[2] Primary care providers can partner with dietitians and/or community-based programs to provide their patients similar care to prevent or delay the onset of T2D. Dietitians were involved in the many facets of the study and were integral in designing and achieving the significant reduction in new cases of diabetes. Through intensive lifestyle intervention, DPP participants achieved a

- mean weight loss of 7% after 1 year and maintained a 5% weight loss at 3 years, and
- mean level of physical activity of 208 minutes/week at 1 year and 189 minutes/week at 3 years.

These results have the potential to reduce the onset of diabetes and treat other medical conditions, such as hypertension and elevated cholesterol levels, increasing the impact of lifestyle intervention on overall health outcomes.

Individuals at risk for T2D include those described in Chapter 16. Special attention can be given to people who are overweight and women who have had gestational diabetes. Children pose difficult challenges that involve public health and school policy issues. Diabetes care providers can contribute greatly to these issues to ensure access to appropriate food and activity throughout the day.

OBESITY TREATMENT

The U.S. has experienced epidemics of obesity, prediabetes, and diabetes in the past decade. Approximately 70% of Americans are overweight or obese. The proportion of Americans who are severely obese has increased by 70% since. Approximately 85% of people diagnosed with T2D are overweight or obese at the time of diagnosis. The risk for cardiometabolic disease and biomechanical complications increases relative to the increase in BMI. Obesity increases insulin resistance and may aggravate hypertension and hyperlipidemia. Aggressive intervention is war-

---

Table 5.7 Components of Intensive Lifestyle Intervention Programs

- Calorie intake deficit achieved through calorie counting or fat gram counting, with strict attention to portion control
- Increased physical activity
- Individual goal setting
- Developing plan-making skills
- Individual or group sessions
- Standardized curriculum
- Follow-up contact during weight-maintenance phase
- Self-monitoring (i.e., food records, physical activity, blood glucose, weight)

ranted to treat obesity in patients diagnosed with diabetes as well as individuals with prediabetes, or those with one or more risk factors for developing diabetes.

Long-term weight maintenance poses a major challenge. Structured, intensive lifestyle-change programs (Table 5.7), similar to those used in the DPP and Look AHEAD (Action for Health in Diabetes) trials, produce more successful weight loss and weight maintenance than conventional treatment consisting of one initial visit followed by two follow-up visits. Look AHEAD, a large National Institutes of Health–sponsored clinical trial that recently concluded, was designed to determine the effects of an intensive lifestyle intervention program on glycemia to prevent cardiovascular events. This study showed that the intensive lifestyle intervention group reported a 5% reduction in body weight at 11 years, and showed significant improvements in fitness levels, A1C, systolic and diastolic blood pressure, HDL cholesterol, and triglyceride levels. LDL cholesterol levels, however, remained unchanged from the control group. The Look AHEAD trial showed that intensive lifestyle intervention allows people with diabetes to lose weight, reduce the need for and cost of medications, reduce the rate of sleep apnea, improve well-being, and in some cases, achieve a diabetes remission. Although study results did not show clear evidence for reduced rates of cardiovascular events, the Look AHEAD study clearly showed that attention to activity and diet can safely reduce health risks commonly associated with diabetes.

Weight-loss medications may be useful in the treatment of overweight individuals with and at risk for T2D and can help achieve 5–10% weight loss when combined with lifestyle change. These medications should be used only in people with diabetes who have BMI >27 kg/m². Gastric surgery can be an effective weight-loss treatment for obesity and may be considered in people with diabetes who have BMI ≥35 kg/m².

The increased prevalence of diabetes in youth, particularly minority adolescents, has become a major concern. Although data are insufficient at present to warrant any specific recommendations for the prevention of T2D in youth, clinical trials are ongoing. A variety of interventions similar to those shown to be effective for prevention of T2D in adults are likely to be beneficial. Family support is essential for the implementation of dietary interventions in young patients to be successful.

INITIATING THERAPY

Nutrition therapy must be goal directed and individualized according to a person's usual food intake and lifestyle. It is not appropriate to prescribe a precise caloric intake or a precise distribution of food. As with medication initiation, it takes a series of visits to develop and refine the food plan. Yet along with nutrition therapy, many knowledge and behavioral decisions are required throughout each day such that additional visits usually are required for the patient to learn how to implement and maintain the food plan in a variety of situations and to incorporate a variety of food choices (see Table 5.8 for time frames for nutrition intervention). Modifying eating patterns is not a simple procedure, yet reasonable, achievable goals can be set and successfully met with the guidance of a skilled nutrition counselor.

When initiating or adjusting MNT, the patient needs to increase the frequency of glucose monitoring to guide changes in food intake, activity, and medications. More frequent glucose monitoring provides the data needed to determine whether

Table 5.8 Time Frames for Nutrition Intervention

Initial workup/assessment (can be part of group diabetes self-management education [DSME]) or separate MNT

■ A series of 3–4 encounters with a registered dietitian (RD) lasting 45–90 minutes, spaced out over 3–6 months, beginning at diagnosis of diabetes or at first referral to an RD.

DSME (can be part of group DSME)

■ Biweekly or monthly sessions for 2–4 months, 30–60 minutes each.
■ Daily or weekly phone calls to discuss glucose records, as needed.

Diabetes self-management support (DSMS)

■ Ongoing support provided by dietitian, diabetes care team, or other resource.
■ Follow-up for therapy evaluation, adjustment, and education.

Diabetes self-management education (DSME) follow-up

■ Review progress with lifestyle behavior-change goals, and assess life-cycle changes, as needed.
■ Children: Minimum follow-up every 3–6 months.
■ Adults: At least one follow-up encounter annually.
■ Intensive insulin therapy requires 4–6 visits a year plus phone contact.

changes to the food plan are necessary or whether adjusting another therapy is more appropriate. The review of glucose records is an important component of MNT as glucose pattern management guides nutrition recommendations.

NUTRITION CARE PROCESS

The nutrition care process includes a continuous four-step process:

STEP ONE: NUTRITION ASSESSMENT

The assessment process includes obtaining, verifying, and interpreting data that are needed to identify and understand nutrition needs. Five categories of data are reviewed: *1)* food and nutrition history; *2)* biochemical data, medical tests, and procedures; *3)* anthropometric measurements; *4)* physical examination findings; and *5)* patient history.

STEP TWO: NUTRITION DIAGNOSIS

The purpose of a diagnosis is to describe the presence of, risk of, or potential for developing a nutritional situation that can be addressed by nutrition therapy.

Diagnoses include a diagnostic label, etiology, and signs and symptoms. Diagnoses are organized into three categories: *1*) clinical, *2*) intake related, or *3*) behavioral–environmental.

STEP THREE: NUTRITION INTERVENTION

Interventions are specific actions to remedy the nutrition diagnosis and include the planning phase as well as the intervention. The focus is on *1*) food or nutrient intake and *2*) nutrition education, nutrition counseling, and coordination of care. There is no gold-standard single strategy or method of nutrition intervention because various methods have been tested and demonstrated to facilitate attainment of nutrition goals. During initial phases of education (soon after diabetes diagnosis), simplified resources are recommended. Subsequently, more complex approaches may be appropriate. Commonly used nutrition interventions are listed in Table 5.9. More than one intervention can be used simultaneously, as needed. Use of various nutrition interventions provides greater flexibility and choices to the person with diabetes and is especially useful for those who have been discouraged or frustrated by previous nutrition instruction methods. The different nutrition interventions have distinctive and varying characteristics of structure and complexity. The choice of a food plan depends on both the dietitian's experience with different strategies and on which approach best meets the individual needs of the patient.

STEP FOUR: NUTRITION MONITORING AND EVALUATION

The purpose of the monitoring and evaluation step is to determine the amount of progress made and whether goals are met. It is a continuous process of observing metabolic outcomes and patient perceptions of how things are going as well as designing additional education and support services to meet instructional and lifestyle needs.

Table 5.9 Nutrition Intervention Options

- Healthy eating guidelines with some portion control guidance
  - Healthy food choices
  - Food guide pyramid
  - Plate method
  - Consistent eating based on one's current eating pattern
- Carbohydrate-focused guidelines
  - Carbohydrate counting—using choices or grams
  - Food lists
  - Carbohydrate counting using insulin-to-carbohydrate ratios
  - Calorie counting
  - Fat gram counting
  - Medically supervised very-low-calorie diets
  - Structured lifestyle change diets
  - Other

Follow-up educational sessions with the dietitian focus on various topics, such as food composition, food labeling, shopping, recipe adaptations, and eating in restaurants. Dietitians guide patients in using food records in conjunction with blood glucose records to observe patterns in blood glucose control. A problem-solving approach is used to analyze individual blood glucose responses to food, activity, and medications. Patients then are able to make adjustments in food intake or insulin dosage to maintain target blood glucose levels. Algorithms for food, medication, and activity can be developed to help manage diabetes on a daily basis. Small careful steps over weeks or months help move the patient toward nutrition goals. Follow-up sessions by the dietitian can be accomplished via clinic visits and telephone conversations to facilitate problem solving. Family members and significant others should be involved in the nutrition education process and are encouraged to follow the same healthy lifestyle recommendations as the person with diabetes.

Contact with a dietitian is recommended at least annually (Table 5.8) to monitor metabolic parameters and assess the appropriateness and effectiveness of the nutrition therapy. When patients experience lifestyle changes, such as schedule changes, marriage, divorce, change of job or home, or pregnancy, nutrition therapy should be reviewed. If nutrition therapy goals are not met, changes can be made in the overall diabetes care and management plan. See Table 5.10 for reasons to refer a patient to a dietitian.

ACCESS TO MNT

Although referrals for diabetes self-management education (DSME) are increasing, the sad fact remains that only ~50% of individuals with diabetes report having attended some type of diabetes self-management class, only 26% report seeing a diabetes educator within the previous year, and only 9% have had at least one visit with a dietitian, despite nutrition therapy being an integral component of diabetes care. Studies of referral patterns indicate that the lack of referral by physicians and other health care professionals remains a major barrier. Poor awareness of the existence and value of medical nutrition is a primary factor, along with misinformation about reimbursement for these services. Promotion of these services is often poor, irregular, or nonexistent. Table 5.10 provides information about how to access dietitians and diabetes education.

Table 5.10 Accessing Dietitians and Diabetes Education

- To find a dietitian, go to the Academy of Nutrition and Dietetics website at www.eatright.org/programs/rdfinder.
- To find a diabetes educator who is a dietitian, go to the American Association of Diabetes Educators (AADE) website at www.diabeteseducator.org and go to "Find a Diabetes Educator" in the "About Diabetes Education" section.
- To find an ADA- or AADE-accredited diabetes education program in your area, go to www.professional.diabetes.org/recognition or www.diabeteseducator.org/diabeteseducation/programs.
- Ask colleagues about dietitians and diabetes education programs in your area.

A recent analysis reported that MNT provided by a registered dietitian could be more cost effective than intensive lifestyle intervention. An RD and a DSME program can help assess your patients' needs.

REIMBURSEMENT FOR DIABETES MNT

Over the past decade, reimbursement and coverage for diabetes MNT have improved greatly. Since January 2002, RDs have been able to bill Medicare Part B for medical nutrition therapy provided to patients with diabetes. Many private-sector insurance plans have adopted similar coverage as Medicare provides. The Medicare benefit allows 3 hours of MNT in the first referral year and 2 hours each subsequent calendar year. In January 2006, the Centers for Medicare and Medicaid Services (CMS) added individual MNT to the list of Medicare tele-health services eligible for reimbursement, and in 2011, CMS added group MNT to reimbursement-eligible services. Medicare does not cover MNT for prediabetes or cardiovascular disease; however, many private payers recognize MNT current procedural terminology codes for diagnoses, such as prediabetes, diabetes, obesity, hyperlipidemia, and hypertension. Following Medicare guidelines for physician referral and authorization of patient visits is key to reimbursement. Use of the electronic health record to document MNT services improves patient care documentation, patient continuity of care, and the process for reimbursement of services provided. Individuals with diabetes should be encouraged to contact their health plan provider to determine their benefits for MNT.

REIMBURSEMENT FOR DSME

Medicare covers DSME for people with diabetes who meet specific eligibility criteria and when it is provided by programs that have been reviewed and recognized by the ADA Education Recognition Program or the American Association of Diabetes Educators. These programs must follow the National Standards for Diabetes Self-Management Education programs. Ten hours of outpatient training are available initially during the first 12 months of applying for this service, and up to 2 hours annually thereafter, with provider referral. Medicare requires that the DSME be provided in groups unless the provider has identified a specific barrier to group education.

Eligible beneficiaries are allowed to use both the MNT and DSME benefit. The only restriction is that the services cannot be provided on the same day.

WHAT TO EXPECT

MNT is effective in lowering A1C, blood pressure, and lipid levels when used without medications, and it improves the effectiveness of medication when needed (Table 5.2). MNT is the initial treatment for diabetes, although at some point in its progression, medication often is needed to support MNT. Continued support and reinforcement of behavioral goals are necessary and usually can be reimbursed as part of established changes in federal and state laws governing health care.

Establishing a referral network to dietitians has become easier as these reimbursement changes occur. Patients ultimately will benefit as they achieve their goals and decrease the risk of developing complications from diabetes, hypertension, or cardiovascular disease. This result is achieved through the implementation of individualized food plans that take into consideration the patient's lifestyle and metabolic needs.

REFERENCES

1. DietaryGuidelines.gov. Dietary guidelines for Americans, n.d. Available at www.health.gov/dietaryguidelines. Accessed 27 April 2013.

2. National Diabetes Information Clearinghouse. Diabetes prevention program, 2013. Available at www.diabetes.niddk.nih.gov/dm/pubs/prevention-program. Accessed 27 April 2013.

BIBLIOGRAPHY

Academy of Nutrition and Dietetics. Disorders of lipid metabolism evidence-based nutrition practice guidelines, 2011. Available at http://adaevidencelibrary.com/topic.cfm?cat=4528. Accessed 27 April 2013.

Academy of Nutrition and Dietetics. Effectiveness of MNT for hypertension, 2008. Available at www.adaevidencelibrary.com/conclusion,cfm?conclusion_statement_id=251204. Accessed 27 April 2013.

Academy of Nutrition and Dietetics. Type 1 and type 2 diabetes evidence-based nutrition practice guidelines for adults, 2008. Available at http://adaevidencelibrary.com/topic.cfm?cat=3253. Accessed 27 April 2013.

American Diabetes Association. Nutrition therapy recommendations for management of adults with diabetes (Position Statement). *Diabetes Care* 2014; 36:3821–3842.

Anderson J. Achievable cost saving and cost-effective thresholds for diabetes prevention lifestyle interventions in people aged 65 years and older: a single-payer perspective. *J Acad Nutr Diet* 2012;112:1747–1754.

Diabetes Prevention Program Research Group, Knowler WC, Fowler SE, Haman RF, Chirstophi CA, Hoffman H. 10 year follow-up of diabetes incidence and weight loss in the Diabetes Prevention Program Outcomes Study. *Lancet* 2009;374:1677–1686.

Franz MJ, Powers MA, Leontos C, Holzmeister LA, Kulkarni K, Mon A, Wedel N, Gradwell E. The evidence for medical nutrition therapy for type 1 and type 2 diabetes in adults. *J Am Diet Assoc* 2010;110:1852–1889.

Franz M, Warshaw H, Pastors JG, Daly A, Arnold M. The evolution of diabetes medical nutrition therapy. *Postgrad Med J* 2003;79:30–35.

Klein S, Sheard NF, Pi-Sunyer X, Daly A, Wylie-Rosett J, Kulkarni K, Clark NG. Weight management through lifestyle modification for the prevention and management of type 2 diabetes: rationale and strategies: a statement of the American Diabetes Association, the North American Association of the Study of Obesity, and the American Society for Clinical Nutrition. *Diabetes Care* 2004;27:2067–2073.

Look AHEAD Research Group. Cardiovascular effects of intensive lifestyle intervention in type 2 diabetes. *N Engl J Med* 2013;369:145–154.

Pastors JG, Warshaw H, Daly A, Franz M, Kulkarni K. Evidence for effectiveness of medical nutrition therapy in diabetes management. *Diabetes Care* 2002;25:608–613.

Powers M. *American Dietetic Association Guide to Eating Right When You Have Diabetes.* Hoboken, NJ, John Wiley & Sons, 2003.

Rickheim P, Weaver TW, Flader JL, Kendall DM. Assessment of group versus individual diabetes education. *Diabetes Care* 2002;25:608–613.

Rosett JW, Delahanty L. An integral role of the dietitian: implications of the Diabetes Prevention Program. *J Am Diet Assoc* 2002;102:1065–1068.

Wolf AM, Conaway MR, Crowther JQ, Hazen KY, Nadler JL, Oneida B, Bovbjerg VE. Translating lifestyle intervention to practice in obese patients with type 2 diabetes: Improving Control with Activity and Nutrition (ICAN) study. *Diabetes Care* 2004;27:1570–1576.

Chapter 6

Exercise

JUDITH G. REGENSTEINER, PhD
TIMOTHY A. BAUER, PhD
EDWARD S. HORTON, MD

Regular physical exercise is a firmly established cornerstone in the treatment of people with diabetes. As with healthy people, there are clear benefits of an exercise program for people with both type 1 diabetes (T1D) and type 2 diabetes (T2D). Regular physical exercise (and physical activity) has been shown to reduce the risk of some chronic health problems and improve psychological outlook in addition to improving sleep quality and overall quality of life. Importantly, in the management of diabetes, regular exercise also can confer substantial benefit for glycemic control, weight management, and the reduction of risk factors for cardiovascular disease.

In prior years, T2D was considered to be a disease affecting only middle-aged and older people, but it now is occurring in adolescents in increasing numbers. Thus, many of the issues of T2D formerly faced by middle-aged or older adults now have to be addressed in youth, as is also the case with T1D. The goals of physical exercise in youth with T2D therefore also must be considered. In spite of the differing issues and needs of young versus old, and T1D versus T2D, regular exercise and physical activity are clearly beneficial to individuals of all ages who have diabetes.

In people with T2D, regular exercise is an important component of treatment and should be prescribed along with appropriate diet and medications as part of a comprehensive treatment program. It has been clearly shown by the Diabetes Prevention Program and the Finnish Diabetes Prevention Study, among others, that regular exercise and physical activity actually can prevent or delay the onset of T2D in many cases, especially when combined with other components of healthy lifestyle behavior. A meta-analysis by Thomas et al. provided evidence that regular moderate-intensity exercise improves metabolic control in T2D even in the absence of weight loss.[1] In many studies, exercise training in people with T2D also has a potent effect in terms of improving exercise performance, including maximal oxygen consumption, and markers of submaximal exercise performance as well as potentially reducing cardiovascular risk. This is important because maintaining or improving exercise performance benefits cardiovascular health and functional ability. Although it is clear that regular exercise has many desirable effects, designing an appropriate exercise program for people with T2D requires a careful assessment of the expected benefits and associated risks in individuals and the inclusion of appropriate monitoring to avoid injuries and other complications.

The goals, benefits, and risks for exercise in those with T1D may be different than for those with T2D, although strong evidence exists for regular physical exercise as part of a healthy lifestyle in these individuals as well as for those with T2D.[2] Data suggest that benefits of regular exercise in T1D include a reduction

DOI: 10.2337/9781580405096.06

in cardiovascular risk and mortality and an improvement in well-being. Therefore, it is recommended that exercise training be used as a key therapy with which to manage T1D. In T1D, exercise poses a metabolic challenge unlike that in healthy people and people with T2D, and it is important to understand the complexities of hormonal regulation of metabolic fuels at rest, during exercise of varying intensities and durations, and during the postexercise recovery period. For example, in people with T1D, exercise may cause a further rise in blood glucose and the rapid development of ketosis, and even in well-controlled patients, vigorous exercise may result in sustained hyperglycemia. The management of insulin dosing is also important. If insulin levels are excessive, hypoglycemia may occur during or after exercise. Because of these problems with regulation of blood glucose and ketones during or after exercise, people with T1D may find it challenging to participate in sports or other recreational activities as well as to manage regular exercise as part of their daily lives. Despite these challenges, however, evidence shows that with good cooperation between patient and health care provider, barriers to exercise can be overcome. The availability of self-monitoring of blood glucose (SMBG) and continuous glucose monitors as well as the increased use of multiple-dose insulin regimens or insulin pumps and exercise-related insulin adjustments have led to the development of individualized strategies for the management of exercise in people with T1D, making it possible for them to safely participate in a wide range of physical activities and thus to have a normal or near-normal lifestyle.

BENEFITS

The overall benefits of regular exercise for people with diabetes are listed in Table 6.1. Moderate-intensity, sustained regular exercise in people with either T1D or T2D may be used to help regulate glucose on a day-to-day basis and may be the mechanism by which regular exercise assists in achieving improved long-term metabolic control.[3] A regular exercise program results in lower fasting and postprandial insulin concentrations, as well as increased insulin sensitivity. In people with T1D, increased insulin sensitivity results in lowered insulin requirements. In people with T2D, the improvement in insulin sensitivity resulting from regular physical exercise may be of major importance in improving long-term glycemic control and may lead to the decreased need for diabetes medications. Several studies have demonstrated that both aerobic and strength-training exercise programs improve insulin sensitivity and glycemic control as measured by improvement in A1C and that both types of exercise training provide benefits.

The benefit of regular exercise for the reduction of cardiovascular risk factors is well documented and includes improvement of the lipid profile, reduction in blood pressure, decreased biomarker findings of subclinical inflammation, and improved endothelial function. Several population studies have demonstrated an inverse correlation between the amount of regular exercise and cardiovascular events; however, these findings are not universal. One prospective randomized controlled trial evaluating the effects of lifestyle intervention (diet and physical activity) on cardiovascular morbidity and mortality in T2D failed to show clinical benefit. Although more definitive work is needed to fully describe the potential

Table 6.1 Benefits of Exercise for People with Diabetes

■ Regular aerobic exercise improves cardiovascular conditioning and reduces cardio-vascular risk factors.
  • Aerobic exercise training may reduce systolic blood pressure.
  • Responses of blood lipids to regular exercise and physical activity may include a reduction in low-density lipoprotein cholesterol.
  • Combined weight loss and regular exercise or physical activity may be more effective than aerobic exercise training alone on lipids.
  • Reduction in markers of inflammation
  • Improved endothelial function
■ Moderate amounts of regular exercise alone are not adequate for weight loss. When coupled with diet management, however, regular exercise helps maintain weight loss and improve body composition.
  • Adjunct to diet for weight reduction
  • Increased fat loss
  • Preservation of lean body mass
■ Regular exercise is associated with improved functional capacity.
■ Aerobic exercise and resistance exercise both improve insulin action, blood glucose control, and fat oxidation and storage in muscle.
■ Increased physical activity and physical fitness can reduce symptoms of depression and improve health-related quality of life.
■ Increased regular exercise and physical activity can improve flexibility.
■ Resistance exercise enhances skeletal muscle mass and strength.

effects of exercise on mortality, the preponderance of findings suggests many clear benefits of regular exercise in people with diabetes.

In addition to improvement in cardiovascular risk factors, regular exercise may be an effective adjunct to diet for weight reduction and weight maintenance. Regular exercise programs alone usually are associated with little or no weight loss and must be combined with caloric restriction to achieve significant weight loss. Numerous studies have demonstrated, however, that regular exercise is an important part of a lifestyle-modification program and is particularly important for weight maintenance after weight-loss goals have been achieved.

Finally, regular exercise improves cardiovascular fitness and physical working capacity and also improves the sense of well-being and quality of life. The ability to carry out physical activities tends to be reduced with age so that maintenance of functional ability is a key benefit of exercise training and physical fitness.

RISKS

Several potential risks are associated with exercise for people with diabetes (Table 6.2). In people with T1D, either hyperglycemia or hypoglycemia can occur during exercise, depending on its intensity and duration as well as on the amount and timing of insulin administration. In addition, late-onset postexercise hypoglycemia can occur 7–11 hours after the completion of the exercise and may persist for up to 24 hours after prolonged, strenuous exercise. High-intensity exercise may result in a

Table 6.2 Risks of Exercise for People with Diabetes

More common risks involving glycemic control:
- ■ Hypoglycemia, if treated with insulin or oral agents (especially in T1D)
  - • Exercise-induced hypoglycemia
  - • Late-onset postexercise hypoglycemia
- ■ Hyperglycemia after very strenuous exercise
- ■ Hyperglycemia and ketosis in insulin-deficient people

Worsening of long-term complications of diabetes:
- ■ Proliferative retinopathy
  - • Vitreous hemorrhage
  - • Retinal detachment
- ■ Nephropathy
  - • Increased proteinuria
- ■ Peripheral neuropathy
  - • Soft tissue and joint injuries
- ■ Autonomic neuropathy
- ■ Impaired response to dehydration
  - • Postural hypotension
- ■ Degenerative joint disease
- ■ Abnormal cardiovascular response to exercise
  - • Decreased maximum aerobic capacity
  - • Slowed heart rate recovery
- ■ Precipitation or exacerbation of manifestations of cardiovascular disease
  - • Angina pectoris
  - • Myocardial infarction
  - • Arrhythmias

Source: Steppel and Horton.[4]

rapid increase in blood glucose that can persist for several hours after exercise is discontinued. Even moderate-intensity exercise may result in hyperglycemia and in the rapid development of ketosis or ketoacidosis in people with T1D who are insulin deficient. These risks make it apparent that careful monitoring of blood glucose is important, particularly in the early phases of beginning a regular exercise regimen. The risks of regular exercise in T2D also include hypoglycemia, but this is much less common than with T1D. Other risks of exercise in all diabetes patients include orthopedic and cardiovascular consequences, but the benefits generally are considered to outweigh the risks. In light of the potential risks of exercise, it is recommended that people with diabetes who are planning to begin a regular exercise program more intensive than walking consult with their health care providers.

Careful screening for underlying cardiac disease is important for all people with diabetes before starting a vigorous regular exercise program that involves an exercise intensity that is unusual for the patient and is greater than that achieved by brisk walking or its equivalent. As noted in Table 6.2, several complications of diabetes may be aggravated by regular exercise, and all people with these complications should be screened before they start an exercise program to avoid exacerbation. The most important of these is proliferative retinopathy because exercise may result in retinal or vitreous hemorrhage.[4]

An ophthalmologist should clear a person with significant diabetic retinopathy before beginning exercise, because exercises that increase blood pressure (e.g., heavy lifting or exercise associated with Valsalva-like maneuvers), may exacerbate the condition. People requiring laser photocoagulation for proliferative retinopathy may need to wait 3–6 months after the procedure before physical exertion. Regular exercise also is associated with increased proteinuria in people with diabetic nephropathy, likely because of changes in renal hemodynamics. It has not been shown, however, that exercise leads to more rapid progression of renal disease, and the use of angiotensin-converting enzyme (ACE) inhibitors does appear to decrease the amount of exercise-induced albuminuria.

People with peripheral neuropathy have an increased risk of soft tissue and joint injuries, and, if autonomic neuropathy is present, the capacity for high-intensity exercise is impaired because of a decreased maximum heart rate and aerobic capacity with exercise as well as a slowed heart rate recovery following exercise. In addition, people with autonomic neuropathy may have impaired responses to dehydration and develop postural hypotension after exercise. With proper selection of the type, intensity, and duration of exercise, most of these complications can be avoided.[4]

GUIDELINES FOR EXERCISE

SCREENING

Before starting a regular exercise program, all people with diabetes should have a complete history and physical examination, with particular attention paid to identifying any long-term complications of diabetes.[4,5] For young, generally healthy people with T1D or T2D, an exercise stress test typically is not needed before starting a mild or moderate-intensity exercise program, such as a brisk walking program. In older individuals, however, particularly those who have increased risk factors for cardiovascular disease, a stress test will be useful to identify silent ischemic heart disease and may identify people who have an exaggerated hypertensive response to exercise or who may develop postexercise orthostatic hypotension. The American College of Sports Medicine (ACSM) recommends exercise testing before initiating physical activity for people with diabetes who meet one of the following criteria: age ≥35 years, duration of diabetes >10 years for T2D or >15 years for T1D, smoking, hypertension, hypercholesterolemia, family history of coronary artery disease in a first-degree relative <60 years, presence of microvascular disease, peripheral artery disease, or autonomic neuropathy.[5] A careful ophthalmologic examination to identify proliferative retinopathy; renal function tests, including screening for albuminuria; and a neurological examination to determine peripheral or autonomic neuropathy should be performed.[4] If abnormalities are found, exercises should be selected that will not pose significant risks for worsening complications or result in injuries. In general, active young people with diabetes of brief duration and no evidence of long-term complications do not require formal exercise prescriptions, although they need specific recommendations regarding strategies for managing exercise and avoiding injuries.

SELECTION OF TYPE OF EXERCISE

If there are no contraindications, the types of exercise a person with diabetes performs can be a matter of personal preference. In general, moderate-intensity *moderate-intensity* [handwritten]

aerobic exercises that involve large muscle groups and that can be sustained for ≥30 minutes are preferred. Examples include walking, cycling, jogging, and organized exercise classes such as aerobics or spin classes. There is evidence that intermittent high-intensity and resistance exercises can be utilized successfully in people with diabetes, once a base level of aerobic and muscular fitness is attained. Most exercise programs for people with diabetes should include a combination of aerobic exercises and resistance (muscular fitness) exercises to achieve the maximum benefits on insulin sensitivity and glycemic control from a regular exercise program.

FREQUENCY, INTENSITY, AND DURATION OF EXERCISE

It generally is recommended that most people with diabetes participate in moderate-intensity exercise for 150 minutes/week.[6] Exercise at least three times a week, however, has been shown to result in significant improvement in cardiovascular fitness, improved glycemic control, and reduction in cardiovascular risk factors in people with T2D. The effect of a single bout of aerobic exercise on insulin sensitivity typically lasts 24–72 hours, depending on the duration and intensity of the exercise. Consequently, for people with diabetes, a common recommendation is to keep the time between exercise sessions to no more than 2 consecutive days. The carryover effect of resistance exercise training may be longer, and resistance training each major muscle group 2–3 days per week is recommended.

The intensity of exercise is important, and there is evidence for a positive dose–response relationship between exercise intensity (as well as frequency) and derived health benefits. The recommendation made in the Physical Activity Guidelines for Americans report recommends that for "substantial health benefits, all adults (ages 18–64) should do at least 150 minutes (2 hours and 30 minutes) a week of moderate-intensity, or 75 minutes (1 hour and 15 minutes) a week of vigorous-intensity aerobic physical activity, or an equivalent combination of moderate- and vigorous-intensity aerobic activity. Aerobic activity should be performed in episodes of at least 10 minutes, and preferably, it should be spread throughout the week. A person who moves toward 300 minutes (5 hours) or more of moderate-intensity activity a week gets even greater benefit."[6]

In addition to the 150 minutes a week of aerobic-type exercise, it is also recommended that adults should perform 2 bouts a week of muscle-strengthening exercise of moderate or high intensity involving all major muscle groups for additional benefits to health. For children and adolescents, it is recommended that they should perform 60 minutes (1 hour) or more of physical activity daily, which should consist mostly of moderate- or vigorous-intensity aerobic physical activity, and should include vigorous-intensity physical activity at least 3 days a week. The 60 minutes a day also should include muscle- and bone-strengthening activity on at least 3 days. These recommendations are in line with those of the American Diabetes and American Heart Associations as well as the ACSM.

Initially, moderate-intensity aerobic exercise—that is, 40 to <60% of aerobic capacity reserve (VO₂R) or heart rate reserve (HRR), should make up the majority of each exercise session, progressing to include periods of more vigorous exercise and higher intensity as training adaptations occur. Exercise intensity that corresponds to a rate of perceived exertion (RPE) of 11–13 on a 6–20 RPE scale also

less reliable in bursts [handwritten]

may be used in conjunction with the VO$_2$R; however, recent evidence suggests people with diabetes may perceive greater exertion at lower work rates than healthy individuals, making the RPE method of assessing exercise intensity potentially less reliable in those with diabetes. The VO$_2$R and HRR can be accessed from supervised exercise testing or obtained using submaximal exercise tests (e.g., 6-minute walk test) and standardized equations.[5] Once the desired exercise intensity is determined for an individual patient, exercise intensity can be monitored conveniently by teaching the patient to measure his or her own pulse periodically during exercise and recording the results. Greater benefits on glucose control may be achieved with higher exercise intensities (>60% VO$_2$R), and vigorous exercise may be added once a regular pattern of exercise is established.

TYPICAL STRUCTURE OF EXERCISE SESSIONS

The general structure of a single exercise training session typically follows a four-phase progression: warm-up, main conditioning or sports-related exercise, cool-down, and stretching or flexibility. Each session should last 20–45 minutes and gradually be increased up to 60 minutes as conditioning improves. The warm-up phase typically consists of 5–10-minutes of light to moderate intensity aerobic and muscular exercise. This phase allows the body to adjust to the neuromuscular, hemodynamic, and bioenergetic requirements of the main conditioning phase. The main conditioning phase consists of the planned aerobic endurance activity or resistance exercise. This represents the main portion of the exercise session, with a focus on dynamic, repetitive exercise involving the large muscle groups within the desired exercise intensity. Following the conditioning phase, a light to moderate-intensity cool-down phase allows for a gradual recovery of exercise hemodynamics (heart rate and blood pressure) toward resting levels. In most cases, a stretching or flexibility phase may be performed of the main muscle groups to enhance and maintain joint range of motion.

For resistance training, the ACSM recommends resistance exercises involving the major muscle groups with a minimum of one set of 8–12 repetitions resulting in near fatigue for most adults. For older adults or adults first starting exercise, a minimum of one set of 10–15 repetitions resulting in near fatigue is recommended. A general plan would be to start with a single set of 10–15 repetitions of each major muscle group two to three times weekly at moderate intensity, gradually increasing to two sets, and finally to three or four sets of repetitions of resistance exercise. The amount of resistance during this progression also should increase as strength improves.

By undertaking a program of regular aerobic exercise equivalent to brisk walking ≥3 days/week and resistance training ≥2 days/week, one can expect improved glucose, blood pressure, and dyslipidemia control as well as better maintenance of weight loss if the program is combined with reduced caloric intake.

PROGRESSION, MONITORING, AND COMPLIANCE

For people with diabetes who have not regularly exercised in the past or who have significant complications of diabetes or other impediments to exercise, supervised exercise programs may be beneficial. Often cardiac rehabilitation programs will be of assistance in supervising exercise programs for people with diabetes, particularly given the increased risk for cardiovascular disease. An increasing number of diabetes treatment centers offer supervised exercise programs for people with either T1D or T2D. Certified personal trainers and supervised community exercise classes are also an option. Many people, however, do not need formal supervision once an initial assessment has been completed and an appropriate exercise plan has been established.

The progression of exercise duration and intensity should begin conservatively in unconditioned adults and in those starting an exercise routine. The general rule is to start slowly and build up gradually as cardiovascular capacity and strength improve. As an example, a 3- to 4-week period of light to moderate-intensity aerobic and flexibility training may be advised for people naive to exercise training before beginning these standardized exercise recommendations. This allows time for mild neuromuscular and anatomical adaptations to occur and for a pattern of regular exercise to be established as a routine. During this initial period, exercise durations and intensity may need to be built up gradually to meet recommendations.

Patient motivation and participation are critical for exercise training success. Several things can be done to improve the patient's motivation and participation on a regular basis. These include choosing activities the patient enjoys, providing a variety in types and settings for exercise, performing exercise at convenient times and locations, encouraging participation in group activities, involving the patient's family and associates for reinforcement, and measuring progress to provide positive feedback. Most important is to begin slowly, build up gradually, and not set excessive or unrealistic goals.

People should be instructed on how to correctly perform exercise activities to avoid injuries or other complications while participating in physical exercise. Feet should be inspected daily and always after exercise for cuts, blisters, and infections. Exercise should be avoided in extreme hot or cold environments and during periods of poor metabolic control. Special guidelines for people taking insulin are described in the following section.

SPECIFIC CONSIDERATIONS FOR EXERCISE AND PHYSICAL ACTIVITY IN DIABETES

EFFECTS OF ACUTE EXERCISE

It is well established that exercise and physical activity cause increased glucose uptake into active muscles balanced by hepatic glucose production, with a greater reliance on carbohydrates to fuel muscular activity as intensity increases. Insulin-stimulated blood glucose uptake into skeletal muscle predominates at rest and is impaired in T2D. Muscular contractions, however, stimulate blood glucose transport via a separate, additive mechanism not impaired by insulin resistance or T2D. Repeated bouts of exercise appear to have a cumulative and beneficial effect on glucose metabolism. It has been well established that a single bout of moderate exercise has a profound effect on glucose metabolism that may last up to ~24–72 hours.

MANAGEMENT OF EXERCISE IN PEOPLE WITH TYPE 1 DIABETES

Whereas changes in blood glucose are small in individuals without diabetes during exercise, several factors may complicate glucose regulation during and after exercise in people with T1D. Plasma insulin concentrations do not decrease normally during exercise, thus upsetting the balance between peripheral glucose utilization and hepatic glucose production.[4] With insulin treatment, plasma insulin concentrations stay the same or may even increase if exercise is undertaken within 1 hour of an insulin injection. Enhanced insulin absorption during exercise is most likely to occur when the insulin injection is given immediately before or within a few minutes of the onset of exercise, particularly when using rapid-onset, short-acting insulin preparations. The longer the interval between injection and onset of exercise, the less significant this effect will be, and the less important it is to choose the site of injection to avoid an exercising area.[4]

The sustained insulin levels during exercise increase peripheral glucose uptake and stimulate glucose oxidation by the exercising muscles. In addition, insulin inhibits hepatic glucose production. When the hepatic glucose production rate cannot match the rate of peripheral glucose utilization, blood glucose concentration falls. During mild to moderate exercise of short duration, this may be a beneficial effect of exercise, but during more prolonged exercise, hypoglycemia may result.[4] If exercise is intense, sympathetic nervous stimulation of hepatic glucose production may result in a rapid and sustained rise in blood glucose concentrations. If there is also insulin deficiency, hepatic ketone production is stimulated, and ketosis or ketoacidosis may occur.

Factors to consider before undertaking exercise are listed in Table 6.3. The variability of conditions under which exercise and physical activity may be performed is great, so probably not all of these factors can be taken into account.

By considering the exercise plan and making adjustments in insulin dosage and food intake, people with T1D can avoid severe hypoglycemia or hyperglycemia. If exercise is of moderate intensity and long duration, blood glucose levels will fall, whereas vigorous exercise of short duration often will cause blood glucose to rise. Attention should be paid to the amount, timing, and site of insulin administration. Food intake before, during, and after exercise should be considered. It is important to measure blood glucose before starting exercise and, if necessary, during and after exercise. With this information, the strategies outlined in Table 6.4 can be used to avoid either hypoglycemia or hyperglycemia.

Usually, a snack containing 20–25 g carbohydrate every 30 minutes is sufficient to provide enough glucose to maintain normal blood levels during prolonged exercise. Carbohydrate requirements will depend on such factors as the intensity and duration of exercise, the level of physical conditioning, the antecedent diet, and the circulating insulin levels.

If the exercise is planned, the insulin dosage schedule may be altered to decrease the likelihood of hypoglycemia. Individuals who take a single dose of intermediate-acting insulin may decrease the dose by 30–35% on the morning before exercise or may change to a split-dose regimen, taking 65% of the usual dose in the morning and 35% before the evening meal. Those who are taking a combination of intermediate- and short-acting insulin may decrease the short-acting insulin by 50% or omit it altogether before exercise; they also may decrease

Table 6.3 Pre-exercise Checklist for People with Type 1 Diabetes

1. Consider the exercise plan.
   What is the duration and intensity of the planned exercise?
   Is the exercise habitual or unusual (e.g., more intense than usual)?
   How does the exercise relate to the level of physical conditioning?
   What is the estimated calorie expenditure?
2. Consider the insulin regimen.
   What is the usual insulin dosage schedule? Should it be decreased?
   What is the interval between injection of insulin and the onset of exercise?
   Should the site of injection be changed to avoid exercising areas?
3. Consider the plan for food intake.
   What is the interval between the last meal and the onset of exercise?
   Should a pre-exercise snack be eaten?
   Should carbohydrate feedings be taken during exercise?
   Will extra food be required after exercise?
4. Check blood glucose.
   If <100 mg/dl (<5.5 mmol/l), eat a pre-exercise snack, and recheck blood glucose
       after 15–30 minutes.
   If 100–250 mg/dl (5.5–14 mmol/l), it should be alright to exercise.
   If >250 mg/dl (>14 mmol/l), check urine ketones.
5. Check urine ketones (if glucose is >250 mg/dl [>14 mmol/l]).
   If negative, it is alright to exercise.
   If positive, take insulin; do not exercise until ketones are negative.

Source: Steppel and Horton.[4]

the intermediate-acting insulin before exercise and take supplemental doses of short-acting insulin later if needed. Many people now are treated with once-daily long-acting insulin glargine or detemir with multiple daily doses of rapid-onset, short-acting insulin (i.e., aspart, lispro, glulisine). In these people, the short-acting insulin dose before exercise may be decreased by 30–50%, and postexercise doses may be adjusted based on glucose monitoring and experience with postexercise hypoglycemia. If insulin infusion devices are used, the basal infusion rate may be decreased during exercise and premeal boluses may be decreased or omitted.[4]

EXERCISE PROGRAMS FOR TREATING TYPE 2 DIABETES

In people with T2D, exercise programs may improve insulin sensitivity and lower average blood glucose concentrations as well as provide the benefits listed in Table 6.1. The increased energy expenditure associated with exercise, when combined with calorie restriction, may support additional goals, including weight loss and weight maintenance. Thus, regular exercise is an important component of treating people with T2D.[7]

People with T2D are usually older and frequently obese, and may have significant long-term complications, making the initiation of an exercise program difficult. In this group of people, exercises that enhance motivation and participation and have a low risk of injury should be selected. Increasing daily activities such as walking, climbing stairs, and other familiar activities is an excellent start.

Table 6.4 Strategies for Avoiding Hypoglycemia and Hyperglycemia with Exercise

1. Eat a meal 1–3 hours before exercise.
2. Take supplemental carbohydrate feedings at least every 30 minutes during exercise if exercise is vigorous and of long duration.
3. Increase food intake for up to 24 hours after exercise, depending on intensity and duration of exercise.
4. Take insulin at least 1 hour before exercise. If <1 hour before exercise, inject in a nonexercising area.
5. Decrease insulin dose before exercise.
6. Alter daily insulin schedule.
7. Monitor blood glucose before, during, and after exercise.
8. Delay exercise if blood glucose is >250 mg/dl (>14 mmol/l) and ketones are present.
9. Learn individual glucose responses to different types of exercise.
10. Continuous glucose monitoring may be a useful tool.

Source: Steppel and Horton.[4]

For the growing group of adolescents who have T2D, exercise is a key treatment. Typically, exercise prescriptions for younger people with T2D can be similar to those for healthy adolescents. As previously mentioned, it is recommended that all youth participate in exercise for 300 minutes/week.

Unlike in people with T1D, problems in glucose regulation do not occur in T2D, with the exception of occasional problems with hypoglycemia in people taking insulin or insulin secretogogues. In people treated with diet alone, supplemental feedings before, during, or after exercise are generally unnecessary.[4]

In people being treated with low-calorie diets, regular exercise generally is well tolerated and does not pose any additional risks if the diet is adequately supplemented with vitamins and minerals and adequate hydration is maintained. In people treated with very-low-calorie diets (600–800 kcal/day), the diet should contain ≥35% of calories as carbohydrate to maintain normal muscle glycogen stores, which are needed to maintain high-intensity exercise. Of note, very-low-calorie diets severely restricted in carbohydrate are compatible with moderate-intensity exercise after an adaptation period of ≥2 weeks. Increasing activity while on a very-low-calorie diet in someone on a hypoglycemic agent will increase the risk of hypoglycemia.

An exercise program for obese people with T2D should start slowly, build up gradually, and include exercises that are familiar to the patient and least likely to cause injuries or worsening of long-term diabetes complications.[4]

REFERENCES

1. Thomas DE, Elliott EJ, Naughton GA. Exercise for type 2 diabetes mellitus. *Cochrane Database Syst Rev* 2006;(3):CD002968.

2. Chimen M, Kennedy A, Nirantharakumar K, Pang TT, Andrews R, Narendran P. What are the health benefits of physical activity in type 1 diabetes mellitus? A literature review. *Diabetologia* 2012;55(3):542–551.

3. Lebovitz HE, Ed. *Therapy for Diabetes Mellitus and Related Disorders, 2nd ed..* Alexandria, VA, American Diabetes Association, 1994.

4. Steppel JH, Horton ES. Exercise for the patient with type 1 diabetes mellitus. In *Diabetes Mellitus: A Fundamental and Clinical Text*. 3rd ed. Le Roth D, Taylor SI, Olefsky JM, Eds. Philadelphia, Lippincott Williams & Wilkins, 2004, p. 671–681.

5. Riebe D (ed). Exercise prescription for other clinical populations: diabetes mellitus. In *ACSM's Guidelines for Exercise Testing and Prescription*. 9th ed. Pescatello LS, Arena R, Riebe D, Thompson PD, Eds. Philadelphia, Lippincott Williams & Wilkins, 2014, p. 278–284.

6. U.S. Department of Health and Human Services. Physical activity guidelines for Americans, 2008. Available at www.health.gov/paguidelines. Accessed 24 March 2014.

7. Colberg SR, Sigal RJ, Fernhall B, Regensteiner JG, Blissmer BJ, Rubin RR, Chasan-Taber L, Albright AL, Braun B. Exercise and type 2 diabetes: the American College of Sports Medicine and the American Diabetes Association: joint position statement executive summary. American College of Sports Medicine; American Diabetes Association. *Diabetes Care* 2010; 33(12):2692–2696.

Chapter 7
Epidemiology of
Type 1 and Type 2 Diabetes

Edward W. Gregg, PhD
Giuseppina Imperatore, MD, PhD
K.M. Venkat Narayan, MD

INTRODUCTION

In an era of generally improving health and life expectancy, diabetes along with obesity has distinguished itself as one of the most challenging chronic public health problems of the present era—with continued increases in prevalence and wide-ranging morbidity and costs that follow. The number of cases of diagnosed diabetes has roughly tripled—from ~7 to 21 million—in the U.S. during the past two decades and also has become a global public health problem, expected to surpass 500 million persons in the world by the year 2030.[1,2] Although treatment options, quality of care, risk of complications, and the evidence base for diabetes prevention have all improved dramatically in recent decades,[3–6] diabetes remains a particularly challenging public health problem—largely because of the heterogeneity of the condition itself, the wide range of preventive services needed to optimize risk reduction, and the complex interaction of genes and environment in the disease's etiology.[7] This chapter describes trends in diabetes and prediabetes, summarizes the dominant risk factors for the conditions at the individual and community level, and reviews the role of epidemiology in the selection of prioritization of individuals for intervention.

MAGNITUDE AND TRENDS OF DIABETES IN U.S. ADULTS

Prevalence of diagnosed diabetes in adults in the U.S. has increased steadily since first reported as 1% of the population, nationally, in 1960.[1,8] Prevalence of diagnosed diabetes increased one percentage point every decade between 1960 and 1990 and then accelerated in the 1990s, leading to a most recent prevalence in 2010 of 8.2% of adults (Figure 7.1).[1,9] When glycemic indicators are incorporated into diabetes estimates to account for persons with undiagnosed diabetes, prevalence is considerably higher, ranging from 11.1% when diabetes is defined by A1C or fasting plasma glucose (FPG), to 13.6% when 2-hour postload glucose is included in the definition.[9–11]

Prevalence of dysglycemia, or "prediabetes," depends heavily on the definition that is used. Prevalence ranges from 14.7% when the traditional definition of impaired glucose tolerance is used (i.e., 2-hour postload glucose >140 mg/dl), to 17.1% when the newly recommended A1C definition (A1C >5.7 to <6.5%) to 29.3% when the American Diabetes Association (ADA)–recommended FPG of 100–126 mg/dl is used. When any of the three glycemic indicators (FPG, A1C, 2-hour glucose) are used, 37.5% of adults have prediabetes.[9,12,13] Although the dif-

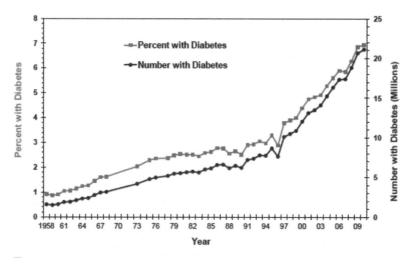

CDC's Division of Diabetes Translation. National Diabetes Surveillance System available at http://www.cdc.gov/diabetes/statistics

Figure 7.1—Number and percentage of U.S. population with diagnosed diabetes, 1958–2010.

ferent glycemic indicators identify different subgroups of the population as having "prediabetes,"[14] each is highly predictive of subsequent diabetes and, ultimately, of risk for retinopathy and other complications.[15–18]

Over the past two decades, prevalence has increased most over time in relative terms among young adults ages 20–34 years (from 0.8% in 1988–1994 to 1.9% in 2005–2010) and increased most in absolute terms in older adults >65 years old (19.8% in 1988–1994 to 28.2% in 2005–2010) (Figure 7.2).[19] Meanwhile, the greatest increase in absolute numbers of people with diabetes is occurring among people of middle age (age 35–64) because of the large numbers of baby boomers (i.e., those born between 1945 and 1960 when the U.S. birth rate was particularly high), who are now moving into an age range associated with high diabetes incidence.[19] The increase in diabetes prevalence also has been accompanied by an increase in prediabetes when defined by A1C or the union of elevated A1C and FPG, but not when defined by FPG alone.[12] The shift in the distribution of A1C levels also has been accompanied by an increase in levels of A1C and fasting insulin levels in the general population.[20]

Diabetes prevalence varies considerably by geographic region in the U.S., with prevalence two to three times as high in the highest quartile of counties than the lowest quartiles (Figure 7.3).[21,22] The highest-prevalence counties in the U.S. are clustered around the Mississippi Delta southern belt extending across Louisiana, Alabama, South Georgia, the coastal regions of the Carolinas, West Virginia, and the Appalachian counties of Tennessee, Kentucky, and Ohio. Several distinct areas, corresponding to areas with Native American reservations, also have nota-

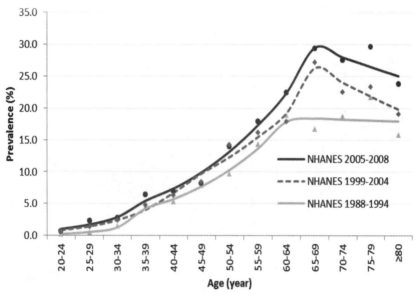

Figure 7.2—Prevalence of total diabetes adjusted for sex, race/ethnicity, and education level, according to year (NHANES 1988–1994; NHANES 1999–2004; NHANES 2005–2008).

bly high prevalence; these include northern Maine, selected areas of North and South Dakota, Montana, Arizona, and New Mexico. More recent county-level estimates of incidence (i.e., as opposed to prevalence) describe similar patterns, and further highlight the Deep South, Oklahoma, Arkansas, Kentucky, and West Virginia as particular problem areas (Figure 7.4).[23] Geographic variation in obesity and physical inactivity tend to mirror diabetes patterns. The Midwestern states of Minnesota, Iowa, Nebraska, and the Dakotas, however, are notable for having many counties with relatively high prevalence of obesity but relatively low diabetes prevalence.

Because of the data limitations in national surveys, combined with the difficulty in defining true diabetes type, most national estimates have combined all types, leaving the ratio of type 1 diabetes (T1D) versus type 2 diabetes (T2D) unclear. Using a crude definition of T1D, diagnoses before age 40 years with the need for insulin since the first year postdiagnosis, ~5% of all diabetes cases are estimated to be T1D.[24] However, the ratio of T1D to T2D varies considerably by age; among youth (<18 years), young adult (18–44 years), middle age (45–64 years), and older adults (>65 years), the proportion of cases that are T1D is estimated to be 80–90%, 10%, 4%, and <1%, respectively. In absolute terms, these estimates correspond to prevalence of T1D of 0.2%, 0.4%, 0.5%, and 0.1% for youth, young adult, middle age, and older adults, respectively.[24,25] Incidence of T1D in the U.S. peaks during adolescence, and across all age-groups is higher in whites than non-whites. Several reports suggest that incidence of T1D has

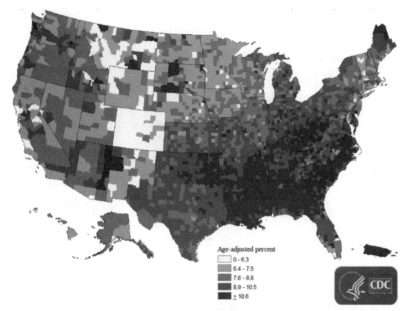

Age-adjusted percent
- 0 - 6.3
- 6.4 - 7.5
- 7.6 - 8.8
- 8.9 - 10.5
- ≥ 10.6

Figure 7.3—Age-adjusted county-level estimates of diagnosed diabetes among adults age ≥20 years, U.S., 2010.

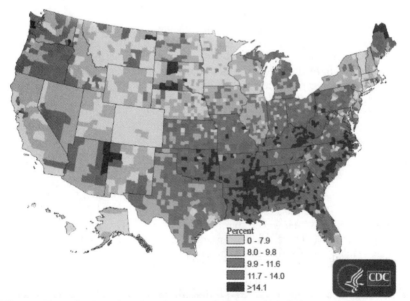

Percent
- 0 - 7.9
- 8.0 - 9.8
- 9.9 - 11.6
- 11.7 - 14.0
- ≥14.1

Figure 7.4—County-level estimates of diagnosed diabetes incidence among adults age ≥20 years, U.S., 2010.

increased by 2–3% per year, and since the 1980s has doubled.[26] This is consistent with increases worldwide, as observed in the DiaMOND registries, as well as by registries in Europe (EURODiab).[27,28]

Although diabetes in youth historically has been defined as T1D, epidemiologic studies suggest that in some ethnic groups, T2D accounts for a large portion of cases of diabetes in youth. In the SEARCH study, prevalence in youth <20 years is 2.2/1,000, of which almost 90% are T1D (1.93/1,000) and the remainder are T2D (0.24/1,000) and other types (0.05/1,000) (Figure 7.5).[25] The ratio of T1D to T2D in youth varies considerably by race and ethnicity. Among diabetes cases in youth, roughly two-thirds of American Indians and Alaska Natives have T2D, whereas about one-fourth of blacks, Hispanics, and Asian-Pacific Islanders cases have T2D, compared with <10% among whites. Although direct data on trends in T2D in youth are lacking, these rates almost certainly have a higher prevalence than in prior decades. Similarly, the prevalence of prediabetes among youth ages 12–17 years increased over the 1999–2010 decade when defined by A1C (from 2.4–4.5%) but not when defined by FPG (12–14.8%).[12] However, the implications of prediabetes for subsequent progression to diabetes and for increased cardiovascular risk are not as clear for youth as they are for adults.

DETERMINANTS OF PREVALENCE: INCIDENCE AND MORTALITY

The diabetes prevalence of the population is determined primarily by the incidence rate, or rate of onset of new cases of diabetes, the survival rate of people with diagnosed diabetes, and changing demographics of the population, which is affected by diverse factors such as migration patterns and changing birth rates. In settings in which the prevalence of only diagnosed diabetes is being assessed, prevalence also is affected by the level of detection of undiagnosed cases.

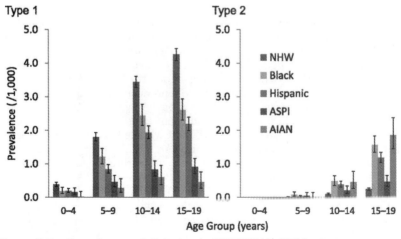

Figure 7.5—Prevalence of diabetes in SEARCH/1,000 by type, age-group, and race or ethnicity. Source: Pettit et al.[25]

The increases in prevalence in the U.S. have been mirrored by increases in the incidence of diagnosed diabetes. Incidence trends were flat through the 1980s and then rose sharply after 1990, increasing by a relative ~5% per year to an absolute incidence in 2011 of ~1% per year.[29] These increases in incidence have occurred in all age-groups, genders, and races or ethnicities. Recent analyses suggest that in the overall population, increases in incidence may have slowed or subsided around the year 2008, coincidental with a slowing of the obesity epidemic recently observed.[30] National incidence data are based on self-reported diagnosis, however, and may be affected by increased detection over time along with changing diagnostic thresholds. Data from at least three regional cohort studies, however, have assessed diabetes incidence using clinic visits and glycemic measurements and have suggested that the increase in incidence of diagnosed diabetes is driven by a true increase in the rate of new cases.[31-33] In the San Antonio Heart Study, 7- to 8-year incidence tripled during the 1980s in both Mexican Americans (from 5.7 to 15.7%) and whites (from 2.6 to 9.4%), whereas in the Framingham Heart Study, incidence roughly doubled from the 1970s to 1990s (from 2 to 3.7% in women and from 2.7 to 5.8% in men).[31,32]

The increases in diabetes prevalence also may have been affected by decreases in mortality of the diabetes population. Recent analyses of data from the National Health Interview Survey showed that all-cause and cardiovascular disease (CVD) mortality in the diabetes population declined by >50%, considerably narrowing the gap in mortality rates between adults with and without diabetes.[34]

DIABETES AS A GLOBAL PROBLEM

Although the U.S. has been noted for its high levels of obesity and diabetes and popular magazines have even labeled it as an "American Epidemic,"[35] diabetes is now recognized as a public health problem in virtually every continent, and by international standards, the U.S. now has prevalence that is considered average relative to the rest of the world.[36-38] Although it is difficult to compare prevalence directly across countries and regions because of the differences in sampling and measurement approaches and population representativeness, several patterns are evident in the global epidemiology of diabetes. Selected islands of the Western Pacific have been acknowledged as having among the highest age-standardized prevalence in the world for several decades, with prevalence exceeding 20% in Kiribati, the Marshall Islands, and Nauru.[38,39] Although nationally representative surveys are lacking, studies in several areas and populations suggest that prevalence is similarly high (~20%) in several countries of the Middle East, including Lebanon, Qatar, South Arabia, Bahrain, and the United Arab Emirates.[40,41] Estimates from several areas of India indicate that it is under a similar threat, and prevalence may exceed that of the U.S.[42] National prevalence is also moderately high (i.e., ranging from 8 to 12%) in China, the U.S., Mexico, Canada, and several countries of Europe.[9-11,43,44] Furthermore, the high prevalence of diabetes in developing countries is no longer restricted to urban areas, and available data indicate that diabetes prevalence in rural parts of low- and middle-income countries has increased several-fold in the past two decades.[45] The combination of moderately high prevalence in India and China and their enormous population sizes means that India and China account for 40% of the world's population of diabetes. Africa consistently has had the lowest prevalence in the world, but it is now projected to have the largest relative increase in prevalence in the upcoming decades.[46]

The diabetes epidemic in lower- and middle-income countries tends to differ from that of high-income countries in several distinct ways. First, the middle-aged segment of the population accounts for a higher proportion of cases in lower- and middle-income countries than in higher-income countries, a difference that has potential economic implications for lower- and middle-income countries because of the potential for diabetes to affect the productivity of the working-age population.[36,37] Second, the proportion of cases that are undiagnosed is appreciably higher in lower- and middle-income countries.[47] Third, the availability of services and essential medications for the prevention of both diabetes and its complications is notably lower than in upper-income countries,[48] leaving rates of the complications and morbidity that result from diabetes concerning and largely unknown.

Previous observations of particularly high diabetes prevalence in populations that have undergone a recent increase in economic well-being have led to the notion that diabetes is associated with wealth and high socioeconomic status in many international settings. Recent systematic reviews, however, suggest that obesity and diabetes increasingly are associated with lower socioeconomic strata in lower- and middle-income countries, similar to what has been observed in higher-income countries.[49] For example, being in the lowest education group was associated with a 41% higher prevalence across 23 studies overall, as well as in stratified analyses in which studies came from middle-income countries in Asia, the Middle East, Latin America, and Africa.

RISK FACTORS FOR DIABETES

Diabetes risk factors can generally be classified into *1*) nonmodifiable risk factors such as demographic factors and genes, *2*) modifiable behavioral or environmental risk factors, *3*) physiological biomarkers that aid in the prediction of diabetes and monitoring of preventive interventions, and *4*) a subset of risk factors that explain the changes in diabetes incidence over time for the population.

Nonmodifiable Risk Factors

Age, sex, race and ethnicity, family history, and genetic factors are the most prominent nonmodifiable risk factors for T2D. Incidence of diagnosed diabetes increases from 0.3% per year among adults ages 18–44 years to 1.1% per year among those ages 45–64 years (i.e., three times as high), to 1.3% among those age 65 years (four times as high).[29] Accordingly, the prevalence of total diabetes increases steeply with age, from 0.2% in youth, 3.6% in young adulthood (ages 20–44 years), 13.5% in middle age (45–64 years), and 26.5% in older adults (≥65 years).[9,12,50] National surveys suggest that prevalence plateaus after age 75 years, but they do not take into account adults living in assisted living and nursing centers, where prevalence has been shown to be higher.[51]

Diabetes prevalence historically has been higher in women than men, in part because of greater female longevity. Incidence of diagnosed diabetes, however, is at least as high in men as in women, surpassed that of women in the mid-2000s, and along with greater reductions in death rates of men compared with women, has made diabetes prevalence of men even with that of women).[1]

Compared with non-Hispanic whites, among whom prevalence of diagnosed diabetes in the overall population (including adults and youth) is 7.6%, age-standardized prevalence is more than twice as high in American Indians (16.1%) and almost twice as high in non-Hispanic blacks (13.3%) and Hispanics (12.7%). Among Hispanics, prevalence is notably higher among Puerto Ricans and Mexicans. Asians have a prevalence that is similar to whites; prevalence is >50% higher than whites among Asian Indians and Filipinos but lower among Chinese Americans.[9,52–54]

T2D is associated strongly with family history and genetics. By 2013, ~80 genetic loci had been identified that collectively explain ~10% of the heritability of diabetes.[55–58] The loci identified carry significant but modest (10–20% elevated) associations with diabetes incidence and most loci have been linked to β-cell function, as opposed to insulin resistance. For a number of major genes, lifestyle modification appears to negate the excess risk conferred by genes, indicating the strong environmental influence even among those with genetic predisposition.[59,60] In a study of 18 single-nucleotide polymorphisms among adults in the Framingham Heart Study, a genotype score was developed that showed that people in the top decile had about two and half times the incidence of adults in the bottom quarter of the genotype score. The genotype score, however, was only slightly more predictive than a conventional risk score composed of self-reported risk factors along with glucose and triglyceride levels.[61,62] Genotype-based scores may become an important part of risk prediction in the future, but this is likely to depend on a better future understanding of how high-risk genes interact with lifestyle and environmental factors.[63]

Modifiable Risk Factors

Obesity is widely recognized as the predominant potentially modifiable risk factor for T2D. Each standard deviation of BMI, or ~3–5 kg/m^2 in most populations, increases risk by 80–90%.[64,65] In the U.S., incidence of diagnosed diabetes ranges from ~0.2% per year among normal-weight adults to ~0.5% (2.2 times as high) among overweight adults to ~1.7% per year among obese adults (i.e., eight times as high). Obesity indicators that capture central obesity more directly, such as the waist circumference, waist-to-hip ratio, and sagittal abdominal diameter, provide a similar or stronger association with subsequent diabetes risk. In a meta-analysis of >32 studies, relative risk of diabetes per standard deviation of obesity-related factors is slightly greater for waist circumference (relative risk ([RR] = 1.87, 95% confidence interval [CI] 1.62–2.15) than BMI (RR = 1.72, 1.47–2.15).[64] Similarly, the European Prospective Investigation into Cancer and Nutrition (EPIC) study found that each standard deviation of waist circumference was associated with a 95% increased diabetes incidence in men (RR = 1.95, 1.83–2.08) and a 143% increased incidence in women (RR = 2.43, 2.23–2.64).[65] In addition, waist circumference was strongly predictive of diabetes incidence within BMI strata, including among overweight and obese persons. More recent studies have found that sagittal abdominal diameter, a simple measure of central obesity, to have a similar association with diabetes incidence.[66] Others have shown that the magnitude of weight change, particularly during young adulthood, and the person-time associated with obesity also are associated strongly with risk.[67]

Increasing physical activity levels have been associated consistently with a reduced incidence of T2D in a dose-response manner.[68–70] Compared with sedentary people, regular participation in moderate physical activity is associated with a ~30% reduction in diabetes incidence.[68,69] About half of the association of physical activity and diabetes risk is explained by more active people having lower levels of obesity. More specific examination of the beneficial attributes of physical activity has shown that total energy and duration of physical activity are particularly associated with diabetes incidence. However, whether vigorous activity, or the level of intensity, affects risk above and beyond total energy expenditure, is less clear. Growing evidence suggests that the levels of sedentary behavior (i.e., the amount of time sitting) is associated with increased diabetes risk above and beyond the impact of levels of moderate leisure-time physical activity like walking.[71,72] Sedentary time is thought to affect insulin sensitivity through physiological effects on muscle and metabolic disuse as well as through the dietary behavior that may accompany sitting.

Several dietary factors may have positive effects on insulin resistance or T2D risk independent of their effects on obesity.[25] Consumption of fruits and vegetables, whole grains and cereal fibers, and other components of the Mediterranean diet (including olive oil, red wine, and moderate dairy intake) have each been found to be protective against diabetes incidence in cohort studies.[73–75] These findings support earlier observations that polyunsaturated and monounsaturated fats may reduce risk, but saturated fats and total intake have been associated with increased risk.[76] The value of a composite Mediterranean diet also has been supported in at least one randomized controlled trial, but the impact may be weaker in the general population than among people with prediabetes or prior CVD.[74,75,77] People with low levels of vitamin D have an increased diabetes risk, and concomitantly, higher levels of vitamin D intake have been associated with a modest (13%) reduction in the risk of diabetes.[78] A trial currently underway will determine whether vitamin D supplementation in people with prediabetes reduces progression to diabetes.[79]

Other factors in the diet, including sugar-sweetened beverages (SSBs), red meat, saturated fat, refined carbohydrates, fast foods, and other components of the "Western" diet are notable for increasing, rather than decreasing, diabetes risk.[80,81] Consumption of SSBs, including soft drinks, sweetened carbonated beverages, and fruit drinks, have more than doubled in the U.S. population over the past two decades and are associated with obesity, insulin resistance, and T2D.[82–84] Potential mechanisms for the association of SSBs with obesity and diabetes include greater compensatory and overall caloric consumption as well as more direct effects of SSBs on insulin resistance through their glycemic properties. Longitudinal evidence to support these hypotheses is limited, however. Data from the Nurses Health study found that women reporting more than seven servings per week of SSB had an 80% greater diabetes risk than those reporting less than one serving per week.[84] Other cohort studies found only modest or null associations with diabetes risk. There are also no data from randomized controlled trials that interventions aimed at changing SSB intake, whether through individual or policy-based approaches, result in appreciable reductions in the incidence of T2D. Consumption of red meat, particularly processed red meat, also is associated with diabetes; systematic reviews have suggested that each serving of red meat per day (~3 ounces) is associated with a 14% increase in diabetes incidence, whereas the people in the highest quintile of red meat consumption have a 32% increased diabetes risk relative to the lowest quintile, adjusted for total intake and dietary quality.[85–87] Several other dietary risk factors, including energy density and glycemic load, also have been examined but have been found to have less consistent associations with diabetes incidence.[88–90]

Birth weight is associated inversely with diabetes risk, reflecting the potential for the quality of prenatal development to influence risk of insulin resistance or β-cell function. Infants born <2 kg in weight have a 50–100% increased risk of diabetes during adulthood compared with normal-weight infants.[91] In some studies, the shape of the relationship of birth weight with diabetes risk has been U-shaped, such that infants of very large birth weight (i.e., >4.5 kg) have an increased risk of adult diabetes as well. The potential public health impact of low birth weight could vary considerably by population, depending on levels of prenatal care and the prevalence of low birth weight.

Socioeconomic factors, including low education, income, and adverse neighborhood and environmental surroundings, each have been associated with the prevalence of diabetes and obesity in the U.S. and may underlie many of the risk factors of diabetes.[1,92] In the U.S., age-adjusted prevalence is 50% higher in people without a high school diploma than in those who have gone to college and poverty level is one of the most important predictors of county-level diabetes prevalence.[93]

Finally, several other factors consistently distinguish people who are at increased risk for subsequent diabetes. Having hypertension, depressive symptoms, being a smoker, dysfunctional sleep, and exposure to environmental pollutants have each been associated with elevated T2D risk while coffee intake and moderate alcohol consumption have each been associated with decreased risk.[94–97] Whether acting on these risk factors with interventions in turn leads to a reduction in diabetes incidence is not known. For example, modification of smoking risk or depressive symptoms, for example, actually may lead to some weight gain and thus counteract the benefit of removing smoking as a diabetes risk factor.[98] Similarly, there is not evidence that treating hypertension or poor sleep influences disease risk, although each is plausible.

Biomarkers to Aid in Prediction and Monitoring

Levels of A1C, FPG, and 2-hour glucose each are associated strongly with subsequent diabetes risk.[99–101] The slope and magnitude of the association of these factors with diabetes risk depend on how diabetes is defined.[102] A1C is more predictive of A1C-defined diabetes, and FPG is more predictive of FPG-based diabetes. In addition, the A1C-based prediabetes definition (5.7%) is less sensitive but has a higher positive predictive value than the FPG-based threshold of FPG 100–125, which selects more people but includes more lower-risk people.[14,103] People with elevated FPG and A1C-based glycemia have higher risk than those identified by just a single marker.[104]

RISK FACTORS IN PREVENTION AND RISK STRATIFICATION

Findings from epidemiologic studies have been used to influence the selection of interventions in diabetes prevention trials and the selection of variables that are used in risk scores to identify good candidates for intervention.[105] The consistent associations of weight gain and physical inactivity observed in epidemiologic studies ultimately led major prevention studies to examine the effect of multicomponent lifestyle intervention on diabetes incidence among people with impaired glucose tolerance.[4] At least six randomized controlled trials conducted in the U.S., Finland, India, China, and Japan demonstrated 30–60% relative reductions in diabetes incidence associated with lifestyle intervention of at least 2 years.[4,5,106–109] Weight loss was greatest in the U.S. trial and post hoc analyses suggested that it was the dominant factor affecting incidence.[110] For intervention participants in the Finnish Diabetes Prevention Study, weight loss was an important factor, but post hoc analyses also showed that the relative risk reduction associated with intervention was explained by the number of intervention goals, including not only weight loss but also physical activity, reduction in fat intake, and increase in fiber intake.[111] The intervention arms in the studies conducted in China, Indian, and Japan were successful in reducing diabetes despite no or modest weight loss.[107,109,112] These trials confirm the efficacy of multicomponent lifestyle interventions in high-risk adults but leave some questions unclear: For example, it is unclear whether the impact of interventions focusing solely on physical activity or diet without an emphasis on weight loss are similarly effective or whether lifestyle interventions targeting persons below the threshold of prediabetes are also effective.

Risk scores have emerged as an important tool to aid in the selection of people who would benefit most from preventive interventions or who should be prioritized for further testing for undiagnosed diabetes.[105,113] Simple risk factor questionnaires, typically based on age, height, weight, sex, race or ethnicity, and history of hypertension or history of gestational diabetes, have been shown to have modest predictability of undiagnosed or subsequent diabetes but are good inexpensive options with which to select people for further testing or monitoring.[105] Inclusion of additional risk factors, including physical inactivity, smoking, and diet quality, or more precise indicators of central obesity, improve predictability but also increase the complexity of the risk scores. The addition of biochemical measures, including fasting glucose A1C, or triglycerides, further improves the predictability of risk scores, but further increases the complexity and cost. Future risk prediction may include more complex multi-element biochemical assays with and without genetic or epigenetic markers, but such tools have not yet been incorporated into practice.[114]

FACTORS EXPLAINING TRENDS IN THE EPIDEMIC

Although many risk factors have been identified for T2D in individuals, it is likely that a smaller subset of these factors has explained the increases in population incidence and prevalence over time. For example, factors like smoking and saturated fat intake may increase diabetes risk but generally have declined over time in the population.[115] Instead, increases in obesity levels affecting virtually all segments of the population appear to have been the most prominent factor driving the increases in diabetes risk. This is supported by ecologic observations that levels of diabetes within obesity strata have been relatively stable but the excess prevalent diabetes cases in later decades have been disproportionately composed of individuals with class II (BMI ≥35 kg/m^2) and class III (BMI ≥40 kg/m^2) obesity.[116] The primary factors explaining the increasing obesity prevalence remains controversial. Total dietary intake, average portion sizes, consumption of refined carbohydrates, corn sugars, and SSBs all have increased in parallel with increases in obesity and diabetes.[117] Levels of leisure-time physical activity have been relatively stable, but levels of occupational activity have declined and sedentary behavior have increased. Sleep quality may have declined over time and contributed to diabetes risk. The dietary and physical activity changes that have occurred could have affected diabetes risk through their effects on obesity as well as by affecting risk of insulin resistance and levels of glycemia independent of obesity. Other trends in behavior and health care, including sleep quality; commonly taken medications, such as selective serotonin reuptake inhibitors for depression and anxiety, which may affect obesity; and statins, which affect diabetes risk, also could have contributed to trends over time, but their contributions have not been quantified. Despite the long list of dietary, behavioral, and pharmacological factors potentially affecting diabetes trends, few studies have examined the impact of policy changes aimed at these factors on diabetes risk.

CONCLUSION

This summary of the epidemiology of diabetes and its risk factors reveals several important conclusions: Prevalence and incidence of diabetes have each increased in the U.S. population, with a particularly steep increase during the 1990s and early 2000s, which has been greatest in relative terms among young adults but greatest in absolute terms in older adults. Increases in prevalence of diagnosed diabetes have been driven by a combination of an increased rate of diabetes, an earlier detection of cases, and declining mortality rates in people with diabetes. The combination of a high diabetes incidence rate with declining mortality rates in the general population has led to large increases in the average person's probability of developing diabetes over a lifetime. Risk of diabetes in individuals is affected by numerous risk factors, most notably central obesity, physical inactivity, family history, age, male sex, and hypertension. Increases in diabetes incidence over time have been affected most by increasing levels of obesity and the changes to dietary behavior and physical activity that have increased obesity levels. Lifestyle changes, including weight reduction through changes in dietary and physical activity levels for people with prediabetes, substantially reduce the risk of progression to diabetes. Changing trends in diabetes incidence likely will require a multitiered strategy consisting of structured lifestyle interventions for people at highest risk and effective policies and community-level changes to alter the risk factor distributions of the population as a whole.

REFERENCES

1. Centers for Disease Control and Prevention. Diabetes surveillance system: diagnosed diabetes; number and percentage of U.S. population with diagnosed diabetes, 2014. Available at www.cdc.gov/diabetes/statistics/prev/national/index.htm. Accessed 1 January 2014.

2. Whiting DR, et al. IDF diabetes atlas: global estimates of the prevalence of diabetes for 2011 and 2030. *Diabetes Res Clin Pract* 2011;94(3):311–321.

3. Ali MK, et al. Achievement of goals in U.S. Diabetes care, 1999-2010. *N Engl J Med* 2013;368(17):1613–1624.

4. Crandall JP, et al. The prevention of type 2 diabetes. *Nat Clin Pract Endocrinol Metab 2008*;4(7):382–393.

5. Knowler WC, et al. Reduction in the incidence of type 2 diabetes with lifestyle intervention or metformin. *N Engl J Med* 2002;346(6):393–403.

6. Gregg EW, Li Y, Wang J, Burrows NR, Ali MK, Rolka DR, Williams DE, Geiss L. Changes in diabetes-related complications in the U.S., 1990–2010. *N Engl J Med* 2014. In press.

7. Kahn SE, Cooper ME, Del Prato S. Pathophysiology and treatment of type 2 diabetes: perspectives on the past, present, and future. *Lancet* 2014 Mar 22;383(9922):1068–1083.

8. U.S. Department of Health, Education, and Welfare. Diabetes reported in interviews. United States July 1957–1959. Health Statistics from the US National Health Survey: Series B-No 21 1960. Available at http://www.cdc.gov/nchs/products/public_health.htm. Accessed 17 July 2013.

9. Centers for Disease Control and Prevention. *National Diabetes Fact Sheet: National Estimates and General Information on Diabetes and Prediabetes in the United States 2011.* Atlanta, GA, Department of Health and Human Services, Centers for Disease Control and Prevention, 2011.

10. Cowie CC, et al. Prevalence of diabetes and high risk for diabetes using A1C criteria in the U.S. population in 1988–2006. *Diabetes Care* 2010;33(3):562–568.

11. Cowie CC, et al. Full accounting of diabetes and pre-diabetes in the U.S. population in 1988–1994 and 2005–2006. *Diabetes Care* 2009;32(2):287–294.

12. Bullard KM, et al. Secular changes in U.S. prediabetes prevalence defined by hemoglobin A1c and fasting plasma glucose: National Health and Nutrition Examination Surveys, 1999-2010. *Diabetes Care* 2013;36(8):2286–2293.

13. James C, et al. Implications of alternative definitions of prediabetes for prevalence in U.S. adults. *Diabetes Care* 2011;34(2):387 391.

14. Gregg EW, et al. Implications of risk stratification for diabetes prevention: the case of hemoglobin A1c. *Am J Prev Med* 2013;44(4Suppl 4):S375–S380.

15. Selvin E, et al. Glycated hemoglobin and the risk of kidney disease and retinopathy in adults with and without diabetes. *Diabetes* 2011;60(1):298–305.

16. Selvin E, et al. Glycated hemoglobin, diabetes, and cardiovascular risk in nondiabetic adults. *N Engl J Med* 2010;362(9):800–811.

17. Colagiuri S, et al. Glycemic thresholds for diabetes-specific retinopathy: implications for diagnostic criteria for diabetes. *Diabetes Care* 2011;34(1):145–150.

18. Cheng YJ, et al. Association of A1C and fasting plasma glucose levels with diabetic retinopathy prevalence in the U.S. population: implications for diabetes diagnostic thresholds. *Diabetes Care* 2009;32(11):2027–2032.

19. Cheng YJ, et al. Secular changes in the age-specific prevalence of diabetes among U.S. adults: 1988–2010. *Diabetes Care* 2013;36(9):2690–2696.

20. Cheng YJ, et al. Recent population changes in HbA(1c) and fasting insulin concentrations among US adults with preserved glucose homeostasis. *Diabetologia* 2010;53(9):1890–1893.

21. County level estimates of diagnosed diabetes—U.S. maps, 2008. Available at http://apps.nccd.cdc.gov/DDT_STRS2/NationalDiabetesPrevalenceEstimates.aspx. Accessed 24 March 2014.

22. Estimated county-level prevalence of diabetes and obesity—United States 2007. *MMWR* 2009;58(45):1259–1263.

23. Centers for Disease Control and Prevention. National diabetes surveillance system, 2013. Available at www.cdc.gov/diabetes/surveillance/index.htm. Accessed 11 March 2009.

24. Menke A, et al. The prevalence of type 1 diabetes in the United States. *Epidemiology* 2013;24(5):773–774.

25. Pettitt DJ, et al. Prevalence of diabetes mellitus in U.S. youth in 2009: the SEARCH for Diabetes in Youth study. *Diabetes Care* 2014;37(2):402–408.

26. Vehik K, et al. Increasing incidence of type 1 diabetes in 0- to 17-year-old Colorado youth. *Diabetes Care* 2007;30(3):503–509.

27. DIAMOND Project Group. Incidence and trends of childhood type 1 diabetes worldwide 1990–1999. *Diabet Med* 2006;23(8):857–866.

28. Patterson CC, et al. Trends in childhood type 1 diabetes incidence in Europe during 1989-2008: evidence of non-uniformity over time in rates of increase. *Diabetologia* 2012;55(8):2142–2147.

29. Centers for Disease Control and Prevention. Crude and age-adjusted incidence of diagnosed diabetes per 1,000 population aged 18–79 years, United States, 1980–2011. Available at www.cdc.gov/diabetes/statistics/prev/national/figage.htm. Accessed 24 September 2012.

30. Flegal KM, et al. Prevalence of obesity and trends in the distribution of body mass index among US adults, 1999-2010. *JAMA* 2012;307(5):491–497.

31. Burke JP, et al. Rapid rise in the incidence of type 2 diabetes from 1987 to 1996: results from the San Antonio Heart Study. *Arch Intern Med* 1999;159(13):1450–1456.

32. Fox CS, et al. Trends in the incidence of type 2 diabetes mellitus from the 1970s to the 1990s: the Framingham Heart Study. *Circulation* 2006;113(25):2914–2918.

33. Burke JP, et al. Impact of case ascertainment on recent trends in diabetes incidence in Rochester, Minnesota. *Am J Epidemiol* 2002;155(9):859–865.

34. Gregg EW, et al. Trends in death rates among U.S. adults with and without diabetes between 1997 and 2006: findings from the National Health Interview Survey. *Diabetes Care* 2012;35(6):1252–1257.

35. Adler J, Kalb C. An American epidemic—diabetes. *Newsweek* 2000;136(10):40–47.

36. Shaw JE, Sicree RA, Zimmet PZ. Global estimates of the prevalence of diabetes for 2010 and 2030. *Diabetes Res Clin Pract* 2010;87(1):4–14.

37. Yach D, Stuckler D, Brownell KD. Epidemiologic and economic consequences of the global epidemics of obesity and diabetes. *Nat Med* 2006;12(1):62–66.

38. International Diabetes Federation. *IDF Diabetes Atlas* (6th ed.). Brussels, International Diabetes Federation, 2103.

39. Chan JC, et al. Diabetes in the Western Pacific region: past, present and future. *Diabetes Res Clin Pract* 2014;103(2):244–255.

40. Majeed A, et al. Diabetes in the Middle-East and North Africa: an update. *Diabetes Res Clin Pract* 2014;103(2):318–322.

41. Mokdad AH, et al. The state of health in the Arab world, 1990-2010: an analysis of the burden of diseases, injuries, and risk factors. *Lancet* 2014;383(9914):309–320.

42. Ramachandran A, Snehalatha C, Ma RC. Diabetes in South-East Asia: an update. *Diabetes Res Clin Pract* 2014;103(2):321–327.

43. Lipscombe LL, Hux JE. Trends in diabetes prevalence, incidence, and mortality in Ontario, Canada 1995-2005: a population-based study. *Lancet* 2007;369(9563):750–756.

44. Xu Y, et al. Prevalence and control of diabetes in Chinese adults. *JAMA* 2013;310(9):948–959.

45. Hwang CK, et al. Rural diabetes prevalence quintuples over twenty-five years in low- and middle-income countries: a systematic review and meta-analysis. *Diabetes Res Clin Pract* 2012;96(3):271–285.

46. Peer N, et al. Diabetes in the Africa region: 2013 update. *Diabetes Res Clin Pract* 2014;103(2):197–205.

47. Beagley J, et al. Global estimates of undiagnosed diabetes in adults. *Diabetes Res Clin Pract* 2014;103(2):150–160.

48. Yusuf S, et al. Use of secondary prevention drugs for cardiovascular disease in the community in high-income, middle-income, and low-income countries (the PURE Study): a prospective epidemiological survey. *Lancet* 2011;378(9798):1231–1243.

49. Agardh E, et al. Type 2 diabetes incidence and socio-economic position: a systematic review and meta-analysis. *Int J Epidemiol* 2011;40(3):804–818.

50. Liese AD, et al. The burden of diabetes mellitus among US youth: prevalence estimates from the SEARCH for Diabetes in Youth Study. *Pediatrics* 2006;118(4):1510–1518.

51. Zhang X, et al. Trends in the prevalence and comorbidities of diabetes mellitus in nursing home residents in the United States: 1995–2004. *J Am Geriatr Soc* 2010;58(4):724–730.

52. Oza-Frank R, Narayan KM. Overweight and diabetes prevalence among US immigrants. *Am J Public Health* 2010;100(4):661–668.

53. Weber MB, et al. Type 2 diabetes in Asians: prevalence, risk factors, and effectiveness of behavioral intervention at individual and population levels. *Ann Rev Nutr* 2012;32:417–439.

54. Lee JW, Brancati FL, Yeh HC. Trends in the prevalence of type 2 diabetes in Asians versus whites: results from the United States National Health Interview Survey, 1997–2008. *Diabetes Care* 2011;34(2):353–357.

55. Morris AP, et al. Large-scale association analysis provides insights into the genetic architecture and pathophysiology of type 2 diabetes. *Nat Genet* 2012;44(9):981–990.

56. Scott RA, et al. Large-scale association analyses identify new loci influencing glycemic traits and provide insight into the underlying biological pathways. *Nat Genet* 2012;44(9):991–1005.

57. McCarthy MI. Genomics, type 2 diabetes, and obesity. *N Engl J Med* 2010;363(24):2339–2350.

58. Billings LK, Florez JC. The genetics of type 2 diabetes: what have we learned from GWAS? *Ann N Y Acad Sci* 2010;1212:59–77.

59. Florez JC, et al. TCF7L2 polymorphisms and progression to diabetes in the Diabetes Prevention Program. *N Engl J Med* 2006;355(3):241–250.

60. Delahanty LM, et al. Genetic predictors of weight loss and weight regain after intensive lifestyle modification, metformin treatment, or standard care in the Diabetes Prevention Program. *Diabetes Care* 2012;35(2):363–366.

61. Bao W, et al. Predicting risk of type 2 diabetes mellitus with genetic risk models on the basis of established genome-wide association markers: a systematic review. *Am J Epidemiol* 2013;178(8):1197–1207.

62. Meigs JB. Prediction of type 2 diabetes: the dawn of polygenetic testing for complex disease. *Diabetologia* 2009;52(4):568–570.

63. Gluckman PD. Epigenetics and metabolism in 2011: epigenetics, the life-course and metabolic disease. *Nat Rev Endocrinol* 2012;8(2):74–76.

64. Vazquez G, et al. Comparison of body mass index, waist circumference, and waist/hip ratio in predicting incident diabetes: a meta-analysis. *Epidemiol Rev* 2007;29:115–128.

65. Langenberg C, et al. Long-term risk of incident type 2 diabetes and measures of overall and regional obesity: the EPIC-InterAct case-cohort study. *PLoS Med* 2012;9(6):e1001230.

66. Pajunen P, et al. Sagittal abdominal diameter as a new predictor for incident diabetes. *Diabetes Care* 2013;36(2):283–288.

67. Schienkiewitz A, et al. Body mass index history and risk of type 2 diabetes: results from the European Prospective Investigation into Cancer and Nutrition (EPIC)-Potsdam Study. *Am J Clin Nutr* 2006;84(2):427–433.

68. Jeon CY, et al. Physical activity of moderate intensity and risk of type 2 diabetes: a systematic review. *Diabetes Care* 2007;30(3):744–752.

69. InterAct Consortium. Physical activity reduces the risk of incident type 2 diabetes in general and in abdominally lean and obese men and women: the EPIC-InterAct Study. *Diabetologia* 2012;55(7):1944–1952.

70. Hu FB, et al. Walking compared with vigorous physical activity and risk of type 2 diabetes in women: a prospective study. *JAMA* 1999;282(15):1433–1439.

71. Lahjibi E, et al. Impact of objectively measured sedentary behaviour on changes in insulin resistance and secretion over 3 years in the RISC study: interaction with weight gain. *Diabetes Metab* 2013;39(3):217–225.

72. Henson J, et al. Associations of objectively measured sedentary behaviour and physical activity with markers of cardiometabolic health. *Diabetologia* 2013;56(5):1012–1020.

73. Carter P, et al. Fruit and vegetable intake and incidence of type 2 diabetes mellitus: systematic review and meta-analysis. *BMJ* 2010;341:c4229:1–8.

74. Romaguera D, et al. Mediterranean diet and type 2 diabetes risk in the European Prospective Investigation into Cancer and Nutrition (EPIC) study: the InterAct project. *Diabetes Care* 2011;34(9):1913–1918.

75. Mozaffarian D, et al. Incidence of new-onset diabetes and impaired fasting glucose in patients with recent myocardial infarction and the effect of clinical and lifestyle risk factors. *Lancet* 2007;370(9588):667–675.

76. Hu FB, Van Dam RM, Liu S. Diet and risk of type II diabetes: the role of types of fat and carbohydrate. *Diabetologia* 2001;44(7):805–817.

77. Salas-Salvado J, et al. Reduction in the incidence of type 2 diabetes with the Mediterranean diet: results of the PREDIMED-Reus nutrition intervention randomized trial. *Diabetes Care* 2011;34(1):14–19.

78. Mitri J, Muraru MD, Pittas AG. Vitamin D and type 2 diabetes: a systematic review. *Eur J Clin Nutr* 2011;65(9):1005–1015.

79. National Institutes of Health. Large study to examine if vitamin D prevents diabetes. Department of Health and Human Services. Available at www.nih.gov/news/health/oct2013/niddk-21.htm. Accessed 24 March 2014.

80. Van Dam RM, et al. Dietary patterns and risk for type 2 diabetes mellitus in U.S. men. *Ann Intern Med* 2002;136(3):201–209.

81. Williams DE, et al. The effect of Indian or Anglo dietary preference on the incidence of diabetes in Pima Indians. *Diabetes Care* 2001;24(5):811–816.

82. Malik VS, et al. Sugar-sweetened beverages and risk of metabolic syndrome and type 2 diabetes: a meta-analysis. *Diabetes Care* 2010;33(11):2477–2483.

83. Schulze MB, et al. Sugar-sweetened beverages, weight gain, and incidence of type 2 diabetes in young and middle-aged women. *JAMA* 2004;292(8):927–934.

84. Hu FB, Malik VS. Sugar-sweetened beverages and risk of obesity and type 2 diabetes: epidemiologic evidence. *Physiol Behav* 2010;100(1):47–54.

85. Pan A, et al. Red meat consumption and risk of type 2 diabetes: 3 cohorts of US adults and an updated meta-analysis. *Am J Clin Nutr* 2011;94(4):1088–1096.

86. Micha R, Wallace SK, Mozaffarian D. Red and processed meat consumption and risk of incident coronary heart disease, stroke, and diabetes mellitus: a systematic review and meta-analysis. *Circulation* 2010;121(21):2271–2283.

87. Interact Consortium. Association between dietary meat consumption and incident type 2 diabetes: the EPIC-InterAct study. *Diabetologia* 2013;56(1):47–59.

88. Patel PS, et al. The prospective association between total and type of fish intake and type 2 diabetes in 8 European countries: EPIC-InterAct Study. *Am J Clin Nutr* 2012;95(6):1445–1453.

89. InterAct Consortium, van den Berg SW, et al. The association between dietary energy density and type 2 diabetes in Europe: results from the EPIC-InterAct Study. *PLoS One* 2013;8(5):e59947.

90. Schulze MB, et al. Glycemic index, glycemic load, and dietary fiber intake and incidence of type 2 diabetes in younger and middle-aged women. *Am J Clin Nutr* 2004;80(2):348–356.

91. Whincup PH, et al. Birth weight and risk of type 2 diabetes: a systematic review. *JAMA* 2008;300(24):2886–2897.

92. Brown AF, et al. Socioeconomic position and health among persons with diabetes mellitus: a conceptual framework and review of the literature. *Epidemiol Rev* 2004;26:63–77.

93. Centers for Disease Control and Prevention. Estimated county-level prevalence of diabetes and obesity—United States 2007. *MMWR* 2009;58(45):1259–1263.

94. Huxley R, et al. Coffee, decaffeinated coffee, and tea consumption in relation to incident type 2 diabetes mellitus: a systematic review with meta-analysis. *Arch Intern Med* 2009;169(22):2053–2063.

95. Kivimaki M, et al. Antidepressant medication use, weight gain, and risk of type 2 diabetes: a population-based study. *Diabetes Care* 2010;33(12):2611–2616.

96. Hectors TL, et al. Environmental pollutants and type 2 diabetes: a review of mechanisms that can disrupt beta cell function. *Diabetologia* 2011;54(6):1273–1290.

97. Cappuccio FP, et al. Quantity and quality of sleep and incidence of type 2 diabetes: a systematic review and meta-analysis. *Diabetes Care* 2010;33(2):414–420.

98. Yeh HC, et al. Smoking, smoking cessation, and risk for type 2 diabetes mellitus: a cohort study. *Ann Intern Med* 2010;152(1):10–17.

99. Zhang X, et al. A1C level and future risk of diabetes: a systematic review. *Diabetes Care* 2010;33(7):1665–1673.

100. Gerstein HC, et al. Annual incidence and relative risk of diabetes in people with various categories of dysglycemia: a systematic overview and meta-analysis of prospective studies. *Diabetes Res Clin Pract* 2007;78(3):305–312.

101. Santaguida PL, et al. Diagnosis, prognosis, and treatment of impaired glucose tolerance and impaired fasting glucose. *Evid Rep Technol Assess* 2005;(128):1–11.

102. Pajunen P, et al. HbA(1c) in diagnosing and predicting type 2 diabetes in impaired glucose tolerance: the Finnish Diabetes Prevention Study. *Diabet Med* 2011;28(1):36–42.

103. Soulimane S, et al. HbA1c, fasting plasma glucose and the prediction of diabetes: Inter99, AusDiab and D.E.S.I.R. *Diabetes Res Clin Pract* 2012;96(3):392–399.

104. Heianza Y, et al. Screening for pre-diabetes to predict future diabetes using various cut-off points for HbA(1c) and impaired fasting glucose: the Toranomon Hospital Health Management Center Study 4 (TOPICS 4). *Diabet Med* 2012;29(9):e279–e285.

105. Noble D, et al. Risk models and scores for type 2 diabetes: systematic review. *BMJ* 2011;343:d7163:1–31.

106. Tuomilehto J, et al. Prevention of type 2 diabetes mellitus by changes in lifestyle among subjects with impaired glucose tolerance. *N Engl J Med* 2001;344(18):1343–1350.

107. Pan XR, et al. Effects of diet and exercise in preventing NIDDM in people with impaired glucose tolerance. The Da Qing IGT and Diabetes Study. *Diabetes Care* 1997;20(4):537–544.

108. Kosaka K, Noda M, Kuzuya T. Prevention of type 2 diabetes by lifestyle intervention: a Japanese trial in IGT males. *Diabetes Res Clin Pract* 2005;67(2):152–162.

109. Ramachandran A, et al. The Indian Diabetes Prevention Programme shows that lifestyle modification and metformin prevent type 2 diabetes in Asian Indian subjects with impaired glucose tolerance (IDPP-1). *Diabetologia* 2006;49(2):289–297.

110. Hamman RF, et al. Effect of weight loss with lifestyle intervention on risk of diabetes. *Diabetes Care* 2006;29(9):2102–2107.

111. Lindstrom J, et al. Determinants for the effectiveness of lifestyle intervention in the Finnish Diabetes Prevention Study. *Diabetes Care* 2008;31(5):857–862.

112. Li G, et al. The long-term effect of lifestyle interventions to prevent diabetes in the China Da Qing Diabetes Prevention Study: a 20-year follow-up study. *Lancet* 2008;371(9626):1783–1789.

113. Lindstrom J, Tuomilehto J. The diabetes risk score: a practical tool to predict type 2 diabetes risk. *Diabetes Care* 2003;26(3):725–731.

114. Meigs JB. Multiple biomarker prediction of type 2 diabetes. *Diabetes Care* 2009;32(7):1346–1348.

115. Centers for Disease Control and Prevention. Ten great public health achievements—worldwide, 2001–2010. *MMWR* 2011;60(24):814–818.

116. Gregg EW, et al. The relative contributions of different levels of overweight and obesity to the increased prevalence of diabetes in the United States: 1976-2004. *Prev Med* 2007;45(5):348–352.

117. Brownell KD, et al. The public health and economic benefits of taxing sugar-sweetened beverages. *N Engl J Med* 2009;361(16):1599–1605.

ACKNOWLEDGMENT

The findings and conclusions in this report are those of the authors and do not necessarily represent the official position of the Centers for Disease Control and Prevention.

Chapter 8

loss of insulin production

Type 1 Diabetes: Pathogenesis and Natural History

Guillermo E. Umpierrez, MD, CDE
Francisco Pasquel, MD
Isabel Errazuriz, MD

Type 1 diabetes (T1D) is a polygenic autoimmune disease characterized by progressive destruction of the insulin-producing β-cells of the pancreatic islets, leading to severe insulin deficiency or absence. The American Diabetes Association recommends classification of patients with diabetes into two groups: a classic form or type 1A diabetes, representing immune-mediated diabetes, and type 1B, a nonautoimmune idiopathic form of T1D.[1] The best marker to distinguish type 1A diabetes from other forms of diabetes is the presence of islet autoantibodies. Typically, autoantibodies reacting with glutamic acid decarboxylase (GAD65), insulin autoantibody (IAA), insulinoma-associated protein 2 autoantibody (IA-2A), and zinc transporter 8 antibody (ZnT8A) are measured.[2] Testing for at least two of these autoantibodies at diagnosis is now considered standard of care in T1D. These antibodies are present at the time of clinical diagnosis in >80–90% of subjects with T1D.[3,4]

T1D is among the most common autoimmune disorders in children and young adults.[3,5] T1D accounts for 5–10% of the total cases of diabetes worldwide.[6] It is the major type of diabetes in youth, accounting for ≥85% of all diabetes cases in youth <20 years of age worldwide.[7] Diagnosis of T1D follows a bimodal incidence pattern with one peak between the ages of 5 and 7 years old and a second peak between the ages of 10–14 years old during puberty.[8] The incidence of T1D in adults is lower than in children, although approximately one-fourth of people with T1D are diagnosed as adults.[9] Around 5–15% of adults initially thought to have type 2 diabetes (T2D) are found to have islet autoantibodies (most often anti-GAD65) associated with T1D and β-cell destruction and accelerated loss of C-peptide secretion.[9,10] Different names have been given to this subgroup of patients, including latent autoimmune disease of the adult (LADA) and slow autoimmune diabetes.

Data from large epidemiologic studies worldwide indicate that the incidence of T1D has been increasing worldwide during the past decades,[11] with a wide geographic variation in disease incidence reported around the world.[12,13] It is most common in Finland and northern Europe (up to >60 cases per 100,000 people each year) where countries have reported increases in incidence between 2.2 and 3.3% per year.[13,14] By contrast, the disorder is uncommon in China, India, Peru, and Venezuela (around 0.1 cases per 100,000 people each year). Currently, in the U.S., T1D affects 1.4 million people,[15] with an incidence that has doubled over the past 20 years affecting ~1 in 300 by 18 years of age.[8] In contrast to many other autoimmune diseases, T1D is one of the few autoimmune diseases that affect men and women equally. Some studies even suggest a greater male-to-female ratio (>1.5) in male adults after the pubertal years in populations of European origin.[16]

DOI: 10.2337/9781580405096.08

The incidence of T1D varies with seasonal changes, with a higher number of cases diagnosed in autumn and winter. Environmental factors early in life also seem to play a role in the development of diabetes later in life. Spring births are associated with a higher chance of having T1D.[3,15]

PATHOPHYSIOLOGY

T1D is a multifactorial disease caused by a combination of events in genetically susceptible individuals (Figure 8.1). Although the pathophysiology of T1D is not completely understood, it results from a combination of three mechanisms leading to islet cell destruction: genetic susceptibility, autoimmunity, and environmental insult(s). Genetically susceptible individuals exposed to an environmental insult such as a virus or allergen can develop autoantibodies to β-islet cells. The disease process leading to the clinical manifestation of T1D in childhood initiates early, in most cases even before the age of 3 years. The progression rate is highly individualized with an estimated duration of the disease process lasting from a few months to >20 years.[17] Autoantibodies in the blood serve only as a marker of autoimmune disease; the damage to the β-islet cells occurs as a result of the autoreactive T-cells produced.[2] Consistent with autoantibodies serving as markers, T1D does not manifest clinically until 80–90% of β-cells have been destroyed, which is typically years after autoantibody appearance.[9]

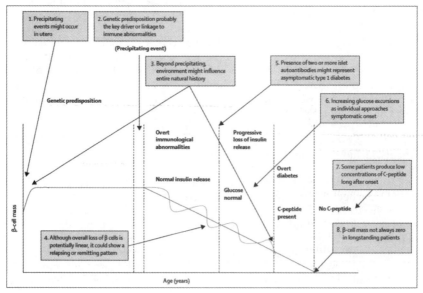

Figure 8.1—The natural history of type 1 diabetes.

Source: Atkinson MA, Eisenbarth GS, Michels AW. Type 1 diabetes. *Lancet* 2014;383:69–82. Reprinted with permission from the publisher.

GENETIC SUSCEPTIBILITY

T1D has a multifactorial inheritance pattern affected by genetic and environmental risk factors. It is a polygenic disorder, with >40 loci known to affect disease susceptibility.[2,3,18] The main genes that have shown the strongest association with T1D include those coding for the major histocompatibility complex (MHC) class II proteins; specifically human leukocyte antigen (HLA) in chromosome 6, in particular the HLA class II. The strongest associations with both susceptibility and protection from type 1A diabetes are HLA DR and DQ molecules. Of the many HLA types, haplotypes DRB1*0401-DQB1*0302 and DRB1*0301-DQB1*0201 confer the greatest susceptibility, and DRB1*1501 and DQA1*0102-DQB1*0602 provide disease resistance.[2,3,18] Approximately 40–50% familial clustering in T1D is attributable to allelic variation in the HLA region. About 2% of newborns in the U.S. are DR3/DR4 heterozygotes compared with 30% of children developing type 1A diabetes. The remaining genetic risk is made up of many diverse genes, each having a small individual impact on genetic susceptibility.[8] Non-HLA genes with increased susceptibility to developing T1D are CTLA4 (cytotoxic T-lymphocyte-associated protein 4), IFIH1 (interferon induced with helicase C domain 1), ITPR3 (inositol 1,4,5-triphosphate receptor 3), IL-2 receptor, and PTPN22 (protein tyrosine phosphatase, nonreceptor type 22).[9]

The majority of T1D cases occur in individuals without a family history of the disease; T1D is strongly influenced by genetic factors, however, with sibling relative risk being one of the highest among common complex diseases.[19] Individuals with a first-degree relative with T1D have a 1 in 20 lifetime risk of developing T1D, compared with a 1 in 300 lifetime risk for the general population. Monozygotic twins have a concordance rate of >50%, whereas dizygotic twins have a concordance rate of 6–10%.[9]

AUTOIMMUNITY

More than 90% of individuals with newly diagnosed T1D have one or more anti-islet cell autoantibodies.[20] There are at least five autoantibodies, including islet cell antibodies (ICA), insulin autoantibodies (IAA), antibodies to the 65 kD isoform of glutamic acid decarboxylase (GAD65), the protein tyrosine phosphatase–related islet antigen 2 molecule (IA-2A), and more recently zinc transporter 8 (ZnT8A), each of which has been shown to be predictive of T1D.[21] The presence of two or more autoantibodies, rather than the overall titer of autoantibodies, is highly predictive of progression to clinical diabetes.[18] These autoantibodies can appear as early as 6 months of age, with a peak incidence before 2 years of age in genetically susceptible individuals;[3] thus, they can be present months to years before symptomatic onset. Although many people are genetically predisposed to the development of T1D, disease development does not occur until there is autoimmune destruction of the β-cells.

A number of theories have been proposed to explain the trigger for autoimmunity against the β-cells of the pancreas; however, the specific mechanism responsible has yet to be elucidated. Autoantibodies appear to develop sequentially. Insulin appears to be the primary autoantigen for disease initiation and molecules such as islet-specific glucose-6-phosphatase catalytic subunit-related protein (IGRP) and chromogranin A have been suggested to promote disease progression. Insulin autoantibodies are often the first expressed autoantibody, especially in young children. Family members who expressed positive islet cell autoantibodies have a 75% 5-year risk of diabetes compared with a 25% 5-year risk in relatives who expressed one of those autoantibodies.[2,22]

About 70–90% of newly diagnosed patients have T1D-associated autoantibodies versus <1% of the general population and 3–4% of relatives of patients with T1D.[23] The younger a person is when T1D-related autoantibodies are found, the more likely they are to develop disease, in particular if they have multiple autoantibodies.[2] For example, a patient with one autoantibody has a 5-year risk of developing T1D of 20–25%, whereas a patient with four autoantibodies has an 80% 5-year risk of developing T1D.[23] Autoantibodies, however, do not appear to have the major etiologic role in the development of T1D. Several studies have identified key roles for cells of the innate immune system (dendritic cells, macrophages, and natural killer cells) along with the adaptive immune response (CD4+ T cells, CD8+ T cells, regulatory T-cells, B-lymphocytes, and plasma cells) in both the initiation and the development of diabetes.[3,15,24] Moreover, β-cells appear to have a potential role in the progression of disease by secreting proinflammatory factors that can attract pathological cells.[24]

ENVIRONMENTAL FACTORS

Epidemiological studies have identified that environmental factors operating early in life appear to trigger the immune-mediated process in genetically susceptible individuals.[25] The large geographic variation in the incidence of childhood diabetes in Europe,[26] seasonal variation, and migrant studies that have reported an increased incidence of T1D when population groups moved from a low-incidence region to a high-incidence area emphasize the role of environmental factors in the pathogenesis of diabetes.[17,19] Potential candidates are viral, microbial, dietary, and anthropometric factors. Such environmental factors may trigger autoimmunity and either speed up or slow down the progression to clinical onset in subjects with persistent islet cell autoimmunity.[25]

Nutritional factors that have been investigated include cow's milk, breast-feeding, wheat gluten, and vitamin D. Some studies have shown a significant association between T1D and a shortened period of breast-feeding and cow's milk exposure before 3–4 months of age[27]; however, evidence regarding early introduction of cow's milk (or protective effects of breast milk consumption) in infants contributing to the development of childhood T1D is equivocal[28] and may depend on genetic susceptibility. Timing of the introduction of cereals and gluten or other foods to the infant diet has been suggested to alter the risk for autoimmunity and development of T1D.[28]

Two prospective studies have reported that the introduction of cereals in infancy <4 months of age may trigger the emergence of early β-cell autoimmu-

[handwritten annotations:]
pancreatitis mass remove → type I
genetic predispose hypertriglyceridemia
hypercholesterem FFA

nity.[29,30] In addition, both gluten-containing and nongluten-containing cereals conferred an increased risk for β-cell autoimmunity. Increased use of vitamin D supplementation during infancy has been associated with a decreased risk of islet autoimmunity in the offspring and reduced risk for childhood T1D.[31] Despite these intriguing associations, there is little firm evidence of the significance of nutritional factors in the etiology of T1D.

Viruses have been implicated in the etiology of T1D following outbreaks of childhood diabetes after mumps epidemics or rubella infections.[17,25] Other in utero infections, including enterovirus, have been proposed to induce β-cell autoimmunity based on findings in Finland and Sweden, which showed that the pregnant sera of mothers with children who developed T1D had higher levels of antibodies to procapsid enterovirus antigens. It currently is thought that although direct virus-induced β-cell injury is rarely severe enough to cause T1D, the viral infection may cause mild β-cell injury and subsequent antigen release.[32]

Increasing epidemiological studies and the report of a meta-analysis indicate that higher birth weight and early childhood weight gain are risk factors for subsequent development of T1D.[33] Maternal gestational diabetes and overweight can lead to antenatal overstimulation of fetal β-cells, higher fetal body weight, and insulin resistance. Surrogate markers of insulin resistance and BMI predict progression to T1D in subjects with islet autoimmunity, and weight gain in early life may predict risk of islet autoimmunity in children with a first-degree relative with T1D.[34] Other studies have reported contradictory results and failed to show that excess body weight and insulin resistance influence autoantibody frequency.[35]

LATENT AUTOIMMUNE DIABETES

In most patients, differentiation between T1D and T2D is straightforward based on phenotypic characteristics, such as age of onset, presence of abdominal obesity and acanthosis nigricans, presence of other autoimmune diseases, family history, severity of hyperglycemia and ketosis, and the need for insulin replacement therapy. People with T1D frequently present with acute symptoms of hyperglycemia (polyuria, polydipsia, weight loss), markedly elevated blood glucose levels with or without ketosis, and presence of islet autoantibodies. Occasionally, the clinical classification between T1D and T2D is not clear at presentation. About 10–15% of patients initially classified as having T2D test positive for at least one of the islet autoantibodies, and this group often is referred to as LADA.[36] This subtype of diabetes is more common in adults than in children[37] with >40% of patients older than 40 years and >20% older than 55 years.[38] These patients share many genetic and immunological similarities with T1D, suggesting that LADA, like typical T1D, is an autoimmune disease. There are differences in autoantibody clustering, T-cell reactivity, and genetic susceptibility and protection between T1D and LADA, implying important differences in the underlying disease processes. Initially, most LADA patients are treated with oral antidiabetic agents, but with progressive β-cell destruction, they require insulin treatment to maintain metabolic control.[36]

CONCLUSION

T1D is a polygenic autoimmune disease characterized by progressive destruction of the insulin-producing β-cells of the pancreatic islets, leading to severe insulin deficiency. T1D accounts for 5–10% of the total cases of diabetes worldwide[6] and the annual incidence of T1D has been increasing by 2–4% in some populations.[13] T1D is a multifactorial disease caused by a combination of autoimmune and environmental factors in genetically susceptible individuals. Genetically susceptible individuals exposed to an environmental insult (virus, nutritional factors) triggers the production of autoantibodies to β-cells. Autoantibodies in the blood serve only as a marker of autoimmune disease; the damage to the β-islet cells occurs as a result of the autoreactive T-cells produced.[2] Increasing evidence from T1D prevention studies suggests that measurement of islet autoantibodies identifies individuals who are at risk for developing T1D. Such testing may be appropriate in high-risk individuals, such as those with prior transient hyperglycemia or those who have relatives with T1D, in the context of clinical research studies. Widespread clinical testing of asymptomatic low-risk individuals cannot currently be recommended, as it would identify few individuals in the general population who are at risk. Individuals who screen positive should be counseled about their risk of developing diabetes. Clinical studies are being conducted to test various methods of preventing or reversing early T1D in subjects with evidence of autoimmunity.

REFERENCES

1. American Diabetes Association. Standards of medical care in diabetes—2014. *Diabetes Care* 2014;37(Suppl 1):S14–S80.

2. Eisenbarth GS. Update in type 1 diabetes. *J Clin Endocrinol Metab* 2007;92(7):2403–2407.

3. Atkinson MA, Eisenbarth GS, Michels AW. Type 1 diabetes. *Lancet* 2014;383(9911):69–82.

4. Padgett LE, Broniowska KA, Hansen PA, Corbett JA, Tse HM. The role of reactive oxygen species and proinflammatory cytokines in type 1 diabetes pathogenesis. *Ann N Y Acad Sci* 2013;1281:16–35.

5. Gale EA. Type 1 diabetes in the young: the harvest of sorrow goes on. *Diabetologia* 2005;48(8):1435–1438.

6. American Diabetes Association. Diagnosis and classification of diabetes mellitus. *Diabetes Care* 2012;35(Suppl 1):S64–S71.

7. Liese AD, D'Agostino RB Jr, Hamman RF, Kilgo PD, Lawrence JM, Liu LL, et al. The burden of diabetes mellitus among US youth: prevalence estimates from the SEARCH for Diabetes in Youth Study. *Pediatrics* 2006;118(4):1510–1518.

8. Maahs DM, West NA, Lawrence JM, Mayer-Davis EJ. Epidemiology of type 1 diabetes. *Endocrinol Metab Clin North Am* 2011;39(3):481–497.

9. Haller MJ, Atkinson MA, Schatz D. Type 1 diabetes mellitus: etiology, presentation, and management. *Pediatr Clin North Am* 2005;52(6):1553–1578.

10. Turner R, Stratton I, Horton V, Manley S, Zimmet P, Mackay IR, et al. UKPDS 25: autoantibodies to islet-cell cytoplasm and glutamic acid decarboxylase for prediction of insulin requirement in type 2 diabetes. U.K. Prospective Diabetes Study Group. *Lancet* 1997;350(9087):1288–1293.

11. Berhan Y, Waernbaum I, Lind T, Mollsten A, Dahlquist G. Thirty years of prospective nationwide incidence of childhood type 1 diabetes: the accelerating increase by time tends to level off in Sweden. *Diabetes* 2011;60(2):577–581.

12. Knip M. Pathogenesis of type 1 diabetes: Implications for incidence trends. *Horm Res Paediatr* 2011;76(Suppl 1):57–64.

13. Dabelea D. The accelerating epidemic of childhood diabetes. *Lancet* 2009; 373(9680):1999–2000.

14. Patterson CC, Dahlquist GG, Gyurus E, Green A, Soltesz G. Incidence trends for childhood type 1 diabetes in Europe during 1989-2003 and predicted new cases 2005-20: a multicentre prospective registration study. *Lancet* 2009; 373(9680):2027–2033.

15. Nokoff N, Rewers M. Pathogenesis of type 1 diabetes: lessons from natural history studies of high-risk individuals. *Ann N Y Acad Sci* 2013;1281:1–15.

16. Soltesz G, Patterson CC, Dahlquist G. Worldwide childhood type 1 diabetes incidence—what can we learn from epidemiology? *Pediatr Diabetes* 2007;8(Suppl 6):6–14.

17. Knip M, Simell O. Environmental triggers of type 1 diabetes. *Cold Spring Harb Perspect Med* 2012;2(7):a007690.

18. Knip M, Siljander H. Autoimmune mechanisms in type 1 diabetes. *Autoimmun Rev* 2008;7(7):550–557.

19. Polychronakos C, Li Q. Understanding type 1 diabetes through genetics: advances and prospects. *Nat Rev Genet* 2011;12(11):781–792.

20. Bingley PJ. Clinical applications of diabetes antibody testing. *J Clin Endocrinol Metab* 2010;95(1):25–33.

21. Siljander HT, Simell S, Hekkala A, Lahde J, Simell T, Vahasalo P, et al. Predictive characteristics of diabetes-associated autoantibodies among children with HLA-conferred disease susceptibility in the general population. *Diabetes* 2009;58(12):2835–2842.

22. Verge CF, Gianani R, Kawasaki E, Yu L, Pietropaolo M, Jackson RA, et al. Prediction of type I diabetes in first-degree relatives using a combination of insulin, GAD, and ICA512bdc/IA-2 autoantibodies. *Diabetes* 1996;45(7):926–933.

23. Winter WE, Harris N, Schatz D. Type 1 diabetes islet autoantibody markers. *Diabetes Technol Ther* 2002;4(6):817–839.

24. Herold KC, Vignali DA, Cooke A, Bluestone JA. Type 1 diabetes: Translating mechanistic observations into effective clinical outcomes. *Nat Rev Immunol* 2013;13(4):243–256.

25. Eringsmark Regnell S, Lernmark A. The environment and the origins of islet autoimmunity and type 1 diabetes. *Diabet Med* 2013;30(2):155–160.

26. EURODIAB ACE Study Group. Variation and trends in incidence of child-hood diabetes in Europe. *Lancet* 2000;355(9207):873–876.

27. Virtanen SM, Knip M. Nutritional risk predictors of beta cell autoimmunity and type 1 diabetes at a young age. *Am J Clin Nutr* 2003;78(6):1053–1067.

28. Norris JM, Beaty B, Klingensmith G, Yu L, Hoffman M, Chase HP, et al. Lack of association between early exposure to cow's milk protein and beta-cell auto-immunity. Diabetes Autoimmunity Study in the Young (DAISY). *JAMA* 1996;276(8):609–614.

29. Norris JM, Barriga K, Klingensmith G, Hoffman M, Eisenbarth GS, Erlich HA, et al. Timing of initial cereal exposure in infancy and risk of islet autoim-munity. *JAMA* 2003;290(13):1713–1720.

30. Ziegler AG, Schmid S, Huber D, Hummel M, Bonifacio E. Early infant feed-ing and risk of developing type 1 diabetes-associated autoantibodies. *JAMA* 2003;290(13):1721–1728.

31. Hypponen E, Laara E, Reunanen A, Jarvelin MR, Virtanen SM. Intake of vita-min D and risk of type 1 diabetes: a birth-cohort study. *Lancet* 2001; 358(9292):1500–1503.

32. Viskari HR, Koskela P, Lonnrot M, Luonuansuu S, Reunanen A, Baer M, et al. Can enterovirus infections explain the increasing incidence of type 1 diabetes? *Diabetes Care* 2000;23(3):414–416.

33. Harder T, Roepke K, Diller N, Stechling Y, Dudenhausen JW, Plagemann A. Birth weight, early weight gain, and subsequent risk of type 1 diabetes: sys-tematic review and meta-analysis. *Am J Epidemiol* 2009;169(12):1428–1436.

34. Couper JJ, Beresford S, Hirte C, Baghurst PA, Pollard A, Tait BD, et al. Weight gain in early life predicts risk of islet autoimmunity in children with a first-degree relative with type 1 diabetes. *Diabetes Care* 2009;32(1):94–99.

35. Barker JM, Goehrig SH, Barriga K, Hoffman M, Slover R, Eisenbarth GS, et al. Clinical characteristics of children diagnosed with type 1 diabetes through intensive screening and follow-up. *Diabetes Care* 2004;27(6):1399–1404.

36. Naik RG, Brooks-Worrell BM, Palmer JP. Latent autoimmune diabetes in adults. *J Clin Endocrinol Metab* 2009;94(12):4635–4644.

37. Graves EJ, Gillium BS. Detailed diagnosis and procedures: National Dis-charge Survey, 1995. National Center for Health Statistics. *Vital Health Stat* 1997;13(133):1–146.

38. Johnson DD, Palumbo PJ, Chu CP. Diabetic ketoacidosis in a community-based population. *Mayo Clin Proc* 1980;55(2):83–88.

Chapter 9

Assessment and Treatment of Patients with Type 1 Diabetes

ANNE PETERS, MD
LORI LAFFEL, MD, MPH

Type 1 diabetes (T1D) remains a lifelong, manageable yet incurable condition, present from diagnosis throughout an individual's life span, except for the handful of patients who have had some sort of pancreas or islet cell transplant to temporize the disease. More than half of individuals with T1D develop it in childhood although increasingly new-onset T1D is diagnosed in adulthood as well.[1] Because of the pervasive nature of T1D, individuals may have to transition through many life changes, from childhood to young adulthood, to middle age, and then to the geriatric age-group, mandating patients, families, and providers similarly to deal with the disease in a developmentally appropriate manner.

Regardless of age, T1D needs to be treated in a consistent disease-specific manner, with patients and providers alike recognizing the management requirements inherent in the insulin-deficient state that defines T1D. People with T1D simply are not the same as individuals with type 2 diabetes (T2D) who happen to need insulin (see Table 9.1). The pathophysiology of T1D, as discussed elsewhere in this book (see Chapter 8), is quite different and although the complications of hyperglycemia are similar between T1D and T2D, the fundamental demands of the disease and its management are unique.

In childhood, management of T1D depends initially on parents and guardians, and a family-based treatment approach forms the basis of pediatric care. Education is directed at both the individual with diabetes as well as parents and guardians. As children grow up and become older teens and then adults, the model of medical care shifts to a focus on the individual patient with autonomous decision making who participates in management decisions and understands the need to identify and treat diabetes-related complications. The key to dealing with children is to understand the needs and capabilities of each child and family and to offer education and medical care that are developmentally appropriate. This process occurs fairly quickly as youth grow from infants to toddlers to school-age children and onward. Puberty occurs during early adolescence and brings physiologic and psychosocial challenges associated with pubertal insulin resistance and changes in the parent-child-family dynamic.[2] Family involvement in diabetes management remains fundamental to successful diabetes care in childhood and to changes to shared management during adolescence as teens become more involved in their diabetes self-care.[3,4] Change is measured in months and years rather than decades during childhood. Although changes occur in adult care, the needs of an adult patient tend to transition much more slowly over many years from young adulthood to middle age and finally to older age. The commonality is that change hap-

DOI: 10.2337/9781580405096.09

pens; the differences are in how quickly providers must adapt to these changes and make adjustments in the patient care plan.

This chapter describes the medical care individuals with T1D should receive throughout the life span. Specific interventions, such as use of technology and insulin, are discussed in detail in other chapters. Care for individuals with T1D occurs in a variety of different settings—from the pediatrician's office to the adult provider's office (which can be in a family practice setting as well as in internist or general practitioner's office) and from a large diabetes center to a small endocrinologist's office or a generalist's office. In each setting, basic principles apply that are related to understanding fundamentals of individualized care and intensive insulin therapy. Although care of the pediatric patient with T1D is overwhelmingly managed by pediatric endocrinologists, adults with T1D are managed either

Table 9.1 Differences in the Treatment Needs of People with Type 1 versus Type 2 Diabetes

Feature	Type 1 diabetes	Type 2 diabetes
Age of onset	Generally younger = generally need to support and educate families, schools, day care, camps; assess and manage growth and development, puberty	Generally older = often comorbidities, polypharmacy, considerations regarding care for older individuals
Weight at diagnosis	Traditionally leaner (however, ~1/3 of youth may be overweight or obese at diagnosis), rates consistent with the prevalence of overweight or obesity in the general population = providing adequate nutrition throughout the life span, eating disorders common	Overweight/obese = weight-loss/lifestyle issues, sleep apnea, joint and back pain, cancer risk
Ethnicity	Often Caucasian, although all racial and ethnic groups are susceptible to T1D	African American, Latino, Native American, Asian, Pacific Islander highest risk
Metabolic syndrome	Present in ~30% = less likely to find additional CVD risk factors; often not found in youth—risk increases with age	Present in ~80% = management of hypertension, dyslipidemia, CVD risk evaluation a major component of management
Association with autoimmune disease	Present (Hashimoto's, celiac disease, others), require frequent surveillance	Absent
Monitoring	Must perform SMBG frequently (4–10 times per day) to maintain BG control and help to avoid and manage extreme glycemic excursions; CGM helpful	On oral agents, SMBG has been shown to have limited benefit, once daily if used; on basal insulin SMBG 1–2 times per day; on basal-bolus therapy SMBG 4 times per day; education needed to benefit from SMBG

by an endocrinologist or in a primary care setting. Thus, it is important to maintain awareness of the strengths and weaknesses of each setting and to promote communication across providers and settings.

INITIAL EVALUATION: NEW-ONSET PATIENT OR PATIENT NEW TO A PROVIDER

The initial step in the care of any patient with T1D is an assessment of disease status and overall health.[5] In addition to understanding an individual's medical situation, however, it is also important to understand the person's psychosocial and educational status. A team approach often works best to complete an assessment

Feature	Type 1 diabetes	Type 2 diabetes
Insulin management	Intensive insulin therapy is standard of care with either multiple daily insulin injections (MDI) or continuous subcutaneous insulin infusion (CSII) with adjustments based on carbohydrate intake, prevailing blood glucose level, physical activity	Basal insulin, basal plus bolus therapy or premixed insulin; carbohydrate counting generally not done; premeal adjustments for high blood glucose levels can be used
Hypoglycemia	Minor episodes frequent and severe episodes occur at higher rates than in T2D; must be addressed at every visit; rate of severe hypoglycemia increases with age	Both minor and severe episodes can occur—using drugs that do not cause hypoglycemia will reduce the risk
Complications	At risk for micro- and macrovascular complications; risk increases with uncontrolled diabetes, age, and longer disease duration; glycemic control has major impact on reduction of risk for microvascular complications (DCCT)	Can develop all complications, macrovascular complications more prevalent than in T1D; disease often begins at older age, potentially shorter duration for development of microvascular complications; role of glucose reduction established in reducing risk for microvascular complications (UKPDS)
Psychosocial issues	Must address emotional needs over a lifetime in many individuals, and for parents and guardians of youth with T1D; about twice the risk of depressive symptomatology and disordered eating behaviors compared with general population of youth; also must address potential fear of hypoglycemia	Must address emotional needs over a lifetime in a few individuals; for most diabetes, begins at an older age with issues associated with aging

Note: CGM = continuous glucose monitoring; CVD = cardiovascular disease; DCCT = Diabetes Control and Complications Trial; SMBG = self-monitoring of blood glucose; UKPDS = U.K. Prospective Diabetes Study.

so that each aspect of care can be fully addressed. Even if a team is not available within the same office, capable multidisciplinary specialists can be identified and referrals can be made as needed. Additionally, with the evolving use of telemedicine, access to diabetes specialists may become easier in those communities (often rural) where services do not physically exist (although reimbursement for such services remains in its developmental stages). All providers, however, who are treating individuals with T1D need to know the key elements of care so that treatment is appropriate and sustained over time.

In the initial assessment, confirmation of the diagnosis of T1D is important. Details regarding autoimmunity (positive antibodies to GAD, IA2, insulin, and zinc channel [ZnT8]) may help confirm the diagnosis because family history and classic phenotypic markers, such as age at onset, race or ethnicity, and BMI, cannot readily distinguish T1D from T2D.[6] Substantial numbers of patients are diagnosed with T1D beyond the pediatric age-group. Correct diagnosis of T1D helps ensure timely and appropriate treatment with insulin to optimize glycemia as early as possible after the diagnosis aimed at reducing risk of long-term complications. Finally, given the expanding availability of genetic testing for monogenic forms of diabetes, reassessment of the diagnosis and search for any unusual characteristics of the patient suggestive of an alternative diagnosis (e.g., age of onset <6 months, supportive of possible neonatal diabetes) should encourage additional work-up.[7,8]

Although an extensive review of T2D in youth is beyond the scope of this chapter (see Chapter 12), recent data published from the Treatment Options of Type 2 Diabetes in Adolescents and Youth (TODAY) study reveal that 10% of youth diagnosed by health care professionals as having T2D have evidence of β-cell autoimmunity and thus likely were misdiagnosed.[9] Similar data arise from studies of adults diagnosed with T2D in which up to 15% of patients may have evidence of autoimmunity, and these individuals may benefit from earlier initiation of insulin.[10] It is not known how many adults with new-onset diabetes have T1D, although there are many more adults living with T1D (1–1.5 million)[11] than children (~170,000),[12] both because children diagnosed with T1D now live into old age and because there are individuals with new-onset T1D that develops during adulthood.

Table 9.2, modified from the *Type 1 Diabetes Sourcebook*, lists the basic elements of the initial evaluation of the patient with T1D. For children and young adults with T1D, less focus may need to be given to diabetic complications, because these are less likely to be present. In older individuals and those with diabetes of longer duration, however, assessment and treatment of diabetic complications[13] may consume a great part of care.

For individuals with new-onset T1D, the focus of care is on teaching basic survival skills and educating the patient and appropriate family members. For infants and children, this is generally a very intense team-based process requiring many resources. Children often are diagnosed following a fairly short period of symptoms and in many settings are hospitalized either for diabetic ketoacidosis (DKA) or for diabetes that is out of control. In other settings, in which the child does not have DKA and resources exist, this can be done as an outpatient. Regardless, the advent of new-onset T1D is often a shock to the entire family and requires attention to the care of the child both at home and at school, with accommoda-

Table 9.2 Initial Evaluation of Patients with New-Onset or Established Type 1 Diabetes

- Diabetes classification to confirm type 1 diabetes.
- Review of symptoms and signs at presentation and initial treatment.
- Diabetes history:
  - Review of previous insulin treatment regimens and response to therapy (A1C records); history of DKA or severe hypoglycemia; treatment preferences and prior difficulty with therapies
  - Current treatment of diabetes, including medications and medication adherence, meal plan, physical activity patterns, and readiness for behavior change; assessment of support systems for self-care
  - Use of insulin, insulin pumps, carbohydrate ratios, correction factors; knowledge of sick-day rules, ketone testing, pump troubleshooting (if applicable), availability and past use of glucagon
  - Results of glucose monitoring including SMBG and CGM and patient's or family's use of data
  - DKA frequency, severity, and cause
  - Hypoglycemic episodes
    - i. Hypoglycemia awareness
    - ii. Any severe hypoglycemia: frequency and cause
    - iii. Whether or not patient has glucagon available and someone to administer it
- A review of symptoms of diabetes, diabetes-focused issues, and diabetes complications:
  - Eating patterns, physical activity habits, nutritional status, and weight history
  - Diabetes education history; health literacy/numeracy assessment
  - Whether or not patient wears medical alert identification
- History of diabetes-related complications:
  - Microvascular: retinopathy, nephropathy, neuropathy (sensory, including history of foot lesions; autonomic, including sexual dysfunction and gastroparesis); documentation of last dilated eye examination
  - Macrovascular: HTN, dyslipidemia, CHD, cerebrovascular disease, PAD
- *Assessment of non–diabetes-related medical issues and medications.*
- *Social history, including patient living situation (alone or with others), school or occupational status (understanding schedules, shiftwork, resources at home and at work/school), smoking, driving, alcohol, or drug use.*
- *For women, an assessment of use of contraceptives or other hormonal use, desire for pregnancy, pregnancy planning, history of prior pregnancies and outcomes.*
- *Family history of type 1 diabetes or other endocrine disorders (in some centers, screening for type of diabetes risk is available for first- and second-degree relatives).*
- *Assessment of patient's (and family's, if pediatric) psychosocial, educational, and nutritional needs. Consider screening for depressive symptomatology.*
- *Physical and laboratory evaluation.*
- *Establishment of an individualized follow-up care plan incorporating a patient's goals and preferences for treatment; provide and clearly articulate blood glucose and A1C goals for patient and ensure consistent goal setting across multidisciplinary team members and with the patient or family. Referral to a certified diabetes educator, registered dietitian, expert in psychological assessment and counseling (master's degree in social work), doctor, exercise physiologist if available, and other medical specialists, as needed.*

Note: CGM = continuous glucose monitoring; CHD = coronary heart disease; DKA = diabetic ketoacidosis; HTN = hypertension; PAD = peripheral arterial disease; SMBG = self-monitoring of blood glucose. Italic type = for both new-onset and established patients; regular type = for new patients with established type 1 diabetes only.

Source: Adapted from Peters A, Laffel L. *American Diabetes Association/JDRF Type 1 Diabetes Sourcebook*. Alexandria, VA, American Diabetes Association, 2013.

tions made for participation in sports and other after-school activities. Additionally, parents, as their child's primary caregiver, must advocate for blood glucose management and acquire the needed skills within a fairly short period of time, often within hours for initial outpatient treatment or within 1–2 days during a hospitalization. Thus, youth with new-onset diabetes and their families require multiple resources from medical personnel, including educators, registered dietitians, and psychologists or social workers for support services.[14]

For adults with new-onset T1D, hyperglycemia may have begun some time before their diagnosis—some individuals initially are treated as though they have T2D before being correctly diagnosed with T1D. Others may be more symptomatic and seek medical care acutely for symptoms of hyperglycemia or even DKA. Regardless of circumstance of diagnosis, adults can choose who to involve in their diabetes management and education and when to involve them, although inclusion of family members or close friends may be beneficial. Some adults are private about having diabetes and do not share the diagnosis with friends or colleagues, whether they are fellow students or coworkers. Adults, as with children, need to be educated about diabetes management as well as nutrition, however, and their psychosocial concerns need to be addressed. It is important to review issues of employment, education, relationships, pregnancy and fertility, intimacy, driving, traveling, and exercise, among other areas. For many adults, key issues revolve around integrating their diabetes self-care into their existing life structure with minimal disruption into their premorbid habits. Obviously, life will need to change, but with appropriate education and support, the impact of T1D can be mitigated.

For an established patient referred with T1D, it is important to understand the history of their diabetes and its treatment, including a careful review of previous episodes of severe hypoglycemia and DKA and recognition of existing micro- or macrovascular complications.[15] If it has been a few years since the diagnosis, review and re-education of diabetes management skills often are needed. In particular, it is important to ensure that older teens and young adults who were diagnosed during childhood have received the necessary education for self-management, as their parents were likely the recipients of the initial diabetes education. Additionally, it is important to review problematic areas in diabetes self-care to address and overcome barriers to adherence. Some patients, when offered an open and accepting dialogue with a new provider, may disclose that they have felt "judged" by previous providers and, as a result, they have negative feelings about their diabetes visits. Others may be sensitive about their eating behaviors and weight and seek a new opportunity to address lifestyle issues along with diabetes management needs. Some may have tried using advanced diabetes technologies in the past, such as insulin pumps or continuous glucose monitoring (CGM) devices, but have stopped using them because of inadequate education, unrealistic expectations, or unanticipated burdens associated with their use. Exploring the reasons for discontinuation is especially useful. For other patients, particularly with respect to past CGM use, discontinuation may have been related to earlier models that were less accurate than modern devices. Patients (and their families for the pediatric population) need to be educated about the multiple treatment options available. On the other hand, if an individual has well-controlled blood glucose levels without excessive hypoglycemia and attains target A1C levels, then simply maintaining the current treatment regimen is often reasonable. For those patients, however, who are poorly controlled or who are interested in exploring new treatment approaches to enhance quality of life, the visit should include opportunities for change.

FOLLOW-UP

Routine follow-up of individuals with T1D generally occurs every 3 months. This frequency can be adapted based on the clinical situation of the individual. New-onset patients, those recently discharged from the hospital for acute or chronic complication management, those changing therapies, or those with additional comorbid medical conditions (e.g., receiving chemotherapy for cancer, steroids for asthma, waxing and waning congestive heart failure, dialysis, or progressive dementia) may need more frequent follow-up. Often, patients with recently diagnosed T1D and their families feel overwhelmed by the demands of diabetes management, the reality of its chronicity, and the initial frequency of diabetes visits for initial education and management. It is important, however, to provide reassurance that follow-up becomes much less intensive once the necessary tasks are mastered and glycemic control is achieved.

A number of other areas require attention during follow-up visits, although such issues may not need to be reviewed at every visit. For example, for youth with T1D, there is a need to discuss the importance of ongoing family involvement in diabetes management tasks throughout childhood with a gradual transition to self-care as the child enters the teenage years.[3-5,9,13] Although youth often have the manual dexterity and technical abilities to use an insulin pump or pen and can draw up and inject insulin, children and even teens generally do not possess the emotional maturity to sustain these behaviors on a daily basis. Thus, sharing diabetes management responsibilities remains a critical area for discussion for pediatric patients and parents/guardians. Additionally, the topic of transitions in care and transfer from pediatric to adult providers is another area that requires discussion, generally beginning during the adolescent years.[16] Discussion around complication screening and management is another topic that requires mention at follow-up visits at times during childhood and often during adulthood. Patients and families also like to learn about new technologies and management approaches as well as research advances at their diabetes visits. Finally, while reviewing blood glucose data, it is important to avoid judging the results; providers must remind patients (and parents) that blood glucose levels always vary.[17] The importance of checking blood glucose levels frequently lies in the opportunity to self-correct out-of-range values quickly. Such messaging helps to reinforce the importance of frequent blood glucose monitoring and to avoid engendering negative emotions at visits for the patients and family members.

At each routine follow-up visit, the goals are essentially the same:

- Review symptoms of uncontrolled diabetes (polys) and occurrence of severe hypoglycemia or ketosis/ketoacidosis.
- Review growth and development for youth and weight and BMI for adults.
- Examine insulin injection or infusion sites and perform foot exam (at frequencies determined by age and risk).

- Assess the patient's glycemic control, including self-monitoring of blood glucose, CGM data, and A1C result.
- Review insulin management plan and readjust as needed, including analysis of pump printouts.
- Assess for educational gaps and address if present.
- Determine frequency and severity of episodes of hypoglycemia, and whether hypoglycemia awareness exists.
- Inquire about lifestyle changes, psychosocial challenges, nutrition, and exercise.

Incorporate open-ended questions into the encounter. For example, "Have you had any difficulties with your diabetes management recently?" or "What has been your greatest challenge with regard to your diabetes care?" rather than ask "Have your blood sugar levels been high?" Goal setting often is useful, particularly because of the numeric quality of the A1C measurement. Reviewing the A1C result (preferably with point of care availability) helps align glycemic goals between the patients and providers. Sometimes patients aim for target levels that are too low (or too high) and need to be readjusted tactfully, especially if hypoglycemia (or hyperglycemia) is occurring too frequently. Providing realistic expectations for change is important—for example, in patients having difficulty checking their glucose levels four to five times daily or getting premeal insulin bolus doses, recommend that the patient try increasing the daily frequency of glucose monitoring or bolus dosing by one time per day before escalating the target monitoring or bolus dosing frequency to the full complement. Discussions related to slowing or escalating goals for nutrition, weight management, exercise, and blood glucose pattern management can help patients and families develop realistic expectations and empower them to succeed. If time allows, offer realistic hope while providing care by reviewing new research findings—for example, related to the artificial pancreas and complications management and prevention. Finally, the "teach back" method of treating patients—having the patients explain to the health care provider what they have just been taught in their own words—can be useful in some settings. This helps ensure that the patient has understood key concepts.

At each visit, therefore, an assessment of the patient should be undertaken, including a review of developmental progress for youth. The assessment begins with a diabetes history, including the previously noted elements. In children and adolescents, a diabetes-focused physical examination should occur with an assessment of normal growth and development. A more comprehensive exam should be performed on all patients yearly with particular subsets of the exam performed at follow-up as needed. Key elements to perform at each exam include the following:

- Height (for youth), weight, BMI, or BMI percentile (for youth)
- Blood pressure (percentile assessment for youth based on sex and height)
- Physical exam (modified for diabetes) to include the following:
  - Examination of injection or infusion sites, with attention to areas of lipohypertrophy or atrophy
  - Thyroid exam (yearly, or more often if indicated clinically)
  - Comprehensive foot exam or visual foot inspection (if needed—youth with T1D generally do not have clinically significant peripheral neuropathy but often fail to report paronychia or tinea pedis, thereby add-

ing clinical value to the foot examination of the pediatric patient). In adults, an annual foot exam is important and visual inspection of the feet is recommended at each visit in individuals with high-risk feet (loss of sensation to 5.07 monofilament testing, foot deformities, absent pulses, or history of prior amputation or ulcer)

- Dilated retinal exam (generally done by an eye care professional starting 5 years after the diagnosis of T1D, 3–5 years in youth with T1D beginning at age 10 years or at the onset of puberty, whichever is earlier)
- In adults, assessment for cardiovascular disease may be indicated with careful examination of vasculature (carotid bruits, pedal pulses, etc.)

■ Laboratory assessments include the following:
  - Quarterly: A1C measurement
  - Annually (or more often if abnormal): Renal function (serum creatinine, urine albumin-to-creatinine ratio [starting 5 years after diagnosis in children]), lipid panel
  - At baseline and then periodically as needed:
    ☐ T1D autoantibodies (AntiGAD/IA2/IAA/ZnT8)—as needed to establish the diagnosis (requested only at onset or in patients carrying a diagnosis of T2D who may need reclassification).
    ☐ Celiac and thyroid antibodies, thyroid-stimulating hormone level. With respect to celiac antibody testing, ensure IgA sufficiency, otherwise IgG celiac antibody testing is needed. Adrenal function assessment as needed in individuals with unexplained hypoglycemia or other concerning symptoms/signs of adrenal insufficiency.

CONCLUSION

Individuals with T1D of all ages should not be treated as though they have T2D; this is rarely a problem in pediatrics as most pediatric patients with diabetes in fact do have T1D. On the other hand, the majority of adults have T2D so it is not uncommon for adults with diabetes to be managed as though they have T2D, even if they may actually have T1D. All patients with T1D, independent of age, have a distinct autoimmune disorder that directs their treatment based on the pathophysiology of the β-cell destruction and need for replacement insulin therapy. Additionally, because T1D is a chronic disorder that can begin early in life, multiple issues are related to growth and development that need to be addressed, as well as the transitions from one distinct model of pediatric care to adult care. Ideally, care is multifaceted, using a team approach that encompasses the impact T1D has on a person's entire life, from eating to exercising to school or work, from socializing to emotional relationships and beyond. In the absence of an established team, good care still can be provided, following the recommendations described in this chapter. Additionally, the Internet can provide a positive source of medical information and support. Increasingly, people with T1D can connect with larger groups of individuals who also have the condition. The need for individualization of care remains central to the process of treating people with T1D, and although progress is still needed, patients can live long, productive, and healthy lives with the currently available management tools and technologies that aid in the daily treatment of T1D.

REFERENCES

1. Haller MJ. Type 1 diabetes in the 21st century: a review of the landscape. In *American Diabetes Association/JDRF Type 1 Diabetes Sourcebook*. Peters A, Laffel L, Eds. Alexandria, VA, American Diabetes Association, 2013, p. 1–18.

2. Amiel SA, Sherrwin RS, Simonson DC, Lauritano AA, Tamborlane WV. Impaired insulin action in puberty: a contributing factor to poor glycemic control in adolescents with diabetes. *N Engl J Med* 1986;315:215–219.

3. Anderson B, Ho J, Brackett J, Finkelstein D, Laffel L. Parental involvement in diabetes management tasks in young adolescents with IDDM: relationships to blood glucose monitoring adherence and metabolic control in young adolescents with IDDM. *J Pediatr* 1997;130:257–265.

4. Laffel LMB, Vangsness L, Connell A, Goebel-Fabbri A, Butler D, Anderson BJ. Impact of ambulatory, family focused teamwork intervention on glycemic control in youth with type 1 diabetes. *J Pediatr* 2003;142:409–416.

5. Siminerio LM, Laffel L, Peters A. Initial evaluation and follow-up. In *American Diabetes Association/JDRF Type 1 Diabetes Sourcebook*. Peters A, Laffel L, Eds. Alexandria, VA, American Diabetes Association, 2013, p. 73–101.

6. Arvan P, Pietropaolo M, Ostrov D, Rhodes C. Islet autoantigens: Structure, function, localization, and regulation. *Cold Spring Harb Perspect Med* 2012; doi: 10.1101/cshperspect.a007658.

7. Ellard S, Bellanné-Chantelot C, Hattersley AT; European Molecular Genetics Quality Network (EMQN) MODY Group. Best practice guidelines for the molecular genetic diagnosis of maturity-onset diabetes of the young. *Diabetologia* 2008;51:546–553.

8. Dabelea D, Pihoker C, Talton JW, D'Agostino RB Jr, Fujimoto W, Klingensmith GJ, Lawrence JM, Linder B, Marcovina SM, Mayer-Davis EJ, Imperatore G, Dolan LM; SEARCH for Diabetes in Youth Study. Etiological approach to characterization of diabetes type: the SEARCH for Diabetes in Youth Study. *Diabetes Care* 2011;34:1628–1633.

9. Klingensmith GJ, Pyle L, Arslanian S, Copeland KC, Cuttler L, Kaufman F, Laffel L, Marcovina S, Tollefsen SE, Weinstock RS, Linder B; TODAY Study Group. The presence of GAD and IA-2 antibodies in youth with a type 2 diabetes phenotype: Results from the TODAY study. *Diabetes Care* 2010;33:1970–1975.

10. Syed MA, Barinas-Mitchell E, Pietropaolo SL, Zhang YJ, Henderson TS, Kelley DE, Korytkowski MT, Donahue RP, Tracy RP, Trucco M, Kuller LH, Pietropaolo M. Is type 2 diabetes a chronic inflammatory/autoimmune disease? *Diabetes Nutr Metab* 2002;15:68–83.

11. American Diabetes Association. Type 1 diabetes. Available at www.diabetes. org/diabetes-basics/type-1. Accessed 31 March 2014.

12. Pettitt DJ, Talton J, Dabelea D, Divers J, Imperatore G, Lawrence JM, Liese AD, Linder B, Mayer-Davis EJ, Pihoker C, Saydah SH, Standiford DA, Hamman RF; for the SEARCH for Diabetes in Youth Study Group. Prevalence of diabetes mellitus in US youth in 2009: The SEARCH for Diabetes in Youth Study. *Diabetes Care* 2014;37:402–408.

13. Diabetes Control and Complications Trial/Epidemiology of Diabetes Interventions and Complications (DCCT/EDIC) Research Group, Nathan DM, Zinman B, Cleary PA, Backlund JY, Genuth S, Miller R, Orchard TJ. Modern-day clinical course of type 1 diabetes mellitus after 30 years' duration: the Diabetes Control and Complications Trial/Epidemiology of Diabetes Interventions and Complications and Pittsburgh Epidemiology of Diabetes Complications experience (1983–2005). *Arch Intern Med* 2009;169(14):1307–1316.

14. Silverstein J, Klingensmith G, Copeland K, Plotnick L, Kaufman F, Laffel L, Deeb L, Grey M, Anderson B, Holzmeister LA, Clark N. Care of children and adolescents with type 1 diabetes: a statement of the American Diabetes Association. *Diabetes Care* 2005;28:186–212.

15. American Diabetes Association. Standards of medical care in diabetes—2014. *Diabetes Care* 2014;37(Suppl 1):S14–80.

16. Peters A, Laffel L; the American Diabetes Association Transitions Working Group. Diabetes care for emerging adults: recommendations for transition from pediatric to adult diabetes care systems: a position statement of the American Diabetes Association, with representation by the American College of Osteopathic Family Physicians, the American Academy of Pediatrics, the American Association of Clinical Endocrinologists, the American Osteopathic Association, the Centers for Disease Control and Prevention, Children with Diabetes, The Endocrine Society, the International Society for Pediatric and Adolescent Diabetes, Juvenile Diabetes Research Foundation International, the National Diabetes Education Program, and the Pediatric Endocrine Society (formerly Lawson Wilkins Pediatric Endocrine Society). *Diabetes Care* 2011;34:2477–2485.

17. Moreland EC, Volkening L, Lawlor M, Chalmers K, Anderson BJ, Laffel L. Ambulatory intervention using a BG monitoring manual improves knowledge, adherence, and glycemic control: results from a randomized clinical trial of high risk adults with diabetes. *Arch Intern Med* 2006;166:689–695.

Chapter 10

Preservation and Prevention Strategies for Type 1 Diabetes

Jay S. Skyler, MD, MACP

B ecause type 1 diabetes (T1D) develops as a consequence of immune damage to pancreatic insulin-secreting β-cells, many studies have attempted to halt the immune processes affecting β-cells. Most of the studies, referred to as preservation studies, have been conducted in recent-onset T1D, in an effort to preserve β-cell function, and with the hope of having a milder course of T1D and perhaps diminishing acute and chronic complications. Other studies, known as prevention studies, have been conducted in individuals identified as having high risk of T1D, with the hope of preventing or delaying the clinical onset of T1D. Two National Institutes of Health clinical trials networks, Type 1 Diabetes TrialNet (TrialNet) and the Immune Tolerance Network (ITN), have conducted the bulk of the studies in recent-onset T1D. These studies have used a relatively standardized trial design, including inclusion criteria and outcome measures, and have used centralized laboratories for measurement of key parameters. The majority of the studies discussed in this chapter have been conducted by TrialNet and ITN. Also included are landmark, well-designed randomized controlled trials.

INTERVENTION STUDIES IN RECENT-ONSET T1D

The first randomized, double-masked, controlled trials with statistically significant power were conducted in the mid-1980s with cyclosporine.[1,2] Two large studies were conducted: *1*) the French Cyclosporin Study, which included 122 patients ages 15–40 years, who had been symptomatic for ≤6 months and were on insulin therapy for ≤2 months;[1] and *2*) the Canadian/European Cyclosporin Study, which included 188 subjects ages 9–35 years, who had been symptomatic for ≤14 weeks and were on insulin therapy for ≤6 weeks.[2] Both trials used as their primary outcome the achievement of remission defined two ways: "complete remission" defined as good metabolic control (fasting glucose <140 mg/dl [7.8 mmol/l]; postprandial glucose <200 mg/dl [11.1 mmol/l]; A1C ≤7.5%) in the absence of insulin treatment; and "partial remission" defined as good metabolic control with insulin dose <0.26 units/kg/day. Both studies found a greater proportion of cyclosporine patients than placebo patients achieving and maintaining remissions. In both studies, cyclosporine could be given for 1 year, with stopping rules in place that led to blinded substitution of placebo for cyclosporine if remission was lost. Although both studies found that cyclosporine had superior efficacy than placebo, the magnitude and duration of benefit did not appear sufficient to justify cyclosporine

     DOI: 10.2337/9781580405096.10

treatment in clinical practice, given the potential of cyclosporine-induced neph-rotoxicity. The importance of the studies, however, was that they demonstrated the impact of immune intervention on the evolution of T1D, in a sense fulfilling Koch's postulate.

Smaller randomized trials were conducted with azathioprine,[3–5] linomide,[6] vaccination with bacillus Calmette–Guérin (BCG) strain of *Mycobacterium bovis*,[7,8] and oral insulin.[9–11] Unfortunately, none of these had sufficient beneficial effect to warrant further evaluation on a larger scale.

Recent trials generally have used preservation of C-peptide as an index of β-cell function.[12] This is now generally accepted as the primary outcome measure in clinical trials of immune intervention strategies.

Anti-CD3 monoclonal antibodies target T-lymphocytes, which are thought to mediate the immune attack on pancreatic islet β-cells. A number of studies have been conducted with anti-CD3 monoclonal antibodies. Two anti-CD3 monoclonal antibodies have been used in T1D clinical trials: *1*) the Fc-mutated CD3–hOKT3g1[Ala-Ala], teplizumab; and *2*) an altered CD3–ChAglyCD3, otelixizumab. An important aspect of treatment with these antibodies is the short duration of treatment (14 days for teplizumab, 6 days for otelixizumab). Several studies have been conducted with these antibodies, and all but one was conducted in patients with recent-onset T1D (within 3 months of diagnosis). In the earliest studies with anti-CD3, initial beneficial effects were reported at 12 months with teplizumab[13] and at 18 months with otelixizumab.[14] Although treatment was for only 14 (teplizumab) or 6 days (otelixizumab), sustained beneficial effects were reported in these studies. In the teplizumab study, C-peptide was preserved at 24 months,[15] and in the otelixizumab study, lower insulin doses were observed at 48 months.[16] An additional study with teplizumab, the Autoimmunity-Blocking Antibody for Tolerance in Recently Diagnosed Type 1 Diabetes (AbATE) trial, gave a second course of treatment after 1 year, with the primary outcome being measured at 2 years.[17] C-peptide was improved in treated subjects versus control subjects at 2 years.[17] In addition, the AbATE trial also compared "responders" (those who maintained C-peptide better than the randomized but untreated comparison group at 24 months) to "nonresponders." In the responders (which was nearly half of patients enrolled), the mean preservation of C-peptide continued at baseline levels for 2 years, whereas there was no difference between nonresponders and control patients, both of which showed progressive decline of C-peptide.[17] In another teplizumab study, the Delay trial, patients were enrolled 4–12 months after T1D diagnosis.[18] Nonetheless, there was improvement in C-peptide 1 year after the treatment with anti-CD3.

Phase 3 trials have been conducted with both teplizumab and otelixizumab. The Protégé study was a Phase 3 trial with teplizumab, involving 516 patients, ages 8–35 years, with recent-onset T1D.[19] Unfortunately, the primary outcome measure used in Protégé was the combination of A1C <6.5% and insulin dose <0.5 units/kg/day. It is unclear how this outcome measure was selected. Moreover, by using a composite outcome, a subject must meet two criteria to be classified, and the selection of a "yes or no" outcome dilutes the effect of two continuous variables. On the other hand, in the Protégé study, in exploratory analyses using the conventional outcome measure of C-peptide, the study results were positive, especially in patients enrolled in the U.S., in younger patients ages 8–17 years, in patients enrolled within 6 weeks of diagnosis, and in those with higher baseline C-peptide.[19] Because of failure to achieve the primary outcome measures in Protégé, a second Phase 3 trial was halted.

The DEFEND-1 and DEFEND-2 trials were Phase 3 trials with otelixizumab, involving 272 and 179 patients, respectively, with recent-onset T1D.[20,21] Surprisingly, rather than using the dosage (a total dose of 48 mg over 6 days) schedule that showed sustained beneficial effects in the Phase 1/2 trial,[14,16] the DEFEND trials used a total dose of only 3.1 mg of anti-CD3, one-sixteenth of that used in the earlier study. There was no difference in C-peptide at 1 year with the dose used. Unfortunately, in an attempt to completely obviate potential adverse effects, the DEFEND trials also obviated beneficial effects.

Anti-CD3 may show the greatest promise of any intervention tested to date, based on the Phase 1/2 trials. Yet, the difficulties encountered during Phase 3 trials conducted to date may result in this promising intervention not being pursued. Fortunately, an additional anti-CD3 study, for prevention of T1D in relatives at very high risk (projected 5-year risk of at least 75%), is currently underway in TrialNet.[22]

Two other interventions have shown a beneficial effect on the preservation of C-peptide—the monoclonal antibody rituximab that targets B-lymphocytes,[23,24] and the T-lymphocyte costimulation blocker abatacept.[25,26]

The anti-CD20 monoclonal antibody, rituximab, was evaluated in 87 subjects (ages 8–40 years) with recent-onset T1D.[23] Intervention consisted of 4 weekly infusions. At 1 year, C-peptide was significantly higher in the rituximab group than in the placebo group, and it declined at a slower rate. The rituximab group also had lower A1C levels and used less insulin. Some of the effects persisted at 2 years.[24] Since rituximab targets B-lymphocytes, these results suggest a potential role for B-lymphocytes in the evolution of T1D.

To be activated, T-lymphocytes need a costimulatory signal in addition to an antigen-driven signal. Abatacept (CTLA4-Ig) modulates costimulation, preventing T-lymphocyte activation. Abatacept was evaluated in 112 subjects (ages 6–36 years) with recent-onset T1D, with monthly infusions administered for 2 years.[25] At 2 years, C-peptide was significantly higher in the abatacept group than in the placebo group. Interestingly, 1 year later, after abatacept had been discontinued, the difference between the groups persisted, although the decline of C-peptide in the abatacept group was parallel to that in the placebo group.[26]

Several interventions have had ambiguous effects, including etanercept, DiaPep277, and alefacept. Etanercept, a blocker of the proinflammatory cytokine tumor necrosis factor, was assessed in a small (18 subjects, ages 7–18 years) 6-month pilot feasibility study.[27] C-peptide generally increased in the etanercept group and decreased in the placebo group. Unfortunately, the study was too small to draw meaningful conclusions.

DiaPep277, a peptide derived from human heat shock protein 60 (Hsp60), has been studied in a number of Phase 2 trials and a Phase 3 trial. It is administered intermittently subcutaneously and is posited to induce anti-inflammatory T-lymphocytes. In one Phase 2 trial, 35 subjects (ages 16–55 years) received either three doses of DiaPep277 or three doses of placebo. C-peptide was higher in the DiaPep277 group than in the placebo group at 10 months[28] and at 18 months.[29] Four additional Phase 2 studies have been reported,[30–32] without clear beneficial effect.

A Phase 3 trial enrolled 457 subjects (ages 16–45 years) with recent-onset T1D.[33] The results are ambiguous because glucagon-stimulated C-peptide at 24 months was improved in the DiaPep277 group versus the placebo group, although there was no difference in mixed-meal tolerance test (MMTT) stimulated C-peptide. A second Phase 3 trial is under way.

Alefacept, which targets effector memory T-lymphocytes, was studied in 49 subjects (ages 12–35 years) in the T1DAL study.[34] The primary outcome was an MMTT-stimulated 2-hour C-peptide level, which was not significantly preserved ($P = 0.65$). The MMTT-stimulated 4-hour C-peptide level, a secondary outcome, did show preservation of C-peptide ($P = 0.019$).

Several other interventions have been evaluated and have not shown beneficial effects. One study evaluated mycophenolate mofetil with or without initial treatment with anti-CD25 (daclizumab) and failed to show a benefit.[35] Three large studies evaluated glutamic acid decarboxylase (GAD) formulated as a vaccine of aluminum hydroxide (GAD-alum), with none showing a beneficial effect,[36–38] although a subgroup in an earlier Phase 2 trial had shown an apparent beneficial effect.[39]

Two studies evaluated agents that interfere with interleukin-1 (IL-1), a proinflammatory cytokine that recruits effector T-lymphocytes in inflamed tissues and that also has direct cytotoxic effects on β-cells. One of these studies used the anti-IL-1β monoclonal antibody canakinumab, while the other used the IL-1 receptor antagonist (IL-1Ra) anakinra. Neither study found a difference in C-peptide in comparison to the placebo group.[40]

Thymoglobulin, a polyclonal antilymphocyte preparation that broadly suppresses immune responses, also failed to show a beneficial effect.[41] Two antigen-specific approaches, one with a soluble altered peptide ligand of the insulin B9-23 peptide,[42] and one with an engineered DNA plasmid-encoding proinsulin,[43] both failed to show convincing beneficial effects.

Finally, a controversial, uncontrolled study evaluated profound immunosuppression and nonmyeloablative autologous hematopoietic stem cell transplantation (AHSCT).[44–46] This study involved 23 subjects (ages 13–31 years) with recent-onset T1D. All subjects were treated with profound immunosuppression (cyclophosphamide and thymoglobulin) and AHSCT. C-peptide levels increased and 20 patients became insulin independent, 12 maintaining insulin independence for a mean 31 months. Unfortunately, because of a lack of a randomized control group, it is impossible to fully interpret this study.

PREVENTION STUDIES

Pancreatic autoantibody-positive individuals are at increased risk of developing T1D. Indeed, those screened at birth for increased genetic risk (human leukocyte antigen [HLA]), who develop two or more pancreatic autoantibodies, will almost all eventually develop T1D.[47] That is true whether screening at birth was done in the general population or in family members of patients with T1D. First-degree family members, however, have a 10- to 20-fold increased risk compared with the general population. Consequently, many studies have screened relatives of patients with T1D for pancreatic autoantibodies to identify candidates for prevention studies. Antibody-positive relatives can be further evaluated and classified by level of risk—for example, those with 5-year risks of T1D of 25–50%, >50%, and >75%. Several prevention studies have been completed.

The Diabetes Prevention Trial-Type 1 (DPT-1) Study Group, the predecessor of TrialNet, conducted two studies concomitantly, evaluating injected (parenteral) insulin in individuals with a projected 5-year risk of >50% ("high risk")[48] and oral insulin in individuals with a projected 5-year risk of 25–50% ("intermediate risk").[49] These studies randomized 339 and 372 subjects, respectively. To identify the 711 eligible and randomized subjects, >100,000 relatives of T1D patients were screened.[49] In the high-risk group, subjects randomized to treatment received twice-daily injections of long-acting insulin (total daily dose of 0.25 units/kg) plus a 96-hour intravenous insulin infusion at baseline and annually thereafter. The randomized control group was a closely observed group that did not receive intervention. In the intermediate-risk group, subjects received either oral insulin capsules (containing 7.5 mg of insulin crystals) or matching placebo. Unfortunately, in both the high-risk and the intermediate-risk trials, the rate of diabetes development was the same in both the treated group and the respective control group. In a post hoc analysis of the oral insulin trial, however, a subgroup showed a beneficial effect of oral insulin.[49,50] That subgroup had higher titers of insulin autoantibodies at the time of enrollment. The projected delay in onset of T1D was 4.5–5 years in subjects with a confirmed baseline insulin autoantibody titer >80 nU/ml,[26] and a projected 10-year delay in those with a confirmed baseline insulin autoantibody titer >300 nU/ml.[50] Even after administration of oral insulin was ceased, effects were maintained.[51] Therefore, TrialNet is conducting an oral insulin trial in individuals with similar characteristics of those in the subgroup who showed potential delay in the development of T1D.[52,53]

The European Nicotinamide Diabetes Intervention Trial (ENDIT) tested nicotinamide in autoantibody relatives of patients with T1D.[54] ENDIT screened >30,000 relatives and randomized 552 individuals. Participants received nicotinamide (1.2 g/m^2 daily, maximum of 3 grams/day) or matching placebo. Unfortunately, the rate of development of diabetes was the same in the nicotinamide and placebo groups.

The Type 1 Diabetes Prediction and Prevention study (DIPP), conducted in Finland, the country with the highest incidence of T1D, screened cord blood from 116,720 consecutively born infants from the general population for the HLA-DQB1 susceptibility alleles for T1D.[55] They found 17,397 newborns with increased genetic risk. Additionally, among 3,430 siblings of infants with increased risk, about half (1,613) also had increased risk alleles. If the families consented, high-genetic-risk individuals were seen every 3–12 months and assessed for diabetes-associated autoantibodies. In those who developed two or more antibodies, they randomized 224 children from the infant cohort, and 40 more from the sibling cohort, to receive nasal insulin or placebo. Unfortunately, the rate of development of diabetes was the same in the nasal insulin and placebo groups.

The Trial to Reduce IDDM in the Genetically at Risk (TRIGR) is a primary prevention study in which subjects were identified by performing HLA typing at birth from cord or heel stick blood from newborns who had a first-degree relative with T1D.[56] TRIGR recruited 5,606 infants, and enrolled 2,160 eligible participants. All mothers were encouraged to breast-feed and, at weaning, began the randomized intervention of formulas based either on hydrolyzed casein or standard cow's milk. TRIGR plans to follow subjects until all children are at least 10 years old, with results anticipated in 2017.

Three other prevention trials are underway. One is assessing whether the GAD-alum vaccine can prevent T1D.[57] A second is testing whether the anti-CD3 monoclonal antibody teplizumab can prevent frank T1D in relatives with >75% 5-year risk of T1D.[58] A third trial is assessing whether abatacept can prevent T1D in relatives with two or more antibodies and normal glucose tolerance.[59]

To date, no prevention study has yet delayed or prevented T1D. As noted, additional prevention studies are underway and a number of prevention strategies are on the horizon. Success may require initiation of therapy from birth or universal vaccination. The key is that all interventions must be safe.

CONCLUSION

This chapter reviewed studies using immune intervention strategies in subjects with T1D or at risk of T1D. To date, none of the interventions are ready for routine clinical use. Clinicians, however, are encouraged to have relatives of their patients screened for diabetes autoantibodies, which can be done at no cost to participants through TrialNet,[60] and to potentially participate in ongoing clinical trials aimed at delay or prevention of T1D. A number of trials also are being conducted in recent-onset T1D, and clinicians should consider referring patients for inclusion in these clinical studies. Given the lack of an intervention that has robust evidence for clinical use, the next generation of trials likely will involve a combination of interventions.[61,62]

REFERENCES

1. Feutren G, Assan R, Karsenty G, Du Rostu H, Sirmai J, Papoz L, Vialettes B, Vexiau P, Rodier M, Lallemand A, Bach JF; for the Cyclosporin/Diabetes French Study Group. Cyclosporin increases the rate and length of remissions in insulin dependent diabetes of recent onset. Results of a multicentre double-blind trial. *Lancet* 1986;2(8499):119–124.

2. The Canadian-European Randomized Control Trial Group. Cyclosporin-induced remission of IDDM after early intervention. Association of 1 yr of cyclosporin treatment with enhanced insulin secretion. *Diabetes* 1988;37:1574–1582.

3. Silverstein J, Maclaren N, Riley W, Spillar R, Radjenovic D, Johnson S. Immunosuppression with azathioprine and prednisone in recent-onset insulin-dependent diabetes mellitus. *N Engl J Med* 1988;319:599–604.

4. Harrison LC, Colman PG, Dean B, Baxter R, Martin FI. Increase in remission rate in newly diagnosed type I diabetic subjects treated with azathioprine. *Diabetes* 1985;34:1306–1308.

5. Cook JJ, Hudson I, Harrison LC, Dean B, Colman PG, Werther GA, Warne GL, Court JM. Double-blind controlled trial of azathioprine in children with newly diagnosed type I diabetes. *Diabetes* 1989;38:779–783.

6. Coutant R, Landais P, Rosilio M, Johnsen C, Lahlou N, Chatelain P, Carel JC, Ludvigsson J, Boitard C, Bougneres PF. Low dose linomide in type 1 juvenile diabetes of recent onset: a randomised placebo-controlled double blind trial. *Diabetologia* 1998;41:1040–1046.

7. Elliott JF, Marlin KL, Couch RM. Effect of Bacillus Calmette-Guerin vaccination on C-peptide secretion in children newly diagnosed with IDDM. *Diabetes Care* 1998;21:1691–1693.

8. Allen HF, Klingensmith GJ, Jensen P, Simoes E, Hayward A, Chase HP. Effect of Bacillus Calmette-Guerin vaccination on new-onset type 1 diabetes: a randomized clinical study. *Diabetes Care* 1999;22:1703–1707.

9. Chaillous L, Lefevre H, Thivolet C, Boitard C, Lahlou N, Atlan-Gepner C, Bouhanick B, Mogenet A, Nicolino M, Carel JC, Lecomte P, Marechaud R, Bougneres P, Charbonnel B, Sai P. Oral insulin administration and residual beta-cell function in recent-onset type 1 diabetes: a multicentre randomised controlled trial. Diabete Insuline Orale group. *Lancet* 2000;356:545–549.

10. Pozzilli P, Pitocco D, Visalli N, Cavallo MG, Buzzetti R, Crino A, Spera S, Suraci C, Multari G, Cervoni M, Manca Bitti ML, Matteoli MC, Marietti G, Ferrazzoli F, Cassone Faldetta MR, Giordano C, Sbriglia M, Sarugeri E, Ghirlanda G. No effect of oral insulin on residual beta-cell function in recent-onset type I diabetes (the IMDIAB VII). IMDIAB Group. *Diabetologia* 2000;43:1000–1004.

11. Ergun-Longmire B, Marker J, Zeidler A, Rapaport R, Raskin P, Bode B, Schatz D, Vargas A, Rogers D, Schwartz S, Malone J, Krischer J, Maclaren NK. Oral insulin therapy to prevent progression of immune-mediated (type 1) diabetes. *Ann N Y Acad Sci* 2004;1029:260–277.

12. Palmer JP, Fleming GA, Greenbaum CJ, Herold KC, Jansa LD, Kolb H, Lachin JM, Polonsky KS, Pozzilli P, Skyler JS, Steffes MW. C-peptide is the appropriate outcome measure for type 1 diabetes clinical trials to preserve beta cell function: report of an ADA Workshop, 21–22 October 2001. *Diabetes* 2004;53:250–264.

13. Herold KC, Hagopian W, Auger JA, Poumian-Ruiz E, Taylor L, Donaldson D, Gitelman SE, Harlan DM, Xu D, Zivin RA, Bluestone JA. Anti-CD3 monoclonal antibody in new-onset type 1 diabetes mellitus. *N Engl J Med* 2002;346:1692–1698.

14. Keymeulen B, Vandemeulebroucke E, Ziegler AG, Mathieu C, Kaufman L, Hale G, Gorus F, Goldman M, Walter M, Candon S, Schandene L, Crenier L, De Block C, Seigneurin JM, De Pauw P, Pierard D, Weets I, Rebello P, Bird P, Berrie E, Frewin M, Waldmann H, Bach JF, Pipeleers D, Chatenoud L. Insulin needs after CD3-antibody therapy in new-onset type 1 diabetes. *N Engl J Med* 2005;352:2598–2608.

15. Herold KC, Gitelman SE, Masharani U, Hagopian W, Bisikirska B, Donaldson D, Rother K, Diamond B, Harlan DM, Bluestone JA. A single course of anti-CD3 monoclonal antibody hOKT3gamma1(Ala-Ala) results in improvement in C-peptide responses and clinical parameters for at least 2 years after onset of type 1 diabetes. *Diabetes* 2005;54:1763–1769.

16. Keymeulen B, Walter M, Mathieu C, Kaufman L, Gorus F, Hilbrands R, Vandemeulebroucke E, Van de Velde U, Crenier L, De Block C, Candon S, Waldmann H, Ziegler AG, Chatenoud L, Pipeleers D. Four-year metabolic outcome of a randomised controlled CD3-antibody trial in recent-onset type 1 diabetic patients depends on their age and baseline residual beta cell mass. *Diabetologia* 2010;53:614–623.

17. Herold KC, Gitelman SE, Ehlers MR, Gottlieb PA, Greenbaum CJ, Hagopian W, Boyle KD, Keyes-Elstein L, Aggarwal S, Phippard D, Sayre PH, McNamara J, Bluestone JA; the AbATE Study Team. Teplizumab (anti-CD3 mAb) treatment preserves C-peptide responses in patients with new-onset type 1 diabetes in a randomized controlled trial: Metabolic and immunologic features at baseline identify a subgroup of responders. *Diabetes* 2013;62:3766–3774.

18. Herold KC, Gitelman SE, Willi SM, Gottlieb PA, Waldron-Lynch F, Devine L, Sherr J, Rosenthal SM, Adi S, Jalaludin MY, Michels AW, Dziura J, Bluestone JA. Teplizumab treatment may improve C-peptide responses in participants with type 1 diabetes after the new-onset period: a randomised controlled trial. *Diabetologia* 2013;56:391–400.

19. Sherry N, Hagopian W, Ludvigsson J, Jain SM, Wahlen J, Ferry RJ Jr, Bode B, Aronoff S, Holland C, Carlin D, King KL, Wilder RL, Pillemer S, Bonvini E, Johnson S, Stein KE, Koenig S, Herold KC, Daifotis AG; Protégé Trial Investigators. Teplizumab for treatment of type 1 diabetes (Protégé study): 1-year results from a randomised, placebo-controlled trial. *Lancet* 2011;378:487–497.

20. Trial of otelixizumab for adults with newly diagnosed type 1 diabetes mellitus (autoimmune): DEFEND-1. NCT00678886. Available at www.ClinicalTrials.gov.

21. Ambery P, Donner TW, Biswas N, Donaldson J, Parkin J, Dayan CM. Efficacy and safety of low-dose otelixizumab anti-CD3 monoclonal antibody in preserving C-peptide secretion in adolescent type 1 diabetes: DEFEND-2, a randomized, placebo-controlled, double-blind, multi-centre study. *Diabet Med* November 16, 2013. [Epub ahead of print].

22. Teplizumab for prevention of type 1 diabetes in relatives "at-risk." NCT01030861. Available at www.ClinicalTrials.gov.

23. Pescovitz MD, Greenbaum CJ, Krause-Steinrauf H, Becker DJ, Gitelman SE, Goland R, Gottlieb PA, Marks JB, McGee PF, Moran AM, Raskin P, Rodriguez H, Schatz DA, Wherrett D, Wilson DM, Lachin JM, Skyler JS; the Type 1 Diabetes TrialNet Anti-CD20 Study Group. Rituximab, B-lymphocyte depletion and preservation of beta-cell function. *N Engl J Med* 2009;361:2143–2152.

24. Pescovitz MD, Greenbaum CJ, Bundy BN, Becker DJ, Gitelman SE, Goland R, Gottlieb PA, Marks JB, McGee PF, Moran AM, Raskin P, Rodriguez H, Schatz DA, Wherrett D, Wilson DM, Skyler JS; the Type 1 Diabetes TrialNet Anti-CD20 Study Group. B-lymphocyte depletion with rituximab and beta-cell function: two-year results. *Diabetes Care* 2014;37:453–459.

25. Orban T, Bundy B, Becker DJ, DiMeglio LA, Gitelman SE, Goland R, Gottlieb PA, Greenbaum CJ, Marks JB, Monzavi R, Moran A, Raskin P, Rodriguez H, Russell WE, Schatz D, Wherrett D, Wilson DM, Skyler JS; the Type 1 Diabetes TrialNet Abatacept Study Group. Co-stimulation modulation with abatacept in patients with recent-onset type 1 diabetes: a randomised double-blind, placebo-controlled trial. *Lancet* 2011;378:412–419.

26. Orban T, Bundy B, Becker DJ, DiMeglio LA, Gitelman SE, Goland R, Gottlieb PA, Greenbaum CJ, Marks JB, Monzavi R, Moran A, Peakman M, Raskin P, Rodriguez H, Russell WE, Schatz D, Wherrett D, Wilson DM, Skyler JS; the Type 1 Diabetes TrialNet Abatacept Study Group. Costimulation modulation with abatacept in patients with recent-onset type 1 diabetes: follow-up one year after cessation of treatment. *Diabetes Care* 2014;37(4):1069–1075.

27. Mastrandrea L, Yu J, Behrens T, Buchlis J, Albini C, Fourtner S, Quattrin T. Etanercept treatment in children with new-onset type 1 diabetes: pilot randomized, placebo-controlled, double-blind study. *Diabetes Care* 2009;32:1244–1249.

28. Raz I, Elias D, Avron A, Tamir M, Metzger M, Cohen IR. β-cell function in new-onset type 1 diabetes and immunomodulation with a heat-shock protein peptide (DiaPep277): a randomised, double-blind, phase II trial. *Lancet* 2001;358:1749–1753.

29. Raz I, Avron A, Tamir M, Metzger M, Symer L, Eldor R, Cohen IR, Elias D. Treatment of new-onset type 1 diabetes with peptide DiaPep277 is safe and associated with preserved beta-cell function: extension of a randomised, doubleblind, phase II trial. *Diabetes/Metab Res Rev* 2007;23:292–298.

30. Lazar L, Ofan R, Weintrob N, Avron A, Tamir M, Elias D, Phillip M, Josefsberg Z. Heat-shock protein peptide DiaPep277 treatment in children with newly diagnosed type 1 diabetes: a randomised, double-blind phase II study. *Diabetes/Metab Res Rev* 2007;23:286–291.

31. Huurman VA, Decochez K, Mathieu C, Cohen IR, Roep BO. Therapy with the hsp60 peptide DiaPep277 in C-peptide positive type 1 diabetes patients. *Diabetes/Metab Res Rev* 2007;23:269–275.

32. Schloot NC, Meierhoff G, Lengyel C, Vándorfi G, Takács J, Pánczél P, Barkai L, Madácsy L, Oroszlán T, Kovács P, Sütö G, Battelino T, Hosszufalusi N, Jermendy G. Effect of heat shock protein peptide DiaPep277 on beta-cell function in paediatric and adult patients with recent-onset diabetes mellitus type 1: two prospective, randomized, double-blind phase II trials. *Diabetes/ Metab Res Rev* 2007;23:276–285.

33. Raz I, Ziegler AG, Linn T, Schernthaner G, Bonnici F, Distiller LA, Giordano C, Giorgino F, deVries L, Mauricio D, Wainstein J, Elias D, Avron A, Tamir M, Eren R, Peled D, Dagan S, Cohen IR, Pozzilli P; the DIA-AID 1 Writing Group. Treatment of recent onset type 1 diabetes patients with DiaPep277: results of a double-blind, placebo-controlled, randomized phase 3 trial. *Diabetes Care* (in press).

34. Rigby MR, DiMeglio LA, Rendell MS, Felner EI, Dostou JM, Gitelman SE, Patel CM, Griffin KJ, Tsalikian E, Gottlieb PA, Greenbaum CJ, Sherry NA, Moore WV, Monzavi R, Willi SM, Raskin P, Moran A, Russell WE, Pinckney A, Keyes-Elstein L, Howell M, Aggarwal S, Lim N, Phippard D, Nepom GT, McNamara J, Ehlers MR; the T1DAL Study Team. Targeting of memory T cells with alefacept in new-onset type 1 diabetes (T1DAL study): 12 month results of a randomised, double-blind, placebo-controlled phase 2 trial. *Lancet Diabetes Endocrinol* 2013;1:284–294.

35. Gottlieb PA, Quinlan S, Krause-Steinrauf H, Greenbaum CJ, Wilson DM, Rodriguez H, Schatz DA, Moran AM, Lachin JM, Skyler JS; the Type 1 Diabetes TrialNet MMF/DZB Study Group. Failure to preserve beta-cell function with mycophenolate mofetil and daclizumab combined therapy in patients with new onset type 1 diabetes. *Diabetes Care* 2010;33:826–832.

36. Wherrett DK, Bundy B, Becker DJ, DiMeglio LA, Gitelman SE, Goland R, Gottlieb PA, Greenbaum CJ, Herold KC, Marks JB, Monzavi R, Moran A, Orban T, Raskin P, Rodriguez H, Russell WE, Schatz D, Wilson DM, Skyler JS; the Type 1 Diabetes TrialNet GAD Study Group. Antigen-based therapy with glutamic acid decarboxylase (gad) vaccine in patients with recent-onset type 1 diabetes: a randomised double-blind trial. *Lancet* 2011;378:319–327.

37. Ludvigsson J, Krisky D, Casas R, Battelino T, Castaño L, Greening J, Kordonouri O, Otonkoski T, Pozzilli P, Robert JJ, Veeze HJ, Palmer J. GAD65 antigen therapy in recently diagnosed type 1 diabetes mellitus. *N Engl J Med* 2012;366:433–442.

38. Diamyd initiates closure of US Phase III study. Press release June 23, 2011. Available at www.diamyd.com/docs/pressClip.aspx?section=investor&ClipID=584435.

39. Ludvigsson J, Faresjö M, Hjorth M, Axelsson S, Chéramy M, Pihl M, Vaarala O, Forsander G, Ivarsson S, Johansson C, Lindh A, Nilsson NO, Aman J, Ortqvist E, Zerhouni P, Casas R. GAD treatment and insulin secretion in recent-onset type 1 diabetes. *N Engl J Med* 2008;359:1909–1920.

40. Moran A, Bundy B, Becker DJ, DiMeglio LA, Gitelman SE, Goland R, Greenbaum CJ, Herold KC, Marks JB, Raskin P, Sanda S, Schatz D, Wherrett D, Wilson DM, Skyler JS; the Type 1 Diabetes TrialNet Canakinumab Study Group; Pickersgill L, de Koning E, Ziegler A-G, Böehm B, Badenhoop K, Schloot N, Bak JF, Pozzilli P, Mauricio D, Donath MY, Castaño L, Wagner A, Lervang HH, Perrild H, Mandrup-Poulsen T; on behalf of the AIDA Study Group. Interleukin-1 antagonism in type 1 diabetes of recent onset: two mul-

ticenter, randomized double-masked, placebo-controlled trials. *Lancet* 2013;381:1905–1915.

41. Gitelman SE, Gottlieb PA, Rigby MR, Felner EI, Willi SM, Fisher LK, Moran A, Gottschalk M, Moore WV, Pinckney A, Keyes-Elstein L, Aggarwal S, Phippard D, Sayre PH, Ding L, Bluestone JA, Ehlers MR; the START Study Team. Antithymocyte globulin therapy for patients with recent-onset type 1 diabetes: a randomized double-blind phase 2 trial. *Lancet Diabetes Endocrinol* 2013;1:306–316.

42. Walter M, Philotheou A, Bonnici F, Ziegler AG, Jimenez R; NBI-6024 Study Group. No effect of the altered peptide ligand NBI-6024 on beta-cell residual function and insulin needs in new-onset type 1 diabetes. *Diabetes Care* 2009;32:2036–2040.

43. Roep BO, Solvason N, Gottlieb PA, Abreu JR, Harrison LC, Eisenbarth GS, Yu L, Leviten M, Hagopian WA, Buse JB, von Herrath M, Quan J, King RS, Robinson WH, Utz PJ, Garren H; BHT-3021 Investigators; Steinman L. Plasmid-encoded proinsulin preserves C-peptide while specifically reducing proinsulin-specific CD8+ T cells in type 1 diabetes. *Sci Trans Med* 2013;5(191):191ra82.

44. Voltarelli JC, Couri CE, Stracieri AB, Oliveira MC, Moraes DA, Pieroni F, Coutinho M, Malmegrim KC, Foss-Freitas MC, Simões BP, Foss MC, Squiers E, Burt RK. Autologous nonmyeloablative hematopoietic stem cell transplantation in newly diagnosed type 1 diabetes mellitus. *JAMA* 2007;297:1568–1576.

45. Couri CE, Oliveira MC, Stracieri AB, Moraes DA, Pieroni F, Barros GM, Madeira MI, Malmegrim KC, Foss-Freitas MC, Simões BP, Martinez EZ, Foss MC, Burt RK, Voltarelli JC. C-peptide levels and insulin independence following autologous nonmyeloablative hematopoietic stem cell transplantation in newly diagnosed type 1 diabetes mellitus. *JAMA* 2009;301:1573–1579.

46. Voltarelli JC, Martinez ED, Burt RK. Autologous nonmyeloablative hematopoietic stem cell transplantation in newly diagnosed type 1 diabetes mellitus. Author's Reply. *JAMA* 2009;302:624–625.

47. Ziegler AG, Rewers M, Simell O, Simell T, Lempainen J, Steck A, Winkler C, Ilonen J, Veijola R, Knip M, Bonifacio E, Eisenbarth GS. Seroconversion to multiple islet autoantibodies and risk of progression to diabetes in children. *JAMA* 2013;309:2473–2479.

48. Diabetes Prevention Trial–Type 1 Study Group. Effects of insulin in relatives of patients with type 1 diabetes mellitus. *N Engl J Med* 2002;346:1685–1691.

49. Skyler JS, Krischer JP, Wolfsdorf J, Cowie C, Palmer JP, Greenbaum C, Cuthbertson D, Rafkin-Mervis LE, Chase HP, Leschek E; Diabetes Prevention Trial–Type 1 Diabetes Study Group. Effects of oral insulin in relatives of patients with type 1 diabetes mellitus. *Diabetes Care* 2005;28:1068–1076.

50. Skyler JS; the Type 1 Diabetes TrialNet Study Group. Update on worldwide efforts to prevent type 1 diabetes. *Ann N Y Acad Sci* 2008;1150:190–196.

51. Vehik K, Cuthbertson D, Ruhlig H, Schatz DA, Peakman M, Krischer JP; DPT-1 and TrialNet Study Groups. Long-term outcome of individuals treated with oral insulin: Diabetes Prevention Trial-Type 1 (DPT-1) oral insulin trial. *Diabetes Care* 2011;34:1585–1590.

52. Skyler JS. Primary and secondary prevention of type 1 diabetes. *Diabet Med* 2013;30:161–169.

53. Oral insulin for prevention of diabetes in relatives at risk for type 1 diabetes mellitus. NCT00419562. Available at www.ClinicalTrials.gov.

54. European Nicotinamide Diabetes Intervention Trial (ENDIT) Group. European Nicotinamide Diabetes Intervention Trial (ENDIT): a randomized controlled trial of intervention before the onset of type 1 diabetes. *Lancet* 2004;363:925–931.

55. Näntö-Salonen K, Kupila A, Simell S, Siljander H, Salonsaari T, Hekkala A, Korhonen S, Erkkola R, Sipilä JI, Haavisto L, Siltala M, Tuominen J, Hakalax J, Hyöty H, Ilonen J, Veijola R, Simell T, Knip M, Simell O. Nasal insulin to prevent type 1 diabetes in children with HLA genotypes and autoantibodies conferring increased risk of disease: a double-blind, randomised controlled trial. *Lancet* 2008;372:1746–1755.

56. TRIGR Study Group; Akerblom HK, Krischer J, Virtanen SM, Berseth C, Becker D, Dupré J, Ilonen J, Trucco M, Savilahti E, Koski K, Pajakkala E, Fransiscus M, Lough G, Bradley B, Koski M, Knip M. The Trial to Reduce IDDM in the Genetically at Risk (TRIGR) study: recruitment, intervention and follow-up. *Diabetologia* 2011;54:627–633.

57. Diabetes prevention–immune tolerance (DIAPREV-IT). NCT01122446. Available at www.ClinicalTrials.gov.

58. Teplizumab for prevention of type 1 diabetes in relatives "at-risk." NCT01030861. Available at www.ClinicalTrials.gov.

59. CTLA4-Ig (abatacept) for prevention of abnormal glucose tolerance and diabetes in relatives at risk for type 1. NCT01773707. Available at www.ClinicalTrials.gov.

60. Type 1 Diabetes TrialNet. Available at www.diabetestrialnet.org. Accessed 20 March 2014.

61. Matthews JB, Staeva TP, Bernstein PL, Peakman M, von Herrath M; ITN-JDRF Type 1 Diabetes Combination Therapy Assessment Group. Developing combination immunotherapies for type 1 diabetes: recommendations from the ITN-JDRF type 1 diabetes combination therapy assessment group. *Clin Exp Immunol* 2010;160:176–184.

62. Skyler JS, Ricordi C. Stopping type 1 diabetes: attempts to prevent or cure type 1 diabetes in man. *Diabetes* 2011;60:1–8.

Chapter 11

Insulin Pump Therapy: Artificial Pancreas

Jennifer L. Sherr, MD
William V. Tamborlane, MD

INSULIN PUMPS

The first successful studies of effectiveness of continuous subcutaneous infusion (CSII) pumps were carried out >30 years ago,[1] but these devices were not used extensively in patients with type 1 diabetes (T1D) until after the Diabetes Control and Complications Trial established the benefits of strict control of diabetes in diabetic complications. Since then, an ever-increasing proportion of adults and children with T1D have been utilizing this therapy. Indeed, the T1D Exchange Clinic Registry recently reported that ~60% of adults and ~50% of children with T1D were using pump therapy.[2] CSII has been shown to be more effective in lowering A1C compared with injection therapy in randomized and nonrandomized studies and to be associated with improved patient satisfaction and reduced frequency of hypoglycemia.

PUMP FEATURES

Insulin pump therapy uses only rapid-acting insulin analogs to deliver 24/7 insulin coverage. A reservoir for the pump is filled with several days' worth of insulin. In conventional pumps, the reservoir attaches to a variable length of tubing, which in turn attaches to a small catheter or steel needle that is inserted into the subcutaneous tissue. Most common sites for insertion include the buttocks, abdomen, upper leg, or hip, and some patients use their arms. Insertion of a new infusion set should be done every 2–3 days or whenever persistently high blood glucose (BG) values indicate a potential site failure. "Patch pumps," like the OmniPod, have both the mechanism to drive the pump and the insulin reservoir in a disposable "pod."[3] This pod is attached to the surface of the skin and includes an integrated catheter, which allows for subcutaneous delivery of the insulin. Insulin doses programmed by the patient throughout the day are delivered by a handheld device, which wirelessly communicates with the patch.

Most currently available insulin pumps are "smart" pumps into which both insulin–to-carbohydrate ratios (ICRs) and insulin sensitivity factors (ISFs), which can be varied by time of day, are programmed into the bolus calculator. When the pump's dose calculator is used for meal boluses, the patient enters the number of carbohydrates that will be consumed and the amount of insulin to be given is calculated based on the programmed ICR for that time of day. The premeal BG value is entered into the pump's dose calculator either manually or by wireless

 DOI: 10.2337/9781580405096.11

transmission from the glucose meter, and a correction dose is calculated according to the ISF depending on how much the glucose level differs from the preset target.

Bolus doses can be administered over a few minutes or as square-wave and dual-wave boluses over longer periods of time. Ideally, bolus doses should be delivered 10–15 minutes before the meal to minimize postmeal excursions.[4] In young children and "picky eaters," or when eating at restaurants, a partial priming bolus of insulin can be given before the meal, followed by additional bolus doses depending on how many carbohydrates actually are consumed during the meal. Current technology allows for the delivery of doses as small as 0.025–0.05 units of insulin.

Basal insulin is delivered through a preprogrammed "basal pattern." This pattern can be made up of multiple different rates, which allow for a waxing and waning pattern of basal insulin delivery. In addition, multiple 24-hour basal patterns can be preprogrammed and stored in the pump's memory. For example, some adolescent patients have a basal pattern for schooldays and one for weekends to account for their tendency wake up much later on weekends and holidays. Finally, a temporary change in the basal rate for a specific period of time can be programmed, which can be an effective tool for dealing with exercise or sick-day management.

EFFICACY AND SAFETY OF PUMP THERAPY

Most randomized clinical trials and nonrandomized clinical outcome studies of CSII versus multiple daily injection therapy (MDI) have been carried out in patients with T1D. The wealth of clinical trial data that have been analyzed indicate that A1C levels or the risk of severe hypoglycemia or both are reduced with the use of CSII versus MDI in adults and children. These findings have been supported by data from large patient registries in the U.S.[2] and Europe.[5] Other benefits of CSII include patient perceptions of greater treatment satisfaction and quality of life during treatment with CSII.

The introduction of continuous glucose monitoring (CGM) devices has further enhanced the effectiveness of insulin pump therapy. Real-time and retrospective analyses of sensor glucose profiles provide patients and clinicians with data regarding patterns of glucose excursions after meals and during the night that generally are not available with BG meter monitoring. These data, in turn, allow for better adjustments of basal rate profiles and bolus dose settings. Nevertheless, use of these devices was impeded by the difficulties and inaccuracies of early models, especially in pediatrics,[6] but has increased with the introduction of better sensors.

The effective use of advances in diabetes technology is not without its challenges for patients and providers. Insulin pumps and CGM are best prescribed by multidisciplinary teams ideally consisting of diabetologists, nurse clinicians, dietitians, and social workers or psychologists. The team needs to provide adequate patient education and training to ensure optimal usage of these technologies. On-call clinicians need to be available at all times to assist patients with device-related problems.

ARTIFICIAL PANCREAS

RATIONALE

Despite major advances in the treatment of T1D over the past 3 decades, too many patients with T1D do not meet glycemic goals.[2] Moreover, patients who are able to achieve target BG and A1C levels are at higher risk for severe hypoglycemic events, as well as being exposed frequently to asymptomatic hypoglycemia, especially during the night.[7] Even under the best of circumstances, the constant demands that patients with T1D have to implement to adequately manage their disease can be overwhelming. Only when the patient can be taken out of the equation and when metabolic control can be maintained with little or no effort, will we have achieved the full potential of recent advances in diabetes technology. Given that the risk from immunosuppressive therapy from islet cell transplantation outweighs the benefits, the most promising therapy for β-cell replacement in patients with T1D is a fully automated, closed-loop (CL) artificial pancreas.

COMPONENTS

Although attempts at fully implanted artificial pancreas systems have not been successful, all that is required for an external CL system are a transcutaneous continuous glucose sensor that measures interstitial glucose concentrations, an external insulin pump that is equipped to receive glucose sensor data, and a computer algorithm that varies the rate of insulin delivery based on glucose sensor outputs. Nevertheless, a number of obstacles must be overcome in combining these components into a semi- or fully automated artificial pancreas that can be used by unsupervised patients at home. The devices have to be managed easily by the patient; glucose sensors have to be more accurate and easier to use; the sensors have to be able to respond to the normal daily activities that affect BG levels; and, most important, safety checks have to be in place to avoid overdelivery of insulin.

FEASIBILITY STUDIES

The feasibility of the CL artificial pancreas has been documented in adults and children during the day and night and has demonstrated an increased time spent in target range.[8,9] Because CL insulin delivery has reduced but not eliminated problems with hypoglycemia, a bihormonal CL artificial pancreas using glucagon as the counterregulatory component is being tested.[10]

Even under CL conditions, meal-related BG excursions frequently exceed target levels. This primarily is due to delays in absorption of insulin from the subcutaneous tissue and because the algorithm extends the meal "bolus" over a period of 2–3 hours.[8] Consequently, a number of studies have been undertaken to explore ways to accelerate the time action profiles of rapid-acting insulin analogs to improve performance of CL and open-loop insulin delivery. Cengiz et al.[11] have reported that warming the skin around the insulin infusion site results in an earlier time-to-peak insulin action (T_{GIRmax}) as compared with control glucose clamps without skin warming. Weinzimer et al.[12] demonstrated that postprandial hyperglycemia also can be ameliorated by "meal announcement"—that is, having the patient administer a partial, premeal priming bolus. In that study,[12] this hybrid, semiautomatic approach led to an earlier rise in plasma insulin levels and a reduction in peak postprandial glucose levels. Although this approach did decrease postprandial hyperglycemia, it requires manual inputs from the patient, and therefore it is not fully autonomous. Another strategy for reducing postmeal hyperglycemia is the administration of premeal injections of pramlintide.[13] Pramlintide is an analog of the naturally occurring β-cell peptide amylin. It works by delaying gastric emptying, thus slowing carbohydrate appearance and by lowering meal-stimulated increases in plasma glucagon levels. This mechanism of action is important given that it is now known that there is a dysregulation of α-cell function even during the very early stages of T1D.

SAFETY ISSUES

The major obstacle to outpatient treatment of T1D patients is that a number of redundant safeguards must be in place to ensure that no patient is injured by overdelivery of insulin due to a system malfunction. The translation of advances in diabetes technology in CL control into clinical practice will be facilitated by the improvement in system hardware and software, some of which are shown in Table 11.1.

Although the main danger of CL control is when the system is prompted to increase insulin delivery in response to increasing sensor glucose levels, there are few concerns regarding the safety of shutting down insulin delivery for relatively brief periods of time in response to low sensor glucose levels. The first step in this direction has been achieved with the introduction of an integrated sensor-augmented pump system, which automatically suspends a pump's basal insulin infusion for 2 hours if sensor glucose levels fall to a preprogrammed threshold level and the patient does not respond to low-glucose alarms. This integrated system has shown to be safe and effective in reducing the amount of time spent in hypoglycemia.[14] Another recent study demonstrated that a random 2-hour period of suspension of the basal insulin infusion is safe and does not result in ketoacidosis even when BG levels are elevated.[15]

Although inpatient CL studies will help to inform the development of the ultimate outpatient devices, the inpatient, hospital setting does not represent the real day-to-day life of patients. Thus, the final test of these systems will be how they perform in the home setting in unsupervised patients. Thus, the most excit-

---

Table 11.1 Safeguards Needed to Mitigate the Risk of Overdelivery of Insulin by CL Systems

- Better and more accurate sensors
- Dual sensors
- Integrity of radio-frequency transmissions
- Preventing computer malfunctions
- Limiting maximal delivery rates
- Improved algorithms to detect failing sensors
- Minimizing the risk of user error

ing development in this field is that a number of outpatient feasibility studies already have been completed successfully .[16,17] Given that all stakeholders, including the JDRF, the National Institutes of Health, device companies, and regulatory agencies, have prioritized the development of a practically applicable CL system, this should be a reality before the next edition of this manuscript. We anticipate that large-scale, long-term, pivotal trials of user-friendly CL systems will be launched by 2015.

REFERENCES

1. Tamborlane WV, Sherwin RS, Genel M, Felig P. Reduction to normal of plasma glucose in juvenile diabetics by subcutaneous administration of insulin with a portable infusion pump. *N Engl J Med* 1979;300:573–578.

2. Beck RW, Tamborlane WV, Bergenstal RR, Miller KM, DuBose SN, Hall CA; for the T1D Exchange Clinic Registry Study Group. The T1D Exchange Clinic Registry: overview of the project and characteristics of initial 20,119 participants. *JCEM* 2012;97:4383–4389.

3. Sherr J, Cengiz E, Tamborlane WV. From pumps to prevention: recent advances in the treatment of type 1 diabetes. *Drug Discovery Today* 2009;14:973–981.

4. Tamborlane WV, Sikes KA. Insulin therapy in children and adolescents. *Endocrinol Metab Clin North Am* 2012;41:145–160.

5. Kapellen TM, Klinkert C, Heidtmann B, Jakisch B, Haberland H, Hofer SE, Holl RW. Insulin pump treatment in children and adolescents with type 1 diabetes: experiences of the German Working Group for Insulin Pump Treatment in Pediatric Patients. *Postgrad Med* 2010;122:98–105.

6. Tamborlane WV, Beck RW, Bode BW, Buckingham B, Chase HP, Clemons R, et al. Continuous glucose monitoring and intensive treatment of type 1 diabetes. *N Engl J Med* 2008;359:1464–1476.

7. Tamborlane WV. Triple jeopardy for hypoglycemia on nights following exercise in youth with type 1 diabetes. *J Clin Endocrinol Metab* 2007;92:815–816.

8. Steil GM, Rebrin K, Darwin C, Hariri F, Saad MF. Feasibility of automating insulin delivery for the treatment of type 1 diabetes. *Diabetes* 2006;55(12):3344–3350.

9. Hovorka R, Allen JM, Elleri D, Chassin LJ, Harris J, Xing D, Kollman C, Hovorka T, Larsen AM, Nodale M, De Palma A, Wilinska ME, Acerini CL, Dunger DB. Manual closed-loop insulin delivery in children and adolescents with type 1 diabetes: a phase 2 randomised crossover trial. *Lancet* 2010;375:743–751.

10. Russell SJ, El-Khatib FH, Nathan DM, Magyar KL, Jiang J, Damiano ER. Blood glucose control in type 1 diabetes with a bihormonal bionic endocrine pancreas. *Diabetes Care* 2012;35:2148–2155.

11. Cengiz E, Weinzimer SA, Sherr JL, Tichy E, Martin M, Carria L, Steffen A, Tamborlane WV. Acceleration of insulin pharmacodynamic profile by a novel insulin infusion site warming device. *Pediatr Diabetes* 2013;14:168–173.

12. Weinzimer SA, Steil GM, Swan KL, Dziura J, Kurtz N, Tamborlane WV. Fully automated closed-loop insulin delivery versus semiautomated hybrid control in pediatric patients with type 1 diabetes using an artificial pancreas. *Diabetes Care* 2008;31:934–939.

13. Weinzimer SA, Sherr JL, Cengiz E, Kim G, Ruiz JL, Carria L, et al. Effect of pramlintide on prandial glycemic excursions during closed-loop control in adolescents and young adults with type 1 diabetes. *Diabetes Care* 2012;35:1994–1999.

14. Choudhary P, Shin J, Wang Y, Evans ML, Hammond PJ, Kerr D, et al. Insulin pump therapy with automated insulin suspension in response to hypoglycemia: reduction in nocturnal hypoglycemia in those at greatest risk. *Diabetes Care* 2011;34:2023–2025.

15. Sherr JL, Palau Collazo M, Cengiz E, Michaud C, Carria L, Steffen AT, Weyman K, Zgorski M, Tichy E, Tamborlane WV, Weinzimer SA. Safety of nighttime 2-hour suspension of basal insulin in pump-treated type 1 diabetes even in the absence of low glucose. *Diabetes Care* 2014;37:773–779.

16. Cobelli C, Renard E, Kovatchev BP, Keith-Hynes P, Ben Brahim N, Place J, et al. Pilot studies of wearable outpatient artificial pancreas in type 1 diabetes. *Diabetes Care* 2012;35:e65–67.

17. Phillip M, Battelino T, Atlas E, Kordonouri O, Bratina N, Miller S, Biester T, Stefanija MA, Muller I, Nimri R, Danne T. Nocturnal glucose control with an artificial pancreas at a diabetes camp. *N Engl J Med* 2013;368(9):824–833.

Chapter 12

Psychosocial and Family Issues in Children with Type 1 Diabetes

Barbara J. Anderson, PhD
David D. Schwartz, PhD, ABPP

D aily treatment of children with diabetes affects everyday behavior in the family, alters family routines, and affects relationships among family members. How the family handles these changes has a significant impact on the effectiveness with which childhood diabetes is managed in the family context. This chapter addresses these issues from a developmental perspective by examining the changing developmental tasks of different-age children and their families. The second half of the chapter focuses on screening for common psychosocial concerns and provides guidance to practitioners for effective management of identified problems from a developmentally informed and family-centered perspective.

FAMILY-CENTERED DIABETES CARE

Because research consistently has documented that the family has a central role in the successful management and healthy outcomes of children and adolescents with type 1 diabetes (T1D), national and international standards of care assert that it is critical for diabetes care to be family-centered from diagnosis onward.[1,2] Parents have the ongoing and challenging task of balancing children's increasing needs for autonomy with the child's need for support with the complex daily regimen demanded of T1D. Parent support is a dynamic process and changes over time, as the child and family develop.[3] Therefore, it is imperative that diabetes clinicians assess for developmentally appropriate parental involvement and support for diabetes management (Table 12.1).

Table 12.1 Recommendations for the Diabetes Treatment Team at Diagnosis

- Give parent time to "grieve the diagnosis," normalize typical adjustment difficulties.
- Keep to a minimum the number of staff providing information and treatment.
- Conduct an initial risk screening (see Table 12.3) to help guide follow-up care.
- Provide all important information in a written format.
- Include all primary caregivers in the diabetes education program.
- In single-parent families, encourage another adult (e.g., grandparent, family friend) to support the parent.

DOI: 10.2337/9781580405096.12

CRISIS AT DIAGNOSIS

The diagnosis of diabetes in a child or adolescent hurls the parent from a secure and known reality into a frightening and foreign world. At diagnosis, parents grieve the loss of their healthy child and cope with such normal distress reactions as shock, disbelief and denial, fear, anger, and extreme blame or guilt. While grieving, however, parents are expected to acquire an understanding of the disease and to master the behavioral skills required to manage diabetes at home to achieve acceptable blood glucose control. At the time of diagnosis, parents should receive the support required from a well-meaning diabetes education and treatment team to begin coping with the emotional distress and to avoid being overwhelmed by unrealistic expectations (Table 12.2). Parents must find a sense of balance and should be encouraged to progress at their own pace, with emotional support offered by staff members or another parent.

DIABETES AND CHILD DEVELOPMENT

Diabetes presents family members with the task of being sensitive to the balance between the child's need for a sense of autonomy and mastery of self-care activities and the need for ongoing family support and involvement. The struggle to balance independence and dependence in relationships between the child and family members presents a long-term challenge and raises different issues for families at different stages of development. Focusing on normal developmental tasks at each stage of the child's growth and development provides the most effective structure with which to address this concern.

INFANTS AND TODDLERS WITH DIABETES: 0–3 YEARS OLD

At this earliest stage of child development, the parent is the only appropriate patient with respect to diabetes management. The primary developmental task during infancy is to achieve a stable, trusting relationship between infant and primary care provider. At this stage of development, two important aspects of diabetes care are *1*) how treatment responsibilities are shared between parents, or in a single-parent family to ensure that the single parent has support and relief from relentless caregiving; and *2*) the prevention of severe hypoglycemic episodes as well as extreme hyperglycemia. The latter issue relates to difficulties in administering and adjusting the small insulin doses needed by most infants and toddlers, as well as the preverbal child's inability to recognize and communicate symptoms of hypoglycemia.

The central task of the child from ages 1 to 3 years old is to establish an initial sense of mastery over the world. Toddlers do not have the cognitive skills to understand why cooperation with the intrusive, sometimes painful, procedures of the diabetic regimen is needed. Thus, injections or finger sticks for blood glucose monitoring may become battlegrounds when the toddler resists and will require significant emotional stamina from the parent. Achieving optimal glycemic control in this age range is further complicated by the young child's finicky eating habits, erratic physical activity, inability to well articulate wants or needs, and

Table 12.2 Developmental Factors in Family Management of Diabetes

Child Age	Views & Understanding of Diabetes	Developmental Considerations	Appropriate Responsibilities
5–8 years	Limited, concrete	Diabetes misconceptions are common	Cooperate with all diabetes-related tasks Tell parents if don't feel well
9–11 years	Matter-of-fact: they understand the details but not the implications	Concerns about fitting in Don't want to be seen as different Concerns about fairness: "It's not fair that I have diabetes; why me?"	Parent begins teaching child how to do some tasks if child is interested Okay for child to ask parent to do it Parent involves child in problem solving (e.g., by thinking aloud)
12–14 years	Complex thinking, but limited ability to apply it to real life	Struggles with sense of self: "Am I normal?" Puberty and growth hormone cause insulin resistance, making diabetes more difficult to manage Moodiness More concern about body image Increased peer pressure Increased conflict with parents	Young teen begins doing tasks with "supervised inter-dependence" Some young teens may not be ready at this age Parent helps young teen work through problems Parent works to limit diabetes conflict
14–17 years	Attain adult-level understanding, but poor judgment and self-control (especially "in the moment" and in social situations), overly focused on present	Increased independence, more time with friends, increased exposure to risks and risky opportunities Less willing to work with parents Take more risks (often for social acceptance)	Teen primary responsibility with continued parent oversight Parent helps teen set goals and problem solve Teen begins communicating with health care team Parent and teen work with diabetes team to plan for life with diabetes after high school Parent slowly fades out monitoring but steps back in if control worsens and asks, "What can I do to help?"
18 and older	Young adults still often lack the organizational/planning skills and make poor choices	Young adults often leave home with little preparation for independence Stage of multiple transitions (economic, geographic, social, emotional) and distractions make focus on diabetes management very challenging Many young adults are lost to follow-up as they transition into adult care	Young adult should be active participant in his or her health care Collaborative relationship with parent should now become collaborative relationship with health care provider Equal communication between patient and health care provider Significant others need diabetes education and contact with health care team

rapid growth. Treatment goals not only must be individualized to provide safe and effective medical treatment but also should permit the young child to master the normal developmental tasks of the toddler period of development.

Recently, continuous subcutaneous insulin infusion (CSII) therapy or "pump" therapy increasingly has been used in very young children with T1D. Several studies have shown that insulin pump therapy is a safe alternative to multiple daily insulin injections and may reduce the rate of severe hypoglycemic reactions among young children,[4-6] improving parents' quality of life. The application of technology to the care of very young children highlights the importance of individualizing treatment plans based on the characteristics of individual children and families. Parents will vary with respect to level of parental education and amount of time they can commit to the training required for pump and continuous glucose monitoring (CGM) therapies.

PRESCHOOL AND EARLY-ELEMENTARY SCHOOL CHILDREN: 4–7 YEARS OLD

Preschool, daycare, or kindergarten may represent the first arena in which both parents and children face the social consequences of diabetes, including the need to educate others about the disease. Separation problems that often appear at this age may be heightened in the child with diabetes. Children who are 4–7 years old are beginning to use cause–effect thinking. Thus, the young child with diabetes may blame himself or herself for having the disease or see injections and restrictions as punishments.

At this stage of development, the parent continues to be the primary recipient of diabetes education and the primary person to interact with the health care team. The child's increasing motor coordination and cognitive skills, however, enable him or her to become a more involved partner in certain aspects of diabetes care tasks. Some children can choose appropriate snacks, select and clean injection sites, and begin to identify symptoms of low blood glucose. The goal is for young elementary school–age children to be drawn positively into their own care without premature and unrealistic expectations for independence while parental control and supervision continue.

Insulin pump therapy increasingly has been used in 4- to 7-year-old children, and by decreasing hypoglycemia, and thus reducing stress for families of young children with diabetes, pump therapy has the potential to improve quality of life for families.[7,8] As with all management issues, the decision to start pump therapy or to use a CGM must be individualized to each family's lifestyle and abilities.

OLDER ELEMENTARY SCHOOL CHILDREN: 8–11 YEARS OLD

The preadolescent child forms close friendships with children of the same sex, strives to gain approval from this peer group, and seriously begins to evaluate himself or herself by comparing abilities to those of peers. Peer conformity often peaks at the latter end of this period,[9] driving some children to hide having diabetes out of fear of seeming "different." Children with diabetes, in the process of making these social comparisons, need to develop a strong positive self-image. Participation in activities with peers and positive self-image are key concepts at this age, and health care providers should emphasize to parents the importance of the child with diabetes participating in a wide range of activities with peers.

Parents should focus on realistic blood glucose goals and safety guidelines for prevention of hypoglycemia. That is, parent and child should be ready to increase monitoring of blood glucose and plan ahead for additional snacks with extra activity. It is important to continue emphasizing the long-term benefits of continued parent–child teamwork in diabetes care. Some children at this age can check blood glucose levels and give injections on occasion without supervision. Health care providers should begin to talk more directly with the child concerning issues and problems with diabetes rather than talking solely to the parents.

In contrast to the lack of large studies with younger children, more research has been conducted on how family environment variables relate to glycemic control among school-age children. One of the first studies of families with children with diabetes <12 years old reported that among school-age patients, more diabetes-related family guidance and control were associated with better metabolic outcomes, and diabetes-related parental warmth and caring were important for optimal outcomes.[10] Another early study documented that school-age children hospitalized with diabetic ketoacidosis (DKA) reported less diabetes-related parental warmth and caring.[11] Finally, family environments that are more structured and rule-governed also are associated with better glycemic control in school-age children with T1D.[12] In a study of parenting styles, regimen adherence, and glycemic control in 4- to 10-year-old children with T1D and their parents, "authoritative parenting" characterized by parental support and affection was related to better regimen adherence and glycemic control.[13] Non–diabetes-specific family factors, such as conflict, stress, and family cohesion, also have been linked to glycemic control and adherence (see Early Adolescence).[14]

Empirical studies support the conclusion that older school-age children who are given greater responsibility for their diabetes management make more mistakes in their self-care, are less adherent, and have poorer metabolic control than those whose parents are more involved.[15] From these studies, it has become increasingly clear that parental involvement in diabetes management is required throughout the school-age developmental period.[4]

EARLY ADOLESCENCE: 12–15 YEARS OLD

At this stage of development, dramatic changes typically occur in five areas:

■ Physical development
■ Family dynamics
■ School experiences
■ Cognitive development
■ Social networks

During all of these normal changes of early adolescence, the change in balance of responsibility for diabetes management tasks between the child and the family continues. It is common for families to change their expectations of the young adolescent and frequently "turn over" all responsibility for diabetes management. The physiological changes of puberty, however, which are associated with insulin resistance in both nondiabetic and diabetic adolescents, can complicate this transition. Reduced sensitivity to insulin probably contributes significantly to the difficulty experienced by many young adolescents in achieving optimal glycemic control.[16]

Young teenagers have an increasing cognitive ability to analyze themselves and the world around them and do not simply accept authority, but rather they examine, criticize, and question. This growing ability leads many young teenagers with diabetes to a new sensitivity about their disease (e.g., for the first time, they may vent their anger about having diabetes at parents). Parents and health care professionals frequently overestimate the young teenager's conceptual understanding of diabetes. Parents also can overestimate the young adolescent's ability to follow through with diabetes care tasks without immediate positive reinforcement and support, mistakenly assuming that long-term good health will provide motivation for adherence to the diabetes treatment plan.

Diabetes can further threaten the young teen's self-confidence. Fluctuating blood glucose levels that defy control contribute to teenagers feeling uneasy in their bodies. Insulin reactions, injections, and blood glucose monitoring can further undermine the teen's ability to feel attractive or normal.

Because puberty causes physiological barriers to controlling blood glucose[16] and because of the psychological and social vulnerabilities of this age, parents should continue involvement in and supervision of insulin administration and blood glucose monitoring throughout early adolescence. Negotiation of continued support and supervision is critical even if the young adolescent initially rejects it. Negative family interactions surrounding diabetes management contribute to adherence and metabolic control problems in adolescents with diabetes. The key is that both young adolescents and parents must redefine their roles and renegotiate a balance of responsibility for diabetes management that is acceptable to both parties.

Families also should be encouraged to begin changing their pattern of relationships with diabetes health care providers. Young teenagers often have issues that they do not feel comfortable discussing in front of parents (e.g., concerns about sexuality). Thus, health care providers should begin seeing parents and young teenagers individually as well as together. Young teenagers can be encouraged to come up with a list of diabetes-related questions or problems they have encountered to discuss with their provider.

Both young adolescents and their parents may benefit from contact with other families coping with similar struggles. Diabetes camps often provide an important forum for peer identification, and peer-group education and support programs may be helpful for their parents. Although young adolescents may demonstrate steady increases in diabetes knowledge and skills, as with school-age children, teens who experience more parent involvement, monitoring, and collaborative teamwork in diabetes management achieve and maintain better diabetes outcomes.[17]

LATER ADOLESCENCE AND YOUNG ADULTHOOD: 16–22 YEARS OLD

As physiological growth and change decrease and stabilize in later adolescence, parent–adolescent conflicts over diabetes self-care also decrease. The central developmental tasks of the older adolescent are outlined in Table 12.2.

Some older teenagers with diabetes who feel overwhelmed with the pressures of high school and the need to plan for the future may ignore their self-care. The poor metabolic control of some older teenagers reflects a chronic unmet need for more family support for self-care tasks. Poor control in a teenager can be a reflection of chaos and dysfunction at home. In these instances, more (not less) parental involvement may be needed. Family counseling can help parents and teenagers negotiate roles with respect to sharing diabetes management responsibilities.

Conflicts over friendships are often the cause of alienation between parents and teenagers. This is especially true when issues of alcohol and drugs, safety (driving), and sexual activity are raised. Unfortunately, adolescents are much more likely to make poor decisions when they are with friends,[18] and this can include decisions about diabetes management (e.g., going out with friends despite not having appropriate diabetes supplies with them). Helping older teenagers understand situations that are riskier for them, and helping them plan for these situations can help reduce some of the risk. On the other hand, peer difficulties and social conflict can have harmful effects on diabetes care.[19] Older teenage girls (and their parents) should receive preconception counseling. They should be educated about the importance of good metabolic control before conception and about the challenges of managing a pregnancy for a woman with T1D.[20]

During this stage of development, physical growth and the upheaval of puberty slow and insulin needs stabilize. Many older adolescent girls continue to be concerned about weight gain caused by insulin dose increases and a meal plan that provides many more calories than needed to meet the requirements of accelerated growth, potentially leading to insulin manipulation (see the section Disordered Eating).

By later adolescence, many teens have reached adult levels of intellectual functioning,[18] making them seem perfectly capable of taking the reins of diabetes management. The development of the frontal lobes—the areas of the brain that underlie judgment, decision making, and impulse control—continues into the mid- to late-20s. At the same time, socially motivated reward-seeking behavior mediated by developmental changes in limbic and striatal brain circuits also increases during this period.[18] A consequence of these divergent rates of normal brain development is that many adolescents may be quite knowledgeable about diabetes but are unable to put their knowledge consistently into practice. Teens are much more likely than adults to act first and think later, especially "in the heat of the moment" and when the action is tied to social reward. On the other hand, teens are more likely to weigh the pros and cons of risky behaviors (such as skipping insulin) and then *choose* the risky alternative under the assumption that "it isn't likely to hurt me this time."[21]

Older adolescents who experience more developmentally appropriate parental involvement, monitoring, and collaborative teamwork in diabetes management may be buffered partially from risky decision making, and they achieve and maintain better diabetes outcomes.[22] Over time, responsibility for diabetes management can be transitioned to them with the option for requesting continued support when needed. Care must be taken, however, when transitioning responsibility to adolescents who exhibit psychopathology, particularly depression,[23] conduct problems,[24] and eating disorders,[25] as these youth face far greater risk of poor diabetes outcomes and excessive health care utilization.

Finally, there is evidence that a negative developmental trajectory around diabetes management during adolescence may persist into early adulthood, accelerating the risk of long-term medical and psychological complications of diabetes.[26] During this period of development, which Levinson et al. (1978) called the "early adult transition,"[27] diabetes health care providers should collaborate with older adolescents and their parents to plan for "life with diabetes after high school."[28] Many adolescents who have lived with diabetes since early childhood have not learned essential diabetes consumer skills, such as understanding their health insurance and any changes that are anticipated in health insurance coverage, ordering diabetes care supplies, checking for expiration dates, and creating a "diabetes safety net."[22]

For some older teens and young adults, competing educational, economic, and social priorities detract from a focused commitment to diabetes management. In contrast to younger teens, many older adolescents and young adults believe they are more or less invulnerable to harm (especially if they have previously avoided serious acute complications of nonadherent behavior[21]). They also may have a tendency to reject adult control, and this further limits receptiveness to changes in diabetes treatment. Therefore, it may be unrealistic to expect the older adolescent and young adult with diabetes to intensify their glycemic control, or even to transition to a new adult diabetes provider without sufficient support and efforts to address any barriers to access to diabetes care.[22]

CLINICAL ISSUES AND SUGGESTIONS FOR ASSESSMENT AND MANAGEMENT

Children and adolescents with T1D are at significantly higher risk for developing an array of psychosocial and mental health concerns. Mental health complications are arguably *the* leading morbidity in children with T1D, with overall prevalence falling roughly between 40–50%.[29,30] Rates of subthreshold problems that do not meet full diagnostic criteria for a mental health disorder are likely even higher. Both the American Diabetes Association[1] and the International Society for Pediatric and Adolescent Diabetes[2] have called for regular psychosocial screening of all patients with T1D, starting at the time of diagnosis and continuing on a regular basis during routine care.

PSYCHOSOCIAL RISK SCREENING AT DIABETES DIAGNOSIS

When a child is newly diagnosed with T1D, it can feel as if the family's whole world has been turned upside-down. Most children and families eventually find their feet and adapt well to life with diabetes, but some do not. Children with adjustment difficulties at the time of diagnosis are at significantly greater risk for subsequent problems with depression and anxiety.[31,32] Children with psychosocial and sociodemographic risk factors at diagnosis (Table 12.3) have greater probability of poorer glycemic control, diabetes-related emergency room visits, and DKA in the first 4 years following diagnosis, with glycemic control being poorest for children with both types of risk.[33]

Table 12.3 Indications for Additional Psychological Support at Diagnosis

■ Single-parent families, families with an unemployed primary caregiver
■ Preexisting child behavior, mood, or social problems
■ Preexisting family conflict, poor communication between family members
■ Anticipated family conflict over diabetes management
■ High parent stress or anxiety
■ Other family member with a serious chronic physical or mental illness
■ Infants and toddlers with T1D

Early identification of high-risk patients is critical to efforts at health promotion. Child behavioral and psychological problems can be targeted for empirically supported therapies with the potential to prevent deterioration in diabetes control as well as reduce presenting concerns,[34] and families with socioeconomic risk can be provided with additional resources and support.[35,36] Many health care providers worry that diabetes diagnosis is the worst time to ask families about their psychological functioning. In fact, most families appreciate having someone talk to them about these issues and help them manage the stress of having a child with a new diagnosis of diabetes. We documented a 97% participation rate in a psychosocial screening conducted at diagnosis, and follow-up interviews found high levels of satisfaction with the service.[37] The Risk Index for Poor Glycemic Control is a nine-item screening tool (available on request) developed to assess psychosocial concerns at the time of diabetes diagnosis. The index has good sensitivity and specificity for identifying moderate- and high-risk patients, with each 1-point increase in score associated with an absolute increase in risk for poor glycemic control of ~10%, making the index a practical tool for use in routine care. (A comprehensive training manual and supervisor's guide for psychosocial risk screening of children and youth newly diagnosed with type 1 diabetes are available for free download at www.mededportal.org/publication/9643.

PSYCHOSOCIAL SCREENING AND MANAGEMENT DURING ROUTINE FOLLOW-UP

It is equally important to screen annually for psychosocial difficulties during regular clinic visits to catch later emerging problems. For example, depression and anxiety often do not arise until 1–2 years after diagnosis,[31] and problems with adherence often first appear 3–4 years after diagnosis.[38] The remainder of this chapter reviews the major psychological complications of diabetes and provides guidance for screening and management of the most prevalent or concerning problems (Table 12.4).

Depression

Depression is among the most common mental health concerns for youth with diabetes, with a prevalence nearly double that of youth in general and much higher rates in girls than boys.[39] It is strongly associated with poor illness management and glycemic control. Diabetes burnout (see Adherence Problems) some-

Table 12.4 Indications for Additional Psychological Support Postdiagnosis

- Failure to master the tasks of normal child or adolescent development
- School-related difficulties (school failure, excessive absences)
- Behavior problems, substance use, problems with the legal system
- Symptoms of depression or anxiety, excessive concern about weight
- Parent–child conflict over diabetes care
- Diabetes burnout, lack of cooperation with management tasks
- Any unexplained episode of DKA postdiagnosis
- Repeated hospitalizations for hypoglycemia in a 1-year period
- Weight loss with chronic hyperglycemia (elevated A1C), especially in adolescent girls
- Life crisis, such as divorce or death of a family member
- Suspicion of child sexual, physical, or emotional abuse or neglect, which should be reported immediately to legal authorities

times can look like depression: During a clinic visit, youths may seem sullen and withdrawn, or act distressed or irritable when diabetes is brought up. Further questioning, however, will reveal that the distress is specific to diabetes and does not extend to other areas of their lives.

How to screen and what to do with identified problems. Peyrot and Rubin (2007)[40] suggest using the following two questions to screen for depression: During the past 2 weeks,

- Have you felt down, depressed, or hopeless?
- Have you lost pleasure or interest in doing things?

A positive response to either question should prompt referral for further assessment, ideally by a pediatric health psychologist who has experience working with youth with diabetes. Psychiatric evaluation would be indicated for more severe symptoms. When referring patients for therapy, it is important to advise parents to seek out practitioners who follow principles of evidence-based practice and use empirically supported treatments, as not all mental health treatments are equally helpful. Cognitive behavioral therapy (CBT) is the only well-established treatment for depression in children, while both CBT and interpersonal therapy are well established for adolescents. Antidepressant medication has proven efficaciousness for moderate and severe depression, especially when coupled with CBT.

Clinicians can help youth with milder symptoms of depression by probing for the youth's thoughts about diabetes. Many children experience hopelessness around diabetes because they have incorrect or unhelpful beliefs or engage in negative self-talk. For example, you can ask, "What do you say to yourself when [a diabetes task] is not going well?"[40] Examples of negative and unrealistic thinking include the following:

- "If I don't get diabetes under control now, I'll never get it under control."
- "Unless I keep my blood glucose between 90 and 110, I'll develop horrible complications."
- "I'll never get my diabetes under control, so why bother?"
- "I'm a failure because my blood glucose levels are so consistently high."

Youth with diabetes can be helped to become aware of any negative self-talk they engage in, and unrealistic or overly black-and-white views can be challenged gently. Information about the normal ups and down of diabetes can be helpful. Many people do not realize that it is common for some children with diabetes to have quite variable blood glucose levels, with the result that the child gets blamed (and blames him or herself) for highs and lows. Children or parents who expect "perfect" control place themselves at risk for failure, frustration, and burnout. Other children and parents fear that complications can result from just a few moderately high blood glucose readings and panic at any out-of-range value. Children with diabetes do best when families view out-of-range numbers as problems to be solved and approach the task in a collaborative manner.

Behavior Problems

Children with diabetes and behavior problems are at high risk for problems with regimen adherence and poor glycemic control. These children are more likely to resist cooperating with parent requests to participate in management tasks such as blood glucose monitoring. The impact of child behavior problems can be especially acute in low-income and single-parent families.[37] In younger children, underlying mood problems or anxiety often manifest as behavior problems and only differentiate over time.[32] Children with behavior problems also tend to have more conflict with parents, another factor strongly associated with poorer diabetes management and control (see below).

How to screen and what to do with identified problems. Our clinic screens for behavior problems by asking parents, "Do you have any concerns about your child's behavior: defying you, not doing what you say, arguing, or fighting?" Affirmative responses are followed up by asking, "Is this a significant concern for you, or do you think it can have a significant impact on your child or diabetes management?"

Discrete, mild behavior problems (e.g., tantrums, whining) potentially can be managed in the office. Clinicians can assess the ABCs—the Antecedent or trigger for the behavior, the Behavior itself, and the Consequence—and then work with the family to change this cycle. The goal is to decrease problem behaviors by removing their rewarding consequences (e.g., the child avoids a blood glucose check by having a tantrum) and increasing desired behaviors through reinforcement (e.g., providing small rewards for cooperating).

Referral to a behavioral health specialist is indicated for children with more significant behavior problems, or behavior problems in the context of less stable family environments. Behavior therapy focused on improving parent behavior management skills has the strongest research support for children, whereas behavioral family therapy has good support for adolescents.[41] Children engaging in risky behaviors such as alcohol or drug use or unsafe sex also should be referred to a mental health expert. CBT, motivational interviewing, and family therapy are all empirically supported interventions for substance abuse.

Family Conflict

Family conflict around diabetes management is one of the strongest predictors of poor adherence and poor glycemic control.[14] High levels of conflict that precede diabetes diagnosis predict poorer glycemic control over the next 4 years.[42] Conversely, children living in supportive family environments with a high level of parent involvement generally have better adherence and glycemic control.[43] Conflict is especially common in families with teenagers, given the developmentally appropriate drive for greater autonomy in adolescence. Research suggests, however, that having a greater *amount* of parent involvement does not lead to greater conflict; instead, it appears to be the *type and quality* of involvement that determines whether it is perceived by the adolescent as helpful or intrusive.[14] How families communicate around diabetes is a major determinant of their ability to work together. When communication is highly negative ("shaming and blaming"), involves sarcasm or yelling, or is dishonest (e.g., lying about blood glucose values), teamwork is nearly impossible to maintain and conflict ensues. Interventions to improve teamwork therefore typically revolve around improving communication.

Diabetes clinicians can foster family teamwork around diabetes management without undermining adolescents' attempts at achieving greater independence. Parents can be encouraged to view teamwork as a way to teach and empower their child to become a more active participant in his or her care. Families can schedule regular meetings to discuss "the week in diabetes" in a calm, open, and respectful manner, and engage in collaborative problem solving around any identified concerns. Some parents argue that their continued involvement keeps the child overly dependent on them, without recognizing that for many youth the problem-solving skills needed for independence need to be taught and practiced, and that maintaining a good working relationship provides parents with the best forum for teaching these skills.

How to screen and what to do with identified problems. Family conflict can be screened by asking the parent and child the following questions:

- Do you have any concerns about conflict in your family (i.e., fighting or arguing between family members)?
- Do you fight with your [parent/child] about following any part of the diabetes management plan (e.g., blood glucose checks, taking insulin, following meal plan, coming to clinic)?

If conflict is restricted to only one adherence behavior, it might provide a good opportunity to help the family problem solve that specific issue. Clinicians can use the following approach to help families manage mild to moderate diabetes-related conflict:

- Help family members define the problem (the more specific, the better).
- Focus on small, incremental changes in *behavior* (not on blood glucose outcomes).
- Agree on a plan, discuss potential barriers, and create a written "contract" outlining everyone's responsibilities and how progress toward goals will be measured.
- Encourage family members to communicate in ways that are positive and supportive (versus critical or judgmental), and to listen to each other.

Families with more general, significant, or intractable conflict can be referred for behavioral family therapy. Interventions such as behavioral family systems therapy[44] and multisystemic therapy[45] have demonstrated clinically significant effects on behavioral and psychological outcomes and more modest improvements in glycemic outcomes. In general, approaches that involve working on communication and problem-solving skills and focus specifically on diabetes-related issues appear to be most effective.[46]

Disordered Eating

In U.S. culture, there is tremendous pressure on youth (especially girls) to stay thin, so weight concerns are almost ubiquitous among teens. For the child with diabetes, weight concerns pose an additional hazard, as many will begin to secretly reduce their insulin as a way to purge calories and lose weight. This self-destructive behavior is a form of bulimia nervosa, and it can cause repeated hospitalizations for DKA. There is evidence that intentional insulin omission may be extremely common. For example, the Hvidøre Study[47] found that more than 90% of 2,062 adolescents with T1D reported intentionally omitting insulin at least once per month to control their weight.

How to screen and what to do with identified problems. Warning signs of disordered eating in youth with diabetes include the following:

- Repeated DKA or unexplained chronic hyperglycemia
- Unrealistic concerns about weight and body image
- Excessive dieting or exercise
- Amenorrhea
- Refusal to give insulin under supervision or let parent see glucometer or pump log

Adolescents with diabetes can be screened routinely for eating disorder with the question, "Do you ever take less insulin than you should?"[48] Affirmative answers can trigger referral to a pediatric psychologist. Unfortunately, there are currently no well-established interventions for bulimia, although CBT has been shown to be promising in nondiabetic girls. For girls with diabetes and disordered eating, a multidisciplinary approach has been recommended involving coordinated care among a psychologist, endocrinologist, nurse educator, and a nutritionist.[48]

Adherence Problems

Adherence to a medical regimen involves more than just following physician instructions; it requires actively maintaining a whole new suite of complex and demanding behaviors that can greatly disrupt children's daily lives. It also places a substantial burden on parents. Therefore, it is not uncommon for children and families to struggle with one or more aspects of the diabetes regimen, with overall prevalence of nonadherence estimated at ~50%.[49] The impact of nonadherence is dramatic. Children who do not complete diabetes-monitoring tasks at recommended levels have much poorer glycemic control. Missing insulin is the primary cause of life-threatening DKA in children with established diabetes.[50] Nonadherence also increases medical costs, largely through increased hospitalizations.[51,52]

Poor adherence is not a characteristic of a patient in isolation; instead, it is a multidimensional problem including the health care team, characteristics of the illness and treatment regimen, patient-related variables, and family interactions.[53] Moreover, adherence is not an "all or none" behavior. Children may be partly adherent (e.g., checking blood glucose once per day instead of four times per day) or adherent to one management task but not another. This is an important clinical consideration, as it is much easier to address a specific behavior than to treat a vague and poorly defined "nonadherence." It is also more acceptable to adolescents. Youth will have less difficulty acknowledging that it is hard for them to do a specific task and to discuss possible solutions; in contrast, simply being told they are "noncompliant" or "doing a poor job" likely will demoralize them further.

Adherence is also a primary determinant of treatment effectiveness, and physicians who do not have reliable information about a patient's level of adherence will find themselves "prescribing in the dark." Children who are not completing management tasks at expected levels often feel guilty and ashamed, or they fear being chastised or punished by parents or health care providers. There is a strong impetus to falsify results or lie about what tasks have been completed. Fostering a supportive atmosphere that allows youth to share management-related problems and mistakes without risk of being blamed is one of the best ways to improve the quality of the information you receive and foster a sense of teamwork around diabetes care.

Diabetes burnout is a common presentation of youth struggling with adherence. Burned-out youth have become overwhelmed with the daily requirements of diabetes management and become frustrated with the challenges of keeping blood glucose within range. They come to feel helpless about controlling diabetes and hopeless about their long-term health, and as a result, their self-care dramatically declines. Children who have prematurely been given too much responsibility for diabetes management are at especially high risk.

Many health care providers, when counseling a teenager with adherence difficulties, will stress the most frightening complications of poor glycemic control (e.g., organ failure, limb loss, death) in the hope that this information will motivate behavior change. Unfortunately, substantial research indicates that these well-meaning efforts are often ineffective and may even backfire. Information intended to "scare teens straight" can result in heightened feelings of vulnerability and avoidance of fear-inducing diabetes-related cues (such as a glucometer or insulin pen). Stressing risks also plays into many teenagers' tendency to weigh the risks of a dangerous behavior against its benefits.[21] Teens frequently will choose a risky behavior that has a low probability of negative outcome (however catastrophic) and a high probability of immediate benefit (in contrast to adults, who tend to categorically avoid serious risk).[21] For example, a teen may decide to reduce her insulin to lose weight, accepting the risk of possible complications in the future. Although it is important to ensure that teens understand potential complications, efforts to foster behavior change are likely to be more effective if they stress the immediate benefits of adherence (e.g., having more energy or better skin) rather than potential long-term consequences.

How to screen and what to do with identified problems. Screening for nonadherence can be challenging, as youth often are motivated to hide adherence difficulties. Still, adherence problems can be screened in the office by asking the child and parent separately:

- How often do you [does your child] check blood glucose?
- Do you [does your child] ever miss taking or receiving an insulin dose?
- Do you [does your child] ever take or receive less insulin than prescribed?

■ Do you [does your child] ever eat more than what is on the meal plan without taking extra insulin?

Checking blood glucose less than three times per day, missing insulin, or eating without covering extra carbohydrates with insulin should trigger additional assessment, either through supportive discussion of potential barriers to completing the behavior at recommended levels or by referral to a pediatric psychologist. Diabetes burnout can be screened by asking the following questions:[40]

■ Do you feel overwhelmed or burned out by the demands of diabetes management?
■ Do you get the support you need from your family for diabetes management?

Ways to help prevent or reduce burnout during routine clinic visits include the following:

■ Acknowledging the difficulties inherent in living with diabetes and taking a positive view of the child's and family's attempts to manage diabetes.
■ Focusing on problem solving to foster self-efficacy for diabetes management.
■ Encouraging family teamwork around diabetes management.

If the child maintains a persistently negative view of diabetes or him- or herself, or the family cannot come together around helping the child manage diabetes, referral to a pediatric psychologist would be recommended. Further assessment also may be warranted if the child has insufficient support for diabetes care. Empirically supported interventions for nonadherence include behavior modification; training in diabetes-specific social skills, coping skills, and problem solving; and stress management. Motivational interviewing and telemedicine also have shown promise. In addition, studies have shown the benefits of preventive strategies, such as an office-based intervention designed to promote parent–teen teamwork in diabetes management (for a review, see[46]).

Neurocognitive Difficulties

Self-management is more challenging for children with neurocognitive difficulties, making support and oversight from their parents and health care providers even more important. Children with poor *executive functioning* (i.e., problems with organization and planning, thinking before acting, and changing behavior in response to consequences or feedback) can have an especially difficult time managing diabetes.[54, 55]

Complicating the situation, children with diabetes are at risk for developing mild to moderate executive dysfunction, attention problems, and slower processing speed as early as 2 years postdiagnosis.[56] The following risk factors are known to increase a child's vulnerability to neurocognitive decline:

■ Early onset of diabetes (i.e., in the first 5–7 years of life)
■ DKA, especially DKA with cerebral edema and recurrent DKA
■ Diabetic retinopathy and other microvascular complications
■ Profound hypoglycemia

Several other risk factors may increase risk for cognitive decline, although findings have been mixed. These include severe hyperglycemia at diagnosis, chronic hyperglycemia, recurrent moderate to severe hypoglycemia, and highly variable blood glucose. Boys appear to be more vulnerable than girls (for reviews, see [56,57]).

How to screen and what to do with identified problems. There are currently no validated scales for screening neurocognitive disability in children with diabetes. Simply asking parents how the child is doing in school often is inaccurate and generally uninformative. We therefore developed a brief screener for cognitive complaints for use in our clinic (Table 12.5). Any response of yes or definite problem should be followed up by asking—

- Is the problem new or has it been evident for a while (e.g., >6 months)?
- Has this problem ever been evaluated by anyone else?
- Does your child receive any special services at school?

Identified problems not currently being treated can trigger referral to an appropriate specialist: a psychologist or neuropsychologist (items 1–6), speech or language pathologist (item 7 in isolation), or occupational therapist (item 8 in isolation). If learning problems (item 2) involve academic skills, you might advise the parent to request an evaluation through the child's school. Long-standing attention problems (item 6) raise concern about possible attention deficit–hyperactivity disorder (ADHD) and can be followed up with a brief symptom inventory such as the Vanderbilt ADHD Diagnostic Rating Scales (available at www.brightfutures.org). Positive screens on the Vanderbilt would support referral for behavioral intervention, environmental changes (e.g., 504 Plan at school), and/or consideration of pharmacological management.

Table 12.5—Cognitive Concerns Screening Questionnaire

Do you [does your child] currently have any difficulty with:	No/None	Maybe/ Some	Yes/Definite Problem
Comprehension or understanding?	☐	☐	☐
Learning new information?	☐	☐	☐
Remembering things she or he has already learned?	☐	☐	☐
Remembering to do things she or he is supposed to do?	☐	☐	☐
Thinking or working more slowly than other children his or her age?	☐	☐	☐
Paying attention or concentrating?	☐	☐	☐
Putting thoughts into words, or saying things that do not make sense?	☐	☐	☐
Fine-motor skills (e.g., handwriting, tying, fastening clothes)?	☐	☐	☐

CONCLUSION

Developmental and family factors have a huge impact on diabetes management during childhood and adolescence. Encouraging a collaborative approach in which level of parental support is matched to a child's developmental readiness has the greatest potential for fostering effective diabetes management while helping inoculate against burnout and other psychological sequelae (Table 12.6). Health care providers can model this approach in their relationship with children and families by communicating clearly, asking questions, listening closely, and working together with the family to identify, problem solve, and work through any difficulties in a collaborative fashion.

Table 12.6—Fostering a Positive Approach to Diabetes

- Encourage family teamwork around diabetes management. Explain that working together provides parents with the best opportunity for teaching independence skills.
- Focus on behaviors not outcomes. People with diabetes can change their behavior, but changing metabolic outcomes may or may not be within their control.
- Encourage realistic expectations. Goals should be reachable. For example, a goal to increase glucose checks from once per day to four times per day is probably unrealistic and sets the child up for failure. Start small and "raise the bar" over time.
- Focus on successes (even small successes) not failures. Build on incremental improvements by providing positive feedback to the child and family for any attempts at improving management. If a child does not realize a goal, consider that it may have been unrealistic for the child at that time or that not enough support was given for success. Help the family identify possible barriers to success.
- Reframe mistakes (e.g., forgetting to take insulin) as opportunities for problem solving.
- Avoid using value-laden language (e.g., "good or bad" blood glucose levels). Children will often hide "bad" results so they do not get in trouble. Counsel families to view all information as good information—without accurate information you are managing diabetes blindly. The only bad information is information that is inaccurate or kept hidden.

REFERENCES

1. Silverstein J, Klingensmith G, Copeland K, Plotnick L, Kaufman F, Laffel L, Deeb L, Grey M, Anderson B, Holzmeister L, Clark N, American Diabetes Association. Care of children and adolescents with type 1 diabetes. *Diabetes Care* 2005;28:186–212.

2. ISPAD Clinical Practice Consensus Guidelines 2009 Compendium. *Pediatr Diabetes* 2009;10(Suppl 12):1–210.

3. Anderson BJ. Children with diabetes mellitus and family functioning: translating research into practice. *J Pediatr Endocrin Metab* 2001;14:645–652.

4. Anderson BJ, Brackett J. Diabetes in children. In *Psychology in Diabetes Care*. 2nd ed. F Snoek, TC Skinner, Eds. West Sussex, U.K., John Wiley & Sons, 2005, p. 1–25.

5. Shehadeh N, Battelino T, Galatzer A, Naveh T, Hadash A, de Vries L, Phillip M. Insulin pump therapy for 1-6 year old children with type 1 diabetes. *Isr Med Assoc J* 2004;6:284–286.

6. Weinzimer SA, Swan KL, Sikes KA, Ahern JH. Emerging evidence for the use of insulin pump therapy in infants, toddlers, and preschool-aged children with type 1 diabetes. *Pediatr Diabetes* 2006;7:15–19.

7. Jeha GS, Karaviti LP, Anderson BJ, Smith EO, Donaldson, S, McGirk TS, Haymond MW. Insulin pump therapy in preschool children with type 1 diabetes mellitus improves glycemic control and decreases glucose excursions and the risk of hypoglycemia. *Diabetes Technol Ther* 2005;7:876–884.

8. Tubina-Rufi N, de Lonlay P, Bloch J, Czernichow P. Remission of severe hypoglycemic incidents in young diabetic children treated with subcutaneous infusion. *Arch Pediatr* 1996;3:969–976.

9. Steinberg L, Monahan K. Age differences in resistance to peer influence. *Dev Psychol* 2007;43:1531–1543.

10. Waller D, Chipman JJ, Hardy BW, Hightower MS, North AJ, Williams SB, Babick AJ. Measuring diabetes-specific family support and its relation to metabolic control: A preliminary report. *J Am Acad Child Psychol* 1986;25:415–418.

11. Marteau TM, Bloch S, Baum JD. Family life and diabetic control. *J Child Psychol Psychiat* 1987;28:823–833.

12. Hauser ST, Jacobson AM, Lavori P, Wolfsdorf JI, Herskowitz RD, Milley JE, Bliss R, Gelfand E, Wertlieb D, Stein J. Adherence among children and adolescents with insulin dependent diabetes mellitus over four-year longitudinal follow-up. II: immediate and long-term linkages with the family milieu. *J Pediat Psychol* 1990;15:527–542.

13. Davis CL, Delamater AM, Shaw KH, LaGreca AM, Eidson MS, Perez-Rodriguez JE. Parenting styles, regimen adherence, and glycemic control in 4-10-year-old children with diabetes. *J. Pediatr Psychol* 2001; 26:123–129.

14. Anderson BJ: Family conflict and diabetes management in youth: clinical lessons from child development and diabetes research. *Diabetes Spectrum* 2004;17:22–26.

15. Wysocki T, Taylor A, Housh BS, Linsheid TR, Yeates KO, Naglieri JA. Deviation from developmentally appropriate self-care autonomy: association with diabetes outcomes. *Diabetes Care* 1996;19:119–125.

16. Amiel SA, Sherwin RS, Simonson DC, Lauritano AA. Tamborlane WV. Impaired insulin action in puberty: a contributing factor to poor glycemic control in adolescent with diabetes. *N Engl J Med* 1986;315:215–219.

17. Laffel LMB, Vangsness L, Connell A, Goebel-Fabbri A, Butler D, Anderson B. Impact of ambulatory family-focused teamwork intervention on glycemic control in youth with type 1 diabetes *J. Pediatr* 2003;142:409-416.

18. Steinberg L. Risk-taking in adolescence: new perspectives from brain and behavioral science. *Curr Dir Psychol Sci* 2007;16:55–59.

19. Palladino DK, Helgeson VS. Friends or foes? A review of peer influence on self-care and glycemic control in adolescents with type 1 diabetes. *J Pediat Psychol* 2012;37(5):591–603.

20. Fischl AF, Herman WH, Sereika SM, Hannan M, Becker D, Mansfield MJ, Freytag LL, Milaszewski K, Botscheller AN, Charron-Prochownik D. Impact of a preconception counseling program for teens with type 1 diabetes (READY-Girls) on patient-provider interaction, resource utilization, and cost. *Diabetes Care* 2010;33:701–705.

21. Reyna VF, Farley F. Risk and rationality in adolescent decision making: implications for theory, practice, and public policy. *Psychol Sci in the Public Interest* 2006;7(1):1–44.

22. Wolpert HA, Anderson BJ, Weissberg-Benchell J. *Transitions in Care: Meeting the Challenges of Type 1 Diabetes in Young Adults*. Alexandria, VA, American Diabetes Association, 2009.

23. McGrady ME, Hood KK. Depressive symptoms in adolescents with type 1 diabetes: associations with longitudinal outcomes: *Diabetes Res & Clin Pract* 2010;88:e35–e37.

24. Northam EA, Matthews LK, Anderson PJ, Cameron FJ, Werther GA. Psychiatric morbidity and health outcomes in type 1 diabetes – perspectives from a prospective longitudinal study. *Diabet Med* 2005;22:152-157.

25. Bryden KS, Neil A, Mayou RA, Peveler RC, Fairburn CG, Dunger DB. Eating habits, body weight, and insulin misuse: a longitudinal study of teenagers and young adults with type 1 diabetes. *Diabetes Care* 1999;22:1956–1960.

26. Bryden KS, Dunger DB, Mayou RA, Peveler RC, Neil HA. Poor prognosis of young adults with type 1 diabetes: a longitudinal study. *Diabetes Care* 2003;26:1052–1075.

27. Levinson DJ. *The Seasons of a Man's Life*. New York, Ballantine, 1978.

28. Peters A, Laffel L. The American Diabetes Association Transitions Working Group. Diabetes care for emerging adults: Recommendations for transition from pediatric to adult diabetes care systems. *Diabetes Care* 2011;34:2477–2488.

29. Cameron FJ, Northam EA, Ambler G, Daneman D. Routine psychological screening in youth with type 1 diabetes and their parents: a notion whose time has come? *Diabetes Care* 2007;30:2716–2724.

30. Cameron, F J, Northam EA. Screening for psychological disorders in youth with type 1 diabetes: who, when, what and how? *Diabetes Management* 2012;2(6):513–520.

31. Grey M, Cameron M, Lipman TH, Thurber FW. Psychosocial status of children with diabetes in the first 2 years after diagnosis. *Diabetes Care* 1995;18:1330–1336.

32. Northam EA, Matthews LK, Anderson PJ, Cameron FJ, Werther GA. Psychiatric morbidity and health outcome in type 1 diabetes: perspectives from a prospective longitudinal study. *Diabet Med* 2005;22:152–157.

33. Schwartz DD, Axelrad ME, Anderson BJ. A psychosocial risk index for poor glycemic control in children and adolescents with type 1 diabetes. *Pediatric Diabetes*. Advance online publication. DOI: 10.1111/pedi. 12084.

34. Winkley K, Landau S, Eisler I, Ismail K. Psychological interventions to improve glycaemic control in patients with type 1 diabetes: systematic review and meta-analysis of randomised controlled trials. *BMJ* 2006;333(7558):65–69.

35. Kazak A. Pediatric psychosocial preventative health model (PPPHM): Research, practice and collaboration in pediatric family systems medicine. *Fam Syst Health* 2006;24:381–395.

36. Schwartz DD, Axelrad ME, Cline VD, Anderson BJ. A model psychosocial screening program for children and youth with newly diagnosed type 1 diabetes: implications for psychologists across contexts of care. *Professional Psychol Res Pract* 2011;42(4):324–330.

37. Schwartz DD, Cline VD, Axelrad ME, Anderson BJ. Feasibility, acceptability, and predictive validity of a psychosocial screening program for children and youth newly diagnosed with type 1 diabetes. *Diabetes Care* 2011;34:326–331.

38. Kovacs M, Goldston D, Obrosky S, Iyengar S. Prevalence and predictors of pervasive non-compliance with medical treatment among youths with insulin-dependent diabetes mellitus. *J Am Acad Child Adol Psychiatry* 1992;31:1112–1119.

39. Hood KK, Huestis S, Maher A, Butler D, Volkening L, Laffel LM. Depressive symptoms in children and adolescents with type 1 diabetes: association with diabetes-specific characteristics. *Diabetes Care* 2006;29:1389–1391.

40. Peyrot M, Rubin RR. Behavioral and psychosocial interventions in diabetes: a conceptual review. *Diabetes Care* 2007;30(10):2433–2440.

41. Eyberg SM, Nelson MM, Boggs SR. Evidence-based psychosocial treatments for child and adolescent with disruptive behavior. *J Clin Child Adolesc Psychol* 2008;37:215–237.

42. Schwartz DD, Axelrad ME, Anderson BJ. A psychosocial risk index for poor glycemic control in children and adolescents with type 1 diabetes. *Pediatric Diabetes 2013*. DOI: 10.1111/pedi.12084.

43. Lewin A B, Heidgerken A D, Geffken G R, Williams LB, Storch E A, Gelfand KM, Silverstein, JH. The relation between family factors and metabolic control: the role of diabetes adherence. *J Pediatr Psychol* 2006;31:174–183.

44. Wysocki T, Harris MA, Buckloh LM, et al. Effects of behavioral family systems therapy for diabetes on adolescents' family relationships, treatment adherence, and metabolic control. *J Pediatr Psychol* 2006;31:928–938.

45. Ellis DA, Frey MA, Narr-King S, Templin T, Cunningham P, Cakan N. Use of multisystemic therapy to improve regimen adherence among adolescents with type 1 diabetes in chronic poor metabolic control: a randomized controlled trial. *Diabetes Care* 2005;28:1604–1610.

46. Anderson B J, Svoren, B, Laffel, L. Initiatives to promote effective self-care skills in children and adolescents with diabetes mellitus. *Disease Management & Health Outcomes* 2007;15(2):101–108.

47. Skovlund SE, de Beaufort C, Skinner TC, Swift P, on behalf of the Hvidøre Study Group. Insulin omission and glycaemic control in adolescents with type 1 diabetes from 21 international centers [Abstract]. Berlin, ISPAD, 2007.

48. Goebel-Fabbri AE. Disturbed eating behaviors and eating disorders in type 1 diabetes: clinical significance and treatment recommendations. *Current Diabetes Reports* 2009;9:133–139.

49. Rapoff MA. *Adherence to Pediatric Medical Regimens.* 2nd ed. New York, Springer, 2010.

50. Wolfsdorf J, Craig ME, Daneman D, Dunger D, Edge J, Lee W, Rosenbloom A, Sperling M, Hanas R. Diabetic ketoacidosis in children and adolescents with diabetes. *Pediatr Diabetes* 2009;10:118–133.

51. Maldonado M, Chong E, Oehl M, Balasubramanyam A: Economic impact of diabetic ketoacidosis in a multiethnic indigent population: analysis of costs based on the precipitating cause. *Diabetes Care* 2006;26:1265–1269.

52. Svoren B, Butler D, Levine B, Anderson B, Laffel L. Reducing acute adverse outcomes in youth with type 1 diabetes mellitus: a randomized controlled trial. *Pediatrics* 2003;112:914–922.

53. Sabaté E. Adherence to Long-Term Therapies: Evidence for Action. Geneva, World Health Organization, 2003.

54. Bagner DM, Williams LB, Geffken GR, Silverstein JH, Storch EA. Type 1 diabetes in youth: the relationship between adherence and executive functioning. *Child Health Care* 2007;36:169–179.

55. McNally K, Rohan J, Pendley JS, Delamater A, Drotar D. Executive functioning, treatment adherence, and glycemic control in children with type 1 diabetes. *Diabetes Care* 2010;33:1159–1162.

56. Northam EA, Rankins D, Cameron FJ. Therapy insight: the impact of type 1 diabetes on brain development and function. *Nat Clin Pract Neurol* 2006:2(2):78–86.

57. McCrimmon RJ, Ryan CM, Frier BM. Diabetes and cognitive dysfunction *Lancet* 2012;379:2291–2299.

Chapter 13

Gestational Diabetes Mellitus: Diagnostic Criteria and Epidemiology

Shubhada Jagasia, MD, MMHC

INTRODUCTION

Gestational diabetes mellitus (GDM) is defined as diabetes diagnosed during pregnancy that is not clearly overt diabetes.[1] Several epidemiologic studies have shown an increased risk of maternal and fetal complications associated with abnormal blood glucoses during pregnancy.[2-6] The recent Hyperglycemia and Adverse Pregnancy Outcomes (HAPO) has suggested that GDM be defined as "the condition of maternal hyperglycemia less severe than that found in overt diabetes but associated with an increased risk of adverse pregnancy outcomes."[7] The incidence of this diagnosis has increased in parallel with that of type 2 diabetes (T2D). Women with GDM have a higher lifetime risk of developing diabetes and preventive efforts at the outset may have a significant impact on disease progression and likely prevention. Recent literature has suggested an increased prevalence of long-term metabolic complications in babies born to women with gestational diabetes, due to which improved glycemic control in pregnancy may have future health implications for both mother and baby.

PREVALENCE

The prevalence varies from 4 to 14%. Studies have shown that over the past several years, the prevalence of GDM has increased by 10–100%, more so in minority ethnicities.[8-10] One study performed in an overweight and obese multiethnic population showed that the GDM incidence was 41.1% overall, 15.1% among Asians and Pacific Islanders, 39.1% among Hispanics, 41.2% among non-Hispanic Whites, 50.4% among non-Hispanic Blacks, and 52.8% among American Indians.[11] Several contextual factors such as age, BMI, racial mix, use of health care services, health insurance status, and availability of GDM preventive resources play an important role. Most GDM studies have used "prevalence" and "incidence" interchangeably, although prevalence has been used more often. Several methodological challenges emerge when population data are reviewed while studying the prevalence of GDM. This includes the definition of GDM,[11] various blood glucose cutoffs used to define this condition, selective versus universal screening,[12] terminology such as incidence and prevalence, data sources used for study, determining ethnicity and race in study populations,[13] lack of availability of reliable maternal height and weight measurements,[14] and changing demographics.[15]

DOI: 10.2337/9781580405096.13

PATHOPHYSIOLOGY

The pathophysiology of GDM is a unique combination of insulin resistance along with an underlying insulin secretory defect. As in patients with T2D, the cause underlying this pathophysiology can be as varied.

In a normal pregnancy, women experience increasing insulin resistance stemming from placental secretion of diabetogenic hormones, including growth hormone, corticotropin-releasing hormone, placental lactogen, and progesterone, as well as increased maternal adipose deposition and weight gain, decreased exercise, and increased caloric intake causing weight gain.[16] In response, they mount increased pancreatic insulin secretion to overcome this normally increasing insulin resistance. Women who lack adequate pancreatic insulin reserve develop gestational diabetes. In addition to the placenta and the pancreas, organs such as the liver, muscle, and adipose tissue also play a causative role (see Figure 13.1). The rise in insulin resistance at the level of the liver causes increased hepatic glucose output, potentiating fasting hyperglycemia, and at the level of the muscle, it causes reduced glucose uptake, potentiating postprandial hyperglycemia.[17,18] The adipose tissue produces increased free fatty acids in response to increased activity of hormone-sensitive lipase and reduced adiponectin,[19] which also promotes lipotoxicity, increased insulin resistance, and decreased insulin secretion from pancreatic

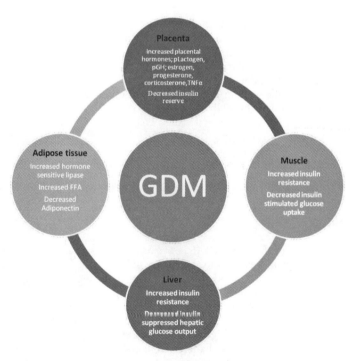

Figure 13.1—The Pathophysiology of GDM

β-cells. Smaller studies have shown that increased circulating leptin levels,[20] inflammatory markers such as TNF-α,[21] and C-reactive proteins[22] may play a causative role. A study showed that the prolactin receptor controls serotonin synthesis, which drives β-cell mass expansion.[23] Fox M1, a transcription factor involved in β-cell replication, is required for the prolactin effect.[24] Suppression of menin (product of MEN 1), which is caused by prolactin elevation, can cause β-cell mass expansion in pregnancy.[24]

In 1952, Jorgen Pederson hypothesized that maternal hyperglycemia produces fetal hyperglycemia and compensatory fetal hyperinsulinemia (Pederson hypothesis).[25] Fetal hyperinsulinemia promotes fetopathy with macrosomia, neonatal hypoglycemia, birth trauma, and possible death, and it may increase the risk of early metabolic complications in the baby's lifetime. This outcome increases the importance of improving glycemic control as soon as possible.

RISK FACTORS

Risk factors for GDM mirror those for T2D and include the following:[26,27]

- A family history of diabetes, especially in first-degree relatives
- Prepregnancy weight ≥110% of ideal body weight or BMI >30 kg/m², significant weight gain in early adulthood and between pregnancies, or excessive gestational weight gain
- Age >25 years
- Previous delivery of a baby >9 lb (4.1 kg)
- Personal history of abnormal glucose tolerance
- Member of a minority ethnic group with higher T2D predisposition (e.g., Hispanic American, African American, Native American, South or East Asian, Pacific Islander)
- Previous unexplained perinatal loss or birth of a malformed child
- Maternal birth weight >9 lb or <6 lb
- Glycosuria at the first prenatal visit
- Polycystic ovary syndrome
- Current use of glucocorticoids
- Essential hypertension or pregnancy-related hypertension
- Metabolic syndrome

SCREENING TESTS

Women with T2D, in the 1940–1950s, were noted to have very large babies and increased perinatal complications in their prior pregnancies. This led to the effort to try to diagnose abnormal blood glucoses in women during pregnancy that were consistent with GDM. In the U.S., Dr. O'Sullivan pioneered the initial glucose testing in pregnancy.[28] However, the methodology of screening and even the mere importance of screening for GDM have been wrought with controversy.[29]

In the past, women lacking high-risk features, such as age >25 years, BMI ≥25 kg/m², first-degree relatives with diabetes, high-risk ethnicity, and history of previous glucose intolerance or adverse pregnancy outcomes, were excluded from screening. Unfortunately, using these selective criteria, only 10% of women would have been excluded, but 3% would have been missed, due to which universal screening is now practiced in all women between 24 and 28 weeks of pregnancy.[30] Screening is recommended as early as at the onset of pregnancy if there are significant risk factors or significant suspicion of underlying diabetes. These risks include severe obesity, first-degree relatives with diabetes, prior history of glucose intolerance or macrosomic baby, or current glycosuria. Retesting for GDM at the usual 24–28 weeks should be pursued for women who have normal testing results earlier in the pregnancy.

Until 2001, the American College of Obstetricians and Gynecologists (ACOG), endorsed that women with low-risk features as noted previously, were less likely to benefit from screening. In 2008, the U.S. Preventive Services Task Force review on screening for gestational diabetes concluded that "evidence was insufficient to assess the balances of benefits and harms of screening for GDM either before or after 24 weeks of gestation." Until 2011, the American Diabetes Association (ADA) had endorsed no screening for women with the earlier mentioned lack of high-risk features. Since 2011, they have endorsed universal screening in all women without a diagnosis of pregestational diabetes. They now recommend a one-step fasting 75-gram glucose tolerance test (GTT) for all women without a prior diagnosis of overt diabetes, as recommended by the International Association of Diabetes in Pregnancy Study Group (IADPSG). The ACOG, based on findings from the National Institutes of Health Consensus Development Conference on diagnosing GSM, have not endorsed this screening methodology. ACOG continues to recommend that screening can be conducted in a one-step or two-step process (Figures 13.2 and 13.3). GTT, though poorly reproducible, with a reproducibility rate of 78%, is still the most practical test currently.[31]

The two-step process includes the performance of a nonfasting 50-gram GTT followed by a 1-hour blood glucose test. Blood glucoses ≥130 mg/dl (90% sensitivity) or ≥140 mg/dl (80% sensitivity) constitute a failed test and the patient pro-

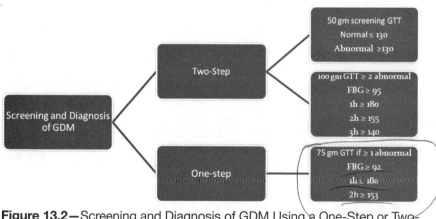

Figure 13.2—Screening and Diagnosis of GDM Using a One-Step or Two-Step Process

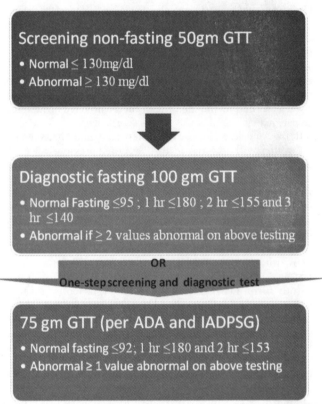

Figure 13.3 — Nonfasting and Fasting Glucose Tolerance Test

ceeds to a diagnostic fasting 100-gram oral GTT (OGTT). Gestational diabetes is diagnosed if ≥2 glucose values are abnormal at the following time-points: fasting ≥95 mg/dl, 1 hour ≥180 mg/dl, 2 hour ≥155 mg/dl, and 3 hour ≥140 mg/dl. On the other hand, recent data have suggested using the one-step combined screening and diagnosis test using a fasting 75-gram GTT. GDM is diagnosed if ≥1 glucose value is abnormal at the following time-points: fasting ≥92 mg/dl, 1 hour ≥180 mg/dl, 2 hour ≥153 mg/dl.

The rising incidence of obesity and decreased rates of screening for diabetes in women during their reproductive years, has led to a rising incidence of diagnosing previously undiagnosed diabetes in pregnant women, which now is called "overt diabetes." This diagnosis is made based on the following criteria:

- Fasting plasma glucose ≥126 mg/dl, or
- A1C ≥6.5% using a standardized assay, or
- Random plasma glucose ≥200 mg/dl that subsequently is confirmed by elevated fasting plasma glucose or A1C

HAPO AND IADPSG

The methods of testing for GDM have remained inconsistent throughout the world. To bring uniformity to the diagnosis of GDM, members of multiple obstetrical and diabetes organizations formed the international consensus group IADPSG. HAPO, a large (21,216 pregnant women) multinational epidemiology study, was performed to study the relationship of 75-gram GTT testing to perinatal outcomes. A large study was required to control for confounders such as weight, ethnicity, age, geographic location, and contributing family history. The major conclusion of the study was that maternal, fetal, and neonatal outcomes were increased in a continuous fashion, as a result of rising maternal glucose levels that were in the previously considered normal range, and there did not appear to be a threshold cutoff for these outcomes. Subsequently, the IADPSG consensus panel concluded that a single-step 75-gram GTT should be performed in all women between 24 and 28 weeks, and a single abnormal value, linked to a hazard ratio of 1.75 for adverse outcomes compared with the mean glucose value, should make the diagnosis. This is projected to increase the prevalence of GDM to 18%, and accordingly, there has been some trepidation and variable acceptance of these criteria.[7]

ALTERNATIVE DIAGNOSTIC TESTS

The hyperosmolarity associated with the GTT solutions frequently leads to gastrointestinal intolerance with nausea and vomiting. This leads to women being unable to tolerate or refusing to undergo standard OGTT, which has led to the development of alternative screening methods. These tests should be used only under exceptional circumstances, or when standard GTT testing is not possible, because their efficacy has not been studied in detail. These methods have not been approved by ADA or ACOG.

Candy such as jelly beans,[32] fixed carbohydrate-containing meals,[33] intravenous (IV) GTT testing,[34] blood glucose monitoring, and A1C testing all have been tried. Some studies have suggested that the A1C test may be used to predict the risk for large-for-gestational-age babies.[35] This may have significant overlap between normal glycemia of a normal pregnancy and the mild and short-lived hyperglycemia of GDM, and it has not been approved by ADA.[36]

COMPLICATIONS ASSOCIATED WITH GDM

Abnormal blood glucoses in pregnancy can be associated with increased maternal and fetal risk. Maternal risk entails an increased likelihood of preeclampsia, polyhydramnios, Cesarean section, and the long-term risk of recurrent gestational diabetes in future pregnancies and T2D over the mother's lifetime.[2,5,37] Fetal complications include macrosomia, shoulder dystocia, birth trauma, fetal hepatosplenomegaly, erythrocytosis, and neonatal hyperbilirubinemia, respiratory distress, hypoglycemia, and intrauterine fetal demise in extreme cases.[3,4,7] In addition, these babies are at a higher future risk of obesity-associated metabolic complications, abnormalities of fine and gross motor function, and inattention and hyperactivity disorders.[38–40]

DIFFERENTIAL DIAGNOSIS

Latent autoimmune diabetes of adult (LADA) and maturity-onset diabetes of the young (MODY) can masquerade as GDM. About 10% of women with GDM may have pancreatic antibodies, indicative of LADA, which can be unmasked in pregnancy because of the associated insulin resistance and dependence on increased insulin secretion.[41] This should be considered in women who are lean, lack a family history of diabetes, present with significant hyperglycemia with associated symptoms or diabetic ketoacidosis, weight loss, and persistent postpartum hyperglycemia. C-peptide levels may be normal secondary to the insidious progression of this disease, but testing for pancreatic antibodies, such as GAD-65 or islet-cell antibodies, can help make the diagnosis.

MODY has several varieties, some of which may be associated with hyperglycemia and may manifest as GDM. Metabolic studies have revealed an abnormality in glucose-mediated insulin secretion in certain forms of MODY.[42] Specific mutational testing helps diagnose this condition and should be considered in women with a family history of diabetes, early age at diagnosis, and persistent postpartum hyperglycemia.[43]

LONG-TERM FOLLOW-UP AND PREVENTION

In Mother

Women with GDM have a high risk of recurrent GDM in subsequent pregnancies and also T2D.[44,45] Given this risk, postpartum fasting 75-gram GTT should be recommended in all patients to assess glycemic control and motivate continued lifestyle modification to achieve ideal body weight.[46] Women should be educated about their risk of recurrent GDM in a future pregnancy.[47,48] Educating women with overt diabetes and GDM to gain weight consistent with Institute of Medicine (IOM) guidelines in pregnancy will help prevent excessive gestational weight gain and enable optimized postpartum weight loss. Screening for postpartum depression should be considered as it may prevent postpartum weight loss.[49] Prevention trials in this subset have shown good efficacy with both lifestyle modification and metformin therapy.[5] Observational studies have shown that exercise before and during pregnancy may reduce the risk of developing GDM. Weight loss of at least 10 lb and surgical weight loss have both shown efficacy in reducing the incidence of gestational diabetes.[50] Only one study has suggested that supplementation with 2 grams myo-inositol plus 200 µg folic acid twice daily from the end of the first trimester of pregnancy in women with a parent with T2D reduced the incidence of GDM to 6% compared with 15.3% in the control group. It is also important that these women get appropriate screening before a future pregnancy to decrease the risk of congenital complications associated with undiagnosed T2D.[51]

In Baby

Babies show evidence of increased adiposity with an intrauterine milieu of hyperglycemia.[52] Fetal hyperinsulinemia may promote obesity and abnormal glucose metabolism from childhood to adulthood.[53,54] The weight and growth of these babies should be followed closely, with efforts being made to reduce excessive weight gain and educate the family about the importance of lifestyle modification. Making the birth weight part of the medical record in babies born to mothers with GDM will help this process.

COSTS ASSOCIATED WITH GDM

An ounce of prevention may truly be better than a pound of cure if we acknowledged the fiscal implications of preventing future diabetes in this high-risk population, inclusive of mother and baby. Intensive lifestyle and pharmacologic interventions have proven to be effective in community settings (e.g., YMCA) and in primary care practices, and the benefits persist for at least 10 years, in addition to being cost-effective.[55] The growing economic and societal burden of diabetes has lent a sense of urgency to prevention.[56] A diagnosis of GDM increases costs related not only to increased Cesarean sections and neonatal unit admissions but also to increased use of resources and costs associated with frequent maternal and fetal monitoring during pregnancy. Preventive interventions have the potential to produce clinical and financial benefits.[56]

REFERENCES

1. Proceedings of the 4th International Workshop-Conference on Gestational Diabetes Mellitus. Chicago, Illinois, USA. 14–16 March 1997. *Diabetes Care* 1998;21(Suppl 2):B1–B167.

2. Dodd JM, et al. Screening for gestational diabetes: the effect of varying blood glucose definitions in the prediction of adverse maternal and infant health outcomes. *Aust N Z J Obstet Gynaecol* 2007;47(4):307–312.

3. Jensen DM, et al. Clinical impact of mild carbohydrate intolerance in pregnancy: a study of 2904 nondiabetic Danish women with risk factors for gestational diabetes mellitus. *Am J Obstet Gynecol* 2001;185(2):413–419.

4. Ferrara A, et al. Pregnancy plasma glucose levels exceeding the American Diabetes Association thresholds, but below the National Diabetes Data Group thresholds for gestational diabetes mellitus, are related to the risk of neonatal macrosomia, hypoglycaemia and hyperbilirubinaemia. *Diabetologia* 2007;50(2):298–306.

5. Sermer M, et al. Impact of increasing carbohydrate intolerance on maternal-fetal outcomes in 3637 women without gestational diabetes. The Toronto Tri-Hospital Gestational Diabetes Project. *Am J Obstet Gynecol* 1995; 173(1):146–156.

6. Hillier TA, et al. Childhood obesity and metabolic imprinting: the ongoing effects of maternal hyperglycemia. *Diabetes Care* 2007;30(9):2287–2292.

7. International Association of Diabetes and Pregnancy Study Group. International Association of Diabetes and Pregnancy Study Group's recommenda-

tions on the diagnosis and classification of hyperglycemia in pregnancy. *Diabetes Care* 2010;33(3):676–682.

8. Ferrara A. Increasing prevalence of gestational diabetes mellitus: a public health perspective. *Diabetes Care* 2007;30(Suppl 2):S141–S146.

9. Dabelea D, et al. Increasing prevalence of gestational diabetes mellitus (GDM) over time and by birth cohort: Kaiser Permanente of Colorado GDM Screening Program. *Diabetes Care* 2005;28(3):579–584.

10. Bardenheier BH, et al. Variation in prevalence of gestational diabetes mellitus among hospital discharges for obstetric delivery across 23 states in the United States. *Diabetes Care* 2013;36(5):1209–1214.

11. Metzger BE, et al. Summary and recommendations of the Fifth International Workshop-Conference on Gestational Diabetes Mellitus. *Diabetes Care* 2007;30(Suppl 2):S251–S260.

12. Ferrara A, et al. An increase in the incidence of gestational diabetes mellitus: northern California, 1991-2000. *Obstet Gynecol* 2004;103(3):526–533.

13. Lawrence JM, et al. Trends in the prevalence of preexisting diabetes and gestational diabetes mellitus among a racially/ethnically diverse population of pregnant women, 1999-2005. *Diabetes Care* 2008;31(5):899–904.

14. Chu SY, et al. Maternal obesity and risk of gestational diabetes mellitus. *Diabetes Care* 2007;30(8):2070–2076.

15. Martin JA, et al. Annual summary of vital statistics: 2006. *Pediatrics* 2008;121(4):788–801.

16. Catalano PM, et al. Gestational diabetes and insulin resistance: role in short- and long-term implications for mother and fetus. *J Nutr* 2003;133(5 Suppl 2):1674S–1683S.

17. Butte NF. Carbohydrate and lipid metabolism in pregnancy: normal compared with gestational diabetes mellitus. *Am J Clin Nutr* 2000;71(5 Suppl):1256S–1261S.

18. Yamashita H, Shao J, Friedman JE. Physiologic and molecular alterations in carbohydrate metabolism during pregnancy and gestational diabetes mellitus. *Clin Obstet Gynecol* 2000;43(1):87–98.

19. Palin MF, Bordignon VV, Murphy BD. Adiponectin and the control of female reproductive functions. *Vitam Horm* 2012;90:239–287.

20. Kautzky-Willer A, et al. Increased plasma leptin in gestational diabetes. *Diabetologia* 2001;44(2):164–172.

21. Winkler G, et al. Tumor necrosis factor system in insulin resistance in gestational diabetes. *Diabetes Res Clin Pract* 2002;56(2):93–99.

22. Retnakaran R, et al. C-reactive protein and gestational diabetes: the central role of maternal obesity. *J Clin Endocrinol Metab* 2003;88(8):3507–3512.

23. Kim H, et al. Serotonin regulates pancreatic beta cell mass during pregnancy. *Nat Med* 2010;16(7):804–808.

24. Zhang H, et al. Gestational diabetes mellitus resulting from impaired beta-cell compensation in the absence of FoxM1, a novel downstream effector of placental lactogen. *Diabetes* 2010;59(1):143–152.

25. Pedersen J. Diabetes and pregnancy; blood sugar of newborn infants during fasting and glucose administration. *Ugeskr Laeger* 1952;114(21):685.

26. Solomon CG, et al. A prospective study of pregravid determinants of gestational diabetes mellitus. *JAMA* 1997;278(13):1078–1083.

27. Hedderson MM, et al. Body mass index and weight gain prior to pregnancy and risk of gestational diabetes mellitus. *Am J Obstet Gynecol* 2008;198(4):409 e1–e7.

28. O'Sullivan JB, Mahan CM. Criteria for the oral glucose tolerance test in pregnancy. *Diabetes* 1964;13:278–285.

29. Landon MB, et al. A multicenter, randomized trial of treatment for mild gestational diabetes. *N Engl J Med* 2009;361(14):1339–1348.

30. Danilenko-Dixon DR, et al. Universal versus selective gestational diabetes screening: application of 1997 American Diabetes Association recommendations. *Am J Obstet Gynecol* 1999;181(4):798–802.

31. Riccardi G, et al. Reproducibility of the new diagnostic criteria for impaired glucose tolerance. *Am J Epidemiol* 1985;121(3):422–429.

32. Lamar ME, et al. Jelly beans as an alternative to a fifty-gram glucose beverage for gestational diabetes screening. *Am J Obstet Gynecol* 1999;181(5 Pt 1):1154–1157.

33. Murphy NJ, et al. Carbohydrate sources for gestational diabetes mellitus screening. A comparison. *J Reprod Med* 1994;39(12):977–981.

34. Posner NA, et al. Simplifying the intravenous glucose tolerance test. *J Reprod Med* 1982;27(10):633–638.

35. Bevier WC, Fischer R, Jovanovic L. Treatment of women with an abnormal glucose challenge test (but a normal oral glucose tolerance test) decreases the prevalence of macrosomia. *Am J Perinatol* 1999;16(6):269–275.

36. Lowe LP, et al. Hyperglycemia and Adverse Pregnancy Outcome (HAPO) study: associations of maternal A1C and glucose with pregnancy outcomes. *Diabetes Care* 2012;35(3):574–580.

37. Pettitt DJ, et al. Gestational diabetes: infant and maternal complications of pregnancy in relation to third-trimester glucose tolerance in the Pima Indians. *Diabetes Care* 1980;3(3):458–464

38. Dabelea D. The predisposition to obesity and diabetes in offspring of diabetic mothers. *Diabetes Care* 2007;30(Suppl 2):S169–S174.

39. Ornoy A. Growth and neurodevelopmental outcome of children born to mothers with pregestational and gestational diabetes. *Pediatr Endocrinol Rev* 2005;3(2):104–113.

40. Clausen TD, et al. High prevalence of type 2 diabetes and pre-diabetes in adult offspring of women with gestational diabetes mellitus or type 1 diabetes: the role of intrauterine hyperglycemia. *Diabetes Care* 2008;31(2):340–346.

41. de Leiva A, Mauricio D, Corcoy R. Diabetes-related autoantibodies and gestational diabetes. *Diabetes Care* 2007;30(Suppl 2):S127–S133.

42. Fajans SS, Bell GI, Polonsky KS. Molecular mechanisms and clinical pathophysiology of maturity-onset diabetes of the young. *N Engl J Med* 2001;345(13):971–980.

43. Weng J, et al. Screening for MODY mutations, GAD antibodies, and type 1 diabetes–associated HLA genotypes in women with gestational diabetes mellitus. *Diabetes Care* 2002;25(1):68–71.

44. Kim C. Gestational diabetes mellitus and risk of future maternal cardiovascular disease. *Expert Rev Cardiovasc Ther* 2010;8(12):1639–1641.

45. Kim C, Newton KM, Knopp RH. Gestational diabetes and the incidence of type 2 diabetes: a systematic review. *Diabetes Care* 2002;25(10):1862–1868.

46. American Diabetes Association. Standards of medical care in diabetes—2012. *Diabetes Care* 2012;35(Suppl 1):S11–S63.

47. Ratner RE. Prevention of type 2 diabetes in women with previous gestational diabetes. *Diabetes Care* 2007;30(Suppl 2):S242–S245.

48. Ratner RE, et al. Prevention of diabetes in women with a history of gestational diabetes: effects of metformin and lifestyle interventions. *J Clin Endocrinol Metab* 2008;93(12):4774–4779.

49. Nicklas JM, et al. Factors associated with depressive symptoms in the early postpartum period among women with recent gestational diabetes mellitus. *Matern Child Health J* 2013 Nov;17(9):1665–1672.

50. Glazer NL, et al. Weight change and the risk of gestational diabetes in obese women. *Epidemiology* 2004;15(6):733–737.

51. Reece EA. Diabetes-induced birth defects. What do we know? What can we do? *Curr Diab Rep* 2012;12(1):24–32.

52. Lawlor DA, et al. Association of existing diabetes, gestational diabetes and glycosuria in pregnancy with macrosomia and offspring body mass index, waist and fat mass in later childhood: findings from a prospective pregnancy cohort. *Diabetologia* 2010;53(1):89–97.

53. Metzger BE. Long-term outcomes in mothers diagnosed with gestational diabetes mellitus and their offspring. *Clin Obstet Gynecol* 2007;50(4):972–979.

54. Kim SY, Sharma AJ, Callaghan WM. Gestational diabetes and childhood obesity: what is the link? *Curr Opin Obstet Gynecol* 2012;24(6):376–381.

55. Diabetes Prevention Program Research Group, et al. 10-year follow-up of diabetes incidence and weight loss in the Diabetes Prevention Program Outcomes Study. *Lancet* 2009;374(9702):1677–1686.

56. Gillespie P, et al. Modeling the independent effects of gestational diabetes mellitus on maternity care and costs. *Diabetes Care* 2013;36(5):1111–1116.

Chapter 14

Gestational Diabetes Mellitus: Management

David A. Sacks, MD

O nce diagnosed, gestational diabetes mellitus (GDM) requires specialized care. To establish the basis for specific interventions, a discussion of the mechanisms of development of selected serious complications of pregnancies in women who have GDM will be followed by a discussion of the approaches to treatment as they relate to attempting to decrease the incidence of these complications. This chapter primarily addresses medical aspects of care. Other guidelines and reviews more thoroughly address issues concerning obstetrical care.[1-3]

WHY TREAT GDM?

Although the question whether to treat GDM may appear to be rhetorical, the dangers posed to both mother and her unborn baby by GDM bear commentary. The prevalence of adverse outcomes in GDM may be lower than that in pregnancies complicated by other forms of diabetes, for example, pregestational types 1 diabetes and type 2 diabetes (T2D), but the types of serious maternal, fetal, perinatal, and neonatal morbidities and mortality are similar if not identical.

CONGENITAL MALFORMATIONS

Nonsyndromic birth defects occur with greater frequency among infants of women who have pregestational diabetes than among infants of women who do not.[4] Because organogenesis is completed for most systems affected by diabetes-associated abnormalities by the seventh week following ovulation (ninth gestational week assuming a 28-day cycle and calculating from the date of onset of last menses), it seems reasonable to assume that anomalous development of a given fetal organ likely is associated with exposure to a teratogen during this early gestational period.[5] Elevated glycated hemoglobin early in pregnancy in diabetic pregnancies complicated by anomalous fetuses bears witness to the association between maternal hyperglycemia and anomalous fetal organ development.[6,7] Whether glucose is itself a teratogen, a cofactor, or merely a marker of activity of the primary teratogen is a subject of debate.[8] The observation, however, that minimizing maternal glucose during organogenesis in a woman who has diabetes is associated with a reduction in the incidence of birth defects to that of the nondiabetic population suggests that the treatments applied to lower maternal glucose inhibit expression of teratogens, whatever they may be.[9]

DOI: 10.2337/9781580405096.14

One meta-analysis documented that women who have GDM have babies with congenital anomalies more frequently than women who do not.[10] Whether this finding is due to some intrinsic (e.g., genetic or metabolic) characteristic of women destined to develop glucose intolerance in the second or third trimester or because some of the patients may have had undiscovered diabetes before pregnancy[11] remains speculative. The weight of evidence is that hyperglycemia is not teratogenic, but rather it provides a permissive milieu for the expression of genes related to the development of certain fetal anomalies. Laboratory work has suggested a variety of possible mechanisms for the development of those birth defects found among infants of women with diabetes. These include endoplasmic reticulum stress, nitrosative stress, phospholipid peroxidation, and activation of families of kinases.[12] The early embryo exists in an anaerobic environment devoid of vascular connections for oxygen supply. In the presence of hyperglycemia, glycolysis and glucose oxidation proceed at an accelerated rate, resulting in oxygen depletion and the production of reactive oxygen species (ROS).[13] Excessive ROS results in decreased expression of the gene Pax3. This in turn results in the derepression of production of the p53 tumor suppressor protein. Increased expression of p53 protein results in apoptosis (programmed cell death) of the epithelial ridges of the neural folds. The cells in the neural crest are essential for the development of a number of structures, including the brain, spinal cord, skull, and jaw, as well as septation of the single cardiac outflow tract, which are all sites of birth defects seen in infants of women with diabetes. Of particular pertinence is the finding in mouse experiments that a glucose concentration of only 250 mg/dl was necessary and sufficient to cause marked decreased expression of Pax3.[14] Thus, it is a tenable hypothesis that early in pregnancy a minimal degree of hyperglycemia in a woman not yet meeting threshold values defining GDM may contribute to the development of fetal anomalies.

A reduction in maternal hyperglycemia early in the first trimester in women with pregestational diabetes has been shown to decrease the incidence of fetal congenital malformations.[9,15] Because most women who either have undiscovered pregestational diabetes or who are destined to develop GDM during pregnancy present for prenatal care after the period of organogenesis, the application of these findings to women at risk for GDM appears quite limited.[16] The use of antioxidants (e.g., vitamins C and E, Cu/Zn superoxide dismutase) has shown promise in laboratory animals, but little human experience has been reported.[17] Folic acid fortification of foodstuffs and supplementation for reproductive-age women has reduced, but not eliminated, neural tube defects in the general population,[18] but it has had little impact on women with diabetes.[19]

STILLBIRTHS

Data regarding the risk of stillbirth in women who have GDM are inconsistent. In comparison with nondiabetic controls, some have reported no difference,[20,21] increased risk,[22-74] and decreased risk[25,76] of intrauterine fetal death. Likely some of these differences can be ascribed to differences in definitions of stillbirth (e.g., by gestational age versus by birth weight), in controlling for confounding variables (e.g., intercurrent medical problems, fetal congenital anomalies), in controlling for gestational age at delivery,[27] and in the definition of gestational diabetes. In 2011, the American Diabetes Association (ADA) changed the definition of GDM from "diabetes diagnosed during pregnancy"[28] to "diabetes diagnosed during pregnancy that is not clearly overt diabetes."[29] The former definition, which is similar to that of the World Health Organization,[30] is inclusive of women who may have had undiagnosed or undetected diabetes before the current pregnancy. Publications defining GDM by this more inclusive definition may include women at heightened risk of fetal demise by virtue of their hyperglycemia being of longer duration than that of the current pregnancy. The report of an increased prevalence of fetal demise in a prior pregnancy in women who have GDM compared with women who do not have GDM[31] is potential evidence of a longer duration of metabolic insult in the former group.

Why fetal demise occurs inexplicably in normally formed infants of women who have diabetes who are in good glycemic control remains largely unexplained. Significantly increased adjusted odds for perinatal mortality at ≥34 weeks' gestation for fasting, 1-, and 2-hour values on glucose tolerance test (GTT) results of women who did not meet criteria defining GDM have been reported.[27] Fetal hyperglycemia accompanied by hypoxia secondary to maternal hyperglycemia resulting in oxidative stress and fetal accumulation of lactic acid has been demonstrated in animal models.[32] Thus, it is a tenable hypothesis that (perhaps transient and undetected) maternal hyperglycemia may result in failure of normal metabolic pathways and in fetal demise.

Prevention of fetal death in GDM poses a clinical challenge. Standard care requires control of maternal glycemia. The addition of antepartum fetal testing toward the latter part of pregnancy, although standard practice in some centers, has not been demonstrated to prevent this tragedy. Three cases of women with well-controlled GDM whose fetal demise was preceded by reassuring antepartum fetal heart rate tests at 37, 38, and 40.5 weeks have been reported.[24] A large (n = 4.2 million nonanomalous births) study compared the weekly risk of fetal and neonatal mortality in women who had GDM compared with those who did not. Included among the findings were the observations that from 36 to 41 weeks the risks of fetal demise were greater and the risks of infant mortality were lower for women who had GDM. From 36 to 38 weeks, the risks of fetal death were not significantly different from the risks of infant death. At 39 and 40 weeks' gestation, however, the relative risk for fetal death was significantly greater than that for neonatal death. From these data one might conclude that elective delivery of a woman with GDM at 38 weeks' gestation may contribute to a decrease in fetal demise. One retrospective study of women with GDM found no significant difference in adverse perinatal outcomes between the group delivered at 38 weeks compared with controls treated expectantly. The one fetal demise occurred at 38-4/7 weeks in a baby in the expectantly managed group, and was associated with a tight double nuchal cord.[33]

RR (relative risk)

FETAL OVERGROWTH

Minimization of excessive fetal growth is probably the most frequently utilized outcome variable for measurement of success of treatment of GDM. The term "excessive fetal growth," however, has no universally accepted definition. "Macrosomia" frequently is used to indicate a minimum birth weight, usually

4,000 or 4,500 grams.[34] Although a definition based on absolute birth weight has the advantages of ease of memorization, measurement, and reproducibility, it fails to consider differences introduced by gestational age. A 4-kilogram neonate at 34 weeks is physically and physiologically very different from one delivered at 38 weeks. Although the concept of large for gestational age (LGA), generally defined as a birth weight ≥90th percentile for gestational age[34] (and sometimes also adjusted for gender or ethnicity), largely neutralizes confounding by gestational age at delivery, it, too, has its limitations. There is no one universally accepted set of reference data of appropriate birth weights at given gestational ages. Some authors use data from their own institutions or regions, whereas others may use published data from national sources.[35] Customized growth curves, which are based on maternal factors (height, weight, ethnicity, parity) as well as ultrasound-generated fetal growth curves[36] may more accurately predict LGA neonates at risk for associated morbidities.[37] Perhaps the most clinically relevant factor absent from using LGA to define fetal overgrowth is that it does not consider differences in body composition between babies of similar weight and gestational age. Infants of women who have diabetes characteristically have a greater percentage of their birth weight as fat weight. Even appropriate for gestational age (AGA) infants of women who have GDM have greater skinfold measures and a greater proportion of their birth weight as fat weight than AGA neonates of women without diabetes.[38] The increase in subcutaneous fat is of clinical concern, in that the cumulative incidence of shoulder dystocia, a rare but unpredictable and potentially disastrous complication of labor, is greater at any birth weight >3,750 grams in pregnancies of diabetic women compared with those of women who do not have diabetes.[39]

There is little doubt that fetal growth and particularly growth in fetal fat has a positive correlation with maternal glycemia. Adjusted for confounders, the odds ratio for birth weight >90th percentile[40] and for newborn skinfold thicknesses (a surrogate measure of subcutaneous fat) >90th percentile was statistically significantly positively correlated with fasting, 1-, and 2-hour values in a multicenter, multinational, blinded observational study.[41] The Pedersen hypothesis[42] posits that excessive fetal growth is due to the transplacental transfer of glucose from maternal to fetal circulations. Fetal glucose stimulates fetal islet cells to produce an abundance of insulin, which in turn drives glucose into the cells of fetal insulin-dependent organs, namely skeletal muscle and fat. Some data, however, suggest that glucose may not be the primary contributor to fetal growth. Maternal insulin resistance, an essential characteristic of GDM, also contributes to elevated maternal free fatty acids and triglycerides. Placental hydrolysis of maternal triglycerides liberates nonesterified (free) fatty acids for transfer to the fetal circulation where they may contribute to fat accretion.[43] A number of findings support this theory. In women who did and did not have GDM, correlations between birth-weight ratios and maternal triglycerides but not with 50-gram glucose screen results were found.[44] In a multivariable regression analysis maternal triglycerides but not post-loading glucose were selected as significantly associated with birth weight.[45] In glucose-tolerant women, first-trimester triglycerides and third-trimester fatty acids had higher correlation coefficients with infant body fat than did any measures of maternal glucose.[46] These data suggest that other metabolic substrates may affect birth weight and body composition, perhaps to a greater extent than does glucose. They also may explain why in two large studies, respectively, 13 and 22% of LGA neonates were born to women who were obese and did not have GDM.[47,48] Like GDM, obesity also is characterized by insulin resistance, but not all obese women develop GDM.[43]

Not all ethnic groups have the same prevalence of GDM, and members of different ethnic groups who have GDM have different prevalence of fetal overgrowth. In the U.S., women of (especially East) Asian extraction were found to have a greater prevalence of GDM than Caucasians, African Americans, and Latinas.[49] Asian women who have GDM are less frequently overweight and obese than women of other ethnicities who have GDM[49-51] and have lower fasting and higher 2-hour postglucose results on 75-gram GTT.[51] Even adjusting for ethnicity, the prevalence of LGA[51] and macrosomia[50] among Asians is <5%. The explanation for the coexistence of maternal hyperglycemia, normal body habitus, and normal neonatal weight in this ethnic group remains speculative. In one study, there were no interethnic differences in the rate of progression of insulin resistance from 15 to 28 weeks, but baseline insulin resistance was greater and the increase in β-cell function was less among East Asians compared with non-Hispanic whites.[52] Whether clinical care of the former group should be altered (e.g., with administration of insulin or metformin early in gestation) requires further investigation.

Fetal overgrowth also is affected by placental structural development and function. The increase in fetal oxygen demands may explain the increase in placental villous and capillary surface areas.[53] Upregulation of placental nutrient transporters by signals of both maternal and fetal origin may explain the accelerated transport of some nutrients to the fetus.[54] Whether such measures as limiting maternal nutrient intake or increasing maternal utilization of substrate with exercise during pregnancy reduces or augments nutrient transplacental transfer remains largely uninvestigated.

PREECLAMPSIA

Defined as hypertension and proteinuria developing in a woman who was normotensive before the 20th week of gestation,[55] preeclampsia does occur more frequently among women who have GDM, independent of such confounders as parity, age, ethnicity, weight, and weight gain.[56] In multivariable analyses, however, obesity, which is often a concomitant of GDM, has been found to have a stronger independent association with preeclampsia than either GDM[56] or maternal glucose concentrations.[57] The proposed mechanisms of development of preeclampsia are similar to those proposed for the development of GDM. These include oxidative stress,[58-60] activation and suppression of adipocytokines, and insulin resistance of a degree greater than that attributable to pregnancy alone.[61] One study found no significant differences between glucose concentrations, insulin concentrations, insulin sensitivity, and glucose clearance among women who had GDM who did and did not develop preeclampsia.[62] Thus, the increased incidence of preeclampsia in women who have GDM remains unexplained. Two randomized controlled trials of treatment with diet and insulin found, however, that women in the treated groups had a significantly lower incidence of preeclampsia.[63,64]

TREATMENT OF GDM DURING PREGNANCY

A number of reviews and meta-analyses examining the benefits and harms of treatment of GDM have been published. Although there is no uniformity of opinion among them about the quality of evidence on which their decisions were based, there is consensus that treatment of GDM with diet or diet and insulin or oral hypoglycemics does reduce the incidence of fetal overgrowth, shoulder dystocia, and preeclampsia. In addition, on the basis of available evidence, it has been concluded that dietary treatment accompanied by blood glucose monitoring serves to decrease the risk of fetal overgrowth for women who have degrees of glucose intolerance less than those defining GDM.[65-69] That treatment also results in an increased frequency of office visits and inductions of labor also was noted.[66,67] The two largest randomized controlled trials of GDM used diet supplemented by insulin, with the second of the two supplementing with insulin if the patient failed to decrease her glucose below designated target values with diet alone.[63,64] Both studies found a decrease in the incidence of LGA neonates in the study group. Only one of these studies[64] reported maternal glycemic results. In that study, a decline in fasting and postprandial glucose during the period of treatment was reported in the group receiving the intervention, but glucose results for controls were not reported.[70] Both studies reported a significantly lower maternal weight gain in their study groups. Thus, it is unclear whether the decreases in adverse outcomes observed were the result of lowering of maternal glycemia, maternal weight restriction, or both.

GLUCOSE CONTROL

Whether glucose is a cause or a covariable of other factors that are responsible for the morbidities associated with GDM, evidence of a reduction in the incidence of these adverse outcomes while focusing on reduction in concentrations of maternal glycemia has been produced.[63,64]

Glucose Targets

Selection of glycemic goals logically should be tied to the relationships between maternal glucose and adverse pregnancy outcomes. One study reported that women who had GDM and who maintained a mean self-monitored blood glucose between 87 and 104 mg/dl had an incidence of LGA neonates that was significantly less than those with higher mean glucose values and not significantly different from those who did not have GDM.[71] Clinicians, however, base their management on self-monitored individual glucose values at different times of day, rather than means. Whether preprandial or postprandial glucose values are more predictive of a given adverse outcomes has been investigated. A study of women without diabetes who underwent a 75-gram GTT found that all fasting glucose values on the GTT >63 mg/dl were significantly associated with LGA neonates, whereas adjusted odds for all 2-hour glucose values were not significantly associated with LGA.[72] A randomized controlled trial of women with GDM who required insulin found that those targeting a fasting capillary glucose of 60–90 mg/dl and a 1-hour postprandial capillary glucose of <140 mg/dl had a lower frequency of LGA neonates than did those using the same fasting glycemic goal and a preprandial target of 60–105 mg/dl alone.[73] Actual glucose values achieved were not reported. The possibility that the group utilizing a more narrow (and lower) range of preprandial glycemia might have achieved the same clinical outcomes as that of the group managed on the basis of postprandial glucose was not studied. Given the continuous positive nature of the relationship between maternal pre- and postloading glucose concentrations and LGA in untreated women,[40] the latter assumption bears investigation. Furthermore, it is possible that different combinations of abnormal glucose values may be associated with different adverse outcomes. For example, in an observational study comparing untreated women who met the International Association of the Diabetes Pregnancy and Study Groups criteria[74] defining GDM with women who did not have GDM, those with normal fasting and elevated postload values were at higher risk for preterm delivery and gestational hypertension, whereas those with elevated fasting and normal postload values were at greater risk of having an LGA infant.[75]

A number of authoritative bodies have proposed glucose target values for purposes of improving perinatal and maternal outcomes. No two are identical (Table 14.1). Most do not specify the method of assay or the medium (plasma, whole blood, capillary) to be assayed, and most do not state when in relation to a meal the timing of the 1- or 2-hour postmeal glucose should begin. None specify the frequency of testing or whether testing at one time of day is more closely related to pregnancy outcomes than is testing at another. Standardization of these parameters, as well as establishment of a quantitative relationship between target values selected and pregnancy outcomes, would help provide meaningful, universally applicable glycemic targets. Glucose values for 57 pregnant woman without diabetes in their third trimester obtained by continuous subcutaneous glucose monitoring were reported in one study. Overall mean fasting (75 mg/dl), preprandial (78 mg/dl), 1-hour postprandial (105 mg/dl), and 2-hour postprandial (97 mg/dl) glucose values were far lower than those glycemic targets recommended in official guidelines (Table 14.1). In addition, preprandial and 1- and 2-hour postprandial glucose values of obese women (respectively 90 mg/dl, 112 mg/dl, and 107 mg/dl) were significantly greater than those of nonobese women. Furthermore, the time to peak glucose for the entire group was 71 minutes and that of the obese women was 88 minutes, both times being intermediate between the 1- and 2-hour measures recommended in standard guidelines.[76] Another review, in which normative pre- and postprandial glucose values were calculated from 12 studies, found weighted mean glucose values of fasting 71 mg/dl, 1-hour 109 mg/dl, and 2-hour 99 mg/dl.[77] Despite the fact that many of the subjects of this study were women under treatment for diabetes in pregnancy, these results are similar to the previously mentioned data from women without diabetes.[76] Whether changes in glycemic targets or timing of testing relative to time of day or time after the last meal would help improve outcome in pregnancies complicated by GDM remains for future investigation.

Glucose Monitoring

Glucose monitoring for GDM has undergone a long evolutionary process. Testing for maternal glycosuria was replaced initially by laboratory blood testing and subsequently by ambulatory self-monitoring of blood glucose (SMBG). In

Table 14.1 Glycemic Goals Recommended by Different Medical Organizations

Organization	Target glucose (mg/dl)					Reason for selection of target/Comments
	Fasting	Preprandial	1-hour post-prandial	2-hour post-prandial	Postprandial (time not stated)	
ACOG[1]	<95		<130–140	<120		Exceeding these values indicates addition of insulin
ADA[85]		≤95	≤140	≤120		Recommended by the 5th International Workshop-Conference on Diabetes*
ADIPS[160]	≤90		≤133*	≤121*		Based on 2 SDs above the mean values for pregnant women without known risk factors.
CDA[161]	<95		<140	<121		Using the targets in the Maternal-Fetal-Medicine-Unit Network study associated with good outcomes
DIPSI[162]	~90**				~120**	Consistent with mean plasma glucose ~105 mg/dl
IDF[163]	60–95	60–105	140	120		
NICE[164]	63-106		<140			If safely achievable
NIDDK[165]	≤95	≤95	≤140	≤120		
SIGN[166]	≥99			≥126		≤35 weeks
	≥99			≥144	>162	>35 weeks

Note: ACOG = American Congress of Obstetricians and Gynecologists; ADA = American Diabetes Association; ADIPS = Australasian Diabetes In Pregnancy Society; CDA = Canadian Diabetes Association; DIPSI = Diabetes in Pregnancy Study Group-India; NICE = National Institute for Health and Care Excellence [UK]; SIGN = Scottish Intercollegiate Guidelines Network; NIDDK = National Institute of Diabetes and Digestive and Kidney Diseases; IDF – International Diabetes Federation.

*Timing for postprandial measures begins after commencing a meal.

**Plasma glucose.

addition to the advantage of offering several data points for patient management, downloaded data from memory-based meters can be used to determine frequency of testing, mean glucose values at different times of day, and comparative data from different times during pregnancy. Unfortunately, the ADA's goal of a glucose meter total error of <10% relative to laboratory-analyzed plasma glucose[78] has not been achieved by all manufacturers.[79] Utilization of these meters requires some degree of training.[80] Reliance should not be placed on patient transcription of SMBG results as they may be inaccurate or falsified.[81,82] The benefit of frequent home glucose monitoring over maternal glucose monitoring only at office visits has been investigated. Nonsignificant differences in maternal glycemia, weight gain, macrosomia, and birth trauma were found between home- and office-monitored groups in one randomized, controlled trial.[83] A cohort study using historic controls, however, found less maternal weight gain and a lower incidence of LGA neonates in the self-monitored group.[84] Although not specifically addressing pregnancy, the ADA has recommended SMBG for patients who require multiple-dose insulin.[85] Others[68,84] have incorporated SMBG into the care plans for all women who have GDM. Whether there is any benefit to continuous glucose monitoring for women who have GDM and who do not require insulin is under investigation.[86]

Dietary Interventions

Dietary interventions to minimize maternal glycemia are the mainstay of and should be the first step in the management of GDM. A major goal of nutritional management of women who have GDM is to provide adequate but not excessive nutrients for maternal and fetal growth. Attempts to limit the supply of nutrients by moderate restrictions on total daily energy (caloric) intake produced no impact on limiting fetal growth.[87-89] Because glucose is a major substrate for fetal growth, the quantity of glucose transferred from maternal to fetal circulations is positively correlated with maternal glucose concentrations, and by definition maternal glucose levels are higher in women who have GDM than in those who do not, strategies have been designed to limit maternal hyperglycemia by changes in dietary content. Limiting total carbohydrates (sugars, starch, and fiber) in one study was associated with a decrease in LGA neonates.[90] Another study, however, found that an *increase* in total carbohydrates in women who have GDM was associated with a *decrease* in the incidence of fetal macrosomia.[91] The failure to distinguish among the types of carbohydrates in the foods ingested may provide a partial explanation for the disparity in findings in these studies. Glucose in simple carbohydrates (as are found in foods containing refined sugars, such as nondiet soft drinks) is most rapidly absorbed while complex carbohydrates (as are found in such foods as whole-grain cereals and pastas) are absorbed more slowly.

The glycemic index (GI) is a quantitative measure of the effect of different foods on blood glucose following ingestion. It is determined in normal test subjects by first calculating the area under the glucose response curve over a 2-hour period following ingestion of a fixed quantity of a specific food. The area under the 2-hour glucose response curve to a 50-gram glucose challenge in the same subject is then measured. The GI of the food then is calculated by dividing the area under the glucose response curve of the food by that of 50 grams of glucose and is expressed as a percent.[92] Results of prospective trials comparing pregnant women randomized to low- versus high-GI foods have reported mixed results. One study of nondiabetic pregnant women randomized at 8 weeks' gestation found significantly lower measures of maternal glucose and insulin and greater insulin sensitivity in late pregnancy in the group consuming a low-GI diet. Newborns of subjects in the latter group had significantly lower birth weight as well as lower lean and fat mass.[93] Another large (*n* = 800) trial investigated pregnant women who had delivered previous babies whose birth weights were ≥4,000 grams. Starting at recruitment (13 weeks), patients were randomized to low GI or no dietary intervention. Women in the low-GI group had less weight gain and lower post–glucose challenge results at 28 weeks. Although birth weight centiles were lower for the low-GI group, the difference did not achieve statistical significance.[94] A lack of differences in newborn weights in a similar trial of women with GDM also has been reported, but interventions were not applied until the gestational age at which the diagnosis of GDM was made (i.e., a mean of 26 weeks).[95] Differences in duration of exposure to the low-GI diet may account for the differences in findings between studies.

A decrease in carbohydrates, whether they are simple or complex, must be accompanied by an increase in other nutrients to maintain caloric intake adequate for pregnancy. An increase in dietary fats has been explored as a means of slowing gastric emptying and thus glucose absorption. A distinction must be made, however, between saturated and unsaturated fats, as the former are associated with increased insulin resistance.[96] Also, as previously noted, there may be a stronger correlation between maternal triglyceride concentrations and neonatal total and fat weight than with maternal glucose.

Dietary advice for pregnant women with GDM covers a wide spectrum of opinion and a narrow spectrum of intervention trials. A review of studies comparing low-moderate with high-moderate GI food; low-GI with high-fiber, moderate-GI diets; calorie-restricted with unrestricted diets; and low- versus high-carbohydrate diets found no significant benefits of any of the diets studied.[97]

Exercise

Exercise improves insulin sensitivity and glucose clearance by a variety of mechanisms. On a molecular level, exercise is associated with increased activity and expression of insulin-signaling proteins and enzymes that participate in skeletal muscle and fat uptake of glucose. Expression of the GLUT4 transporter molecule, required for insulin-dependent transport of glucose from the extracellular fluid to skeletal muscle and fat cells, is increased during exercise.[98,99] A theoretical concern is that during aerobic exercise even of moderate intensity blood along with its oxygen content is shunted away from the uterus. The exercise-associated decrease in uterine blood flow, however, has been reported to be partially compensated by exercise-related hemoconcentration and redistribution of maternal blood flow away from the myometrium and to the cotyledons. Furthermore, both peak lactate levels and oxygen debt are lower following maximal exercise during pregnancy compared with exercise during the nonpregnant state.[100] A review of seven trials of exercise intervention in women who had GDM found a reduction in maternal glucose concentrations and a decrease in insulin use in the patients who added exercise to diet therapy. None reported an effect on birth weight.[101] Another prospective randomized trial found, however, that among women with

GDM, birth weight was reduced significantly in the exercise group.[102] The length of exposure to exercise may have accounted for the difference in findings. In the former report, exercise therapy was not introduced before 24 weeks,[101] whereas in the latter, exercise was introduced for all patients between 10 and 12 weeks (i.e., before the time the diagnosis of GDM was made).[102]

Medication

For some years, standard care of GDM has included the introduction of hypoglycemic medication when dietary or diet and exercise changes failed to lower glucose below desired thresholds (Table 14.1). Insulin was the first such medication and remains the mainstay of medical treatment of persistent maternal hyperglycemia. More recently, some have added insulin to prevent excessive fetal growth for women who have GDM.[103–106] A purported virtue of insulin is that unlike oral medications it was thought to not pass the placental barrier. In vitro studies, however, have demonstrated that insulin lispro does transfer to cord blood when given in higher therapeutic doses.[107]

In individuals without diabetes, pancreatic β-cells respond to secretagogues (glucose, amino acids, incretins, and vagal stimuli) with the acute production and release of insulin. Insulin secreted in lower concentrations during normal between-meal periods is sufficient to prevent hypoglycemia. Efforts have been made to mimic this basal-bolus cycle by combinations of insulin and insulin analogs. The latter are synthetic insulins altered by making changes in physical or structural properties of the insulin molecule to either increase or decrease the duration of hypoglycemic effect. The properties of these analogs are summarized in Table 14.2.[108] Although glargine has been shown to have increased mitogenic potential in vitro in breast cancer and osteosarcoma cells, it has not been reported to have tumorigenic or teratogenic potential in human pregnancies.[109]

The use of oral hypoglycemics for the management of GDM is of relatively recent advent. In 2000, a randomized controlled trial found glyburide in doses up

Table 14.2 Insulin Analogs and Their Pharmacokinetics

Insulin	Trade name	Manufacturer	Onset (h)	Peak (h)	Duration (h)
Rapid-acting					
Lispro	Humalog	Eli Lilly	0.2–0.5	0.5–2	3–4
Aspart	Novolog	Novo Nordisk	0.2–0.5	0.5–2	3–4
Glulisine	Apidra	Sanofi-Aventis	0.2–0.5	0.5–2	3–4
Intermediate-acting					
Isophane insulin (NPH)	Humulin N Novolin N	Eli Lilly Novo Nordisk	1.5–4	4–10	Up to 20
Long-acting					
Glargine	Lantus	Sanofi-Aventis	1–3	No peak	Up to 24
Detemir	Levemir	Novo Nordisk	1–3	No peak	Up to 24

to 20 mg/day to be as effective as multiple-dose insulin administration in the treatment of women who had GDM. There were no differences in mean maternal glycemia, the incidence of LGA neonates, or neonatal morbidities between those treated with glyburide and those treated with insulin.[110] Subsequently a small (*n* = 64) randomized trial reported similar findings.[111] A retrospective analysis of data comparing women who had GDM who were treated with glyburide (*n* = 2,073) with those who received insulin (*n* = 8,609) found a greater proportion of macro-somic neonates among the former.[112] The pharmacokinetics of glyburide during pregnancy are different from those in the nonpregnant state. Glyburide taken during pregnancy takes 30–60 minutes to be detected in maternal blood, and peaks 2–3 hours after administration. Glucose concentration begins to increase within minutes of starting a meal. Thus for treatment of GDM, glyburide should be taken 30–60 minutes before beginning a meal. Glyburide causes a decrease in glucose in a non–insulin-dependent fashion. Therefore, taking the drug and not following it with a meal increases the risk of hypoglycemia. During pregnancy, the drug is cleared by the liver within 8–10 hours. Therefore, the woman who has repeated hyperglycemia after the evening meal may benefit from a second dose of glyburide 30–60 minutes before that meal. Finally, although earlier studies sug-gested that glyburide crosses the placenta minimally,[110] subsequent investigation found a ratio of 0.7 of cord-to-maternal plasma concentrations of the drug. Although compared with insulin treatment of diabetes the incidence of neonatal hypoglycemia in glyburide-treated women with GDM is not significantly differ-ent, the effects on fetal programming of future metabolic function are unknown.[113]

Metformin is an oral hypoglycemic that decreases gut absorption of glucose, decreases insulin resistance, and enhances glucose uptake in insulin-dependent cells. Unlike glyburide, it is secreted actively into renal tubules. Given the increase in renal blood flow and glomerular filtration during pregnancy, the clearance of metformin is increased in pregnancy. Because of its increased clearance as well as the normal increase in pregnancy-related insulin resistance, it has been speculated that a dose greater than that required in the nonpregnant state may be necessary to be as effective in reducing glucose levels during pregnancy. Metformin is found in cord blood in concentrations from one-half to greater than that found in mater-nal blood.[114] In randomized trials of women with GDM comparing metformin with insulin, most subjects required the addition of insulin to maintain glucose targets. Most reported less maternal weight gain with metformin than with insulin alone, and there were no significant differences in birth weight between the two groups (Table 14.3).

Restricting Weight Gain

The Institute of Medicine (IOM) guidelines for weight gain during pregnancy are based on estimates of that weight gain within each category of maternal pre-pregnancy BMI, which is associated with the lowest prevalence of Cesarean deliv-ery, preterm delivery, small for gestational age or LGA, childhood obesity, and maternal postpartum weight retention (Table 14.4).[115] Recommendations specific to pregestational or gestational diabetes were not included in these guidelines. Large population-based studies from which the data of women known to have diabetes were deleted,[116,117] or in which the data were adjusted for maternal glyce-mia,[118,119] found independent positive relationships between the prevalence of

Table 14.3 Comparative Trials of Metformin and Insulin in GDM

Ref.	Type	n	Metformin vs. other	Maternal Needed addi- tional insulin	Weight gain	Neonatal Birth weight	Macro/LGA
167	Cohort	592	Met(+Ins) vs. Diet(+Ins)	21 vs. 37% OR 0.46 (0.32–0.66)			Met < Diet OR 0.56 (0.33–0.99)
168	Case Control	200	Met vs. Ins	NA	Met < Diet	NS	NS
169	RCT	200	Met vs. Ins	NA		NS	NS
170	RCT	751	Met(+Ins) vs. Ins	46%	Met < Ins	NS	NS
171	RCT	100	Met(+Ins) vs. Ins	32%	NS	NS	NS
172	RCT	160	Met(+Ins) vs. Ins	14%	Met < Ins	Met < Ins	Met < Ins
173	RCT	94	Met(+Ins) vs. Ins	26%	Met < Ins	NS	NS

RCT = Randomized controlled trial. OR = Odds ratio. NA = Not assessed.
NS = Not statistically significant.

Table 14.4 Institute of Medicine Recommended Weight Gain for Pregnancy

Prepregnancy BMI	Total Weight Gain Range in kg	Range in lb	Rates of Weight Gain* 2nd and 3rd Trimesters Mean (range) in kg/week	Mean (range) in lb/week
Underweight (< 18.5 kg/m²)	12.5–18	28–40	0.51	1
Normal weight (18.5-24.9 kg/m²)	11.5–16	25–35	0.42	1
Overweight (25.0-29.9 kg/m²)	7–11.5	15–25	0.28	0.6
Obese (≥ 30.0 kg/m²)	5–9	11–20	0.22	0.5

Note: *Calculations assume a 0.5–2 kg (1.1–4.4 lb) weight gain in the first trimester.

Source: Rasmussen KM, Yaktine AL. *Weight Gain During Pregnancy: Reexamining the Guidelines.* Washington, DC: Institute of Medicine and National Research Council of the National Academies, 2009.

LGA and maternal prepregnancy BMI and incremental weight gain within each BMI category, respectively. In general, the magnitude of association of the adjusted odds ratio for excessive weight gain with LGA decreased with progressive increases in BMI category. In other words, the odds of having an LGA neonate for a woman whose weight gain was in excess of that recommended by the IOM was greater if she were of normal weight than if she were obese. In addition, increased neonatal fat mass of offspring of nondiabetic women was found to be related incrementally with prepregnancy BMI[120] and with categories of weight gain within BMI groups.[120,121] Similar data were reported for women with GDM, whose progressive increase in BMI category,[122,123] as well as excessive weight gain within each category,[122-124] was associated with excessive birth weight.

In women who had at least two pregnancies complicated by GDM, pregnancy weight gain but not BMI category was associated with birth weight.[125] In another study, weight gain to 24 weeks was significantly greater among overweight and obese women with GDM than among those who did not have GDM. Together these studies suggest that although overweight and obese women with GDM gain more weight than their counterparts without diabetes, restricting their weight gain may reduce the incidence of large neonates.[126] Although no intervention studies specifically targeting women with GDM have been reported, a number of individual studies and reviews have examined the effects of lifestyle (primarily dietary) changes on pregnancy outcomes in unselected or overweight and obese obstetric populations. Most randomized trials have found that the group receiving the intervention had less gestational weight gain but no impact on birth weight.[127-131] Adherence to instructions is a problem, as some subjects reported either not having received instructions or having received incorrect advice about weight gain.[132,133] In studies confined to women who were overweight and obese, significant decreases in gestational weight gain but no decreases in the incidence of fetal macrosomia,[134] LGA,[135] or birth weight[136] were reported.

In both women who do and those do not have GDM, gestational weight loss in overweight and obese women has been associated with a reduction in the frequency of LGA neonates. Particularly in overweight women, however, pregnancy weight loss also has been associated with an increased risk of small-for-gestational-age neonates.[137-140] Given these findings plus the negative association between (presumably fasting-associated) maternal ketonemia and intellectual performance in children of women with diabetes,[141] weight loss during pregnancy seems ill-advised.

DELIVERY

The timing of delivery for a woman who has GDM involves two primary considerations. Awaiting delivery until the onset of spontaneous labor carries with it the risk of excessive fetal growth and thus the increased risk of shoulder dystocia, as well as the small risk of fetal demise. Delivery before term carries with it the risk of prematurity as well as that of Cesarean delivery for a failed induction of labor. Expert opinions differ, with the ADA suggesting that "[p]rolongation of gestation past 38 weeks increases the risk of fetal macrosomia without reducing Cesarean rates, so that delivery during the 38th week is recommended,"[142] whereas the American Congress of Obstetricians and Gynecologists recommends that "[w]hen glucose control is good and no other complications supervene, there is no good evidence to support routine delivery before 40 weeks."[1] Data from a large (n = 193,028 GDM births) database suggests, however, that although the risk of infant death for delivery at 36 weeks exceeds that of expectant management, at 39 weeks the risk of fetal demise in the expectant management group exceeds that of the risk of delivery, although the absolute risks with either management plan are low.[143]

POSTPARTUM CARE

TESTING FOR GLUCOSE INTOLERANCE

In each of two large population-based studies, the recurrence risk of GDM in the first subsequent pregnancy was reported as 41%.[144,145] Women who had GDM in a first pregnancy and were found to not have the disease in the second pregnancy had a lower recurrence risk, 23%, in their third pregnancy.[145] Factors positively associated with an increased risk of recurrence include maternal age, ethnicity (e.g., Latina, Pacific Islander, Middle Eastern, African American, and Asian descent), and longer interpregnancy interval. The risk of development of nongestational diabetes (usually T2D) is also higher for women who have had prior GDM, with observed rates of 18% in women followed for 9 years[146] and up to 70% in women observed up to 28 years postindex pregnancy.[147] In the former study, the rate of development of T2D 9 months after pregnancy was 3.7%.[146]

The current recommendation of the ADA is that all women found to have GDM should be rescreened 6–12 weeks following delivery with either the fasting glucose or 2-hour 75-gram GTT. In two studies, women who had GDM and were tested with GTTs within 3–6 months postpartum were found to have a prevalence of 6.5%[148] and 11%[149] of overt diabetes. In the latter study, 10% of women with overt diabetes and 38% with prediabetes had a normal fasting glucose. It seems well advised, therefore, to perform the complete 2-hour GTT rather than a fasting glucose analysis, unless the patient refuses the test. The ADA recommends that following a pregnancy complicated by GDM, women not found to have persistent diabetes or prediabetes (impaired glucose tolerance or impaired fasting glucose) should be retested for glucose intolerance every 3 years or more often for the rest of their lives.[85]

FAMILY PLANNING

A woman who has had GDM is at substantial increased risk of development of recurrent GDM and overt diabetes, and both of these entities have potentially serious consequences for mother and offspring. A collaborative effort between mother and caregiver to ensure optimal metabolic control before undertaking pregnancy seems warranted. Family planning is an essential component of pregnancy preparation. According to the Centers for Disease Control and Prevention, diabetes is a condition for which there is no restriction for the use of any contraceptive method.[150] In contrast with a global decrease in unintended pregnancies, the unintended pregnancy rate has remained stable in the U.S. since 1994, accounting for 49% of all pregnancies.[151] Although substantial economic and social barriers to the use of effective family planning methods exist, the one modifiable factor is the caregiver's discussion and provision of contraception to women of reproductive age. For the woman with prior GDM, that burden falls on all professionals responsible for her care, including primary care physicians, endocrinologists, obstetricians and gynecologists, diabetes educators, midwives, and nurse practitioners.[152]

BREAST-FEEDING

Besides the benefits attributed to breast-feeding for all women and their newborns, specific benefits accrue to women who have GDM and their offspring. Among women who had GDM such measurements as fasting and 2-hour glucose insulin areas under the curve during a postpartum GTT were found to be lower among breast-feeding compared with non–breast-feeding mothers.[153,154] The effects of lactation on metabolism may vary with duration of lactation. One study reported improvement in maternal glucose and insulin secretion and sensitivity among women who breast-fed for >10 months, compared with those who breast-fed for <10 months.[155] A 19-year follow-up study of women who had had GDM found that those women who breast-fed for >3 months had the lowest risk of development of T2D, and that women who breast-fed had a fivefold longer latency period before developing overt diabetes than those who did not.[156] Although little has been written about the effects of oral hypoglycemic agents on breast-milk production and content, what evidence exists suggests minimal amounts of these drugs are found in breast milk.[157]

There is a paucity of data on the effect of breast-feeding limited to children of women who had GDM. In one such report, the trajectory of childhood increase in BMI was significantly slower for breast-fed compared with non–breast-fed infants of women with diabetes, despite the absence of differences in BMI at birth.[158] In another study, the prevalence of childhood overweight was lower for children of women who breast-fed for 3–6 months than for those of mothers who breast-fed for 0–3 months, but prolonging breast-feeding beyond 6 months did not further decrease children's excessive growth.[159]

LONG-TERM INTERVENTIONS

Although a discussion of efforts to limit the long-term adverse effects and sequelae of GDM on mothers and their offspring is beyond the scope of this chapter, it should be acknowledged that the results of these efforts likely will have application to the care of women who have other forms of metabolic dysfunction.

CONCLUSION

Many of the complications of pregnancy associated with pregestational diabetes also are seen in association with GDM. Indeed, GDM is likely a *forme fruste* of

T2D. Treatments beginning during pregnancy and those initiated postpartum may have lifelong positive effects on the health of both the mother who has GDM and on her children.

REFERENCES

1. American College of Obstetricians and Gynecologists. Gestational diabetes. ACOG Practice Bulletin Number 30, September 2001. *Obstet Gynecol* 2001;98:525–538.

2. Coustan DR. Clinical chemistry review: gestational diabetes mellitus. *Clin Chem* 2013;59:1310–1321.

3. Landon MB, Gabbe SG. Gestational diabetes mellitus. *Obstet Gynecol* 2011;118:1379–1393.

4. Kucera J. Rate and type of congenital anomalies among offspring of diabetic women. *J Reprod Med* 1971;7:73–82.

5. Mills JL, Baker L, Goldman AS. Malformations in infants of diabetic mothers occur before the seventh gestational week. Implications for treatment. *Diabetes* 1979;28:292–293.

6. Miller E, Hare JW, Cloherty JP, et al. Elevated maternal hemoglobin A1c in early pregnancy and major congenital anomalies in infants of diabetic mothers. *N Engl J Med* 1981;304:1331–1334.

7. Hanson U, Persson B, Thunell S. Relationship between haemoglobin A1C in early type 1 (insulin-dependent) diabetic pregnancy and the occurrence of spontaneous abortion and fetal malformation in Sweden. *Diabetologia* 1990;33:100–104.

8. McCarter RJ, Kessler, II, Comstock GW. Is diabetes mellitus a teratogen or a coteratogen? *Am J Epidemiol* 1987;125:195–205.

9. Fuhrmann K, Reiher H, Semmler K, Fischer F, Fischer M, Glockner E. Prevention of congenital malformations in infants of insulin-dependent diabetic mothers. *Diabetes Care* 1983;6:219–223.

10. Balsells M, Garcia-Patterson A, Gich I, Corcoy R. Major congenital malformations in women with gestational diabetes mellitus: a systematic review and meta-analysis. *Diabetes/Metab Res Rev* 2012;28:252–257.

11. Allen VM, Armson BA, Wilson RD, et al. Teratogenicity associated with pre-existing and gestational diabetes. *J Obstet Gynaecol Can* 2007;29:927–944.

12. Zhao Z, Reece EA. New concepts in diabetic embryopathy. *Clin Lab Med* 2013;33:207–233.

13. Clapes S, Fernandez T, Suarez G. Oxidative stress and birth defects in infants of women with pregestational diabetes. *MEDICC Review* 2013;15:37–40.

14. Zabihi S, Loeken MR. Understanding diabetic teratogenesis: where are we now and where are we going? Birth defects research Part A. *Clin Mol Ter* 2010;88:779–790.

15. Goldman JA, Dicker D, Feldberg D, Yeshaya A, Samuel N, Karp M. Pregnancy outcome in patients with insulin-dependent diabetes mellitus with preconceptional diabetic control: a comparative study. *Am J Obstet Gynecol* 1986;155:293–297.

16. Sacks DA. Preconception care for diabetic women: background, barriers, and strategies for effective implementation. *Curr Diabetes Rev* 2006;2:147–161.

17. Reece EA, Wu YK, Zhao Z, Dhanasekaran D. Dietary vitamin and lipid therapy rescues aberrant signaling and apoptosis and prevents hyperglycemia-induced diabetic embryopathy in rats. *Am J Obstet Gynecol* 2006;194:580–585.

18. Jagerstad M. Folic acid fortification prevents neural tube defects and may also reduce cancer risks. *Acta Paediatr* 2012;101:1007–1012.

19. Correa A, Gilboa SM, Botto LD, et al. Lack of periconceptional vitamins or supplements that contain folic acid and diabetes mellitus-associated birth defects. *Am J Obstet Gynecol* 2012;206:218 e1–13.

20. Lapolla A, Dalfra MG, Bonomo M, et al. Gestational diabetes mellitus in Italy: a multicenter study. *Eur J Obstet Gynecol Reprod Biol* 2009;145:149–153.

21. Fadl HE, Ostlund IK, Magnuson AF, Hanson US. Maternal and neonatal outcomes and time trends of gestational diabetes mellitus in Sweden from 1991 to 2003. *Diabet Med* 2010;27:436–441.

22. O'Sullivan JB, Charles D, Mahan CM, Dandrow RV. Gestational diabetes and perinatal mortality rate. *Am J Obstet Gynecol* 1973;116:901–904.

23. Keshavarz M, Cheung NW, Babaee GR, Moghadam HK, Ajami ME, Shariati M. Gestational diabetes in Iran: incidence, risk factors and pregnancy outcomes. *Diabetes Res Clin Pract* 2005;69:279–286.

24. Girz BA, Divon MY, Merkatz IR. Sudden fetal death in women with well-controlled, intensively monitored gestational diabetes. *J Perinatol* 1992; 12:229–233.

25. Karmon A, Levy A, Holcberg G, Wiznitzer A, Mazor M, Sheiner E. Decreased perinatal mortality among women with diet-controlled gestational diabetes mellitus. *Int J Gynaecol Obstet* 2009;104:199–202.

26. Ohana O, Holcberg G, Sergienko R, Sheiner E. Risk factors for intrauterine fetal death (1988-2009). *J Matern Fetal Neonatal Med* 2011;24:1079–1083.

27. Wendland EM, Duncan BB, Mengue SS, Schmidt MI. Lesser than diabetes hyperglycemia in pregnancy is related to perinatal mortality: a cohort study in Brazil. *BMC Pregnancy Childbirth* 2011 Nov 11;11:92. doi: 10.1186/1471-2393-11-92

28. American Diabetes Association. Standards of medical care in diabetes—2010. *Diabetes Care* 2010;33(Suppl 1):S11–S61.

29. American Diabetes Association. Standards of medical care in diabetes—2011. *Diabetes Care*;34(Suppl 1):S11–S61.

30. Alberti KG, Zimmet PZ. Definition, diagnosis and classification of diabetes mellitus and its complications. Part 1: diagnosis and classification of diabetes mellitus. Provisional report of a WHO consultation. *Diabet Med* 1998;15:539–553.

31. Aberg A, Rydhstrom H, Kallen B, Kallen K. Impaired glucose tolerance during pregnancy is associated with increased fetal mortality in preceding sibs. *Acta Obstet Gynecol Scand* 1997;76:212–217.

32. Dudley DJ. Diabetic-associated stillbirth: incidence, pathophysiology, and prevention. *Obstet Gynecol Clin North Am* 2007;34:293–307, ix.

33. Rayburn WF, Sokkary N, Clokey DE, Moore LE, Curet LB. Consequences of routine delivery at 38 weeks for A-2 gestational diabetes. *J Matern Fetal Neonatal Med* 2005;18:333–337.

34. American College of Obstetricians and Gynecologists. Fetal macrosomia. ACOG Practice Bulletin No. 22, November 2000; reaffirmed 2013. *Obstet Gynecol* 2000;96:1–11

35. Alexander GR, Himes JH, Kaufman RB, Mor J, Kogan M. A United States national reference for fetal growth. *Obstet Gynecol* 1996;87:163–168.

36. Gardosi J. Customised assessment of fetal growth potential: implications for perinatal care. *Arch Dis Child Fetal Neonatal Ed* 2012;97:F314–F317.

37. Larkin JC, Speer PD, Simhan HN. A customized standard of large size for gestational age to predict intrapartum morbidity. *Am J Obstet Gynecol* 2011;204:499 e1–10.

38. Catalano PM, Thomas A, Huston-Presley L, Amini SB. Increased fetal adiposity: a very sensitive marker of abnormal in utero development. *Am J Obstet Gynecol* 2003;189:1698–1704.

39. Langer O, Berkus MD, Huff RW, Samueloff A. Shoulder dystocia: should the fetus weighing greater than or equal to 4000 grams be delivered by cesarean section? *Am J Obstet Gynecol* 1991;165:831–837.

40. Metzger BE, Lowe LP, Dyer AR, et al. Hyperglycemia and adverse pregnancy outcomes. *N Engl J Med* 2008;358:1991–2002.

41. Hyperglycemia and Adverse Pregnancy Outcome (HAPO) Study: associations with neonatal anthropometrics. *Diabetes* 2009;58:453–459.

42. Pedersen J. Diabetes and pregnancy. Blood Sugar of Newborn Infants. Copenhagen, Danish Science Press, 1952.

43. Catalano PM, Hauguel-De Mouzon S. Is it time to revisit the Pedersen hypothesis in the face of the obesity epidemic? *Am J Obstet Gynecol* 2011;204:479–487.

44. Knopp RH, Magee MS, Walden CE, Bonet B, Benedetti TJ. Prediction of infant birth weight by GDM screening tests. Importance of plasma triglyceride. *Diabetes Care* 1992;15:1605–1613.

45. Di Cianni G, Miccoli R, Volpe L, et al. Maternal triglyceride levels and newborn weight in pregnant women with normal glucose tolerance. *Diabet Med* 2005;22:21–25.

46. Harmon KA, Gerard L, Jensen DR, et al. Continuous glucose profiles in obese and normal-weight pregnant women on a controlled diet: metabolic determinants of fetal growth. *Diabetes Care* 2011;34:2198–2204.

47. Catalano PM, McIntyre HD, Cruickshank JK, et al. The Hyperglycemia and Adverse Pregnancy Outcome Study: associations of GDM and obesity with pregnancy outcomes. *Diabetes Care* 2012;35:780–786.

48. Black MH, Sacks DA, Xiang AH, Lawrence JM. The relative contribution of prepregnancy overweight and obesity, gestational weight gain, and IADPSG-defined gestational diabetes mellitus to fetal overgrowth. *Diabetes Care* 2013;36:56–62.

49. Hedderson M, Ehrlich S, Sridhar S, Darbinian J, Moore S, Ferrara A. Racial/ethnic disparities in the prevalence of gestational diabetes mellitus by BMI. *Diabetes Care* 2012;35:1492–1498.

50. Esakoff TF, Caughey AB, Block-Kurbisch I, Inturrisi M, Cheng YW. Perinatal outcomes in patients with gestational diabetes mellitus by race/ethnicity. *J Matern Fetal Neonatal Med* 2011;24:422–426.

51. Wong VW. Gestational diabetes mellitus in five ethnic groups: a comparison of their clinical characteristics. *Diabet Med* 2012;29:366–371.

52. Morkrid K, Jenum AK, Sletner L, et al. Failure to increase insulin secretory capacity during pregnancy-induced insulin resistance is associated with ethnicity and gestational diabetes. *Eur J Endocrinol* 2012;167:579–588.

53. Vambergue A, Fajardy I. Consequences of gestational and pregestational diabetes on placental function and birth weight. *World Journal of Diabetes* 2011;2:196–203.

54. Lager S, Powell TL. Regulation of nutrient transport across the placenta. *Journal of Pregnancy* 2012;2012:179827. doi: 10.1155/2012/179827. Epub 2012 Dec 10. Review.

55. Report of the National High Blood Pressure Education Program Working Group on High Blood Pressure in Pregnancy. *Am J Obstet Gynecol* 2000;183:S1–S22.

56. Schneider S, Freerksen N, Rohrig S, Hoeft B, Maul H. Gestational diabetes and preeclampsia—similar risk factor profiles? *Early Human Dev* 2012;88:179–184.

57. Yogev, Chen, Hod, et al. Hyperglycemia and Adverse Pregnancy Outcome (HAPO) study: preeclampsia. *Am J Obstet Gynecol* 2010;202:255 e1–7.

58. Harlev A, Wiznitzer A. New insights on glucose pathophysiology in gestational diabetes and insulin resistance. *Curr Diab Rep* 2010;10:242–247.

59. Karacay O, Sepici-Dincel A, Karcaaltincaba D, et al. A quantitative evaluation of total antioxidant status and oxidative stress markers in preeclampsia and gestational diabetic patients in 24-36 weeks of gestation. *Diabetes Res Clin Pract* 2010;89:231–238.

60. Zavalza-Gomez AB. Obesity and oxidative stress: a direct link to preeclampsia? *Arch Gynecol Obstet* 2011;283:415–422.

61. Parretti E, Lapolla A, Dalfra M, et al. Preeclampsia in lean normotensive normotolerant pregnant women can be predicted by simple insulin sensitivity indexes. *Hypertension* 2006;47:449–453.

62. Montoro MN, Kjos SL, Chandler M, Peters RK, Xiang AH, Buchanan TA. Insulin resistance and preeclampsia in gestational diabetes mellitus. *Diabetes Care* 2005;28:1995–2000.

63. Crowther CA, Hiller JE, Moss JR, McPhee AJ, Jeffries WS, Robinson JS. Effect of treatment of gestational diabetes mellitus on pregnancy outcomes. *N Engl J Med* 2005;352:2477–2486.

64. Landon MB, Spong CY, Thom E, et al. A multicenter, randomized trial of treatment for mild gestational diabetes. *N Engl J Med* 2009;361:1339–1348.

65. Han S, Crowther CA, Middleton P. Interventions for pregnant women with hyperglycaemia not meeting gestational diabetes and type 2 diabetes diagnostic criteria. *Cochrane Database Syst Rev* 2012;1:CD009037.

66. Hartling L, Dryden DM, Guthrie A, Muise M, Vandermeer B, Donovan L. Benefits and harms of treating gestational diabetes mellitus: a systematic review and meta-analysis for the U.S. Preventive Services Task Force and the National Institutes of Health Office of Medical Applications of Research. *Ann Intern Med* 2013;159:123–129

67. Alwan N, Tuffnell DJ, West J. Treatments for gestational diabetes. *Cochrane Database Syst Rev* 2009:CD003395.

68. Horvath K, Koch K, Jeitler K, et al. Effects of treatment in women with gestational diabetes mellitus: systematic review and meta-analysis. *BMJ* 2010;Apr 1;340:c1395. doi: 10.1136/bmj.c1395.

69. Falavigna M, Schmidt MI, Trujillo J, et al. Effectiveness of gestational diabetes treatment: a systematic review with quality of evidence assessment. *Diabetes Res Clin Pract* 2012;98:396–405.

70. Durnwald CP, Mele L, Spong CY, et al. Glycemic characteristics and neonatal outcomes of women treated for mild gestational diabetes. *Obstet Gynecol* 2011;117:819–827.

71. Langer O, Levy J, Brustman L, Anyaegbunam A, Merkatz R, Divon M. Glycemic control in gestational diabetes mellitus—how tight is tight enough: small for gestational age versus large for gestational age? *Am J Obstet Gynecol* 1989;161:646–653.

72. Kerenyi Z, Tamas G, Kivimaki M, et al. Maternal glycemia and risk of large-for-gestational-age babies in a population-based screening. *Diabetes Care* 2009;32:2200–2205.

73. de Veciana M, Major CA, Morgan MA, et al. Postprandial versus preprandial blood glucose monitoring in women with gestational diabetes mellitus requiring insulin therapy. *N Engl J Med* 1995;333:1237–1241.

74. Metzger BE, Gabbe SG, Persson B, et al. International Association of Diabetes and Pregnancy Study Groups recommendations on the diagnosis and classification of hyperglycemia in pregnancy. *Diabetes Care* 2010;33:676–682.

75. Black MH, Sacks DA, Xiang AH, Lawrence JM. Clinical outcomes of pregnancies complicated by mild gestational diabetes mellitus differ by combinations of abnormal oral glucose tolerance test values. *Diabetes Care* 2010;33:2524–2530.

76. Yogev Y, Ben-Haroush A, Chen R, Rosenn B, Hod M, Langer O. Diurnal glycemic profile in obese and normal weight nondiabetic pregnant women. *Am J Obstet Gynecol* 2004;191:949–953.

77. Hernandez TL, Friedman JE, Van Pelt RE, Barbour LA. Patterns of glycemia in normal pregnancy: should the current therapeutic targets be challenged? *Diabetes Care* 2011;34:1660–1668.

78. American Diabetes Association. Self-monitoring of blood glucose. *Diabetes Care* 1994;17:81–86.

79. Kuo CY, Hsu CT, Ho CS, Su TE, Wu MH, Wang CJ. Accuracy and precision evaluation of seven self-monitoring blood glucose systems. *Diabetes Technol Ther* 2011;13:596–600.

80. Kazlauskaite R, Soni S, Evans AT, Graham K, Fisher B. Accuracy of self-monitored blood glucose in type 2 diabetes. *Diabetes Technol Ther* 2009;11:385–392.

81. Mazze RS, Shamoon H, Pasmantier R, et al. Reliability of blood glucose monitoring by patients with diabetes mellitus. *Am J Med* 1984;77:211–217.

82. Kendrick JM, Wilson C, Elder RF, Smith CS. Reliability of reporting of self-monitoring of blood glucose in pregnant women. *J Obstet Gynecol Neonatal Nurs* 2005;34:329–334.

83. Homko CJ, Sivan E, Reece EA. The impact of self-monitoring of blood glucose on self-efficacy and pregnancy outcomes in women with diet-controlled gestational diabetes. *Diabetes Educ* 2002;28:435–443.

84. Hawkins JS, Casey BM, Lo JY, Moss K, McIntire DD, Leveno KJ. Weekly compared with daily blood glucose monitoring in women with diet-treated gestational diabetes. *Obstet Gynecol* 2009;113:1307–1312.

85. American Diabetes Association. Standards of medical care in diabetes—2013. *Diabetes Care* 2013;36(Suppl 1):S11–S66.

86. Voormolen DN, DeVries JH, Franx A, Mol BW, Evers IM. Effectiveness of continuous glucose monitoring during diabetic pregnancy (GlucoMOMS trial); a randomised controlled trial. *BMC Pregnancy Childbirth* 2012 Dec 27;12:164. doi: 10.1186/1471-2393-12-164.

87. Rae A, Bond D, Evans S, North F, Roberman B, Walters B. A randomised controlled trial of dietary energy restriction in the management of obese women with gestational diabetes. *Aust N Z J Obstet Gynaecol* 2000;40:416–422.

88. Dornhorst A, Nicholls JS, Probst F, et al. Calorie restriction for treatment of gestational diabetes. *Diabetes* 1991;40(Suppl 2):161–164.

89. Algert S, Shragg P, Hollingsworth DR. Moderate caloric restriction in obese women with gestational diabetes. *Obstet Gynecol* 1985;65:487–491.

90. Major CA, Henry MJ, De Veciana M, Morgan MA. The effects of carbohydrate restriction in patients with diet-controlled gestational diabetes. *Obstet Gynecol* 1998;91:600–604.

91. Romon M, Nuttens MC, Vambergue A, et al. Higher carbohydrate intake is associated with decreased incidence of newborn macrosomia in women with gestational diabetes. *J Am Diet Assoc* 2001;101:897–902.

92. Jenkins DJ, Wolever TM, Taylor RH, et al. Glycemic index of foods: a physiological basis for carbohydrate exchange. *Am J Clin Nutr* 1981;34:362–366.

93. Clapp JF. Maternal carbohydrate intake and pregnancy outcome. *Proc Nutr Soc* 2002;61:45–50.

94. Walsh JM, McGowan CA, Mahony R, Foley ME, McAuliffe FM. Low glycaemic index diet in pregnancy to prevent macrosomia (ROLO study): randomised control trial. *BMJ* 2012 Aug 30;345:e5605. doi: 10.1136/bmj.e5605

95. Louie JC, Markovic TP, Perera N, et al. A randomized controlled trial investigating the effects of a low-glycemic index diet on pregnancy outcomes in gestational diabetes mellitus. *Diabetes Care* 2011;34:2341–2346.

96. Hernandez T L AM, Chartier-Logan C, Friedman JE, Barbour LA. Strategies in the nutritional management of gestational diabetes. *Clin Obstet Gynecol.* In press.

97. Han S, Crowther CA, Middleton P, Heatley E. Different types of dietary advice for women with gestational diabetes mellitus. *Cochrane Database Syst Rev* 2013;3:CD009275.

98. Frosig C, Rose AJ, Treebak JT, Kiens B, Richter EA, Wojtaszewski JF. Effects of endurance exercise training on insulin signaling in human skeletal muscle: interactions at the level of phosphatidylinositol 3-kinase, Akt, and AS160. *Diabetes* 2007;56:2093–2102.

99. Golbidi S, Laher I. Potential mechanisms of exercise in gestational diabetes. *J Nutr Metab* 2013;2013:285948. doi: 10.1155/2013/285948. Epub 2013 Apr 9.

100. Wolfe LA, Weissgerber TL. Clinical physiology of exercise in pregnancy: a literature review. *J Obstet Gynecol Can* 2003;25:473–483.

101. Ruchat SM, Mottola MF. The important role of physical activity in the prevention and management of gestational diabetes mellitus. *Diabetes Metab Res Rev* 2013;29:334–346.

102. Barakat R, Pelaez M, Lopez C, Lucia A, Ruiz JR. Exercise during pregnancy and gestational diabetes-related adverse effects: a randomised controlled trial. *Br J Sports Med* 2013;47:630–636.

103. Buchanan TA, Kjos SL, Montoro MN, et al. Use of fetal ultrasound to select metabolic therapy for pregnancies complicated by mild gestational diabetes. *Diabetes Care* 1994;17:275–283.

104. Kjos SL, Schaefer-Graf U, Sardesi S, et al. A randomized controlled trial using glycemic plus fetal ultrasound parameters versus glycemic parameters to determine insulin therapy in gestational diabetes with fasting hyperglycemia. *Diabetes Care* 2001;24:1904–1910.

105. Schaefer-Graf UM, Kjos SL, Fauzan OH, et al. A randomized trial evaluating a predominantly fetal growth-based strategy to guide management of gestational diabetes in Caucasian women. *Diabetes Care* 2004;27:297–302.

106. Bonomo M, Cetin I, Pisoni MP, et al. Flexible treatment of gestational diabetes modulated on ultrasound evaluation of intrauterine growth: a controlled randomized clinical trial. *Diabet Metab* 2004;30:237–244.

107. Boskovic R, Feig DS, Derewlany L, Knie B, Portnoi G, Koren G. Transfer of insulin lispro across the human placenta: in vitro perfusion studies. *Diabetes Care* 2003;26:1390–1394.

108. Borgono CA, Zinman B. Insulins: past, present, and future. *Endocrinol Metab Clin North Am* 2012;41:1–24.

109. Pollex E, Moretti ME, Koren G, Feig DS. Safety of insulin glargine use in pregnancy: a systematic review and meta-analysis. *Ann Pharmacother* 2011;45:9–16.

110. Langer O, Conway DL, Berkus MD, Xenakis EM, Gonzales O. A comparison of glyburide and insulin in women with gestational diabetes mellitus. *N Engl J Med* 2000;343:1134–1138.

111. Tempe A, Mayanglambam RD. Glyburide as treatment option for gestational diabetes mellitus. *J Obstet Gynaecol Res* 2013;39:1147–1152.

112. Cheng YW, Chung JH, Block-Kurbisch I, Inturrisi M, Caughey AB. Treatment of gestational diabetes mellitus: glyburide compared to subcutaneous insulin therapy and associated perinatal outcomes. *J Matern Fetal Neonatal Med* 2012;25:379–384.

113. Caritis SN, Hebert MF. A pharmacologic approach to the use of glyburide in pregnancy. *Obstet Gynecol* 2013;121:1309–1312.

114. Eyal S, Easterling TR, Carr D, et al. Pharmacokinetics of metformin during pregnancy. *Drug Metab Dispos* 2010;38:833–840.

115. Rasmussen KM, Yaktine AL. Weight Gain During Pregnancy: Reexamining the Guidelines. Washington, DC, Institute of Medicine and National Research Council of the National Academies, 2009.

116. Dietz PM, Callaghan WM, Sharma AJ. High pregnancy weight gain and risk of excessive fetal growth. *Am J Obstet Gynecol* 2009;201:51 e1–6.

117. Park S, Sappenfield WM, Bish C, Salihu H, Goodman D, Bensyl DM. Assessment of the Institute of Medicine recommendations for weight gain during pregnancy: Florida, 2004-2007. *Matern Child Health J* 2011;15:289–301.

118. Hedderson MM, Weiss NS, Sacks DA, et al. Pregnancy weight gain and risk of neonatal complications: macrosomia, hypoglycemia, and hyperbilirubinemia. *Obstet Gynecol* 2006;108:1153–1161.

119. Simas TA, Waring ME, Liao X, et al. Prepregnancy weight, gestational weight gain, and risk of growth affected neonates. *J Womens Health (Larchmt)* 2012;21:410–417.

120. Waters TP, Huston-Presley L, Catalano PM. Neonatal body composition according to the revised institute of medicine recommendations for maternal weight gain. *J Clin Endocrinol Metab* 2012;97:3648–3654.

121. Josefson JL, Hoffmann JA, Metzger BE. Excessive weight gain in women with a normal pre-pregnancy BMI is associated with increased neonatal adiposity. *Pediatric Obesity* 2013;8:e33–36.

122. Ouzounian JG, Hernandez GD, Korst LM, et al. Pre-pregnancy weight and excess weight gain are risk factors for macrosomia in women with gestational diabetes. *J Perinatol* 2011;31:717–721.

123. Ray JG, Vermeulen MJ, Shapiro JL, Kenshole AB. Maternal and neonatal outcomes in pregestational and gestational diabetes mellitus, and the influence of maternal obesity and weight gain: the DEPOSIT study. Dia-

betes Endocrine Pregnancy Outcome Study in Toronto. *QJM* 2001;94:347–356.

124. Park JE, Park S, Daily JW, Kim SH. Low gestational weight gain improves infant and maternal pregnancy outcomes in overweight and obese Korean women with gestational diabetes mellitus. *Gynecol Endocrinol* 2011;27:775–781.

125. Hutcheon JA, Platt RW, Meltzer SJ, Egeland GM. Is birth weight modified during pregnancy? Using sibling differences to understand the impact of blood glucose, obesity, and maternal weight gain in gestational diabetes. *Am J Obstet Gynecol* 2006;195:488–494.

126. Gibson KS, Waters TP, Catalano PM. Maternal weight gain in women who develop gestational diabetes mellitus. *Obstet Gynecol* 2012;119:560–565.

127. Asbee SM, Jenkins TR, Butler JR, White J, Elliot M, Rutledge A. Preventing excessive weight gain during pregnancy through dietary and lifestyle counseling: a randomized controlled trial. *Obstet Gynecol* 2009;113:305–312.

128. Kinnunen TI, Raitanen J, Aittasalo M, Luoto R. Preventing excessive gestational weight gain—a secondary analysis of a cluster-randomised controlled trial. *Eur J Clin Nutr* 2012;66:1344–1350.

129. Skouteris H, Hartley-Clark L, McCabe M, et al. Preventing excessive gestational weight gain: a systematic review of interventions. *Obes Rev* 2010;11:757–768.

130. Thangaratinam S, Rogozinska E, Jolly K, et al. Effects of interventions in pregnancy on maternal weight and obstetric outcomes: meta-analysis of randomised evidence. *BMJ* 2012 May 16;344:e2088. doi: 10.1136/bmj.e2088.

131. Tanentsapf I, Heitmann BL, Adegboye AR. Systematic review of clinical trials on dietary interventions to prevent excessive weight gain during pregnancy among normal weight, overweight and obese women. *BMC Pregnancy Childbirth* 2011 Oct 26;11:81. doi: 10.1186/1471-2393-11-81.

132. Stotland NE, Haas JS, Brawarsky P, Jackson RA, Fuentes-Afflick E, Escobar GJ. Body mass index, provider advice, and target gestational weight gain. *Obstet Gynecol* 2005;105:633–638.

133. Cogswell ME, Scanlon KS, Fein SB, Schieve LA. Medically advised, mother's personal target, and actual weight gain during pregnancy. *Obstet Gynecol* 1999;94:616–622.

134. Thornton YS, Smarkola C, Kopacz SM, Ishoof SB. Perinatal outcomes in nutritionally monitored obese pregnant women: a randomized clinical trial. *JAMA* 2009;101:569–577.

135. Oteng-Ntim E, Varma R, Croker H, Poston L, Doyle P. Lifestyle interventions for overweight and obese pregnant women to improve pregnancy outcome: systematic review and meta-analysis. *BMC Med* 2012 May 10;10:47. doi: 10.1186/1741-7015-10-47.

136. Quinlivan JA, Julania S, Lam L. Antenatal dietary interventions in obese pregnant women to restrict gestational weight gain to Institute of Medicine recommendations: a meta-analysis. *Obstet Gynecol* 2011;118:1395–1401.

137. Yee LM, Cheng YW, Inturrisi M, Caughey AB. Gestational weight loss and perinatal outcomes in overweight and obese women subsequent to diagnosis of gestational diabetes mellitus. *Obesity (Silver Spring)* 2013 Dec;21(12):E770–4. doi: 10.1002/oby.20490. Epub 2013 Jul 5.

138. Hinkle SN, Sharma AJ, Dietz PM. Gestational weight gain in obese mothers and associations with fetal growth. *Am J Clin Nutr* 2010;92:644–51.

139. Beyerlein A, Schiessl B, Lack N, von Kries R. Associations of gestational weight loss with birth-related outcome: a retrospective cohort study. *BJOG* 2011;118:55–61.

140. Katon J, Maynard C, Reiber G. Attempts at weight loss in U.S. women with and without a history of gestational diabetes mellitus. *Women's Health Issues* 2012;22:e447–e453.

141. Rizzo T, Metzger BE, Burns WJ, Burns K. Correlations between antepartum maternal metabolism and child intelligence. *N Engl J Med* 1991;325:911–916.

142. American Diabetes Association. Gestational diabetes mellitus. *Diabetes Care* 2004;27(Suppl 1):S88–S90.

143. Rosenstein MG, Cheng YW, Snowden JM, Nicholson JM, Caughey AB. Risk of stillbirth and infant death stratified by gestational age. *Obstet Gynecol* 2012;120:76–82.

144. Getahun D, Fassett MJ, Jacobsen SJ. Gestational diabetes: risk of recurrence in subsequent pregnancies. *Am J Obstet Gynecol* 2010;203:467 e1–e6.

145. Khambalia AZ, Ford JB, Nassar N, Shand AW, McElduff A, Roberts CL. Occurrence and recurrence of diabetes in pregnancy. *Diabet Med* 2013;30:452–456.

146. Feig DS, Zinman B, Wang X, Hux JE. Risk of development of diabetes mellitus after diagnosis of gestational diabetes. *Can Med Assoc J* 2008;179:229–234.

147. Kim C, Newton KM, Knopp RH. Gestational diabetes and the incidence of type 2 diabetes: a systematic review. *Diabetes Care* 2002;25:1862–1868.

148. Weijers RN, Bekedam DJ, Goldschmidt HM, Smulders YM. The clinical usefulness of glucose tolerance testing in gestational diabetes to predict early postpartum diabetes mellitus. *Clin Chem Lab Med* 2006;44:99–104.

149. McClean S, Farrar D, Kelly CA, Tuffnell DJ, Whitelaw DC. The importance of postpartum glucose tolerance testing after pregnancies complicated by gestational diabetes. *Diabet Med* 2010;27:650–654.

150. Centers for Disease Control and Prevention. U.S. medical eligibility criteria for contraceptive use, 2010. *MMWR Early Release* 2010;59: Available at http://www.cdc.gov/mmwr/pdf/rr/rr59e0528.pdf.

151. Finer LB, Zolna MR. Unintended pregnancy in the United States: incidence and disparities, 2006. *Contraception* 2011;84:478–485.

152. Kerlan V. Postpartum and contraception in women after gestational diabetes. *Diabetes Metab* 2010;36:566–574.

153. Kjos SL, Henry O, Lee RM, Buchanan TA, Mishell DR, Jr. The effect of lactation on glucose and lipid metabolism in women with recent gestational diabetes. *Obstet Gynecol* 1993;82:451–455.

154. Gunderson EP, Hedderson MM, Chiang V, et al. Lactation intensity and postpartum maternal glucose tolerance and insulin resistance in women with recent GDM: the SWIFT cohort. *Diabetes Care* 2012;35:50–56.

155. Chouinard-Castonguay S, Weisnagel SJ, Tchernof A, Robitaille J. Relationship between lactation duration and insulin and glucose response among women with prior gestational diabetes. *Eur J Endocrinol* 2013;168:515–523.

156. Ziegler AG, Wallner M, Kaiser I, et al. Long-term protective effect of lactation on the development of type 2 diabetes in women with recent gestational diabetes mellitus. *Diabetes* 2012;61:3167–3171.

157. Feig DS, Briggs GG, Koren G. Oral antidiabetic agents in pregnancy and lactation: a paradigm shift? *Ann Pharmacother* 2007;41:1174–1180.

158. Crume TL, Ogden LG, Mayer-Davis EJ, et al. The impact of neonatal breast-feeding on growth trajectories of youth exposed and unexposed to diabetes in utero: the EPOCH Study. *Int J Obes (Lond)* 2012;36:529–534.

159. Zhao YL, Ma RM, Huang YK, Liang K, Ding ZB. [Effect of breastfeeding on childhood overweight in the offspring of mothers with gestational diabetes mellitus]. *Zhongguo dang dai er ke za zhi = Chinese journal of contemporary pediatrics* 2013;15:56–61.

160. Nankervis A MH, Moses R, Ross GP, Callaway L, Porter C, Jeffries W, Boorman C, De Vries B for the Australasian Diabetes in Pregnancy Society. Australasian Diabetes In Pregnancy Society (ADIPS) Consensus Guidelines for the Testing and Diagnosis of Gestational Diabetes Mellitus in Australia. 2013. Available at www.adips.org.

161. Canadian Diabetes Association Clinical Practice Guidelines Expert Committee. Clinical practice guidelines. Diabetes and pregnancy. *Can J Diabetes* 2013;37:S168–S183.

162. Seshiah V, Das AK, Balaji V, Joshi SR, Parikh MN, Gupta S. Gestational diabetes mellitus—guidelines. *J Assoc Physicians India* 2006;54:622–628.

163. Koivisto VA. Meal-time blood sugar control in pregnancy. *Diabetes Voice*, volume 49. Brussels, International Diabetes Federation ID, Ed. International Diabetes Federation, 2008.

164. National Institute for Health and Care Excellence. Diabetes in Pregnancy. NICE Clinical Guidelines, No. 63. London, Royal College of Obstetricians and Gynaecologists Press, 2008.

165. National Diabetes Information Clearinghouse. *Gestational Diabetes.* National Institute of Diabetes and Digestive and Kidney Diseases (NIDDK), U.S. Department of Health and Human Services, Washington, DC, 2007.

166. Scottish Intercollegiate Guidelines Network. *Management of Diabetes. A National Clinical Guideline.* Scottish Intercollegiate Guidelines Network; 2010, p. 1–170.

167. Gandhi P, Bustani R, Madhuvrata P, Farrell T. Introduction of metformin for gestational diabetes mellitus in clinical practice: has it had an impact? *Eur J Obstet Gynecol Reprod Biol* 2012;160:147–150.

168. Balani J, Hyer SL, Rodin DA, Shehata H. Pregnancy outcomes in women with gestational diabetes treated with metformin or insulin: a case-control study. *Diabet Med* 2009;26:798–802.

169. Mesdaghinia E, Samimi M, Homaei Z, Saberi F, Moosavi SG, Yaribakht M. Comparison of newborn outcomes in women with gestational diabetes mellitus treated with metformin or insulin: a randomised blinded trial. *Int J Prev Med* 2013;4:327–333.

170. Rowan JA, Hague WM, Gao W, Battin MR, Moore MP. Metformin versus insulin for the treatment of gestational diabetes. *N Engl J Med* 2008; 358:2003–2015.

171. Ijas H, Vaarasmaki M, Morin-Papunen L, et al. Metformin should be considered in the treatment of gestational diabetes: a prospective randomised study. *BJOG* 2011;118:880–885.

172. Niromanesh S, Alavi A, Sharbaf FR, Amjadi N, Moosavi S, Akbari S. Metformin compared with insulin in the management of gestational diabetes mellitus: a randomized clinical trial. *Diabetes Res Clin Pract* 2012;98:422–429.

173. Spaulonci CP, Bernardes LS, Trindade TC, Zugaib M, Vieira Francisco RP. Randomized trial of metformin vs insulin in the management of gestational diabetes. *Am J Obstet Gynecol* 2013 Jul;209(1):34.e1–7. doi: 10.1016/j.ajog.2013.03.022. Epub 2013 Mar 21.

Chapter 15

Management of Pregnant Women with Type 1 and Type 2 Diabetes

ELISABETH R. MATHIESEN, MD, DMSc
LENE RINGHOLM, MD, PhD
PETER DAMM, MD, DMSc

Type 1 diabetes (T1D) complicates up to 0.3% of all pregnancies and the prevalence of type 2 diabetes (T2D) in pregnancy is rising to comparable levels in the U.S. and many other countries. Pregnancies complicated with preexisting diabetes have an increased risk of malformations, preeclampsia, preterm delivery, macrosomia, and neonatal morbidity as well as perinatal mortality. The degree of glycemic control at conception and during pregnancy as well as the presence or absence of late diabetes complications, such as increased albumin levels (>30 mg/24 h), nephropathy, and hypertension, greatly influence the likelihood for a favorable outcome for the mother and the fetus. This main message is the same for both T1D and T2D and other types of diabetes. This chapter handles the two types of diabetes in a similar way, and unless otherwise specified, they are discussed jointly as diabetes.

GLYCEMIC CONTROL AND PREGNANCY OUTCOME

In the first weeks of pregnancy, poor diabetes control increases the risk of congenital malformations and miscarriages. Later in pregnancy, high blood glucose levels may bring about other serious consequences. Because glucose, in contrast to insulin, crosses the placenta from the mother to the fetus, high maternal plasma glucose levels stimulate the fetus to overproduce insulin, which may cause excessive fetal growth and therefore result in increased risk of shoulder dystocia, birth injury, and need for Cesarean delivery.

In addition, high maternal glucose levels are associated with preeclampsia, preterm delivery, and immature lung function as well as sudden unexplained fetal death late in pregnancy. The risk of preeclampsia is lowest in women with optimal glycemic control and rises as A1C increases. The risk of preeclampsia in women with T1D is increased specifically in the presence of albumin levels >30 mg/24 hours, nephropathy, or hypertension. Overall, the risk of an adverse outcome is halved with each percentage reduction in A1C achieved before pregnancy. This information could be a useful motivating factor to achieve glycemic goals and to reassure women that any improvement of blood glucose regulation is genuinely helpful, irrespective of the final value achieved.

DOI: 10.2337/9781580405096.15

PRECONCEPTION CARE AND COUNSELING

Treatment of women with diabetes must begin before gestation. Consequently, any regular visit to the physician by a reproductive-age woman with diabetes, from teenage to middle age, should be considered a preconception visit (Table 15.1). These contacts provide an important opportunity to discuss the patient's contraceptive needs and her thoughts and concerns about a future pregnancy. Important regular assessments include measurements of blood pressure, dilated eye examinations, and assessments of kidney function and urine albumin excretion. A1C testing should be performed routinely and self-monitoring of blood glucose (SMBG) should be taught, if needed. The desired outcome of glycemic control in the preconception phase of care is to lower A1C as close to normal as possible (<7%, International Federation of Clinical Chemistry [IFCC] 52 mmol/mol is considered acceptable), while focusing on the risk of severe hypoglycemia to achieve maximum fertility and optimal embryo and fetal development. Poor glycemic control during the period of organogenesis (the first 7 weeks after conception) significantly increases the risk of congenital malformations and early pregnancy loss. Because much of this period may pass before the woman is aware that she is pregnant, preconception planning and excellent glycemic control are critical.

Daily folic acid supplementation should be advised. There is no consensus on the dose of folic acid; at least 400 μg/day is recommended in Denmark, 600 μg/day in the U.S, and up to 5 mg/day is recommended in other countries. The patient must understand that smoking and alcohol are discouraged strongly during pregnancy.

Kidney function needs to be examined by urinary excretion of albumin, blood pressure, and measurement of serum creatinine to evaluate whether albuminuria or overt diabetic nephropathy is present. If so, antihypertensive treatment including inhibitors of the renin angiotensin system should be given to normalize albumin excretion and blood pressure before pregnancy, if possible. This class of antihypertensive agents may give rise to congenital malformations and impaired fetal development. Therefore, these drugs need to be changed, before or in early pregnancy, to antihypertensive agents that are suitable for use in pregnancy, such as methyldopa, labetalol, or nifedipine.

Because of an increased risk of sight-threatening retinopathy progression during pregnancy, retinopathy needs to be assessed before pregnancy as described in the section Pregnancy Counseling and Late Diabetes Complications.

Table 15.1 Recommendations for Pregnancy Planning

- Use safe contraception in the planning phase
- Achieve an A1C level as near to normal levels as possible (<7%, ~50 mmol/mol)
- Supplement with folic acid
- Ensure appropriate antihypertensive therapy
- Treat possible thyroid dysfunction
- Revise other medical treatment (such as cholesterol-lowering agents)
- Monitor and treat late diabetes complications (e.g., nephropathy and retinopathy)
- Reduce the risk of severe hypoglycemia

From Ringhom et al., 2012. Reprinted with permission from the publisher.

Thyroid dysfunction is prevalent in women with T1D and screening for thyroid dysfunction with thyroid-stimulating hormone (TSH) is indicated in these women. Hypo- or hyperthyroidism should be treated accordingly.

Assessment of other medical treatment is also recommended. Subjects with diabetes often receive cholesterol-lowering agents, which should be stopped before conception, if possible. The use of safe contraception in the planning phase is recommended. Women who obtain these goals before pregnancy have a risk of fetal anomalies or early fetal death close to the background population.

PREGNANCY COUNSELING AND LATE DIABETES COMPLICATIONS

A dilated eye examination before conception and in the first trimester is advised to evaluate retinal function and the risk of progression to sight-threatening retinopathy. Women without prior diabetic retinopathy usually will not develop clinically significant retinopathy during pregnancy. Very few women who have background retinopathy at the start of pregnancy experience a clinically significant progression to proliferative retinopathy or macular edema. Proliferative retinopathy treated by laser photocoagulation and in a stable state before pregnancy generally will remain so. In contrast, women with untreated active proliferative retinopathy should be advised to postpone pregnancy until this condition is treated properly and has remained stable for at least 6 months. Long-term optimal glycemic control decreases the risk of diabetic retinopathy progression. However, intensification of insulin therapy with an abrupt improvement in glycemic control has been associated with a temporary worsening of diabetic retinopathy. Poor glycemic control and elevated blood pressure in early pregnancy increases the risk of retinopathy progression in pregnancy.

Proliferative retinopathy can be treated with laser photocoagulation and clinically significant macular edema by intraocular injections of steroid if significant deterioration of vision has occurred.

Elevated serum creatinine >200 µmol/l increases the risk of pregnancy-induced deterioration of maternal kidney function that may lead to kidney failure. In women with serum creatinine <200 µmol/l, however, well-controlled hypertension and albumin excretion <2,000 mg/24h, maternal kidney function usually will remain stable during pregnancy with low risk of fetal complications. Women with kidney involvement often are treated with blockers of the renin angiotensin system as angiotensin-converting-enzyme (ACE) inhibitor or angiotensin receptor inhibitors. These drugs are not regarded as safe in pregnancy, and in women who are planning pregnancy, a shift to drugs compatible with pregnancy such as methyldopa, labetalol, and dihydropyradine should be performed before pregnancy or when pregnancy is confirmed at the latest. Women with albumin levels 30–299 mg/24 h or diabetic nephropathy have markedly increased risk of developing preeclampsia and preterm delivery. In these women, tight antihypertensive control during pregnancy reduces the urinary albumin excretion and thereby also reduces the risk of these complications. A blood pressure target <135/85 mmHg and a urinary albumin excretion target <300 mg/24 h have been evaluated in observational studies and a marked reduction in the prevalence of preeclampsia and preterm delivery using these targets and aggressive antihypertensive treatment has been demonstrated (Table 15.1). The ADA position statement recommends a blood pressure of 110–129/65–79 mmHg during pregnancy in women with chronic hypertension before pregnancy.

Women with diabetes and established coronary disease have an increased risk of maternal death during pregnancy, and therefore, pregnancy generally is not recommended in these women.

MATERNAL GLUCOSE CONTROL DURING PREGNANCY

Both women with T1D and with T2D are at risk of severe hypoglycemia during pregnancy. Death resulting from maternal hypoglycemia has been described. In addition, because of the risk of traffic accidents, driving is forbidden at glucose levels <70 mg/dl (3.9 mmol/l) in many countries. Several large randomized controlled trials in pregnant women with diabetes have successfully targeted preprandial plasma glucose levels between ~70 and 110 mg/dl (4 and 6 mmol/l) and postprandial plasma glucose levels between ~70 and 140 mg/dl (4 and 8 mmol/l). Therefore, we recommend following the treatment targets indicated in Table 15.2. The goal for A1C is <6% (42 mmol/l) in pregnancy.

MONITORING DURING PREGNANCY

During pregnancy, women with T1D should use SMBG to assess glycemic control in the fasting state, before each meal, and 1–2 hours after meals. Testing at 2:00–3:00 a.m. may be encouraged in women at high risk of severe nocturnal hypoglycemia. Continuous glucose monitoring (CGM) can be used in pregnancy and may help diagnose episodes with nocturnal hypoglycemia that are missed with SMBG. Careful systematic recording of mild and severe episodes of hypoglycemia is advisable.

Table 15.2 Recommendations during Pregnancy

- Maintain preprandial glucose levels of 4–6 mmol/l (~70–110 mg/dl)
- Maintain postprandial glucose levels of 4–8 mmol/l (~70–140 mg/dl)
- Avoid severe hypoglycemia
- Aim for an A1C <6% (~40 mmol/mol) in second part of pregnancy
- Supplement with folic acid during the first 12 weeks
- Administer appropriate antihypertensive treatment to obtain blood pressure <135/85 mmHg and albumin-to-creatinine ratio <300 mg/mmol
- Aim for a blood pressure goal in chronic hypertension of 110–129/65–79 mmHg
- Treat thyroid dysfunction
- Revise other medical treatment (such as cholesterol-lowering agents)
- Conduct eye examination for signs of retinopathy and treatment given, if necessary
- Ensure close obstetrical surveillance

From Ringhom et al., 2012. Reprinted with permission from the publisher.

A1C testing should be obtained at the patient's first prenatal visit to assess previous glycemic control and thereafter every 2 weeks throughout pregnancy as a supplement to SMBG.

Women should be instructed to test for ketones any time glucose levels exceed 240 mg/dl (aproximately 13 mmol/l). The risk of developing diabetic ketoacidosis is increased in pregnant women with T1D and can be fatal for the fetus.

Screening for thyroid dysfunction with plasma TSH is indicated when planning pregnancy and at first pregnancy visit in all women with diabetes. The presence of hypo- or hyperthyroidism during pregnancy in women with diabetes is more commen than in nondiabetic pregnant women and should be monitored and treated accordingly. Daily folic acid supplementation during the first 12 gestational weeks according to local guidelines should be assessed (600 µg/day in the U.S.).

NUTRITIONAL NEEDS

The daily nutritional needs of pregnant women with diabetes should be based on a nutrition assessment by a dietitian. SMBG values, ketone tests, appetite, and weight gain can be used to develop and evaluate an individualized meal plan.

The caloric content of the meal plan may focus on restricting weight gain to the American Institute of Medicine (IOM) recommendations for weight gain in normal pregnancy (Table 15.3). The caloric content of the meal plan therefore may be reduced in women who are obese, who demonstrate early excessive weight gain, or who have a sedentary lifestyle. Recent literature suggests that this can be

Table 15.3 New Recommendations for Total and Rate of Weight Gain During Pregnancy, by Prepregnancy BMI

Prepregnancy BMI	Total Weight Gain		Rates of Weight Gain* (second and third trimester)	
	Range in kg	Range in lbs	Mean (range) in kg/week	Mean (range) in lbs/week
Underweight (<18.5 kg/m²)	12.5–18	28–40	0.51 (0.44–0.58)	1 (1–1.3)
Normal weight (18.5–24.9 kg/m²)	11.5–16	25–35	0.42 (0.35–0.50)	1 (0.8–1)
Overweight (25.0–29.9 kg/m²)	7–11.5	15–25	0.28 (0.23–0.33)	0.6 (0.5–0.7)
Obese (≥30.0 kg/m²)	5–9	11–20	0.22 (0.17–0.27)	0.5 (0.4–0.6)

* Calculations assume a 0.5–2 kg (1.1–4.4 lbs) weight gain in the first trimester.

Source: Weight gain during pregnancy: reexamining the guidelines. Available at http://www.iom.edu/Reports/2009/weight-gain-during-pregnancy-Reexamining-the-Guidelines.aspx. Accessed August 2013. Reprinted with permission.

done without significant ketonuria, but intermittent control of ketonemia or ketonuria is advisable.

The individual daily food plan must include an appropriate caloric level, adequate consumption of protein, fats, and micronutrients and at least 175 g/day of carbohydrate. A distribution of carbohydrate intake that will promote optimal glycemic control and avoidance of hypoglycemia and ketonemia around the clock is advisable. For most patients, this may include 10% of the daily caloric intake; 10% of the carbohydrates should be consumed at breakfast, 30% at lunch, and 30% at dinner. The remaining 30% of calories can be distributed among several snacks, particularly a bedtime snack to decrease the risk of nocturnal hypoglycemia. Patients with persistently elevated midmorning glucose levels despite adjustments of insulin dose may reduce the caloric or fat content of breakfast and redistribute the calories to lunch and dinner. Fat may slow digestion, resulting in elevated blood glucose levels later than when carbohydrate alone is eaten. The presence of regular morning ketonuria with normal glucose levels indicates the need to increase the carbohydrate content of the bedtime snack to 20–30 grams of carbohydrate with low glycemic index. In general, low–glycemic index food is preferred in comparison with high–glycemic index food, and carbohydrate counting in combination with flexible insulin therapy may improve glycemic control.

Attention should be drawn to providing sufficient intake of iron, calcium, iodine, folic acid, vitamin D, and other vitamins, since these vitamins and minerals are important for all pregnant women. Regarding the lipids, consumption of n-6 and n-3 fatty acids is recommended, while saturated fats and trans fats should be limited. A protein intake of at least 1.1 g/kg/day is recommended.

PHYSICAL ACTIVITY DURING PREGNANCY

The general recommendations for all pregnant women apply. This includes 0.5–1 hour of light physical activity such as walking, cycling, or swimming daily. Walking after a meal reduces the postprandial increase in plasma glucose level. Glucose monitoring before and during physical activity is important in insulin-treated pregnant women. A snack of 10–30 grams of carbohydrate before undertaking physical activity and a reduction of the fast-acting meal insulin to accompany the exercise may be required.

INSULIN TREATMENT DURING PREGNANCY

An insulin regimen tailored to the patient's needs can be developed based on SMBG, the meal plan, and the exercise regimen.

The risk of hypoglycemia in early pregnancy in women with diabetes could be increased because of accelerated utilization of glucose by the developing fetus that draws glucose across the placenta from the maternal bloodstream during periods of fasting. Accordingly, the risk of hypoglycemia is highest between meals and during sleep. Severe hypoglycemia occurs most frequently in the first trimester, during which the incidence is five times higher than in the year preceding pregnancy in T1D.

Risk factors for severe hypoglycemia in T1D include a history of severe hypoglycemia before pregnancy, impaired hypoglycemia awareness, longer duration of diabetes, A1C ≤6.5% (IFCC ≤48 mmol/mol) in early pregnancy, and a higher total daily insulin dose. At present, the evidence from human studies suggests that maternal hypoglycemia is mainly a problem for the mother, although adverse fetal effects have not been documented.

Preventive measures to reduce the risk of severe hypoglycemia during pregnancy include early identification of high-risk patients who are characterized by self-estimated impaired hypoglycemia awareness or a history of severe hypoglycemia the year preceding pregnancy. Focus on reducing insulin doses at 8–16 weeks is needed, and supplementary insulin should be used with caution in early pregnancy.

In women with T1D, insulin needs gradually may rise 50–100% from around 16 weeks, and the total insulin dose at the time of delivery may double or even triple that of prepregnancy. Mainly, the prandial insulin dose needs to be increased. Basal-bolus therapy (primarily rapid-acting insulin at main meals supplemented with long-acting insulin once or twice daily) is used widely in pregnancy. Many women with T1D now use insulin pumps with a bolus guide based on a target plasma glucose value and estimation of carbohydrate ratio and insulin sensitivity. Because of the pregnancy-induced changes in insulin sensitivity, these settings in the bolus guide need to be changed almost every week throughout pregnancy. A gradual reduction in the average carbohydrate ratio from 10 to 3 grams per unit insulin in pregnant women with T1D has been described. Likewise, the insulin sensitivity gradually declines from 2 to 1 mmol/l per unit insulin during pregnancy. Recommendations for changes in these pump settings during pregnancy have been suggested (Table 15.4).

Rapid-acting insulin analogs lispro and aspart as well as the long-acting analog detemir are approved by the U.S. Food and Drug Administration (FDA) as category B and can be used in pregnancy. Although the basal insulin glargine is FDA pregnancy category C, there have been several observational reports of the use of insulin glargine in pregnancy without any indications for increased maternal or perinatal morbidity.

For women who are well controlled on a long-acting analog before pregnancy, the theoretical benefit of switching to neutral protamine Hagedorn insulin (which has a long track record of safety in pregnancy) must be weighed against the risks of a deterioration in glycemic control or increased number of hypoglycemic events with a change in insulin regimen during a vulnerable time of pregnancy.

In general, if glucose levels remain elevated pre- or postprandially, the corresponding insulin dose should be increased by 10–20%. Although glycemic goals are lower, strategies for titrating insulin doses in pregnant women are similar to those used outside of pregnancy.

CONTINUOUS SUBCUTANEOUS INSULIN INFUSION PUMP THERAPY

Patients who have used insulin pump therapy before pregnancy should continue on this program. It is also possible to initiate insulin pump treatment during pregnancy in selected patients if they have the necessary expertise.

Insulin pump therapy in pregnancy may offer several advantages over multiple daily injections. Most important, quick titration of both basal insulin and bolus insulin to achieve the stringent goals of pregnancy without hypoglycemia is relatively easily accomplished. In times of morning sickness in the first trimester, the

Table 15.4 Practical Approach to the Expected Adjustments in Insulin Pump Settings During Pregnancy. The 2012 Copenhagen Recommendations

Basal rates:

- Usually reduced between 8–16 weeks
- Increased from 16 weeks and onward
- Adjustments are based on the fasting and preprandial plasma glucose values

Bolus calculator settings:

- Target plasma glucose set at 86 mg/dl (4.8 mmol/l)
- Carbohydrate-to-insulin ratio:
  - Focus on the need for reduction, especially after 16 weeks
  - Adjustments are based on postprandial plasma glucose levels
  - Boluses are given at all meals and when snacking
  - A fourfold decline in the carbohydrate-to-insulin ratio is common
  - Bolus insulin can be taken 15–30 minutes before the meals, especially in late gestation
- Insulin sensitivity factor:
  - Focus on the need for reduction, especially after 16 weeks
  - Adjustments often follow the adjustments in carbohydrate-to-insulin ratio

Source: Mathiesen JM, Secher AL, Ringholm L, Norgaard K, Hommel E, Andersen HU, Damm P, Mathiesen ER. Changes in basal rates and bolus calculator settings in insulin pumps during pregnancy in women with type 1 diabetes. *Journal of Maternal-Fetal & Neonatal Medicine* 2013. Reprinted with permission from the publisher.

patient can rely on her basal infusion and postpone the bolus until after the meal. The insulin pump also allows the nocturnal basal infusion to be decreased early in pregnancy to reduce the risk of nocturnal hypoglycemia. A practical approach to the expected adjustments in insulin pumps settings during pregnancy can be seen in Table 15.4.

Insulin pump therapy is not without risks during pregnancy. Most importantly, in the case of interruption of insulin delivery, rapid development of ketoacidosis may occur. All pregnant patients on insulin pumps must at each clinic visit be instructed on how to troubleshoot hyperglycemia and change the infusion set and insulin reservoir if hyperglycemia (>270 mg/dl [>15 mmol/l]) does not respond to a correction bolus. In addition, changing of the infusion site every 2 days often is needed in addition to rotation of the sites away from the abdominal area in the third trimester. Surprisingly, insulin pump therapy during pregnancy has not been documented to be better than basal-bolus therapy with respect to either maternal or fetal outcomes.

The fetus is vulnerable to the development of maternal ketoacidosis, and this must be avoided as much as possible. Treatment of ketoacidosis can follow usual guidelines, but a 100–200% higher dose of insulin might be needed.

ORAL HYPOGLYCEMIC TREATMENT DURING PREGNANCY

In recent years, interest has been generated in the application of oral hypoglycemic agents to control maternal hyperglycemia during pregnancy, especially in gestational diabetes and T2D. Many of the oral antidiabetic agents may cross the placenta, and induction of neonatal hypoglycemia by using these agents has been described. In addition to exposing the fetus to antidiabetic drugs, epigenetic changes with possible negative impact later in life might be induced. Our knowledge of the long-term effects of oral antidiabetic agents in offspring is limited. Many clinicians therefore are reluctant to prescribe drugs that are not tested carefully in the pregnant population. Most of the literature has focused on metformin and glyburide, and these two drugs will be discussed briefly.

Metformin

Metformin's principal site of action is the liver, where it reduces excessive hepatic glucose production by decreasing gluconeogenesis and increasing glycogenesis. At the level of skeletal muscle, it enhances glucose uptake and glycogen synthesis. In vitro studies have shown that metformin readily crosses the placenta. A randomized controlled trial comparing metformin with insulin in women with gestational diabetes found no significant differences regarding a composite outcome, including prematurity, birth trauma, neonatal hypoglycemia, and respiratory distress. A large proportion of women receiving metformin also needed insulin. Observational studies in women with T2D also suggest that metformin can be used. Teratogenicity has not been reported with metformin. On the basis of this information, some national guidelines (e.g., in the U.K.) have allowed the use of metformin in pregnancy but the FDA still does not recommend the use of metformin during pregnancy or lactation. At present, there are a few reports of low concentrations of metformin in breast milk and no hypoglycemia in infants of lactating mothers taking metformin.

Glyburide

Sulfonylureas, the class of hypoglycemic drugs to which glyburide belongs, act by stimulating the β-cell to increase the release of insulin. In vitro studies have found minimal transplacental transfer of glyburide. Teratogenicity has not been reported with glyburide and breast-feeding is regarded as safe with glyburide. In a randomized trial in women with gestational diabetes receiving either glyburide or insulin, the pregnancy outcome was similar and several cohort studies using the drug without adverse effect have been published. The addition of insulin treatment often is needed. The FDA lists glyburide in pregnancy as category C, and glyburide should be used during pregnancy only if the potential benefit justifies the risk to the fetus.

OUTPATIENT CARE

Most women with diabetes may be managed as outpatients throughout gestation. Failure to maintain acceptable glucose levels, worsening hypertension, or infectious complications may necessitate hospitalization.

Clinic visits can be scheduled at bimonthly intervals early in pregnancy if glycemic control is good, and at 1- to 2-week intervals during the first trimester if improvement in glycemic control is needed. At each visit, the patient's SMBG meter, logbook, or uploaded data should be reviewed; problems with hyperglycemia or hypoglycemia should be discussed; and the patient's weight gain and blood pressure should be checked. Many find the determination of A1C at each pregnancy visit to be a perfect way of giving the patient and caregiver immediate feedback on how close the woman is to her glycemic target.

If background retinopathy has been detected, repeated ophthalmologic examinations should be obtained in the second or third trimester; proliferative retinopathy requires more intensive follow-up. If rapid normalization of blood glucose is needed, monthly visits to the ophthalmologist can be considered for prompt detection of development of neovascularization.

When microalbuminuria or diabetic nephropathy is present, renal function should be evaluated by urinary albumin excretion (albumin-to-creatinin ratio or 24-hour excretion) and blood pressure at each visit, and serum creatinine should be measured one to three times throughout the pregnancy.

Severe autonomous neuropathy may lead to relentless vomiting, which may require intravenous fluid replacement and, in rare cases, parenteral nutrition.

Preterm delivery is frequent in diabetic pregnancies, and urinary tract infections may contribute to this. A urine analysis should be performed in the first trimester to exclude asymptomatic urinary tract infections during pregnancy.

ASSESSMENT OF FETAL CONDITION

The risk for abnormalities increases proportionally to the degree of elevation of A1C measured in early pregnancy covering 3–8 gestational weeks. Therefore, the risk of fetal anomalies can be estimated at the first prenatal visit based on the A1C value.

All women should be offered an ultrasound scanning of the fetal anatomy at 14–21 weeks in an attempt to diagnose clinically significant anomalies. In women with a high risk of fetal cardiac anomalies (such as those with poor first trimester glycemic control), this examination can be supplemented by assessment of fetal cardiac structure by echocardiography around 20 weeks. These scans should be performed and interpreted by specialists in fetal medicine.

Significant advances have been made in the ability to assess fetal growth and well-being. In the third trimester, attention should be directed toward the assessment of fetal growth and well-being. Several approaches should be used to assess fetal condition to prevent sudden intrauterine death in late pregnancy.

ASSESSMENT OF FETAL GROWTH

Fetal growth assessment with serial ultrasound examinations may be warranted 2–3 times during the third trimester in all women with diabetes and more often in those at risk for fetal growth restriction (women with nephropathy or hypertension) or excessive fetal growth (women with poor glycemic control). Delivery by Cesarean section should be considered if the ultrasound suggests excessive fetal size. In women with diabetes, the risk of shoulder dystocia is around fourfold increased due to excessive central fat deposition, and many centers recommend Cesarean section if the estimated fetal weight exceeds 4,000 grams.

ASSESSMENT OF FETAL WELL-BEING

Maternal monitoring of fetal activity is a simple yet valuable screening approach in high-risk pregnancies often used in diabetic pregnancy. Daily assessment of fetal movements may start at 28 weeks.

The nonstress test or antenatal cardiotocography is a screening technique that is performed easily in an outpatient setting and usually requires 20 minutes registration. A normal reactive response is considered a reassuring finding. The nonstress test may be performed 1–2 times/week from 32–34 weeks.

Because normal fetal activity and a reactive nonstress test rarely are associated with an intrauterine unexplained fetal death, the primary value of the surveillance is to allow the clinician to delay delivery safely while the fetus gains further maturity. Some centers use surveillance with ultrasound examinations of fetal blood flow as routine examinations. There is limited documentation, however, that this helps in addition to daily fetal activity registration and regular nonstress testing.

Although the insulin requirement often decreases gradually by 10–20% during the last weeks of pregnancy, a sudden drop in the insulin requirement can be a sign of placental dysfunction, indicating a thorough examination to confirm the well-being of the fetus.

The woman with diabetes, therefore, should notifiy her diabetes specialist and obstetrician of any increase in hypoglycemia or decline in daily insulin dose of >20% to alert her provider that increasing fetal surveillance may be relevant. When fetal evaluation is reassuring, the techniques utilized for antepartum fetal surveillance enable most patients to have their checkups at an outpatient clinic. Nevertheless, hospitalization may be necessary if the patient has nephropathy or hypertension, if she does not adhere to the treatment regimen, or when fetal jeopardy is suspected.

LABOR AND DELIVERY

Continuous intrapartum cardiotocography is mandatory. Labor should be allowed to progress as long as cervical dilation and descent follow the established curves for normal labor. Any evidence of an arrest pattern should alert the physician to the possibility of cephalopelvic disproportion and fetal macrosomia.

MATERNAL GLUCOSE LEVELS DURING DELIVERY

Maintenance of normal maternal glucose levels (70–130 mg/dl [4–7 mmol/l]) during labor and delivery is important and monitoring of plasma glucose every hour is recommended (Table 15.5).

Table 15.5 Recommendations During and After Delivery

- Monitor plasma glucose every hour during delivery
- Maintain plasma glucose of 70–120 mg/dl (4–7 mmol/l) during delivery
- Ensure close obstetric surveillance during labor and delivery
- Ensure close observation of the newborn for morbidity, including hypoglycemia
- Monitor the maternal insulin requirement immediately after delivery; a decline to ~60% of the prepregnancy dose is expected
- Note that ACE inhibitors captopril and enalapril are considered safe during lactation
- Treat thyroid dysfunction during lactation, as warranted

From Ringhom et al., 2012. Reprinted with permission from the publisher.

A combination of intravenous glucose and intravenous insulin infusion can be used to maintain glucose levels in the target range. Following are intravenous insulin infusion rates that have been deemed safe and effective in maintaining maternal glucose levels during labor. They are used with a 10% dextrose solution at a rate of 80 ml/hour and with hourly capillary blood glucose monitoring:

- Constant 1 U/hour with a SMBG level of 3.4–7.8 mmol/l (61–140 mg/dl)
- Increase to 1.5 U/hour for SMBG 7.9–9.9 mmol/l (140–180 mg/dl)
- Increase to 2 U/hour for SMBG of 10.0–12.2 mmol/l (180–220 mg/dl)
- Increase to 3 U/hour for SMBG >12.2 mmol/l (220 mg/dl)

An alternative strategy is to continue with the patient's usual subcutaneous insulin treatment in reduced doses (approximately one-third) in combination with intravenous glucose infusion of 3 grams/hour during active labor. In patients treated with a subcutaneous insulin pump, the basal rate can be continued during active labor, at a reduced dose.

If a Cesarean section is planned in the early morning, the patient's usual morning rapid-acting insulin dose should be omitted. Instead, a long-acting insulin dose can be given. Because of the rapid decline in insulin dose after removal of the placenta, the dose might be calculated as one-third of the individual pregnant woman's insulin requirement during the following 8–12 hours, and only small doses of insulin may be required for the remainder of the day. If using an insulin pump, the basal insulin may be continued at low rates (e.g., 80% of usual dose). After surgery, glucose levels should be monitored every 1–2 hours, and an intravenous solution containing 5% dextrose should be continued until the mother is eating.

TIMING OF DELIVERY

Today, delivery can be safely awaited until 38–40 weeks in most women with diabetes. Labor then may be induced or the onset of spontaneous labor may be awaited. Most centers will not recommend waiting beyond term. Maintenance of excellent glycemic control is important, and all parameters of antepartum fetal surveillance should remain normal.

In the clinical setting, labor often is induced at 38–39 weeks because of a "relatively big baby" and to avoid stillbirth close to term. However, iatrogenic preterm delivery may be relevant because of preeclampsia or excessive fetal growth.

As is the case in women without diabetes, antenatal glucocorticoid treatment is indicated to enhance lung maturity for preterm delivery at 24–33 weeks' gestation. Administration of high-dose corticosteroids will cause hyperglycemia in the woman if insulin dose is not increased appropriately. This is best done using an algorithm increasing insulin dose immediately from the beginning of the steroid treatment. In general, an increase in the present insulin dose of 50% in addition to supplementation with rapid-acting insulin according to the SMBG levels can be recommended. The increased insulin requirement levels out within 4–7 days.

POSTPARTUM CARE

The newborn needs close observation for morbidity, including neonatal hypoglycemia. The elevated maternal glucose levels and the following fetal hyperinsulinemia can lead to neonatal hypoglycemia, when the infant no longer receives glucose from the mother because of inappropriate downregulation of the fetal insulin production in the first hours of life. Early feeding every 3 hours the first 24 hours is recommended in many centers to prevent neonatal hypoglycemia. Breast-feeding may reduce the risk of the infant to develop obesity as well as T1D and is strongly recommended to be initiated as soon as possible.

Because the risk of maternal hypoglycemia also is considerable, the goal for maternal plasma glucose returns to prepregnancy levels (70–180 mg/dl [5.0–10.0 mmol/l]). In the immediate postpartum period, the mother's insulin requirements are usually lower than her prepregnancy needs, often corresponding to around one-third of the insulin dose in late pregnancy. The expected insulin dose after delivery therefore can be set in advance to one-third of the dose in late pregnancy. This dose often is around 60% of the dose before pregnancy. A lower insulin requirement during nighttime in the breast-feeding woman must be reflected, but otherwise the usual distribution between long- and rapid-acting insulin doses in the nonpregnant women can guide the set of the individual insulin doses.

The doses should be adjusted based on SMBG. Insulin requirements gradually increase over the next weeks following delivery. In women who are breast-feeding, the insulin dose requirement is still around 10% lower than before pregnancy, with wide individual variations.

A few days after delivery, ongoing antihypertensive treatment can be reduced or stopped in many cases. Transition to types of drugs used outside pregnancy must be considered. ACE inhibitors, such as captopril and enalapril, can be used during lactation.

Treatment for thyroid dysfunction often needs to be changed after delivery. Immediately after delivery, possible treatment for hypothyroidism often can be reduced to the dose used before pregnancy and TSH can be reassessed after 1–2 months.

CONCLUSION

Pregnancy in women with diabetes increases the risk of adverse outcomes for mother and offspring. The careful preconception counseling is important with a particular focus on glycemic control, indications for antihypertensive therapy, screening for diabetic nephropathy, diabetic retinopathy, and thyroid dysfunction, as well as a review of other medications. Supplementation with folic acid should be initiated before conception to minimize the risk of fetal malformations. Obtaining and maintaining tight control of blood glucose and blood pressure before and during pregnancy is crucial for optimizing outcomes; however, the risk of severe hypoglycemia during pregnancy is a major obstacle. Rapid-acting insulin analogs and insulin detemir are considered to be safe to use in pregnancy, and studies on insulin glargine are reassuring. Immediately following delivery, the insulin requirement declines dramatically, and during breast-feeding, remains lower than the dose before pregnancy.

BIBLIOGRAPHY

American Diabetes Association. *Medical Management of Pregnancy Complicated by Diabetes.* 5th ed. Coustan DR, Ed. Alexandria, VA, American Diabetes Association, 2013.

American Diabetes Association. *Medical Management of Type 1 Diabetes.* 6th ed. Kaufman FR, Ed. Alexandria, VA, American Diabetes Association, 2012.

American Diabetes Association. Preconception care of women with diabetes (position statement). *Diabetes Care* 2013;34(Suppl 1):S41–S42.

Cordua S, Secher AL, Ringholm L, Damm P, Mathiesen ER. Real-time continuous glucose monitoring during labour and delivery in women with type 1 diabetes—observations from a randomized controlled trial. *Diabet Med* 2013;30(11):1374–1381.

Damm JA, Asbjörnsdóttir B, Callesen NF, Mathiesen JM, Ringholm L, Pedersen BW, Mathiesen ER. Diabetic nephropathy and microalbuminuria in pregnant women with type 1 and type 2 diabetes. *Diabetes Care* 2013;36(11):3489–3494.

Inkster ME, Fahey TP, Donnan PT, Leese GP, Mires GJ, Murphy DJ. Poor glycated haemoglobin control and adverse pregnancy outcomes in type 1 and type 2 diabetes mellitus: systematic review of observational studies. *BMC Pregnancy Childbirth* 2006;6:30.

Kitzmiller JL, Block JM, Brown FM, Catalano PM, Conway DL, Coustan DR, Gunderson EP, Herman WH, Hoffman LD, Inturrisi M, Jovanovic LB, Kjos SI, Knopp RH, Montoro MN, Ogata ES, Paramsothy P, Reader DM, Rosenn BM, Thomas AM, Kirkman MS. Managing preexisting diabetes for pregnancy: summary of evidence and consensus recommendations for care. *Diabetes Care* 2008;31:1060–1079.

Management of diabetes from preconception to the postnatal period: Summary of NICE guidance. *BMJ* 2008;336:714–717.

Mathiesen JM, Secher AL, Ringholm L, Norgaard K, Hommel E, Andersen HU, Damm P, Mathiesen ER. Changes in basal rates and bolus calculator settings in insulin pumps during pregnancy in women with type 1 diabetes. *Journal of Maternal-Fetal & Neonatal Medicine* 2013.

Ringholm L, Mathiesen ER, Kelstrup L, Damm P. Glycemic control and antihypertensive therapy in women with type 1 diabetes: from pregnancy planning to the breastfeeding period. *Nat Rev Endocrinol* 2012;8:659–667.

Weight gain during pregnancy: Reexamining the guidelines. Available at http://www.iom.edu/Reports/2009/weight-Gain-during-pregnancy-Reexamining-the-Guidelines.aspx. Accessed August 2013.

Chapter 16

Type 2 Diabetes: Pathogenesis and Natural History

JACK L. LEAHY, MD

INTRODUCTION

Type 2 diabetes (T2D) is part of a worldwide health crisis of noncommunicable disease that is replacing pandemics and infectious diseases as the greatest threat to public health. In the U.S., 8.3% of the population (25.8 million) is affected with diabetes and another 35% with prediabetes at a cost of $245 billion in 2012.[1] Racial disparities account for even higher rates, in particular Mexican Americans, African Americans, and Native Americans.[2] Globally, the incidence rate is predicted to increase from 382 million in 2014 to 592 million in 2035, with developing nations particularly affected. Some reasons are obvious—our modern lifestyles of high-calorie diets and physical inactivity, with the most dramatic effects in children resulting in an epidemic of obesity and metabolic syndrome.[3,4] This same concept is used for developing nations—urbanization causing a shift away from the physical labor and food shortages of agrarian and nomadic lives. Not surprisingly, a complete understanding for the diabetes epidemic is more complex, with key findings from epidemiologists, geneticists, clinical physiologists, and basic researchers having provided a working model that is reviewed in this chapter (Figure 16.1) and many excellent reviews.[5-9]

NATURAL HISTORY OF TYPE 2 DIABETES

The clinical picture of T2D is well known: slow rise in blood glucose values over many years from normal glucose tolerance to prediabetes and diabetes. Typically, obesity and other elements of the metabolic syndrome such as hypertension and a metabolic pattern of hyperlipidemia are present along with a family history. Once hyperglycemia is present, a progressive nature to the diabetes usually occurs, with the U.K. Prospective Diabetes Study (UKPDS) having identified that the clinical indicator of that progression is a loss of response to therapy requiring additional pharmaceuticals, and sooner or later insulin.[10]

Insight into this clinical picture came when it was shown that two distinct pathogenic elements are present in virtually all people with T2D—resistance to the effect of insulin on its target tissues, skeletal muscle, adipose, and liver, and impaired secretion of the glucoregulatory hormones insulin and glucagon. People with prediabetes showed the same dual-pathogenic pattern.[11,12] Determining which came first, insulin resistance or β-cell dysfunction, however, posed technical challenges in terms of who to study. It subsequently was shown in people at presumed

DOI: 10.2337/9781580405096.16

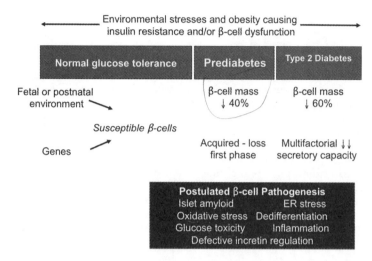

Figure 16.1—Proposed sequence of the key pathological features of T2D as discussed in this review. ER, endoplasmic reticulum.

high risk for T2D, while they still were normoglycemic (high-risk ethnic groups, both parents with T2D, women with polycystic ovary syndrome or prior gestational diabetes), also in cross-sectional and longitudinal studies of insulin resistance and β-cell function across a wide range of glycemia, that insulin resistance is present when glucose values are still within the normal glucose tolerance range,[13–16] with factors such as obesity, lack of exercise, and high-fat diets playing a major role. Thereafter, insulin resistance worsens minimally or not at all as glucose levels rise.[6,17] In contrast, the temporal details for β-cell dysfunction were more difficult to identify related to technical challenges and misinterpretations of measured insulin levels. An important advance was the understanding that the insulin response to a meal is normally biphasic, and a characteristic feature of evolving T2D is absence of first-phase insulin secretion causing postmeal hyperglycemia (i.e., the clinical definition of impaired glucose tolerance [IGT]).[18,19] In contrast, later insulin secretion (second phase) is supernormal because of the hyperglycemia.[20,21] Thus β-cell dysfunction also predates T2D and is related more to defective kinetics of insulin secretion than the overall quantity of secretion. Recent studies have confirmed that β-cell dysfunction is present before the glucose level rises out of the normal range.[22–26] In addition, there is a dynamic pattern for β-cell function after diabetes is present that contrasts with the mostly unchanging insulin resistance—the early-on postmeal hyperinsulinemia that keeps glucose values near-normal despite the insulin resistance (*β-cell compensation*) is followed by a slow sustained fall of insulin levels (*β-cell failure*) after T2D is present, accounting for the progressive rise in glycemia and failing response to therapy that characterizes longstanding T2D.[5–9]

An important technical advance for fully mapping out the pathophysiological patterns in T2D came with calculating the *disposition index*, which is a way to gauge the correctness of a subject's insulin responses for their measured level of insulin sensitivity, using curves of these parameters mapped out in large numbers of subjects without diabetes.[27,28] Plotting subjects with varying degrees of glucose tolerance allows the roles of β-cell dysfunction and insulin resistance to be identified.[5] A well-known study using this method was performed in 48 normally glucose-tolerant Pima Indians (an ethnic group with a high rate of T2D) who were studied prospectively for an average of 5 years.[29] Seventeen developed T2D (*progressors*) and 31 maintained normal glucose tolerance (*nonprogressors*). The groups were matched for obesity and insulin resistance. Despite a high level of insulin resistance, the nonprogressors stayed on the disposition curve throughout the study, showing perfect β-cell compensation. The progressors instead progressively fell away from the β-cell function side of the curve—insulin sensitivity changed only minimally over the 5 years of the study—confirming that the cause for the rise in glycemia from normal glucose tolerance to IGT and overt T2D was worsening β-cell function. Another key finding was that the progressors were already off the curve at the start of the study, consistent with β-cell dysfunction being present in susceptible individuals when they still are normally glucose tolerant. A representation of this pathogenic schema is shown in Figure 16.2.

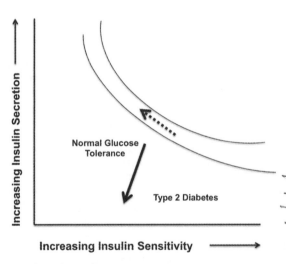

Figure 16.2—Schema based on the results from many studies of the relationship between insulin sensitivity (on the x-axis) and insulin secretion (on the y-axis) in people who develop T2D. The curved lines show the normal relationship between these parameters, termed the "disposition index." The dotted arrow represents subjects who undergo metabolic stresses, such as obesity, ageing, pregnancy, or modern diet and inactivity habits, without any rise in their blood glucose levels. Multiple studies have shown they remain on the disposition curve, showing intact β-cell compensation. The solid line represents subjects who go on to develop T2D, typically falling below the curve while still normally glucose tolerant, and with a deterioration in β-cell function rather than a worsening insulin sensitivity as the basis for their developing T2D. These findings reinforce key issues discussed in the text: β-cell function is the major determinant of the blood glucose level in people who are at risk for T2D, and β-cell dysfunction is present before blood glucose values rise into the prediabetes range.[5]

To summarize, these various experimental approaches support a uniform understanding of the natural history of T2D. Major derangements in tissue insulin sensitivity and β-cell function are both present before glucose values are abnormal by current criteria. As such, those at risk rarely are identified because of their "normal" glucose value along with the lack of clinical tools in an office setting to measure insulin sensitivity or β-cell function. Indeed, the artificiality of the official cutoff between normoglycemia and prediabetes was demonstrated by a report that showed an eightfold higher rate of subsequent T2D with fasting glucose values at the high range of normal (>87 mg/dl vs. <81 mg/dl) when hypertriglyceridemia and obesity were present.[30]

Also both defects are key to the diabetes risk—the "two-hit hypothesis." Insulin resistance is a common risk factor for T2D, but unless β-cells are compromised in some fashion, the diabetes risk is low. In turn, the risk in people with compromised β-cells depends on whether environmental or metabolic risk factors are present that cause their insulin demands to reach unobtainable levels. At that point, the sequence of pathogenic events that culminate in overt T2D is initiated and is followed by a slow continuous decline in β-cell function that causes worsening of glycemia and a progressive loss of response to therapy.

This model provides a framework for how to lower the diabetes risk by improving β-cell function or insulin sensitivity in high-risk individuals, while still normally glucose tolerant. Many studies have shown that insulin sensitization through lifestyle intensification[31,32] or thiazolidinediones[33] lessens the conversion of prediabetes to T2D. One expects a better approach in the future will be methods that precisely define the mechanistic basis for early β-cell dysfunction in the individual, paired with interventions that restore normal compensation responses, thereby eliminating the diabetes risk. As such, important investigation into the causes and molecular basis for the β-cell susceptibility and metabolic risk factors that make up this schema is ongoing as detailed in the following section.

DEFECTIVE β-CELL COMPENSATION IN PEOPLE AT RISK FOR T2D

The first stage of T2D in Figure 16.1 is compromised β-cells related to a defective compensation system[34]—the terminology often used today is *susceptible β-cells*. A common prediction is that the cause is an inadequate number of normally functioning β-cells, in part because many of the genetic loci linked to T2D act in signaling pathways that affect β-cell development, proliferation, or survival.[35] Also a study of autopsy-obtained human pancreas reported a 40% reduced β-cell volume in subjects with prediabetes versus weight-matched subjects without diabetes,[36] and another that measured β-cell mass across a wide range of BMI in Europeans without diabetes found a high level of variability (three- to fourfold) at any BMI,[37] fueling speculation that those at the lowest range are at risk for diabetes. Further support is provided by the glucose intolerance that developed in healthy donors of half of their pancreas for transplantation to relatives with type 1 diabetes.[38]

An alternate mechanism is inadequate insulin secretion unrelated to changes in β-cell mass. Kinetic changes in insulin secretion—absent first phase,[18,21] and an impaired pulsatile pattern of insulin secretion[39,40]—are the characteristic β-cell defects that predate T2D. Also, experimental interventions have shown recovery of first-phase insulin secretion within a few days, presumably well before the possibility of β-cell mass reexpansion.[41,42] Further implicating dysfunctional β-cells is a study that infused intralipid for 4 days into patients without diabetes to investigate lipotoxicity[43]—high levels of fatty acids impairing insulin secretion. In subjects without a family history of T2D, insulin secretion to meals and a glucose challenge increased as expected in response to the insulin insensitivity that occurs with a lipid infusion. The opposite occurred in subjects with a strong family history of T2D—their insulin secretory responses fell, although the basis for the dichotomy is unknown.

A third area of interest is defects within the incretin system. Incretin hormones are the gut peptides—glucagon-like peptide-1 (GLP-1) and glucose-dependent insulinotropic polypeptide (GIP)—released with eating that are key initiators and regulators of mealtime insulin and glucagon secretion.[44] A characteristic feature of T2D is a reduced incretin effect related to resistance to incretin hormone–induced insulin secretion[45,46] and a lowered expression of β-cell receptors for GIP and GLP-1.[47] This defect is presumed not only to impair mealtime insulin secretion but also to cause defective lowering of glucagon levels with eating.[48] Support for this defect being present before overt T2D is an impaired incretin effect having been reported in people without diabetes who are first-degree relatives of people with T2D[49] and subjects with IGT.[50] Also, many of the susceptibility genes identified for T2D interact in some way with the incretin system.[51]

MOLECULAR MECHANISMS OF β-CELL SUSCEPTIBILITY

Genetic Predisposition

The importance of genetics was proven 40 years ago in a study of identical twins that showed close to a 100% concordance rate for T2D, while it was much lower for T1D.[52] Heritability for β-cell function also has been demonstrated.[53] It has long been predicted that major breakthroughs will come with uncovering the genetic basis for T2D. Recent advancements in gene-probing technology, however, have identified >60 susceptibility loci for T2D, but as yet, none promises to revolutionize diabetes prevention, diagnosis, or therapy.[54,55] Complicating issues are the large number of loci, and all are of modest effect—10% to <30% increased risk of diabetes. It was hoped that ethnic-based differences in diabetes risk would be explained by genetic patterns. Instead, there mostly has been consistency across ethnic populations, although studies are beginning to identify novel loci in high-risk populations, the significance of which remains to be determined.[56,57]

There have been surprises. Almost all of the identified T2D loci seem to impact the β-cell—development, proliferation, survival, and function.[35] The lack of genes linked to insulin signaling, obesity, and insulin resistance was initially unexpected, but in part reflects the studies having been conducted mostly in people with T2D and matched controls who were similarly obese but without diabetes; obesity, insulin resistance, and insulin clearance loci now are being identified.[58,59] Another issue relates to most of the loci having been identified using genome-wide association scans (GWAS) that study many hundreds of thousands to more than a million small nucleotide sequences within the whole genome of affected people looking for single nucleotide polymorphism (SNP) patterns that track with the disease. This agnostic approach has identified many loci without known functions for blood glucose regulation, with investigation of their biological roles having provided new insight into the workings of the glucose homeostasis system. For instance, transcription factor 7-like 2 (TCF7L2) is the gene with the strongest diabetes risk.[60] When first identified, it was unknown to diabetes researchers, but now it is linked to the canonical Wnt signaling pathway of β-cell development and function,[61] modulating β-cell expression of GIP and GLP-1 receptors,[47] and insulin granule fusion.[62] Finally, a recent development is the concept that identifying protective genes for T2D is another approach to better understand the genetic basis for diabetes risk.[63]

So we have a plethora of susceptibility loci for T2D, and geneticists are predicting we can expect many more as technology evolves to probe noncoding areas and epigenetic regulators of gene expression—potentially many hundreds. Thus, it is anyone's guess where genetics eventually will take us. The reader is referred to excellent reviews on this topic.[35,64]

Other Mechanisms of Susceptible β-Cells

A potential cause with worldwide public health implications is inadequate prenatal diabetes care or malnutrition during pregnancy that imprints offspring with a heightened risk of diabetes and obesity. A similar concept is malnutrition in young children. This idea is supported by long-term epidemiology studies of offspring from mothers with diabetes[65] and of children born during periods of starvation from wars or famines,[66] showing high rates of diabetes and obesity. Animal models of intrauterine growth retardation[67] or highly restrictive diets in pregnancy or newborn pups[68] have shown long-term reductions in β-cell mass and function with a heightened diabetes risk. Of particular concern is the potential for epigenetic changes that lead to transmission of this risk to future generations.[69-72]

A growing research topic is diabetes susceptibility from food additives, air pollution, and environmental toxins, with β-cell–mediated mechanisms under investigation.[73-76] Also of current interest are metabolic regulatory effects of gut microflora—the species balance varies with nutrient intake patterns and antibiotics—on cellular energy expenditure, obesity, endotoxins and cellular inflammation, and levels of gut peptides such GLP-1and GLP-2.[77-80] Finally, an active area of investigation is central nervous system (CNS)–related regulation of peripheral metabolism and β-cell function.[81-83]

ENVIRONMENTAL RISK FACTORS

When a β-cell predisposition for glucose intolerance is present, the next stage relates to the metabolic stress environment. Many risk factors are known (Figure 16.3). Most understandable is the association of T2D with physical inactivity, high-calorie diets, aging, and our modern lifestyle in general. Also obvious are pharmaceuticals, such as corticosteroids, thiazides, and β-blockers, that negatively affect glucose homeostasis. Other associations with high rates of diabetes are sleep deprivation including sleep apnea, poverty, and various forms of mental illness.[84-86]

The general concept is that these factors negatively affect glucose homeostasis by worsening of the insulin resistance. This schema is oversimplistic, however, with the more likely possibility of complex multifaceted metabolic effects. For instance, high-fat and high-calorie diets not only cause obesity-related insulin resistance, but also elicit adipokine, fatty acid, and CNS-related negative impacts on energy homeostasis, insulin sensitivity, and β-cell mass and function.[87,88]

A number of protective factors also are known, although how they act is poorly understood.[5] The Nurses Health Survey confirmed the expected associations of obesity and lack of physical activity with T2D, but it also showed protection with moderate alcohol and abstinence from smoking.[89] Many studies have confirmed the protective effect of alcohol,[90] and other protective factors including a moderate use of caffeine[91] or chocolate,[92] and eating brown rice versus white rice.[93]

This schema implies that the diabetes risk can be lowered by altering the balance between positive and negative environmental risk factors—conceptually much easier from a public health perspective than trying to prevent or reverse the underlying β-cell dysfunction. For instance, a worldwide observation has been that the migration of nomadic or indigenous populations to urban environments invariably results in an explosion of diabetes and obesity. A dramatic example of the reversibility of the disadvantageous metabolic factors was studies of Australian Aborigines who returned to the bush and their prior way, with reversal of obesity and diabetes.[94]

RELATIONSHIP BETWEEN OBESITY AND INSULIN RESISTANCE

The strongest risk factor for T2D is obesity, with double-digit higher rates in both men and women with obese versus nonobese BMI levels.[95,96] Assessing risks based on BMI can be misleading, however, as intra-abdominal fat is more associated with insulin resistance and risk of diabetes than subcutaneous fat depots,[97]

Environmental Factors Affecting Diabetes Risk

RISK FACTORS	PROTECTIONS
• Obesity	• Modest alcohol
• High-fat/-calorie diets	• Modest caffeine
• Inactivity	• Chocolate
• Malnutrition	• Brown rice versus white rice
• Emotional stress/depression	
• Poverty	
• Low socioeconomic status	
• Sleep disorders	
• Pharmaceuticals	

Figure 16.3—Environmental risk factors and protections for T2D as discussed in this chapter.

which is why the obesity criterion in the metabolic syndrome is based on waist circumference rather than BMI. Also, ectopic fat stores—liver, skeletal muscle, epicardial, and pancreas—are most linked to organ dysfunction.[98,99] Additionally, there are ethnic differences—insulin resistance and high intra-abdominal fat deposits have been found in Asians at modest BMI levels.[100] Another confounder is obese individuals with relatively normal insulin sensitivity and cardiovascular risk factors, the *metabolically healthy obese*,[101,102] and people with a high degree of metabolic dysregulation at a normal BMI.[103] The goal of metabolomics is to identify markers of dysmetabolism or cardiovascular risk that are independent of a person's clinical phenotype.

Historically, fat stores were considered metabolically inert and simply a storage site for the concentrated energy within fat. As such, a conundrum was how obesity negatively affected insulin sensitivity in terms of inhibiting insulin-mediated glucose clearance into target tissues, primarily skeletal muscle. The past decade has seen a redefining of our understanding of adipose biology and pathophysiology. One surprise is that fat is necessary for normal glucose metabolism, as reflected in the profound insulin resistance of lipodystrophy syndromes[104] and very similar metabolic derangements in mouse models with genetic ablation of fat that are reversed with fat transplants.[105] Part of the explanation is that adipocytes are now known to synthesize and release numerous peptides that affect metabolic homeostasis systems (*adipokines*), with dysregulation proposed to play a direct role in the development of insulin resistance and T2D.[106–108] Leptin is an 18-kilodalton cytokine-like molecule that plays an important regulatory role in appetite and energy expenditure.[109] Adiponectin positively affects insulin sensitivity through anti-inflammatory and direct insulin-sensitizing effects, with countless studies showing lowered adiponectin levels in obesity, metabolic syndrome, and T2D.[110,111] A recent focus is retinol binding protein-4 as a proinflammatory factor causing insulin resistance,[112,113] although that remains controversial.[114]

Our current understanding for obesity-related insulin resistance is based on a multifaceted schema.[115] One element is an excess release of fatty acids related to the adipose insulin resistance—fatty acid infusions in healthy humans have been shown to cause impairment of tissue insulin sensitivity related to the generation of proinflammatory cytokines and lipid metabolites that disrupt target tissue cellular insulin signaling.[116] Another key pathogenic factor is an adipose proinflammatory state; expansion of fat stores causes macrophages that reside within adipose to undergo activation and expansion, with secretion of powerful cytokines and immune regulatory molecules such as tumor necrosis factor-α and several interleukins (IL) that also disrupt insulin signaling.[117,118]

ONSET OF HYPERGLYCEMIA

The next stage in the development of T2D is the progression to clinical hyperglycemia—a time when the β-cell compensation to insulin resistance wanes so hyperglycemia appears. This is the most understudied aspect of T2D pathogenesis. There remains no clear answer as to why β-cells that have compensated reasonably well, often for decades, fail.

One idea termed *β-cell exhaustion* implies that the insulin resistance–induced compensatory hyperinsulinemia in susceptible subjects when they are still normoglycemic eventually has a negative impact on some aspect of β-cell biology so that insulin output can no longer be maintained at a high level. There is support from animal studies and humans for this concept. Careful mapping of the stages to T2D in rhesus monkeys found that hyperinsulinemia related to hyperresponsiveness of glucose-induced insulin secretion was the first identifiable event.[119] Similarly, a high fasting insulin level independent of insulin resistance is an important risk factor for T2D in Pima Indians.[120] Most influential are the studies of inhibitors of insulin secretion (diazoxide, somatostatin, novel K_{ATP}-channel openers), the so-called *β-cell rest strategies*, which have shown paradoxical increases in β-cell function in animals and humans with T2D.[121–123] Many mechanisms have been proposed, with the most common being that the early insulin hypersecretion depletes the pool of readily releasable insulin granules, thereby lowering insulin secretory responses.

A second idea relates to modest hyperglycemia or some other form of dysmetabolism of the evolving diabetes, directly causing defects in the blood glucose regulatory system—so-called *acquired abnormalities*.[5] This concept was first proposed based on studies that intensively treated glycemia in people with T2D and unexpectedly noted improved β-cell function;[41] later studies also showed improvement in insulin resistance. The beneficial effects are unrelated to any specific treatment[124] and appear to be most effective early in the disease. Notable are recent studies showing long-term recovery of glucose tolerance and improved β-cell function in Chinese patients with newly diagnosed T2D after short-term insulin therapy.[125,126]

A particularly informative study was performed in subjects with an average 8-year duration of T2D who were placed on an insulin pump for 3 weeks with excellent blood glucose control.[127] When studied 2 days after stopping the pump, there were large increases in insulin secretion, normalization of hepatic glucose production, and lessening of insulin resistance from the prepump baseline. These results provided an answer to what had been a major dilemma—this triad of defective β-cell function along with peripheral and hepatic insulin resistance made up the classic hyperglycemia-causing defects in T2D, but no known biology linked these organs. The concept has evolved that irrespective of the genetic and environmental factors present in any patient, as glucose intolerance develops so too do the acquired abnormalities causing the same clinical phenotype in all patients. Support for this concept playing a role in the transition from normoglycemia to early diabetes includes studies that have shown that the characteristic insulin secretory defect in T2D—lowered first-phase insulin secretion—is present with fasting glucose levels between 100 and 115 mg/dl.[128] This abnormality also is reversed after just 20 hours of normoglycemia in people with T2D.[42] Collectively, these findings suggest that a dysmetabolism (likely hyperglycemia)-based onset of defective first-phase insulin secretion is part of the transition to IGT.

PROGRESSIVE DECLINE IN β-CELL FUNCTION IN ESTABLISHED TYPE 2 DIABETES

The final stage is the progressive waning of β-cell function causing hyperglycemia to worsen and the need to advance therapy. Many mechanisms are proposed that accelerate β-cell destruction or impair insulin secretion in established T2D;

it must be kept in mind that they are based mostly on models (diabetic animals or *in vitro* cellular systems) because of the inability to safely perform human pancreas biopsies. Also, although the number of studies using tissue from people with T2D is growing (isolated islets from brain-dead donors or autopsy pancreas sections), one must remain cautious as to how well they replicate the *in vivo* situation. Fundamental questions persist. Is the progressive loss of function related to a decline in the number of β-cells or cellular function? It is clear from autopsy specimens that the β-cell mass is reduced in T2D on average 50%,[36,129] with increased β-cell apoptosis.[36,130,131] One study reported a 40% lowering of pancreatic β-cell volume in impaired fasting glucose and 60% in T2D, possibly supporting a progressive decline.[36] Also, a recent focus has been on an increased mass of glucagon-secreting α-cells in T2D.[129] The lack of noninvasive islet-cell mass monitoring, however, makes it impossible to map out the temporal profiles for any of these. Alternatively worsening β-cell function without any loss of β-cell mass is a well-established pathogenic mechanism in diabetic animals.[132,133] Another key issue is whether the progressive β-cell dysfunction comes from multiple different mechanisms or a single mechanism in most patients. The following sections discuss many of the proposed causes for the dysfunctional β-cells in T2D (Figure 16.4)— how they interrelate, when they begin, and how they worsen over the course of the disease are all unknown.

Islet Amyloid

Islets of people with T2D often contain amyloid plaques with distorted and shrunken β-cells.[134] Interest in amyloid-induced β-cell destruction markedly increased when it was shown that nonhuman primates develop age-related diabetes and islet amyloid at the same time.[135] A major breakthrough came with identifying the amyloid protein, now termed islet-associated polypeptide (IAPP) or

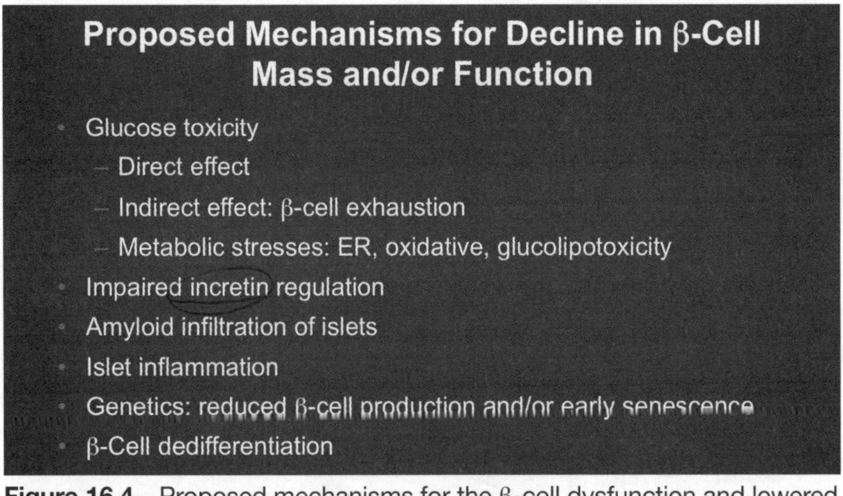

Proposed Mechanisms for Decline in β-Cell Mass and/or Function

- Glucose toxicity
  - Direct effect
  - Indirect effect: β-cell exhaustion
  - Metabolic stresses: ER, oxidative, glucolipotoxicity
- Impaired incretin regulation
- Amyloid infiltration of islets
- Islet inflammation
- Genetics: reduced β-cell production and/or early senescence
- β-Cell dedifferentiation

Figure 16.4—Proposed mechanisms for the β-cell dysfunction and lowered β-cell mass in T2D as discussed in this chapter. ER, endoplasmic reticulum.

amylin. It is a β-cell–specific polypeptide that normally is packaged in insulin granules and cosecreted with insulin.[5] The 25– to 28–amino acid sequence is the amyloidogenic portion. Rodents lack that sequence, so transgenic mice that overexpress human IAPP have been created, with many developing islet amyloid, β-cell apoptosis, and diabetes.[136,137] Current interest has shifted from the extracellular plaques to the toxic effects of small intracellular microfibrils of IAPP. Proposed mechanisms are direct mitochondrial damage,[138,139] endoplasmic reticulum or oxidative stress,[140,141] or IAPP-enhanced IL-1β production and inflammation.[142]

Glucose Toxicity

The concept of glucose toxicity implies a direct effect of a high glucose level to impair some aspect of β-cell function or viability. It originally was proposed because of studies that showed improved β-cell function after intensive blood glucose control in people with T2D.[41] Support came from animal studies that showed experimental hyperglycemia was associated with impaired glucose-induced insulin secretion,[143,144] as well as from an intervention that lowered the glucose level without changing the insulin level and was able to restore glucose-regulated insulin secretion.[145] Many defects in β-cell signaling, gene expression, glucose and other fuel metabolism, and β-cell architecture have been linked to chronic high glucose.[146–148] Although much of the focus has been on β-cell dysfunction, high glucose levels enhancing β-cell death also are likely.[149,150] The related concept of hyperglycemia acting indirectly through insulin hypersecretion to cause β-cell dysfunction (*β-cell exhaustion*) has been discussed previously.

ER Stress

Endoplasmic reticulum (ER) stress refers to a defect in the folding, packaging, or export of newly formed proteins from the ER, either because of impairments in the complex biology of this process, or because protein synthesis is increased to a point at which it overwhelms the unfolded protein response. Unfolded or misfolded proteins accumulate, and in its extreme, results in ER swelling and cellular apoptosis. Islet β-cells are especially vulnerable because of the wide swings in insulin production and secretion that occur in everyday life—it is estimated that β-cells have the capacity to produce as many as 1 million insulin molecules every minute. β-Cell ER stress is believed to be a major pathogenic mechanism in human diabetes.[151–153] Mice with missense mutations in proinsulin develop diabetes, with β-cell apoptosis and morphological evidence of ER stress.[154] Also a number of rare proinsulin mutations causing human neonatal diabetes recently were described that are presumed to stem from the same mechanism.[155] Considerable research is ongoing into ER stress in T2D based on in vitro studies of β-cells or islets cultured with fatty acids, cytokines, or IAPP fibrils. Additionally, many rodent models of T2D have shown evidence for β-cell ER stress.[156] Particularly influential is a study of isolated islets from people with T2D incubated for 24 hours at high glucose (200 mg/dl); in this study, ER stress markers developed as opposed to the lack of these markers in islets from people without diabetes.[157]

Nutrient Excess: Oxidative Stress and Glucolipotoxicity

Oxidative stress refers to the excess production of reactive oxygen species from mitochondrial metabolism because of a high glucose level with or without excess fatty acids, resulting in cellular dysfunction or death. A related term is glucolipotoxicity, although multiple mechanisms of β-cell dysfunction and death have been proposed for this concept.[158,159] β-Cells are presumed particularly vulnerable because of a high metabolic rate and a low level of intrinsic antioxidants.[160] Animals with diabetes have provided the strongest evidence for the cytotoxic role of β-cell oxidative stress. β-Cell–specific overexpression of glutathione peroxidase in db/db mice improved β-cell mass and function, and reversed their diabetes.[161] Also, an oral glutathione peroxidase mimetic markedly improved glycemia and β-cell mass and function in Zucker fatty rats with diabetes.[162] Interest regarding oxidative stress and (gluco)lipotoxicity recently has shifted away from cytotoxicity toward more impacting β-cell signaling pathways and β-cell function.[163] Particularly influential is the study by Del Guerra et al. that correlated their finding of a high concentration of oxidative stress markers in islets from people with T2D to defective glucose-induced insulin secretion and then showed markedly improved glucose-stimulated insulin secretion after 24 hours of glutathione.[164] Collectively, these findings have created interest in β-cell oxidative stress as a drug target for T2D.[165]

Islet Inflammation

One of the newer ideas is chronic inflammation in β-cells causing insulin secretory dysfunction or β-cell apoptosis in T2D.[117,166,167] This idea is based on several discoveries. Macrophage infiltrates have been found in islets of animals and humans with T2D.[168] Islet and ductal cells when exposed to hyperglycemia and metabolic stresses, such as free fatty acids or IAPP, express cytokines (prominently IL-1β) and antagonists (IL-1 receptor antagonist) to regulate activation of cytokine-responsive signaling pathways.[169,170] It has been proposed that extrinsic and intrinsic cytokines overwhelm the islet's immune system defenses and activate the NLR family PYR-containing 3 (NLRP3) inflammasome, resulting in production of reactive oxygen species, β-cell dysfunction, and death.[142] The most cited evidence for this concept is trials of IL-1β antagonists or blocking antibodies in animals and humans with T2D that improved β-cell function and glycemia.[171,172]

β-Cell Dedifferentiation

A variation on glucose toxicity is an altered pattern of transcriptional expression of β-cell genes—not only a reduced expression of key β-cell genes but also an aberrant expression of genes not normally present in β-cells that could negatively affect β-cell function or viability—resulting from chronic hyperglycemia that was termed *β-cell dedifferentiation*.[173-175] A more recent use of that term is based on a highly discussed paper that found disruption of the β-cell signaling pathways in diabetic β-cells related to FoxO1 resulted in dedifferentiation of β-cells to progenitor cells, which can redifferentiate into glucagon-containing α-cells.[176]

CONCLUSION

The pathological sequence for T2D (Figure 16.1) entails many stages. A predisposition centered within the β-cell appears to be mandatory, with environmental and genetic factors affecting insulin secretion or the development and mass of β-cells. The actual diabetes risk then depends on numerous common environmental factors that stress the glucose homeostasis system, either through a worsening of insulin resistance or by further impairing insulin secretion. Chief among them is obesity, with a complex biology and pathophysiology that links excess adipose stores to insulin resistance, altered β-cell function, and dysmetabolism. The main determinant of an individual's risk, however, is the adequacy of their β-cell compensation system to counter the environmental stresses. Healthy β-cells are amazingly adept at preserving euglycemia even with the poor lifestyle practices and emotional stresses of modern society. Alternatively, those who develop T2D have both insulin resistance and β-cell defects long before glucose values are obviously abnormal—when the metabolic demands exceed their capacity for β-cell compensation, the pathogenic sequence to T2D is initiated. A particularly important research topic is to discover the biologic basis for susceptible β-cells; many genetic and environmental causes are being investigated, and it is inevitable that important discoveries will be made with the potential to identify novel intervention strategies. An important unknown is what initiates the transition from adequate β-cell compensation to the beginning of β-cell failure? At this point, once glucose control starts to fail and the earliest stages of T2D appear, the acquired defects within the glucose homeostasis system occur. Initially, mealtime glycemia is impaired because of a reduction in first-phase insulin secretion. As the blood glucose rises, likely in concert with excess fatty acids or other aspects of obesity and insulin resistance, β-cell function further deteriorates along with a worsening of target organ insulin sensitivity and the onset of excessive hepatic glucose production. Blood glucose levels now reach full-blown T2D.[5] Over time, the β-cell mass and insulin secretory capacity continue to decline, causing the progressive hyperglycemia and waning response to therapy that is characteristic of T2D. This review has summarized current dogma and research topics concerning the various stages of T2D. It is important, however, to realize that many questions remain, and much more will need to be learned before this illness finally is unraveled. Still, the speed of discovery and technology is intensifying, and it is only a matter of time before the cellular basis for T2D will be clarified and understood in exact detail.

REFERENCES

1. American Diabetes Association. Economic costs of diabetes in the U.S. in 2012. *Diabetes Care* 2013;36:1033–1046.

2. Zhang Q, Wang Y, Huang ES. Changes in racial/ethnic disparities in the prevalence of type 2 diabetes by obesity level among US adults. *Ethn Health* 2009;14:439–457.

3. Hedley AA, Ogden CL, Johnson CL, Carroll MD, Curtin LR, Flegal KM. Prevalence of overweight and obesity among US children, adolescents and adults, 1999–2002. *JAMA* 2004;291:2847–2850.

4. Weiss R, Dziura J, Burgert TS, Tamborlane WV, Taksali SE, Yeckel CW, Allen K, Lopes M, Savoye M, Morrison J, Sherwin RS, Caprio S. Obesity

and the metabolic syndrome in children and adolescents. *N Engl J Med* 2004;350:2362–2374.

5. Leahy JL. Pathogenesis of type 2 diabetes. In *Type 2 Diabetes Mellitus. An Evidence-Based Approach to Practical Management.* Feinglos MN, Bethel MA, Eds. Totawa, NJ, Humana Press, 2008, p. 17–33.

6. DeFronzo RA. Banting Lecture. From the triumvirate to the ominous octet: a new paradigm for the treatment of type 2 diabetes mellitus. *Diabetes* 2009;58:773–795.

7. Ferrannini E. The stunned beta cell: a brief history. *Cell Metab* 2010;11:349–352.

8. Leahy JL, Pratley RE. What is type 2 diabetes mellitus? Crucial role of maladaptive changes in beta cell and adipocyte biology. *Translational Endocrinol Metab* 2011;2:9–42.

9. Kahn SE, Cooper ME, Del Prato S. Pathophysiology and treatment of type 2 diabetes: perspectives on the past, present, and future. *Lancet* 2013;383:1068–1083.

10. Turner RC, Cull CA, Frighi V, Holman RR. Glycemic control with diet, sulfonylurea, metformin, or insulin in patients with type 2 diabetes mellitus: progressive requirement for multiple therapies (UKPDS 49). U.K. Prospective Diabetes Study (UKPDS) Group. *JAMA* 1999;281:2005–2012.

11. Abdul-Ghani MA, DeFronza RA. Pathophysiology of prediabetes. *Curr Diab Rep* 2009;9:193–199.

12. Ferrannini E, Gastaldelli A, Iozzo P. Pathophysiology of prediabetes. *Med Clin North Am* 2011;95:327–339.

13. Martin BC, Warram JH, Krolewski AS, Bergman RN, Soeldner JS, Kahn CR. Role of glucose and insulin resistance in development of type 2 diabetes mellitus: results of a 25-year follow-up study. *Lancet* 1992;340:925–929.

14. Lillioja S, Mott DM, Howard BV, Bennett PH, Yki-Järvinen H, Freymond D, Nyomba BL, Zurlo F, Swinburn B, Bogardus C. Impaired glucose tolerance as a disorder of insulin action. Longitudinal and cross-sectional studies in Pima Indians. *N Engl J Med* 1988;318:1217–1225.

15. Lillioja S, Mott DM, Spraul M, Ferraro R, Foley JE, Ravussin E, Knowler WC, Bennett PH, Bogardus C. Insulin resistance and insulin secretory dysfunction as precursors of non-insulin-dependent diabetes mellitus. Prospective studies of Pima Indians. *N Engl J Med* 1993;329:1988–1992.

16. Dunaif A, Finegood DT. Beta-cell dysfunction independent of obesity and glucose intolerance in the polycystic ovary syndrome. *J Clin Endocrinol Metab* 1996;81:942–947.

17. Stancáková A, Javorský M, Kuulasmaa T, Haffner SM, Kuusisto J, Laakso M. Changes in insulin sensitivity and insulin release in relation to glycemia and glucose tolerance in 6,414 Finnish men. *Diabetes* 2009;58:1212–1221.

18. Calles-Escandon J, Robbins DC. Loss of early phase of insulin release in humans impairs glucose tolerance and blunts thermic effect of glucose. *Diabetes* 1987;36:1167–1172.

19. Luzi L, DeFronzo RA. Effect of loss of first-phase insulin secretion on hepatic glucose production and tissue glucose disposal in humans. *Am J Physiol* 1989;257:E241–E246.

20. Perley MJ, Kipnis DM. Plasma insulin responses to oral and intravenous glucose: studies in normal and diabetic subjects. *J Clin Invest* 1967;46:1954–1962.

21. Mitrakou A, Kelley D, Mokan M, Veneman T, Pangburn T, Reilly J, Gerich J. Role of reduced suppression of glucose production and diminished early insulin release in impaired glucose tolerance. *N Engl J Med* 1992;326:22–29.

22. Gastaldelli A, Ferrannini E, Miyazaki Y, Matsuda M, DeFronzo RA; San Antonio Metabolism Study. Beta-cell dysfunction and glucose intolerance: results from the San Antonio Metabolism (SAM) Study. *Diabetologia* 2004;47:31–39.

23. Fukushima M, Usami M, Ikeda M, Nakai Y, Taniguchi A, Matsuura T, Suzuki H, Kurose T, Yamada Y, Seino Y. Insulin secretion and insulin sensitivity at different stages of glucose tolerance: a cross-sectional study of Japanese type 2 diabetes. *Metabolism* 2004;53:831–835.

24. Osei K, Rhinesmith S, Gaillard T, Schuster D. Impaired insulin sensitivity, insulin secretion, and glucose effectiveness, predict future development of impaired glucose tolerance and type 2 diabetes in pre-diabetic African Americans. *Diabetes Care* 2004;27:1439–1446.

25. Cnop M, Vidal J, Hull RL, Utzschneider KM, Carr DB, Schraw T, Scherer PE, Boyko EJ, Fujimoto WY, Kahn SE. Progressive loss of beta-cell function leads to worsening glucose tolerance in first-degree relatives of subjects with type 2 diabetes. *Diabetes Care* 2007;30:677–682.

26. Tabák AG, Jokela M, Akbaraly TN, Brunner EJ, Kivimäki M, Witte DR. Trajectories of glycaemia, insulin sensitivity, and insulin secretion before diagnosis of type 2 diabetes: an analysis from the Whitehall II study. *Lancet* 2009;373:2215–2221.

27. Bergman RN, Phillips LS, Cobelli C. Physiologic evaluation of factors controlling glucose tolerance in man: measurement of insulin sensitivity and beta-cell glucose sensitivity from the response to intravenous glucose. *J Clin Invest* 1981;68:1456–1467.

28. Kahn SE, Prigeon RL, McCulloch DK, Boyko EJ, Bergman RN, Schwartz MW, Neifing JL, Ward WK, Beard JC, Palmer JP. Quantification of the relationship between insulin sensitivity and beta-cell function in human subjects. Evidence for a hyperbolic function. *Diabetes* 1993;42:1663–1672.

29. Weyer C, Bogardus C, Mott DM, Pratley RE. The natural history of insulin secretory dysfunction and insulin resistance in the pathogenesis of type 2 diabetes mellitus. *J Clin Invest* 1999;104:787–794.

30. Tirosh A, Shai I, Tekes-Manova D, Israeli E, Pereg D, Shochat T, Kochba I, Rudich A; Israeli Diabetes Research Group. Normal fasting plasma glucose levels and type 2 diabetes in young men. *N Engl J Med* 2005;353:1454–1462.

31. Knowler WC, Barrett-Connor E, Fowler SE, Hamman RF, Lachin JM, Walker EA, Nathan DM; Diabetes Prevention Program Research Group. Reduction in the incidence of type 2 diabetes with lifestyle intervention or metformin. *N Engl J Med* 2002;346:393–403.

32. Tuomilehto J, Lindström J, Eriksson JG, Valle TT, Hämäläinen H, Ilanne-Parikka P, Keinänen-Kiukaanniemi S, Laakso M, Louheranta A, Rastas M, Salminen V, Uusitupa M; Finnish Diabetes Prevention Study Group. Prevention of type 2 diabetes mellitus by changes in lifestyle among subjects with impaired glucose tolerance. *N Engl J Med* 2001;344:1343–1350.

33. DeFronzo RA, Tripathy D, Schwenke DC, Banerji M, Bray GA, Buchanan TA, Clement SC, Henry RR, Hodis HN, Kitabchi AE, Mack WJ, Mudaliar S, Ratner RE, Williams K, Stentz FB, Musi N, Reaven PD; ACT NOW Study. Pioglitazone for diabetes prevention in impaired glucose tolerance. *N Engl J Med* 2011;364:1104–1115.

34. Cavaghan MK, Ehrmann DA, Polonsky KS. Interactions between insulin resistance and insulin secretion in the development of glucose intolerance. *J Clin Invest* 2000;106:329–333.

35. McCarthy MI. Genomics, type 2 diabetes, and obesity. *N Engl J Med* 2010;363:2339–2350.

36. Butler AE, Janson J, Bonner-Weir S, Ritzel R, Rizza RA, Butler PC. Beta-cell deficit and increased beta-cell apoptosis in humans with type 2 diabetes. *Diabetes* 2003;52:102–110.

37. Rahier J, Guiot Y, Goebbels RM, Sempoux C, Henquin JC. Pancreatic beta-cell mass in European subjects with type 2 diabetes. *Diabetes Obes Metab* 2008;10(Suppl 4):32–42.

38. Kumar AF, Gruessner RW, Seaquist ER. Risk of glucose intolerance and diabetes in hemipancreatectomized donors selected for normal preoperative glucose metabolism. *Diabetes Care* 2008;31:1639–1643.

39. O'Rahilly S, Turner RC, Matthews DR. Impaired pulsatile secretion of insulin in relatives of patients with non-insulin-dependent diabetes. *N Engl J Med* 1988;318:1225–1230.

40. Schmitz O, Pørksen N, Nyholm B, Skjaerbaek C, Butler PC, Veldhuis JD, Pincus SM. Disorderly and nonstationary insulin secretion in relatives of patients with NIDDM. *Am J Physiol* 1997;272:E218–E226.

41. Turner RC, McCarthy ST, Holman RR, Harris E. Beta-cell function improved by supplementing basal insulin secretion in mild diabetes. *BMJ* 1976;1:1252–1254.

42. Vague P, Moulin JP. The defective glucose sensitivity of the B cell in non insulin dependent diabetes. Improvement after twenty hours of normoglycaemia. *Metabolism* 1982;31:139–142.

43. Kashyap SR, Belfort R, Berria R, Suraamornkul S, Pratipranawatr T, Finlayson J, Barrentine A, Bajaj M, Mandarino L, DeFronzo R, Cusi K. Discordant effects of a chronic physiological increase in plasma FFA on insulin signaling in healthy subjects with or without a family history of type 2 diabetes. *Am J Physiol* 2004;287:E537–E546.

44. Campbell JE, Drucker DJ. Pharmacology, physiology, and mechanisms of incretin hormone action. *Cell Metab* 2013;17:819–837.

45. Holst JJ, Knop FK, Vilsbøll T, Krarup T, Madsbad S. Loss of incretin effect is a specific, important, and early characteristic of type 2 diabetes. *Diabetes Care* 2011;34(Suppl 2):S251–S257.

46. Nauck MA, Vardarli I, Deacon CF, Holst JJ, Meier JJ. Secretion of glucagon-like peptide-1 (GLP-1) in type 2 diabetes: what is up, what is down? *Diabetologia* 2011;54:10–18.

47. Shu L, Matveyenko AV, Kerr-Conte J, Cho JH, McIntosh CH, Maedler K. Decreased TCF7L2 protein levels in type 2 diabetes mellitus correlate with downregulation of GIP- and GLP-1 receptors and impaired beta-cell function. *Hum Mol Genet* 2009;18:2388–2399.

48. Dunning BE, Gerich JE. The role of alpha-cell dysregulation in fasting and postprandial hyperglycemia in type 2 diabetes and therapeutic implications. *Endocr Rev* 2007;28:253–283.

49. Meier JJ, Hücking K, Holst JJ, Deacon CF, Schmiegel WH, Nauck MA. Reduced insulinotropic effect of gastric inhibitory polypeptide in first-degree relatives of patients with type 2 diabetes. *Diabetes* 2001;50:2497–2504.

50. Faerch K, Vaag A, Holst JJ, Glümer C, Pedersen O, Borch-Johnsen K. Impaired fasting glycaemia vs impaired glucose tolerance: similar impairment of pancreatic alpha and beta cell function but differential roles of incretin hormones and insulin action. *Diabetologia* 2008;51:853–861.

51. Müssig K, Staiger H, Machicao F, Häring H-U, Fritsche A. Genetic variants affecting incretin sensitivity and incretin secretion. *Diabetologia* 2010;53:2289–2297.

52. Barnett AH, Eff C, Leslie RD, Pyke DA. Diabetes in identical twins. A study of 200 pairs. *Diabetologia* 1981;20:87–93.

53. Elbein SC, Hasstedt SJ, Wegner K, Kahn SE. Heritability of pancreatic beta-cell function among nondiabetic members of Caucasian familial type 2 diabetic kindreds. *J Clin Endocrinol Metab* 1999;84:1398–1403.

54. Meigs JB, Shrader P, Sullivan LM, McAteer JB, Fox CS, Dupuis J, Manning AK, Florez JC, Wilson PW, D'Agostino RB Sr, Cupples LA. Genotype score in addition to common risk factors for prediction of type 2 diabetes. *N Engl J Med* 2008;359:2208–2219.

55. Lyssenko V, Jonsson A, Almgren P, Pulizzi N, Isomaa B, Tuomi T, Berglund G, Altshuler D, Nilsson P, Groop L. Clinical risk factors, DNA variants, and the development of type 2 diabetes. *N Engl J Med* 2008;359:2220–2232.

56. Tabassum R, Chauhan G, Dwivedi OP, Mahajan A, Jaiswal A, Kaur I, Bandesh K, Singh T, Mathai BJ, Pandey Y, Chidambaram M, Sharma A, Chavali S, Sengupta S, Ramakrishnan L, Venkatesh P, Aggarwal SK, Ghosh S, Prabhakaran D, Srinath RK, Saxena M, Banerjee M, Mathur S, Bhansali A, Shah VN, Madhu SV, Marwaha RK, Basu A, Scaria V, McCarthy MI; DIAGRAM; INDICO; Venkatesan R, Mohan V, Tandon N, Bharadwaj D. Genome-wide association study for type 2 diabetes in Indians identifies a new susceptibility locus at 2q21. *Diabetes* 2013;62:977–986.

57. SIGMA Type 2 Diabetes Consortium, Williams AL, Jacobs SB, Moreno-Macías H, Huerta-Chagoya A, Churchhouse C, Márquez-Luna C, García-Ortíz H, Gómez-Vázquez MJ, Burtt NP, Aguilar-Salinas CA, González-Villalpando C, Florez JC, Orozco L, Haiman CA, Tusié-Luna T, Altshuler D. Sequence variants in SLC16A11 are a common risk factor for type 2 diabetes in Mexico. *Nature* 2014;506:97–101.

58. Loos RJ, Yeo GS. The bigger picture of FTO—the first GWAS-identified obesity gene. *Nat Rev Endocrinol* 2014;10:51–61.

59. Tamaki M, Fujitani Y, Hara A, Uchida T, Tamura Y, Takeno K, Kawaguchi M, Watanabe T, Ogihara T, Fukunaka A, Shimizu T, Mita T, Kanazawa A, Imaizumi MO, Abe T, Kiyonari H, Hojyo S, Fukada T, Kawauchi T, Nagamatsu S, Hirano T, Kawamori R, Watada H. The diabetes-susceptible gene SLC30A8/ZnT8 regulates hepatic insulin clearance. *J Clin Invest* 2013;123:4513–4524.

60. Grant SF, Thorleifsson G, Reynisdottir I, Benediktsson R, Manolescu A, Sainz J, Helgason A, Stefansson H, Emilsson V, Helgadottir A, Styrkarsdottir U, Magnusson KP, Walters GB, Palsdottir E, Jonsdottir T, Gudmundsdottir T, Gylfason A, Saemundsdottir J, Wilensky RL, Reilly MP, Rader DJ, Bagger Y, Christiansen C, Gudnason V, Sigurdsson G, Thorsteinsdottir U, Gulcher JR, Kong A, Stefansson K. Variant of transcription factor 7–like 2 (TCF7L2) gene confers risk of type 2 diabetes. *Nat Genet* 2006;38:320–323.

61. Liu Z, Habener JF. Wnt signaling in pancreatic islets. *Adv Exp Med Biol* 200;654:391–419.

62. da Silva Xavier G, Loder MK, McDonald A, Tarasov AI, Carzaniga R, Kronenberger K, Barg S, Rutter GA. TCF7L2 regulates late events in insulin secretion from pancreatic islet beta-cells. *Diabetes* 2009;58:894–905.

63. Flannick J, Thorleifsson G, Beer NL, Jacobs SB, Grarup N, Burtt NP, Mahajan A, Fuchsberger C, Atzmon G, Benediktsson R, Blangero J, Bowden DW,

Brandslund I, Brosnan J, Burslem F, Chambers J, Cho YS, Christensen C, Douglas DA, Duggirala R, Dymek Z, Farjoun Y, Fennell T, Fontanillas P, Forsén T, Gabriel S, Glaser B, Gudbjartsson DF, Hanis C, Hansen T, Hreidarsson AB, Hveem K, Ingelsson E, Isomaa B, Johansson S, Jørgensen T, Jørgensen ME, Kathiresan S, Kong A, Kooner J, Kravic J, Laakso M, Lee JY, Lind L, Lindgren CM, Linneberg A, Masson G, Meitinger T, Mohlke KL, Molven A, Morris AP, Potluri S, Rauramaa R, Ribel-Madsen R, Richard AM, Rolph T, Salomaa V, Segrè AV, Skärstrand H, Steinthorsdottir V, Stringham HM, Sulem P, Tai ES, Teo YY, Teslovich T, Thorsteinsdottir U, Trimmer JK, Tuomi T, Tuomilehto J, Vaziri-Sani F, Voight BF, Wilson JG, Boehnke M, McCarthy MI, Njølstad PR, Pedersen O, Groop L, Cox DR, Stefansson K, Altshuler D. Loss-of-function mutations in SLC30A8 protect against type 2 diabetes. *Nat Genet* 2014 [Epub ahead of print].

64. Stolerman ES, Florez JC. Genomics of type 2 diabetes mellitus: implications for the clinician. *Nat Rev Endocrinol* 2009;5:429–436.

65. Fetita LS, Sobngwi E, Serradas P, Calvo F, Gautier JF. Consequences of fetal exposure to maternal diabetes in offspring. *J Clin Endocrinol Metab* 2006;91:3718–3724.

66. Whincup PH, Kaye SJ, Owen CG, Huxley R, Cook DG, Anazawa S, Barrett-Connor E, Bhargava SK, Birgisdottir BE, Carlsson S, de Rooij SR, Dyck RF, Eriksson JG, Falkner B, Fall C, Forsén T, Grill V, Gudnason V, Hulman S, Hyppönen E, Jeffreys M, Lawlor DA, Leon DA, Minami J, Mishra G, Osmond C, Power C, Rich-Edwards JW, Roseboom TJ, Sachdev HS, Syddall H, Thorsdottir I, Vanhala M, Wadsworth M, Yarbrough DE. Birth weight and risk of type 2 diabetes: a systematic review. *JAMA* 2008;300:2886–2897.

67. Simmons RA, Templeton LJ, Gertz SJ. Intrauterine growth retardation leads to the development of type 2 diabetes in the rat. *Diabetes* 2001;50:2279–2286.

68. Patel MS, Srinivasan M, Laychock SG. Metabolic programming: role of nutrition in the immediate postnatal life. *J Inherit Metab Dis* 2009;32:218–228.

69. Seki Y, Williams L, Vuguin PM, Charron MJ. Minireview: Epigenetic programming of diabetes and obesity: animal models. *Endocrinology* 2012; 153:1031–1038.

70. Lillycrop KA, Burdge GC. Epigenetic mechanisms linking early nutrition to long term health. *Best Pract Res Clin Endocrinol Metab* 2012;26:667–676.

71. Dayeh TA, Olsson AH, Volkov P, Almgren P, Rönn T, Ling C. Identification of CpG-SNPs associated with type 2 diabetes and differential DNA methylation in human pancreatic islets. *Diabetologia* 2013;56:1036–1046.

72. Guénard F, Deshaies Y, Cianflone K, Kral JG, Marceau P, Vohl MC. Differential methylation in glucoregulatory genes of offspring born before vs. after maternal gastrointestinal bypass surgery. *Proc Natl Acad Sci U S A* 2013; 110:11439–11444.

73. Carpenter DO. Environmental contaminants as risk factors for developing diabetes. *Rev Environ Health* 2008;23:59–74.

74. Rajagopalan S, Brook RD. Air pollution and type 2 diabetes: mechanistic insights. *Diabetes* 2012;61:3037–3045.

75. Corkey BE. Diabetes: Have we got it all wrong? Insulin hypersecretion and food additives: cause of obesity and diabetes? *Diabetes Care* 2012;35:2432–2437.

76. Thayer KA, Heindel JJ, Bucher JR, Gallo MA. Role of environmental chemicals in diabetes and obesity: a National Toxicology Program workshop review. *Environ Health Perspect* 2012;120:779–789.

77. Musso G, Gambino R, Cassader M. Obesity, diabetes, and gut microbiota. The hygiene hypothesis expanded? *Diabetes Care* 2010;33:2277–2284.

78. Qin J, Li Y, Cai Z, Li S, Zhu J, Zhang F, Liang S, Zhang W, Guan Y, Shen D, Peng Y, Zhang D, Jie Z, Wu W, Qin Y, Xue W, Li J, Han L, Lu D, Wu P, Dai Y, Sun X, Li Z, Tang A, Zhong S, Li X, Chen W, Xu R, Wang M, Feng Q, Gong M, Yu J, Zhang Y, Zhang M, Hansen T, Sanchez G, Raes J, Falony G, Okuda S, Almeida M, LeChatelier E, Renault P, Pons N, Batto JM, Zhang Z, Chen H, Yang R, Zheng W, Li S, Yang H, Wang J, Ehrlich SD, Nielsen R, Pedersen O, Kristiansen K, Wang J. A metagenome-wide association study of gut microbiota in type 2 diabetes. *Nature* 2012;490:55–60.

79. Karlsson FH, Tremaroli V, Nookaew I, Bergström G, Behre CJ, Fagerberg B, Nielsen J, Bäckhed F. Gut metagenome in European women with normal, impaired and diabetic glucose control. *Nature* 2013;498:99–103.

80. Karlsson F, Tremaroli V, Nielsen J, Bäckhed F. Assessing the human gut microbiota in metabolic diseases. *Diabetes* 2013;62:3341–3349.

81. Thaler JP, Yi CX, Schur EA, Guyenet SJ, Hwang BH, Dietrich MO, Zhao X, Sarruf DA, Izgur V, Maravilla KR, Nguyen HT, Fischer JD, Matsen ME, Wisse BE, Morton GJ, Horvath TL, Baskin DG, Tschöp MH, Schwartz MW. Obesity is associated with hypothalamic injury in rodents and humans. *J Clin Invest* 2012;122:153–162.

82. Osundiji MA, Evans ML. Brain control of insulin and glucagon secretion. *Endocrinol Metab Clin North Am* 2013;42:1–14.

83. Tarussio D, Metref S, Seyer P, Mounien L, Vallois D, Magnan C, Foretz M, Thorens B. Nervous glucose sensing regulates postnatal β cell proliferation and glucose homeostasis. *J Clin Invest* 2014;124:413–424.

84. Mallon L, Broman JE, Hetta J. High incidence of diabetes in men with sleep complaints or short sleep duration: a 12-year follow-up study of a middle-aged population. *Diabetes Care* 2005;28:2762–2767.

85. Calkin CV, Gardner DM, Ransom T, Alda M. The relationship between bipolar disorder and type 2 diabetes: more than just co-morbid disorders. *Ann Med* 2013;45:171–181.

86. Sinnige J, Braspenning J, Schellevis F, Stirbu-Wagner I, Westert G, Korevaar J. The prevalence of disease clusters in older adults with multiple chronic diseases: a systematic literature review. *PLoS One* 2013;8:e79641.

87. Sandoval DA, Obici S, Seeley RJ. Targeting the CNS to treat type 2 diabetes. *Nat Rev Drug Discov* 2009;8:386–398.

88. Vogt MC, Brüning JC. CNS insulin signaling in the control of energy homeostasis and glucose metabolism—from embryo to old age. *Trends Endocrinol Metab* 2013;24:76–84.

89. Hu FB, Manson JE, Stampfer MJ, Colditz G, Liu S, Solomon CG, Willett WC. Diet, lifestyle, and the risk of type 2 diabetes mellitus in women. *N Engl J Med* 2001;345:790–797.

90. Koppes LL, Dekker JM, Hendriks HF, Bouter LM, Heine RJ. Moderate alcohol consumption lowers the risk of type 2 diabetes: a meta-analysis of prospective observational studies. *Diabetes Care* 2005;28:719–725.

91. van Dam RM, Hu FB. Coffee consumption and risk of type 2 diabetes: a systematic review. *JAMA* 2005;294:97–104.

92. Buitrago-Lopez A, Sanderson J, Johnson L, Warnakula S, Wood A, Di Angelantonio E, Franco OH. Chocolate consumption and cardiometabolic disorders: systematic review and meta-analysis. *BMJ* 2011;343:d4488.

93. Sun Q, Speigelman D, van Dam RM, Holmes MD, Malik VS, Willett WC, Hu FB. White rice, brown rice, and risk of type 2 diabetes in US men and women. *Arch Intern Med* 2010;170:961–969.

94. O'Dea K. Marked improvement in carbohydrate and lipid metabolism in diabetic Australian aborigines after temporary reversion to traditional lifestyle. *Diabetes* 1984;33:596–603.

95. Colditz GA, Willett WC, Rotnitzky A, Manson JE. Weight gain as a risk factor for clinical diabetes mellitus in women. *Ann Intern Med* 1995;122:481–486.

96. Chan JM, Rimm EB, Colditz GA, Stampfer MJ, Willett WC. Obesity, fat distribution, and weight gain as risk factors for clinical diabetes in men. *Diabetes Care* 1994;17:961–969.

97. Ebbert JO, Jensen MD. Fat depots, free fatty acids, and dyslipidemia. *Nutrients* 2013;5:498–508.

98. Yki-Jarvinen H. Fat in the liver and insulin resistance. *Ann Med* 2005;37:347–356.

99. Morelli M, Gaggini M, Daniele G, Marraccini P, Sicari R, Gastaldelli A. Ectopic fat: the true culprit linking obesity and cardiovascular disease? *Thromb Haemost* 2013;110:651–660.

100. Tong J, Boyko EJ, Utzschneider KM, McNeely MJ, Hayashi T, Carr DB, Wallace TM, Zraika S, Gerchman F, Leonetti DL, Fujimoto WY, Kahn SE. Intra-abdominal fat accumulation predicts the development of the metabolic syndrome in non-diabetic Japanese-Americans. *Diabetologia* 2007;50:1156–1160.

101. Kramer CK, Zinman B, Retnakaran R. Are metabolically healthy overweight and obesity benign conditions? A systematic review and meta-analysis. *Ann Intern Med* 2013;159:758–769.

102. Roberson LL, Aneni EC, Maziak W, Agatston A, Feldman T, Rouseff M, Tran T, Blaha MJ, Santos RD, Sposito A, Al-Mallah MH, Blankstein R, Budoff MJ, Nasir K. Beyond BMI: the "metabolically healthy obese" phenotype & its association with clinical/subclinical cardiovascular disease and all-cause mortality: a systematic review. *BMC Public Health* 2014;14:doi: 10.1186/1471-2458-14-14.

103. Oliveros E, Somers VK, Sochor O, Goel K, Lopez-Jimenez F. The concept of normal weight obesity. *Prog Cardiovasc Dis* 2014;56:426–433.

104. Garg A. Clinical review: Lipodystrophies: genetic and acquired body fat disorders. *J Clin Endocrinol Metab* 2011;96:3313–3325.

105. Savage DB. Mouse models of inherited lipodystrophy. *Dis Model Mech* 2009;2:554–562.

106. Harwood HJ Jr. The adipocyte as an endocrine organ in the regulation of metabolic homeostasis. *Neuropharmacology* 2012;63:57–75.

107. Sahin-Efe A, Katsikeris F, Mantzoros CS. Advances in adipokines. *Metabolism* 2012;61:1659–1665.

108. Cao H. Adipocytokines in obesity and metabolic disease. *J Endocrinol* 2014;220:T47–59.

109. Gautron L, Elmquist JK. Sixteen years and counting: an update on leptin in energy balance. *J Clin Invest* 2011;121:2087–2093.

110. Kadowaki T, Yamauchi T, Kubota N, Hara K, Ueki K, Tobe K. Adiponectin and adiponectin receptors in insulin resistance, diabetes, and the metabolic syndrome. *J Clin Invest* 2006;116:1784–1792.

111. Lee B, Shao J. Adiponectin and energy homeostasis. *Rev Endocr Metab Disord* 2013 October 30 [Epub ahead of print].

112. Graham TE, Yang Q, Blüher M, Hammarstedt A, Ciaraldi TP, Henry RR, Wason CJ, Oberbach A, Jansson PA, Smith U, Kahn BB. Retinol-binding protein 4 and insulin resistance in lean, obese, and diabetic subjects. *N Engl J Med* 2006;354:2552–2563.

113. Norseen J, Hosooka T, Hammarstedt A, Yore MM, Kant S, Aryal P, Kiernan UA, Phillips DA, Maruyama H, Kraus BJ, Usheva A, Davis RJ, Smith U, Kahn BB. Retinol-binding protein 4 inhibits insulin signaling in adipocytes by inducing proinflammatory cytokines in macrophages through a c-Jun N-terminal kinase- and toll-like receptor 4–dependent and retinol-independent mechanism. *Mol Cell Biol* 2012;32:2010–2019.

114. Kotnik P, Fischer-Posovszky P, Wabitsch M. RBP4: a controversial adipokine. *Eur J Endocrinol* 2011;165:703–711.

115. Samuel VT, Shulman GI. Mechanisms for insulin resistance: common threads and missing links. *Cell* 2012;148:852–571.

116. Boden G. Obesity, insulin resistance and free fatty acids. *Curr Opin Endocrinol Diabetes Obes* 2011;18:139–143.

117. Donath MY, Shoelson SE. Type 2 diabetes as an inflammatory disease. *Nat Rev Immunol* 2011;11:98–107.

118. Gregor MF, Hotamisligil GS. Inflammatory mechanisms in obesity. *Annu Rev Immunol* 2011;29:415–445.

119. Hansen BC, Bodkin NL. Beta-cell hyperresponsiveness: earliest event in development of diabetes in monkeys. *Am J Physiol* 1990;259:R612–R617.

120. Weyer C, Hanson RL, Tataranni PA, Bogardus C, Pratley RE. A high fasting plasma insulin concentration predicts type 2 diabetes independent of insulin resistance: evidence for a pathogenic role of relative hyperinsulinemia. *Diabetes* 2000;49:2094–2101.

121. Greenwood RH, Mahler RF, Hales CN. Improvement in insulin secretion in diabetes after diazoxide. *Lancet* 1976;1:444–447.

122. Laedtke T, Kjems L, Porksen N, Schmitz O, Veldhuis J, Kao PC, Butler PC. Overnight inhibition of insulin secretion restores pulsatility and proinsulin/insulin ratio in type 2 diabetes. *Am J Physiol Endocrinol Metab* 2000;279:E520–E528.

123. Song SH, Rhodes CJ, Veldhuis JD, Butler PC. Diazoxide attenuates glucose-induced defects in first-phase insulin release and pulsatile insulin secretion in human islets. *Endocrinology* 2003;144:3399–3405.

124. Kosaka K, Kuzuya T, Akanuma Y, Hagura R. Increase in insulin response after treatment of overt maturity-onset diabetes is independent of the mode of treatment. *Diabetologia* 1980;18:23–28.

125. Li Y, Xu W, Liao Z, Yao B, Chen X, Huang Z, Hu G, Weng J. Induction of long-term glycemic control in newly diagnosed type 2 diabetic patients is associated with improvement of beta-cell function. *Diabetes Care* 2004;27:2597–2602.

126. Weng J, Li Y, Xu W, Shi L, Zhang Q, Zhu D, Hu Y, Zhou Z, Yan X, Tian H, Ran X, Luo Z, Xian J, Yan L, Li F, Zeng L, Chen Y, Yang L, Yan S, Liu J, Li M, Fu Z, Cheng H. Effect of intensive insulin therapy on beta-cell function and glycaemic control in patients with newly diagnosed type 2 diabetes: a multicentre randomised parallel-group trial. *Lancet* 2008;371:1753–1760.

127. Garvey WT, Olefsky JM, Griffin J, Hamman RF, Kolterman OG. The effect of insulin treatment on insulin secretion and insulin action in type II diabetes mellitus. *Diabetes* 1985;34:222–234.

128. Brunzell JD, Robertson RP, Lerner RL, Hazzard WR, Ensinck JW, Bierman EL, Porte D Jr. Relationships between fasting plasma glucose levels and insulin secretion during intravenous glucose tolerance tests. *J Clin Endocrinol Metab* 1976;42:222–229.

129. Yoon KH, Ko SH, Cho JH, Lee JM, Ahn YB, Song KH, Yoo SJ, Kang MI, Cha BY, Lee KW, Son HY, Kang SK, Kim HS, Lee IK, Bonner-Weir S. Selective beta-cell loss and alpha-cell expansion in patients with type 2 diabetes mellitus in Korea. *J Clin Endocrinol Metab* 2003;88:2300–2308.

130. Marchetti P, Del Guerra S, Marselli L, Lupi R, Masini M, Pollera M, Bugliani M, Boggi U, Vistoli F, Mosca F, Del Prato S. Pancreatic islets from type 2 diabetic patients have functional defects and increased apoptosis that are ameliorated by metformin. *J Clin Endocrinol Metab* 2004;89:5535–5541.

131. Lupi R, Del Prato S. β-Cell apoptosis in type 2 diabetes: quantitative and functional consequences. *Diabetes Metab* 2008;34(Suppl 2):S56–S64.

132. Peyot ML, Pepin E, Lamontagne J, Latour MG, Zarrouki B, Lussier R, Pineda M, Jetton TL, Madiraju SR, Joly E, Prentki M. Beta-cell failure in diet-induced obese mice stratified according to body weight gain: secretory dysfunction and altered islet lipid metabolism without steatosis or reduced beta-cell mass. *Diabetes* 2010;59:2178–2187.

133. Fontés G, Zarrouki B, Hagman GK, Latour MG, Semache M, Roskens V, Moore PC, Prentki M, Rhodes CJ, Jetton TL, Poitout V. Glucolipotoxicity age-dependently impairs beta cell function in rats despite a marked increase in beta cell mass. *Diabetologia* 2010;53:2369–2379.

134. Opie EL. The relation of diabetes mellitus to lesions of the pancreas: hyaline degeneration of the islands of Langerhans. *J Exp Med* 1900–1901;5:527–540.

135. Guardado-Mendoza R, Davalli AM, Chavez AO, Hubbard GB, Dick EJ, Majluf-Cruz A, Tene-Perez CE, Goldschmidt L, Hart J, Perego C, Comuzzie AG, Tejero ME, Finzi G, Placidi C, La Rosa S, Capella C, Halff G, Gastaldelli A, DeFronzo RA, Folli F. Pancreatic islet amyloidosis, beta-cell apoptosis, and alpha-cell proliferation are determinants of islet remodeling in type-2 diabetic baboons. *Proc Natl Acad Sci U S A* 2009;106:13992–13997.

136. Janson J, Soeller WC, Roche PC, Nelson RT, Torchia AJ, Kreutter DK, Butler PC. Spontaneous diabetes mellitus in transgenic mice expressing human islet amyloid polypeptide. *Proc Natl Acad Sci U S A* 1996;93:7283–7288.

137. Verchere CB, D'Alessio DA, Palmiter RD, Weir GC, Bonner-Weir S, Baskin DG, Kahn SE. Islet amyloid formation associated with hyperglycemia in transgenic mice with pancreatic beta cell expression of human islet amyloid polypeptide. *Proc Natl Acad Sci U S A* 1996;93:3492–3496.

138. Janson J, Ashley RH, Harrison D, McIntyre S, Butler PC. The mechanism of islet amyloid polypeptide toxicity is membrane disruption by intermediate-sized toxic amyloid particles. *Diabetes* 1999;48:491–498.

139. Gurlo T, Ryazantsev S, Huang CJ, Yeh MW, Reber HA, Hines OJ, O'Brien TD, Glabe CG, Butler PC. Evidence for proteotoxicity in beta cells in type 2 diabetes: toxic islet amyloid polypeptide oligomers form intracellularly in the secretory pathway. *Am J Pathol* 2010;176:861–869.

140. Zraika S, Hull RL, Udayasankar J, Aston-Mourney K, Subramanian SL, Kisilevsky R, Szarek WA, Kahn SE. Oxidative stress is induced by islet amyloid formation and time-dependently mediates amyloid-induced beta cell apoptosis. *Diabetologia* 2009;52:626–635.

141. Matveyenko AV, Gurlo T, Daval M, Butler AE, Butler PC. Successful versus failed adaptation to high-fat diet-induced insulin resistance: the role of IAPP-induced endoplasmic reticulum stress. *Diabetes* 2009;58:906–916.

142. Masters SL, Dunne A, Subramanian SL, Hull RL, Tannahill GM, Sharp FA, Becker C, Franchi L, Yoshihara E, Chen Z, Mullooly N, Mielke LA, Harris J, Coll RC, Mills KH, Mok KH, Newsholme P, Nuñez G, Yodoi J, Kahn SE, Lavelle EC, O'Neill LA. Activation of the NLRP3 inflammasome by islet amyloid polypeptide provides a mechanism for enhanced IL-1β in type 2 diabetes. *Nat Immunol* 2010;11:897–904.

143. Leahy JL, Cooper HE, Deal DA, Weir GC. Chronic hyperglycemia is associated with impaired glucose influence on insulin secretion. A study in normal rats using chronic in vivo glucose infusions. *J Clin Invest* 1986;77:908–915.

144. Leahy JL, Bonner-Weir S, Weir GC. Minimal chronic hyperglycemia is a critical determinant of impaired insulin secretion after an incomplete pancreatectomy. *J Clin Invest* 1988;81:1407–1414.

145. Rossetti L, Shulman GI, Zawalich W, DeFronzo RA. Effect of chronic hyperglycemia on in vivo insulin secretion in partially pancreatectomized rats. *J Clin Invest* 1987;80:1037–1044.

146. Leahy JL. Detrimental effects of chronic hyperglycemia on the pancreatic β-cell. In *Diabetes Mellitus: A Fundamental and Clinical Text*. LeRoith D, Olefsky JM, Taylor S, Eds. Philadelphia, Lippincott, 2004, p. 115–127.

147. Prentki M, Nolan CJ. Islet beta cell failure in type 2 diabetes. *J Clin Invest* 2006;116:1802–1812.

148. Weir GC, Marselli L, Marchetti P, Katsuta H, Jung MH, Bonner-Weir S. Towards better understanding of the contributions of overwork and glucotoxicity to the beta-cell inadequacy of type 2 diabetes. *Diabetes Obes Metab* 2009;11(Suppl 4):82–90.

149. Koyama M, Wada R, Sakuraba H, Mizukami H, Yagihashi S. Accelerated loss of islet beta cells in sucrose-fed Goto-Kakizaki rats, a genetic model of non-insulin-dependent diabetes mellitus. *Am J Pathol* 1998;153:537–545.

150. McKenzie MD, Jamieson E, Jansen ES, Scott CL, Huang DC, Bouillet P, Allison J, Kay TW, Strasser A, Thomas HE. Glucose induces pancreatic islet cell apoptosis that requires the BH3–only proteins Bim and Puma and multi-BH domain protein Bax. *Diabetes* 2010;59:644–652.

151. Fonseca SG, Gromada J, Urano F. Endoplasmic reticulum stress and pancreatic β-cell death. *Trends Endocrinol Metab* 2011;22:266–274.

152. Back SH, Kaufman RJ. Endoplasmic reticulum stress and type 2 diabetes. *Annu Rev Biochem* 2012;81:767–93.

153. Montane J, Cadavez L, Novials A. Stress and the inflammatory process: a major cause of pancreatic cell death in type 2 diabetes. *Diabetes Metab Syndr Obes* 2014;7:25–34.

154. Oyadomari S, Koizumi A, Takeda K, Gotoh T, Akira S, Araki E, Mori M. Targeted disruption of the Chop gene delays endoplasmic reticulum stress-mediated diabetes. *J Clin Invest* 2002;109:525–532.

155. Støy J, Edghill EL, Flanagan SE, Ye H, Paz VP, Pluzhnikov A, Below JE, Hayes MG, Cox NJ, Lipkind GM, Lipton RB, Greeley SA, Patch AM, Ellard S, Steiner DF, Hattersley AT, Philipson LH, Bell GI; Neonatal Diabetes International Collaborative Group. Insulin gene mutations as a cause of permanent neonatal diabetes. *Proc Natl Acad Sci U S A* 2007;104:15040–14044.

156. Chan JY, Luzuriaga J, Bensellam M, Biden TJ, Laybutt DR. Failure of the adaptive unfolded protein response in islets of obese mice is linked with abnormalities in β-cell gene expression and progression to diabetes. *Diabetes* 2013;62:1557–1568.

157. Marchetti P, Bugliani M, Lupi R, Marselli L, Masini M, Boggi U, Filipponi F, Weir GC, Eizirik DL, Cnop M. The endoplasmic reticulum in pancreatic beta cells of type 2 diabetes patients. *Diabetologia* 2007;50:2486–2494.

158. Poitout V, Amyot J, Semache M, Zarrouki B, Hagman D, Fontés G. Gluco-lipotoxicity of the pancreatic beta cell. *Biochim Biophys Acta* 2010;1801:289–298.

159. Prentki M, Madiraju SR. Glycerolipid/free fatty acid cycle and islet β-cell function in health, obesity and diabetes. *Mol Cell Endocrinol* 2012;353:88–100.

160. Robertson R, Zhou H, Zhang T, Harmon JS. Chronic oxidative stress as a mechanism for glucose toxicity of the beta cell in type 2 diabetes. *Cell Biochem Biophys* 2007;48:139–146.

161. Harmon JS, Bogdani M, Parazzoli SD, Mak SS, Oseid EA, Berghmans M, Leboeuf RC, Robertson RP. β-cell-specific overexpression of glutathione peroxidase preserves intranuclear MafA and reverses diabetes in db/db mice. *Endocrinology* 2009;150:4855–4862.

162. Mahadevan J, Parazzoli S, Oseid E, Hertzel AV, Bernlohr DA, Vallerie SN, Liu CQ, Lopez M, Harmon JS, Robertson RP. Ebselen treatment prevents islet apoptosis, maintains intranuclear Pdx-1 and MafA levels, and preserves β-cell mass and function in ZDF rats. *Diabetes* 2013;62:3582–3588.

163. Guo S, Dai C, Guo M, Taylor B, Harmon JS, Sander M, Robertson RP, Powers AC, Stein R. Inactivation of specific β cell transcription factors in type 2 diabetes. *J Clin Invest* 2013 [Epub ahead of print].

164. Del Guerra S, Lupi R, Marselli L, Masini M, Bugliani M, Sbrana S, Torri S, Pollera M, Boggi U, Mosca F, Del Prato S, Marchetti P. Functional and molecular defects of pancreatic islets in human type 2 diabetes. *Diabetes* 2005;54:727–735.

165. Robertson RP. Antioxidant drugs for treating beta-cell oxidative stress in type 2 diabetes: glucose-centric versus insulin-centric therapy. *Discov Med* 2010;9:132–137.

166. Donath MY, Böni-Schnetzler M, Ellingsgaard H, Kalban PA, Ehses JA. Cytokine production by islets in health and diabetes: cellular origin, regulation and function. *Trends Endocrinol Metab* 2010;21:261–267.

167. Donath MY, Dalmas É, Sauter NS, Böni-Schnetzler M. Inflammation in obesity and diabetes: Islet dysfunction and therapeutic opportunity. *Cell Metab* 2013;17:860–872.

168. Ehses JA, Perren A, Eppler E, Ribaux P, Pospisilik JA, Maor-Cahn R, Gueripel X, Ellingsgaard H, Schneider MK, Biollaz G, Fontana A, Reinecke M, Homo-Delarche F, Donath MY. Increased number of islet-associated macrophages in type 2 diabetes. *Diabetes* 2007;56:2356–2370.

169. Böni-Schnetzler M, Boller S, Debray S, Bouzakri K, Meier DT, Prazak R, Kerr-Conte J, Pattou F, Ehses JA, Schuit FC, Donath MY. Free fatty acids induce a proinflammatory response in islets via the abundantly expressed interleukin-1 receptor I. *Endocrinology* 2009;150:5218–5229.

170. Maedler K, Sergeev P, Ris F, Oberholzer J, Joller-Jemelka HI, Spinas GA, Kaiser N, Halban PA, Donath MY. Glucose-induced beta cell production of IL-1beta contributes to glucotoxicity in human pancreatic islets. *J Clin Invest* 2002;110:851–860.

171. Larsen CM, Faulenbach M, Vaag A, Vølund A, Ehses JA, Seifert B, Mandrup-Poulsen T, Donath MY. Interleukin-1–receptor antagonist in type 2 diabetes mellitus. *N Engl J Med* 2007;356:1517–1526.

172. Larsen CM, Faulenbach M, Vaag A, Ehses JA, Donath MY, Mandrup-Poulsen T. Sustained effects of interleukin-1 receptor antagonist treatment in type 2 diabetes. *Diabetes Care* 2009;32:1663–1668.

173. Cavelti-Weder C, Babians-Brunner A, Keller C, Stahel MA, Kurz-Levin M, Zayed H, Solinger AM, Mandrup-Poulsen T, Dinarello CA, Donath MY. Effects of gevokizumab on glycemia and inflammatory markers in type 2 diabetes. *Diabetes Care* 2012;35:1654–1662.

174. Jonas JC, Sharma A, Hasenkamp W, Ilkova H, Patanè G, Laybutt R, Bonner-Weir S, Weir GC. Chronic hyperglycemia triggers loss of pancreatic beta cell differentiation in an animal model of diabetes. *J Biol Chem* 1999;274:14112–14121.

175. Laybutt DR, Sharma A, Sgroi DC, Gaudet J, Bonner-Weir S, Weir GC. Genetic regulation of metabolic pathways in beta-cells disrupted by hyperglycemia. *J Biol Chem* 2002;277:10912–10921.

176. Weir GC, Aguayo-Mazzucato C, Bonner-Weir S. β-cell dedifferentiation in diabetes is important, but what is it? *Islets* 2013 [Epub ahead of print].

177. Talchai C, Xuan S, Lin HV, Sussel L, Accili D. Pancreatic β cell dedifferentiation as a mechanism of diabetic β cell failure. *Cell* 2012;150:1223–1234.

Chapter 17

Obesity and Type 2 Diabetes

Catherine M. Champagne, PhD, RDN, LDN
Frank L. Greenway, MD
William T. Cefalu, MD

INTRODUCTION

Overweight and obesity are chronic conditions that continue to be recognized as global epidemics. As currently defined, overweight and obesity are assessed by use of BMI, as overweight is defined as a BMI of 25 kg/m² to 29.9 kg/m², whereas obesity is defined as a BMI >30 kg/m².[1] Current estimates suggest that ~70% of the U.S. population is considered overweight, whereas ~35% are now considered obese.[2,3] Although the prevalence of overweight in the U.S. over the past 10 years appears to be slowing or leveling off, it appears the prevalence of more severe obesity continues to rise.[2,3] Interestingly, dynamic models suggest that the U.S. prevalence of obesity may be stabilizing and may plateau, and this will be independent of current preventive strategies.[4] Specifically, it is suggested that the prevalence of overweight, obesity, and extreme obesity may plateau by the year 2030 at 28, 32, and 9%, respectively.[4]

Given the current prevalence of obese and overweight individuals, the concern remains that these two conditions will continue to contribute greatly to chronic diseases and represent major public health challenges.[1] Obesity is well known to be significantly associated with the traditional risk factors for cardiovascular disease (CVD; i.e., hypertension, dyslipidemia, type 2 diabetes [T2D]). In addition, it is clearly associated with the nontraditional risk factors as well (i.e., fibrinogen and inflammatory markers). An obese individual has a greater risk for cancer, gastrointestinal diseases, arthritis, diabetes, and CVD.[4,5] The presence of these conditions greatly increases the costs of care. As outlined in the recently published guidelines, when compared with normal-weight individuals, obese patients are reported to incur 46% increased inpatient costs, have 27% more physician visits, and spend 80% more on prescription drugs.[1,6] The cost attributed to the disease as of 2008 was ~$147 billion.[1,6]

PATHOPHYSIOLOGY

Obesity is viewed as developing in any given individual secondary to an imbalance in energy balance. The concept of "energy balance" is not new and implies that food consumption (i.e., "energy intake") needs to match energy output (i.e., "energy expenditure") to maintain a stable body weight.[5,7,8] Several major determinants of energy expenditure consist of the following: 1) thermogenic effect of food (TEF), which represents the amount of energy utilized by ingestion and digestion of food we consume; 2) physical activity; and 3) resting metabolic rate

DOI: 10.2337/9781580405096.17

(RMR) determined in large measure by the amount of lean body mass.[5,9] Hyperphagia, a low metabolic rate, low rates of fat oxidation, and an impaired sympathetic nervous activity characterize animal models of obesity.[9] Similar metabolic factors have been found to characterize humans who are susceptible to weight gain. Specifically, at least four metabolic parameters have been found to be predictive of weight gain in the Pima Indian population, a population in which obesity is extremely prevalent and weight gain is common among young adults.[9] These factors were described as being a low metabolic rate, low spontaneous physical activity, low sympathetic nervous system (SNS) activity, and low fat oxidation.

In clinical terms, we have defined obesity as an excessive amount of body fat and the increase in adiposity through multiple mechanisms contributing to an increased prevalence of CVD risk factors, an increase in medical illness, and premature death. The fundamental problem underlying development of obesity is an alteration in energy balance of the individual, and obesity develops over time when an individual consumes more calories on a daily basis than is expended. Development of obesity is not such a simple process, however, and the obesity epidemic appears to be the result of a normal physiology (genetic variability) in a pathoenvironment.[9,10] Over the recent past, there have been many changes in our environment that promote obesity. As currently understood, many individuals, even when faced with factors predisposing to obesity as part of an obesogenic environment, have managed to resist obesity. Thus, there appears to be evidence that the variable susceptibility to obesity in response to environmental factors is undoubtedly modulated by specific genes.[5,10,11] Furthermore, there has been considerable research and understanding as to mechanisms that contribute to its development. In this regard, we now recognize that research has revealed molecular, cellular, and physiologic systems that are complex and highly integrated, and key regulators of energy balance and insulin signaling have been elucidated. It also has been determined that there is a dynamic interplay between the adipose tissue and other key tissues in the body, such as liver, muscle, and regulatory centers of the brain. Altered regulation of this integrated and coordinated system inevitably leads to accumulation of body fat, insulin resistance, and the development of associated cardiovascular risk factors.[5]

CLINICAL CLASSIFICATION

Body weight and BMI have been the traditional clinical assessments used to define obesity and to classify obesity into specific risk categories. The BMI simply represents the relationship between a patient's weight and height and is derived by *1*) calculating either the weight (in kg) and dividing by the height (in meters squared), or *2*) calculating weight (in pounds) times 704 divided by height in inches squared.[7] The risk calculation obtained from the BMI is obtained from data collected from large population-based studies that assessed the relationship between body weight and mortality and provides the clinician a mechanism for identifying patients at high risk for complications associated with obesity.[5,12,13]

Assessing obesity by use of BMI clearly has served as an important clinical tool, but it has been recognized for many years that assessing adiposity by evaluating the specific distribution of the body fat (e.g., central or abdominal obesity) is an even more important assessment.[5] Assessing total body adiposity can be obtained with use of dual-energy X-ray absorptiometry scans to obtain total body fat. Body fat distribution can be performed by obtaining simple anthropometric measurements (i.e., waist circumference, the waist–hip ratio, or skinfold thickness). For research purposes, and to specifically define the specific fat depots (i.e., abdominal visceral and abdominal subcutaneous fat), more precise imaging techniques, such as computed tomography (CT) scans or magnetic resonance imaging (MRI), are routinely used.[14,15] Thus, with use of these techniques, the relationship between specific adipose tissue depots (e.g., visceral fat depots) and cardiovascular risk factors (i.e., insulin sensitivity) and CVD has been obtained in both cross-sectional and longitudinal studies.[16]

In addition to assessing specific abdominal fat depots, the use of MRI and magnetic resonance and spectroscopy (MRS) techniques has demonstrated the important role of "ectopic" lipids in the pathophysiology of metabolic dysfunction.[17] Specifically, over the recent past, it is clear adipose tissue is not simply a passive energy depot but is clearly a dynamic "endocrine organ."[18] Adipose tissue is well known to modulate metabolism by means of a complex cross talk of adipocytes with their microenvironment.[18] The observed "dysfunctional adipose tissue," is characterized by adipocyte hypertrophy, macrophage infiltration, impaired insulin signaling, and insulin resistance.[18] Inflammatory adipokines and excessive amounts of free fatty acids are released, and these compounds are reported to enhance ectopic fat deposition. Specifically, in addition to lipid accumulation in adipose tissue, obesity is associated with increased lipid storage in ectopic tissues, such as skeletal muscle, liver, and pancreatic β-cells.[18,19] Currently, measurement of ectopic lipids is not readily clinically available but can be measured histologically with muscle and liver biopsies or chemically by determining lipid intermediates in biopsies, as well as by assessing lipid content with imaging techniques (i.e., CT scan, MRI).

COMORBIDITIES

The association between obesity and cardiometabolic risk factors, such as dyslipidemia and hypertension, is not in question.[20,21] For example, obese subjects with T2D are reported to have increased triglyceride levels along with low HDL levels and atherogenic LDL particles.[22] Hypertension is also a common comorbidity observed in individuals with obesity and T2D and is observed to be a major risk factor for CVD and microvascular complications.[23,24] The presence of these complications is reported to lead to additional complications in patients with T2D.[23,25] Individuals with newly diagnosed T2D are reported to have a 25% increase in risk of CVD, emanating from numerous contributors.[26]

Given the association of obesity, T2D, and cardiovascular risk factors, it is now well appreciated that modest weight loss (5–10% from baseline) appears to be achievable and sustainable and is associated with significant health benefits.[27] For example, as recently reviewed by Ryan and Bray, the Look AHEAD study, an observation of >2,500 subjects with diabetes in an intensive lifestyle intervention, demonstrated the ability to produce modest weight loss and sustain it over 1 years.[27] As reported, weight loss had benefits in regard to reducing risk factors and improving sleep apnea, urinary incontinence, mobility, and symptoms of depression.[27] Importantly, the intervention appeared to have significant economic benefits as it reduced medication use and costs.[27] As also reviewed, given this beneficial effect of modest weight loss and the impact of obesity on morbidity and health care costs, reimbursement is now provided by the Center for Medicare and Medicaid Services for up to 14 sessions of intensive behavioral therapy for obesity, when delivered by primary care physicians.[27]

Therefore, it is clear that the primary strategy for prevention and treatment of the obese patient with T2D is lifestyle modification through changes in diet and physical activity. The American Diabetes Association's (ADA's) goals and recommendations for achieving diet and lifestyle change are available elsewhere.[23] In addition to moderate weight loss, the ADA suggests that management of the overweight patient with T2D should focus on control of glycemia with the use of antidiabetic therapy.[23] Clinicians, however, now have at their disposal a large list of medications to treat T2D that improve glycemic control and can provide weight loss or can be considered weight neutral. Given this strategy, it is clear that the approach to management of obesity in T2D has evolved significantly. Lifestyle and enhanced physical activity clearly remain the cornerstone for management, but the recent results and benefits achieved by surgery are impressive. Finally, clinicians now have medications specifically marketed to achieve weight loss in individuals with T2D.

Even in patients with established diabetes, intensive management of the metabolic syndrome will reduce the higher risk of CVD. Most individuals affected by the metabolic syndrome are overweight or obese and, as such, weight reduction represents the principal goal of most intervention studies.[23-26] It has been well noted that weight loss is associated with significant improvement in the clinical abnormalities of the metabolic syndrome, such as blood glucose, lipid profile, and blood pressure.[26] Even a moderate weight reduction of 7% in 4 weeks can improve the metabolic syndrome despite persistence of a high BMI,[27] and the greater the weight reduction, the greater the improvement in CVD risk factors. Likewise, effective lifestyle interventions should increase insulin sensitivity and high-density lipoprotein cholesterol (HDL-C) levels, and should decrease triglyceride, glucose concentrations, and blood pressure.

LIFESTYLE MODIFICATION: DIABETES PREVENTION

The literature describes the effectiveness of lifestyle intervention in preventing the development of T2D in high-risk individuals with impaired glucose tolerance (IGT). Dietary modification (i.e., reduction in energy) and increased physical activity were the main lifestyle interventions, which resulted in subjects losing weight (~5%). The progression from IGT to T2D over a defined period (3–6 years) of observation in the intervention group versus a comparison group was the primary outcome for the studies.[28-30]

THE DA QING IGT AND DIABETES STUDY

In the Da Qing IGT and Diabetes Study, 577 Chinese adults with IGT were randomized to one of three treatment groups (diet only, exercise only, or diet plus exercise) or a control group.[28] The diet-only group was encouraged to reduce their weight if BMI was ≥25 kg/m² (61% of all participants) with a goal of 23 kg/m². The exercise group was instructed to increase their level of leisure-time activity by at least 1–2 units (i.e., 1 unit equaled 30 minutes slow walking, 10 minutes slow running, or 5 minutes swimming) per day. The third group was a diet-plus-exercise group. Subjects were evaluated every 2 years for 6 years. At year 6, the diet, exercise, and diet-plus-exercise groups had a reduction in risk of developing T2D (31, 46, and 42%, respectively). The importance of this study is that it established the feasibility of implementing a successful lifestyle modification program in an outpatient clinic setting.

A follow-up to the Da Qing Study in 2006 on the subjects with IGT assessed the long-term effect of the lifestyle interventions on T2D and other related health conditions.[31] Compared with control participants, those in the diet-plus-exercise lifestyle intervention group had a 43% lower incidence of T2D up to 14 years after the initial 6-year active intervention (years 1986–1992) was completed. The onset of diabetes also was delayed almost 4 years. No significant differences were found between intervention and control groups for CVD incidence and mortality and all-cause mortality, indicating that benefits from lifestyle intervention could be maintained long-term following completion of an active intervention.

THE FINNISH DIABETES PREVENTION STUDY

The Finnish Diabetes Prevention Study examined the effects of an intensive modification program in 522 middle-age and overweight Finnish subjects with IGT.[29] Subjects were randomized to either intensive lifestyle intervention or control groups. The lifestyle intervention goals included reductions in weight (≥5%), total fat intake (<30% of energy), and saturated fat intake (<10% of energy). Dietary fiber intake (≥15 grams/1,000 kcal) was increased and moderate exercise (≥30 minutes/day by both aerobic and resistance training) was promoted. After the first year, weight, waist circumference, glucose, insulin, triglycerides, and blood pressure in the intervention group all were reduced from baseline values. Body weight decreased on average 4 kg (5%) in the intervention group and 1 kg (1%) in the control group. At year 2, the lifestyle intervention group continued to have a greater weight loss than the control group. After 4 years, the cumulative incidence of diabetes was 11% in the intervention group and 23% in the control group. The risk of diabetes was reduced significantly by 58% in the lifestyle group. During the overall follow-up period of 7 years (4 years of active intervention), the incidence of diabetes rates still was lower in the intervention (4.3% per 100 person-years) versus control (7.4% per 100 person-years) groups.[32] This result indicated a 43% reduction in the relative risk of diabetes. Most important, the beneficial effects of lifestyle intervention were maintained after discontinuation of the study.[32]

DIABETES PREVENTION PROGRAM

The Diabetes Prevention Program (DPP) is the largest study in the U.S. to examine the effectiveness of a lifestyle modification program designed to prevent or delay the development of T2D in people with IGT.[30] This multicenter trial randomized 3,234 subjects with IGT to one of three interventions (1,082 to placebo, 1,073 to metformin, and 1,079 to the intensive lifestyle intervention). The goals of the intensive lifestyle intervention were ≥7% weight loss and 150 minutes of physical activity per week (moderate intensity, such as brisk walking). The intensive lifestyle group received individual counseling on a low-fat, low-calorie diet and motivational support (Table 17.1). After an average follow-up of 2.8 years, the lifestyle intervention group reduced the incidence of diabetes by 58% when compared with the placebo group. DPP participants on metformin medication also reduced their incidence of diabetes (31%), but not as much as those in the lifestyle intervention group. In addition, the lifestyle intervention group had a significantly greater average weight loss (5.6 kg) than the metformin (2.1 kg) and placebo (0.1 kg) groups. Thirty-eight percent of the lifestyle participants achieved at least a 7% weight loss and 58% met the physical activity goal.

Another important highlight of the DPP study was the impact of intensive lifestyle intervention, metformin, and placebo on components of the metabolic syndrome and risk factors for CVD.[33] When compared with the metformin and placebo groups, the lifestyle intervention group reduced the prevalence of dyslip-

Table 17.1 The Diabetes Prevention Program Intervention Sessions

Session 1A:	Welcome to the Lifestyle Balance Program
Session 1B:	Getting Started Being Active
Session 1B:	Getting Started Losing Weight
Session 2 or 5:	Move Those Muscles
Session 3 or 6:	Being Active: A Way of Life
Session 4 or 2:	Be a Fat Detective
Session 5 or 3:	Three Ways to Eat Less Fat
Session 6 or 4:	Healthy Eating
Session 7 or 8:	Take Charge of What's Around You
Session 8 or 7:	Tip the Calorie Balance
Session 9:	Problem Solving
Session 10:	Four Keys to Healthy Eating Out
Session 11:	Talk Back to Negative Thoughts
Session 12:	The Slippery Slope of Lifestyle Change
Session 13:	Jump Start Your Activity Plan
Session 14:	Make Social Cues Work for You
Session 15:	You Can Manage Stress
Session 16:	Ways to Stay Motivated

Note: The 16 sessions listed were carried out over a period of 24 weeks in individual visits with participants.
Source: Adapted from the Diabetes Prevention Program's Lifestyle Change Program Manual of Operations. Available from http://www.bsc.gwu.edu/dpp/lifestyle/dpp_duringcore.pdf. Accessed 23 March 2014.

idemia, LDL phenotype B (i.e., smaller, denser, and more atherogenic LDL particle), and hypertension. The intensive lifestyle group also saw reductions in systolic and diastolic blood pressure and triglyceride levels and increases in HDL-C when compared with the other groups. After 3 years, the need for antihypertensive and lipid-lowering medications among subjects assigned to the intensive lifestyle intervention was reduced.[33]

Ten years following the randomization in the DPP, the DPP Outcomes Study (DPPOS) found that the diabetes incidence was reduced by 34% in the lifestyle intervention group and 18% in the metformin group compared with the placebo group.[34] The DPPOS results indicate that high-risk individuals can delay or prevent developing T2D by losing weight through a diet low in fat and calories and regular physical activity. The interpretation after 10 years of observation was that although the former placebo and metformin groups had incidences of diabetes equal to the former lifestyle group, the cumulative incidence of diabetes was still lowest in the lifestyle group; these benefits thus can persist on a fairly long-term basis.[34]

LIFESTYLE MODIFICATION: DIABETES

LOOK AHEAD

The Look AHEAD (Action for Health in Diabetes) trial was designed to address the question of whether or not a lifestyle intervention designed to achieve weight loss via caloric restriction and increased physical activity could decrease cardiovascular morbidity and mortality in overweight and obese individuals with diabetes.[35] Although the trial was stopped early because the rate of cardiovascular events was not reduced in these individuals, there were other benefits to those in the lifestyle intervention. Weight loss was greater in the intervention group compared with the control group both at 1 year and at study end, glycated hemoglobin was reduced, and fitness improved, along with other cardiovascular risk factors (except LDL cholesterol [LDL-C]).[35]

Perri[36] has described the Look AHEAD trial as the largest and longest randomized controlled trial of a behavioral intervention for weight loss. He noted that although non-Hispanic whites had the larger weight losses in year 1, the assessments at 4 and 8 years showed comparable weight reductions for other ethnic groups in the study, specifically African Americans, Hispanic, and American Indian and other ethnicities. In addition, weight loss for men and women were comparable, but older participants lost more weight (which also may have been a result of the aging process).[36]

Perhaps one of the most striking benefits of lifestyle modification as reported in the Look AHEAD trial is remission of T2D.[37] Gregg et al. noted that along with the weight loss and fitness increases, the intensive lifestyle intervention participants were significantly more likely to experience either partial or complete remission during the first year (prevalence 11.5%) and at year 4 (prevalence 7.3%) compared with a lesser prevalence in the diabetes support and education group at either time point (prevalence 2%).[37] Over the entire study, however, the absolute remission rates were modest.

LIFESTYLE MODIFICATION: OBESITY AND THE METABOLIC SYNDROME

DIET AND WEIGHT LOSS

A weight loss of at least 7% has been suggested to improve the metabolic syndrome.[27] Dansinger compared four popular diets (i.e., Atkins, Ornish, Weight Watchers, and Zone) in 160 overweight and obese participants with known hypertension, dyslipidemia, or fasting hyperglycemia in a randomized controlled trial.[38] CVD risk factor outcome measures were assessed at baseline, 2, 6, and 12 months. After 1 year, all four diets produced moderate, but statistically significant, effects on weight loss, as well as other CVD risk factors such as total cholesterol (except Akins and Zone diets), LDL-C (except Atkins diet), HDL-C (except Ornish diet), LDL-C/HDL-C ratio, insulin (except Atkins diet), and C-reactive protein (except Zone diet). This moderate effect may have been due to poor long-term compliance with the diets.

Another landmark study on the effects of macronutrient-altered diets, POUNDS LOST, included 811 overweight participants randomized to one of four treatments varying in either protein or fat.[39] The main conclusion from this study was that reduction of calories resulted in clinically meaningful weight loss regardless of which macronutrients were emphasized. Resting energy expenditure decreased significantly after weight loss, but also was not related to diet composition.[40] A substudy in ~25% of the subject population by Bray et al.,[41] however, found that the low-fat diet was associated with significant changes in body composition and energy expenditure compared with the high-fat diet.

The popular Mediterranean-style diet was evaluated in a study of 190 women by Esposito et al.[42] Seventy-five women with a carbohydrate intake ≤50% of energy intake were compared with 115 women with a carbohydrate intake >50% of energy and included a follow-up for 2 years.[42] After 2 years, those consuming a low-carbohydrate diet lost significantly more weight and had lower adiponectin and triglyceride levels than women consuming a high-carbohydrate diet.[42]

Weight loss has been shown to improve CVD risk factors; however, the benefits will not remain unless the weight loss is maintained. Behavioral weight-loss clinical trials, such as the Trial of Hypertension Prevention Phase II (TOHP II),[43] STOP Regain,[44] and Weight Loss Maintenance (WLM),[45] all demonstrated the ability to maintain weight loss on a long-term basis. In particular, the WLM trial found that 71% of the study participants remained at or below their entry level weight 30 months after a 6-month behavioral weight-loss program by providing only brief monthly personal-contact sessions with the majority by telephone contact.[45]

PHYSICAL ACTIVITY AND PHYSICAL ACTIVITY AND DIET COMBINED

Independent of dietary changes, physical activity has been shown to decrease abdominal visceral and subcutaneous fat in healthy, overweight, and obese men and women.[46,47] Joseph et al. evaluated the effects of a 6-month weight-loss (250–350 kcal/day caloric restriction) and low-intensity aerobic exercise (i.e., walking) program on body composition and metabolic parameters in obese postmenopausal women with and without the metabolic syndrome.[48] After the 6-month program, they found reductions in weight, fat mass, visceral and subcutaneous abdominal tissues, triglycerides, C-reactive protein, tumor necrosis factor-α, and glucose concentrations in women with the metabolic syndrome. Resolution of the metabolic syndrome was best predicted by reductions in fat mass. Furthermore, the HERITAGE Family Study found that after 20 weeks of supervised aerobic exercise training (cycle ergometer), 30.5% of their obese subjects no longer had metabolic syndrome.[49] There were also decreases in their waist circumference and improvement in their metabolic profile (triglycerides, HDL-C, blood pressure, and fasting plasma glucose concentrations). Another significant study conducted by Lofgren et al.[50] in 70 overweight, obese premenopausal women found that 10 weeks of increased low-impact physical activity (walking) and consumption of a low-energy diet led to significant reductions in weight, BMI, waist circumference, total fat mass, trunk fat mass, and insulin and leptin levels. Importantly, after the intervention, some subjects with metabolic syndrome no longer had the syndrome.

LIFESTYLE MODIFICATION: BENEFITS OF A HEALTHY DIET

The diets with the most science behind them are those used in the DPP[30] and the Dietary Approaches to Stop Hypertension (DASH) trials. The DPP diet focused primarily on preventing diabetes, while the DASH diet was found to help control high blood pressure, improve blood lipid profile, and reduce cancer risk (Table 17.2).[51] An interesting side note is that the DASH diet has been ranked as the best diet overall by a panel of nationally recognized experts in diet, nutrition, obesity, food psychology, diabetes, and heart disease convened by *U.S. News & World Report*.[52] In 2014, the DASH diet was voted the best diet for diabetes, the best diet overall, and the best diet for healthy eating. The DASH diet has now been named the best overall diet for 4 consecutive years (2011–2014).[53] Both the DPP intervention trial and the DASH dietary strategies were built around healthy choices and nutrients that help prevent or manage diabetes.

Other benefits of healthy diets include improvement in hypertensive status. The DASH-Sodium trial was designed as a diet-based plan for modification of blood pressure and evaluated different levels of dietary sodium (high, 3.5 g/day; intermediate, 2.3 g/day; and low, 1.2 g/day) combined with the DASH[51] diet (fruits, vegetables, low-fat dairy products) versus a standard U.S. diet (control) in 412 adults with prehypertension or stage-1 hypertension.[54] Compared with the control group, the DASH diet significantly improved blood pressure at each sodium level. Implementation of the DASH diet in the PREMIER study resulted in decreased blood pressure; additionally, total cholesterol, homeostatic model assessment index for insulin sensitivity (HOMA-IR), and fasting insulin were improved in individuals with prehypertension or stage-1 hypertension, regardless of metabolic syndrome status.[55]

Popular low-carbohydrate diets have been shown to lower triglyceride concentrations and raise HDL-C levels more than conventional diets and the opposite effect has been documented with high-carbohydrate diets.[56-60] The effects on blood

Table 17.2 The DASH Eating Plan

Food group	No. servings @ 2,000 kcal	No. servings @ 1,600 kcal	Serving sizes
Grains*	6–8	6	1 slice bread 1 ounce dry cereal 1/2 cup cooked rice, pasta, or cereal
Vegetables	4–5	3–4	1 cup raw leafy vegetable 1/2 cup cut-up raw or cooked vegetable 1/2 cup vegetable juice
Fruits	4–5	4	1 medium fruit 1/4 cup dried fruit 1/2 cup fresh, frozen, or canned fruit 1/2 cup fruit juice
Fat-free or low-fat milk and milk products	2–3	2–3	1 cup milk or yogurt 1 1/2 ounces cheese
Lean meats, poultry, and fish	≤6	3–6	1 ounce cooked meats, poultry, or fish 1 egg
Nuts, seeds, and legumes	4–5 per week	3 per week	1/3 cup or 1 1/2 ounces nuts 2 Tbsp peanut butter 2 Tbsp or 1/2 ounce seeds 1/2 cup cooked legumes (dry beans and peas)
Fats and oils	2–3	2	1 tsp soft margarine 1 tsp vegetable oil 1 Tbsp mayonnaise 2 Tbsp salad dressing
Sweets and added sugars	≤5 per week	0	1 Tbsp sugar 1 Tbsp jelly or jam 1/2 cup sorbet, gelatin 1 cup lemonade

Note:
*Whole grains are recommended for most grain servings as a good source of fiber and nutrients.
Source: Adapted from www.nhlbi.nih.gov/health/public/heart/hbp/dash/new_dash.pdf. Accessed 12 February 2014.

lipids with the DASH diet have been mixed. Obarzanek et al.[61] reported lower total cholesterol, LDL-C, and HDL-C in DASH participants, but no effect on triglycerides. Conversely, Azadbakht et al.[62] found beneficial effects of a DASH eating plan in a randomized controlled outpatient trial of 116 patients with metabolic syndrome. Compared with the control group, individuals consuming the DASH diet were found to have increased HDL-C and lower triglycerides after 6 months.[62]

Diets high in soy protein and Mediterranean-type diets also have been shown to improve lipid and inflammatory disease markers. In one study, increased consumption of soy protein (~47 g/day) reduced total cholesterol by 9.3%, LDL-C by 12.9%, and triglycerides by 10.5%, while increasing HDL-C by 2.4%.[63] Esposito et al.[64] conducted a randomized trial comparing the Mediterranean-style diet to a control diet in 180 adults with metabolic syndrome. At the end of the 2 years when compared with the control group, those patients following the Mediterranean-style diet had a lower body weight and significantly reduced serum concentrations of high-sensitivity C-reactive protein and interleukin-6 (IL-6), IL-7, and IL-18; they decreased insulin resistance and improved endothelial function score.

BOTANICAL, PHARMACEUTICAL, AND SURGICAL APPROACHES

BOTANICALS

Current estimates are that ~40% of U.S. adults use complementary and alternative medicine (CAM), regardless of the absence of conclusive evidence of the effectiveness of these compounds on health status.[65] Nguyen et al. have suggested that based on a survey of >23,000 adults, those reporting use of CAM were more likely to rate their health as excellent; however, they suggested that large-scale randomized trials are needed to establish a causal relationship.[65] Reports are that the most commonly used CAM therapies consist of nonvitamin, nonmineral, and natural products (especially derived from botanicals) because they are perceived to be less toxic with fewer side effects than synthetic products.[66]

Some have suggested that botanicals be used to treat or prevent metabolic syndrome.[67] The suggestion is that plant-derived compounds consist of many biologically active components, producing a more synergistic effect than that derived from single compounds; in particular, bitter melon, blueberries, cinnamon, fenugreek, grape seed, hawthorn, hoodia, and Russian tarragon have been reported to beneficially affect diabetes, hypertension, obesity status, and blood cholesterol status.[67] A randomized controlled trial comparing a blueberry supplemented smoothie with a placebo smoothie found an improvement in insulin sensitivity in obese, insulin-resistant adults with prediabetes.[68]

Bell et al.[69] studied patterns of complementary therapy use in 71 older adults with diabetes living in a rural area. Among the most commonly reported therapies were food and beverages (50.7%) and herbs (11.3%), but the authors suggested that further research is needed to understand both the motivation as well as the pattern of use by these patients with diabetes.

Clearly, research is needed in this area because marketing messages by manufacturers may not necessarily reflect valid scientific research.

PHARMACEUTICALS

Lifestyle interventions provide recommended strategies to improve the metabolic syndrome. Although lifestyle changes can provide benefits for the management of the syndrome, these changes are often difficult to implement and maintain. When lifestyle modifications are unsuccessful, pharmacological intervention may be the next approach.

Obesity Drugs Approved for Short-Term Use

Before 1985 when the National Institutes of Health consensus conference declared obesity to be a chronic disease, obesity was considered to be the result of bad habits.[70] Psychologists suggested that new habits were like riding a bicycle and could be learned over a period up to 12 weeks and the training wheels removed. Obesity drugs before 1985 were tested and approved by the U.S. Food and Drug Administration (FDA) for up to 12 weeks of use to aid in retraining eating habits. This created a situation in which drugs like phentermine, diethylpropion, phendimetrazine, and benzphetamine were approved only for up to 12 weeks' use even though we now appreciate obesity as a chronic disease. These four drugs all stimulate release of norepinephrine, reduce appetite, and are stimulants. Because of concern about the potential for abuse of a stimulant medication, these drugs are placed in Drug Enforcement Administration (DEA) schedules. Phentermine and diethylpropion are in schedule IV, the schedule with a low potential for abuse, whereas phendimetrazine and benzphetamine are in schedule III, a category for a greater potential for abuse. Munro et al.[71] presented a study comparing intermittent and continuous treatment with phentermine. The intermittent group was treated every other month with phentermine and the alternate months with placebo. Although the weight-loss curve was smoother with continuous phentermine, both the continuous and intermittent groups achieved the same weight loss at 36 weeks.[71] Thus, use of these drugs on an every-other-month basis has been suggested as a way to use them in compliance with the package insert. Potential side effects of these drugs are similar; relate to their stimulation of norepinephrine release; and include tachycardia, hypertension, restlessness, insomnia, dry mouth, and tremor. A meta-analysis concluded that phentermine caused a 3.6 kg greater weight loss than placebo, and diethylpropion caused a 3 kg weight loss in excess of a placebo.[72] Weight loss is thought to be similar with all of four of these drugs that reduce appetite through the stimulation of norepinephrine release. For that reason, phentermine and diethylpropion usually are preferred over phendimetrazine and benzphetamine because they are regulated in the DEA schedule with the lowest potential for abuse.

Obesity Drugs Approved for Long-Term Use

Three obesity drugs presently are approved for long-term use: orlistat, lorcaserin, and phentermine-topiramate in combination. Each of these drugs will be briefly reviewed.

Orlistat. Orlistat is a lipase inhibitor that causes dietary fat to be excreted as oil in the stool and should be taken with a diet containing 30% fat. Orlistat is prescribed at a dose of 120 mg three times a day with meals by prescription and is available over the counter at 60 mg three times a day with meals. A meta-analysis concluded that weight loss with orlistat was 2.9 kg greater than placebo at 12 months.[72] The nonprescription dose of orlistat provides ~80% of the weight loss seen with the prescription dose. Orlistat 120 mg three times a day was also effective in subjects with T2D, and glycohemoglobin was reduced a significant 0.4% over a

6-month period.[73] Orlistat was evaluated in a 4-year trial in 3,305 subjects who were randomized to lifestyle changes with or without orlistat 120 mg three times a day. The risk of conversion to diabetes from IGT was reduced by 37% ($P = 0.0032$).[74] Orlistat is not absorbed to any significant degree and the side effects relate to the fat in the stool, including abdominal cramps, flatus with discharge, oily spotting, and fecal incontinence. Because of the potential for the loss of fat-soluble vitamins, orlistat is to be taken with a vitamin supplement.[75]

Lorcaserin. Lorcaserin is an agonist of the serotonin (5-HT) 2c receptor in the hypothalamus. Unlike fenfluramine, which was a nonspecific serotonin agonist, lorcaserin has selectivity for the 2c receptor and did not significantly increase valvulopathy in the clinical trials. Lorcaserin at 10 mg twice a day gave a 3.3% greater weight loss than placebo, but the 0.5% reduction of glycohemoglobin in subjects with diabetes was disproportionate to the weight loss. Although fenfluramine combined with phentermine gave a 15% weight loss, whether phentermine and lorcaserin will perform similarly presently is untested.[76] Lorcaserin was well tolerated, with side effects being headache, dizziness, fatigue, nausea, dry mouth, and constipation.[77] Lorcaserin is in DEA schedule IV.[78]

Phentermine-Topiramate. Phentermine causes a decrease in food intake by stimulating the release of norepinephrine in the hypothalamus. Topiramate reduces appetite by augmenting the neurotransmitter γ-aminobutyrate, modulating voltage-gated ion channels, inhibiting excitatory glutamate receptors, and inhibiting carbonic anhydrase. A controlled-release formulation of phentermine-topiramate in doses of 3.75/23, 7.5/46, and 15/92 mg is approved for the treatment of obesity. The dosage should begin at the low dose for 14 days and be escalated to the mid-dose. If a 3% weight loss is not achieved on the mid-dose of the medication by 12 weeks, the medication should be discontinued or increased to the high dose. If a 5% weight loss is not achieved after 12 weeks on the high dose, the medications should be discontinued. Discontinuation should be preceded by taking a dose every other day for a week to avoid seizures. Weight loss was 3.5, 6.2, and 9.3% greater than placebo in the low, mid, and high doses, respectively.[79,80] The glycohemoglobin in diabetic subjects was reduced 0.3% more than placebo in the mid- and high-dose groups. There are warnings for this combination drug because of the potential for fetal toxicity (cleft lip and cleft palate), elevations in heart rate, suicidal ideation, acute glaucoma, mood and sleep disorders, cognitive impairment, metabolic acidosis, kidney stones, and seizures on rapid discontinuation. Patients treated with this combination should have a baseline chemistry profile to include bicarbonate, creatinine, potassium, and glucose repeated periodically during treatment in addition to ensuring adequate contraception. Adverse events occurring in >5% of patients include paraesthesias, dizziness, dysguesia, insomnia, constipation, and dry mouth.[81]

Obesity Drugs in Late Development

Two obesity drugs were submitted as new applications to the FDA in December 2013: liraglutide and bupropion-naltrexone.

Liraglutide. Liraglutide is a glucagon-like peptide-1 agonist approved at the 1.8 mg dose for the treatment of diabetes. A 3 mg dose given daily has been evaluated for the treatment of obesity. Liraglutide 3 mg/day gave a 5.8 kg greater weight loss than placebo at 1 year. Liraglutide 2.4–3 mg/day at 2 years reduced the prevalence of prediabetes and metabolic syndrome by 52 and 59%, respectively.[82] The common side effects included nausea and vomiting that was mild to moderate and transient. Present warnings on liraglutide include a notation of increased pancreatitis and increased thyroid C-cell tumors in rodents without an established risk in humans.[83]

Bupropion-Naltrexone. Bupropion stimulates pro-opiomelanocortin (POMC) neurons to release α-melanocyte stimulating hormone (MSH), which increases metabolic rate and decreases food intake. Naltrexone blocks a μ-opioid receptor on POMC neurons, which otherwise would act as a brake on MSH secretion. Bupropion has an indication for the treatment of depression and smoking cessation. Naltrexone has an indication for the treatment of alcohol and opioid addiction. As one might expect from a combination of two drugs to treat addictions, it has an effect on suppressing food cravings. Bupropion-Naltrexone, both in a sustained-release formulation, come in two dosage forms, 360/32 and 360/16 mg/day given in divided doses twice a day, which give weight losses in excess of placebo at 1 year of 4.8 and 3.7% respectively.[84] Bupropion/naltrexone 360/32 mg/day reduced glycohemoglobin 0.5% more than placebo in diabetic individuals.[85] Bupropion carries warnings about increased suicidal ideation common to all depression drugs, seizure risk, increased blood pressure, and neuropsychiatric reactions.[86] The combination was generally well tolerated. Most frequent side effects were consistent with the known side effects of the two component medications and included nausea, constipation, and vomiting. The nausea and vomiting were usually mild to moderate and resolved with continued use of the medication.

Surgical Treatment of Obesity

Three forms of obesity surgery commonly are employed: laparoscopic gastric banding (lap-band), the Roux-en-Y gastric bypass (bypass), and laparoscopic sleeve gastrectomy (sleeve). Each of these surgeries will be briefly reviewed.

Laparoscopic Gastric Banding. The lap-band is the only approved medical device for the treatment of obesity in the U.S. (Figure 17.1). Lap-band is indicated for the treatment of obesity with a BMI >35 kg/m² and for a BMI >30 kg/m² with at least one obesity-related medical problem. The operation is attractive because it does not permanently alter the anatomy of the gastrointestinal tract, but it requires extensive follow-up to properly adjust the band. The lap-band has been most successful in Australia, where medical physicians do the band adjustment. In the U.S., the adjustment follow-up is more challenging because adjustments typically are left to the surgeons, who prefer to spend their time in the operating room. Ten-year follow-up of gastric banding shows a maximal weight loss of ~20% at 1–2 years with maintenance of a 15% weight loss at 10 years.[87] Remission of diabetes is ~50% compared with 85% for the sleeve and bypass.[88] Reoperation rates for the lap-band are greater than for the gastric bypass (14 vs. 16%).[89] The popularity of the lap-band has been decreasing in recent years in the U.S. because of inferior weight loss, more complex follow-up, a lower remission of diabetes, and a greater need for reoperation from band-related complications.

Gastric Bypass. The gastric bypass has been considered the gold-standard obesity operation (Figure 17.2). It gives a 35% weight loss at 1–2 years and maintains a 30% weight loss at 10 years.[87] This surgery alters the normal anatomy more than

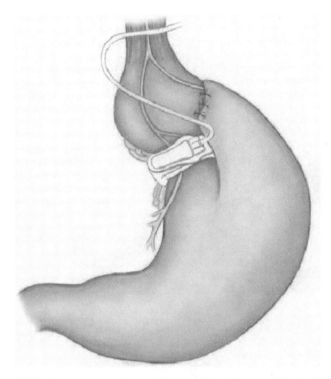

Figure 17.1—Laparoscopic gastric banding. *Source:* Runkel N, et al. Bariatric surgery. *Dtsch Arztebl Int* 2011;108(20);341–346. Reprinted with permission from the publisher.

the other two operations, has a higher mortality and rate of operative complications, and creates more severe metabolic abnormalities than lap-bands or the sleeve. As with all obesity operations, however, the mortality rate is <1%. Remission of diabetes is ~85%.[88] Metabolically, the gastric bypass is associated with a need for protein, iron, and vitamin supplementation as well as a need for calcium and vitamin D to maintain bone health.[90]

Sleeve Gastrectomy. Sleeve gastrectomy is the newest of the three bariatric procedures (Figure 17.3), but now data are available for >5 years of follow-up. Sleeve gastrectomy is gaining rapidly in popularity because of similar weight loss and a similar remission in T2D to that seen with the gastric bypass at a lower cost.[91,92] The metabolic complications are less than the gastric bypass, but vitamin supplementation and monitoring of iron calcium and vitamin D for bone health still are recommended. The operation is likely to continue to grow in popularity, because compared with the gastric bypass, it is less complex to perform, has a lower mortality rate, and has a lower rate of complications.[90]

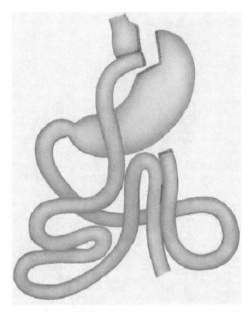

Figure 17.2—Laparoscopic Roux-en-Y gastric bypass. *Source:* Runkel N, et al. Bariatric surgery. *Dtsch Arztebl Int* 2011;108(20);341–346. Reprinted with permission from the publisher.

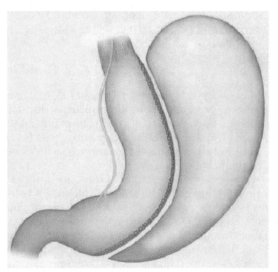

Figure 17.3—Laparoscopic gastric banding. *Source:* Runkel N, et al. Bariatric surgery. *Dtsch Arztebl Int* 2011;108(20);341–346. Reprinted with permission from the publisher.

CONCLUSION

Diabetes and metabolic syndrome are complex conditions that involve the treatment of multiple associated risk factors. Lifestyle modification can help to manage or prevent these conditions. The evidence briefly reviewed in this chapter demonstrates the efficacy of modifying diet and increasing physical activity to reduce diabetes, prevent diabetes, and treat metabolic syndrome and associated risk factors, primarily through weight reduction. Diet and physical activity changes to lose weight and sustain weight loss are essential. One of the main challenges is long-term maintenance of lifestyle changes because only long-term changes can result in positive benefits. The reality is that these lifestyle changes may not be implemented, leading to other strategies to lose weight and improve health status, namely drugs and, in more difficult cases, weight-loss surgery. Physicians and health care professionals need to prioritize lifestyle change strategies as part of their medical practice but also realize that further interventions may well be needed.

REFERENCES

1. Jensen MD, Ryan DH, Apovian CM, Loria CM, Ard JD, Millen BE, Comuzzie AG, Nonas CA, Donato KA, Pi-Sunyer FX, Hu FB, Stevens J, Hubbard VS, Stevens VJ, Jakicic JM, Wadden TA, Kushner RF, Wolfe BM, Yanovski SZ. 2013 AHA/ACC/TOS guideline for the management of overweight and obesity in adults: a report of the American College of Cardiology/American Heart Association Task Force on Practice Guidelines and The Obesity Society. *J Am Coll Cardiol.* 2013 Nov 7;pii: S0735-1097(13)06030-0.

2. Flegal KM, Carroll DM, Kit BK, Ogden CL. Prevalence of obesity and trends in the distribution of body mass index among US adults. 1999–2010. *JAMA* 2012;307:491–497.

3. Ogden CL, Carroll MD, Curtin LR, Lamb MM, Flegal KM. Prevalence of high body mass index in US children and adults. *JAMA* 2010;303:242–249.

4. Thomas DM, Weedermann M, Fuemmeler BF, Martin CK, Dhurandhar NV, Bredlau C, Heymsfield SB, Ravussin E, Bouchard C. Dynamic model predicting overweight, obesity, and extreme obesity prevalence trends. *Obesity* 2013 June 26 [Epub ahead of print].

5. Greenway FL and Cefalu WT. Obesity and its treatment in type 2 diabetes. In *Type 2 Diabetes Mellitus: An Evidence-Based Approach to Practical Management.* Feinglos MN, Bethel MA, Eds. Totowa, NJ, Humana Press, 2008, p. 333–350.

6. Finkelstein EA, Trogdon JG, Cohen JW, Dietz W. Annual medical spending attributable to obesity: payer-and service-specific estimates. *Health Aff* 2009;28(5):w822–831.

7. Klein S, Wadden T, Sugerman HJ. AGA technical review on obesity. *Gastroenterology* 2002;123:882–932.

8. Bouchard C. The biological predisposition to obesity: beyond the thrifty genotype scenario. *Int J Obes* 2007;31(9):1337–1339.

9. Galgani J, Ravussin E. Energy metabolism, fuel selection and body weight regulation. *Int J Obes* 2008;32(Suppl 7):S109–119.

10. Bouchard C. Genetics and the metabolic syndrome. *Int J Obes Relat Metab Disord* 1995;19(Suppl 1):S52–59.

11. Liese AD, Mayer-Davis EJ, Haffner SM. Development of the multiple metabolic syndrome: an epidemiologic perspective. *Epidemiol Rev* 1998;20:157–172.

12. Troiano RP, Frongillo EA Jr, Sobal J, Levitsky DA. The relationship between body weight and mortality: a quantitative analysis of combined information from existing studies. *Int J Obes Relat Metab Disord* 1996;20:63–75.

13. Calle EE, Thun MJ, Petrelli JM, Rodriguez C, Heath CW Jr. Body-mass index and mortality in a prospective cohort of U.S. adults. *N Engl J Med* 1999;341:1097–1105.

14. Rosenquist KJ, Pedley A, Massaro JM, Therkelsen KE, Murabito JM, Hoffmann U, Fox CS. Visceral and subcutaneous fat quality and cardiometabolic risk. *JACC Cardiovasc Imaging* 2013;6(7):762–771.

15. Addeman BT, Kutty S, Perkins TG, Soliman AS, Wiens CN, McCurdy CM, Beaton MD, Hegele RA, McKenzie CA. Validation of volumetric and single-slice MRI adipose analysis using a novel fully automated segmentation method. *J Magn Reson Imaging* 2014 Jan 15. doi: 10.1002/jmri.24526. [Epub ahead of print]

16. Britton KA, Massaro JM, Murabito JM, Kreger BE, Hoffmann U, Fox CS. Body fat distribution, incident cardiovascular disease, cancer, and all-cause mortality. *J Am Coll Cardiol* 2013;62(10):921–925.

17. Thomas EL, Parkinson JR, Frost GS, Goldstone AP, Doré CJ, McCarthy JP, Collins AL, Fitzpatrick JA, Durighel G, Taylor-Robinson SD, Bell JD. The missing risk: MRI and MRS phenotyping of abdominal adiposity and ectopic fat. *Obesity* 2012;20(1):76–87.

18. Cusi K. The role of adipose tissue and lipotoxicity in the pathogenesis of type 2 diabetes. *Curr Diab Rep* 2010;10(4):306–315.

19. Borén J, Taskinen MR, Olofsson SO, Levin M. Ectopic lipid storage and insulin resistance: a harmful relationship. *J Intern Med* 2013;274(1):25–40.

20. Henry RR, Chilton R, Garvey WT. New options for the treatment of obesity and type 2 diabetes mellitus (narrative review). *J Diabetes Complications* 2013;27(5):508–518.

21. National Institutes of Health, National Heart, Lung, & Blood Institute. Clinical guidelines on the identification, evaluation, and treatment of over-

weight and obesity in adults—the evidence report. *Obes Res* 1998;6(Suppl 2):51S–209S.

22. Subramanian S, Chait A. Hypertriglyceridemia secondary to obesity and diabetes. *Biochim Biophys Acta*. 2012 May;1821(5):819–825.

23. American Diabetes Association. Standards of medical care in diabetes—2014. *Diabetes Care* 2014;37(Suppl 1):S14–S80.

24. Chobanian AV, Bakris GL, Black HR, Cushman WC, Green LA, Izzo JL Jr, Jones DW, Materson BJ, Oparil S, Wright JT Jr, Roccella EJ; National Heart, Lung, and Blood Institute Joint National Committee on Prevention, Detection, Evaluation, and Treatment of High Blood Pressure; National High Blood Pressure Education Program Coordinating Committee. The seventh report of the Joint National Committee on Prevention, Detection, Evaluation, and Treatment of High Blood Pressure: the JNC 7 report. *JAMA* 2003;289(19):2560–2572. [Erratum in *JAMA* 2003;290(2):197.]

25. Eckel RH, Kahn SE, Ferrannini E, Goldfine AB, Nathan DM, Schwartz MW, Smith RJ, Smith SR; Endocrine Society; American Diabetes Association; European Association for the Study of Diabetes. Obesity and type 2 diabetes: what can be unified and what needs to be individualized? *Diabetes Care* 2011;34(6):1424–1430.

26. Dalle GR, Calugi S, Centis E, Marzocchi R, El Ghoch M, Marchesini G. Lifestyle modification in the management of the metabolic syndrome: achievements and challenges. *Diabetes Metab Syn Obes* 2010;3:373–385.

27. Look AHEAD Research Group. Cardiovascular effects of intensive lifestyle intervention in type 2 diabetes. *N Engl J Med* 2013;369(2):145–154.

28. Pan XR, Li GW, Hu YH, et al. Effects of diet and exercise in preventing NIDDM in people with impaired glucose tolerance. The Da Qing IGT and Diabetes Study. *Diabetes Care* 1997;20:537–544.

29. Tuomilehto J, Lindstrom J, Eriksson JG, et al. Prevention of type 2 diabetes mellitus by changes in lifestyle among subjects with impaired glucose tolerance. *N Engl J Med* 2001;344:1343–1350.

30. Knowler WC, Barrett-Connor E, Fowler SE, et al. Reduction in the incidence of type 2 diabetes with lifestyle intervention or metformin. *N Engl J Med* 2002;346:393–403.

31. Li G, Zhang P, Wang J, et al. The long-term effect of lifestyle interventions to prevent diabetes in the China Da Qing Diabetes Prevention Study: a 20-year follow-up study. *Lancet* 2008;371:1783–1789.

32. Lindstrom J, Ilanne-Parikka P, Peltonen M, et al. Sustained reduction in the incidence of type 2 diabetes by lifestyle intervention: follow-up of the Finnish Diabetes Prevention Study. *Lancet* 2006;368:1673–1679.

33. Ratner R, Goldberg R, Haffner S, et al. Impact of intensive lifestyle and metformin therapy on cardiovascular disease risk factors in the Diabetes Prevention Program. *Diabetes Care* 2005;28:888–894.

34. Diabetes Prevention Program Research Group; Knowler WC, Fowler SE, et al. 10-year follow-up of diabetes incidence and weight loss in the Diabetes Prevention Program Outcomes Study. *Lancet* 2009;374:1677–1686.

35. Look AHEAD Research Group; Wing RR, Bolin P, Brancati FL, Bray GA, Clark JM, Coday M, Crow RS, Curtis JM, Egan CM, Espeland MA, Evans M, Foreyt JP, Ghazarian S, Gregg EW, Harrison B, Hazuda HP, Hill JO, Horton ES, Hubbard VS, Jakicic JM, Jeffery RW, Johnson KC, Kahn SE, Kitabchi AE, Knowler WC, Lewis CE, Maschak-Carey BJ, Montez MG, Murillo A, Nathan DM, Patricio J, Peters A, Pi-Sunyer X, Pownall H, Reboussin D, Regensteiner JG, Rickman AD, Ryan DH, Safford M, Wadden TA, Wagenknecht LE, West DS, Williamson DF, Yanovski SZ. Cardiovascular effects of intensive lifestyle intervention in type 2 diabetes. *N Engl J Med* 2013;369(2):145–154.

36. Perri MG. Effects of behavioral treatment on long-term weight loss: lessons learned from the Look AHEAD Trial. *Obesity* 2014;22(1):3–4.

37. Gregg EW, Chen H, Wagenknecht LE, Clark JM, Delahanty LM, Bantle J, Pownall HJ, Johnson KC, Safford MM, Kitabchi AE, Pi-Sunyer FX, Wing RR, Bertoni AG; for the Look AHEAD Research Group. Association of an intensive lifestyle intervention with remission of type 2 diabetes. *JAMA* 2012;308(23):2489–2496.

38. Dansinger ML, Gleason JA, Griffith JL, Selker HP, Schaefer EJ. Comparison of the Atkins, Ornish, Weight Watchers, and Zone diets for weight loss and heart disease risk reduction: a randomized trial. *JAMA* 2005;293:43–53.

39. Sacks FM, Bray GA, Carey VJ, Smith SR, Ryan DH, Anton SD, McManus K, Champagne CM, Bishop LM, Laranjo N, Leboff MS, Rood JC, de Jonge L, Greenway FL, Loria CM, Obarzanek E, Williamson DA. Comparison of weight-loss diets with different compositions of fat, protein, and carbohydrates. *N Engl J Med* 2009;360:859–873.

40. de Jonge L, Bray GA, Smith SR, Ryan DH, de Souza R, Loria CM, Champagne CM, Williamson D, Sacks FM. Effect of diet composition and weight loss on resting energy expenditure in the POUNDS LOST study. *Obesity* 2012;20(12):2384–2389.

41. Bray GA, Smith SR, DeJonge L, de Souza R, Rood J, Champagne CM, Laranjo N, Carey V, Obarzanek E, Loria CM, Anton SD, Ryan DH, Greenway FL, Williamson D, Sacks FM. Effect of diet composition on energy expenditure during weight loss: the POUNDS LOST study. *Int J Obes* 2012;36(3):448–455.

42. Esposito K, Ciotola M, Giugliano D. Low-carbohydrate diet and coronary heart disease in women. *N Engl J Med* 2007;356:750; author reply 750–752.

43. Stevens VJ, Obarzanek E, Cook NR, et al. Long-term weight loss and changes in blood pressure: results of the Trials of Hypertension Prevention, phase II. *Ann Intern Med* 2001;134:1–11.

44. Wing RR, Tate DF, Gorin AA, Raynor HA, Fava JL. A self-regulation program for maintenance of weight loss. *N Engl J Med* 2006;355:1563–1571.

45. Svetkey LP, Stevens VJ, Brantley PJ, et al. Comparison of strategies for sustaining weight loss: the Weight Loss Maintenance randomized controlled trial. *JAMA* 2008;299:1139–1148.

46. Donnelly JE, Hill JO, Jacobsen DJ, et al. Effects of a 16-month randomized controlled exercise trial on body weight and composition in young, overweight men and women: the Midwest Exercise Trial. *Arch Intern Med* 2003;163:1343–1350.

47. Irwin ML, Yasui Y, Ulrich CM, et al. Effect of exercise on total and intra-abdominal body fat in postmenopausal women: a randomized controlled trial. *JAMA* 2003;289:323–330.

48. Joseph LJ, Prigeon RL, Blumenthal JB, Ryan AS, Goldberg AP. Weight loss and low-intensity exercise for the treatment of metabolic syndrome in obese postmenopausal women. *J Gerontol A Biol Sci Med Sci.* 2011 Sep;66(9):1022–1029.

49. Katzmarzyk PT, Leon AS, Wilmore JH, et al. Targeting the metabolic syndrome with exercise: evidence from the HERITAGE Family Study. *Med Sci Sports Exerc* 2003;35:1703–1709.

50. Lofgren IE, Herron KL, West KL, et al. Weight loss favorably modifies anthropometrics and reverses the metabolic syndrome in premenopausal women. *J Am Coll Nutr* 2005;24:486–493.

51. Appel LJ, Moore TJ, Obarzanek E, Vollmer WM, Svetkey LP, Sacks FM, Bray GA, Vogt TM, Cutler JA, Windhauser MM, Lin PH, Karanja N; for the DASH Collaborative Research Group. A clinical trial of the effects of dietary patterns on blood pressure. *N Engl J Med* 1997;336(16):1117–1124.

52. U.S. News & World Report. Find the best diet for you. Available at http://health.usnews.com/best-diet. Accessed 8 February 2014.

53. Wilson J. Paleo diet ranks last on "best diets" list. Available at www.cnn.com/2014/01/07/health/best-diets-ranked/index.html?hpt=he_c1. Accessed 8 February 2014.

54. Sacks FM, Svetkey LP, Vollmer WM, et al. Effects on blood pressure of reduced dietary sodium and the Dietary Approaches to Stop Hypertension (DASH) diet. DASH-Sodium Collaborative Research Group. *N Engl J Med* 2001;344:3–10.

55. Lien LF, Brown AJ, Ard JD, et al. Effects of PREMIER lifestyle modifications on participants with and without the metabolic syndrome. *Hypertension* 2007;50:609–616.

56. Foster GD, Wyatt HR, Hill JO, et al. A randomized trial of a low-carbohydrate diet for obesity. *N Engl J Med* 2003;348:2082–2090.

57. Nordmann AJ, Nordmann A, Briel M, et al. Effects of low-carbohydrate vs low-fat diets on weight loss and cardiovascular risk factors: a meta-analysis of randomized controlled trials. *Arch Intern Med* 2006;166:285–293.

58. Stern L, Iqbal N, Seshadri P, et al. The effects of low-carbohydrate versus conventional weight loss diets in severely obese adults: one-year follow-up of a randomized trial. *Ann Intern Med* 2004;140:778–785.

59. Garg A, Grundy SM, Unger RH. Comparison of effects of high and low carbohydrate diets on plasma lipoproteins and insulin sensitivity in patients with mild NIDDM. *Diabetes* 1992;41:1278–1285.

60. Abbasi F, McLaughlin T, Lamendola C, et al. High carbohydrate diets, triglyceride-rich lipoproteins, and coronary heart disease risk. *Am J Cardiol* 2000;85:45–48.

61. Obarzanek E, Sacks FM, Vollmer WM, et al. Effects on blood lipids of a blood pressure-lowering diet: the Dietary Approaches to Stop Hypertension (DASH) Trial. *Am J Clin Nutr* 2001;74:80–89.

62. Azadbakht L, Mirmiran P, Esmaillzadeh A, Azizi T, Azizi F. Beneficial effects of a Dietary Approaches to Stop Hypertension eating plan on features of the metabolic syndrome. *Diabetes Care* 2005;28:2823–2831.

63. Anderson JW, Johnstone BM, Cook-Newell ME. Meta-analysis of the effects of soy protein intake on serum lipids. *N Engl J Med* 1995;333:276–282.

64. Esposito K, Marfella R, Ciotola M, et al. Effect of a Mediterranean-style diet on endothelial dysfunction and markers of vascular inflammation in the metabolic syndrome: a randomized trial. *JAMA* 2004;292:1440–1446.

65. Nguyen LT, Davis RB, Kaptchuk TJ, Phillips RS. Use of complementary and alternative medicine and self-rated health status: results from a national survey. *J Gen Intern Med* 2010;26(4):399–404.

66. Barnes PM, Bloom B, Nahin RL. Complementary and alternative medicine use among adults and children: United States, 2007. *Natl Health Stat Report* 2008:1–23.

67. Graf BL, Raskin I, Cefalu WT, Ribnicky DM. Plant-derived therapeutics for the treatment of metabolic syndrome. *Curr Opin Investig Drugs* 2010;11:1107–1115.

68. Stull AJ, Cash KC, Johnson WD, Champagne CM, Cefalu WT. Bioactives in blueberries improve insulin sensitivity in obese, insulin-resistant men and women. *J Nutr* 2010;140:1764–1768.

69. Bell RA, Quandt SA, Grzywacz JG, Neiberg R, Altizer KP, Lang W, Arcury TA. Patterns of complementary therapy use for symptom management for older rural adults with diabetes. *J Evidence-Based Complementary Alternative Med* 2013;18(2):93–99.

70. National Institutes of Health, Consensus Development Conference Statement. Health implications of obesity. *Ann Intern Med* 1985;103(1):147–151.

71. Munro JF, MacCuish AC, Wilson EM, Duncan LJP. Comparison of continuous and intermittent anorectic therapy in obesity. *BMJ* 1968;1:352–356.

72. Li Z, Magilone M, Tu W, Mojica W, Arterburn D, Shugarman LR, Hilton L, Suttorp M, Solomon V, Shekelle PG, Morton SC. Meta-analysis: pharmacologic treatment of obesity. *Ann Intern Med* 2005;142(7):532–546.

73. Shi YF, Pan CY, Hill J, Gao Y. Orlistat in the treatment of overweight or obese Chinese patients with newly diagnosed type 2 diabetes. *Diabet Med* 2005;22(12):1737–1743.

74. Torgerson JS, Hauptman J, Boldrin MN, Sjostrom L. Xenical in the prevention of diabetes in obese subjects (XENDOS) study: a randomized study of orlistat as an adjunct to lifestyle changes for the prevention of type 2 diabetes in obese patients. *Diabetes Care* 2004;27(1):155–161.

75. Xenical (orlistat) capsule. Available at http://dailymed.nlm.nih.gov/dailymed/lookup.cfm?setid=5bbdc95b-82a1-4ba5-8185-6504ff68cc06. Accessed 9 February 2014.

76. Weintraub M, Sundaresan PR, Madan M, Schuster B, Balder A, Lasagna L, Cox C. Long-term weight control study. I (Weeks 0 to 34). The enhancement of behavior modification, caloric restriction, and exercise by fenfluramine plus phentermine versus placebo. *Clin Pharmacol Ther* 1992; 51(5):586–594.

77. Smith SR, Weissman NJ, Anderson CM, Sanchez M, Chuang E, Stubbe S, Bays H, Ahanahan WR. Behavioral modification and lorcaserin for overweight and obesity management (BLOOM) study group. *N Engl J Med* 2010;363(3):245–256.

78. Belviq prescribing information. Available at www.belviq.com/pdf/Belviq_Prescribing_information.pdf. Accessed 9 February 2014.

79. Gadde KM, Allison DB, Ryan DH, Peterson CA, Troupin B, Schwiers ML, Day WW. Effects of low-dose, controlled-release phentermine plus topiramate combination on weight and associated comorbidities in overweight and obese adults (CONQUER): a randomized, placebo-controlled, phase 3 trial. *Lancet* 2011;377(9774):1341–1352.

80. Allison DB, Gadde KM, Garvey WT, Peterson CA, Schwiers ML, Najarian T, Tam PY, Troupin B, Day WW. Controlled-release phentermine/topiramate in severely obese adults: a randomized controlled trial (EQUIP). *Obesity* 2012;20(2):330–342.

81. Qsymia prescribing information. Available at www.qsymia.com/pdf/prescribing-information.pdf. Accessed 9 February 2014.

82. Astrup A, Carraro R, Finer N, Harper A, Kunesova M, Lean ME, Niskanen L, Rasmussen MF, Rissanen A, Rossner S, Savolainen MJ, Van Gaal L; NN8022-1807 investigators. Safety, tolerability and sustained weight loss over 2 years with the once-daily human GLP-1 analog, liraglutide. *Int J Obes* 2012;36(6):843–854.

83. Victoza (liraglutide) prescribing information. Available at www.accessdata. fda.gov/drugsatfda_docs/label/2010/022341lbl.pdf. Accessed 9 February 2014.

84. Greenway FL, Fujioka K, Plodkowski RA, Mudaliar S, Guttadauria M, Erickson J, Kim DD, Dunayevich E; COR-1 study group. Effect of naltrexone plus bupropion on weight loss in overweight and obese adults (COR-1): a multicenter, randomized, double-blind, placebo-controlled, phase 3 trials. *Lancet* 2010;376(9741):595–605.

85. Hollander P, Gupta AK, Plodkowski R, Greenway F, Bays H, Burns C, Klassen P, Fujioka K; COR-Diabetes study group. Effects of naltrexone sustained-release/bupropion combination therapy on body weight and glycemic parameters in overweight and obese patients with type 2 diabetes. *Diabetes Care* 2013;36(12):4022–4029.

86. Wellbutrin (bupropion hydrochloride) prescribing information. Available at http://us.gsk.com/products/assets/us_wellbutrin_tablets.pdf. Accessed 9 February 2014.

87. Sjostrom L, Marbro K, Sjostrom D et al. Effects of bariatric surgery on mortality in Swedish obese subjects. *N Engl J Med* 2007;357(8):741–752.

88. Runkel, N, Colombo-Berkmann M, Huttl TP, Tigges H, Mann O, Sauerland S. Bariatric surgery. *Dtsch Arxtebl Int* 2011;108(20):341–346.

89. Tice JA, Karliner L, Walsh L, Petersen AJ, Feldman MD. Gastric banding or bypass? A systematic review comparing the two most popular bariatric procedures. *Am J Med* 2008;121(10):885–893.

90. Heber D, Greenway FL, Kaplan LM, Livingston E, Salvador J, Still C; Endocrine Society. Endocrine and nutritional management of the post-bariatric surgery patient: an Endocrine Society Clinical Practice Guideline. *J Clin Endocrinol Metab* 2010;95(11):4823–4843.

91. Peterli R, Borbely Y, Kern B, Gass M, Peters T, Thurnheer M, Schultes B, Laederach K, Bueter M, Schiesser M. Early results of the Swiss Multicenter Bypass or Sleeve Study (SM-BOSS): a prospective randomized trial comparing laparoscopic sleeve gastrectomy and Roux-en-Y gastric bypass. *Ann Surg* 2013;258(5):690–694.

92. Jimenez A, Cassamitjana R, Flores L, Viaplana J, Corcelles R, Lacy A, Vidal J. Long-term effects of sleeve gastrectomy and Roux-en-Y gastric bypass surgery on type 2 diabetes mellitus in morbidly obese subjects. *Ann Surg* 2012;256(6):1023–1029.

Chapter 18
Obesity and Type 2 Diabetes in Children

Michelle Y. Rivera-Vega, MD
Ingrid Libman, MD, PhD
Silva Arslanian, MD

INTRODUCTION

Over the past few decades the trajectory of childhood obesity has resulted in escalating rates of type 2 diabetes (T2D) in youth. Obesity, in particular abdominal adiposity, is associated strongly with insulin resistance in children. The insulin resistance is compensated by increased insulin secretion from a healthy pancreatic β-cell, resulting in the hyperinsulinemia frequently observed in obese people. In individuals at risk for T2D, there is impairment in this compensatory response secondary to a failing β-cell, resulting initially in impaired glucose tolerance (IGT) or prediabetes, which ultimately may progress to T2D, if left without intervention. T2D, whether in adults or children, is the byproduct of genetic, environmental, social, cultural, and lifestyle factors resulting in obesity and its comorbidities.

Results from the 2007–2008 National Health and Nutrition Examination Survey (NHANES) indicate that ~16.9% of children and adolescents age 2–19 years are obese, which is defined as having a gender-specific BMI for age ≥95th percentile.[1] Data from 2010, however, demonstrated a slight decrease to 14.9%.[1] The distribution by age-group is as follows: 10.4% of 2- to 5-year-olds, 19.6% of 6- to 11-year-olds, and 18.1% of 12- to 19-years-olds.[2] Racial and ethnic disparities in obesity prevalence among U.S. children and adolescents are quite significant. In 2007–2008, the prevalence of obesity was higher among Mexican American adolescent boys (26.8%) than among non-Hispanic white adolescent boys (16.7%) and also among non-Hispanic black adolescent girls (29.2%) than among non-Hispanic white adolescent girls (14.5%).[2]

Studies from the two previous decades indicated that depending on location, 8–45% of new pediatric cases of diabetes have T2D.[3] The SEARCH for Diabetes in Youth study, a multiethnic, population-based study, estimated that ~3,700 youth, age <20 years, in the U.S. are diagnosed yearly with T2D, with higher incidence in minority populations.[4] A more recent study using prediction models with an annual increase of 2.3% in the incidence of T2D estimated that by 2010 22,820 youth age <20 years had T2D and that by 2050 this number would quadruple, with Hispanics representing 50% of all youth with T2D.[5] The TODAY (Treatment Options for Type 2 Diabetes in Adolescents and Youth) study revealed that 31.5% of youth in the study were non-Hispanic blacks, 41.1% were Hispanics, 19.6% were non-Hispanic whites, 6.1% were American Indians, and 1.7% were Asians.[6]

DOI: 10.2337/9781580405096.18

DEFINITION

T2D (formerly known as non–insulin-dependent diabetes mellitus or adult-onset diabetes) is a metabolic disorder characterized by hyperglycemia with varying degrees of insulin resistance and relative insulin deficiency. This is in contrast to type 1 diabetes (T1D), in which there is an absolute insulin deficiency due in most cases to an autoimmune-mediated destruction of the islet cells.[7] Obesity is the hallmark of T2D, with up to 85% of affected children in North America being overweight or obese at diagnosis.

PATHOPHYSIOLOGY OF TYPE 2 DIABETES IN YOUTH

The coupling between insulin action or sensitivity and insulin secretion is a key factor regulating the maintenance of normal glucose homeostasis. As mentioned, to maintain glucose tolerance, a decrease in insulin sensitivity is compensated by an increase in insulin secretion. Both insulin resistance (hepatic and peripheral) and insulin deficiency are the key components in the pathogenesis of T2D. Recent studies demonstrate that the disposition index (DI), a measure of β-cell function relative to insulin sensitivity, is highest among children with normal glucose tolerance, lower among those with IGT, and lowest in those with T2D.[8] In obese adolescents, alterations in β-cell function appear to manifest even in the presence of normal glucose tolerance. As demonstrated by our group, the impairment in β-cell function relative to insulin sensitivity, the DI, is apparent even within the nondiabetic fasting plasma glucose range[9] and within the normal glucose tolerance range during an oral glucose tolerance test (OGTT).[10] Furthermore, in obese youth with impaired fasting glucose (IFG) or IGT, first-phase insulin secretion is impaired around 40–50% while in youth with T2D it is ~75% impaired.[11,12] This impairment in β-cell function also is evident in the prediabetes A1C category of 5.7 to <6.5%.[13] Youth with T2D also have hepatic and peripheral insulin resistance, with ~50% lower *in vivo* insulin sensitivity compared with equally obese peers without diabetes. When the impairment in β-cell function is expressed relative to the degree of insulin resistance, there is an ~85% deficiency in β-cell function relative to insulin sensitivity in youth with T2D of short duration.[14] Moreover, our data and TODAY data demonstrate that there is on average ~20–35% decline per year in β-cell function in youth with T2D, portending the need for early institution of insulin therapy.[15,16]

RISK FACTORS FOR TYPE 2 DIABETES

OBESITY

Obesity, through its association with impaired insulin action or insulin resistance, is a major risk factor for T2D in youth.[17] Besides total body adiposity, abdominal fat distribution and ectopic fat are major correlates of insulin resistance in childhood. Among obese youth pair-matched for age, pubertal stage, BMI, and total body fat, those with severe insulin resistance had higher visceral fat and waist-to-hip ratio and lower high-density lipoprotein (HDL) than those with lesser degrees of insulin resistance. More important, the former group had a lower DI, indicative of a heightened risk for T2D manifested in impaired β-cell insulin secretion relative to insulin sensitivity.[18] Moreover, in youth with IGT, intramyocellular and intra-abdominal lipid accumulation is linked closely to the development of severe peripheral insulin resistance.[19] Recent cross-sectional studies demonstrated an association between high hepatic fat content and impaired glucose metabolism and metabolic syndrome in obese youth.[20]

GENETIC SUSCEPTIBILITY

The cross-talk between β-cell insulin secretion and insulin sensitivity, although still not well characterized, is dependent on multiple factors, including genetics and environment. There is definite evidence that genes play a role in the development of T2D. Most youth with T2D regardless of ethnic background have a first- or second-degree relative with T2D. Our studies demonstrate that the genetic heritability of T2D manifests metabolically in the first decade of life by impaired insulin sensitivity and β-cell function relative to insulin sensitivity in healthy youth with a family history of T2D compared with those without a family history of diabetes.[14] This metabolically evident genetic susceptibility when combined with environmental factors conducive to obesity and a sedentary lifestyle ultimately may translate to T2D. Indeed, adults who have one parent with T2D have ~30–40% lifetime risk of developing diabetes, and those who have both parents with T2D have a 70% risk.[21] Moreover, risk of developing T2D is two- to fourfold increased in an individual who has a sibling with T2D compared with the normal population. A genome-wide associated study in adults identified >64 genetic variants associated with T2D and 53 genetic variants associated with glycemic traits of fasting glucose, fasting insulin, and 2-hour OGTT glucose concentration.[22] However, the pathophysiologic role of these variants remains unknown. Genetic data are lacking in pediatric T2D.

ETHNICITY

In the U.S., minority ethnic populations, including African Americans, Native Americans, Pima Indians, Pacific Islanders, and Hispanics, represent the group with the highest incidence of pediatric T2D. Pima Indian adolescents have the highest prevalence rate of 50.9 per 1,000.[23] SEARCH incidence data, per 100,000 person-years, show the highest incidence of 49.4 in 15- to 19-year-old American Indians, followed by Asian/Pacific Islanders of 22.7, followed by African Americans of 19.4, and Hispanics of 17.[4] The SEARCH data from 2002 revealed the highest prevalence rate in American Indians (1.74 per 1,000 youth) followed by African Americans (1.05 per 1,000 youth), and lowest in non-Hispanic whites (0.12 per 1,000 youth).[24] New prediction models, however, revealed that by 2010 the prevalence of T2D was highest in non-Hispanic blacks (0.63 per 1,000 youth) followed by American Indians (0.50 per 1,000 youth), and was lowest among non-Hispanic whites (0.11 per 1,000 youth) and that such differences will persist by the year 2050. The most widely accepted explanation for the heightened risk of T2D in minority populations is lower insulin sensitivity compared with their white peers.[14,25]

INTRAUTERINE EXPOSURE

Intrauterine exposure to hyperglycemia predisposes the fetus to T2D later in life. This relationship was first described in the Pima Indians when offspring of women who had diabetes during pregnancy were more obese and had a higher prevalence of T2D during childhood.[26] Other studies show that teenage offspring of mothers with diabetes compared with offspring of mothers who are normally glucose tolerant have significantly higher BMI, higher 2-hour glucose and insulin concentrations during an OGTT, and higher rates of IGT (~20%).[27] Most recently, the SEARCH study demonstrated that up to 47.2% of children with T2D had a prior exposure to maternal diabetes and obesity in utero.[28]

LIFESTYLE

Our present-day, highly technologically driven society creates an obesogenic environment, characterized by low levels of physical activity and abundant consumption of calorically dense and easily available fast foods and drinks of low nutritional value. This energy surplus is stored as fat, leading to obesity. Lifestyle modification is a primary target for the prevention of obesity and T2D.

INSULIN RESISTANCE PHENOTYPE

Puberty, polycystic ovary syndrome (PCOS), metabolic syndrome, and acanthosis nigricans are all linked to insulin resistance in childhood.[17] Childhood T2D typically manifests at midpuberty. Insulin sensitivity is ~30% lower in pubertal adolescents compared with prepubertal children.[29] It is likely that insulin resistance during adolescence may precipitate the imbalance between insulin action and secretion in a child with a predisposition to T2D.

Rates of IGT (30%) and T2D (3.7%) are higher in girls with PCOS,[30] a condition characterized with oligo/anovulation, signs of hyperandrogenism, and laboratory evidence of hyperandrogenemia. Insulin resistance is an integral component of the syndrome and is present in overweight and normal-weight women with PCOS. Data from our group demonstrate that obese adolescents with PCOS have 50% lower in vivo insulin sensitivity compared with equally obese control girls of similar body composition and abdominal adiposity.[31] Moreover, PCOS adolescents with IGT compared with normal glucose tolerance have decreased first-phase insulin secretion, 50% impairment in β-cell function relative to insulin sensitivity, and increased hepatic glucose production, all metabolic precursors of T2D.[32]

Acanthosis nigricans has been associated with hyperinsulinemia, insulin resistance, and higher BMI, suggesting that acanthosis nigricans may be a harbinger of the metabolic syndrome in obese children.[33] TODAY data demonstrated that 85.6% of youth diagnosed with T2D had acanthosis nigricans at diagnosis.[6] Therefore, the presence of acanthosis nigricans on examination should raise suspicion for increased risk for T2D.

DIAGNOSIS

The diagnostic criteria for diabetes are the same for children and adults and are based on fasting blood glucose, random blood glucose, and OGTT. Any one of these is diagnostic. Each, however, should be confirmed on a subsequent day by any one of the three mentioned methods (Table 18.1).[34]

Metabolic stages between normal glucose homeostasis and diabetes constitute prediabetes or IGT and IFG. IGT is defined as a plasma glucose value of 140–199 mg/dl during an OGTT. The American Diabetes Association (ADA) defines IFG as a fasting glucose value of 100–125 mg/dl.[34] The International Diabetes Federation and the World Health Organization (WHO) use 110 mg/dl as the cutoff.[35]

Recently, the ADA endorsed the use of A1C as a screening test. An A1C level ≥6.5% (on two occasions) is used to diagnose diabetes in adults, and the same diagnostic criteria are being used for pediatric patients. However, these recommendations were based on studies in adults, and a subsequent report concluded that a single measurement of A1C ≥6.5% had high specificity (99%) but only 75% sensitivity for detecting diabetes mellitus in the pediatric population.[36] In a multiethnic cohort of obese children and adolescents without diabetes, OGTT and A1C measurements were compared as a diagnostic tool. According to OGTT criteria, 62% were identified as T2D versus 1% with A1C ≥6.5%.[37]

Even though the hallmark of youth with T2D is obesity, the escalating rates of obesity in youth with T1D are making the clinical diagnosis of T2D and the distinction between obese T1D and the former difficult.[38] Therefore, analysis of pancreatic autoantibodies may be necessary in some cases when the clinical picture is not clear.

SCREENING FOR TYPE 2 DIABETES IN YOUTH

An estimated ~25% of adults with diabetes are undiagnosed.[39] It is not known if this is similar in children. There is evidence that at the time of diagnosis of T2D

Table 18.1 ADA Criteria for Diagnosis of Prediabetes and Type 2 Diabetes

	Prediabetes	Diabetes
FPG*	100–125 mg/dl 5.6–6.9 mmol/l	≥126 mg/dl ≥7.0 mmol/l
OGTT* after 75 g glucose load	140–199 mg/dl 7.8–11 mmol/l	≥200 mg/dl ≥11.1 mmol/l
A1C**	5.7–6.4 %	≥6.5%

Note: FPG = fasting plasma glucose; OGTT = oral glucose tolerance test.
*FPG and OGTT guidelines for gestational diabetes mellitus (GDM) are different.
**A1C does not apply to the diagnosis of T1D or GDM.
Source: American Diabetes Association. Revisions to the standards of medical care in diabetes—2014. *Diabetes Care* 2014;37(Suppl 1):S14–S80.

in youth, there is an increased incidence of comorbidities, for which the ADA recommends screening such as blood pressure measurements, fasting lipid profile, albuminuria assessment, and dilated eye exam at the time of diagnosis.[7] Therefore, the ADA has developed guidelines for T2D screening in youth who are overweight and who have two or more risk factors for diabetes (Table 18.2). For children who do not fully meet the screening criteria, clinical judgment should be exercised. Furthermore, the ADA recommends using fasting plasma glucose, 2-hour plasma glucose after OGTT, or A1C as the screening test, whereas the WHO recommends an OGTT as the screening tool. Recent studies compared the cost-effectiveness of these methods, and despite higher cost for the 2-hour OGTT, it had the highest effectiveness in diagnosing diabetes versus A1C.[40] The ADA recommends screening children every 3 years beginning at 10 years of age or at onset of puberty if they are overweight or obese (BMI >85th percentile) and have two or more risk factors.[34]

CLINICAL PRESENTATION

The clinical presentation of youth with T2D is a wide spectrum from minimal symptomatology to severe symptoms. Some youth are diagnosed incidentally during a routine medical checkup when they are found to have glycosuria against the backdrop of obesity and a strong family history of T2D. Others present with polyuria, polydipsia with or without weight loss, blurry vision, and monilial vaginitis in females, with or without severe hyperglycemia. Up to 13% of youth with T2D present in diabetic ketoacidosis (DKA)[41] and some patients may present with hyperglycemic-hyperosmolar nonketotic syndrome (HHNK).[42] HHNK syndrome is a life-threatening condition with reported case-fatality of 37%.[42]

The presence of DKA in an obese child complicates the distinction between T2D and autoimmune T1D in an obese child. With the escalating rates of obesity

Table 18.2 Screening for Youth Type 2 Diabetes

Overweight status
   BMI >85th percentile for age and gender
   Weight for height >85th percentile
   Weight >120% of ideal for height

Plus any two of the following risk factors
   Family history of T2D in a first- or second-degree relative
   High-risk race/ethnicity (Native American, African American, Latino, Asian American, Pacific Islander)
   Signs of insulin resistance on physical exam or conditions associated with insulin resistance
   Maternal history of diabetes or gestational diabetes during the child's gestation

Source: American Diabetes Association. Standards of medical care in diabetes—2013. *Diabetes Care* 2013;36(Suppl 1):S11–S66.

in the general population, children with autoimmune T1D also are becoming obese.[43] The overlap in the clinical presentation between obese adolescents with T2D and obese youths with autoimmune T1D makes the clinical distinction difficult. Up to 33% of youth with T2D have ketonuria at diagnosis, and 5–25% present with DKA.[2,44] DKA also may occur during acute intercurrent illness and should not be used as a criterion on which to base the diagnosis of T1D versus T2D.[45] Furthermore, not infrequently, adolescents who are clinically diagnosed with T2D have evidence of islet cell autoimmunity,[46] which has been reported to be as high as 32% for two antibodies.[47] In the TODAY study, 9.7% of youth clinically diagnosed with T2D had positive autoantibodies (glutamic decarboxyl-ase-65 and tyrosine phosphatase autoantibodies)[6] diagnostic of autoimmune T1D. Our studies demonstrate that obese youth clinically diagnosed with T2D who have evidence of islet cell autoimmunity have severe insulin deficiency and β-cell failure compared with youth with T2D and negative islet cell autoantibodies.[9,15,48] Additionally, the former group is not as insulin resistant as the latter; supporting the notion that T2D is characterized by an inherent genetic–epigenetic insulin resistance that is not present in obese youth with autoimmune T1D.[48] Therefore, the absence of diabetes autoimmune markers should be a prerequisite for the diagnosis of T2D in obese children and adolescents.[3]

ACUTE COMPLICATIONS

Acute complications in adolescents with T2D include DKA and less frequently HHNK syndrome. The latter is characterized by blood glucose >600 mg/dl and serum osmolality >330 mOsm/l, mild acidosis (bicarbonate >15 mmol/l), and mild ketonuria (<15 mg/dl).[42] No prospective data are available to guide the treatment of children and adolescents with HHNK; nonetheless, experience from adult data indicates that all patients with HHNK should be admitted to an intensive care unit.[49] The management includes fluid resuscitation until peripheral perfusion is restored along with electrolyte replacement and correction. Insulin therapy should be considered when serum glucose is no longer declining (<50mg/dl/hour) with fluid administration alone.[49]

CHRONIC COMPLICATIONS

Youth with T2D routinely are seen in clinic three to four times a year. Education provided by the physicians, diabetes educators, nurses, and dietitians remains important in subsequent visits. Besides an emphasis on lifestyle modifications, glucose homeostasis, and social and behavior evaluation, physicians should screen for complications. Children and adolescents with T2D are at risk for comorbid conditions, including hypertension, dyslipidemia, nephropathy, subclinical evidence of cardiovascular disease (CVD), and nonalcoholic fatty liver disease (NAFLD). These disorders may present before the diagnosis of T2D and, like T2D, they are associated with excessive weight gain.

HYPERTENSION

Primary hypertension was once uncommon in the pediatric population, but with increasing prevalence of obesity, it has become the most common cause of hypertension in adolescents.[50] In the SEARCH data, 17–32% of patients had hypertension at the time of diagnosis with T2D.[50] The TODAY data show that of the 699 randomized cohort between 10 and 17 years of age, 11.6% were hypertensive at baseline and 33.8% were hypertensive by the end of the study after an average follow-up of 3.9 years.[51] Regardless of treatment, the prevalence of hypertension increased over time in TODAY, with the greatest risk factors being male gender and higher BMI, the latter pointing to the critical role that obesity plays.[51] For the proper monitoring and early detection of hypertension in youth with T2D, blood pressure should be measured at each health care visit. The diagnosis of prehypertension or hypertension is based on blood pressure obtained on three separate occasions, as defined by the National High Blood Pressure Education Group, and evaluation is based on height, sex, and age-specific percentile tables.[52] A systolic or diastolic blood pressure between the 90th and 95th percentile is considered as prehypertension. A systolic or diastolic blood pressure ≥95th percentile is stage 1 hypertension. Stage 2 hypertension is classified when systolic or diastolic blood pressure is >95th percentile plus 5 mmHg. The goal for blood pressure control is for both systolic and diastolic blood pressure to be <90th percentile.[52]

For children with diabetes and prehypertension, nonpharmacologic treatment is indicated, consisting of diet, salt restriction, exercise, and weight reduction. If prehypertension is not responsive to these measures within 3–6 months, pharmacologic therapy should be initiated.[7] Angiotensin-converting enzyme (ACE) inhibitors are first-line therapy, as they have been shown in adults to reduce the risk for renal disease.[7] Other options include angiotensin II receptor blockers (ARBs), calcium channel blockers, and diuretics, but their use is based on adult data. Therapy should be initiated at the lowest recommended dose and increased until the goal of blood pressure <90th percentile. Serum creatinine and potassium should be checked monthly during the first 2–3 months as ACE inhibitors and ARBs can cause hyperkalemia. ACE inhibitors are teratogenic, and therefore patients should be counseled on contraception while on therapy.[53] In patients with stage 2 hypertension, referral to a specialist with expertise in pediatric hypertension should be considered.

DYSLIPIDEMIA

Various studies in different populations reveal high rates of dyslipidemia in youth with T2D. The SEARCH data show 22% hypercholesterolemia and 29% hypertriglyceridemia rates. Data from Australia demonstrate 32 and 53%, respectively, and the Canadian First Nations' children data demonstrate 75 and 65%, respectively.[54,55,56] These rates are significantly higher in youth with T2D compared with T1D.[55] The TODAY study, consistent with prior reports, revealed that by the time of diagnosis, 16.7% of youth with T2D had low HDL, 21% had high triglycerides (TGs), and only 71.9% had optimal LDL concentrations.[57] This dyslipidemia worsened over time with an increase in LDL, apoB, TGs, and non-HDL cholesterol over 12 months and then stabilized over the following 24 months.[57] Although the treatment group did not affect LDL, apoB, or non-HDL cholesterol, treatment differences were identified in small dense LDL, TGs, and HDL.[57] The genesis of atherosclerosis begins in childhood with autopsy evidence of aortic and coronary atherosclerosis seen before 20 years of age.[58] Because youth with T2D are at a heightened risk for CVD, with dyslipidemia posing a major threat besides diabetes and hypertension, the ADA in association with the American Academy of Pediatrics (APP) developed guidelines for screening and treatment of dyslipidemia in pediatric T2D (Table 18.3). [44,59]

Once metabolic control is established, a fasting lipid profile should be obtained at diagnosis of T2D and should be repeated at least every 2 years. The goal includes LDL cholesterol (LDL-C) <100 mg/dl (2.6 mmol/l), HDL cholesterol (HDL-C) >35 mg/dl (0.9 mmol/l), and TGs <150 mg/dl (1.7 mmol/l). Initial treatment modalities for dyslipidemia include dietary changes, weight reduction, increasing physical activity, and glucose homeostasis. The American Heart Association (AHA) step 2 diet—daily intake of dietary cholesterol <200 mg/day and saturated fat <7% of the total calories—is suggested as an initial lifestyle modification.[59] Follow-up fasting lipid profile should be obtained at 3 months and at 6 months after the beginning of nonpharmacologic therapy. If after 6 months of nonpharmacologic therapy, LDL-C is >160 mg/dl (4.4 mmol/l), or between 130 and 159 mg/dl (3.36 and 4.14 mmol/L) in a patient with risk factors, drug therapy is recommended in children >10 years of age. HMG-CoA reductase inhibitors (statins) are the first-line therapy; main side effects include hepatic and renal dysfunction and renal injury. The ADA recommends that elevated TG >150 mg/dl be managed with maximizing glycemic control and weight reduction. The TODAY data found that TGs were lower in the metformin-plus-lifestyle-treatment groups versus the metformin-only group.[57] In cases of TG >1,000 mg/dl, fibric acid medication is suggested because of increased risk of pancreatitis.

Table 18.3 Management of Dyslipidemia in Youth with Type 2 Diabetes

Goals		
LDL	<100 mg/dl	
HDL	>35 mg/dl	
TG	<150 mg/dl	
Treatment strategies		
LDL	100–129 mg/dl	Maximize non-pharmacological therapy
LDL	130–159 mg/dl	Consider pharmacological therapy based on risk factors (blood pressure, family history, smoking)
LDL	≥160 mg/dl	Start pharmacologic treatment
Pharmacologic therapy		
LDL	≥160 mg/dl	Statins ± resins
TG	>1,000 mg/dl	Fibric acid derivatives

Source: Flint A, Arslanian S. Treatment of type 2 diabetes in youth. *Diabetes Care* 2011;34(Suppl 2):S177–S183.

NONALCOHOLIC FATTY LIVER DISEASE

NAFLD is the most common cause of liver disease in children and is common in children with T2D. Serum alanine aminotransferase is elevated more than twice normal in ~20% of youth with T2D.[60] Abnormalities include hepatic steatosis and nonalcoholic steatohepatitis (NASH). NASH may lead to fibrosis, cirrhosis, and liver failure if untreated. In the TODAY study, youth with liver enzymes >2.5 times the upper limit of normal (ULN) at screening were excluded, but 3.3% of participants had liver enzymes 1.5–2.5 times ULN at baseline.[6] Routine care of children and adolescents with T2D should include abdominal examination for hepatomegaly and monitoring of serum aminotransferase concentrations. Consultation with a gastroenterologist should be considered if hepatic abnormalities persist after weight reduction or if advanced liver disease is present.

MICROVASCULAR COMPLICATIONS

Studies have demonstrated that youth with T2D and poor glycemic control are at increased risk for microvascular complications, including retinopathy, nephropathy, and neuropathy.[61,62]

Retinopathy

Recent data from the SEARCH study estimated a 42% prevalence of diabetic retinopathy in children with T2D with a mean time since diagnosis of 7.2 years versus 17% in patients with T1D.[63] In contrast, the TODAY study revealed a prevalence of 13.7% in youth with T2D with a mean time since diagnosis of 4.9 years.[64] Previous studies in Pima Indians showed that the risk of developing retinopathy was lower in those diagnosed before 20 years of age compared with those diagnosed later in life.[65] Youth with T2D should be screened by direct ophthalmoscopy of dilated fundi by trained personnel at the time of diagnosis and annually.

Nephropathy

Youth with T2D have higher rates of albuminuria >30mg/24 hours as well as increased incidence and progression of nephropathy compared with those with T1D with similar disease duration.[60] Persistent albumin excretion between 30 and 300 mg/day (20–200 mcg/minute) is the first stage of nephropathy. Albumin levels >30mg/24 hours was present in 14–22% of adolescents with T2D.[60] In the SEARCH study, 22% of youth with T2D had albuminuria >30 mg/24 hours,[66] fairly close to the Australian data of 28%.[54] In TODAY, albuminuria >30 mg/24 hours was present in 6.3% of youth at baseline, and increased to 16.6% by the end of the study.[51] Higher levels of A1C were significantly related to risk of developing albuminuria >30 mg/24 hours, with no differences between treatment arms, sex, or race.[51] Among Pima Indians, the incidence of end-stage renal disease is 25 per 1,000 patient-years in youth-onset T2D versus older-onset T2D.[67] Canadian First Nations Children with T2D have a fourfold increased risk of renal failure versus youth with T1D.[68] Against this backdrop of increased risk of nephropathy in adolescents with T2D, the recommendation is to screen annually for albuminuria by measuring the albumin-to-creatinine ratio in random urine sample.[69] Patients with positive results should have repeat screening on at least two occasions during the subsequent 6 months.[7] Treatment includes tight glycemic control, and the use of ACE inhibitors or ARBs.

Neuropathy

Data are limited on the frequency of neuropathy among adolescents with T2D, but adult data suggest that 10–18% have evidence of nerve damage at the time of diagnosis.[61] Data need to be generated in youth with T2D.

MACROVASCULAR COMPLICATIONS

Adolescents with T2D are at increased risk of macrovascular complications, due to the combined effects of long-standing obesity, compounded with diabetes, dyslipidemia, and hypertension. Our early studies demonstrated that youth with T2D have significantly increased pulse-wave velocity, indicative of increased arterial stiffness, compared with obese and normal-weight healthy peers, suggestive of premature aging of the cardiovascular system.[70] Moreover, the SEARCH study demonstrated that youth with T2D had worse arterial stiffness than similar youth with T1D and that increased central adiposity and blood pressure were associated with arterial stiffness, independent of diabetes type.[71]

OTHER COMORBIDITIES

Management of T2D goes beyond the treatment of metabolic abnormalities and the prevention of complications. The SEARCH study found the prevalence of depressed mood to be higher among males with T2D than those with T1D and to be higher among females with comorbidities than those without comorbidities.[72] Health care professionals should be astute in recognizing possible comorbidities, and once identified, appropriate referrals should be made. Because T2D usually is related to obesity, screening for signs of obstructive sleep apnea, with associated pulmonary hypertension, orthopedic problems, pancreatitis, cholecystitis, and pseudotumor cerebri should be made.[69]

TREATMENT

The treatment of youth T2D necessitates a multifaceted approach to alleviate both the insulin resistance and β-cell failure, achieve glycemic control, and prevent acute and chronic complications.[44] This could be achieved only through a diabetes team that includes the patient, family, physician, behavioral specialist, nurse educator, dietitian, and school personnel. This approach should focus on family-based behavioral lifestyle intervention together with pharmacotherapy, with the objectives of weight loss or prevention of continued weight gain, adoption of healthier lifestyle habits, normalization of glycemia, and control of comorbidities such as hypertension, dyslipidemia, nephropathy, and hepatic steatosis.[44,69] Efforts should be geared to individualize therapy in T2D not only based on phenotype and genotype but also based on ethnic or cultural beliefs and traditions.[73] Until recently, and before the TODAY study results were unveiled, few data were available to guide treatment. Most pediatric recommendations were based on studies in adults with T2D.

The TODAY study compared the efficacy of three treatment regimens, metformin alone, metformin plus intensive lifestyle intervention, or metformin plus rosiglitazone, to achieve durable glycemic control in children and adolescents, 10–17 years of age, with recent-onset T2D. Of the 699 randomly assigned participants, 45.6% reached the primary outcome of glycemic failure over an average follow-up of 3.86 years. Rates of glycemic failure were 51.7, 38.6, and 46.6% for metformin alone, metformin plus rosiglitazone, and metformin plus lifestyle intervention, respectively. Metformin plus rosiglitazone was superior to metformin alone; metformin plus lifestyle intervention was intermediate but not significantly different from metformin alone.[16] Because of concerns about cardiovascular and other adverse effects, however, rosiglitazone currently is not being used and is not Food and Drug Administration (FDA)-approved in pediatric T2D.

LIFESTYLE MODIFICATION: NUTRITION AND ACTIVITY

Weight reduction and individualized nutrition therapy is important because all youth in North America with T2D are overweight or obese. In children, the decision on whether to recommend weight reduction or weight maintenance depends on the age of the patient, the degree of obesity, and the presence of secondary comorbidities. Initially, the patient and family should be encouraged to maintain the child's weight, and after successful maintenance, gradual weight loss is recommended, aiming at a BMI <85th percentile. Ideally, care should include guidance by a nutritionist with the elimination of sugar-containing beverages and high-fat, high-calorie foods and the establishment of a regular meal schedule, portion control, and improvement in food choices.[42]

Increased physical activity independent of weight loss carries health benefits. We recently demonstrated in obese adolescents boys that both aerobic and resistance exercise without weight loss are effective in reducing abdominal and intrahepatic fat, and aerobic exercise also was associated with significant improvement in insulin sensitivity.[74] Recommended exercise goals include decreasing sedentary behaviors, such as time spent watching television and using the computer, and increasing energy expenditure through incorporating active daily lifestyle habits, such as using the stairs and walking as a mode of transportation.[44,75] Such lifestyle modifications should be family centered because studies in obese nondiabetic youth show better short- and long-term outcome when the intervention involves both the child and the family.[44,76] Physical activity recommendations should be coordinated among the patient, the family, and the health care team, particularly the behavioral psychologist, and be individualized and specific to the patient's need and abilities.[77]

Despite the overall belief that lifestyle intervention could be beneficial in glycemic control in youth with T2D, the TODAY study revealed that the addition of intensive lifestyle intervention to metformin was not superior to metformin alone in maintaining glycemic durability nor in achieving better weight loss.[16] At 6 months, the proportion of participants with meaningful weight loss in the metformin plus lifestyle intervention group (31.2%) was not significantly different from the metformin-alone group (24.3%).[16] Furthermore, the average change in percent overweight at 24 months was similar between the metformin-plus-lifestyle-intervention group (–5.02 percentage points) and the metformin-alone group (–4.42 percentage points). Additional analyses are being performed to examine the reasons behind these observations.

PHARMACOLOGIC THERAPY OF YOUTH TYPE 2 DIABETES

According to International Society for Pediatric and Adolescent Diabetes (ISPAD) guidelines, pharmacologic therapy in youth with T2D should be initiated in an asymptomatic patient who fails to reach glycemic control 3 months after initiation of lifestyle modifications or in symptomatic patients at presentation.[69] In our practice, we initiate metformin or insulin therapy, depending on the severity of the hyperglycemia, at the time of diagnosis along with lifestyle modifications (Figure 18.1). At the present time, the only agents approved by the FDA for the treatment of T2D in children are metformin and insulin.

Insulin should be used in patients who present with severe hyperglycemia (≥200 mg/dl or A1C >8–8.5%) or who are in ketosis or ketoacidosis. Insulin treatment will rapidly reverse the metabolic abnormalities and should be continued until ketosis resolves and plasma glucose returns to near-normal levels. In patients who are able to achieve normoglycemia, insulin can be weaned carefully with close monitoring of home blood glucose meter levels. In adults with newly diagnosed T2D, there is evidence that aggressive reduction of glycemia, particularly with insulin, can result in sustained remission.[78] In pediatrics, short-term use of insulin (<16 weeks) in poorly controlled adolescents with T2D, using premixed 70/30 insulin given twice daily, was associated with significant improvement in A1C without significant changes in BMI or hypoglycemia. This effect lasted for 12

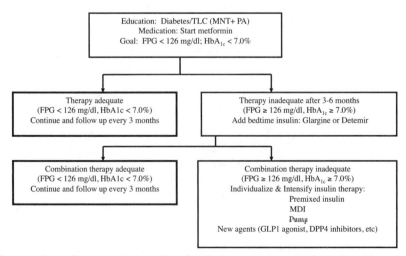

Figure 18.1—Proposed algorithm for the management of youth with T2D.[44]

months after insulin was discontinued without additional medications,[44,79] suggestive of improved β-cell function. Insulin regimens should be individualized based on patient characteristics, family dynamics, and adherence.

Metformin can be started once ketosis resolves. Metformin is a biguanide that mainly improves hepatic insulin resistance and lowers hepatic glucose production and, to a lesser degree, improves peripheral insulin sensitivity. As stated earlier, the only FDA-approved oral treatment for youth with T2D is metformin.[80] In a randomized placebo-controlled trial of metformin in adolescents with new-onset T2D, metformin treatment resulted in a significantly lower A1C after 16 weeks, compared with placebo (7.5% vs. 8.6%).[44,81] In addition, fasting plasma glucose improved by −42.9 mg/dl (−2.4 mmol/l) compared with an increase of +21.4 mg/dl (+1.2 mmol/l) with placebo. Moreover, there were no safety issues or untoward effects of metformin. This study led to the FDA approving metformin in youth with T2D, and both the ADA and ISPAD guidelines recommended metformin as the first-line oral antidiabetic drug.[3,44,69]

The initial dose of metformin is usually 500–1,000 mg/day, to be increased to a maximum of 1,000 mg twice a day in a period of 2–4 weeks. Before starting metformin therapy, we recommend to measure baseline creatinine and liver enzymes, and if the liver enzymes levels are 2.5 times the ULN, metformin should not be initiated or should be initiated with close and frequent monitoring of the liver enzymes. Metformin is contraindicated in patients with impaired renal function, cirrhosis, hepatitis, and lactic acidosis. Patients planning to have elective surgeries or imaging studies with contrast should stop metformin 24 hours before and resume 48 hours after, provided there are no complications.

Despite the short-term beneficial glycemic effects of metformin, the TODAY study showed that over an average follow-up of 3.86 years, more than half the patients on metformin had glycemic failure, defined by either A1C ≥8% for 6 months or by an inability to wean from temporary insulin therapy within 3 months of acute metabolic decompensation.[16] Previous studies also have shown that most youth with T2D are able to maintain A1C for up to ~2 years after diagnosis, following which A1C levels escalate.[36] These observations could be explained by the findings that β-cell function deteriorates rapidly in youth with T2D, on average 20–35% per year, compared with 7–11% in adults.[16] Furthermore, both β-cell function and A1C at randomization were important predictors of glycemic failure in TODAY. For every 0.5% increase in A1C at the time of randomization, the odds ratio increased to 1.83, and for every doubling of β-cell function, the odds ratio decreased to 0.84 (0.74–0.95).[16] These observations point to the importance of early diagnosis, while a still-significant β-cell reserve is left and before far advanced hyperglycemia, for the successful maintenance of glycemic durability with treatment.

Sulfonylureas (glimepiride, glyburide, and glipizide) are insulin secretagogues routinely used in adults, none of which are currently FDA-approved in pediatric T2D. The efficacy of glimepiride in pediatric patients was evaluated in a 26-week multinational clinical trial compared with metformin with no significant difference in A1C reduction between the two groups.[82] Other medications used in the treatment of adult T2D include α-glucosidase inhibitors, dipeptidyl peptidase-IV inhibitors, glucagon-like peptide-1 agonists, amylin analogs, and inhibitors of the selective sodium-glucose transporter-2, none of which are approved or even tested yet in youth, but with promising results in adults.

MEDICAL AND SURGICAL THERAPY OF OBESITY

Pharmacologic therapy for pediatric obesity should be selective under medical supervision and after an adequate trial of lifestyle modifications. Currently, only one medication is approved for weight loss in adolescents. Orlistat is a gastrointestinal lipase inhibitor, which has been shown to reduce body weight over 1 year in adolescents and is approved by the FDA for adolescents >12 years. Potential side effects include fat-soluble vitamin deficiencies, diarrhea, and flatulence. Off-label uses of medications that have been associated with weight loss include metformin, topiramate, and fluoxetine, but they have not been studied in depth and are not recommended until more data become available.

Weight-loss surgery occasionally is used in the treatment of severe obesity in adolescents, improving their metabolic and psychosocial health. A limited study of 11 severely obese adolescents (BMI 50 ± 5.9 kg/m^2) demonstrated a 91% remission of diabetes after 1 year of surgery, but the patients remained obese.[83] Considering the very small study size and the short duration of observation, one must exercise caution before adopting such an approach for the treatment of T2D in youth until results from larger and longer well-controlled studies become available.[44] Preliminary evidence indicates that bariatric surgery may reduce lifetime health care expenditures for obese individuals, although a comparison of the cost of bariatric surgery versus lifetime medical treatment has not yet been studied.[84] Despite health and financial benefits, bariatric surgery poses some risk, including risks of attenuated linear growth and nutritional deficiencies, which need to be studied in more depth.

CONCLUSION

The trajectory of childhood obesity has given rise to adult diseases presenting in youth, such as T2D, along with escalating comorbidities and complications of nephropathy, dyslipidemia, and premature aging of the cardiovascular system. This, against the backdrop of the gloomy results of the TODAY study showing very high rates of glycemic failure on metformin, the only FDA-approved medication, and the aggressive course of the disease for β-cell failure and complications, demonstrates the urgent need for effective and safe pharmacotherapy in those with established diabetes, and the dire societal need for the prevention of diabetes for those at risk. The burden for the latter does not fall on the health care profession, but rather starts with the family, the school, the neighborhood, the society, the food industry, health care policy makers, economists, and the government. The successful antismoking campaign should be the launching pad for a successful obesity prevention campaign starting in utero.

REFERENCES

1. Ogden CL, Carroll MD, Kit BK, Flegal KM. Prevalence of obesity and trends in body mass index among US children and adolescents, 1999-2010. *JAMA* 2012;307(5):483–490.

2. National Diabetes Statistics, 2011. Available at www.cdc.gov/diabetes/pubs/pdf/ndfs_2011.pdf.

3. American Diabetes Association. Type 2 diabetes in children and adolescents. *Diabetes Care* 2000;23(3):381–389.

4. Dabelea D, Bell RA, D'Agostino RB Jr, Imperatore G, Johansen JM, Linder B, Liu LL, Loots B, Marcovina S, Mayer-Davis EJ, Pettitt DJ, Waitzfelder B. Incidence of diabetes in youth in the United States. *JAMA* 2007; 297(24):2176–2724.

5. Imperatore G, Boyle JP, Thompson TJ, Case D, Dabelea D, Hamman RF, Lawrence JM, Liese AD, Liu LL, Mayer-Davis EJ, Rodriguez BL, Standiford D. Projections of type 1 and type 2 diabetes burden in the U.S. population aged <20 years through 2050. *Diabetes Care* 2012; 35(12):2515–2520.

6. TODAY Study Group, Copeland K, Zietler P, et al. Characteristics of adolescents and youth with recent onset type 2 diabetes: the TODAY cohort at baseline. *J Clin Endocrinol Metab* 2011;96(1):159–167.

7. American Diabetes Association. Standards of medical care—2013. *Diabetes Care* 2013;36(Suppl 1):Sl1–S66.

8. Bacha F, Gungor N, Lee S, Arslanian SA. In vivo insulin sensitivity and secretion in obese youth: what are the differences between normal glucose tolerance, impaired glucose tolerance, and type 2 diabetes? *Diabetes Care* 2009; 32(1):100–105.

9. Tfayli H, Lee SJ, Arslanian S. Declining beta cell function relative to insulin sensitivity with increasing fasting glucose levels in the nondiabetic range in children. *Diabetes Care* 2010;33(9):224–230.

10. Burns SF, Bacha F, Lee S, Tfayli H, Arslanina S. Declining B cell function relative to insulin sensitivity with escalating OGTT 2-h glucose concentrations in the nondiabetic through the diabetic range in overweight youth. *Diabetes Care* 2011;34 (9):2033–2040.

11. Bacha F, Lee S, Gungor N, Arslanian S. From pre-diabetes to type 2 diabetes in obese youth: pathophysiological characteristics along the spectrum of glucose dysregulation. *Diabetes Care* 2010;33(10):2225–2231.

12. Gungor N, Bacha F, Saad S, Janosky J, Arslanian S. Youth type 2 diabetes: insulin resistance, beta cell failure, or both? *Diabetes Care* 2005;28(3):638–644.

13. Sjaadra LA, Michaliszyn SF, et al. HbA1c diagnostic categories and B-cell function relative to insulin sensitivity in overweight/obese adolescents. *Diabetes Care* 2012;35(12):2559–2563.

14. Arslanian S, Bacha F, Saad R, Gungor N. Family history of type 2 diabetes is associated with decreased insulin sensitivity and an impaired balance between insulin sensitivity and insulin secretion in white youth. *Diabetes Care* 2005;28(1):115–119.

15. Bacha F, Gungor N, Lee S, Arslanian SA. Progressive deterioration of β-cell function in obese youth with type 2 diabetes. *Pediatr Diabetes* 2013;14(2):106–111.

16. TODAY Study group. Effects of metformin, metformin plus rosiglitazone and metformin plus lifestyle on insulin sensitivity and β-cell function in TODAY. *Diabetes Care* 2013;36(6):1749–1757.

17. Levy-Marchal C, Arslanian S, Cutfiels W, et al. Insulin Resistance in Children Consensus Conference Group. Insulin resistance in children: consensus, perspective and future directions. *J Clin Endocrinol Metab* 2010;95(12):5189–5198.

18. Bacha F, Saad R, Gungor N, Arslanian SA. Are obesity-related metabolic risk factors modulated by the degree of insulin resistance in adolescents? *Diabetes Care* 2006;29(7):1599–1604.

19. Weiss R, Dufor S, Takasali SE, et al. Prediabetes in obese youth: a syndrome of impaired glucose tolerance, severe insulin resistance, and altered myocellular and abdominal fat partitioning. *Lancet* 2003;362(9388):951–957.

20. Kim G, Giannini C, Caprio S, et al. Longitudinal effects of MRI-measure hepatic steatosis on biomarkers of glucose homeostasis and hepatic apoptosis in obese youth. *Diabetes Care* 2013;36(1):130–136.

21. Meigs JB, Cupples LA, Wilson PW. Parental transmission of type 2 diabetes: the Framingham Offspring Study. *Diabetes* 2000;49(12):2201–2207.

22. Heon S, Soo K. Genetics of type 2 diabetes and potential clinical implications. *Arch Pharmacol Res* 2013;36:167–177.

23. Fagot-Campagna A, Pettitt DJ, Narayan KM, et al. Type 2 diabetes among North American children and adolescents: an epidemiologic review and a public health perspective. *J Pediatr* 2000;136(5):664–672.

24. SEARCH for Diabetes in Youth Study Group, Liese AD, D'Agostino RB Jr, et al. The burden of diabetes mellitus among US youth: prevalence estimates from the SEARCH for Diabetes in Youth Study. *Pediatrics* 2006;118(4):1510–1518.

25. Goran MI, Bergman RN, Cruz ML, Watanabe R. Insulin resistance and associated compensatory responses in African-American and Hispanic children. *Diabetes Care* 2002;25(12):2184–2190.

26. Dabelea D, Knowler WC, Pettitt DJ. Effects of diabetes in pregnancy on offspring: follow up research in the Pima Indians. *J Matern Fetal Med* 2000;9(1):83–88.

27. Silverman BL, Metzger BE, Cho NH, Loeb CA. Impaired glucose tolerance in adolescent offspring of diabetic mothers. Relationship to fetal hyperinsulinism. *Diabetes Care* 1995;18(5):611–617.

28. Dabelea D, Mayer-Davis EJ, Lamichhane A, D'Agostino RJ, Hamman R. Association of intrauterine exposure to maternal diabetes and obesity with

type 2 diabetes in youth. The SEARCH case-control study. *Diabetes Care* 2008;31(7):1422–1426.

29. Amiel SA, Sherwin RS, Simonson DC, Lauritano AA, Tamborlane WV. Impaired insulin action in puberty. A contributing factor to poor glycemic control in adolescents with diabetes. *New Engl J Med* 1986;315(4):215–219.

30. Palmert MR, Gordon CM, Kartashov AI, Legro RS, Emans SJ, Dunaif A. Screening for abnormal glucose tolerance in adolescents with polycystic ovary syndrome. *J Clin Endocrinol Metab* 2002;87(3):1017–1023.

31. Lewy VD, Danadian K, Arslanian S. Early metabolic abnormalities in adolescents girls with polycystic ovarian syndrome. *J Pediatr* 2001;138(1):38–44.

32. Arslanian S, Lewy VD, Danadian K. Glucose intolerance in obese adolescents with polycystic ovary syndrome: roles of insulin resistance and beta-cell dysfunction and risk of cardiovascular disease. *J Clin Endocrinol Metab* 2001;86(1):66–71.

33. Guran T, Turan S, Bereket A. Significance of acanthosis nigricans in childhood obesity. *J Paediatr Child Health* 2008;44(6):338–341.

34. American Diabetes Association. Revisions to the standards of medical care in diabetes 2014. *Diabetes Care* 2014;37(Suppl 1):S14–S80.

35. World Health Organization. Definition and diagnosis of diabetes mellitus and intermediate hyperglycaemia. Report of a WHO/IDF consultation 2005. Available at http://whqlibdoc.who.int/publications/2006/9241594934_eng.pdf.

36. Lee JM, Wu EL, Tarini B, Herman WH, Yoon E. Diagnosis of diabetes using hemoglobin A1c: should recommendations in adults be extrapolated to adolescents? *J Pediatr* 2011;158(6):947–952.

37. Nowicka P, Santoro N, Liu H, Lartaud D, Shaw MM, Goldberg R, Guandalini C, Savoye M, Rose P, Caprio S. Utility of hemoglobin A(1c) for diagnosing prediabetes and diabetes in obese children and adolescents. *Diabetes Care* 2011;34(6):1306–1311.

38. Libman IM, Becker DJ. Coexistence of type 1 and type 2 diabetes mellitus: "double" diabetes? *Pediatr Diabetes* 2003;4(2):110–113.

39. National Diabetes Information Clearinghouse. Available at www.diabetes.niddk.nih.gov. 2011:1–12.

40. Wu EL, Kazzi N, Lee J. Cost-effectiveness of screening strategies for identifying pediatric diabetes mellitus and dysglycemia. *JAMA Pediatr* 2013;167(1):32–39.

41. Sapru A, Gitelman SE, Flori H, et al. Prevalence and characteristics of type 2 diabetes mellitus in 9-18 year old children with diabetic ketoacidosis. *J Pediatric Endocrinol Metab* 2005;18(9):865–872.

42. Rosenbloom AL. Hyperglycemic hyperosmolar state: an emerging pediatric problem. *J Pediatr* 2010;156(2):180–184.

43. Libman IM, Pietropaolo M, Arslanian SA, LaPorte RE, Becker DJ. Changing prevalence of overweight children and adolescents at onset of insulin treated diabetes. *Diabetes Care* 2003;26(10):2871–2875.

44. Flint A, Arslanian S. Treatment of type 2 diabetes in youth. *Diabetes Care* 2011;34(Suppl 2):S177–S183.

45. Rewers A, Klingensmith G, Davis C., et al. Presence of diabetic ketoacidosis at diagnosis of diabetes mellitus in youth: the Search for Diabetes in Youth Study. *Pediatrics* 2008;121(5):e1258–1266.

46. Gilliam LK, Brooks-Worrell BM, Palmer JP, Greenbaum CJ, Pihoker C. Autoimmunity and clinical course in children with type 1, type 2 and type 1.5 diabetes. *J Autoimm* 2005;25(3):244–250.

47. Brooks-Worrell BM, Palmer JP, Greenbaum CJ, Pihoker C. Autoimmunity to islet proteins in children diagnosed with new-onset diabetes. *JCEM* 2004;89(5):2222–2227.

48. Tfayli H, Bacha F, Arslanian S. Phenotypic type 2 diabetes in obese youth: insulin sensitivity and secretion in islet cell antibody negative vs. positive patients. *Diabetes* 2009;58(3):738–744.

49. Zietler P, Haqq A, Rosenbloom A. Drugs and Therapeutics Committee of the Lawson Wilkins Pediatric Endocrine Society. Hyperglycemic hyperosmolar syndrome in children: pathophysiological considerations and suggested guidelines for treatment. *J Pediatr* 2011;158(1):9–14.

50. Rodriguez BL, Dabelea D, Liese AD, et al. Prevalence and correlates of elevated blood pressure in youth with diabetes mellitus: the SEARCH for Diabetes in Youth study. *J Pediatr* 2010;157(2):245–251.

51. TODAY Study Group. Rapid rise in hypertension and nephropathy in youth with type 2 diabetes. *Diabetes Care* 2013;36(6):1735–1741.

52. National High Blood Pressure Education Program Working Group on High Blood Pressure in Children and Adolescents. The fourth report on the diagnosis, evaluation and treatment of high blood pressure in children and adolescents. *Pediatrics* 2004;114:555–576.

53. Blowey DL. Update on the pharmacologic treatment of hypertension in pediatrics. *J Clin Hypertens* 2012;14(6):383–387.

54. Eppens MC, Craig ME, Cusumano J, et al. Prevalence of diabetes complications in adolescents with type 2 compared with type 1 diabetes. *Diabetes Care* 2006;29(6):1300–1306.

55. Kershnar AK, Daniels SR, Imperatore G, et al. Lipid abnormalities are prevalent in youth with type 1 and type 2 diabetes: the SEARCH for Diabetes in Youth study. *J Pediatr* 2006;149(3):314–319.

56. Sellers EA, Yung G, Dean HJ. Dyslipidemia and other cardiovascular risk factors in a Canadian First Nation pediatric population with type 2 diabetes mellitus. *Pediatr Diabetes* 2007;8(6):384–390.

57. TODAY Study Group. Lipid and inflammatory cardiovascular risk worsens over 3 years in youth with type 2 diabetes. *Diabetes Care* 2013;36(6):1758–1764.

58. Berenson GS, Srinivasan SR, Bao W, et al. Association between multiple cardiovascular risk factors and atherosclerosis in children and young adults. The Bogalusa Heart Study. *New Engl J Med* 1998;338(23):1650–1656.

59. Maahs D, Wadwa RP, Bishop F, et al. Dyslipidemia in youth with diabetes: to treat or not to treat? *J Pediatr* 2008;153(4):458–465.

60. Pinhas-Hamiel O, Zeitler P. Acute and chronic complications of type 2 diabetes mellitus in children and adolescents. *Lancet* 2007;26:369(9575):1823–1831.

61. Dart AB, Martens PJ, Sellers EA, et al. Earlier complications in youth with type 2 diabetes. *Diabetes Care* 2014:37(2):436–443.

62. Constantino M, Wu T, Wong J, et al. Long term complications and mortality in young onset diabetes. *Diabetes Care* 2013;36(12):3863–3869.

63. Mayer-Davis EJ, Davis C, Saadine J, et al. Diabetic retinopathy in the SEARCH for Diabetes in Youth cohort: a pilot study. *Diabetic Med* 2012;29(9):1148–1152.

64. TODAY Study Group. Retinopathy in youth with type 2 diabetes participating in the TODAY clinical trial. *Diabetes Care* 2013;36(6):1772–1774.

65. Krakoff J, Limdsay RS, Looker HC, Nelson RG, Hanson RL, Knowler WC. Incidence of retinopathy and nephropathy in youth onset compared with adult onset type 2 diabetes. *Diabetes Care* 2003;26(1):76–81.

66. Maahs DM, Snively BM, Bell RA, et al. Higher prevalence of elevated albumin excretion in youth with type 2 than type 1 diabetes: the SEARCH for Diabetes in Youth study. *Diabetes Care* 2007;30(10):2593–2598.

67. Pavkov ME, Bennett PH, Knowler WC, et al. Effect of youth-onset type 2 diabetes mellitus on incidence of end stage renal disease and mortality in young and middle age Pima Indians. *JAMA* 2006;26:296(4):421–426.

68. Dart AB, Sellers EA, Martens PJ, Rigatto C, Brownell MD, Dean HJ. High burden of kidney disease in youth-onset type 2 diabetes. *Diabetes Care* 2012;35(6):1265–1271.

69. Rosenbloom AL, Silverstein JH, Amemiya S, et al. Type 2 diabetes in children and adolescents. ISPAD Clinical Practice Consensus Guidelines. *Pediatr Diabetes* 2009:10(Suppl 12):17–32.

70. Gungor N, Thompson T, Sutton-Tyrrell K, et al. Early signs of cardiovascular disease in youth with obesity and type 2 diabetes. *Diabetes Care* 2005;28(5):1219–1221.

71. Wadwa P, Urbina E, Anderson A, et al. Measures of arterial stiffness in youth with type 1 and type 2 diabetes. *Diabetes Care* 2010;33(4):881–886.

72. Lawrence JM, Standiford DA, Loots B, et al. Prevalence and correlates of depressed mood among youth with diabetes: the SEARCH for Diabetes in Youth study. *Pediatrics* 2006;117(4):1348–1358.

73. Smith RJ, Nathan DM, Arslanian SA, et al. Individualizing therapies in type 2 diabetes mellitus based on patient characteristics: what we know and what we need to know. *J Clin Endocrinol Metab* 2010;95(4):1566–1574.

74. Lee S, Bacha F, Arslanian S, et al. Effects of aerobic versus resistance exercise without caloric restriction on abdominal fat, intrahepatic lipid, and insulin sensitivity in obese adolescent boys: a randomized, controlled trial. *Diabetes* 2012;61(11):2787–2795.

75. Wilfey DE, Tibbs TL, Van Buren DJ, Epstein LH, et al. Lifestyle interventions in the treatment of childhood overweight: a meta-analytic review of randomized controlled trials. *Health Psychol* 2007;26(5):521–532.

76. McLean N, Griffin S, Toney K, Hardeman W. Family involvement in weight control, weight maintenance and weight loss intervention: a systematic review of randomized trials. *Int J Obes* 2003;27(9):987–1005.

77. Centers for Disease Control and Prevention. Physical activity facts, 2013. Available at www.cdc.gov/healthyyouth/physicalactivity/facts.

78. Bretzel RG, Nuber U, Landgraf W, Owens DR, Bradley C, Linn T. Once-daily basal insulin glargine vs. thrice-daily pandrial insulin lispro in people with type 2 diabetes on oral hypoglycemic agents (APOLLO): an open randomized controlled trial. *Lancet* 2008;371(9618):1073–1084.

79. Sellers EA, Dean HJ. Short term insulin therapy in adolescents with type 2 diabetes mellitus. *J Pediatr Endocrinol Metab* 2004;17(11):1561–1564.

80. Weigensberg MJ, Goran MI. Type 2 diabetes in children and adolescents. *Lancet* 2009;373(9677):1743–1744.

81. Jones KL, Arslanian S., Peterokova VA, et al. Effect of metformin in pediatric patients with type 2 diabetes: a randomized controlled trial. *Diabetes Care* 2002;25(1):89–94.

82. Gottschalk M, Danne T, Vlajnic A, et al. Glimepiride versus metformin as monotherapy in pediatric patients with type 2 diabetes: a randomized, single blind comparative study. *Diabetes Care* 2007;30(4):790–794.

83. Inge TH, Miyano G, Bean J, et al. Reversal of type 2 diabetes mellitus and improvements in cardiovascular risk factors after surgical weight loss in adolescents. *Pediatrics* 2009;123(1):214–222.

84. Stefater MA, Jenkins T, Inge TH. Bariatric surgery for adolescents. *Pediatr Diabetes* 2013;14(1):1–12.

Chapter 19

Psychosocial Issues Related to Type 2 Diabetes

Deborah Young-Hyman, PhD

OVERVIEW

The psychosocial burden of type 2 diabetes (T2D) is underreported, understudied, and increasing. Examination of psychosocial barriers to effective management of T2D are essential as the T2D epidemic increases in all segments of the population and among all age-groups. Effective disease management must include addressing psychosocial issues.

- Psychological and diabetes morbidity are reciprocal. Patients with psychiatric disorders have higher rates of T2D diagnoses than individuals without mental illness, less effective disease management, and poorer glycemic control. Diagnosis of T2D has been associated with poor mental health, disability, and reduced quality of life, risk factors for poor medical outcomes. The incidence of depression in patients with T2D is estimated to be two to three times that of the healthy population. To achieve treatment goals, comorbid diabetes and mental health problems need simultaneous treatment. Ongoing psychosocial monitoring and care are an integral part of treatment success.
- A majority of T2D diagnoses are weight related. Therefore, the foundation treatment for T2D involves lifestyle and behavior modification. Failed attempts at weight management can result in low self- and body-esteem, and low self-efficacy for leading a healthy lifestyle. Stigmatization associated with being overweight or obese is associated with poor psychological adjustment and quality of life, adding risk for poor disease management.
- Beyond access to and resources for medical care, adherence to self-management behaviors (taking medications, monitoring health indicators, healthy eating, routine physical activity) is the foundation for treatment success. In addition to psychosocial barriers, adherence to the self-care regimen can be compromised by diabetes-specific physiologic processes that impair regulation of appetite and satiety, compromised by other comorbid diseases and their treatment, and impeded by weight-related physical disability. Patients' success in self-care will be aided by education regarding how these conditions affect their ability to carry out their treatment regimen, rather than by patient and provider assuming noncompliance.
- Living with T2D over the life course will be affected by issues specific to an individual's developmental stage and social context. Successful daily

 DOI: 10.2337/9781580405096.19

management of T2D affects interpersonal relationships, tasks of daily living, role functions, and allocation of personal and family resources.

- To achieve treatment success, individuals must adjust to the patient role, learning to navigate the health care system that requires detailed communication with providers, assumption of self-care responsibilities, and obtaining financial resources for care. Self-management of disease may be a novel paradigm to patients, and it is best accomplished by ongoing diabetes education, support, and communication between patient and provider to ensure a shared understanding of regimen requirements.
- Assessing patient knowledge, attitudes, and motivation and health care provider estimation of a patient's abilities to carry out the diabetes care regimen—and identifying provider and interpersonal supports—are part of routine psychosocial care. This knowledge will help the clinician tailor and facilitate a successful care regimen.
- An ecological patient-centered chronic disease approach, factoring the patient's sociocultural environment into treatment recommendations, is more likely to facilitate effective treatment and produce better medical outcomes, especially as T2D is diagnosed disproportionately in minority populations. Promoting health literacy is an important part of patient care.

This chapter will enable the reader to achieve the following:

1. Identify common psychological comorbid conditions known to affect ability to cope with disease management and outcomes.
2. Identify common behavioral issues associated with disease management and outcomes.
3. Summarize what is known about sociocultural and life course issues affecting disease management.
4. Summarize the use of psychological criteria and contraindications for intensive management, use of polypharmacy, and initiation of insulin and other needle-based therapies, including insulin pump use.
5. Summarize special issues of children and adolescents diagnosed with T2D.
6. List recommended evaluation and treatment methods and their incorporation into routine diabetes care.

COMMON PSYCHOLOGICAL CONDITIONS COMORBID WITH T2D

The most common psychological comorbidity documented in individuals with T2D is depression, including subclinical symptoms and those reaching the level of major depression.[1] Depression is estimated at two to three times more likely in an individual with diabetes than in the general population and is associated with poor medical outcomes.[2,3]

Depression comorbid with diabetes can be psychologically based or secondary to disease morbidity. Effects are bidirectional.[4] After adjusting for pathophysiologic markers of risk for T2D, among multiple ethnicities, depression has been found to be predictive of diagnosed disease[5] and after controlling for markers of the metabolic syndrome and other psychosocial risk factors, depression (and

Depression is the most common symptom of psychological distress in all patients with diabetes. Some depression is normal in the context of diagnosis, occurrence of complications, difficulty following medical advice, or accessing care. Depressive symptoms can be expected to fluctuate and should be monitored so that services can be provided when depressive symptoms become clinically significant and interfere with a patient's ability to carry out self-management behaviors.

comorbid anxiety) has been shown to be predictive of disease onset.[6] In patients with T2D, depressive symptoms are associated with higher weight,[7] poorer adherence to self-care behaviors,[8] and higher disability related to activities of daily living.[9] Diagnosed depression also has been associated with increased rates of dementia[10] and advanced complications.[11] Anxiety symptoms are known to co-occur with depression, associated with poor diabetes self-efficacy and poorer adherence.[6] According to a meta-analysis of anxiety symptoms in adults with T1D and T2D, 14% had symptoms that reached the level of generalized anxiety disorder and 40% had elevated anxiety symptoms, with no difference in prevalence found between patients with T1D or T2D.[12] Thus, depressive and anxiety symptoms have the potential to impede achieving treatment goals and should be comanaged with the physiologic disease. Depressive symptoms associated with diagnosis or change in medical status are expected, but they usually do not reach the level of diagnosable psychiatric illness. Patients who are already vulnerable or have previously been diagnosed and treated for psychiatric illness can be expected to have worsening of symptoms at diagnosis or at onset of complications.[13]

Patients often are diagnosed with T2D after a prolonged period of trying to lose weight and "predisease," with consequent low disease-related self-efficacy and self-esteem. Disease burden is increased further increased by societal stigmatization of overweight or obesity and as patients understand the negative health consequences of their being overweight. Psychological vulnerability and poor self-efficacy related to weight management pertain to difficulty changing lifestyle, fatalism about weight and poor health, depression secondary to inability to affect weight or health, and adoption of maladaptive weight management behaviors (see the following section).[14] Patients having difficulty controlling glucose and weight can be expected to experience cognitive impairment,[15] especially if sleep apnea is present.[16] Those with poor long-term control, complications, and associated comorbid disease (such as cardiovascular disease) have been documented to be less productive in the workforce, more likely to be on disability, and more likely to have signs of dementia.[9,17]

Alcohol consumption, use of recreational drugs, and misuse of prescription drugs can significantly impair a patient's judgment and ability to carry out self-management behaviors, with the potential to effect glycemic control.[18] Alcohol consumption also can promote accretion of abdominal fat, thereby increasing insulin resistance[19] and difficulty controlling glycemia. The prevalence of current alcohol use in the population with diabetes is estimated to be ~50–60%, based on epidemiological surveys of treatment-seeking populations.[20] Prevalence of patients with T2D who are alcoholic or addicted to prescription pain medication or "street" drugs is not well characterized. Some studies have found relatively high rates of alcohol abuse and dependence (28 and 13%, respectively).[21] Engler and Ramsey[22] found 13% of their patients with T2D met National Institute on Alcohol Abuse and Alcoholism criteria for at-risk drinking, and 11% of the 13% met criteria for alcohol dependence.[22] High rates of alcohol abuse might be expected because of the known association between the common physiologic and reward pathways between alcohol use and development of T2D.[23] Misuse of prescription drugs, particularly opioids, has increased in the general population[24] and might also increase in the population with T2D as the prevalence of T2D increases, the population ages, and complications develop. Peripheral neuropathy often is treated with opioids after first-line drugs such as antidepressants do not adequately control pain.[25] Medication for pain can make patients with T2D who have advanced disease vulnerable to cognitive and motor impairment, further affecting disease management. Monitoring use and misuse of alcohol and of pain medication may help to explain nonadherence and poor success in obtaining desired metabolic outcomes.

Disordered eating behavior (DEB) is a common maladaptive behavior identified in patients with diabetes and is defined as weight-management behavior that is extreme; disrupts daily living; and is driven by concerns about weight, size, appearance, and self-esteem.[1] Concerns can be realistic or disproportionate to actual weight and size. Binge-eating disorder (BED) is the most common DEB documented in patients with T2D, making glycemic and weight control more difficult. BED and other types of DEB are associated with a higher incidence of complications.[26] Symptoms of BED include eating large amounts of food in a short period of time and purging of calories by vomiting, extreme exercise, use of laxatives, or misuse of other medications affecting appetite or weight, particularly insulin. Insulin misuse is reported less commonly in the population of patients with T2D (compared with patients with T1D), but as the diagnosis of T2D increases in teen and young adult women, and treatment with insulin is introduced earlier in the disease course,[7] incidence of insulin misuse for weight control can be expected to increase. Better glycemic control secondary to treatment with insulin likely will result in difficulty controlling weight gain. Patients with T2D who associate insulin use with unwanted weight gain are more likely to refuse or misuse insulin.[27]

Diagnosable eating disorder rates in patients with T2D are low or estimated to be comparable to the general population.[26] True prevalence of diagnosable eating disorders, however, is not known in part because behavior that is consis-

---

Control of food intake is a central component of successful diabetes treatment. Because T2D usually is associated with being overweight, most patients' relationship with food intake will be conflicted. Failed attempts at weight loss can result in low self- and body-esteem, and low self-efficacy for healthy eating. In addition, a majority of individuals with diabetes can be expected to have difficulty regulating caloric intake because of disease-related alterations in their physiology and prescription of medications that alter glucose level, appetite, and satiety. Thus, the need for medical nutrition therapy is universal and ongoing.

tent with DEB is prescribed as part of the diabetes treatment regimen. A prime example for patients with T2D is dietary restraint.[28,29] Furthermore, answers indicating risk for DEB on questionnaires standardized in the general population have been shown to be highly influenced by having diabetes, resulting in the potential for misinterpretation of total and subscale scores by clinicians.[30] Complicating the etiology of DEB-like behavior, derangements in physiology associated with the disease will disrupt cues of hunger and satiety, making food intake more difficult to control.[31,32] On the basis of a recent review of the literature, it is becoming evident that appetite modulators such as leptin, ghrelin, brain-derived neurotrophic factor, and endocannabinoids also affect nonhomeostatic cognitive, emotional, and reward components of food intake, suggesting that changes in the physiology of appetite modulators may play a role in the pathophysiology of DEBs.[33] Education regarding DEB, as distinct from prescribed treatment behaviors regarding food intake, and from disrupted eating (disregulated hunger and satiety cues associated with disruption in appetite modulators), needs to be incorporated into diabetes education and routine medical nutrition therapy.[28,34] Given preliminary evidence that clinicians may misattribute patient responses on screening tools to eating pathology, care should be taken to evaluate the etiology of patient focus on food, weight, and weight-management behavior and to map attempts to control weight in response to the pathophysiology of the disease, treatment effects, and behaviors that are prescribed as part of diabetes care. This can be accomplished by assessing weight history, eating behavior, and attitudes about size and weight when a patient is diagnosed or presents for treatment and by providing ongoing assessment regarding the patient's ability to control appetite and weight in relation to medication dosing and blood glucose fluctuations.

Among anxiety symptoms, needle phobia has long been considered an important psychological phenomenon affecting T2D patients' willingness to intensify their treatment using insulin. The prevalence of needle phobia in patients with T2D is not known as there have been no systematic population prevalence studies of this phenomenon among patients with T1D or T2D. Recent studies, however, have indicated that diabetes education and skills acquisition reduce patients' reticence to using needle-based therapies.[35] The issue of needle phobia is particularly relevant because new needle-administered pharmacotherapies are available to help patients control blood glucose, reduce caloric intake, and improve appetite regulation and thereby weight status.[32,36] Fear of hypoglycemia may occur once insulin is started,[3] although the frequency of this phenomenon in the population of patients with T2D is not well documented due to varying clinical criteria.[37] Some anxiety about health status after diagnosis is normative, as is anxiety about well-being and functional status when complications occur.[13] Monitoring for disabling levels of anxiety that interfere with diabetes care tasks is indicated in ongoing care. Common, however, is a sense of fatalism regarding disease outcomes, as T2D has strong heritability,[38] and many patients assume they will have the same disease course as relatives, affecting willingness to intensify treatment and affecting associated quality of life. Patients may be reticent to tell care providers they will not adhere to the prescribed regimen because of fears or anxiety about use of needles, side effects of treatment (weight gain in particular), burden of care[39] or their sense of fatalism about medical outcomes.[38]

Major psychiatric illnesses, particularly schizophrenia and bipolar disorder, have been associated with higher rates of T2D diagnosis than rates found among individuals without mental illness.[40] Possible causes are sedentary behavior and psychotropic medications. Antipsychotic use in youth and adults has been associated with higher rates of T2D diagnosis than in referent populations that do not use these drugs.[41] Complexity of treatment regimen should be considered in the context of intellectual limitations (including impaired judgment), interaction of psychotropic medications, and availability of supports to ensure that treatment is accurately and adequately carried out. Conversely, patients with major psychiatric illness may be undertreated because of the same concerns. In both situations, thorough mental status and mental health history taking can inform the clinician of needed supports to enhance the likelihood of achieving standards of care.

Psychological function should be evaluated at diagnosis or as a patient enters the health care system and should be monitored as part of routine care. Brief screening tools usually take no more than 10–15 minutes and provide the clinician with timely actionable information. Methods of administration include paper and pencil, computer interface, or telephone administered. Scoring algorithms indicate when a patient endorses a clinically significant level of distress or symptoms, indicating the need for further assessment by a mental health professional familiar with diabetes and its treatment (see Table 19.1). When using screening tools, caution must be used in interpretation of results for minority populations given the lack of standardization that takes into account specific cultural and religious values that could produce response bias.[42] Measurement of the functional health status of the individual also will help interpretability of screening results (Table 19.1).

TREATMENT RECOMMENDATIONS

Following are treatment recommendations for common psychological conditions comorbid with T2D:

- Psychological function, particularly depressive, anxiety, and eating-disordered symptoms and the presence of major psychiatric disorders, including impaired judgment or cognitive function, should be evaluated at diagnosis or as a patient enters the health care system, and monitored as part of routine care.
- Standardized screening measures of psychological or psychiatric symptoms should be incorporated into routine management visits, providing the clinician with indicators of current function, the ability to track changes in mental status related to disease state or life course, and flags for further evaluation and referral.
- Immediate referral for further psychological evaluation is indicated if significant depression, suicidal or homicidal ideation with intent to act, clinically significant DEB, or obvious impairment of judgment or cognitive functioning are identified.
- If major psychiatric impairment is identified, appropriate pharmacologic, interpersonal therapy, and supervised medical management is indicated. Identification of interpersonal as well as financial supports are essential, as mental health functioning will significantly affect a patient's ability to self-manage their disease.

BEHAVIORAL ISSUES ASSOCIATED WITH DISEASE MANAGEMENT: ADHERENCE AND BEHAVIOR MONITORING

Adherence to a medical regimen is defined as carrying out a clearly explained and expected set of treatment behaviors.[43] For patients with T2D, adherence to healthy lifestyle behaviors and to prescribed medication regimen[44] is a central issue contributing to treatment success.

Behavioral nonadherence is most frequent regarding nutrition intake and physical activity, followed by medication.[45] Reasons can include lack of education regarding the disease and its treatment, low health literacy, lack of belief in the health benefits of specific behaviors, and functional disability due to worsening disease.[46] Changing lifestyle behaviors, particularly patterns of food intake and physical activity, require ongoing intervention, including social and medical sys-

---

Table 19.1 Validated Psychosocial Screening and Evaluation Tools*

Depression:
Beck Depression Inventory–II (Beck, 1996)
Children's Depression Inventory (Kovacs, 1992)
Patient Health Questionnaire (PHQ-9, Depression portion; Kroenke, Spitzer, and Williams, 2001)
Centre for Epidemiologic Studies Depression Scale (CES-D; Radloff, 1977)

Anxiety:
Generalized Anxiety Disorder 7-Item Scale (GAD-7; Spitzer, Kroenke, Williams, and Lowe, 2006)
Hamilton Anxiety Scale (HAM-A; Hamilton, 1959)
Zung Self-Rating Anxiety Scale (SAS; Zung, 1971)

Psychiatric Symptoms:
Symptom Checklist-90-R (SCL-90-R; Derogatis, 1994)
Structured Clinical Interview for DSM Disorders (SCID-5-RV; American Psychiatric Pub. Inc., 2014)

Life Stress:
Family Environment Scale (FES; Moos and Moos, 1981)
Perceived Stress Scale (PSS; Cohen and Williamson, 1983)

Mental Status:
Mini-Mental State Examination, 2nd ed. (MMSE; PAR, 2010)

Eating Behavior:
Eating Disorder Examination-Questionnaire (EDE-Q; Fairburn and Beglin, 1994)
Diabetes Eating Problem Survey–Revised (DEPS-R; Markowitz, 2010)
Diabetes Treatment and Satiety Scale (DTSS-20; Young-Hyman, 2011)

*Sources for Table 19.1 begin on p. 311.

tem support, as goals are set, achieved, and modified. Difficulty changing habits includes the need for new patterns of behavior to be learned and rehearsed by the patient and to be supported by the patient's medical care team and nonmedical interpersonal environment.

Diabetes is self-managed and requires self and external behavioral monitoring. Corrective action is taken based on biologic indicators of glycemia and disease-related comorbidities. Behavioral monitoring is introduced as soon as diagnosis is established: self-report of food intake, physical activity, symptoms, medication dosing, and preferably results of blood glucose tests. The need to self-monitor and share results with care providers may be novel for the patient; the roles of patient and provider change, making the patient central to ongoing disease management.[47] This chronic care paradigm is different from the accustomed acute care model utilized in most medical treatment.[48] For example, the usefulness of blood glucose testing has been questioned in the population with T2D. When examined,

Diabetes Distress:
Problem Areas in Diabetes Scale (PAID-R; Polonsky, 2000)
Diabetes Distress Scale (DDS17; Polonsky, 2005)

Diabetes Self-Efficacy:
Diabetes Empowerment Scale (DES; Anderson, Funnell, Fitzgerald, and Marrero, 2000)

Health Related Quality of Well-Being:
SF-36® Health Survey and SF-12® Health Survey (Ware, 1992)
Centers for Disease Control and Prevention Health-Related Quality of Life Surveillance
   Program (CDC HRQOLB; 2012)

Health Literacy:
Test of Functional Health Literacy Assessment (TOFHLA; Cavanaugh, Huizinga, and
   Wallston et al., 2008)
Literacy Assessment for Diabetes (LAD; Nath et al., 2001, 2001)

Diabetes Knowledge:
Audit of Diabetes (ADKnowl; Celerier et al,, 2009)
Diabetes Knowledge Test (DKT; Michigan Diabetes Research and Training Center, 1998)
Diabetes Self-Management Assessment Report Tool (D-SMART; Peyrot et al., 2007)

Diabetes Self-Care Behaviors/Adherence:
Diabetes Self-Care Profile (DSCP; Welch, 2011)
Self-Management Profile for Type 2 Diabetes (SMP-T2D; Peyrot et al., 2012)
Self-Care Inventory–Revised (SCI-R; Weinger et al,, 2005)

Hypoglycemia:
Hypoglycemic Fear Survey–II (Gonder-Frederick, 2011)

*Sources for Table 19.1 begin on p. 311.

The Importance of Adherence

Adherence to—

- Healthy lifestyle behaviors and medication regimen and
- Behavioral monitoring

will facilitate successful treatment.

Services that improve—

- Availability of financial resources, social support, and medical personnel;
- Diabetes knowledge and self-care skills;
- Behavioral feedback facilitating regimen change; and
- Belief in the efficacy of treatment behaviors

will improve adherence and medical outcomes.

---

however, lack of usefulness often can be attributed to limited or no feedback to patients regarding test results. Thus, unless the paradigm of behavioral monitoring with immediate feedback regarding efficacy of the behavior is implemented, and the patient is educated to what that information provides to them and the practitioner (gauging treatment effects), patients may be nonadherent. Nonadherence to behavioral monitoring, however, must be evaluated in the context of skills, education, and financial resources to obtain, for example, testing supplies.[47] In the role of patient, individuals may be reticent to talk about nonadherence to their care providers, because of being judged a "bad patient."[39,49] Less-than-ideal patient–provider communication has been implicated in poor adherence.[45]

As T2D disproportionately affects lower socioeconomic status individuals, lack of availability, affordability, and accessibility of medical resources decrease the likelihood of adherence to the prescribed regimen, causing patient and provider frustration and reduced expectations for successful treatment. These issues should be part of ongoing assessment.[50] Care paradigms such as virtual care, the "patient-centered medical home," and third-party payment for preventive and ongoing ancillary services may help to overcome these obstacles. Insurance coverage for prevention services will greatly enhance supports for behavior change. The Patient Protection and Affordable Care Act and the Health Care and Education Affordability Act of 2010 contain specific directives regarding obesity treatment, prevention services, and care for weight-related diabetes that include education, medication, and supplies.

TREATMENT RECOMMENDATIONS

Following are the treatment recommendations for behavioral issues associated with disease management:

- Monitoring of self-management behaviors accompanied by skills training, education about treatment effectiveness, and how to use the feedback to improve medical outcomes[51] should be initiated at time of diagnosis and updated as the management regimen changes.

- Expectations for adherence to a prescribed regimen will be tempered by knowledge of the patient's health literacy (see the section Health Literacy), resources, and life circumstances. This information can be obtained using an in-depth medical history and supplemented by screening tools that assess diabetes knowledge, general and disease-related quality of life, life events, and financial resources (see Table 19.1).
- The agreed-upon treatment regimen, decided collaboratively by patient and provider, should be based on medical need and feasibility. Significant others may be needed to endorse and provide instrumental support for the "self-care contract."
- If a patient is not receptive to the treatment regimen indicated by their disease state, talk therapy and re-education is suggested before significant regimen changes are made, new medications are introduced, or adjunctive treatment is begun. Assessing life events and daily routine may provide added information regarding barriers to adherence to the medical regimen and to adoption of a healthy lifestyle.

SOCIOCULTURAL AND LIFE COURSE ISSUES INTERACTING WITH DISEASE MANAGEMENT

As tasks related to disease management are incorporated into a patient's life, disruption of tasks of daily living, family routine, work schedule, and role functions can be expected, especially if diabetes is not well controlled or if complications occur.[17] Conversely, daily responsibilities can be expected to affect compliance with regimen requirements, such as frequency of medication dosing or clinic attendance. Loss of job or spouse, change in marital status, incarceration, pregnancy, and other major life events—positive or negative—affect a patient's ability to carry out disease management tasks and maintain ongoing medical care.[52] Ethnic culture, religious beliefs, and living environment also represent opportunities for or barriers to success in self-care. Thus, patient and provider expectations for requirements of self-care should be tailored to the patient's life circumstances, with the expectation that alternative means of access to and supports for medical care must be considered.[53]

Patient perception of social role functions can affect disease management. Adult women often view themselves as caretakers for others, whereas men stereotypically prioritize job tasks and function over self-care. Shifting focus to themselves requires patients to prioritize themselves as "in need" and allocate time to medical management.[54] Concern about revealing a diagnosis can negatively affect self-management, especially if inadequate or inaccurate information about diabe-

---

Patients can be educated to expect that medical management will require integration into tasks of daily living, interpersonal role and job functions, and allocation of financial resources. A patient's social and cultural milieu should be taken into account to maximize a patient's ability to incorporate care into their lifestyle.

Patient–provider communication about the incorporation of treatment behaviors into daily living includes "how-to" strategies. Development of how-to strategies will be facilitated by obtaining a social and mental health history from the patient and by including family members in the assessment.

---

tes and its treatment are prevalent in the patient's social environment. Employers may be hesitant to hire individuals diagnosed with diabetes because of the potential for lost productivity, although illegal to do so.[55] Fears about job loss could result in patients hiding diagnosis or abandoning self-care behaviors during work hours.[46]

Particularly for midlife adults, changes in role functions to accommodate disease management may cause distress about self-concept and conflict between family members as emotional, instrumental, and financial resources are reallocated to the needs of the patient. Relationships within the family may shift as children and other family members participate in caretaking or feel the need to change their lifestyle to accommodate the patient's altered lifestyle needs. Alternatively, a spouse or persons in the patient's social support network may have difficulty or be unwilling to change their own behavior or lifestyle to facilitate management of diabetes within the home. A term, "misguided helping," has been coined to describe others' attempts to help a patient comply with treatment requirements in a manner that is not helpful to either the patient or the caring individual.[56] The burden of primary caretaking of a chronically ill patient has been shown to result in poorer health and quality of life for the caretaker.[57] Emotional and practical spousal or family support, however, has been shown to be associated with better patient adherence[58] and quality of life for the patient and spouse.[59]

Conflict around developmental tasks and disease management is common during adolescence, when teens' developmental tasks center around gaining autonomy, and management of diabetes requires greater parental involvement and health care provider monitoring (see the section Special Issues of Childhood and Adolescence). Including family members in treatment has been advocated for children and teens with T1D,[60] and this treatment paradigm also applies to youth and teens with T2D. In general, inclusion of social support networks in a patient's resources to manage their disease can be expected to improve medical outcomes.[61]

Elderly patients with T2D often are undertreated and underserved because of actual or perceived physical and cognitive limitations and lack of social, financial, and instrumental supports.[62] The elderly may need treatment accommodations, such as large-font written materials, adaptive medication dosing devices, and tailored exercise and nutrition programs. Elderlies (individuals past middle age and approaching old age) more often have comorbid diseases requiring complex treatment regimens, polypharmacy, and the potential for drug interactions.[63] Cognitive and motor limitations may result in the need for direct supervision of regimen behaviors. Practical issues for patients at this life stage may involve obtaining adaptive devices for the home, obtaining caretaker support, identifying resources for the costs of care, ensuring functional health, and demonstrating the ability to independently carry out medical management, including attending doctor and clinic visits.[57] For elderlies, a family member or caretaker present during medical visits will increase the likelihood of integrated care that is carried out accurately.[46] Thus, monitoring of knowledge, attitudes, and well-being for people participating in primary caretaking for elderly patients with T2D is indicated, as is the provision of diabetes education and clinician support, and when distress is identified, psychological intervention.[64]

Religious and cultural beliefs can influence patients to adopt a variety of roles in and attitudes about medical care and outcomes. Optimistic bias, the tendency to minimize the possibility of negative outcomes, may confer risk or protective effects on medical outcomes depending on whether it results in a patient seeking information and executing protective behaviors.[65] Religiosity, however, has been shown to be a predictor of better psychological adjustment to illness and to predict better medical outcomes, particularly in minority populations.[66,67]

Minority race and ethnicity are strong predictors of poor control in adults with T2D. Minority and poor patients have been shown to be more likely to live in neighborhoods that have less access to healthy and affordable food and that lack facilities for safely carrying out physical activity.[68,69] These patients have been found to be undertreated relative to other populations with diabetes,[70] having less access to medical resources to achieve accepted standards of care.[71] Furthermore, regimen prescriptions that are counter to cultural or religious beliefs may be perceived as conflicting with the patient's value system. Patients may view behavior, such as dietary restrictions, as putting them at odds with their culture or social milieu (e.g., church supper). Health literacy in minority groups tends to be lower, impeding effective management,[72] and there is broad recognition of need for cultural tailoring of care systems for minority patients.[73] Community-based services provided by culturally equivalent providers have shown promise in improving medical outcomes in patients with T2D.[74]

Health literacy significantly contributes to a patient's ability to successfully carry out their treatment regimen. Health literacy pertains to access to information, comprehension of educational materials, mastery of self-management tasks, understanding the requirements of the prescribed treatment regimen, and how these behaviors affect disease outcomes. Thus, method of presentation, reading level of materials, and cultural specificity of information and language will affect whether a patient will derive accurate information and facilitate mastery of skills to adequately carry out the care regimen.[75] A key component of health literacy resides in patient–caregiver communication. Specific and precise transmission of the requirements of the care regimen, and the patient's ability to

---

Health literacy is patients' ability to understand and effectively use culturally sensitive and tailored information provided to them to help manage their disease and improve access to medical care. Updating health literacy continues as new treatments become available and the patient's health status evolves.

accurately report requirements will enhance the likelihood that the treatment regimen will be carried out accurately.[76] If the patient does not comprehend instructions or indicates low efficacy or mastery for specific tasks, reeducation, skills training, or simplification of the regimen is indicated *until* mastery of regimen behaviors occurs. Accomplishing care tasks may involve nonmedical caretaker help to achieve mastery. Experience with treatment failure can discourage both patient and provider, and negatively affect expectations for achieving treatment goals. To prevent this, as with other methods of facilitating adherence, timely feedback to correct misinformation or poorly executed self-management behaviors must be provided. Burnout and poor medical outcomes are thereby less likely. Cultural specificity of materials is preferable for all patients, but it is essential in populations who have not acculturated significantly to mainstream U.S. culture, including the use of the medical care system, or those individuals who do not speak and read English.[77,78]

Finances are central to patient adherence to the care regimen. Lack of resources is often a direct barrier to successful care. Increased availability of insurance coverage is expected to reduce this barrier as restrictions against preexisting conditions are removed.[79,80] In regards to medication, insurance-based and pharmaceutical programs can help make medications more available and affordable. However, current levels of coverage for diabetes education and nutrition education based on Medicare guidelines[81] are less than optimal to support the ongoing behavior and regimen change needed to maintain good glycemic control in a majority of the population with T2D, independent of patient-based issues of adherence. In particular, although electronic means can facilitate exchange of information between patient and provider, reimbursement for provider time during which regimen changes can be discussed and implemented is limited. The Affordable Care Act includes several provisions that directly address gaps in diabetes prevention, screening, care, and treatment. As more health coverage is provided by the Patient Protection and Affordable Care Act and the Health Care and Education Affordability Act of 2010, pharmaceutical programs are being phased out, which previously facilitated achieving standards of care for underserved and minority populations. Despite changes in coverage, finances will remain a significant barrier to achieving glycemic goals and should be addressed during management visits.

To effectively accomplish tailoring a regimen to a patient's lifestyle, the clinician can use life events and quality of well-being screening questionnaires to obtain relevant information (see Table 19.1). Barriers to achieving standards of care need to be acknowledged and discussed between the patient and provider so that optimal treatment is initiated and maintained (see the sections Patient–Provider Communication, Health Literacy). If initiation of an optimal regimen is delayed because of psychosocial barriers, worsening disease course and the need for more complex treatment can be expected to compound disease burden and difficulty in achieving desired medical outcomes.[82] Provider concerns about burden of self-care need to be balanced against the potential benefits of optimizing treatment early in disease course.[83] Optimization of treatment also becomes a topic of patient education so that this approach is incentivized, based on the potential to preserve health and quality of well-being.[82]

TREATMENT RECOMMENDATIONS

Following are recommendations to address sociocultural and life course issues that interact with disease management:

- Inclusion of significant others during medical management visits, regardless of patient age, can alert the practitioner to psychosocial issues affecting the patient's ability to carry out diabetes care tasks, particularly success in lifestyle changes and adherence to the medical regimen.
- For youth diagnosed with T2D, medical management evaluation should include parents or family caregivers. Adult-monitored self-management should be encouraged.
- Diagnosis during adulthood has the potential to disrupt social role functions for the patient. Obtaining a social history that includes role functions such as job history and finances will aid the practitioner in tailoring the regimen to best fit the patient's lifestyle. Social and physical environment should be included in the assessment.
- Inclusion of family and social supports into routine care may be necessary for the elderly because of loss of cognitive functions and mobility. Ongoing screening of these functions is needed (see Table 19.1).
- Models of care are recommended that address psychosocial barriers. They include collaborative care, the patient medical home, and distance medical management. Collaborative care and the patient medical home emphasize coordination of treatment for multiple outcomes and centralized management of information, which has the potential to reduce burden of care for the patient. Distance management can be expected to improve access to care. Use of electronic communication has the potential to reduce the need for in-person visits and further reduce burden of illness.
- In addition to patient knowledge and skill mastery, beliefs about the efficacy of treatment should be evaluated as part of treatment initiation and regimen intensification (see Table 19.1).
- Regimen modification needs to be proactive as lifestyle accommodations are made, rather than reactive to treatment failure.

PSYCHOLOGICAL AND BEHAVIORAL CRITERIA AND CONTRAINDICATIONS FOR INTENSIVE MANAGEMENT: POLYPHARMACY, INITIATION OF INSULIN, AND OTHER NEEDLE-BASED THERAPIES

Patient motivation, self-efficacy, and mastery of necessary skills are known predictors of treatment success.[84] These indicators should be evaluated and facilitated and skill mastery should be monitored as intensification is undertaken. Conversely, when patients lack these beliefs and skills, intensification should be undertaken with caution and with increased monitoring by medical care providers.

The potential impact of major psychiatric disorders that impair judgment, reasoning, or motor function or that require medications that impair a patient's cognitive or motor abilities should be evaluated during the process of treatment

Monitoring of Psychological Status

- Diabetes-specific screening tools can be used to assess the need for further evaluation of diabetes-related distress.
- Monitoring of mental well-being should be integrated into routine care.
- When screening indicates clinically significant distress, refer to a mental health professional familiar with diabetes treatment for further evaluation.
- Integrated care can facilitate better medical and mental health outcomes.
- Multidisciplinary team care that monitors periods of expected distress can help prevent worsening of mental health problems.

implementation and intensification. If initial screening by medical history or screening measures indicates current or past history of major depression, thought or personality disorders, major anxiety disorders (such as obsessive–compulsive disorder), or limited or impaired intellectual functioning (such as diagnoses on the autism spectrum, developmental delay, or dementia),[1] further psychological or psychiatric evaluation is indicated. Untreated or inadequately treated psychiatric illness will affect a patient's ability to self-manage the disease, indicating the need for external oversight of the treatment regimen. When diagnosed psychiatric illness is comorbid with diabetes, resources are needed for simultaneous management of both conditions to reduce risk for poor medical outcomes. The collaborative care model that incorporates monitoring of and treatment for mental health conditions into diabetes care has been found to be effective in improving medical and psychological outcomes for the diabetes population.[85]

Patient attitudes, beliefs, and knowledge about treatment recommendations are important to evaluate as treatment is initiated or changed.[86] A gap can exist between provider recommendations and patient motivation or self-efficacy to adopt care recommendations. Patients often are reticent to tell care providers they are unwilling or unable to implement care behaviors.

It is important for patient and providers to share a collaborative chronic illness framework for diabetes management. A chronic illness framework defines management as patient centered, ongoing, expected to change over time, and requiring complex lifestyle-based interventions. Initiation of suboptimal treatment regimens because of psychosocial barriers has the potential to increase a patient's sense of failure and burden of treatment. A "treatment to failure" approach—that is, we will try this, and if it fails, we will use more-intensive treatment modalities— has the potential reduce patient willingness to take an active role in their own care. Conversely, intensifying treatment early in the disease course (with appropriate supports) has the potential to slow disease progression and empower patients by improving disease-based efficacy and self-esteem.

Negative attitudes about burdens of care, side effects of medications, and unwillingness to make suggested lifestyle changes are contraindications to initiation of the planned regimen. For example, a majority of patients with T2D are unable to obtain glycemic targets with first-line oral agents in addition to a diet and exercise regimen.[7] When intensification of treatment is sought by the medical care provider or family members—for example, initiation of insulin—but is not supported by the patient, resolution of negative attitudes and beliefs is an expected component of care. If not resolved, treatment failure will reinforce negative attitudes about treatment efficacy and will potentiate nonadherence. Negative attitudes for patients with T2D often pertain to needle-based therapies, particularly insulin and other hormonal or incretin therapies that have the potential to affect appetite and a patient's ability to control caloric intake,[87] to restructuring of lifestyle, to avoidance of treatment side effects, and to prioritization of disease management, especially in youths, adolescents, and young adults. Negative attitudes about insulin use have been associated with experiencing hypoglycemia, having low pain tolerance, or fearing high costs and with concerns about weight gain, especially for women.[88]

Adoption of realistic attitudes about treatment intensification necessitates patient understanding of how treatment achieves glycemic control. Patients do not need to understand the pathophysiology of the disease, but rather how treatment behaviors directly affect indicators of disease state such as blood glucose, weight, lipids, and other cardiovascular function indicators. This education will help the patient and provider avoid a "treatment to failure approach" (i.e., when this treatment fails, we will intensify your care, requiring you to do more to take care of your diabetes). In other words, treatment will now increase disease burden. This approach has the potential to make the patient feel as if they have failed. In many cases, the individual has not been able to carry out the regimen as prescribed (nutrition, physical activity, and pharmacotherapy) or the patient is being undertreated based on medical need, despite adhering to recommended care. When anticipatory steps are taken to frame diabetes management as an ongoing changing process, addressing patient and provider attitudes and expectations for implementation of the care regimen, and patients clearly understand the medical efficacy of a treatment approach and potential for improved well-being, adoption of the regimen is more likely.[89] For example, there are special circumstances, such as use of an insulin pump during pregnancy, when women will "suspend" negative attitudes about using a pump because of increased motivation for glycemic control (i.e., protecting the neonate).[90] Intensification may be accepted under these circumstances but may not maintained once the pregnancy is over. Conversely, although insulin needs will decrease, women may view this more intensive form of therapy positively after pregnancy because it provides them with lifestyle flexibility after the birth of their child.[90] If, however, a patient does not understand the medical efficacy of the prescribed regimen, or is intransigent in their attitudes, intensification should be approached with caution. Continuity of care and availability of a treatment *team* can facilitate accomplishment of these tasks and prevent provider and patient burnout.[88]

TREATMENT RECOMMENDATIONS

Following are treatment recommendations to address psychological and behavioral criteria and contraindications for intensive management:

- Baseline evaluation of knowledge, motivation, and skill mastery is recommended *before* the process of intensification of the treatment regimen is begun.
- Evaluation of baseline psychological functioning is recommended *before* increasing regimen burden.
- Identification of social and instrumental supports is needed *before* intensification begins. This includes updating diabetes education, assessing availability of talk therapy and pharmacotherapy and reimbursement for costs of care, agreement to a contract for self-care by the patient and their significant others, and availability of care provider resources to provide medical monitoring for timely and appropriate changes to the regimen.
- Patient and provider attitudes about and expectations for self-care need to be assessed and reconciled in an ongoing manner to prevent patients being labeled as "bad patients."
- With appropriate supports, optimal treatment should be initiated early in disease course to prevent treatment failure, patient, and provider burnout.

SPECIAL ISSUES OF CHILDREN AND ADOLESCENTS WITH T2D

Youth are now being diagnosed with T2D as young as 7–8 years old (also see Chapter 18).[91] Youth diagnosed with T2D are usually significantly overweight and have a strong family history of the disease. In addition to genetic transmission of risk for the disease, ecological transmission of risk conferred by cultural, physical, and family environment occurs. Overweight and obesity in the U.S. has become normative, with two-thirds of adults overweight or obese, and as of 2010, more than one-third of children and adolescents overweight or obese.[92] Overweight and obese children often have overweight/obese parents.[93] Therefore sociocultural (familial and environmental) issues will need to be addressed to successfully treat T2D in youth.

To help cope with the life changes a youth must make after diagnosis, the family is an essential partner in treatment. Parental or caretaker roles will moderate depending on the age of the child. In addition to the concrete help primary caretakers provide—meals, medications, and opportunities to lead a healthy lifestyle—parental attitudes about the disease; parental role in care; and assessment of their child's ability to carry out treatment behaviors needs to be evaluated and monitored.

Family cohesion and clearly defined roles of individual family members in a child's diabetes care have been shown to be associated with better adherence in

---

Family members may not understand that T2D diagnosed in youth is the same disease with the same potential for negative health consequences as that diagnosed during adulthood. Earlier diagnosis in the life course may seem different because children look healthy and may not feel sick. Diabetes education to correct this misinformation needs to include the family, other caretakers, and the youth.

> Families with multiple members and generations diagnosed with T2D
> may have a set of attitudes (family mythologies) about the disease and
> its inevitability. Attitudes such as "We all are big in my family" and "We
> die young from diabetes" have the potential to affect adoption of medi-
> cal management behaviors and lifestyle changes. These mythologies
> must be identified and addressed as part of diabetes education.

youth with T1D and better medical outcomes (A1C).[94] Issues regarding parental involvement, however, can be complicated in "T2D families" because multiple generations of family members may have, and have had, the disease. For example, adult family members with the disease may not believe their child has the same disease, hold their child to the same standards of care, or may have heightened anxiety as they watch older family members develop complications and experience reduced quality of life. Family mythologies about the disease can affect how disease treatment is carried out in the home environment.

Although treatment dynamics are well studied in families with a child with T1D, to date, family interactions have not been well characterized in the youth population with T2D. When parental attitudes about healthy children's weight and size are evaluated, parents have been shown to underestimate their child's overweight status and the health risks of overweight.[95] These findings have been demonstrated in all ethnicities, but they occur more frequently in African American and Latino populations, which are at highest risk for development of T2D. Parents may under- or overestimate health risks of diabetes based on optimistic bias,[96] disease progression of family members with diabetes, or attitudes toward treatment. Family mythology around weight and size ("We are all big in my family") and the inevitability of diabetes will affect caretaker and youth attitudes about care behaviors and fatalism about disease outcomes. Presence of other members of the family or individuals in the home with T2D presents role models regarding disease management for the child, conferring risk or protective influence. A systems approach to care suggests that inclusion of household members in care will maximize likelihood for treatment success.[97,98]

Youth who grow up overweight, who have struggled to lose weight, and who have been warned about or have "predisease" also may develop fatalistic attitudes about developing diabetes. Children and adolescents, however, typically do not have concerns about their health, often do not feel sick before diagnosis,[91] and based on cognitive development, do not necessarily have the capacity to consider the future health consequences of their behavior.[99] Thus, treatment of youth with T2D must be shared among the child, family members, and significant others.

Major developmental issues for youth are socialization and peer acceptance, and for teens, satisfaction with body image and the drive for autonomy. Desire for peer acceptance and "sameness" can negatively affect adherence with the care regimen.[100] The need to follow a nutrition plan potentially places youth and teens at risk for noncompliance in the school setting and in the home if individuals are not following the same dietary restrictions or if the nutrition environment is not conducive to weight loss. Children do not have primary control over the food that is available to them in the home environment and will form eating patterns and taste preferences based on maternal food intake, family preferences, and local culture.[101,102] Other developmental issues specific to adolescence include increasing insulin resistance and adiposity due to pubertal development,[103] making weight and glucose more difficult to control. Changes in body habitus can contribute to body image dissatisfaction, which in turn can contribute to low self-efficacy and low self-esteem.[104] Adolescence is also known to be a period of decreasing physical activity for teens, especially girls.[105] Screen time is associated directly with overweight.[106] The combination of increasing screen time and decreasing physical activity places teens at risk for poorly controlled weight-related diabetes.[107]

Youth with T2D are at higher risk for depression, subclinical and diagnosed.[108] Adolescence, with or without diabetes, is known to be a time of frequently reported but transient depressive symptoms.[109] Preexisting psychological vulnerability may be exacerbated by diagnosis, treatment failure, or weight-related stigmatization. Lack of future orientation, a developmental task to be accomplished during adolescence, accompanied by other risk factors, may help explain nonadherence to the care regimen during adolescence, especially when teens with T2D do not "feel sick." Conversely, successful treatment associated with weight gain may exacerbate risk for the development of DEB. As with young adult women, binging behavior is the most prevalent behavior found in teens with T2D.[28]

For all youth with T2D, supportive monitoring and provision of consistent resources in the family environment will facilitate success in adjusting to illness and achieving successful treatment outcomes. Family conflict around allocation of resources, familial roles regarding supervision of the care regimen, and monitoring of self-care behaviors will potentiate poor adjustment to illness and could contribute to adoption of maladaptive weight-management behaviors. Conversely, families receiving continuing education and ongoing guidance regarding integration of treatment into the family environment will, in most cases, achieve better adjustment of their child (or adult family member) to the diagnosis[56] and better medical outcomes while successfully balancing the developmental tasks of childhood and adolescence.

One of the most difficult clinical issues a practitioner may face is the discrepancy between recommended treatment regimen for the child and that which a parent or caretaker with T2D is following. Caregivers may not understand, or want to understand (optimistic bias), that their child has the same disease, and that treatment, though dependent on the length and state of the disease, is the same. Expectations for a healthy lifestyle apply to all family members and, if possible, coordinated care of adults and youth in a family that has multiple members with T2D will normalize expectations for a healthy lifestyle and adherence to the medical regimen.

Although the American Diabetes Association has a position statement on diabetes care in the school setting,[110] the psychosocial needs of youth and adolescents with T2D within the school environment may go unaddressed because medication is usually taken at home, an Individualized Educational Plan often is not initiated based on medical need, and nutrition intake and physical activity are not designated as medical treatment within the school environment. It remains, however, that overweight and poor glycemic control can be expected to interfere with optimal cognitive performance (such as the effects of sleep apnea) and issues such as bullying and ostracism may occur for overweight or obese students.[111] Adolescents with a chronic disease are known to miss more school than healthy counterparts and have poorer academic performance.[112] Thus, these issues—the needs and treatment of youth with T2D in the school setting—are both under-recognized and understudied. The practitioner can play an important role in educating parents and caregivers to services needed for their children and can serve as an advocate in the school environment, educating teachers and students about the health risks of overweight and T2D. Education regarding the care of students with T2D and alerting school personnel to issues of bullying and poor academic performance has the potential to contribute to better adjustment to illness and greater adherence to the care regimen for youth with T2D.

TREATMENT RECOMMENDATIONS

Following are treatment recommendations to address special issues faced by children and adolescents with T2D:

- For all youth with diabetes, family member inclusion in education, medical management, and psychological support is essential.
- For youth who have other family members with T2D, family-based treatment is recommended, along with coordination of care providers so that adherence to the care regimen can be maximized in the home environment.
- For adolescents with T2D, adult-monitored self-management is recommended, with expectations that the adolescent will take increasing responsibility for self-care, with adult supervision and monitoring by medical care providers.
- Parents should be encouraged to meet with their child's school principal and counselor when a diagnosis of T2D is made to educate school personnel to the health risks of overweight, explain the need for their child to manage lifestyle behaviors (food intake and physical activity) within the school environment, and discuss expectations for school performance.
- Monitoring of depressive symptoms and disordered eating behavior should be a routine part of care so that preventive measures can be taken if elevations in symptoms occur or persist.
- Monitoring for the occurrence of weight- or diabetes-related bullying and social ostracism in the school setting is recommended.
- Teens will need help structuring opportunities to increase physical activity, decrease screen time, and improve skills to modify dietary intake.

REFERENCES

1. American Psychiatric Association. *Diagnostic and Statistical Manual of Mental Disorders.* 5th ed. Washington, DC, APA, 2013.

2. de Groot M, et al. Depression among adults with diabetes: prevalence, impact, and treatment options. *Diabetes Spect* 2010;23:15–18.

3. Wild D, et al. A critical review of the literature on fear of hypoglycemia in diabetes: implications for diabetes management and patient education. *Patient Educ Couns* 2007;68:10–15.

4. Golden S, et al. Examining a bidirectional association between depressive symptoms and diabetes. *JAMA* 2008;299(23):2751–2759.

5. Golden S, et al. Depression and type 2 diabetes mellitus: the multiethnic study of atherosclerosis. *Psychosom Med* 2007;69:529–536.

6. Engum A. The role of depression and anxiety in onset of diabetes in a large population-based study. *J Psychosom Res* 2007;62:31–38.

7. Nathan D, et al. Medical management of hyperglycemia in type 2 diabetes: a consensus algorithm for the initiation and adjustment of therapy. *Diabetes Care* 2009;32(1):193–203.

8. Gonzalez J, et al. Symptoms of depression prospectively predict poorer self-care in patients with type 2 diabetes. *Diabet Med* 2008;25(9):1–10.

9. Black S, MarKides K, Ray L. Depression predicts increased incidence of adverse health outcomes in older Mexican Americans with type 2 diabetes. *Diabetes Care* 2003;26(10):2822–2828.

10. Katon W, et al. Association of depression with increased risk of dementia in patients with type 2 diabetes. *Arch Gen Psychiatry* 2012;69(4):410–417.

11. Lin E, et al. Depression and advanced complications of diabetes. *Diabetes Care* 2010;33(2):264–269.

12. Grigsby A, et al. Prevalence of anxiety in adults with diabetes: a systematic review. *J Psychosom Res* 2002;53(6):1053–1060.

13. Rubin R, Peyrot M. Psychosocial adjustment to diabetes and critical periods of psychological risk. In *Psychosocial Care for People with Diabetes*. Young-Hyman D, Peyrot M, Eds. Alexandria, VA, American Diabetes Association, 2012, p. 219–228.

14. Schwarzer R, Fuchs R. Self-efficacy and health behaviours. In *Predicting Health Behaviour: Research and practice with social cognition models*. Conner M, Norman P, Eds. Buckingham, U.K., Open University Press, 1995, p. 163–196.

15. Rizzo M, et al. Relationships between daily acute glucose fluctuations and cognitive performance among aged type 2 diabetic patients. *Diabetes Care* 2010;33(10):2169–2174.

16. Marc-André Bédardab JM, Richerb F, Rouleaub I, Maloa J. Obstructive sleep apnea syndrome: pathogenesis of neuropsychological deficits. *J Clin Exp Neuropsychol* 1991;13(6):950–964.

17. Rubin R, Peyrot M. Quality of life and diabetes. *Diabetes Metab Res Rev* 1999;15(3):205–218.

18. Ahmed A, Karter A, Liu J. Alcohol consumption is inversely associated with adherence to diabetes self-care behaviours. *J Diabet Med* 2006;23:795–802.

19. Suter P, Vetter R, Vetter W. Alcohol consumption: a risk factor for abdominal fat accumulation in men. *Addict Biol* 1997;2:101–103.

20. Ghitza U, Wu L, Ta B. Integrating substance abuse care with community diabetes care: implications for research and clinical practice. *Substance Abuse and Rehabilitation* 2013;4:3–10.

21. Fleming M, Mundt M. Carbohydrate-deficient transferrin: validity of a new alcohol biomarker in a sample of patients with diabetes and hypertension. *J Am Board Fam Pract* 2004;17:247–255.

22. Engler P, Ramsey S. Diabetes and alcohol use: detecting at-risk drinking. *J Fam Pract* 2011;60(12):e1–e6.

23. Cullmann M, Hilding A, Östenson C. Alcohol consumption and risk of pre-diabetes and type 2 diabetes development in a Swedish population. *Diabet Med* 2012;29(4):441–452.

24. Manubay J, Muchow C, Sullivan M. Prescription drug abuse: epidemiology, regulatory issues, chronic pain management, with narcotic analgesics. *Prim Care* 2012;38(1):71–90.

25. Dworkin R, O'Connor A. Treatment of neuropathic pain: an overview of recent guidelines. *Am J Med* 2009;122(10):S22–S32.

26. Meneghini L, Spadola J, Florez H. Prevalence and associations of binge eating disorder in a multiethnic population with type 2 diabetes. *Diabetes Care* 2006;29(12):2760.

27. Nam S, Chesla C, Janson S. Factors associated with psychological insulin resistance in individuals with type 2 diabetes. *Diabetes Care* 2010;33(8):1747–1749.

28. Young-Hyman D, Davis C. Disordered eating behavior in individuals with diabetes: importance of context, classification and evaluation. *Diabetes Care* 2010;33:683–689.

29. Delahanty L, et al. Pretreatment, psychological, and behavioral predictors of weight outcomes among lifestyle intervention participants in the Diabetes Prevention Program (DPP). *Diabetes Care* 2013;36:34–40.

30. Powers M, et al. Determining the influence of type 1 diabetes on two common eating disorder questionnaires. *Diabetes Educ* 2013;39:387–396.

31. Lutz T. Control of food intake and energy expenditure by amylin: therapeutic implications. *Int J Obesity* 2009;33(Suppl 1):s24–s27.

32. Chapman I, et al. Effect of pramlintide on satiety and food intake in obese subjects and subjects with type 2 diabetes. *Diabetologia* 2005;48:838–848.

33. Monteleone P, Maj M. Dysfunctions of leptin, ghrelin, BDNF and endocannabinoids in eating disorders: beyond the homeostatic control of food intake. *Psychoneuroendocrinology* 2013;38:312–330.

34. Morris S, Wylie-Rosett J. Medical nutrition therapy: a key to diabetes management and prevention. *Clin Diabetes* 2010;28:12–18.

35. Stotland N. Overcoming psychological barriers in insulin therapy. *Insulin* 2006;1(1):38–45.

36. Bloomgarden Z, et al. Current issues in GLP-1 receptor agonist therapy for type 2 diabetes. *Endocr Pract* 2012;18(Suppl 3):6–36.

37. Hajos T, et al. Towards defining a cut-off score for elevated fear of hypoglycemia on the Hypoglycemia Fear Survey Worry subscale in patients with type 2 diabetes. *Diabetes Care* 2013;37:102–108.

38. Egede L, Ellis C. Development and psychometric properties of the 12 item diabetes fatalism scale. *J Gen Intern Med* 2009;25(1):61–66.

39. Beverly E, et al. Look who's (not) talking: diabetic patients' willingness to discuss self-care with physicians. *Diabetes Care* 2012;35(7):1466–1472.

40. Regenold W, et al. Increased prevalence of type 2 diabetes mellitus among psychiatric inpatients with bipolar I affective and schizoaffective disorders independent of psychotropic drug use. *J Affective Disord* 2002;70(1):19–26.

41. Bobo W, et al. Antipsychotics and the risk of type 2 diabetes mellitus in children and youth. *JAMA Psychiatry* 2013;70(10):1067–1075.

42. Reynolds C, Suzuki L. Bias in psychological assessment. In *Handbook of Psychology*. 2nd ed. Weiner I, Ed. New York, John Wiley & Sons, 2013, p. 882–113.

43. World Health Organization. *Adherence to Long-Term Therapies: Evidence for Action*. Geneva, WHO, 2003.

44. Rubin R. Adherence to pharmacologic therapy in patients with type 2 diabetes mellitus. *Am J Med* 2005;118(Suppl 5A):27S–34S.

45. Johnson S. Adherence to medical regimens. In *Psychosocial Care for People with Diabetes*. Young-Hyman D, Peyrot M, Eds. Alexandria, VA, American Diabetes Association, 2012, p. 117–130.

46. Hill-Briggs F. Diabetes-related functional impairment and disability. In *Psychosocial Care for People with Diabetes*. Young-Hyman D, Peyrot M, Eds. Alexandria, VA, American Diabetes Association, 2012, p. 273–289.

47. Stetson B, et al. Monitoring in diabetes self-management: issues and recommendations for improvement. *Popul Health Manag* 2011;14:189–197.

48. Wagner E, et al. Improving chronic illness care: translating evidence into action. *Health Aff* 2001;20(6):64–78.

49. Bennett Johnson S. Adherence to medical regimens. In *Psychosocial Care for People with Diabetes.* Young-Hyman D, Peyrot M, Eds. Alexandria, VA, American Diabetes Association, 2012, p. 117–130.

50. National Institutes of Health, Office of Behavioral and Social Sciences Research. Adherence. Available at http://obssr.od.nih.gov/scientific_areas/health_behaviour/adherence/index.aspx. Accessed 10 March 2014.

51. Clark C, et al. The National Diabetes Education Program, changing the way diabetes is treated: comprehensive diabetes care. *Diabetes Care* 2001; 24(4):617–618.

52. Kuh D, Ben Shlomo Y. *A Life Course Approach to Chronic Disease Epidemiology.* Oxford, U.K., Oxford University Press, 2004.

53. Case Management Society of America. Standards of practice for case management, 2010. Available at www.cmsa.org/portals/0/pdf/memberonly/StandardsOfPractice.pdf. Accessed 10 March 2014.

54. Pearson M, et al. *Patient Self-Management Support Programs: An Evaluation.* Santa Monica, CA, Agency for Healthcare Research and Quality, U.S. Department of Health and Human Services, 2007.

55. U.S. Equal Employment Opportunity Commission. Available at www.eeoc.gov. Accessed 10 March 2014.

56. Mayberry L, Osborn C. Family support, medication adherence, and glycemic control among adults with type 2 diabetes. *Diabetes Care* 2012; 35(6):1239–1245.

57. Trief P. Lifespan development issues for adults. In *Psychosocial Care for People with Diabetes.* Young-Hyman D, Peyrot M, Eds. Alexandria, VA, American Diabetes Association, 2012, p. 251–272.

58. DiMatteo M. Social support and patient adherence to medical treatment: a meta-analysis. *Health Psychol* 2004;32(2):207–218.

59. Hemphill, R. *Disease-Related Collaboration and Adjustment Among Couples Coping with Type 2 Diabetes.* (Electronic Thesis or Dissertation). 2013. Retrieved from https://etd.ohiolink.edu. Accessed 10 March 2014.

60. Katz M, et al. Impact of type 1 diabetes mellitus on the family is reduced with the medical home, care coordination, and family-centered care. *J Pediatrics* 2012;160(5):861–867.

61. Gallant M. The influence of social support on chronic illness self-management: a review and directions for research. *Health Educ Behav* 2003;30(2):170–195.

62. Kristine Yaffe MCF, Nathan Hamilton MA, Schwartz AV, Simonsick EM, Satterfield S, Cauley JA, Rosano C, Launer LJ, Strotmeyer ES, Harris TB. Diabetes, glucose control, and 9-year cognitive decline among older adults without dementia. *JAMA Neurology* 2012;69(9):1170–1175.

63. Elsawy B, Higgins K. The geriatric assessment. *Am Fam Physician* 2011;83(1):48–56.

64. Reinhard S, et al. Supporting family caregivers in providing care. In *Patient Safety and Quality: An Evidence-Based Handbook for Nurses.* Hughes R, Ed. Rockville, MD, Agency for Healthcare Research and Quality, 2008, p. 1–64.

65. Weinstein N, Lyon J. Mindset, optimistic bias about personal risk and health-protective behaviour. *Br J Health Psychol* 2010;4(4):289–300.

66. Becker G, Gates R, Newsom E. Self-care among chronically ill African Americans: culture, health disparities, and health insurance status. *Am J Public Health* 2004;94(12):2066–2073.

67. Coruh B, Avele H, Pugh M, Mulligan T, Pugh M, Mulligan T. Does religious activity improve health outcomes? A critical review of the recent literature. *Explore* 2005;1(3):186–191.

68. Marrero D, Trief P. Lifestyle modification: Exercise. In *Psychosocial Care for People with Diabetes.* Young-Hyman D, Ed. Alexandria, VA, American Diabetes Association, 2012, p. 147–158.

69. Wylie-Rosett J, Delahanty L. Lifestyle modification: Nutrition. In *Psychosocial Care for People with Diabetes.* Young-Hyman D, Ed. Alexandria, VA, American Diabetes Association, 2012, p. 131–146.

70. Harris M, et al. Racial and ethnic differences in glycemic control of adults with type 2 diabetes. *Diabetes Care* 1999:22:403–408.

71. Anderson R. Into the heart of darkness: reflections on racism and diabetes care. *Diabetes Educ* 1998;24:689–692.

72. Harris M, et al. Racial and ethnic differences in glycemic control of adults with type 2 diabetes. *Diabetes Care* 1999;22:403–408.

73. Rosal M, et al. Randomized trial of a literacy-sensitive, culturally tailored diabetes self-management intervention for low-income Latinos: Latinos en Control. *Diabetes Care* 2011;34(4):838–844.

74. Hunt C, Grant J, Appel S. An integrative review of community health advisors in type 2 diabetes. *J Community Health* 2011;36(5):883–893.

75. Cavanaugh K. Health literacy in diabetes care: explanation, evidence and equipment. *Diabetes Manag* 2011;1(2):191–199.

76. Yannakoulia M. Eating behavior among type 2 diabetic patients: a poorly recognized aspect in a poorly controlled disease. *Rev Diabet Stud* 2006;3(1):11–16.

77. Dressler W. Health in the African American community: accounting for health inequalities. *Med Anthropol Q* 1993;73:325–345.

78. Solis J, et al. Acculturation, access to care, and use of preventive services by Hispanics: findings from HHANES 1982–84. *Am J Public Health* 1990;80(Suppl):11–19.

79. U.S. Department of Health and Human Services. Patient Protection and Affordable Care Act (8/25/2010). Available at www.hhs.gov/healthcare/rights/law/patient-protection.pdf. Accessed 10 March 2014.

80. U.S. Department of Health and Human Services. About the law. Available at www.hhs.gov/healthcare/rights. Accessed 10 March 2014.

81. Centers for Medicare & Medicare Services. Medicare's Coverage of Diabetes Supplies & Services. Available at www.medicare.gov/pubs/pdf/11022.pdf. Accessed 10 March 2014.

82. National Diabetes Education Program, U.S. Department of Health and Human Services. Guiding principles for diabetes care: for health care professionals. (NDEP-16, 2011). Available at http://ndep.nih.gov. Accessed10 March 2014.

83. American Diabetes Association. Executive summary: standards of medical care in diabetes—2013. *Diabetes Care* 2013;36(Suppl 1):S4–S10.

84. Steinsbekk A, et al. Group based diabetes self-management education compared to routine treatment for people with type 2 diabetes mellitus. A systematic review with meta-analysis. *BMC Health Serv Res* 2012;12:213–232.

85. Unützer J, et al. The collaborative care model: an approach for integrating physical and mental health care in Medicaid health homes. Available at http://medicaid.gov/State-Resource-Center/Medicaid-State-Technical-Assistance/Health-Homes-Technical-Assistance/Downloads/HH-IRC-Collaborative-5-13.pdf. Accessed 10 March 2014.

86. Madden T, Ellen PS, Ajzen I. A comparison of the theory of planned behavior and the theory of reasoned action. *Pers Soc Psychol Bull* 1992;18(1):3–9.

87. Bloomgarden Z. Incretin concepts. *Diabetes Care* 2010;33(2):e20–e25.

88. Polonsky W, et al. Psychological insulin resistance in patients with type 2 diabetes. *Diabetes Care* 2005;28(10):2543–2545.

89. Bloomgarden Z. Approaches to treatment of type 2 diabetes. *Diabetes Care* 2008;31(8):1697–1703.

90. Simmons D, et al. Use of insulin pumps in pregnancies complicated by type 2 diabetes and gestational diabetes in a multiethnic community. *Diabetes Care* 2001;24(12):2078–2082.

91. Alberti G, et al. Type 2 diabetes in the young: the evolving epidemic. The International Diabetes Federation Consensus Workshop. *Diabetes Care* 2004;27(7):1798–1811.

92. Hedley AA, et al. Prevalence of overweight and obesity among US children, adolescents, and adults, 1999-2002 [see comment]. *JAMA* 2004;291(23):2847–2850.

93. Agras W, Mascola A. Risk factors for childhood overweight. *Curr Opin Pediatr* 2005;17:648–652.

94. Silverstein J, et al. Care of children and adolescents with type 1 diabetes: a statement of the American Diabetes Association. *Diabetes Care* 2005; 28(1):186–212.

95. Young-Hyman D, et al. Care giver perception of children's obesity-related health risk: a study of African American families. *Obesity Res* 2000;8(3):241–254.

96. Weinstein N. Unrealistic optimisms about susceptibility to health problems: conclusions from a community-wide sample. *J Behav Med* 1987;10(5):481–500.

97. Mulvaney S, et al. Parent perceptions of caring for adolescents with type 2 diabetes. *Diabetes Care* 2009;29(5):993–997.

98. Bradshaw B. The role of the family in managing therapy in minority children with type 2 diabetes mellitus. *J Pediatr Endocrinol Metab* 2002;15(Suppl 1):547–551.

99. Steinberg L. A social neuroscience perspective on adolescent risk-taking. *Dev Rev* 2008;28(1):78–106.

100. Suris J, Michaud P, Viner R. The adolescent with a chronic condition. Part I: developmental issues. *Arch Dis Child* 2004;89:938–942.

101. Forestell C, Mennella J. Early determinants of fruit and vegetable acceptance. *Pediatrics* 2007;120:1247–1254.

102. Benton D. Role of parents in the determination of the food preferences of children and the development of obesity. *Int J Obesity* 2004;28:858–869.

103. Moran A, et al. Insulin resistance during puberty: results from clamp studies in 357 children. *Diabetes* 1999;48:2039–2044.

104. Croll J. Body image and adolescents. In *Guidelines for Adolescent Nutrition Services*. Stang J, Story M, Eds. Minneapolis, MN, University of Minnesota, 2005, p. 155–166.

105. Kimm S, et al. Decline in physical activity in black girls and white girls during adolescence. *N Engl J Med* 2002;347(10):709–715.

106. Eisenmann J, Bartee R, Wang M. Physical activity, TV viewing, and weight in U.S. youth: 1999 Youth Risk Behavior Survey. *Obesity Res* 2002;10(5):379–385.

107. Raynor H, et al. Sedentary behaviors, weight, and health and disease risks. *J Obesity* 2012:1–3.

108. Anderson B, et al. Depressive symptoms and quality of life in adolescents with type 2 diabetes. *Diabetes Care* 2011;34:2205–2207.

109. National Institute of Mental Health. Depression in Children and Adolescents (Fact Sheet). Available at www.nimh.nih.gov/health/publications/depression-in-children-and-adolescents/index.shtml. Accessed 10 March 2014.

110. American Diabetes Association. Diabetes care in the school and day care setting. *Diabetes Care* 2011;34(Suppl 1):S70–S74.

111. Puhl R, Luedicke J. Weight-based victimization among adolescents in the school setting: emotional reactions and coping behaviors. *J Youth Adolescence* 2012;41(1);27-40.

112. Yeo M, Sawyer S. Chronic illness and disability. *BMJ* 2005;330:721–723.

ACKNOWLEDGMENT

The views and opinions expressed in this manuscript are those of the author and do not reflect the view of the National Institutes of Health, Department of Health and Human Services.

SOURCES FOR TABLE 19.1

American Psychiatric Association. *Structured Clinical Interview for DSM Disorders (SCID-5-RV).* Available from www.scid4.org. Accessed 14 March 2014.

Anderson RM, Funnell MM, Fitzgerald JJ, Marrero, DG. The diabetes empowerment scale: a measure of psychosocial self-efficacy. *Diabetes Care* 2000;23:739–743.

Beck AT, Steer RA, Ball R, Ranieri W. Comparison of Beck Depression Inventories-IA and -II in psychiatric outpatients. *Pers Assess* 1996;67(3):588–597.

Gonder-Frederick L, Schmidt, KM, Vajda KA, Greear ML, Singh H, Shepard JA, Cox DJ. Psychometric properties of the Hypoglycemia Fear Survey-II for adults with type 1 diabetes. *Diabetes Care* 2011:34(4):801–806.

Cavanaugh KL. Health literacy in diabetes care: explanation, evidence and equipment. *Diabetes Manag* 2011;1(2):191–199.

Cavanaugh K, Huizinga MM, Wallston KA, et al. Association of numeracy and diabetes control. *Ann Intern Med* 2008;148(10):737–746.

Celerier S, Plowright R, Reaney M, Bradley C. Linguistic validation, including cultural adaptation, of an updated ADKNOLW, diabetes knowledge questionnaire for international use. *Value in Health* 2009:A411–A412.

Cohen S, Kamarck T, Mermelstein R. A global measure of perceived stress. *J Health Social Behav* 1983;24:385–396.

Fairburn CG, Beglin SJ. Eating Disorder Examination Questionnaire (EDE-Q 6.0). In *Cognitive Behavior Therapy and Eating Disorders,* Fairburn CG, Ed. New York, Guilford Press, 2008, p. 309–313.

Fitzgerald JT, Anderson RM, Funnell MM, Hiss RG, Hess GE, Davis WK, Barr PA. The reliability and validity of a brief diabetes knowledge test." *Diabetes Care* 1998;21(5):706–710.

Folstein MF, Folstein SE. *Mini-Mental® State Examination, 2nd Edition™ (MMSE®-2™)*. Lutz, FL, Psychological Assessment Resources, 2010.

Hamilton M. The assessment of anxiety states by rating. *Br Med Psychol* 1959; 32:50–55.

Kovacs M. *Children's Depression Inventory Manual*. North Tonawanda, NY, Multi-Health Systems, 1992.

Kroenke K, Spitzer RL, Williams JBW. The PHQ-9: validity of a brief depression severity measure. *J Gen Intern Med* 2001;16(9):606–613.

Markowitz JT, Butler DA, Volkening LK, Antisdel JE, Anderson BJ, Laffel LMB. Brief screening tool for disordered eating in diabetes: internal consistency and external validity in a contemporary sample of pediatric patients with type 1 diabetes. *Diabetes Care* 2010;33(3):495–500.

Moos R, Moos B. *Family Environment Scale Manual: Development, Applications, Research*. 3rd ed. Palo Alto, CA, Consulting Psychologist Press, 1994.

Nath CR, Sylvester ST, Yasek V, Gunel E. Development and validation of a literacy assessment tool for person with diabetes. *Diabetes Educ* 2001;27(6):857–864.

National Computer Systems. *Symptom Checklist-90-R: Administration, Scoring, and Procedures Manual*. 3rd ed. Minneapolis, MN, National Computer Systems.

Peyrot M, Bushnell DM, Best JH, Martin ML, Cameron A, Patrick DL. Development and validation of the Self-Management Profile for Type 2 Diabetes (SMP-T2D). *Health Qual Life Outcomes* 2012 Oct 5;10:125.

Peyrot M, Peeples M, Tomky D, Charron-Prochownik D; AADE Outcomes Project. Development of the American Association of Diabetes Educators (AADE) Diabetes Self-Management Assessment Report Tool (D-SMART). *Diabetes Educ* 2007;33 818–827.

Polonsky WH, Anderson BJ, Lohrer PA, Welch G, Jacobson AM, Aponte JE, Schwartz CE. Assessment of diabetes-related distress. *Diabetes Care* 1995 Jun;18(6):754–760.

Polonsky WH, Fisher L, Earles J, Dudl RJ, Lees J, Mullan J, Jackson RA. Assessing psychosocial distress in diabetes: development of the diabetes distress scale. *Diabetes Care* 2005 Mar;28(3):626–631.

Radloff LS. The DESC-D Scale: a self-report depression scale for research in the general population. *Applied Psychological Measurement* 1977;1(3):385–401.

Spitzer RI, Kroenke K, Williams JBW. A brief measure for assessing generalized anxiety disorder. *Arch Intern Med* 2006;166:1092–1097.

Ware JE, Sherbourne CD. The MOS 36-item short-form health survey (SF-36). I. Conceptual framework and item selection. *Medical Care* 1992;30(6):473–483.

Weinger K, Butler HA, Welch GW, LaGreca AM. Measuring diabetes self-care: a psychometric analysis of the Self-Care Inventory–Revised with adults. *Diabetes Care* 2005;28(6):1346–1352.

Welch G, Zagarins SE, Feinberg RG, Garb JL. Motivational interviewing delivered by diabetes educators: does it improve blood glucose control among poorly controlled type 2 diabetes patients? *Diabetes Res Clin Pract* 2011 Jan;91(1):54–60.

Young-Hyman D, Davis C, Looney S, Grigsby C, Peterson C. Development of the Diabetes Treatment and Satiety Scale (DTSS-20). *Diabetes* 2011;60 (Suppl 1):A218.

Zung WWK. A rating instrument for anxiety disorders. *Psychosomatics* 1971;12(6):371–379.

Chapter 20

Prevention Strategies for Type 2 Diabetes

Asqual Getaneh, MD, MPH
Vanita R. Aroda, MD

INTRODUCTION

The rising prevalence of type 2 diabetes (T2D) and advances in its prevention in the past 20 years have injected a sense of urgency in the call for prevention efforts.[1–5] Distinct factors make diabetes a prime target for prevention: 1) Diabetes is preceded by a long hyperglycemia state distinct from undiagnosed diabetes that can be detected early; 2) Simple diagnostic tests can identify this preclinical phase, and 3) effective and acceptable interventions are available to prevent diabetes. The preclinical phase is termed "prediabetes" by several bodies including the International Expert Committee, and "intermediate hyperglycemia" by the World Health Organization (WHO). For the purposes of this chapter, we will refer to this preclinical phase as prediabetes.

THE PREVALENCE OF PREDIABETES

The number of people living with prediabetes worldwide is expected to increase from 316 million in 2013 to 471 million by 2035.[6] Prevalence estimates in the Middle East (6.7–17.7%), Africa (7.3–13.2%), and South and East Asia (2.7–19%) are similar, but in some pockets exceed rates in Europe (5.1–9.9%) and the U.S. (13.5%).[6,9–11] Many of the prevalence estimates for Africa, Asia, the Middle East, and Latin America, however, are extrapolated from limited surveys within populations and better data are needed to accurately gauge the burden of prediabetes.[6,9–11]

DIABETES RISK ASSESSMENT

Prediabetes is defined by glucose states that meet the American Diabetes Association (ADA) or WHO criteria for impaired fasting glucose (IFG), impaired glucose tolerance (IGT), or elevated A1C 5.7–6.4%.[12–14] There is some overlap among these dysglycemia states,[15–32] reflecting relative influence of interrelated yet distinct pathophysiologic mechanisms.[33–36] But, there is no agreement on the choice of a single best test for prediabetes screening.[2,37–39] Nonetheless, each criterion identifies individuals with greater risk for diabetes[40–45]and micro- and macrovascular outcomes[46–68] than normal glucose states. Some studies have shown differences among test criteria in risk for incident diabetes[40] and for micro-[49] and macrovascular[60,61,63,64] outcomes. However, a meta-analysis of 18 studies has not demonstrated significant differences.[58] More importantly, progression to diabetes

DOI: 10.2337/9781580405096.20

is linear without a distinct cut point for FPG[47] and A1C.[42,46,68] According to one report, the development of retinopathy also is not associated with a clear FPG threshold,[47] unlike the bimodal distribution suggested by earlier studies.[38,39] A large meta-analysis of 102 prospective studies and two large cohort studies have shown linear and direct associations of FPG with cardiovascular disease (CVD) mortality,[67] CVD events,[46,65,66] and all-cause mortality.[65]

Given the prevalence of prediabetes and the linear risk of macrovascular and possibly microvascular diseases, identifying high-risk groups using any of the ADA or WHO screening criteria could result in substantial benefit. The ADA recommends screening adults without any risk factors starting at age 45 years and at age 18 years for overweight individuals if they have at least one additional risk factor.[37] These risk factors include family history of diabetes, belonging to a high-risk ethnic group, prediabetes, a history of gestational diabetes, polycystic ovarian syndrome, CVD, hypertension, dyslipidemia, physical inactivity, and signs of insulin resistance, such as acanthosis nigricans and severe obesity.[37] If screening test results are normal, testing should be repeated at 3-year intervals.[37] The Task Force on Diabetes and Cardiovascular Diseases of the European Society of Cardiology and the European Association for the Study of Diabetes (ESC-EASD) guideline advocates a two-step approach for prediabetes screening: *1)* identifying at-risk individuals utilizing cost-efficient tools that include demographic and clinical characteristics and previous laboratory exams or a questionnaire such as the Finnish Diabetes Risk Assessment (FINDRISK) tool, and *2)* glucose testing of a subgroup identified as high risk during the first step.[2]

Several assessment tools have been proposed that incorporate clinical and epidemiologic characteristics to accurately identify those at increased risk for diabetes. A recent review distills the number of tools that are most feasible in routine clinical settings to six:[69] the Atherosclerosis Risk in Communities (ARIC) risk calculator, the Australian Diabetes Risk Assessment Tool (AusDrisk), the Cambridge Risk Score, the FINDRISK, the San Antonio Heart Study risk score, and the QDScore. The FINDRISK is the only tool extensively evaluated. It incorporates age, BMI, waist circumference, use of antihypertensive medicines, history of elevated blood glucose, physical activity, and dietary fruits and vegetables intakes;[70] and it predicts with 85% accuracy the 10-year risk of diabetes in asymptomatic individuals.[71] The Canadian Diabetes Risk Assessment Questionnaire (CANRISK) is based on the FINDRISK and includes additional risk factors, such as gender, ethnicity, education level, and history of elevated blood pressure.[72] CANRISK was validated in two cross-sectional convenience sample studies.[73]

Prevention trials have used a combination of clinical and epidemiologic risk factors and prediabetes blood test criteria to enroll participants: The Finnish Diabetes Prevention Study (DPS) used elements of FINDRISK and IGT,[74] and the U.S. Diabetes Prevention Program (DPP) used IGT and FPG 95–125 mg/dl and BMI of $\geq$24 kg/m^2, or $\geq$22 kg/m^2 for Asian Americans.[75] Further research could fine-tune risk assessment tools and diagnostic tests for better precision in predicting clinically meaningful glucose dysregulation.

DIABETES PREVENTION: EVIDENCE FROM TRIALS

There is solid evidence from several prospective randomized controlled trials (RCTs) and cohort studies among diverse groups that diabetes can be delayed or prevented among individuals identified using risk categories and prediabetes criteria.[74,76–80] These and other trials have demonstrated that lifestyle intervention and selected classes of drugs result in a reduction of incident diabetes among individuals with prediabetes (Tables 20.1 and 20.2).[79,81–90]

LIFESTYLE INTERVENTION

Several of the randomized controlled prevention trials have combined dietary and physical activity counseling and widely varying degrees of behavior modification counseling and incentives to effect change in lifestyle.[74,76–80] The DPS,[74] the DPP,[78] and the Study on Lifestyle Intervention and Impaired Glucose Tolerance Maastricht[81] encouraged 150 minutes or more of weekly moderate-intensity physical activity; the Indian Diabetes Prevention Program (IDPP)[81] and the Japanese trial encouraged 210 minutes or more weekly exercise;[80] and the Da Qing study encouraged general increase in leisure-time physical activity (LTPA).[76] In the Swedish Malmö feasibility study, participants had access to 120-minute weekly sessions of physical activity.[77] The DPS and the DPP also provided supervised exercise sessions.[74,78] The latter studies targeted weight-loss averages of 7 and 5% of body weight, respectively, and achieving a BMI goal of ≤ 25 kg/m^2 for the DPS participants.[74,78] The Japanese and Da Qing trials encouraged weight loss to reach a target BMI of 23 and 22 kg/m^2, respectively.[76,80] These cut points are consistent with the consensus that the proportion of Asians who experience increased risk of T2D at a lower BMI range is substantial. Dietary interventions when explicitly stated included reduced overall calories and dietary fat (20–30% of calories),[74,76,78] 55–60% calories from carbohydrates and 10–15% from protein,[74,78] high fiber intake,[74,79,80] and a greater proportion of vegetable intake.[79,80]

Behavior modification counseling was provided in both the DPP and DPS.[74,78] Participants were encouraged to set personal weight, exercise, and dietary goals using stages of change, motivational interviewing, and self-efficacy principles. They were counseled on stimulus control and self-monitoring behaviors correlated with weight control and physical activity.[91] The DPP problem-solving toolbox included incentives, personal trainers, cookbooks, and exercise tapes to prevent relapse.[91] The DPP also had lifestyle intervention curriculum tailored to five ethnic groups with flexibility for individualized goal setting. These approaches take elements from several behavior change theoretical models: the transtheoretical, social cognitive theory, planned behavior change, and relapse prevention models.[91]

When compared with control groups, those who participated in the lifestyle intervention arms in diabetes prevention trials had a statistically significant reduction of incident diabetes (45.2–67.4%) (Table 20.1).[74–80]

Over time, in the three RCTs that published long-term findings, the benefit of lifestyle intervention remained, but its magnitude diminished.[92–94] In the Da Qing trial, an average of 14 years after intervention ended the diabetes risk reduction

Table 20.1 Diabetes Prevention Programs with Lifestyle Intervention: Design, Methods, and Outcomes

	U.S. DPP 1996–2001	Finnish DPS 1993–2003	Da Qing China 1986–1992	Swedish Malmö 1974–1985	Indian DPP 2001–2002	Japan Prevention Trial
N	3,234	522	577	415	531	458 (males)
Design	RCT 27 sites	RCT 5 sites	RCT, cluster 33 sites	Nonrandomized 1 site	RCT	RCT
Diagnostic test	IGT & FPG >95 mg/dl	IGT	IGT	IGT	IGT	IGT
Mean age ± SD	50.6+/−10.7	55+/−7	45+/−9.1	45.9	35–55	51.5
BMI, kg/m² (SD)	34 (6.7)	31.3 (4.6)	25.8 (3.8)	26.6 (3.1) Intervention; 26.7 (4.0) Control	25.8	23.8
Follow-up (yrs)	2.8	3.2	4.51–4.62	5.0	2.5	3.64
Interventions	Lifestyle Metformin Troglitazone	Lifestyle	Diet alone Exercise alone Diet and exercise	Lifestyle	Lifestyle Metformin	Lifestyle
Goal: weight	7% weight loss	>5% weight loss	BMI = 23 kg/m²	Not stated	Not stated	BMI <24 kg/m² for control <22 kg/m² for intervention
Goal: diet	500–1,000 kcal/day <25% kcal from fat	<30% kcal from fat <10% saturated fat >fiber /1,000 kcal	25–30 kcal/kg 55–65% carbohydrate 10–15% protein 25–30% fat lower cal if BMI >25	Decrease simple carbohydrates and saturated fats, substitute PUFAs, increase complex carbohydrates Reduce calories if obese	Portion control, decrease fat, high fruit, vegetable fiber	Portion control, decrease fat, high fruit, vegetable fiber

(continued)

Table 20.1 Diabetes Prevention Programs with Lifestyle Intervention: Design, Methods, and Outcomes *(continued)*

	U.S. DPP 1996–2001	Finnish DPS 1993–2003	Da Qing China 1986–1992	Swedish Malmö 1974–1985	Indian DPP 2001–2002	Japan Prevention Trial
Exercise	150 minutes/week	30 minutes moderate intensity daily	Increase LTPA by 30 minutes of light or 20 minutes of moderate intensity	Not stated	>210 minutes/week moderate intensity	210–280 minutes/week moderate intensity
Tracking	Goal setting, self-monitoring, food records, exercise logs, weight	Goal setting, self-monitoring, food records, exercise logs, weight	Goal setting, no self-monitoring or logging		Goal setting, no logging or self-monitoring	Goal setting, no logging or self-monitoring, self-weighing weekly
Counseling	16 core curriculum sessions, individual and group first 24 weeks, lifestyle coaches	Quarterly visits with review of food records and 7 visits per year with nutritionist; 3 in first 6 weeks	Individual counseling quarterly and group counseling once weekly for 1 month and then quarterly	Small-group or individual counseling monthly for 6 months, 60-minute activity sessions twice/week under the guidance of a physiotherapist	Individual counseling session at baseline and every 6 months	Detailed instruction on lifestyle every 3–4 months
Follow-up	Every 2 months face-to-face group or individual, phone call in between	Quarterly	One group session quarterly		Every 6 months, phone contact after 2 weeks then monthly	Every 3–4 months

	U.S. DPP 1996–2001	Finnish DPS 1993–2003	Da Qing China 1986–1992	Swedish Malmö 1974–1985	Indian DPP 2001–2002	Japan Prevention Trial
Diet and exercise	Twice-weekly session, including personal training, self-monitoring weight, fat, calories	Supervised exercise offered free				
Outcomes	(3 years) 28.9% controls 14.4% lifestyle 21.7% metformin	(4 years) 23% control 11% lifestyle	(6 years) 67.7% control 43.8% diet 41.1% exercise 46.0% diet and exercise	(6 years) 28.6% control 10.6% lifestyle	(3 years) 55% control 39.3% lifestyle 40.5% metformin 39.5% lifestyle and metformin	(4 years) 9.3% control 3.0% lifestyle
Risk reduction intervention vs. control	(3 years) 58% lifestyle	(6 years) 58% lifestyle	(6 years) 31% diet 46% exercise 42% diet and exercise	(6 years) 63% lifestyle	(3 years) 45.2% lifestyle	(4years) 67.4% lifestyle
Long-term, mean follow-up	(7 years) 34% lifestyle 18% metformin	(7 years) 43%	(14 years) 14%	N/A	N/A	N/A

Note: DPP = Diabetes Prevention Program; DPS = Diabetes Prevention Study; FPG = fasting plasma glucose; IGT = impaired glucose tolerance; LTPA = leisure-time physical activity; N/A = not available; PUFAs = polyunsaturated fatty acids; RCT = randomized controlled trial.

Table 20.2 Diabetes Prevention Trials with Pharmacotherapy: Design and Outcomes

	Population*	Design	Follow-up (years)	Outcome relative risk reduction (RRR)	Long-term RRR	Adverse effects
DPP	$N = 3,234$ Age 50.6 BMI 34 kg/m^2 IGT with FPG >95 mg/dl	RCT Lifestyle ($n = 1,073$) Metformin ($n = 1,079$)	2.8	31%	18%	Mild diarrhea
IDPP	$N = 532$ Age 45.9 BMI 25.2 kg/m^2	RCT Metformin	2.5	25.4%	N/A	Not reported
DREAM	$N = 5,269$ Age 54.7 BMI 30.9 kg/m^2 IFG or IGT	RCT Rosiglitazone Ramipril	3	No significant risk reduction	N/A	No significant difference for Ramipril
ACT NOW	$N = 602$ Age 53.3 BMI 34 kg/m^2 IGT	RCT Pioglitazone	2.4	72%	N/A	Edema (12.9 vs. 6.7%)
IDPP	$N = 401$ Age 45.3 BMI 25.9 kg/m^2 IGT	RCT Pioglitazone	3	No significant risk reduction	N/A	
STOP-NIDDM	$N = 1,429$ Age 54 BMI 31 kg/m^2 IGT	RCT Acarbose	3.3	25%	N/A	Flatulence (15.9 vs. 6.1%) Bloating (9.5 vs. 2.3%)
Kawamori	$N = 1,780$ Age 55.7 BMI 25.76 kg/m^2 IGT	RCT Voglibose	3	40.5%	N/A	Mild gastrointestinal symptoms

	Population*	Design	Follow-up (years)	Outcome relative risk reduction (RRR)	Long-term RRR	Adverse effects
Glipizide	N = 37 IGT	RCT Glipizide		80%	N/A	Hypoglycemia symptoms (41 vs. 32%)
NAVIGATOR	N = 9,306 Age 63.7 BMI 30.4 kg/m²	RCT Nateglinide	5	No significant risk reduction	N/A	Hypoglycemia
NAVIGATOR	N = 9,306 Age 63.7 BMI 30.4 kg/m²	RCT Valsartan	5	No significant risk reduction	N/A	Nasopharyngitis, back pain, arthralgia hypotension
Tenenbaum	N = 339 Obese Age 42–74	RCT Bezafibrate	6.3	59%	N/A	
XENDOS	N = 3,277 Age 43 BMI 37.3 kg/m²	RCT Orlistat	4	37.3%	N/A	Mild to moderate gastrointestinal events
Heymsfield	N = 675 Age 43.9 & 44.3 I/C BMI 35.6 kg/m², 35 kg/m² I/C Obese	RCT Orlistat IGT		39%	N/A	

Note: ACT NOW = Actos Now for Prevention of Diabetes study; DPP = Diabetes Prevention Program; DREAM = Diabetes Reduction Assessment with Ramipril and Rosiglitazone Medication; IDDP = Indian Diabetes Prevention Program; I/C = intervention/control; IGT = impaired glucose tolerance; N/A = not available; NAVIGATOR = Nateglinide and Valsartan in Impaired Glucose Tolerance Outcomes Research; RCT = randomized controlled trial; STOP-NIDDM = Study to Prevent Non-Insulin-Dependent Diabetes Mellitus; XENDOS = Xenical in the Prevention of Diabetes in Obese Subjects.

*Mean age and BMI unless stated as range.

was 43% compared with 51% during the active intervention period.[92] The relative risk reduction in the DPS at the end of 4 years of intervention (hazard ratio [HR] = 0.55; 95% confidence interval [CI] 0.41–0.75) was greater compared with the cumulative risk reduction (HR = 0.614; 95% confidence interval [CI] 0.478–0.789) at 13 years.[93] In the DPP, differences narrowed between the lifestyle intervention and metformin or placebo arms in the observational phase, primarily due to fewer incident diabetes observed in the metformin (7.8 to 4.9 cases/100 person-years) and placebo (11 to 5.6 cases/100 person-years) arms and the increase in the lifestyle intervention arm (4.8 cases/100 person-years to 5.9/100 person-years).[94]

Lifestyle interventions are effective to the extent to which they are followed. Poor adherence to behavior changes has been identified as a determinant for diabetes prevention programs' lack of short-term benefit and the diminishing long-term benefit.[93–100] In the short term, participants in the DPP who self-monitored their dietary intake were more likely to lose 7% of their weight and reach their activity goals, and those who met their activity goals were more likely to achieve their weight-loss goals.[96] The DPS post hoc analysis of data among 487 men and women showed that those who increased their moderate to vigorous or strenuous structured LTPA had a 63–65% reduction of diabetes incidence. Although attenuated by diet or body weight (relative risk [RR] = 0.63; CI 0.35–1.13) for strenuous LTPA, this benefit remained statistically significant for vigorous LTPA (RR = 0.51; CI 0.26–0.97).[99]

PHARMACOPREVENTION

Since the first article on drug prevention appeared in 1975,[100] several trials have evaluated the effectiveness of several classes of medicines in reducing risk of diabetes (Table 20.2). Larger trials, the DPP ($N = 3234$) and the IDPP1 ($N = 531$), included participants randomized to a metformin arm.[78,79] Both trials demonstrated a significant reduction in incident diabetes in individuals treated with metformin (DPP: HR = 0.69; CI 0.57–0.84 and IDPP1: RRR (relative risk reduction) 26.4%; CI:19.1–35.1).[78,79] During the DPP's observational period (10 years), risk reduction was sustained although the magnitude diminished (18 vs. 31%).[94]

Studies of thiazolidinediones have demonstrated greater magnitude of benefit in diabetes risk reduction compared with studies that evaluated biguanides or α-glucosidase inhibitors.[78,79,83,85,91,100–102] In the DPP, after 2 years of follow-up, individuals who were randomized to the troglitazone arm had a 75% risk reduction compared with individuals in the placebo arm.[83] The incidence of diabetes was far lower (2 per 100 person-years) compared with rates for lifestyle intervention, metformin, or placebo arms (5.1, 6.7, 12 per 100 person-years, respectively).[83] In subsequent studies, both rosiglitazone and pioglitazone reduced the incidence of diabetes (62 and 72%, respectively).[103,104] About half (50.5%) in the rosiglitazone arm reverted to normal glycemia compared with about a third (30.3%) in the placebo arm.[103] These proportions were similar for pioglitazone.[84]

In the Study to Prevent Non-Insulin-Dependent Diabetes Mellitus (STOP-NIDDM), which randomized 1,368 individuals, after 2.2 years of follow-up, acarbose, an α-glucosidase inhibitor, was associated with a significant risk reduction compared with placebo in progression to diabetes (HR = 0.75; CI 0.63–0.90).[85] In contrast, a smaller study ($N = 301$) conducted in China did not show a statistically significant benefit (9.45 vs. 5.6%, P = 0.245) after 16 weeks of treatment with acarbose.[102]

The report on insulin secretagogues in diabetes prevention is mixed. In one study, after 18 months of follow-up, glipizde was associated with lower prevalence of diabetes (7 vs. 31%).[87] Nateglinide, a rapid-acting nonsulfonylurea insulin secretagogue, did not show any effect on diabetes risk reduction compared with placebo in the Nateglinide and Valsartan in Impaired Glucose Tolerance Outcomes Research study (NAVIGATOR).[105]

NAVIGATOR is also the only large-scale prospective RCT designed to investigate the effect of an angiotensin-receptor blocker (ARB) on the incidence of diabetes.[106] In this study, valsartan was associated with a 14% reduction of incident diabetes (P <0.001) over 5 years.[106] Other trials that included ARB treatment in their assignment were examined in post hoc analyses for effect on diabetes prevention and have found a trend towards benefit.[107-110]

Angiotensin-converting enzyme (ACE) inhibitors also have been evaluated for diabetes prevention. No benefit was observed from ramipril, an angiotensin enzyme inhibitor, compared to placebo in an RCT (HR = 1.16; CI 1.07–1.27; P = 0.001).[111] This finding was contrary to findings in several other retrospective analyses.[112-114]

Most recently the effects of fibric acid were investigated in a trial of 339 obese individuals ages 42–74 years, randomized to bezafibrate 400 mg or placebo. Development of diabetes in a median follow-up period of 6.3 years was lower in the bezafibrate treatment group (27.1 vs. 37%; P = 0.01, corresponding to a relative risk reduction of 0.59; CI 0.39–0.91).[88]

Given the epidemiologic and physiologic correlation between obesity and diabetes, two trials have evaluated the effect of antiobesity drugs on diabetes prevention. Xenical in the Prevention of Diabetes in Obese Subjects (XENDOS) randomized 3,277 individuals in Sweden to orlistat or placebo arms.[89] After 4 years of follow-up, the cumulative incidence of diabetes was 6.2% in the treatment arm compared with 9% in the placebo arm, corresponding to HR = 0.627 (CI 0.455–0.863), although this study was limited by high dropout rates in both the treatment and placebo arms.[89] A similar finding was observed in a retrospective evaluation of data from 675 obese individuals mean age 44 years randomized in the orlistat or placebo arms.[90] Diabetes risk reduction was correlated with weight loss.[89,90]

A meta-analysis of 20 trials concluded that the relative risk reduction associated with thiazolidinediones was greatest (64%), compared with α-glucosidase inhibitors (40%) and biguanides (27%).[115] There was no effect from sulfonylureas and glinides.[115] The numbers needed to treat were 11 for thiazolidinediones and 14 for both α-glucosidase inhibitors and biguanides to reduce the incidence of diabetes by 9 and 7%, respectively.[115] The effectiveness of metformin, thiazolidinediones, and α-glucosidase inhibitors is partly attributed to early treatment or "masking" of diabetes, given the relatively higher rate of diabetes in the treatment arms after the withdrawal of medicines.[85,95,116-118] Residual reduction of incident diabetes, however, points to other mechanisms.[115]

It remains to be determined whether reducing diabetes risk translates into cardiovascular risk reduction. Most studies in diabetes prevention were not powered to detect differences in cardiovascular or mortality outcomes, and the trials that have thus far reported on cardiovascular outcomes showed no significant long-term benefit from lifestyle intervention. In the DPS, after 10 years of follow-up, the differences in cardiovascular morbidity (22.9 vs. 22.0 per 1,000 person-years) and cardiovascular mortality (2.2 vs. 3.8 per 1,000 person-years) were not statistically significant between the intervention and control arms.[119] In the Da Qing trial, the 17% risk reduction of CVD deaths after 14 years of follow-up in the lifestyle intervention arm also was not statistically significant (HR = 0.83; CI 0.48–1.10), and there was no mortality benefit.[92] Unlike acarbose in the STOP-NIDDM trial, which led to a 49% relative risk reduction in cardiovascular events, no other drug intervention has shown cardiovascular benefit.[85] In STOP-NIDDM, however, a disproportionate number dropped out in the acarbose arm (30%) than in the placebo arm (19%), tempering the enthusiasm for its robust result.[85] In addition, concern over side effects and intolerance has been expressed in the adaption of pharmacoprevention. The rate of side effects is greater for thaizolidinediones compared with α-glucosidase inhibitors and metformin due to associated bone fracture in women and reported cardiovascular adverse effects.[119]

TRANSLATION OF DIABETES PREVENTION PROGRAMS TO REAL-WORLD SETTINGS

Increasingly greater attention is drawn to demonstrating effectiveness of diabetes prevention programs in usual-care or community settings. Several studies have examined feasibility and short-term benefits of low-intensity programs in real-world settings. Seventeen European countries are participating in a collaboration for the Development and Implementation of a European Guideline and Training Standards for Diabetes Prevention (IMAGE).[4] IMAGE provides diabetes prevention tools and practical guidelines targeting physicians, educators, policy makers, and other health or health care–related stakeholders. It also has developed a training curriculum and a web portal for training and quality control standards for prevention programs.[4] Linked with this initiative is the Diabetes in Europe-Prevention using Lifestyle Physical Activity and Nutritional Intervention (DE-PLAN) project.[120]

Reports from programs that implemented DE-PLAN have shown feasibility and short-term effectiveness.[121-123] In DE-PLAN, high-risk individuals identified using FINDRISK are enrolled in group or individual-based lifestyle intervention programs in primary care settings.[120] In Spain, after a 4.2-year median follow-up, 18.3% in the intervention group compared with 28.8% in the standard group developed diabetes, correlating with a RRR of 36.5%.[121] In Greece after 1 year, the number of people with IFG or IGT decreased from 68 to 53.6% in the intervention group.[122] In Finland, in programs across 400 primary care centers, data available for 2,798 after an average of 14 months follow-up showed that diabetes prevention programs could be adapted to the primary care setting.[123] Almost a fifth (18%) lost 5% of their body weight, and this was correlated with a 69% diabetes risk reduction.[123] Those who lost 2.5–5 pounds had a 29% RRR of diabetes compared with a 10% rise in diabetes in those who gained weight.[123]

The adoption of the DPP was assessed in a meta-analysis of 28 studies in usual-care settings.[124] Weight loss was the major target goal. Four of the studies were RCTs, 20 were single group pre–post studies, the remaining were nonrandomized or cluster-randomized studies. Median study duration ranged from 3 to 12 months. Of the 3,797 participants, complete follow-up data were available and analyzed on 2,916 participants, mean age of 55.1 years and BMI of 34 kg/m^2. The majority (70.9%) were non-Hispanic white and women (69.9%). The mean weight change among all the studies at 12 months was –3.99% (95% CI –5.16 to –2.83). Participants who adhered to core program elements achieved the highest weight loss, but there was no benefit in diabetes risk reduction. Of note, programs delivered by lay workers had similar benefits as programs delivered by health professionals.[124]

Similarly, trained lifestyle coaches led a 16-week group-based program in pilot sites at YMCAs in the U.S. in a collaborative program between United Health plan, the Centers for Disease Control and Prevention (CDC), and the YMCA.[125] During the pilot phase 92 individuals who had a BMI of ≥24 kg/m^2, at least two diabetes risk factors, and capillary blood glucose of 110–199 mg/dl were randomized into group-based DPP or brief counseling groups.[125] The pilot phase lasted for about a year and showed that implementing a modified DPP that was delivered by health coaches was feasible.[125] At the end of the pilot period, 72% of the 92 participants were enrolled in an 8-month lifestyle maintenance intervention program. Results from the latter program showed significant weight loss from baseline (–3.6 and –6% in the DPP-based vs. brief advice groups).[126] Now 17 YMCAs have joined the effort across the country and both the YMCA and the CDC have established training programs for lifestyle coaches that focus on nutrition, physical activity, and behavior change.[128] Given that there are 2,700 YMCAs in the U.S., it is possible that the program could have wide-reaching effect. The CDC has expanded these efforts by bringing together public and private partnerships to support and establish local evidence-based lifestyle change programs for people at risk of T2D.[127] Others have reported on the feasibility of low-intensity diabetes prevention programs in usual-care or community settings from data among diverse populations.[128–132]

COST

There has been significant debate on the cost-effectiveness of implementing diabetes prevention programs.[133] Part of this debate stems from methodological variations of cost analyses; the use of data from a limited number of trials; and to a lesser extent, the diversity in settings, components, and length of the programs from which cost-effectiveness estimates were derived. Different models used for estimating cost-effectiveness have disparate conclusions. Eddy et al. using the Archimedes model to estimate incremental cost-effectiveness ratio (ICER) projecting into a 30-year period concluded that implementing large-scale lifestyle interventions was not cost-effective at $62,600/quality-adjusted life-years (QALYs) societal cost and $143,000/QALY health plan cost, and thus advocated delaying intervention to diagnosis of diabetes.[134] This contrasts with Hermann et al.'s estimates of ICER of $29,900/QALY societal cost, using Markov's model and 70 years' projection.[135] In a more recent analysis using only the 10-year DPP data without projected estimates, the authors confirmed the assertion that lifestyle intervention is cost-effective at $4,365/QALY societal cost and $10,037/QALY health systems cost.[136] In this analysis, metformin is cost-saving compared with being cost-effective in Eddy et al.'s analyses.[134,136]

The per capita direct medical cost estimates from the DPP over 10 years were $4,572 for lifestyle intervention and $2,281 for metformin treatment compared with $752 for placebo, much lower than the medical cost of care for diabetes.[136] These estimates correspond to the cumulative QALYs accrued over 10 years, 6.89 for lifestyle, 6.79 for metformin, and 6.74 for placebo.[138]

A systematic review on cost-effectiveness of various ADA recommendations concluded that intensive lifestyle intervention at $1,600/QALY was "very cost-effective" and prevention with metformin at $26,000/QALY was "cost-effective" compared with standard recommendation and placebo, respectively.[137] The authors of this review included eight studies, seven of which were rated excellent, on the prevention of diabetes and three on screening for undiagnosed diabetes, and considered interventions that cost <$25,000/QALY "very cost-effective" and $25,000–50,000/QALY as "cost-effective."[137]

There are a few favorable reports on cost-effectiveness of diabetes prevention programs in various settings. In Australia, a semi-Markov, second-order Monte Carlo model for four health states, "normal," "IGT," "type 2 diabetes," and "dead," showed a cost-saving of $289 ($4,296) for lifestyle intervention, and an added cost of $1,217 ($4,411) for metformin per individual lifetime compared with controls. ICER per QALY gained for metformin versus control was $10,142.[138] Further models for five European countries, Australia, Germany, United Kingdom, Switzerland, and France, estimated the ICER at $8,300/QALY.[139] The cost estimates from the IDPP were much lower given the economic setting.[140] For different scenarios using physicians or group sessions in three degrees of sensitivities, the ICER estimates ranged from $753–$955 for lifestyle intervention, $965–$1,093 for metformin, and $1,028–$1,287 for drug and lifestyle combination intervention.[140]

Interventions in group settings and those that used trained nonphysician workers were more cost-effective in usual-care or community settings. Compared with costs in the DPP trial setting, a community-based group lifestyle weight-loss program among individuals at risk for diabetes was less costly ($850 in direct medical costs over 2 years vs. $2,631 for the DPP).[141]

Other considerations that could improve cost-effectiveness estimates are better adherence to intervention,[135] age at start of intervention,[142] targeting high-risk population groups,[141] and specifically individuals with hypertension.[143] In the DPP over 10 years the differential per capita cost of care in individuals who were adherent to lifestyle intervention ($4,250) and metformin ($3,251) were lower compared with the placebo arm. The corresponding accrued QALY's were 6.80, 6.74, and 6.67 for the lifestyle intervention, metformin, and placebo groups, respectively.[144]

CONCLUSION

Diabetes is a preventable disease that has an easily identifiable preclinical phase and cost-effective methods of prevention. Evidence is accumulating that diabetes prevention programs from trial settings can be adapted to usual-care or community settings. Future studies could establish whether these programs are effective in preventing diabetes and, more important, that diabetes risk reduction is correlated with reduction in CVD risks and improvement in long-term health outcomes. Consider the following summary statements:

- The worldwide prevalence of prediabetes is rising.
- Populations at risk can be identified using risk assessment tools that screen for clinical and demographic characteristics. Currently, only one, the FINDRISK, has been validated extensively.
- Despite differences in diagnostic test agreements, existing screening criteria identify populations at-risk and provide ample opportunity for the provision of preventive care.
- Lifestyle measures that institute dietary changes and exercise regimen are effective in delaying onset or preventing incident diabetes.
- Several medicines in different classes have been shown to reduce incident diabetes. The best evidence is available for metformin, thiazolidinediones, and acarbose.
- Side effects and intolerances of pharmacoprevention should be balanced with the benefit of prevention.
- Evidence is accumulating that instituting diabetes prevention programs in real-world settings is feasible and effective.
- There is no evidence to date that diabetes prevention is associated with long-term reduction of micro- or macrovascular outcomes.
- The preponderance of evidence shows that diabetes prevention efforts that institute lifestyle modification programs are cost-effective.
- Clear cost-effectiveness for pharmacoprevention has not been demonstrated conclusively, although data from the Diabetes Prevention Program Outcomes Study suggest cost-effectiveness of metformin over the long term.

ACKNOWLEDGMENT

This activity was supported in part by a KL2 award from the Georgetown–Howard Universities Center for Clinical and Translational Science, supported by the National Center for Advancing Translational Sciences, 8KL2TR000102.

REFERENCES

1. Eckel RH, Kahn R, Robertson RM, Rizza RA. ADA/AHA Scientific Statement. Preventing cardiovascular disease and diabetes: a call to action from the American Diabetes Association and the American Heart Association. *Circulation* 2006;113:2943–2946.

2. Ryden L, Standl E, Bartnik M, Van den Berghe G, Betteridge J, De Boer Menko-Jan, Cosentino F, Jonsson B, Laakso M, Malmberg K, Priori S,

Östergren J, Tuomilehto J, Thrainsdottir I. Guidelines on diabetes, pre-diabetes, and cardiovascular diseases: full text. The Task Force on Diabetes and Cardiovascular Diseases of the European Society of Cardiology (ESC) and the European Association for the Study of Diabetes (EASD). *Eur Heart J* 2007;9:C3–C74.

3. Singh RB, Rastogi SS, Rao PV, Das S, Madhu SV, Das AK, Sahay BK, Fuse SM, Beegom R, Sainani GS, Shah NA. Diet and lifestyle guidelines and desirable levels of risk factors for the prevention of diabetes and its vascular complications in Indians: a scientific statement of the International College of Nutrition. Indian Consensus Group for the Prevention of Diabetes. *J Cardiovasc Risk* 1997;4(3):201–208.

4. Paulweber B, Valensi P, Lindström J, Lalic N, Greaves C, McKee M; on behalf of the IMAGE Study Group. A European evidence-based guideline for the prevention of type 2 diabetes. *Metab Res* 2010;32(Suppl 1):S3–S36.

5. Valensi P, Schwarz PEH, Hall M, Felton AM, Maldonato A, Mathieu C. Prediabetes essential action: a European perspective. *Diabetes Metab* 2005;31:606–620.

6. International Diabetes Federation. *IDF Diabetes Atlas.* 6th ed. Brussels. International Diabetes Federation, 2013.

7. Ramachandran A, Mary S, Yamuna A, Murugesan N, Snehalatha C. High prevalence of diabetes and cardiovascular risk factors associated with urbanization in India. *Diabetes Care* 2008;31(5):893–898.

8. Hall V, Thomsen RW, Henriksen O, Lohse N. Diabetes in sub Saharan Africa 1999–2011: epidemiology and public health implications. A systematic review. *BMC Public Health* 2011;11:564. Available from http://www.biomedcentral.com/1471-2458/11/564. Accessed 18 March 2013.

9. Asfour MG, Lambourne A, Soliman A, Al-Behlani S, Al-Asfoor D, Bold A, Mahtab H, King H. High prevalence of diabetes mellitus and impaired glucose tolerance in the Sultanate of Oman: results of the 1991 national survey. *Diabet Med* 1995;12:1122–1125.

10. Karim A, Ogbeide DO, Siddiqui S, Al-Khalifa IM. Prevalence of diabetes mellitus in a Saudi community. *Saudi Med J* 2000;21(5):438–442.

11. Escobedo J, Buitron LV, Velasco MF, Ramirez JC, Hernandez R, Macchia A, Pellegrini F, Schargrodsky H, Boissonnet C, Champagne BM; on behalf of the CARMELA Study Investigators. High prevalence of diabetes and imipaired fasting glucose in urban Latin America: the CARMELA Study. *Diabet Med* 2009;26:864–871.

12. World Health Organization. *Definition and Diagnosis of Diabetes Mellitus and Intermediate Hyperglycemia.* Geneva, World Health Organization, 2006.

13. American Diabetes Association. Diagnosis and classification of diabetes mellitus. *Diabetes Care* 2010;33(Suppl 1):S62–S69.

14. World Health Organization. *Use of Glycated Haemoglobin (HA1c) in the Diagnosis of Diabetes Mellitus.* Geneva, World Health Organization, 2011. Available at http://www.who.int/diabetes/publications/report-hba1c_2011.pdf. Accessed 18 March 2013.

15. DECODE Study Group on behalf of the European Diabetes Epidemiology Study Group. Will new diagnostic criteria for diabetes mellitus change phenotype of patients with diabetes? Reanalysis of European epidemiological data. *BMJ* 1998;317:371–375.

16. Qiao Q, Hu G, Tuomilehto J, Nakagami T, Balkau B, Borch-Johnsen K, Ramachandran A, Mohan V, Lyer SR, Tominaga M, Kiyohara Y, Kato I, Okubo K, Nagai M, Shibazaki S, Yang Z, Tong Z, Fan Q, Wang B, Chew SK, Tan BY, Heng D, Emmanuel S, Tajima N, Iwamoto Y, Snehalatha C, Vijay V, Kapur A, Dong Y, Nan H, Gao W, Shi H, Fu F; DECODA Study Group. Age- and sex-specific prevalence of diabetes and impaired glucose regulation in 11 Asian cohorts. *Diabetes Care* 2003;26:1770–1780.

17. Mann DM, Carson AP, Shimbo D, Fonesca V, Fox V, Muntner P. Impact of A1C screening criterion on the diagnosis of pre-diabetes among U.S. adults. *Diabetes Care* 2010;33:2190–2195.

18. Cowie CC, Rust KF, Byrd-Holt DD, Eberhardt MS, Flegal KM, Engelgau MM, Saydah SH, Williams DE, Geiss LS, Gregg EW. Prevalence of diabetes and impaired fasting glucose in adults in the U.S. population: National Health and Nutrition Examination Survey 1999–2000. *Diabetes Care* 2006;29(6):1263–1268.

19. Marini MA, Succurro E, Castaldo E, Cufone S, Arturi F, Sciacqua A, Lauro R, Hribal ML, Pericone F, Sesti G. Cardiometabolic risk profiles and carotid atherosclerosis in individuals with prediabetes identified by fasting glucose, postchallenge glucose and hemoglobin A1c criteria. *Diabetes Care* 2012;35(5):1144–1149.

20. Christensen DL, Witte DR, Kaduka L, Jorgensen ME, Borch-Johnsen K, Mohan V, Shaw JE, Tabak AG, Vistisen D. Moving to an A1C-based diagnosis of diabetes has a different impact on prevalence in different ethnic groups. *Diabetes Care* 2010;33:580–582.

21. Olson DE, Rhee MK, Herrick K, Ziemer DC, Twombly JG, Phillips LS. Screening for diabetes and pre-diabetes with proposed A1C-based diagnostic criteria. *Diabetes Care* 2010;33:2184–2189.

22. Araneta MR, Grandinetti A, Chang HK. A1c and diabetes diagnosis among Filipino Americans, Japanese Americans and Native Hawaiians. *Diabetes Care* 2010;33:2626–2628.

23. Kramer CK, Araneta MRG, Barrett-Connor E. A1c and diabetes diagnosis: the Rancho Bernardino Study. *Diabetes Care* 2010;33:101–103.

24. Pinelli NR, Jantz AS, Martin ET, Jaber LA. Sensitivity and specificity of glycated hemoglobin as a diagnostic test for diabetes and prediabetes in Arabs. *J Clin Endocrionol Metab* 2011;96(10):E1680–1683.

25. Balding EA, Dyal L, Schoterman L, Lok DJ, Stoel I, Gerding MN, Gerstein HC, Tijssen GJ. Strategies to detect abnormal glucose metabolism in people at high risk of cardiovascular disease from the ORIGIN (Outcome Reduction with Glargine Intervention) trial population. *J Diabetes* 2011;3(3):232–237.

26. Hu Y, Liu W, Chen Y, Zhang M, Wang L, Shou H, Wu P, Teng X, Dong Y, Shou JW, Xu H, Aheng J, Li S, Tao T, Hu Y, Jia Y. Combined use of fasting plasma glucose and glycated hemoglobin A1c in the screening of diabetes and impaired glucose tolerance. *Acta Diabetol* 2010;47(3):231–236.

27. Qiao Q, Hu G, Tuomilehto J, Nakagami T, Balkau B, Borch-Johnsen K, Ramachandran A, Mohan V, Lyer SR, Tominaga M, Kiyohara Y, Kato I, Okubo K, Nagai M, Shibazaki S, Yang Z, Tong Z, Fan Q, Wang B, Chew SK, Tan BY, Heng D, Emmanuel S, Tajima N, Iwamoto Y, Snehalatha C, Vijay V, Kapur A, Dong Y, Nan H, Gao W, Shi H, Fu F; DECODA Study Group. Age- and sex-specific prevalence of diabetes and impaired glucose regulation in 11 Asian cohorts. *Diabetes Care* 2003;26:1770–1780.

28. Shaw JE, Zimmet PZ, de Courten M, Dowse GK, Chitson P, Gareeboo H, Hemraj F, Fareed D, Tuomilehto J, Alberti KG. Impaired fasting glucose or impaired glucose tolerance. What best predicts future diabetes in Mauritius? *Diabetes Care* 1999;22:399–402.

29. Herman WH, Yong MA, Uwaifo G, Haffner S, Kahn SE, Horton ES, Lachin JM, Mntez MG, Brenneman T, Barrett-Connor E; for the Diabetes Prevention Program Research Group. Differences in A1C by race and ethnicity among patients with impaired glucose tolerance in the Diabetes Prevention Program. *Diabetes Care* 2007;30:2453–2457.

30. Kramer CK, Araneta MRG, Barrett-Connor E. A1c and diabetes diagnosis the Rancho Bernardino Study. *Diabetes Care* 2010;33:101–103.

31. van't Riet E, Alssema M, Rijkelijkhuizen JM, Kostense PJ, Nijpels G, Dekker JM. Relationship between A1C and glucose levels in the general Dutch population: the New Hoorn Study. *Diabetes Care* 2010;33:61–66.

32. Zhou X, Pang Z, Gao W, Wang S, Zhang L, Ning G, Qiao Q. Performance of an A1c and fasting capillary blood glucose for screening newly diagnosed diabetes and pre-diabetes defined by an oral glucose tolerance test in Qingdao. *Diabetes Care* 2009;33:545–550.

33. Abdul-Ghani MA, DeFronzo RA. Pathophysiology of prediabetes. *Curr Diab Rep* 2009;9:193–199.

34. Abdul-Ghani MA, Jenkinson CP, Richardson DK, Tripathy D, DeFronzo RA. Insulin secretion and action in subjects with impaired fasting glucose and impaired glucose tolerance: results from the Veterans Administration Genetic Epidemiology Study. *Diabetes* 2006;55:1430–1435.

35. Meyer C, Pimenta W, Woerle HJ, Van Haeften T, Szoke E, Mitrakou A, Gerich J. Different mechanisms for impaired fasting glucose and impaired postprandial glucose tolerance in humans. *Diabetes Care* 2006;29:1909–1914.

36. Faerch K, Vaag A, Holst JJ, Hansen T, Jorgensen T, Borch-Johnsen K. Natural history of insulin sensitivity and insulin secretion in the progression from normal glucose tolerance to impaired fasting glycemia and impaired glucose tolerance: the Inter99 study. *Diabetes Care* 2009;32:439–444.

37. American Diabetes Association. Clinical practice recommendations. *Diabetes Care* 2014;37:S1–S155.

38. McCance DR, Hanson RL, Charles M-A, Jacobsson LTH, Pettitt DJ, Bennett PH, Knowler WC. Comparison of tests for glycated haemoglobin and fasting and two hour plasma glucose concentrations as diagnostic methods for diabetes. *BMJ* 1994;308:1323–1328.

39. Engelgau MM, Thompson TJ, Herman WH, Boyle JP, Aubert RE, Kenny SJ, Badran A, Sous ES, Ali MA. Comparison of fasting and 2-hour glucose and HbA1c levels for diagnosing diabetes: diagnostic criteria and performance revised. *Diabetes Care* 1997;20:785–791.

40. Gerstein HC, Santaguida P, Raina P, Morrison KM, Balion C, Hunt D, Yazdi H, Booker L. Annual incidence and relative risk of diabetes in people with various categories of dysglycemia: a systematic overview and meta-analysis of prospective studies. *Diabetes Res Clin Pract* 2007;78:305–312.

41. Shimazaki T, Kadowaki T, Ohyama Y, Ohe K, Kubota K. Hemoglobin A1c (HbA1c) predicts future drug treatment for diabetes mellitus: a follow-up study using routine clinical data in a Japanese university hospital. *Transl Res* 2007;149:196–204.

42. Pradhan AD, Rifai N, Buring JE, Ridker PM. Hemoglobin A1c predicts diabetes but not cardiovascular disease in nondiabetic women. *Am J Med* 2007;120:720–727.

43. Zhang X, Gregg EW, Williamson DF, Barker LE, Thomas W, Bullard KM, Imperatore G, Williams DE, Albright AL. A1C level and future risk of diabetes: a systematic review. *Diabetes Care* 2010;33:1665–1673.

44. Larson H, Lindgarde F, Berglund G, Ahren B. Prediction of diabetes using ADA or WHO criteria in post-menopausal women: a 10-year follow-up study. *Diabetologia* 2004;43:1224–1228.

45. Pajunen P, Peltonen M, Eriksson JG, Ilanne-Parikka P, Aunola S, Keinänen-Kiukaanniemi S, Uusitupa M, Tuomilehto J, Lindström J; Finnish Diabetes Prevention Study. HbA(1c) in diagnosing and predicting Type 2 diabetes in impaired glucose tolerance: the Finnish Diabetes Prevention Study. *Diabet Med* 2011;28(1):36–42.

46. Selvin E, Steffes MW, Zhu H, Matsushita K, Wagenknecht L, Pankow J, Coresh J, Brancati FL. Glycated hemoglobin, diabetes, and cardiovascular risk in nondiabetic adults. *N Engl J Med* 2010;362:800–811.

47. Wong TY, Liew G, Tapp RJ, Schmidt MI, Wang JJ, Mitchell P, Klein R, Kleing BE, Zimmet P, Shaw J. Relation between fasting glucose and retinopathy

for diagnosis of diabetes: three population-based cross-sectional studies. *Lancet* 2008;371(9614):736–743.

48. Klein R, Barrett-Connor EL, Blunt BA, Wingard DL. Visual impairment and retinopathy in people with normal glucose status, impaired glucose tolerance, and newly diagnosed NIDDM. *Diabetes Care* 1991;14:914–918.

49. Massin P, Lange C, Tichet J, Erginay SA, Cailleau M, Eschewege E, Balkau B. Hemoglobin A1c and fasting plasma glucose levels as predictors of retinopathy at 10 years: the French DESIR Study. *Arch Ophthalmol* 2011;129(2):188–195.

50. Karadeniz S, Kir N, Yilmaz MT, Ongor E, Dinccag N, Basar D, Akarcay K, Satman I, Devrim AS. Alteration of visual function in impaired glucose tolerance. *Eur J Ophthalmol* 1996;6:59–62.

51. Singleton JR, Smith AG, Bromberg MB. Increased prevalence of impaired glucose tolerance in patients with painful sensory neuropathy. *Diabetes Care* 2001;24:1448–1453.

52. Sumner CJ, Sheth S, Griffin JW, Cornblath DR, Polydefkis M. The spectrum of neuropathy in diabetes and impaired glucose tolerance. *Neurology* 2003;60:108–111.

53. Franklin GM, Kahn LB, Bender J, Marshall JA, Hamman RF. Sensory neuropathy in non-insulin-dependent diabetes mellitus. The San Luis Valley Diabetes Study. *Am J Epidemiol* 1990;131:633–643.

54. Mykkanen L, Haffner SM, Kuusisto J, Pyorala K, Laakso M. Microalbuminuria precedes the development of NIDDM. *Diabetes* 1994;43:552–557.

55. Metcalf PA, Baker JR, Scragg RK, Dryson E, Scott AJ, Wild CJ. Microalbuminuria in a middle-aged workforce: effect of hyperglycemia and ethnicity. *Diabetes Care* 1993;16:1485–1493.

56. Tapp RJ, Tikellis G, Wong TY, Harper CA, Zimmet PZ, Shaw JE; Australian Diabetes Obesity and Lifestyle Study Group. Longitudinal association of glucose metabolism with retinopathy: results from the Australian Diabetes Obesity and Lifestyle (AusDiab) study. *Diabetes Care* 2008;31(7):1349–1354.

57. Coutinho M, Gerstein HC, Wang Y, Yusuf S. The relationship between glucose and incident cardiovascular events. A metaregression analysis of published data from 20 studies of 95,783 individuals followed for 12.4 years. *Diabetes Care* 1999;22:233–240.

58. Ford ES, Zhao G, Li C. Pre-diabetes and the risk for cardiovascular disease: a systematic review of the evidence. *J Am Coll Cardiol* 2010;55:1310–1317.

59. Saydah SH, Miret M, Sung J, Varas C, Gause D, Brancati FL. Postchallenge hyperglycemia and mortality in a national sample of U.S. adults. *Diabetes Care* 2001;24:1397–1402.

60. Tominaga M, Eguchi H, Igarashi K, Kato T, Sekikawa A. Impaired glucose tolerance is a risk factor for cardiovascular disease, but not impaired fasting glucose: the Funagata Diabetes Study. *Diabetes Care* 1999;22:920–924.

61. The DECODE Study: Group for the European Diabetes Epidemiology Group. Glucose tolerance and cardiovascular mortality: comparison of fasting and two hour diagnostic criteria. *Arch Intern Med* 2001;161:397–405.

62. Kuller LH, Velentgas P, Barzilay J, Beauchanp NJ, O'Leary DH, Savage PJ. Diabetes mellitus: subclinical cardiovascular disease and risk of incident cardiovascular disease and all-cause mortality. *Arterioscler Thromb Vasc Biol* 2000;20:823–829.

63. Meigs JB, Nathan DM, D'Agostino RB Sr, Wilson PW; Framingham Offspring Study. Fasting and postchallenge glycemia and cardiovascular disease risk: the Framingham Offspring Study. *Diabetes Care* 2002;25:1845–1850.

64. Smith NL, Barzilay JI, Shaffer D, Savage PJ, Heckbert SR, Kuller LH, Kronmal RA, Resnick HE, Psaty BM. Fasting and 2-hour postchallenge serum glucose measures and risk of incident cardiovascular events in the elderly: the Cardiovascular Health Study. *Arch Intern Med* 2002;162:209–216.

65. Khaw KT, Wareham N, Bingham S, Luben R, Welch A, Day N. Association of hemoglobin A1c with cardiovascular disease and mortality in adult: the European Prospective Investigation into Cancer in Norfolk. *Ann Intern Med* 2004;141(6):413–420.

66. The Emerging Risk Factors Collaboration. Diabetes mellitus, fasting blood glucose concentration, and risk of vascular disease: a collaborative meta-analysis of 102 prospective studies. *Lancet* 2010;375(9733):2215–2222.

67. Asia Pacific Cohort Study Collaboration. Blood glucose and risk of cardiovascular disease in the Asia Pacific Region. *Diabetes Care* 2004;27(12):2836–2842.

68. Tirosh A, Shai I, Tekes-Manova D, Israeli E, Pereg D, Shochat T, Kochba I, Rudich A; Israeli Diabetes Research Group. Normal fasting plasma glucose levels and type 2 diabetes in young men. *N Engl J Med* 2005;353:1454–1462.

69. Noble D, Marthur R, Dent T, Meads C, Greenhalgh T. Risk models and scores for type 2 diabetes: systematic review. *BMJ* 2011;343:d7163. Available at http://www.bmj.com/content/343/bmj.d7163.pdf%2Bhtml. Accessed 20 June 2013.

70. Lindström J, Tuomilehto J. The diabetes risk score: a practical tool to predict type 2 diabetes risk. *Diabetes Care* 2003;26:725–731.

71. Saaristo T, Peltonen M, Lindström J, Saarikoski L, Sundvall J, Eriksson JG, Tuomilehto J. Cross-sectional evaluation of the Finnish Diabetes Risk score: a tool to identify undetected type 2 diabetes, abnormal glucose tolerance and metabolic syndrome. *Diabetes Vasc Dis Res* 2005;2:67–72.

72. Public Health Agency of Canada. *The Canadian Diabetes Risk Assessment Questionnaire: CANRISK.* Ottawa, ON, The Agency, 2009. Available at www.dia-

betes.ca/documents /for-professionals/NBI CANRISK.pdf. Accessed 30 June 2013.

73. Robinson CA, Agarwal G, Nerenberg K. Validating the CANRISK prognostic model for assessing diabetes risk in Canada's multi-ethnic population. *Chronic Dis Inj Can* 2011;32:19–31.

74. Tuomilehto J, Lindström J, Eriksson JG, Valle TT, Hamalainen H, Ilanne-Parikka P, Keinänen-Kiukaanniemi S, Laakso M, Louheranta A, Rastas M, Salminen V, Uusitupa M; Finnish Diabetes Prevention Study Group. Prevention of type 2 diabetes mellitus by changes in lifestyle among subjects with impaired glucose tolerance. *N Engl J Med* 2001;344:1343–1350.

75. Diabetes Prevention Program Research Group. Strategies to identify adults at high risk for type 2 diabetes. The Diabetes Prevention Program. *Diabetes Care* 2005;28(1):138–144.

76. Pan SR, Li GW, Hu YH, Wang JX, Yang WY, An ZX, Hu ZX, Lin J, Xiao JZ, Cao HB, Liu PA, Jiang XG, Jiang YY, Wang JP, Zheng H, Zhang H, Bennett PH, Howard BV. Effects of diet and exercise in preventing NIDDM in people with impaired glucose tolerance. The Da Qing IGT and Diabetes Study. *Diabetes Care* 1997;20(4):537-44.

77. Eriksson KF, Lindgiirde E. Prevention of type 2 (non-insulin-dependent) diabetes mellitus by diet and physical exercise. The 6-year Malmö Feasibility study. *Diabetologia* 1991;34:891–898.

78. Knowler WC, Barrett-Connor E, Fowler SE, Hamman RF, Lachin JM, Walker EA, Nathan DM. The Diabetes Prevention Program Research Group. Reduction in the incidence of type 2 diabetes with lifestyle intervention or metformin. *N Engl J Med* 2002;346:393–403.

79. Ramachandran A, Snehalatha C, Mary S, Mukesh B, Bhaskar AD, Vigay V. Indian Diabetes Prevention Programme (IDPP). The Indian Diabetes Prevention Programme shows that lifestyle modification and metformin prevent type 2 diabetes in Asian Indian subjects with impaired glucose tolerance (IDPP-1). *Diabetologia* 2006;49(2):289–297.

80. Kosaka K, Noda M, Kuzuya T. Prevention of type 2 diabetes by lifestyle intervention: a Japanese trial in IGT males. *Diabetes Res Clin Pract* 2005;67(2):152–162.

81. Roumen C, Corpeleijn E, Feskens EJM, Mensink M, Saris WH, Blaak EE. Impact of 3-year lifestyle intervention on postprandial glucose metabolism: the SLIM study. *Diabet Med* 2008;25:597–605.

82. Penn L, White M, Oldroyd J, Walker M, Alberti KG, Mathers JC. Prevention of type 2 diabetes in adults with impaired glucose tolerance; the European diabetes prevention RCT in Newcastle upon Tyne UK. *BMC Public Health* 2009;9:342.

83. Knowler WC, Hamman RF, Edelstein SL, Barrett-Connor E, Ehrmann DA, Walker EA, Fowler SE, Nathan DM, Kahn SE. Diabetes Prevention Pro-

gram. Prevention of type 2 diabetes with troglitazone in the Diabetes Prevention Program. *Diabetes* 2005;54(4):1150–1156.

84. DeFronzo RA, Tripathy D, Schwenke DC, Banerji M, Bray GA, Buchanan TA, Clement SC, Henry RR, Hodis HN, Kitabchi AE, Mack WJ, Mudaliar S, Ratner RE, Williams K, Stentz FB, Musi N, Reaven PD; ACT NOW Study. Pioglitazone for diabetes prevention in impaired glucose tolerance. *N Engl J Med* 2011;364(12):1104–1115.

85. Chiasson JL, Josse RG, Gomis R, Hanefeld M, Karasik A, Laakso M; STOP-NIDDM Trial Research Group. Acarbose for prevention of type 2 diabetes mellitus: the STOP-NIDDM randomised trial. *Lancet* 2002;359(9323):2072–2077.

86. Kawamori R, Tajima N, Iwamoto Y, Kashiwagi A, Shimamoto K, Kaku K; Voglibose Ph-3 Study group. Voglibose for prevention of type 2 diabets mellitus: a randomized double –blind trial in Japanese individuals with impaired glucose tolerance. *Lancet* 2009;373(9675):1607–1613.

87. Eriksson JG, Lehtovirta M, Ehrnstrom B, Slamela S, Groop L. Long term beneficial effects of glipizide treatment on glucose tolerance in subjects with impaired glucose tolerance. *J Intern Med* 2006;259(6):553–560.

88. Tenenbaum A, Motro M, Fisman EZ, Adler Y, Shemesh J, Tanne D, Leor J, Boyko V, Schammenthal E, Behar S. Effect of bezafibrate on incidence of type 2 diabetes mellitus in obese patients. *Eur Heart J* 2005;26:2032–2038.

89. Torgerson JS, Hauptman J, Boldrin MN, Sjostrom L. XENical in the prevention of Diabetes in Obese Subjects (XENDOS) study: a randomized study of orlistat as an adjunct to lifestyle changes for the prevention of type 2 diabetes in obese patients. *Diabetes Care* 2004;27:155–161.

90. Heymsfield SB, Segal KR, Hauptman J, Lucas CP, Boldrin MN, Rissanen A, Wilding JP, Sjöström L. Effects of weight loss with orlitstat on glucose tolerance and progression to type 2 diabetes in obese adults. *Arch Intern Med* 2000;160:1321–1326.

91. Baker MK, Simpson K, Lloyd B, Bauman AE, Singh MA. Behavioral strategies in diabetes prevention programs: a systematic review of randomized controlled trials. *Diabetes Res Clin Pract* 2011;91(1):1–12.

92. Li G, Zhang P, Wang J, Gregg EW, Yang W, Gong Q, Li H, Li H, Jiang Y, An Y, Shuai Y, Zhang B, Zhang J, Thompson TJ, Gerzoff RB, Roglic G, Hu Y, Bennett PH. The long-term effect of lifestyle interventions to prevent diabetes in the China Da Qing Diabetes Prevention Study: a 20-year follow-up study. *Lancet* 2008;371(9626):1783–1799.

93. Lindström J, Peltonen M, Eriksson JG, Ilanne-Parikka P, Aunola S, Keinänen-Kiukaanniemi S, Uusitupa M, Tuomilehto J; Finnish Diabetes Prevention Study (DPS). Improved lifestyle and decreased diabetes risk over 13 years: long-term follow-up of the randomised Finnish Diabetes Prevention Study (DPS). *Diabetologia* 2013;56(2):284–293.

94. Diabetes Prevention Program Research Group. 10-year follow-up of diabetes incidence and weight loss in the Diabetes Prevention Program Outcomes Study. *Lancet* 2009;374(9702):1677–1686.

95. Perreault L, Pan Q, Mather KJ, Watson KE, Hamman RF, Kahn SE; Diabetes Prevention Program Research Group. Effect of regression from prediabetes to normal glucose regulation on long-term reduction in diabetes risk: results from the Diabetes Prevention Program Outcomes Study. *Lancet* 2012;379(9833):2243–2251.

96. Wing RR, Hamman RF, Bray GA, Delahanty L, Edelsteing SL, Hill JO, Horton ES, Hoskin MA, Kriska A, Lachin J, Mayer-Davis EJ, Pi-Sunyer X, Regensteiner JG Wylie-Roselt J; Diabetes Prevention Program Research. Achieving weight and activity goals among Diabetes Prevention Program lifestyle participants. *Obes Res* 2004;12(9):1426–1434.

97. Roumen C, Feskens EJ, Corpeleijn E, Mensink M, Saris WH, Blaak EE. Predictors of lifestyle intervention outcome and dropout: the SLIM study. *Eur J Clin Nutr* 2001;65(10):1141–1147.

98. Lindahl B, Nilsson TK, Borch-Johnsen K, Roder ME, Soderberg S, Widman L, Hallmans G, Jansson JH. A randomized lifestyle intervention with 5-year follow-up in subjects with impaired glucose tolerance: pronounced short-term impact but long-term adherence problems. *Scand J Public Health* 2009;37(4):434–442.

99. Laaksonen DE, Lindström J, Lakka TA, Eriksson JG, Niskanen L, Wikström K, Aunola S, Keinänen-Kiukaanniemi S, Laakso M, Valle TT, Ilanne-Parikka P, Louheranta A, Hämäläinen H, Rastas M, Salminen V, Cepaitis Z, Hakumäki M, Kaikkonen H, Härkönen P, Sundvall J, Tuomilehto J, Uusitupa M; Finnish Diabetes Prevention Study. Physical activity in the prevention of type 2 diabetes: the Finnish Diabetes Prevention Study. *Diabetes* 2005;54(1):158–165.

100. Neumann VI, Michaelis D, Schulz B, Wulfert P, Heinke P. Results of long-term biguanide therapy as a preventive measure in protodiabetes. *Endokrinologie* 1975;64(3):290–298.

101. Buchanan TA, Xiang AH, Peters RK, Kjos SL, Marroquin A, Goico J, Ochoa C, Tan S, Berkowitz K, Hodis HN, Azen SP. Preservation of pancreatic beta-cell function and prevention of type 2 diabetes by pharmacological treatment of insulin resistance in high-risk Hispanic women. *Diabetes* 2002;51:2796–2803.

102. Pan CY, Gao Y, Chen JW, Luo BY, Fu ZZ, Lu JM, Guo SH, Cheng H. Efficacy of acarbose in Chinese subjects with impaired glucose tolerance. *Diabetes Res Clin Pract* 2003;61(3):183–190.

103. DREAM (Diabetes REduction Assessment with ramipril and rosiglitazone Medication) Trial Investigators. Effect of rosiglitazone on the frequency of diabetes in patients with impaired glucose tolerance or impaired fasting glucose: a randomised controlled trial. *Lancet* 2006;368:1096–1105.

104. Xiang AH, Peters RK, Kjos SL, Marroquin A, Goico J, Ochoa C, Kawakubo M, Buchanan TA. Effect of pioglitazone on pancreatic beta-cell function and diabetes risk in Hispanic women with prior gestational diabetes. *Diabetes* 2006;55:517–522.

105. NAVIGATOR (Nateglinide and Valsartan in Impaired Glucose Tolerance Outcomes Research) Study Group. Effect of nateglinide on the incidence of diabetes and cardiovascular events. *N Engl J Med* 2010;362:1463–1476.

106. NAVIGATOR Study Group. Effect of Valsartan on the incidence of diabetes and cardiovascular events. *N Engl J Med* 2010;362:1477–1490.

107. The Telmisartan Randomised AssessmeNT Study in ACE iNTolerant subjects with cardiovascular Disease (TRANSCEND) Investigators. Effects of the angiotensin receptor blocker telmisartan on cardiovascular events in high-risk patients intolerant to angiotensin-converting enzyme inhibitors: a randomised controlled trial. *Lancet* 2008;372:1174–1183.

108. Dahlöf B, Devereux RB, Kjeldsen SE, Julius S, Beevers G, de Faire U, Fyhrquist F, Ibsen H, Kristiansson K, Lederballe-Pedersen O, Lindholm LH, Nieminen MS, Omvik P, Oparil S; for the LIFE Study Group. Cardiovascular morbidity and mortality in the Losartan Intervention for Endpoint Reduction in Hypertension Study (LIFE): a randomized trial against atenolol. *Lancet* 2002;359:995–1003.

109. Arase Y, Suzuki F, Suzuki Y, Akuta N, Kobayashi M, Kawamura Y, Yatsuji H, Sezaki H, Hosaka T, Hirakawa M, Saito S, Ikeda K, Kobayashi M, Kumada H, Kobayashi T. Losartan reduces the onset of type 2 diabetes in hypertensive Japanese patients with chronic hepatitis C. *J Med Virol* 2009;81(9):1584–1590.

110. Aksnes TA, Kjeldsen SE, Rostrup M, Omvik P, Hua TA, Julius S. Impact of new onset diabetes mellitus on cardiac outcomes in the Valsartan Antihypertensive Long-Term Use Evaluation (VALUE) trial population. *Hypertension* 2007;50:467–473.

111. DREAM Trial Investigators. Effect of ramipril on the incidence of diabetes. *N Engl J Med* 2006;355:1551–1562.

112. Wright JT Jr, Harris-Haywood S, Pressel S, Barzilay J, Baimbridge C, Baeis C, Basile JN, Black HR, Dart R, Gupta AK, Hamilton BP, Einhorn PT, Haywood LJ, Jafri SZ, Louis GT, Wheltaon PK, Scott CL, Simmons DL, Stanford C, Davis BR. Clinical outcomes by race in hypertensive patients with and without the metabolic syndrome: antihypertensive and Lipid-Lowering Treatment to Prevent Heart Attack Trial (ALLHAT). *Arch Intern Med* 2008;168:207–217.

113. Zidek W, Schrader J, Lüders S, Matthaei S, Hasslacher C, Hoyer J, Bramlage P, Sturm CD, Paar WD. First-line antihypertensive treatment in patients with pre-diabetes: rationale, design and baseline results of the ADaPT investigation. *Cardiovasc Diabetol* 2008. Published online Jul 24;7:22. doi: 10.1186/1475-2840-7-22. Accessed 10 June 2013.

114. Niklason A, Hedner T, Niskanen L, Lanke J; Captopril Prevention Project Study Group. Development of diabetes is retarded by ACE inhibition in hypertensive patients: a subanalysis of the Captopril Prevention Project (CAPPP). *J Hypertens* 2004;22(3):645–652.

115. Phung OJ, Sood NA, Sill BE, Coleman CI. Oral anti-diabetic drugs for the prevention of type 2 diabetes. *Diabet Med* 2011;28(8):948–964.

116. Gerstein HC, Yusuf S, Bosch J, et al., DREAM (Diabetes Reduction Assessment with Ramipril and Rosiglitazone Medication) Trial Investigators: effect of rosiglitazone on the frequency of diabetes in patients with impaired glucose tolerance or impaired fasting glucose: a randomized controlled trial. *Lancet* 2006;368:1096–1105.

117. van de Laar FA, Lucassen PLBJ, Akkermans RP, van de Lisdonk EH, De Grauw WJC. Alpha glucosidase inhibitors for people with impaired glucose tolerance or impaired fasting blood glucose. *Cochrane Database of Systematic Reviews* 2006;4CD005061.

118. Diabetes Prevention Program Research Group. Effects of withdrawal from metformin on the development of diabetes in the Diabetes Prevention Program. *Diabetes Care* 2003;26:977–980.

119. Uusitupa, M, Peltonen M, Lindström J, Sirkka A, Ilanne-Parikka P, Keinänen-Kiukaanniemi S; for the Finnish Diabetes Prevention Study Group. Ten-year mortality and cardiovascular morbidity in the Finnish Diabetes Prevention Study: secondary analysis of the randomized trial. *PLoS One* 4(5):e5656. Published online May 21, 2009. doi:10.1371/journal.pone.0005656. Accessed 18 June 2013.

120. Schwartz PE, Lindström J, Kissimova-Scarbeck K, Szybinski Z, Barengo NC, Peltonen M, Tuomilehto J; DE-PLAN project. The European perspective of type 2 diabetes prevention: Diabetes in Europe—Prevention Using Lifestyle, Physical Activity and Nutritional Intervention (DE-PLAN) project. *Exp Clin Endorinol Diabetes* 2008;116:167–172.

121. Costa B, Barrio F, Cabré JJ, Piñol JL, Cos X, Solé C, Bolíbar B, Basora J, Castell C, Solà-Morales O, Salas-Salvadó J, Lindström J, Tuomilehto J; DE-PLAN-CAT Research Group. Delaying progression to type 2 diabetes among high-risk Spanish individuals is feasible in real-life primary health-care settings using intensive lifestyle intervention. *Diabetologia* 2012;55(5):1319–1328.

122. Makrilakis K, Liatis S, Grammatikou S, Perrea D, Katsilambros N. Implementation and effectiveness of the first community lifestyle intervention programme to prevent type 2 diabetes in Greece. The DE-PLAN study. *Diabet Med* 2010;27(4):459–465.

123. Saaristo T, Moilanen L, Korpi-Hyövälti E, Vanhala M, Saltevo J, Niskanen L, Jokelainen J, Peltonen M, Oksa H, Tuomilehto J, Uusitupa M, Keinänen-Kiukaanniemi S. Lifestyle intervention for prevention of type 2 diabetes in

primary health care: one-year follow up of the Finnish National Diabetes Prevention Program (FIN-D2D). *Diabetes Care* 2010;33:2146–2151.

124. Ali MK, Echouffo-Tcheugui JB, Williamson D. How effective were life style interventions in real-world settings that were modeled after the Prevention Program? *Health Affairs* 2013;31(1):67–75.

125. Ackermann RT, Finch EA, Brizendnie E, Shou H, Marrero DG. Translating the Diabetes Prevention Program in to the community: the DEPLOY pilot study. *Am J Prev Med* 2008;35(4):357–363.

126. Ackermann RT, Finch EA, Caffre HM, Lipscomb ER, Hays LM, Saha C. Long-term effects of a community-based lifestyle intervention to prevent type 2 diabetes: the DEPLOY extension pilot study. *Chronic Illn* 2011;7(4):279–290.

127. National Diabetes Prevention Program. Centers for Disease Control and Prevention. Available at www.cdc.gov/diabetes/prevention/about.htm. Accessed 16 November 2013.

128. Ockene IS, Tellez TL, Rosal MC, Reed GW, Mordes J, Merriam PA, Olendzki BC, Handelman G, Nicolosi R, Ma Y. Outcomes of a Latino community-based intervention for the prevention of diabetes: the Lawrence Latino Diabetes Prevention Project. *Am J Public Health* 2012;102(2):336–342.

129. Johnson M, Jones R, Freeman C, Woods HB, Gillett M, Goyder E. Can diabetes prevention programmes be translated effectively into real-world settings and still deliver improved outcomes? A synthesis of evidence. *Diabet Med* 2013;30:3–15.

130. Ma J, Yank V, Xiao L, Lavori PW, Wilson SR, Rosas LG, Stafford RS. Translating the Diabetes Prevention Program lifestyle intervention for weight loss into primary care: a randomized trial. *JAMA Intern Med* 2013;173(2):113–121.

131. Aldana SG, Barlow M, Smith R, Yanowitz FG, Adams T, Loveday L, Arbuckle J, LaMonte MJ. The Diabetes Prevention Program: a worksite experience. *AAOHN J* 2005;53(11):499–505.

132. Watanabe M, Yamaoka K, Yokotsuka M, Tango T. Randomized controlled trial of a new dietary education program to prevent type 2 diabetes in a high-risk group of Japanese male workers. *Diabetes Care* 2003;26(12):3209–3214.

133. Narayan KM, Thompson TJ, Boyle JP, Beckles GL, Engelgau MM, Vinicor F, Williamson DF. The use of population attributable risk to estimate the impact of prevention and early detection of type 2 diabetes on population-wide mortality risk in US males. *Health Care Manag Sci* 1999;2(4):223–227.

134. Eddy DM, Schlessinger L, Kahn R. Clinical outcomes and cost-effectiveness of strategies for managing people at high risk for diabetes. *Ann Intern Med* 2005;143:251–264.

135. Herman WH, Hoerger TJ. Brandle M, Hicks K, Sorensen S, Zhang P, Hamman RF, Ackermann RT, Engelgau MM, Ratner RE; for the Diabetes Pre-

vention Program Research Group. The cost-effectiveness of lifestyle modification or metformin in preventing type 2 diabetes in adults with impaired glucose tolerance. *Ann Intern Med* 2005;142;323–332.

136. Diabetes Prevention Program Research Group. The 10-year cost-effectiveness of lifestyle intervention or metformin for diabetes prevention: an intent-to-treat analysis of the DPP/DPPOS. *Diabetes Care* 2012;35(4):723–730.

137. Li R, Zhang P, Baker LW, Chowdhury FM, Zhang X. Cost-effectiveness of interventions to prevent and control diabetes mellitus. A systematic review. *Diabetes Care* 2010;22:1872–1894.

138. Palmer AJ, Tucker DM. Cost and clinical implications of diabetes prevention in an Australian setting: a long-term modeling analysis. *Prim Care Diabetes* 2012;6(2):109–121.

139. Palmer AJ, Roze S, Valentine WJ, Spinas GA, Shaw JE, Zimmet PZ. Intensive lifestyle changes or metformin in patients with impaired glucose tolerance: modeling the long-term health economic implications of the diabetes prevention program in Australia, France, Germany, Switzerland and the United Kingdom. *Clin Ther* 2004;26(2):304–321.

140. Ramachandran A, Snehalatha C, Yamuna A, Mary S, Ping Z. Cost-effectiveness of the interventions in the primary prevention of diabetes among Asian Indians: within-trial results of the Indian Diabetes Prevention Program. *Diabetes Care* 2007;30:2548–2552.

141. Lawlor MS, Blackwell CS, Isom SP, Katula JA, Vitolins MZ, Morgan TM, Goff DC. Cost of a group translation of the Diabetes Prevention Program: healthy living partnerships to prevent diabetes. *Am J Preventive Med* 2013;44(4):S381–S389.

142. Neumann A, Schowarz P, Lindholm L. Estimating the cost-effectiveness of lifestyle intervention programmes to prevent diabetes based on an example from Germany: Markov modeling. *Cost Eff Resour Alloc* 2011;9(1):17. Published online Nov 18, 2011. doi: 10.1186/1478-7547-9-17. Accessed 16 November 2013.

143. CDC Diabetes Cost-Effectiveness Study Group, Centers for Disease Control and Prevention. The cost-effectiveness of screening for type 2 diabetes. *JAMA* 1998;280(20):1757–1763.

144. Herman WH, Edelstein SL, Ratner RE, Montez MG, Achermann RT, Orchard TJ, Foulkes MA, Zhang P, Saudek CD, Brown MB; The Diabetes Prevention Program Research Group. Effectiveness and cost-effectiveness of diabetes prevention among adherent participants. *Am J Manag Care* 2013:19(3):194–202.

Chapter 21
Metformin
Clifford J. Bailey, PhD

In 1995, metformin was introduced in the U.S. for the treatment of hyperglycemia in patients with type 2 diabetes (T2D), having been used in Europe since
the early 1960s. It acts to counter insulin resistance and has several potential
benefits against risk factors for vascular disease that are independent of glycemic
control. It may also be of use for other conditions associated with insulin resistance,
such as polycystic ovarian syndrome (PCOS), and is receiving attention for possible
antineoplastic properties.

Metformin is a member the class of drugs known as biguanides, which are
guanidine derivatives (Figure 21.1). Guanidine is found in the plant *Galega officinalis* (goat's rue or French lilac), which was used in medieval Europe as a treatment
for diabetes. Other biguanides, notably phenformin and buformin, were introduced for the treatment of T2D but were withdrawn because of a significant incidence of associated lactic acidosis. Metformin does not have this risk if
appropriately prescribed and now is used widely as a monotherapy and in combination with other blood glucose–lowering agents.

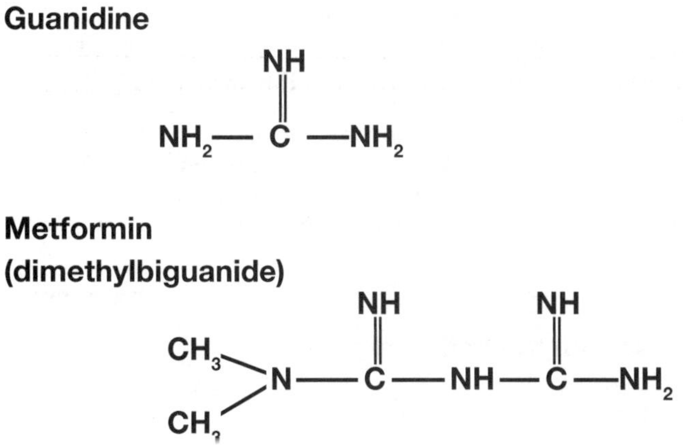

Guanidine

**Metformin
(dimethylbiguanide)**

Figure 21.1—Structures of guanidine and metformin.

DOI: 10.2337/9781580405096.21

MODE OF ACTION AND RATIONALE FOR USE

Key features of the therapeutic effect of metformin in patients with T2D are as follows:

- Metformin counters insulin resistance; it does not stimulate insulin secretion.
- Metformin decreases mainly fasting (and also postprandial) hyperglycemia in patients with T2D.
- Monotherapy with metformin does not cause hypoglycemia.
- The antidiabetic action of metformin requires some circulating insulin.
- Metformin treatment does not cause weight gain and can assist modest weight loss in overweight patients with T2D.
- Metformin treatment often improves the lipid profile.
- Metformin treatment can improve other vascular risk factors (e.g., it can increase fibrinolysis).
- Metformin has been shown to reduce vascular mortality when used as initial antidiabetic therapy in overweight and obese patients with T2D.

BLOOD GLUCOSE LOWERING

Metformin is an antihyperglycemic agent (rather than a hypoglycemic agent); when used as monotherapy, it lowers blood glucose concentrations in patients with T2D without causing overt hypoglycemia. Also, it has little effect on blood glucose concentrations in individuals without diabetes. Although the antihyperglycemic efficacy of metformin requires the presence of insulin, metformin does not stimulate insulin secretion. Some effects of metformin are mediated via increased insulin action (so-called insulin-sensitizing effects), and some are not directly insulin dependent.

The main blood glucose–lowering effects of metformin are summarized in Table 21.1. Fasting hyperglycemia is reduced predominantly by decreased hepatic glucose production, principally because of reduced gluconeogenesis but also through reduced glycogenolysis. At therapeutic concentrations, metformin suppresses hepatic gluconeogenesis by potentiating the effect of insulin and increasing the activity of adenosine monophosphate (AMP)-activated protein kinase. Metformin also can reduce hepatic extraction of lactate. The rate of glycogenolysis is decreased by reducing the effect of glucagon and impeding the activity of hepatic glucose-6-phosphatase.

Table 21.1 Mechanisms for the Antihyperglycemic Effect of Metformin

- Suppression of hepatic glucose production
- Increased insulin-mediated muscle glucose uptake
- Increased intestinal glucose utilization

Insulin-mediated glucose uptake and utilization by skeletal muscle is enhanced during treatment with metformin. Euglycemic-hyperinsulinemic clamp studies in patients with T2D typically have noted an increase in glucose uptake by ~20%, although this is not a consistent finding and appears to be influenced by the severity of the diabetic state, extent of weight reduction, and duration of therapy. Metformin increases the translocation of insulin-sensitive glucose transporters into the cell membrane and promotes the insulin- and glucose-sensitive transport properties of glucose transporters. The increased cellular uptake of glucose is associated with increased glycogen synthase activity and glycogen deposition.

Insulin-independent effects of metformin also contribute to a lowering of blood glucose. High concentrations of metformin—for example, in the walls of the intestine—can suppress the respiratory chain at complex I, reduce the ATP:AMP ratio and favor anaerobic metabolism. This promotes energy consumption through increased glucose turnover, particularly glucose-to-lactate-to-glucose recycling in the splanchnic bed, which may benefit both the blood glucose–lowering and weight-stabilizing effects of metformin. Although basal insulin levels usually are decreased slightly during metformin therapy, prandial insulin responses often are maintained relative to the glycemic excursion, which possibly are associated with deferred absorption of glucose more distally along the intestinal tract and increased secretion of glucagon-like peptide-1 (GLP-1). Metformin also has been reported to reduce hypertriglyceridemia and improve the glucose–fatty acid (Randle) cycle. Thus, metformin exerts a variety of different actions to a modest extent that contribute cumulatively to the glucose-lowering effect.

NONGLYCEMIC EFFECTS

In addition to its antihyperglycemic actions, metformin has been reported to counter several cardiometabolic risk factors and markers attributed to the "metabolic syndrome," as summarized in Table 21.2. While reducing insulin resistance, metformin therapy can lower fasting hyperinsulinemia, prevent weight gain, improve the lipid profile, and decrease certain thrombotic factors. Such actions potentially could reduce vascular risk.

Circulating concentrations of triglycerides and LDL cholesterol usually are reduced by metformin in individuals with raised levels, but there is little or no effect when these parameters are already within the normal range. HDL cholesterol concentrations are slightly raised in some individuals during metformin therapy.

Several actions of metformin oppose the procoagulant state of T2D (e.g., fibrinolytic activity is increased, sensitivity to platelet-aggregating agents is decreased, and plasminogen activator inhibitor-1 [PAI-1] levels are decreased). The U.K. Prospective Diabetes Study (UKPDS) found that use of metformin as initial antidiabetic therapy in overweight patients with T2D reduced macrovascular complications and increased survival compared with equivalent glycemic control by other agents (sulfonylureas or insulin) during a mean follow-up of 10 years. Other studies have reported a lower rate of major cardiovascular events among patients with T2D receiving metformin compared with other glucose-lowering therapies.

Despite occasional claims to the contrary, most studies and clinical experience have found no significant effect of metformin on blood pressure. There have been

Table 21.2 Effects of Metformin to Counter Insulin Resistance (Metabolic) Syndrome

Features of the insulin resistance syndrome	Effects of metformin to counter insulin resistance syndrome
Insulin resistance	Counters insulin resistance (e.g., suppress hepatic glucose production and enhance muscle glucose uptake)
Hyperinsulinemia	Reduces fasting hyperinsulinemia
Abdominal obesity	Typically stabilizes body weight; reduces weight gain and can facilitate weight loss
IGT or T2D	Reduces progression of IGT to T2D; improves glycemic control in T2D
Dyslipidemia (↑VLDL-TG, ↑LDL-C, ↓HDL-C)	Modest improvement of lipid profile often seen in dyslipidemic patients
Hypertension	Little or no effect on blood pressure in most studies
Procoagulant state	Some antithrombotic activity (e.g., decreases in PAI-1, fibrinogen, and platelet aggregation)
Atherosclerosis	Evidence for antiatherogenic activity from preclinical studies and lower rate of major cardiovascular events in clinical studies

Note: HDL-C = HDL cholesterol; IGT = impaired glucose tolerance; LDL-C = LDL cholesterol; T2D = type 2 diabetes; VLDL-TG = very-low-density lipoprotein triglyceride.

preliminary reports, however, that metformin can reduce hepatic steatosis and reduce some proinflammatory markers associated with T2D. Evidence also suggests that metformin is helpful in the treatment of PCOS and can help to reinstate menstruation and fertility. Possible antineoplastic activity of metformin associated with a reduction of hyperinsulinemia and altered cellular energy metabolism is under investigation.

Thus, the rationale for use of metformin to treat patients with T2D is its antihyperglycemic efficacy and its activity against insulin resistance, with reductions in several cardiovascular risk factors. Metformin may be preferred for obese patients because it does not cause weight gain, although it shows similar antihyperglycemic efficacy in nonobese patients.

TREATMENT

Metformin (proprietary name Glucophage) is available in two tablet formulations: the standard (now called immediate-release [IR]) formulation and the extended-release (XR) formulation. The therapeutic effects of the two formulations are essentially the same, but the XR formulation is absorbed more slowly and can be given as once-daily dosing. A liquid formulation of metformin (500 mg/ml), oral powder (500 mg sachet) that dissolves in water, and various generic tablet formulations of standard (IR) and extended-release (XR) metformin are available. Pharmacokinetic aspects of metformin are summarized in Table 21.3.

Table 21.3 Pharmacokinetic Aspects of Metformin

Variable	Comment
Bioavailability	50–60%; absorbed mainly from the small intestine; estimated time to maximal plasma concentration 0.9–2.6 hours for standard (IR) formulation, 4–8 hours for XR formulation
Plasma concentration	Maximal 1–2 µg/ml ($\sim 10^{-5}$ mol/l) 1–2 hours after an oral dose of 500–1,000 mg for standard (IR) formulation; maximal concentration is $\sim$20% lower (but area under the curve is similar) at same dose of XR formulation; negligible binding to plasma proteins
Plasma elimination half-life	~6 hours
Metabolism	Not measurably metabolized
Elimination	~90% of absorbed drug is eliminated in urine in 24 hours; multiexponential pattern involving glomerular filtration and tubular secretion
Tissue distribution	Distributed in most tissues at concentrations similar to those in peripheral plasma; higher concentrations in liver and kidney; highest concentration in salivary glands and intestinal wall

INDICATIONS

Metformin is indicated as monotherapy for the treatment of hyperglycemia in patients with T2D who do not achieve appropriate target levels of glycemic control with nonpharmacological therapy, such as diet, exercise, and health education (Table 21.4). It also can be used in combination with an insulin-releasing agent (sulfonylurea, meglitinide, GLP-1 receptor agonist or dipeptidyl peptidase-4 [DPP-4] inhibitor), α-glucosidase inhibitor, thiazolidinedione, sodium-glucose cotransporter inhibitor, or insulin. Metformin is helpful in patients who require weight stabilization or weight loss or who are vulnerable to hypoglycemia. Potential benefits against various atherogenic risk factors associated with insulin resistance (Table 21.2) are not specific indications but are usefully taken into account in the selection of metformin.

Elderly patients can be given metformin with appropriate adherence to the contraindications, especially renal function. Children also can receive metformin up to a maximum dose of 2,000 mg daily, although studies have not been conducted in subjects <10 years of age. Use in the elderly and in children warrants frequent monitoring.

STARTING METFORMIN

Starting metformin therapy assumes attention to contraindications (detailed in the following) and appropriate monitoring of glycemic control, initially using fasting plasma glucose (FPG) and, subsequently, A1C.

Table 21.4 Clinical Use of Metformin

Indications	As monotherapy or in combination with other oral antidiabetic agents or insulin in patients with T2D inadequately controlled by diet, exercise, and health education
Usage	500, 850, and 1,000 mg standard (IR) tablets, 500 mg dosage of liquid formulation or oral powder: take with meals; increase dose slowly; monitor glycemic control; typical clinical therapeutic dose 1,500–2,000 mg/day; maximal dose 2,550 mg/day
Use in children aged >10 years (maximal dose 2,000 mg/day in children)	500, 750, and 1,000 mg XR tablet: take with evening meal; increase dose slowly; monitor glycemic control; maximal dose 2,000 mg/day
Contraindications and warnings	Renal and hepatic disease; cardiac or respiratory insufficiency; any hypoxic condition; severe infection; alcohol abuse; history of lactic acidosis; temporarily discontinue during use of intravenous radiographic contrast agents; pregnancy
Side effects	Gastrointestinal symptoms and metallic taste, which improve with dose reduction; may impair absorption of vitamin B12 and folic acid; the gastrointestinal symptoms may be lessened with the use of extended release formulation (Metformin XR 500 mg is on the cost-reduced lists [$4.00])
Adverse reactions	Risk of lactic acidosis in patients with a contraindication; hypoglycemia can occur when taken in combination with another antidiabetic drug or during alcohol abuse
Precautions	Check for contraindications; check hemoglobin and serum creatinine or estimated glomerular filtration rate (eGFR) periodically; possible interaction with cimetidine therapy

Standard (IR) metformin should be taken with meals, starting with one 500 or 850 mg tablet (or 500 mg liquid or powder formulation) at breakfast or other main meal. The dose then can be increased one tablet at a time at 4- to 14-day intervals, leading to two or three divided doses with the main meals, until the desired level of blood glucose control is achieved or the maximum tolerated dose is reached. A total dose of three or four 500 mg tablets (or equivalent dosage forms) or two to three 850 mg tablets often is required, with the maximum dose being 2,550 mg daily.

Gastrointestinal side effects are not uncommon during initiation of therapy. These include abdominal discomfort, diarrhea, nausea, anorexia, and a metallic taste. These symptoms are usually transient, remit with dose reduction, and are minimized by gradual dose escalation and administration with meals. Gastrointestinal side effects often are ameliorated with the use of the XR formulation. Note that the metformin 500 mg IR and XR are the same cost.

XR metformin usually is given once daily with the evening meal or occasionally twice daily with the breakfast and evening meals. The XR tablets (500 and 750 mg) always should be taken whole so that the inner- and outer-polymer compartments are undisturbed and continued slow release of metformin is provided for up to 24 hours. The XR tablets may be preferred to reduce initial gastrointestinal side effects.

CONTRAINDICATIONS AND WARNINGS

Metformin is contraindicated in patients with impaired renal function (e.g., serum creatinine ≥1.5 mg/dl in men or ≥1.4 mg/dl in women). In older individuals, in whom serum creatinine is not a reliable measure of renal function, metformin is contraindicated if creatinine clearance is moderately impaired (e.g., <60 ml/minute/1.73 m^2). Renal function should be checked at least yearly during metformin therapy. In some countries outside of the U.S., metformin therapy can be initiated in patients with an eGFR (calculated by the MDRD equation) in the range 60–45 ml/minute/1.73 m^2, and therapy can be continued (if appropriate) with dosage adjustment and frequent monitoring while the eGFR is in the range 45–30 ml/minute/1.73 m^2, usually with specialist supervision. It is suggested that metformin be temporarily discontinued for about 48 hours during or after use of an intravascular contrast medium until normal renal function is evidently reestablished.

Any hypoxic state should be regarded as a contraindication for metformin—notably chronic congestive heart failure, acute heart failure, severe respiratory insufficiency, septicemia, and other conditions with hypoperfusion or hypoxemia. Significant liver disease, history of lactic acidosis, alcohol abuse, or other disturbances of liver function likely to prevent normal hepatic lactate metabolism should be considered as contraindications for metformin.

At present, the product label notes that administration of metformin is not recommended during pregnancy or lactation because of insufficient clinical data. Animal studies and recent clinical trials, however, support earlier clinical experience that metformin is not associated with increased complications in gestational diabetes compared with insulin therapy. Metformin is not teratogenic in animals, and no adverse effects on the fetus or nursing infant are apparent. In consequence, metformin often is used in gestational diabetes provided there are no other contraindications.

Metformin should be discontinued temporarily in favor of insulin administration during severe acute illnesses and major surgical procedures. Metformin is not effective as a primary treatment for type 1 diabetes (T1D).

SIDE EFFECTS OF TREATMENT

Lactic acidosis is a rare but serious adverse event associated with metformin therapy. Extensive worldwide experience indicates that the incidence is ~0.03 cases per 1,000 patient-years of treatment, with a mortality of ~50%. Many of these cases have occurred when the drug was prescribed inappropriately, hence the importance of adequate renal function for the drug to be eliminated and the avoidance of hypoxemia and conditions that compromise lactate metabolism. Lactic acidosis can occur in patients with diabetes unrelated to metformin therapy.

The most common side effects of metformin are the gastrointestinal disturbances described earlier. Although these often resolve with time or with use of XR formulation, dose reduction, gradual titration, and administration with meals, ~5–10% of patients do not tolerate a full therapeutic dose of metformin (e.g., 2,000 mg/day).

Long-term therapy with metformin is associated with a small decrease in the absorption of vitamin B12 and occasionally folate; however, development of anemia from this cause is rare, can be associated with poor diet, and usually is reversed by vitamin B12 supplementation.

Severe hypoglycemia is unlikely with metformin unless administered with another antidiabetic agent. In general, the blood glucose–lowering effect of metformin is additive to that of other oral antidiabetic agents while adequate β-cell function remains. Metformin usually increases the hypoglycemic effect of insulin. Use of metformin in combination with other antidiabetic agents requires appropriate adjustments of dosage based on glucose monitoring. Introduction of drugs that tend to increase blood glucose concentrations, such as corticosteroids, may necessitate dosage adjustment or require the addition of another antidiabetic medication.

Other clinically important drug interactions have not been identified with metformin. Metformin shows little binding to plasma proteins; it is not metabolized and is eliminated unchanged in the urine by glomerular filtration and tubular secretion. Thus, care should be taken if initiating therapies affecting renal function, such as antihypertensives, diuretics, and nonsteroidal anti-inflammatory drugs. Increased metformin levels can occur with cimetidine, which shares the same transporter in the renal tubules, and other cationic drugs theoretically could compete with metformin elimination. Minor pharmacokinetic interactions occur with furosemide and nifedipine.

EXPECTED RESULTS

H2 antagonist

The reduction of hyperglycemia and improvement in glycemic control achieved with oral antihyperglycemic drugs is influenced by many factors, including the level of initial hyperglycemia, the pathophysiological status of β-cell function and insulin resistance, and the mechanism of drug action. The therapeutic action of metformin improves sensitivity to low or moderate concentrations of insulin and therefore requires adequate remaining β-cell function.

Typically, the antihyperglycemic effect of metformin is evident throughout the range of mild to moderately severe fasting hyperglycemia (110–275 mg/dl [6.1–15.5 mmol/l] or A1C 7–12%). In clinical trials involving a broad spectrum of patients with T2D, metformin treatment produced an average lowering of FPG by 55 mg/dl (3.1 mmol/l) and A1C by 1.5%. The absolute drop in plasma glucose and A1C will be greater at higher starting levels of hyperglycemia (e.g., FPG 275 mg/dl [15.5 mmol/l] and A1C 12%) than at lower levels (e.g., FPG 150 mg/dl [8.3 mmol/l] and A1C 8%). It is likely, however, that a smaller proportion of patients will achieve target levels of glycemic control (e.g., A1C <7%) when the starting level of hyperglycemia is high.

The effect of metformin appears to be predominantly on fasting hyperglycemia, with a small effect on the meal-stimulated incremental rise in plasma glucose. A meta-analysis comparing metformin monotherapy with sulfonylurea monotherapy revealed that the two classes of drugs have comparable potency in reducing hyperglycemia and A1C.

Additional benefits ascribed to metformin therapy during trials with T2D include a lack of weight gain or a small weight loss (mean reduction of 1–2 kg). Depending on the extent of initial dyslipidemia, there is often a small decrease in plasma LDL cholesterol and triglycerides (of ~10% in several trials) and a decrease in PAI-1. Severe episodes of hypoglycemia do not occur during metformin monotherapy, and fasting insulin concentrations are reduced slightly.

SINGLE-TABLET COMBINATIONS CONTAINING METFORMIN

Because the cellular mechanism of action of metformin is different from that of other oral antidiabetic agents, its blood glucose–lowering efficacy is generally additive when combined with these agents, provided that adequate β-cell function remains. Single-tablet combinations of metformin with a sulfonylurea (e.g., glyburide or glipizide), with a thiazolidinedione (e.g., pioglitazone or rosiglitazone), or with a DPP-4 inhibitor (e.g., sitagliptin, saxagliptin, linagliptin, or alogliptin) now are available (Table 21.5). The indication for use of a single-tablet fixed-dose combination is normally as second line when one of the agents alone is unable to achieve or maintain adequate glycemic control: A single-tablet fixed-dose combination then reduces the tablet burden of two agents given separately. The range of dosage strengths available as single-tablet fixed-dose combinations includes most of the dosages that could be achieved as separate tablets. Initial pharmacologic therapy with a single-tablet fixed-dose combination might be considered for glucose lowering in patients with substantial hyperglycemia. The precautions and contraindications for the single-tablet fixed-dose combinations include those that apply to each of the individual active ingredients.

Table 21.5 Single-Tablet Combinations That Contain Metformin

Name	Constituents	Tablet strengths (mg)
Glucovance	Metformin + glyburide	250/1.25, 500/2.5, 500/5.0
Metaglip	Metformin + glipizide	250/2.5, 500/2.5, 500/5.0
Avandamet*	Metformin + rosiglitazone	500/2, 500/4, 1,000/2, 1,000/4
Actoplus Met	Metformin + pioglitazone	500/15, 850/15
Janumet	Metformin XR + sitagliptin	500/50, 1,000/50
Kombiglyze	Metformin XR + saxagliptin	500/5, 1,000/2.5, 1,000/5.0
Jentadueto	Metformin + linagliptin	500/2.5, 850/2.5, 1,000/2.5
Kazano	Metformin + alogliptin	500/12.5, 1,000/12.5

Note: *Limited availability due to risk evaluation and mitigation strategy in the U.S.

GLUCOVANCE

Glucovance is a single-tablet combination of metformin with the sulfonylurea glyburide. It was introduced in the U.S. in 2000. Glucovance can be used as initial antidiabetic drug therapy when substantial hyperglycemia persists after nonpharmacological interventions. Glucovance is convenient for patients transferring to a combination of metformin and glyburide because of inadequate glycemic control after monotherapy with one of these agents. Also, patients already receiving metformin and glyburide as separate tablets can be switched conveniently to Glucovance. Additionally, so-called triple therapy can be given using Glucovance plus the thiazolidinedione pioglitazone (rosiglitazone can be considered only if already being prescribed through a restricted access program).

Mode of Action and Rationale for Use

The two antidiabetic components of Glucovance, namely metformin and glyburide, act simultaneously to exert their individual blood glucose–lowering effects as described above. Provided there is adequate β-cell function, the blood glucose–lowering efficacy of the two components is approximately additive. This applies similarly whether metformin and glyburide are given as separate tablets or as Glucovance. However, there is evidence that the formulation of Glucovance may enhance the cumulative efficacy of metformin and glyburide, mainly to improve postprandial glycemic control.

Most patients with T2D exhibit some degree of both insulin resistance and defective β-cell function. These two pathogenic facets of T2D are addressed concurrently by Glucovance: metformin counters the insulin resistance and glyburide stimulates insulin secretion. Although the single-tablet combination of Glucovance offers the additional therapeutic benefits attributed individually to metformin and glyburide, it also carries all of the contraindications of the two compounds. When used in combination, the effects of the two compounds are not mutually exclusive (e.g., the presence of metformin will reduce the extent of weight gain associated with glyburide, but the occurrence of hypoglycemia is likely to increase). Thus, the rationale for use of Glucovance in the treatment of T2D is the additive blood glucose–lowering efficacy of metformin and glyburide, which act by complementary mechanisms to address insulin resistance and defective function. Glucovance enables these agents to be given simultaneously in a convenient single-tablet formulation.

Treatment

Glucovance is available at three strengths of glyburide/metformin: 1.25 mg/250 mg, 2.5 mg/500 mg, and 5 mg/500 mg. Tablets should be swallowed whole. Pharmacokinetic features are generally the same as for the two agents given in separate tablets, except that the peak circulating concentration of the glyburide component is achieved earlier (~1–3 hours compared with 4–8 hours) depending on food consumption (for glyburide). This reflects the distribution of the glyburide particle size in the Glucovance formulation, which includes a high proportion of small particles.

As initial antidiabetic drug therapy, Glucovance can be started if glycemic control is inadequate with nonpharmacological measures. Contraindications for both metformin and glyburide must be respected, and monitoring of FPG is required for gradual dose escalation until the desired glycemic control is achieved. It is recommended that patients begin with the lowest-strength tablet (1.25 mg glyburide/250 mg metformin). If the starting A1C level is >9%, it is usually appropriate to begin with this strength tablet twice daily with the morning and evening meals. If the starting A1C level is between 8 and 9%, begin with this strength tablet once daily with breakfast. Titrate up to twice daily, and then increase one tablet at a time to the next strength level, changing the morning tablet first. The suggested maximal daily dose is 10 mg glyburide/2,000 mg metformin in divided doses. Do not begin with the high-strength tablet (5 mg/500 mg) to reduce risk of hypoglycemia. Patients with a starting A1C <8% may be more appropriately treated with a single oral antidiabetic agent.

As second-line therapy in patients inadequately controlled on a maximally effective amount of either glyburide or metformin, it is recommended to select a starting dose of Glucovance that contains a lower amount of glyburide or metformin than is already being taken. For example, a patient inadequately controlled on 2,000 mg metformin might start Glucovance at 2.5 mg/500 mg twice daily and then increase one tablet at a time. Although a maximal suggested daily dose is 10 mg/2,000 mg, a dose of 20 mg/2,000 mg is permitted when used as second-line therapy.

In patients already taking a combination of glyburide (or another sulfonylurea) and metformin as separate tablets, it is convenient to switch to a similar dosage regimen of Glucovance, but do not exceed the daily amounts of glyburide (or equivalent of another sulfonylurea) and metformin already being taken.

For patients inadequately controlled on Glucovance, a thiazolidinedione can be added (so-called triple therapy). This addition may help patients to achieve the desired glycemic target, while there is remaining β-cell function. Patients with severe and rapidly escalating hyperglycemia, often with unintentional weight loss, should be considered for insulin therapy.

Glucovance can be used in the elderly provided there is careful and frequent monitoring, avoiding the highest doses. Glucovance has not been studied in children and is not recommended during pregnancy and lactation. It is reemphasized that the contraindications and precautions associated with the use of metformin and glyburide separately must be observed with Glucovance. Likewise, the side effects of each drug should be borne in mind when using Glucovance, and gradual dose titration with monitoring is especially important to reduce the risk of hypoglycemia.

Expected Results

In T2D, the blood glucose–lowering effect of oral antidiabetic agents is influenced by many features of the disease process (as noted in the metformin section of this chapter), particularly the extent of starting hyperglycemia. Previous experience with the use of metformin and glyburide in combination as separate tablets has shown that the blood glucose–lowering effect of the two agents is approximately additive.

A 26-week trial conducted for registration purposes found that initial drug therapy with Glucovance in patients with T2D who had a starting A1C 7–11% and FPG ≤240 mg/dl reduced A1C by ~1.5% and FPG by ~40 mg/dl. The effect was generally greater among individuals with a starting hyperglycemia in the upper part of the range, and two-thirds of patients achieved a target A1C of <7%. A greater reduction in blood glucose was achieved in groups treated with Glucovance at a lower mean dose of each of the two active agents than in parallel groups treated with glyburide or metformin alone. Indeed, the Glucovance group treated with the 1.25 mg/250 mg strength tablets had a greater mean improvement in glycemic control than groups treated with glyburide or metformin as single therapies, and the average dosage of Glucovance contained about one-half of the dosage of glyburide or metformin as the single therapies. In particular, there was a greater improvement in the postprandial glucose excursion with Glucovance. This improvement may reflect the pharmacokinetic attribute of an initially rapid release of glyburide from the Glucovance tablet. The postprandial insulin response was greater than that with metformin alone but similar to that with glyburide alone. Weight gain was greater compared with metformin alone, and there was little effect on the lipid profile. Fewer hypoglycemic symptoms were reported with the lowest strength of Glucovance than glyburide alone, but the higher strength of Glucovance was prone to more hypoglycemic symptoms, especially in patients with lower A1C levels (hence, the recommendation to initiate drug therapy with the 1.25 mg/250 mg strength of Glucovance).

An open-label study of patients with either a starting A1C >11% or FPG >240 mg/dl (>13.3 mmol/l) began with the 2.5 mg/500 mg strength Glucovance. After 26 weeks, there was a mean reduction of FPG from 283 to 161 mg/dl (15.7–8.9 mmol/l), with an average A1C of 7.1%, and this response was sustained to 52 weeks.

As second-line therapy, a 16-week study found that in patients inadequately controlled on a sulfonylurea, transfer to Glucovance and titration of the dosage enabled improvements in FPG, postprandial glucose, and A1C. For example, in patients with an A1C of ~9.5% on a maximal or near-maximal dose of glyburide, transfer to Glucovance reduced mean A1C by 1.7–1.9%, whereas continuation therapy with a sulfonylurea alone or switching to metformin alone was not effective.

METAGLIP

Metaglip is a single-tablet combination of metformin with the sulfonylurea glipizide. It was introduced in the U.S. in 2002 for use in the treatment of T2D as initial antidiabetic drug therapy or for progression to a combination of metformin and glipizide if glycemic control was inadequate after monotherapy with metformin or glipizide (or another sulfonylurea) alone. Also, patients already taking a combination of metformin and glipizide as separate tablets can be switched to Metaglip for convenience.

Metaglip can be used in a similar manner to Glucovance (except the triple-therapy indication) and provides an appropriate combination where glipizide is already used or is preferred as the sulfonylurea to give in combination with metformin.

Mode of Action and Rationale for Use

The mode of action and rationale for use of Metaglip follow the same principles as those for Glucovance.

Treatment

Metaglip is available at three strengths of glipizide/metformin: 2.5 mg/250 mg, 2.5 mg/500 mg, and 5 mg/500 mg. Pharmacokinetic features are generally the same as the two agents given together in separate tablets, which are also almost identical to the agents given alone. The procedures for use of Metaglip (metformin/glipizide) are essentially the same as those of Glucovance (metformin/glyburide).

Expected Results

Several studies in T2D have shown that the blood glucose–lowering effects of metformin and glipizide are approximately additive, provided there is adequate β-cell function remaining.

Initial drug therapy with Metaglip (2.5 mg/250 mg and 2.5/500) has been studied in patients with T2D during a 24-week trial for registration purposes. Patients had an average starting FPG of 203–210 mg/dl and A1C of ~9.1%, and Metaglip therapy produced mean decreases in FPG by 54–56 mg/dl and A1C by 2.1%. Thus, appropriate titration of the lower-strength tablets (2.5 mg/250 mg) gave similar results to the higher-strength tablets (2.5 mg/500 mg) in this study. These improvements in glycemic control were greater than those achieved with either glipizide alone (decreased A1C by 1.7%) or metformin alone (decreased A1C by 1.4%). Moreover, the amounts of glipizide and metformin given with the lower-strength Metaglip tablets were less than one-half of the amounts of these agents taken by the groups receiving each agent alone. The Metaglip groups also showed greater improvements in postprandial glucose excursion than groups treated with either glipizide or metformin alone. Metaglip was associated with a small decrease in body weight (by 0.4–0.5 kg), which was less than the decrease in body weight with metformin alone (by 1.9 kg). No clinically significant effects of Metaglip or its separate component drugs were observed on lipid parameters in this study. More reports of hypoglycemic symptoms and finger-stick blood glucose values ≤50 mg/dl were made by patients taking Metaglip (7.6 and 9.3% of patients taking the lower- and higher-strength tablets, respectively) compared with metformin alone (0%) and glipizide alone (2.9%). Metaglip was discontinued by 2.6% of patients because of hypoglycemic symptoms. Gastrointestinal symptoms, including diarrhea, occurred more often than in the group taking metformin alone, and 1.2% of patients on Metaglip discontinued because of gastrointestinal symptoms.

As second-line therapy, an 18-week study noted that patients inadequately controlled on either a sulfonylurea or metformin alone achieved an additional decrease in mean A1C by ~1% when taking Metaglip. Improvements in FPG and postprandial glucose also were noted with Metaglip, but body weight loss was trivial (–0.3 kg) compared with metformin alone (–2.7 kg), and there were no significant changes in lipids.

AVANDAMET

Avandamet is a single-tablet combination of metformin with the thiazolidinedione rosiglitazone. The dosage strengths (in mg) are rosiglitazone/metformin 2/500, 4/500, 2/1,000, 4/1,000. Avandamet was introduced in the U.S. in 2002 as a second-line oral antidiabetic drug therapy for patients with T2D. In 2011, concerns about cardiovascular risks associated with rosiglitazone resulted in Avandamet becoming subject to a risk evaluation and mitigation strategy (REMS). On the basis of new information, however, the U.S. Food and Drug Administration is removing the REMS prescribing and dispensing restrictions for rosiglitazone medicines. The main rationale for use of Avandamet is convenient treatment of T2D with a single-tablet combination of metformin and rosiglitazone to address insulin resistance by complementary actions with minimal risk of hypoglycemia.

Use of Avandamet is similar to the use of a single-tablet metformin-pioglitazone combination described in the following section.

ACTOPLUS MET

Actoplus Met is a single-tablet combination of metformin with the thiazolidinedione pioglitazone, introduced in the U.S. in 2005 as a second-line oral antidiabetic drug therapy for patients with T2D. Actoplus Met can be used in patients who are inadequately controlled by monotherapy with metformin or pioglitazone. Patients already receiving metformin and pioglitazone as separate tablets can switch to the single-tablet formulation if it is more convenient.

Mode of Action and Rationale for Use

Metformin has been used widely in combination therapy with a thiazolidinedione: The two classes of agents show approximately additive blood glucose–lowering effects when used in combination, provided there is adequate β-cell function. Each improves insulin sensitivity, but by different and complementary mechanisms. Pioglitazone stimulates the nuclear receptor peroxisome proliferator–activated receptor-γ and mainly increases peripheral glucose uptake. As described earlier in this chapter, metformin predominantly reduces hepatic glucose production. Because neither agent stimulates insulin secretion, hypoglycemia is uncommon and usually mild, even when the agents are used in combination. Each agent has been reported to influence several cardiovascular risk factors associated with the "metabolic syndrome," in part by reducing insulin resistance.

The main rationale for use of Actoplus Met is convenient treatment of T2D with a single-tablet combination of metformin and pioglitazone to address insulin resistance by complementary actions with minimal risk of hypoglycemia.

Treatment

Actoplus Met is available at two strengths of pioglitazone/metformin: 15 mg/500 mg and 15 mg/850 mg. Pharmacokinetic characteristics of each agent are unaltered by the other, and the single-tablet combination shows similar characteristics to the individual components coadministered as separate tablets.

Actoplus Met normally is used to treat T2D when monotherapy with metformin or pioglitazone alone does not achieve adequate glycemic control. When starting Actoplus Met, it is important to respect the contraindications and cautions for both metformin and pioglitazone. Because pioglitazone can cause edema and increase the risk of congestive heart failure in some patients, Actoplus Met is contraindicated in patients with New York Heart Association classes III or IV heart failure. Actoplus Met also is contraindicated in patients with impaired renal function and other exclusions that apply to metformin. Risk of bone fracture associated with pioglitazone, particularly in older women, also should be considered.

Patients inadequately controlled on metformin monotherapy typically will start Actoplus Met at a similar daily dose of metformin plus 15–30 mg pioglitazone daily, given in divided doses that coincide where possible with the previous metformin regimen. For patients inadequately controlled on pioglitazone monotherapy, start Actoplus Met with a similar daily dose of pioglitazone plus 1,000 mg metformin daily in divided doses, although it may be prudent to introduce metformin at 500 mg daily (with breakfast) for the first few days. If starting Actoplus Met in drug-naïve patients with T2D, begin with 15 mg/500 mg once or twice daily with meals. Titrate the dosage gradually (see previous advice for metformin), bearing in mind that there is a slow onset of the pioglitazone component effect: Monitor FPG and other parameters as required for each component drug.

To switch a patient from a combination of pioglitazone and metformin as separate tablets, use the nearest equivalent daily dose of Actoplus Met. The maximum recommended daily dose of Actoplus Met is 45 mg pioglitazone/2,550 mg metformin in divided doses.

Expected Results

Adding pioglitazone to metformin as separate tablets has demonstrated their additive blood glucose–lowering efficacy. A 24-week trial in patients with T2D inadequately controlled on metformin found that the addition of pioglitazone at 30 or 45 mg daily reduced A1C by 0.8 and 1%, respectively, from baseline. There is little peer-reviewed published evidence regarding the use of the single-tablet combination of pioglitazone and metformin (Actoplus Met), and use of the combination largely is based on experience gained using the separate tablets. In addition to its glucose-lowering effect without risk of significant hypoglycemia, introduction of the combination is likely to cause a small increase in body weight (e.g., 1–2 kg) in patients who previously have not received pioglitazone. These patients also may show a modest reduction of triglycerides and free fatty acids.

Note that a particularly rapid increase in weight on initiation of Actoplus Met warrants investigation for edema and any signs of heart failure. Pioglitazone has been reported to increase the incidence of nonvertebral bone fractures in women and pioglitazone-containing medicines are not recommended in patients with active bladder cancer and only with caution in patients with a history thereof.

JANUMET, KOMBIGLYZE, JENTADUETO, AND KAZANO

Janumet, Kombiglyze, Jentadueto, and Kazano are each single-tablet fixed-dose combinations of metformin with an inhibitor of the enzyme DPP-4. Janumet (metformin + sitagliptin) was introduced in the U.S. in 2007, Kombiglyze (metformin + saxagliptin) in 2010, Jentadueto (metformin + linagliptin) in 2011, and Kazano (metformin + alogliptin) in 2013. Each is indicated to treat patients with T2D with inadequate glycemic control after monotherapy with metformin or the respective DPP-4 inhibitor alone. Also, patients already taking a combination of metformin and one of these DPP-4 inhibitors can be switched to the respective fixed-dose combination for convenience.

Each of the single-tablet fixed-dose combinations of metformin plus a DPP-4 inhibitor can be used in a similar manner to the metformin-sulfonylurea combinations of Glucovance or Metaglip, although combinations of metformin with a DPP-4 inhibitor are unlikely to cause significant hypoglycemia or weight gain.

Mode of Action and Rationale for Use

Metformin and DPP-4 inhibitors act additively to lower blood glucose by complementary mechanisms. Metformin counters insulin resistance (described earlier), and DPP-4 inhibitors act primarily to address defective islet function. DPP-4 inhibitors selectively inhibit activity of the circulating and cell-surface enzyme DPP-4. DPP-4 normally causes rapid degradation of the incretin hormones GLP-1 and glucose-dependent insulinotropic polypeptide (GIP). Thus, inhibition of DPP-4 activity prevents the rapid degradation of GLP-1 and GIP, thereby enhancing endogenous incretin activity. This is associated with increased glucose-induced insulin secretion. Raised circulating concentrations of active GLP-1 also suppress glucagon secretion and may slow the rate of gastric emptying and exert a small satiety effect. There is preliminary evidence that metformin might facilitate an increase in GLP-1 concentrations.

Because the effects of DPP-4 inhibitors on insulin and glucagon secretion are glucose dependent, there is low risk of significant hypoglycemia, and the potential effects on satiety and gastric emptying may contribute to weight neutrality. Moreover, metformin substantially lowers basal glycemia, whereas DPP-4 inhibitors particularly reduce prandial glucose excursions.

Although the various DPP-4 inhibitors each reduce DPP-4 activity to a similar extent, and exhibit a similar glucose-lowering efficacy, there are differences in their pharmacokinetic profiles. Sitagliptin is not appreciably metabolized or protein bound. It has little effect on P450 isoenzymes and is eliminated mostly unchanged in the urine, reducing the risk of drug interactions. Saxagliptin is metabolized in the liver by P450 CYP3A4/5 to active metabolites with >50% renal elimination. Linagliptin and alogliptin are not appreciably metabolized: The former is eliminated via the liver and the latter mostly via the kidneys. These differences have considerable implications for use of DPP-4 inhibitors without metformin in patients with renal impairment (when each agent requires a dose reduction except linagliptin). Use of the fixed-dose combinations with metformin, however, precludes use in renal impairment due to the contraindication with metformin.

Treatment

The available dosage strengths of the various fixed-dose combinations of metformin with a DPP-4 inhibitor provide most of the suitable dosage options available as separate tablets, and coadministration of the two types of agents does not interfere with their pharmacokinetic properties.

Starting a metformin plus DPP-4 inhibitor fixed-dose combination normally assumes that appropriate targets for glycemic control are not achieved with nonpharmacological therapy or with one antidiabetic agent (metformin or DPP-4 inhibitor) alone. Nonpharmacological measures should continue to be reinforced throughout any program of diabetes management. The contraindications of both metformin and the DPP-4 inhibitor must be respected, and FPG monitoring is required for gradual dose escalation until the desired glycemic control is achieved. Introduction and titration of a fixed-dose metformin plus DPP-4 inhibitor combination follows the general principles set out for metformin. In patients inadequately controlled on metformin or a DPP-4 inhibitor alone, the starting dose of the fixed-dose combination should equate where possible (but not exceed) the daily dose of either metformin or the DPP-4 inhibitor already being taken. For patients already taking a combination of metformin and a DPP-4 inhibitor as separate tablets, a switch to the fixed-dose combination should use the nearest equivalent dosage regimen. Patients aiming for tight glycemic control who are close to an A1C target of ~7% can be given a metformin plus DPP-4 fixed-dose combination with little risk of serious hypoglycemia. Patients susceptible to or experiencing episodes of hypoglycemia with a sulfonylurea or meglitinide combined with metformin may be at less risk of hypoglycemia with a metformin plus DPP-4 inhibitor combination. Patients exhibiting persistently severe and escalating hyperglycemia, often with unintentional weight loss, should be considered for insulin therapy.

Expected Results

Evidence for the blood glucose–lowering efficacy of metformin plus DPP-4 combinations is based mostly on studies with these agents as separate tablets. In patients with T2D that is inadequately controlled (e.g., A1C ~8.0%) with metformin, the addition of a DPP-4 inhibitor for 24 weeks reduced A1C by about 0.6–0.8 %. The 2-hour postprandial glucose concentration was reduced about 50 mg/dl (2.8 mmol/l).

All of these studies have resulted in a low incidence of hypoglycemia and no weight gain or sometimes a small weight loss. The incidence of gastrointestinal side effects was similar for the combination as for the respective dose of metformin monotherapy.

BIBLIOGRAPHY

Bailey CJ. Treating insulin resistance in type 2 diabetes with metformin and thiazolidinediones. *Diabetes Obesity Metab* 2005;7:675–691.

Bailey CJ, Campbell IW. United Kingdom Prospective Diabetes Study: Implications for metformin. *Br J Cardiol* 2002;9:115–119.

Bailey CJ, Krentz AJ. Oral antidiabetic agents. In *Textbook of Diabetes*. 4th ed. Holt RIG, Cockram C, Flyvberg A, Goldsten B, Eds. Blackwell, U.K., Oxford, 2010, p. 452–477.

Bailey CJ, Turner RC. Drug therapy: metformin. *N Engl J Med* 1996;334:574–579.

Cusi K, DeFronzo RA. Metformin: a review of its metabolic effects. *Diabetes Rev* 1998;6:89–130.

DeFronzo RA, Goodman AM, Multicenter Metformin Study Group. Efficacy of metformin in patients with non-insulin-dependent diabetes mellitus. *N Engl J Med* 1995;333:541–549.

Garber AJ, Larsen J, Schneider SH, Piper BA, Henry D. Simultaneous glyburide/metformin therapy is superior to component monotherapy as an initial pharmacological treatment for type 2 diabetes. *Diabetes Obes Metab* 2002;4:201–208.

Goldstein BJ, Feinglos MN, Lunceford JK, Johnson J, Williams-Herman DE. Effect of initial combination therapy with sitagliptin, a dipeptidyl peptidase-4 inhibitor, and metformin on glycemic control in patients with type 2 diabetes. *Diabetes Care* 2007;30:1979–1987.

Howlett HCS, Bailey CJ. A risk-benefit assessment of metformin in type 2 diabetes mellitus. *Drug Safety* 1999;20:489–503.

Misbin RI, Green L, Stadel BV, Gueriguian JL, Gubbi A, Fleming GA. Lactic acidosis in patients with diabetes treated with metformin. *N Engl J Med* 1997;338:285–286.

U.K. Prospective Diabetes Study Group. Effect of intensive blood-glucose control with metformin on complications in overweight patients with type 2 diabetes (UKPDS 34). *Lancet* 1998;352:854–865.

Chapter 22
Insulin Secretagogues: Sulfonylureas and Glinides

Giulio R. Romeo, MD
Martin J. Abrahamson, MD
Allison B. Goldfine, MD

This chapter addresses advances in our understanding of mechanisms of action of nonincretin insulin secretagogues belonging to the sulfonylurea (SU) and glinide classes, their efficacy in type 2 diabetes (T2D), common side effects, and impact on cardiovascular disease outcomes.

SUs were the first class of oral glucose-lowering medications to be introduced into clinical practice in the 1950s, and since then, they have been a mainstay of pharmacological therapy for blood glucose control in patients with T2D. Despite extensive clinical experience, questions now arise regarding their role in diabetes management relative to newer agents both as monotherapy and as "add-ons" to other agents, and their relative safety profile compared with alternative diabetes treatments remains under debate. Detailed understanding of cellular and molecular mechanisms of action of SUs, including genetic variants that may influence clinical response, and results from "head-to-head" trials of SUs compared with alternative pharmacologic agents have helped shed light on these questions and brought to focus distinctive features of different SUs that may render some more desirable than others in clinical practice.

Similar to SUs, D-phenylalanine and meglitinide family members (henceforth referred to as "glinides") are rapid-onset, short-acting oral antidiabetic medications that elicit early-phase insulin release and thereby decrease postprandial glucose excursions. Glinides are well tolerated and approved as monotherapy or in combination with insulin sensitizers. Because of their unique pharmacokinetic properties, glinides are effective options for T2D management in selected patient populations, including the elderly.

It is important to understand proper use of drugs that stimulate insulin secretion. Hypoglycemia can be a serious consequence of their inappropriate use. In parallel, these drugs are ineffective in lowering blood glucose in patients who have a marked reduction or total loss of functioning β-cells.

PHARMACOLOGIC PROPERTIES AND MECHANISMS OF ACTION OF SULFONYLUREAS AND GLINIDES

Pharmacokinetic features differ among different SUs and glinides clinically available—their average peak action and half-life are provided in Table 22.1. At the cellular level, SUs and glinides similarly exert their hypoglycemic effects by eliciting a series of ionic events that result in closure of pancreatic ATP-sensitive

DOI: 10.2337/9781580405096.22

K-channels (K_{ATP}) and a rise in intracellular calcium (*i*Ca) concentration, which triggers insulin secretion from the pancreatic β-cell (Figure 22.1).[1,2] The K_{ATP} channel on β-cells is composed of the SU receptor 1 (SUR1), which is the regulatory subunit and functions as the binding site for SUs, and the inward-rectifier potassium ion channel (Kir6.2), which forms the channel pore. Specifically, the pancreatic K_{ATP} channel is composed of four SUR1 subunits and four Kir6.2 subunits. SUR1 is a member of the ATP-binding cassette superfamily and has three transmembrane domains. The binding of SUs to SUR1 results in closure of the K_{ATP} channel, increased concentrations of intracellular potassium, depolarization of the β-cell membrane, and subsequent opening of plasma membrane voltage-gated calcium channels. The increase in calcium ion influx into the β-cell and resultant increased binding of *i*Ca to calmodulin activates myosin-light chain kinase, thereby causing movement of insulin-containing secretory granules to the cell surface and insulin release into the circulation.

Under fasting conditions, most of the K_{ATP} channels are open, and potassium is extruded actively from the β-cell. After a meal, increased plasma glucose concentrations and transport of glucose into β-cells via the GLUT2 transporter leads to a rise in intracellular ATP/ADP ratio causing K_{ATP} channels to close. In turn, this activates the previously mentioned cascade of events, resulting in physiologic postprandial insulin secretion.

Table 22.1—Characteristics of Specific Insulin Secretagogues

Drug	Dose Range (mg)	Peak Level (h)	Half-Life (h)	Metabolites	Excretion
Sulfonylureas					
Tolbutamide	500–3,000	3–4	4.5–6. 5	Inactive	Kidney
Chlorprop-amide	100–500	2–4	36	Active or unchanged	Kidney
Glipizide	2.5–40	1–3	2–4	Inactive	Kidney (80%), feces
Glipizide-XL	5–20	Constant		Inactive	Kidney (80%), feces
Glyburide	1.25–20	~4	10	Weakly active	Kidney (50%), feces (50%)
Glyburide, micronized formulation	1.5–12	2–3	~4	Weakly active	Kidney (50%), feces (50%)
Glimepiride	1–8	2–3	9	Inactive	Kidney (60%), feces (40%)
Nonsulfonylurea Insulin Secretagogues					
Repaglinide	0.5–4/meal	1	1	Inactive	Feces
Nateglinide	60–120/meal	1. 8	1. 4	Weakly active	Kidney (80%), feces

[handwritten margin note: caused prolong hypoglycemia × Crcl < 50]

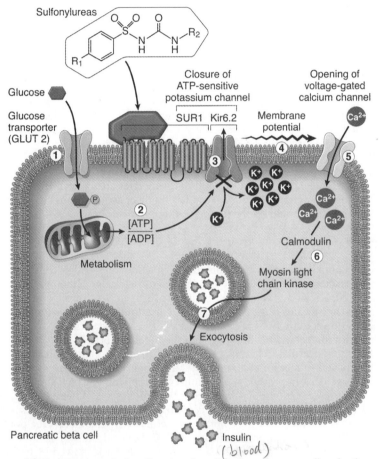

Figure 22.1—Key events in stimulus-insulin secretion coupling in the pancreatic β-cell.

Under fasting conditions, most of the K_{ATP} channels are open, and potassium is extruded actively from the β-cell. Within minutes after a meal, glucose enters the pancreatic β-cell via Glucose Transporter (GLUT)-2 (step 1) and is phosphorylated to glucose-6-phosphate by glucokinase. Metabolism of intracellular glucose via glycolysis/tricarboxylic acid cycle generates ATP and increases the ATP/ADP ratio (step 2), which in turn results in the closure of K_{ATP} channels on the plasma membrane (step 3). The K_{ATP} channel is composed of the sulfonylurea (SU) receptor 1 (SUR1) regulatory subunit, which functions as the binding site for SUs, and the inward-rectifier potassium ion channel (Kir6.2), which forms the channel pore. Similarly to the increase of the ATP/ADP ratio, the binding of SUs to SUR1 results in closure of the K_{ATP} channels, increased concentrations of intracellular potassium, and depolarization of the β-cell membrane (step 4). The subsequent opening of plasma membrane voltage-gated calcium channels and influx of calcium into the β-cell (step 5) lead to the formation of the calcium/calmodulin complex and activation of myosin-light chain kinase (step 6). In turn, myosin-light chain kinase triggers a complex series of cytoskeletal rearrangements (step 7), causing movement of insulin-containing secretory granules to the cell surface and insulin release into the circulation. Illustration by James A. Perkins, MS, MFA.

POTENTIATION OF GLUCOSE-MEDIATED INSULIN SECRETION

Recently, another β-cell target has been identified for some SUs. It is an exchange protein directly activated by cAMP 2 (Epac2). Epac2 potentiates adenosine 3',5'-monophosphate regulated insulin secretion.[3] In animal models, Epac2 was found to be especially important in early-phase glucose-induced insulin release. Glipizide, glyburide, tolbutamide, and chlorpropamide, but not gliclazide, directly interact with Epac2, as seen in fluorescence resonance energy transfer and binding experiments.[3] Notably, Epac2 is required for incretin action and now is being investigated as a target for antidiabetic drug development.

Glinides cause glucose-induced insulin secretion by binding to SUR1 on β-cells, but the precise binding site(s) and pharmacokinetic characteristics differ from SUs (Table 22.1). Although binding properties alter pharmacokinetics of different insulin secretagogues, their similar mode of action means effects are not additive, and they should not be prescribed simultaneously.

EXTRAPANCREATIC EFFECTS OF SUS

K_{ATP} channels are present and functional in a number of other cells, including neurons, cardiomyocytes, and vascular smooth muscle cells. Although the combination of SUR1/Kir6.2 is found in neurons as it is in β-cells, the combinations differ in other tissues (e.g., SUR2A/Kir6.2 predominates in cardiomyocytes). Depending on selectivity, SUs can interact with extrapancreatic K_{ATP} channels, in general with lower binding affinities than the β-cell isoform.

During myocardial ischemia, cardiac K_{ATP} channels open and lead to potassium efflux and reduction in action potential, thus increasing risk for reentrant arrhythmias. SUs can prevent K_{ATP} channels from opening, which should protect against ventricular arrhythmias in the postischemic period. Whether SUs modify the risk of postischemic arrhythmias remains controversial, however. The more concerning consequence of SUs binding to cardiac K_{ATP} channels is the potential impact of SU on ischemic preconditioning (IP) (discussed later). IP refers to myocardial protection conferred by brief periods of ischemia followed by periods of reperfusion that reduce the magnitude of subsequent myocardial injury.[4]

With regard to effects of SUs on neurons, increasing experimental evidence suggests K_{ATP} channels are important in the hypothalamic-liver circuitry regulating hepatic glucose production. Specifically, activation of the K_{ATP} channel in the hypothalamic mediobasal nucleus, which harbors the same isoform on pancreatic β-cells, can lower hepatic glucose production[5] and may control adaptation to hypoglycemia.[6,7]

INFLUENCE OF POLYMORPHISMS OF SUs TARGET GENES ON CLINICAL RESPONSE

Although clinical variables, such as a decline in β-cell function and degree of insulin resistance, are major determinants of response to SUs, polymorphisms of K_{ATP} channel subunits and of drug-metabolizing genes may affect SU binding and clearance, thereby influencing clinical outcomes and the risk of adverse events.

SUs are indicated specifically for patients with diabetes because of insulin deficiency caused by abnormalities of ATP generation or the inability of ATP to close the β-cell K_{ATP} channel. Examples include some forms of neonatal diabetes and maturity-onset diabetes of the young (MODY)-3 due to abnormalities of the hepatic nuclear factor-1α gene. In patients with MODY-3, the inability of the normal regulatory pathways to close the K_{ATP} channel can be bypassed by using sulfonylureas to directly close the channel by binding to the SUR receptor, thereby restoring adequate insulin secretion.

Genetic variants of *KCNJ11*, the gene encoding for Kir6.2, and *ABCC8*, the gene encoding SUR1, also may modulate SU response. The most widely studied polymorphism of *KCNJ11* is the glutamate to lysine substitution at position 23 (E23K). This polymorphism is emerging as a T2D risk allele in some studies and is associated with decreased insulin secretion in humans,[8] and possibly decreased glyburide-induced insulin release.[9] Of note, E23K is in strong linkage disequilibrium with the *ABCC8* Ser1389Ala polymorphism: most carriers of a *KCNJ11* K23 risk allele also carry an *ABCC8* Ala1369 risk allele, with the K23/A1369 haplotype occurring in ~20% of T2D patients. The K23/A1369 double variant confers increased sensitivity to gliclazide, as compared with wild-type E23/S1369 K_{ATP} channels.[10] Studies on the clinical importance of K_{ATP} channel polymorphisms on SU response have been contradictory, however, possibly because of the heterogeneity of the study population, ethnicity, or sample size. For instance, in newly diagnosed T2D patients enrolled in the U.K. Prospective Diabetes Study (UKPDS), the *KCNJ11* E23K variant was not associated significantly with response to SU therapy.[11]

The impact of variants of other candidate genes on SUs also has been investigated. Two single-nucleotide polymorphisms (rs12255372 G>T and rs7903146 C>T) of the T2D susceptibility gene *TCF7L2*, which is a transcription factor involved in glucose homeostasis and lipid metabolism, were studied in the Genetics of Diabetes Audit and Research Tayside (GoDARTS) population.[12] Both polymorphisms were associated with a significantly increased odds ratio of SU failure, which was defined as failure to attain HbA_{1c} <7% over the first 12 months after SU prescription.

Polymorphisms of drug-metabolizing enzymes (e.g., *CYP2C9*3* Isoleucine 359 to Leucine) also could affect clinical response and the risk of SU-induced hypoglycemia. Clearance of all SUs is reduced in patients carrying the *CYP2C9*3* allele.[13] Although the majority of *CYP2C9* pharmacogenomic studies have been conducted in healthy volunteers, a provocative small study of 20 T2D patients treated with SUs and admitted to the emergency department with hypoglycemia showed the *CYP2C9*3/*3* variant was associated with a fivefold increased odds ratio of a severe hypoglycemic event, as compared with other *CYP2C9* genotype groups.[14]

Together, these studies generate intriguing new hypotheses to interpret interindividual variability in SUs response and side effects. Whether similar molecular and genetic variations affect actions of glinides has been less carefully studied to date. Additional investigation in large prospective randomized trials is needed to clarify whether this information can be used to predict SU effectiveness or failure and side-effect risk profiles, and to individualize therapy by guiding selection of a specific SU or the choice of SUs versus other antidiabetic medications.

USE AND EFFICACY OF SULFONYLUREAS

As the first available oral agent to treat T2D, SUs have been a mainstay of treatment, either as monotherapy or, more recently, as an add-on to other diabetes medications—usually metformin. Insulin secretagogues, like all diabetes pharmacotherapies, should be administered in conjunction with dietary and exercise management. Contraindications for use of nonincretin insulin secretagogues are provided in Table 22.2. Insulin secretagogue therapy should be instituted with a low dose and increased at weekly intervals based on glycemic response until the maximal benefit is achieved. Not all people with T2D respond to antihyperglycemic actions of SUs (primary failure), and many patients who respond well initially may have a loss of effective antihyperglycemic response after several years of treatment (secondary failure).

The American Diabetes Association (ADA) and the European Association for the Study of Diabetes (EASD) and other societies agree that metformin generally is the first-line oral agent for T2D treatment. For those with reduced renal function or who experience side effects, SUs and glinides continue to be tier 1 drugs and have many advantages compared with newer agents approved by the U.S. Food and Drug Administration or insulin. SUs are effective alone and in combination with other glucose-lowering agents, and reduce HbA_{1c} by ~1.5%.[15-17] The Multicenter Metformin Study Group[16] included a subgroup of T2D patients in poor control (mean HbA_{1c} 8.5%) with mean diabetes duration of ~8 years who were treated with glyburide in combination with metformin over a period of 29 weeks. As seen in multiple studies, treatment with metformin and glyburide results in greater glycemic reduction than either agent alone, supporting combined use when a single agent is inadequate.

Most SUs have equal efficacy, but glinides are somewhat less effective in lowering HbA_{1c}. A systematic review of placebo-controlled randomized trials on oral antidiabetic agents (including three with glipizide, two with glimepiride, and one with glyburide) show SUs lower A1C by ~1.0–1.25%, whereas glinides decrease HbA_{1c} by 0.5–0.7%, compared with placebo.[17] The six studies with SUs allowed dose adjustments, had a follow-up periods ranging between 12 and 56 weeks, and examined effects of SU treatment either as monotherapy or in combination with

Table 22.2 Contraindications for Insulin Secretagogue Therapy

- Type 1 diabetes or pancreatic diabetes
- Pregnancy

Although not FDA approved for use during pregnancy, glyburide has proven safe and efficacious in patients with gestational diabetes who decline insulin treatment. The effects of glyburide in the management of gestational diabetes are currently being evaluated in a nonrandomized open-label clinical trial (ClinicalTrials.gov Identifier: NCT01947699).

- Major surgery
- Severe infections, stress, or trauma
- History of severe adverse reaction to a sulfonylurea or similar compound (sulfa drug) (does not exclude repaglinide)
- Predisposition to severe hypoglycemia (e.g., patients with significant liver or kidney disease)

other oral medications. Another meta-analysis of placebo-controlled, double-masked randomized trials directly addressed the effects of SUs on HbA_{1c} as monotherapy versus as an add-on to background therapy (another oral agent or insulin) versus background therapy alone. Importantly, only studies with fixed-dose SUs were included.[18] In the nine trials examining SU monotherapy, the HbA_{1c} level was 1.51% lower than the placebo group (trial length ranging between 12 and 36 weeks). When combined with other oral agents (primarily metformin or insulin), SUs decreased HbA_{1c} by 1.6% and by 0.46%, respectively, compared with background therapy. Thus, treatment with SUs in the short term is at least as effective in lowering HbA_{1c} as newer antidiabetic agents, while being markedly less expensive.

How do SUs compare with other antidiabetic medications as an add-on to metformin? The Glycemia Reduction Approaches in Diabetes: A Comparative Effectiveness (GRADE) study now under way (www.ClinicalTrials.gov Identifier: NCT01794143) will examine efficacy and durability of four major classes of anti-diabetic medications, including SUs (specifically, glimepiride) in metformin-treated patients with duration of T2D <5 years and HbA_{1c} of 6.8–8.5%. The main outcome of this National Institute of Diabetes and Digestive and Kidney Diseases (NIDDK)–sponsored unmasked trial will be primary glycemic failure, defined as $HbA_{1c} \geq 7\%$, over an anticipated observation period of ~5 years.[19] There are few adequately powered "head-to-head" trials comparing SUs with other antidiabetic drugs, when added to metformin. In the Liraglutide Effect and Action in Diabetes (LEAD)-2 study, glimepiride showed a comparable mean HbA_{1c} decrease of 1.0% with the two higher dosages of the glucagon-like peptide-1 analog liraglutide, when added to metformin over a 26-week follow-up period. T2D patients enrolled in this double-masked, placebo-controlled, parallel-group trial had a mean diabetes duration of ~7 years with mean HbA_{1c} of 8.4%.[20] Not unexpectedly, incidence of minor hypoglycemia was higher with glimepiride (~17%) than with liraglutide and placebo (both ~3%), whereas gastrointestinal side effects were three- to four-fold more common with liraglutide. Overall safety, efficacy, and side effect profiles of alternative pharmacologic options continue to drive selection of second- and third-line agents when intensification of glycemic management is needed.

When trials with multiple doses of SUs are examined, a decreased incremental-magnitude dose-response improvement in HbA_{1c} is seen when administered above half-maximal SU dosage. These findings support the notion that combination therapy at low doses may maximize the efficacy–adverse events ratio.

PRIMARY AND SECONDARY FAILURE WITH SUs

The majority of trials examining SU efficacy have been limited to <1 year in duration. Yet, T2D is a progressive disease, primarily because of a steady decline in β-cell function (Table 22.3). Thus, initial lack of response to SUs (primary failure) and decline in response over time with continued treatment (secondary failure) can be viewed in part as a function of β cell "reserve," although other factors also contribute to diminished efficacy.

In the UKPDS, treatment with SUs (primarily glyburide or chlorpropamide) led to an HbA_{1c} <7% in 50% of patients at 3 years, 34% at 6 years, and only 24% at 9 years.[21] A similar pattern was observed in the A Diabetes Outcome Progres-

Table 22.3 Common Causes of Secondary Sulfonylurea Failure

Patient-related factors

- Overeating and weight gain
- Poor patient compliance
- Lack of physical activity
- Stress
- Intercurrent illnesses

Disease-related factors

- Decreasing β-cell function
- Increasing insulin resistance

Therapy-related factors

- Inadequate drug dosage
- Desensitization to chronic sulfonylurea exposure
- Impaired absorption of drug due to hyperglycemia
- Concomitant therapy with diabetogenic drugs

sion Trial (ADOPT) trial. To compare cumulative incidence of monotherapy failure of rosiglitazone, glyburide, and metformin, ADOPT enrolled patients with a relatively short duration of T2D (<2 years for ~95% of participants) and mean HbA$_{1c}$ of ~7.3%.[22] At 5 years, secondary failure, defined as confirmed fasting plasma glucose (FPG) >180 mg/dl, was 15% with rosiglitazone, 21% with metformin, and 34% with glyburide. The percentage of patients with HbA$_{1c}$ <7% at 4 years was 40% with rosiglitazone, 34% with metformin, and 26% with glyburide. Within the first 6 months, however, glyburide had the greatest effect on FPG and HbA$_{1c}$ reduction, and these parameters were comparable to rosiglitazone and metformin through the first 2–3 years of the study. Mechanistic insight for the different durability of glyburide and metformin can be gleaned from studies in islets isolated from people with T2D, in which β-cell apoptosis was reduced by metformin,[23] and increased by glyburide.[24]

Although ADOPT showed shorter durability of glycemic effects with glyburide, as compared with metformin and rosiglitazone, it confirmed the rapid onset of action of SUs. This is a key advantage of SU pharmacotherapy. Because the post-trial 10-year follow-up of the UKPDS subjects showed that *early* tight glucose control was associated with persistent risk reduction in microvascular complications, despite the loss of between-group differences in HbA$_{1c}$,[25] there is clearly a benefit in achieving tight glycemic control as soon after diagnosis of T2D as possible. In addition, a decrease in risk of myocardial infarction (MI) and death from any cause was emergent with extended follow-up. This information underscored the beneficial impact of intensive T2D control early after diagnosis, similar to findings of The Diabetes Control and Complications Trial (DCCT)-Epidemiology of Diabetes Interventions and Complications (EDIC) in type 1 diabetes

(T1D) patients.[26] These findings, however, also underscore the need for vigilance in monitoring for progressive dysglycemia and when this occurs, change in therapeutic approach should be initiated without delay.

ADOPT clearly demonstrated that none of the three drugs proved satisfactory as monotherapy in the long term. Thus, early institution of combination therapy, with drugs used at lower-than-maximal doses and with diverse sites of action, is increasingly advocated as an alternative approach to monotherapy at maximal doses or as serial add-on therapy. Plausible postulated benefits would be lower frequency of side effects with use of submaximal doses of medications and the potential for modifying rates of β-cell failure when insulin sensitizers are used in combination with SUs. Ongoing trials are evaluating long-term efficacy and disease-modifying effects of other low-dose combination therapies.

USE AND EFFICACY OF GLINIDES AS ADD-ON AND MONOTHERAPY

Both repaglinide, a carbamoylbenzoic acid derivative related to meglitinide, and nateglinide, a derivative of phenylalanine, have rapid oral absorption with peak plasma levels occurring at 1 hour for repaglinide and ~1.5 hours for nateglinide, and a short half-life of 1.5–1.8 hours for both. Such pharmacokinetic features explain the almost exclusive effect on postprandial glucose excursions and may contribute to the decreased risk of hypoglycemia noted in many, although not all, studies.

When nateglinide was used as monotherapy in a randomized, double-masked trial, patients receiving nateglinide for 12 weeks exhibited a 0.7% mean percentage HbA_{1c} decrease from baseline, compared with placebo.[29] Similar outcomes have been obtained with repaglinide monotherapy in treatment-naïve patients as well as in patients previously treated with other oral antidiabetic drugs.[30] When compared head-to-head in a randomized, parallel-group, open-label 16-week trial, repaglinide resulted in greater reductions of HbA_{1c} than nateglinide (–1.57 versus –1.04%, respectively; $P = 0.002$), with HbA_{1c} values <7% achieved by 54% of repaglinide-treated patients versus 42% for nateglinide. These results were achieved with a median final dose of 6.0 mg/day for repaglinide and 360 mg/day for nateglinide. Increased efficacy with repaglinide treatment was accompanied by more weight gained at the end of the 16-week period (~1.8 versus 0.7 kg, respectively). At least one episode of hypoglycemia occurred in 7% percent of repaglinide-treated patients (plasma glucose <50 mg/dl) versus none with nateglinide. No differences in side effects, such as upper-respiratory infections, headache, and diarrhea, were noted.[31]

Both repaglinide and nateglinide are approved in combination with other antidiabetic drugs. When used in combination with metformin over 2 years, nateglinide was well tolerated and decreased HbA_{1c} by 1.2% from 7.8 to 6.6%, as did the parallel study of glyburide with metformin. The frequency of mild and severe hypoglycemia was significantly higher with glyburide than with nateglinide.[79]

Thus, glinides represent a useful option in patient populations at high risk of hypoglycemia (e.g., the elderly) or with erratic meal intake. The largely distinct routes of clearance of repaglinide (primarily hepatic) and nateglinide (primarily renal) may guide the choice of which glinide should be instituted in an individual patient.

Information regarding the durability of effects of glinides is limited in patients with T2D. Of interest, in persons with impaired glucose tolerance, nateglinide did not modify incidence of progression to T2D.[32]

EFFECTS OF SUs AND GLINIDES ON CARDIOVASCULAR OUTCOMES

Concerns regarding cardiovascular risk associated with SU treatment were first raised in the 1970s following the University Group Diabetes Program Study (UGDPS), which showed a higher incidence of cardiovascular mortality with tolbutamide compared with insulin or placebo.[33] Of note, UGDPS patients allocated to tolbutamide had higher baseline cardiac risk than those on placebo.

One hypothesis regarding the cardiovascular safety signal observed with tolbutamide in the UGDPS and in other studies with glyburide[34] relates to the affinity of these SUs for the cardiac K_{ATP} channel, which may oppose the protective mechanism of ischemic preconditioning. Newer SUs, such as gliclazide and glimepiride, exhibit higher selectivity for the K_{ATP} channel on β-cells than older SUs,[35] which is consistent with a lack of effect on ischemic preconditioning found in both human[36] and experimental models[37] compared with glyburide. Higher binding affinity of glyburide to K_{ATP} channels on cardiomyocytes, as compared with other SUs, may explain this difference.[35] Although randomized comparisons among SUs on hard cardiovascular outcomes are lacking, T2D patients admitted for acute MI who had been chronically treated with gliclazide or glimepiride had fewer arrhythmias, fewer ischemic complications, and lower early mortality than patients on glyburide.[38]

Despite potentially concerning results of the UGDPS and the mechanistic hypothesis on ischemic preconditioning, many other long-term trials demonstrate either neutral or beneficial cardiovascular outcomes with SUs. The UKPDS showed a nonsignificant 16% risk reduction for MI in T2D patients receiving SUs.[21] As mentioned, the post-trial 10-year follow-up showed an emergent risk reduction for MI and death from any cause over time in participants previously randomized to SUs.[25] Likewise, in the Action in Diabetes and Vascular Disease: Preterax and Diamicron Modified Release Controlled Evaluation (ADVANCE) trial, modified-release gliclazide was associated with a decreased rate of primary endpoints at 5 years, combining major macrovascular and microvascular events.[39]

Effects of SUs on cardiovascular outcomes as compared with other antidiabetic drugs remain controversial. Institution of monotherapy with SUs (glipizide or glyburide) in a cohort study of veterans with mean HbA_{1c} 7.2% was associated with an increased hazard ratio for the primary endpoint (a composite of acute MI, stroke, or death), as compared with metformin monotherapy.[40] This study could not clarify whether the difference was the result of enhanced cardiovascular disease risk with SUs, or a more obvious benefit afforded by metformin, or both. On the other hand, the Bypass Angioplasty Revascularization Investigation 2 Diabetes (BARI 2D) did not reveal significant differences in rates of death and major cardiovascular events in T2D patients with coronary artery disease treated with insulin-sensitizing agents versus an insulin-provision therapeutic approach, with 50% of the latter group treated with SUs.[41] Finally, SU treatment was associated with a trend toward fewer serious cardiovascular events than metformin in ADOPT, although the trial was not powered to study cardiovascular endpoints.[22]

With regard to effects of glinides on cardiovascular events, the NAVIGATOR trial demonstrated nateglinide did not reduce rates of cardiovascular outcomes (or incidence of T2D) compared with placebo over a 5-year period in a cohort with impaired glucose tolerance and established cardiovascular disease or cardiovascular risk factors.[32] In this study, all patients were on lifestyle modification program and ~40% were treated with statins at baseline.

The evidence indicates that SUs as a class are not clearly associated with increased adverse CV risk, although there may be relevant differences between older and newer medications, and concerns persist that cardiovascular effects may not be favorable when compared with other agents.

CLASS-SPECIFIC VERSUS DRUG-SPECIFIC COMMON SIDE EFFECTS

The major concerns regarding insulin secretagogue therapy are hypoglycemia and weight gain.

HYPOGLYCEMIA

Severe hypoglycemia (i.e., requiring ambulance or hospital treatment) occurs in ~1 in every 100 people treated with a SU each year versus 1 in every 2,000 treated with metformin and 1 in every 10 treated with insulin.[42] This is an important issue in terms of quality of life, risk of falls, and coma (especially in the elderly), as well as health care costs.

In the UKPDS, the mean percentage of patients per year with one or more episodes of hypoglycemia was 17.7% for glyburide and 11.0% for chlorpropamide, whereas the rate of severe hypoglycemia was ~0.5% per year with both medications.[21] Insulin secretagogues with longer half-life appear to have greater hypoglycemic risk. A meta-analysis of parallel, randomized controlled trials showed a 52% greater risk of experiencing at least one episode of hypoglycemia with glyburide when compared with other secretagogues (RR 1.52 [95% confidence interval, CI 1.21–1.92]).[43] When the analysis was limited to studies comparing glyburide with other SUs, the relative risk with glyburide was 1.44 for overall hypoglycemic events and 4.69 for major hypoglycemic events. Chronic kidney disease (CKD) enhances the risk of hypoglycemia in patients treated with glyburide because of the increased formation of weakly active metabolites.

A meta-analysis of the effect of secretagogues *in combination with metformin*, which included three trials with SUs and two with glinides, confirmed increased risk of overall hypoglycemia with SUs when used with metformin. In addition, the risk of hypoglycemia with nateglinide (RR 7.9, 95% CI 1.45–43.2) was not lower than with SUs as suggested in other studies. Importantly, this meta-analysis did not distinguish mild from severe hypoglycemia.[44]

Glucose potentiation of insulin secretion remains important and both SUs and glinides induce less insulin secretion at relative hypoglycemia.[45] This feature may contribute to the relative infrequency of severe hypoglycemia with use of these agents, which induce insulin secretion.

The risk and consequences of hypoglycemia are not distributed uniformly across the spectrum of diabetic patients. In the elderly, frequency of hypoglycemic events of all severities in response to secretagogues (and insulin) is increased. An increasing appreciation of the impact of hypoglycemia in the elderly is represented in the 2012 Beers criteria issued by the American Geriatrics Society. This updated version recommended that glyburide and chlorpropamide (as well as sliding-scale insulin) be avoided in the geriatric patient population.[46]

WEIGHT GAIN

Weight gain is noted in almost all studies involving T2D patients receiving chronic SU or glinide therapy. In the UKPDS, SU therapy aimed at achieving intensive blood glucose control was associated with ~5.5 kg increase in body weight.[21] Weight gain in patients treated with glyburide monotherapy in ADOPT amounted to ~2.5 kg over the first year, but stabilized after that time.[22] Overall, no significant differences among SUs have been noted.

Weight gain is lower when SUs are combined with other antihyperglycemic agents, such as acarbose or metformin. Some studies suggest repaglinide is associated with less weight gain than SU treatment in pharmacotherapy-naïve patients.[47]

EFFECTS OF OTHER DRUGS ON INSULIN SECRETAGOGUE ACTIONS

Many commonly used drugs can potentiate insulin secretagogue effects and precipitate hypoglycemia or antagonize insulin secretagogue effects and worsen glycemic control. Table 22.4 lists some of the more important interactions. Alcohol and high-dose aspirin interactions may lead to prolonged and severe hypoglycemia.

Table 22.4—Drug Interactions with Sulfonylureas

Increase hypoglycemia

- Drugs that displace sulfonylurea from albumin-binding sites (e.g., aspirin, fibrates, trimethoprim)
- Competitive inhibitors of sulfonylurea metabolism (e.g., alcohol, H2 blockers, anticoagulants)
- Inhibitors of urinary excretion of sulfonylureas (e.g., probenecid, allopurinol)
- Concomitant use of drugs with hypoglycemic properties (e.g., alcohol, aspirin)
- Antagonists of endogenous counterregulatory hormones (e.g., β-blockers, sympatholytic drugs)

Worsen glycemic control

- Drugs that increase sulfonylurea metabolism (e.g., barbiturates, rifampin)
- Agents that antagonize sulfonylurea action (e.g., β-blockers)
- Inhibitors of insulin secretion or action (e.g., thiazides and loop diuretics, β-blockers, corticosteroids, estrogens, phenytoin)

β-Blockers interfere with both the recognition and counterregulatory responses to hypoglycemia. Anticoagulants are competitive inhibitors of SU metabolism, and when both classes of drugs are used, doses of both may have to be reduced appropriately.

Any concomitant drug treatment in a patient on or to be started on insulin secretagogue therapy must be evaluated for possible drug interactions. Because SUs with high intrinsic activity are given in smaller quantities and have somewhat different binding characteristics, they are likely to have fewer drug interactions than those with low intrinsic activity.

Repaglinide metabolism may be inhibited by antifungal agents, such as ketoconazole and miconazole; antibacterial agents, such as erythromycin; and agents that block glucuronidation, such as gemfibrozil. Drugs that increase cytochrome P_{450} enzyme system 3A4 may increase repaglinide metabolism in the liver. Such drugs include thiazolidinediones (TZDs) and barbiturates. Repaglinide does not alter metabolism of digoxin, warfarin, or theophylline. Its interactions with agents that increase hypoglycemia or worsen glycemic control are similar to those of SUs (Table 22.3). Treating patients with repaglinide who are on other medications may require dose adjustments.

THE ROLE OF SUs AND GLINIDES IN MANAGEMENT OF T2D

The role of SUs and glinides in the management of T2D lies in several key factors: *1*) efficacy and durability, *2*) safety, *3*) cost, and *4*) comparison with other antidiabetic drugs.

EFFICACY AND DURABILITY

SUs are highly efficacious both as monotherapy and in combination with many other glucose-lowering therapies, especially within the first few years after onset of T2D. Despite shorter durability than metformin, the rapid onset of action and tight blood glucose control achieved with SUs early in the course of T2D may result in long-term prevention of the development of micro- and macrovascular complications.[25]

SAFETY

Cardiovascular safety with SU treatment has been debated over decades. Multiple randomized studies with extended follow-up, however, have not confirmed a detrimental effect on cardiovascular risk when using newer SUs.[39,41] Distinct effects of newer SUs on cardiovascular outcomes may be one of the factors guiding the choice toward a specific SU.

Although increased risk of hypoglycemia is shared by all secretagogues, relative risk may be higher with glyburide and first generation SUs. These drugs should be avoided in patients at highest risk for hypoglycemia, such as the elderly, those with poor nutrition or who commonly miss meals, or those who have concomitant renal, hepatic, or cardiovascular disease. In these patients, shorter-acting insulin secretagogues may be safer. Attention should be paid to the different clearance properties of the specific agents in patients with underlying liver or kidney diseases.

COST

SUs remain one of the most affordable treatments for T2D. Given the increasing economic impact of diabetes nationally, emphasis on cost-effective treatment is important for chronic diseases like T2D, and the relative low cost of SUs is a major advantage when compared with newer classes of oral antidiabetic agents.

COMPARISON WITH OTHER ANTIDIABETIC MEDICATIONS

Although metformin remains the first-line pharmacologic agent of choice for patients who have adequate renal function and do not experience side effects of treatment, selection of additional agents must be individualized based on age, weight, and comorbidities, such as coronary heart disease, heart failure, chronic kidney disease, liver dysfunction, and hypoglycemic risk. Long-term safety profiles are better understood with SUs than for newly approved antidiabetic therapeutic alternatives. Better understanding of pharmacogenomics may help better guide the selection of the specific SU for a given patient, or be able to differentiate responders from nonresponders, or those at increased risk, to better inform use. In the meantime, SUs and glinides remain appropriate treatment alternatives in our armamentarium to manage T2D.

REFERENCES

1. Seino S, Takahashi H, Takahashi T, Shibasaki T. Treating diabetes today: a matter of selectivity of sulphonylureas. *Diabetes, Obesity & Metabolism* 2012;14(Suppl 1):9–13.

2. Lebovitz HE, Melander A. Sulfonylureas: basic aspects and clinical uses. In *International Textbook of Diabetes Mellitus*. 3rd ed. DeFronzo RA, Keen H, Zimmet P, Eds. Colchester, U.K., Wiley, 2004.

3. Zhang CL, Katoh M, Shibasaki T, Minami K, Sunaga Y, Takahashi H, Yokoi N, Iwasaki M, Miki T, Seino S. The cAMP sensor Epac2 is a direct target of antidiabetic sulfonylurea drugs. *Science* 2009;325:607–610.

4. Murry CE, Jennings RB, Reimer KA. Preconditioning with ischemia: a delay of lethal cell injury in ischemic myocardium. *Circulation* 1986;74:1124–1136.

5. Go EH, Kyriakidou-Himonas M, Berelowitz M. Effects of glipizide GITS and glibenclamide on metabolic control, hepatic glucose production, and insulin secretion in patients with type 2 diabetes. *Diabetes Metab Res Rev* 2004;20:225–231.

6. Pocai A, Lam TK, Gutierrez-Juarez R, Obici S, Schwartz GJ, Bryan J, Aguilar-Bryan L, Rossetti L. Hypothalamic K(ATP) channels control hepatic glucose production. *Nature* 2005;434:1026–1031.

7. Kishore P, Boucai L, Zhang K, Li W, Koppaka S, Kehlenbrink S, Schiwek A, Esterson YB, Mehta D, Bursheh S, Su Y, Gutierrez-Juarez R, Muzumdar R, Schwartz GJ, Hawkins M. Activation of K(ATP) channels suppresses glucose production in humans. *J Clin Invest* 2011;121:4916–4920.

8. Florez JC, Jablonski KA, Kahn SE, Franks PW, Dabelea D, Hamman RF, Knowler WC, Nathan DM, Altshuler D. Type 2 diabetes-associated missense polymorphisms KCNJ11 E23K and ABCC8 A1369S influence progression to diabetes and response to interventions in the Diabetes Prevention Program. *Diabetes* 2007;56:531–536.

9. Sesti G, Laratta E, Cardellini M, Andreozzi F, Del Guerra S, Irace C, Gnasso A, Grupillo M, Lauro R, Hribal ML, Perticone F, Marchetti P. The E23K variant of KCNJ11 encoding the pancreatic beta-cell adenosine 5'-triphosphate-sensitive potassium channel subunit Kir6.2 is associated with an increased risk of secondary failure to sulfonylurea in patients with type 2 diabetes. *J Clin Endocrinol Metab* 2006;91:2334–2339.

10. Hamming KS, Soliman D, Matemisz LC, Niazi O, Lang Y, Gloyn AL, Light PE. Coexpression of the type 2 diabetes susceptibility gene variants KCNJ11 E23K and ABCC8 S1369A alter the ATP and sulfonylurea sensitivities of the ATP-sensitive K(+) channel. *Diabetes* 2009;58:2419–2424.

11. Gloyn AL, Hashim Y, Ashcroft SJ, Ashfield R, Wiltshire S, Turner RC. Association studies of variants in promoter and coding regions of beta-cell ATP-sensitive K-channel genes SUR1 and Kir6.2 with type 2 diabetes mellitus (UKPDS 53). *Diabet Med* 2001;18:206–212.

12. Pearson ER, Donnelly LA, Kimber C, Whitley A, Doney AS, McCarthy MI, Hattersley AT, Morris AD, Palmer CN. Variation in TCF7L2 influences therapeutic response to sulfonylureas: a GoDARTs study. *Diabetes* 2007;56:2178–2182.

13. Kirchheiner J, Roots I, Goldammer M, Rosenkranz B, Brockmoller J. Effect of genetic polymorphisms in cytochrome p450 (CYP) 2C9 and CYP2C8 on the pharmacokinetics of oral antidiabetic drugs: clinical relevance. *Clinical Pharmacokinetics* 2005;44:1209–1225.

14. Holstein A, Plaschke A, Ptak M, Egberts EH, El-Din J, Brockmoller J, Kirchheiner J. Association between CYP2C9 slow metabolizer genotypes and severe hypoglycaemia on medication with sulphonylurea hypoglycaemic agents. *Br J Clin Pharmacol* 2005;60:103–106.

15. Nathan DM, Buse JB, Davidson MB, Ferrannini E, Holman RR, Sherwin R, Zinman B. Medical management of hyperglycemia in type 2 diabetes: a consensus algorithm for the initiation and adjustment of therapy: a consensus statement of the American Diabetes Association and the European Association for the Study of Diabetes. *Diabetes Care* 2009;32:193–203.

16. DeFronzo RA, Goodman AM. Efficacy of metformin in patients with non-insulin-dependent diabetes mellitus. The Multicenter Metformin Study Group. *N Engl J Med* 1995;333:541–549.

17. Sherifali D, Nerenberg K, Pullenayegum E, Cheng JE, Gerstein HC. The effect of oral antidiabetic agents on A1C levels: a systematic review and meta-analysis. *Diabetes Care* 2010;33:1859–1864.

18. Hirst JA, Farmer AJ, Dyar A, Lung TW, Stevens RJ. Estimating the effect of sulfonylurea on HbA1c in diabetes: a systematic review and meta-analysis. *Diabetologia* 2013;56:973–984.

19. Nathan DM, Buse JB, Kahn SE, Krause-Steinrauf H, Larkin ME, Staten M, Wexler D, Lachin JM. Rationale and design of the glycemia reduction approaches in diabetes: a comparative effectiveness study (GRADE). *Diabetes Care* 2013;36:2254–2261.

20. Nauck M, Frid A, Hermansen K, Shah NS, Tankova T, Mitha IH, Zdravkovic M, During M, Matthews DR. Efficacy and safety comparison of liraglutide, glimepiride, and placebo, all in combination with metformin, in type 2 diabetes: the LEAD (liraglutide effect and action in diabetes)-2 study. *Diabetes Care* 2009;32:84–90.

21. UK Prospective Diabetes Study (UKPDS) Group. Intensive blood-glucose control with sulphonylureas or insulin compared with conventional treatment and risk of complications in patients with type 2 diabetes (UKPDS 33). *Lancet* 1998;352:837–853.

22. Kahn SE, Haffner SM, Heise MA, Herman WH, Holman RR, Jones NP, Kravitz BG, Lachin JM, O'Neill MC, Zinman B, Viberti G. Glycemic durability of rosiglitazone, metformin, or glyburide monotherapy. *N Engl J Med* 2006;355:2427–2443.

23. Marchetti P, Del Guerra S, Marselli L, Lupi R, Masini M, Pollera M, Bugliani M, Boggi U, Vistoli F, Mosca F, Del Prato S. Pancreatic islets from type 2 diabetic patients have functional defects and increased apoptosis that are ameliorated by metformin. *J Clin Endocrinol Metab* 2004;89:5535–5541.

24. Maedler K, Carr RD, Bosco D, Zuellig RA, Berney T, Donath MY. Sulfonylurea induced beta-cell apoptosis in cultured human islets. *J Clin Endocrinol Metab* 2005;90:501–506.

25. Holman RR, Paul SK, Berthel A, Matthews DR, Neil HAW. 10-year follow-up of intensive glucose control in type 2 diabetes. *N Engl J Med* 2008;359:1577–1589.

26. Nathan DM, Cleary PA, Backlund JY, Genuth SM, Lachin JM, Orchard TJ, Raskin P, Zinman B. Intensive diabetes treatment and cardiovascular disease in patients with type 1 diabetes. *N Engl J Med* 2005;353:2643–2653.

27. Zinman B, Harris SB, Neuman J, Gerstein HC, Retnakaran RR, Raboud J, Qi Y, Hanley AJ. Low-dose combination therapy with rosiglitazone and metformin to prevent type 2 diabetes mellitus (CANOE trial): a double-blind randomised controlled study. *Lancet* 2010;376:103–111.

28. Retnakaran R, Qi Y, Harris SB, Hanley AJ, Zinman B. Changes over time in glycemic control, insulin sensitivity, and beta-cell function in response to

low-dose metformin and thiazolidinedione combination therapy in patients with impaired glucose tolerance. *Diabetes Care* 2011;34:1601–1604.

29. Schwarz SL, Gerich JE, Marcellari A, Jean-Louis L, Purkayastha D, Baron MA. Nateglinide, alone or in combination with metformin, is effective and well tolerated in treatment-naive elderly patients with type 2 diabetes. *Diabetes Obes Metab* 2008;10:652–660.

30. Moses RG, Gomis R, Frandsen KB, Schlienger JL, Dedov I. Flexible meal-related dosing with repaglinide facilitates glycemic control in therapy-naive type 2 diabetes. *Diabetes Care* 2001;24:11–15.

31. Rosenstock J, Hassman DR, Madder RD, Brazinsky SA, Farrell J, Khutory-ansky N, Hale PM. Repaglinide versus nateglinide monotherapy: a randomized, multicenter study. *Diabetes Care* 2004;27:1265–1270.

32. Holman RR, Haffner SM, McMurray JJ, Bethel MA, Holzhauer B, Hua TA, Belenkov Y, Boolell M, Buse JB, Buckley BM, Chacra AR, Chiang FT, Charbonnel B, Chow CC, Davies MJ, Deedwania P, Diem P, Einhorn D, Fonseca V, Fulcher GR, Gaciong Z, Gaztambide S, Giles T, Horton E, Ilkova H, Jenssen T, Kahn SE, Krum H, Laakso M, Leiter LA, Levitt NS, Mareev V, Martinez F, Masson C, Mazzone T, Meaney E, Nesto R, Pan C, Prager R, Raptis SA, Rutten GE, Sandstroem H, Schaper F, Scheen A, Schmitz O, Sinay I, Soska V, Stender S, Tamas G, Tognoni G, Tuomilehto J, Villamil AS, Vozar J, Califf RM. Effect of nateglinide on the incidence of diabetes and cardiovascular events. *N Engl J Med* 2010;362:1463–1476.

33. Goldner MG, Knatterud GL, Prout TE. Effects of hypoglycemic agents on vascular complications in patients with adult-onset diabetes. 3. Clinical implications of UGDP results. *JAMA* 1971;218:1400–1410.

34. Scognamiglio R, Avogaro A, Vigili de Kreutzenberg S, Negut C, Palisi M, Bagolin E, Tiengo A. Effects of treatment with sulfonylurea drugs or insulin on ischemia-induced myocardial dysfunction in type 2 diabetes. *Diabetes* 2002;51:808–812.

35. Geisen K, Vegh A, Krause E, Papp JG. Cardiovascular effects of conventional sulfonylureas and glimepiride. *Horm Metab Res* 1996;28:496–507.

36. Klepzig H, Kober G, Matter C, Luus H, Schneider H, Boedeker KH, Kiowski W, Amann FW, Gruber D, Harris S, Burger W. Sulfonylureas and ischaemic preconditioning; a double-blind, placebo-controlled evaluation of glimepiride and glibenclamide. *Eur Heart J* 1999;20:439–446.

37. Mocanu MM, Maddock HL, Baxter GF, Lawrence CL, Standen NB, Yellon DM. Glimepiride, a novel sulfonylurea, does not abolish myocardial protection afforded by either ischemic preconditioning or diazoxide. *Circulation* 2001;103:3111–3116.

38. Zeller M, Danchin N, Simon D, Vahanian A, Lorgis L, Cottin Y, Berland J, Gueret P, Wyart P, Deturck R, Tabone X, Machecourt J, Leclercq F, Drouet E, Mulak G, Bataille V, Cambou JP, Ferrieres J, Simon T. Impact of type of preadmission sulfonylureas on mortality and cardiovascular outcomes in dia-

betic patients with acute myocardial infarction. *J Clin Endocrinol Metab* 2010;95:4993–5002.

39. Patel A, MacMahon S, Chalmers J, Neal B, Billot L, Woodward M, Marre M, Cooper M, Glasziou P, Grobbee D, Hamet P, Harrap S, Heller S, Liu L, Mancia G, Mogensen CE, Pan C, Poulter N, Rodgers A, Williams B, Bompoint S, de Galan BE, Joshi R, Travert F. Intensive blood glucose control and vascular outcomes in patients with type 2 diabetes. *N Engl J Med* 2008;358:2560–2572.

40. Roumie CL, Hung AM, Greevy RA, Grijalva CG, Liu X, Murff HJ, Elasy TA, Griffin MR. Comparative effectiveness of sulfonylurea and metformin monotherapy on cardiovascular events in type 2 diabetes mellitus: a cohort study. *Ann Intern Med* 2012;157:601–610.

41. Group TBDS. A randomized trial of therapies for type 2 diabetes and coronary artery disease. *N Engl J Med* 2009;360:2503–2515.

42. Leese GP, Wang J, Broomhall J, Kelly P, Marsden A, Morrison W, Frier BM, Morris AD. Frequency of severe hypoglycemia requiring emergency treatment in type 1 and type 2 diabetes: a population-based study of health service resource use. *Diabetes Care* 2003;26:1176–1180.

43. Gangji AS, Cukierman T, Gerstein HC, Goldsmith CH, Clase CM. A systematic review and meta-analysis of hypoglycemia and cardiovascular events: a comparison of glyburide with other secretagogues and with insulin. *Diabetes Care* 2007;30:389–394.

44. Phung OJ, Scholle JM, Talwar M, Coleman CI. Effect of noninsulin antidiabetic drugs added to metformin therapy on glycemic control, weight gain, and hypoglycemia in type 2 diabetes. *JAMA* 2010;303:1410–1418.

45. Aldhahi W, Armstrong J, Bouche C, Carr RD, Moses A, Goldfine AB. Beta-cell insulin secretory response to oral hypoglycemic agents is blunted in humans in vivo during moderate hypoglycemia. *J Clin Endocrinol Metab* 2004;89:4553–4557.

46. American Geriatrics Society. Updated Beers Criteria for potentially inappropriate medication use in older adults. *J Am Geriatr Soc* 2012;60:616–631.

47. Marbury T, Huang WC, Strange P, Lebovitz H. Repaglinide versus glyburide: a one-year comparison trial. *Diabetes Res Clin Pract* 1999;43:155–166.

ACKNOWLEDGMENT

The authors thank Dr. Harold Lebowitz for his efforts on the previous edition and for materials carried forward.

① PPARG is a nuclear hormone receptor and transcription factor that is essential for adipogenesis and glucose homestatis.

② pleiotropic actions of TZD: one gene influence multiple, seeming unrelated phenotyped traits.

Chapter 23

Future Use of Thiazolidinediones in Type 2 Diabetes: Practical Lessons

Kwame Osei, MD, FACE, FACP
Trudy Gaillard, PhD, RN, CDE

INTRODUCTION

Type 2 diabetes (T2D) is characterized by insulin resistance and β-cell dysfunction. These abnormalities result in the hyperglycemia and carbohydrate intolerance in patients with T2D. The severity of the pathogenic abnormalities varies considerably among individuals. The disease has a heterogeneous presentation within ethnic and racial groups. In general, the insulin resistance appears to antecede the development of T2D or hyperglycemia for decades. Insulin resistance alone, however, is inadequate and insufficient to cause hyperglycemia and T2D.[1–3] In this context, several authorities believe that the primary foundation for the pathophysiology of the hyperglycemia, although debatable, is centered on the β-cell dysfunction. In fact, the ability and the integrity of the β-cell secretion (including its phasic insulin secretion) to compensate for the insulin resistance determine the glucose tolerance status of the patient. Therefore, both the quantitative and qualitative components of the β-cell dysfunction are prerequisites for developing T2D.[6–9]

For the past two decades, thiazolidinediones (TZDs) have been introduced into the diabetes market for the treatment of T2D with the primary goal of reducing insulin resistance. This has been a welcome addition to the therapeutic armamentarium for the management of patients with T2D.[2–4] The primary targets for TZDs are the insulin-sensitive tissues—namely, adipose tissue, skeletal muscles, and the liver. In this regard, the primary mechanism of action of TZDs in patients with T2D is to enhance carbohydrate metabolism through insulin sensitization.[2–4] This has been attributed to increasing tissue glucose uptake in these target tissues. Indeed, it has been well established that TZDs increase adipogenesis and increase fat deposits in the fat cells. Although the mechanism remains debatable, TZDs potentially stimulate adipose cell (precursor or stem) proliferation.

The molecular mechanisms of TZDs have been attributed to the binding and interaction of TZDs with the nuclear peroxisome proliferator–activated receptor (PPAR) ligand receptor, and their ability to modulate the activity of multiple genes and protein synthesis. These processes of activation of PPAR and protein synthesis account for the delayed actions of these agents on glucose metabolism. Most important, TZDs have variable and pleiotropic effects in addition to their metabolic effects by several other regulatory pathways that are unrelated to glucose metabolism. These include inhibition of androgen synthesis and production (e.g., in polycystic ovarian syndrome), anti-inflammatory properties (highly sensitive C-reactive protein [hsCRP]), and renal handling of salt water. Depending on

DOI: 10.2337/9781580405096.23

the ligand subtype, TZDs are involved in lipid and lipoprotein metabolism with variable potencies and benefits. This partly could explain the variable cardiovascular outcomes in clinical trials in patients with T2D.

HISTORICAL PERSPECTIVE OF TZDS

The advent of TZDs introduced a new paradigm of care and the first true insulin sensitizer in the care of patients with T2D. The first TZD, troglitazone, was introduced to the market in 1997. Troglitazone demonstrated its beneficial effects on lowering serum glucose levels, increasing insulin sensitivity, and reducing serum free fatty acid (FFA) and triglyceride concentration. Troglitazone, however, was associated with serious hepatotoxicity and hence was withdrawn from the market in 2000. The next generation of TZDs was the introduction of rosiglitazone and pioglitazone in 2000, which demonstrated less hepatotoxicity, suggesting that the liver toxicity of TZDs was not a class effect. TZDs, however, continued to be associated with fluid retention, edema, and increasing heart failure when compared with placebo or control groups. Furthermore, recent reports have found TZD to be associated with osteoporosis and atypical fractures in postmenopausal women, which appear to be class effects found with both rosiglitazone and pioglitazone.[9-11]

MECHANISMS OF ACTION OF TZDS

The mechanisms of actions of TZDs have been studied extensively in both humans and experimental animals with and without T2D. These studies were based on the pleotropic effects on several genes resulting in multiple biological effects. In this regard, TZDs modulate the action of PPAR-γ and -α. In general, the PPARs are a family of nuclear receptors that regulate gene expression in response to the binding of certain fatty acids. Depending on the tissue and metabolic environment, however, the downstream effects on gene regulation can either be positive (activation or upregulation) or negative (repression or downregulation), depending on the ligand that binds to the receptor.[2-4] In this regard, PPAR-γ subtype primarily is expressed in adipose tissue but remains debatable in the skeletal muscles. In this context, several researchers have shown that TZDs play a crucial role in adipocyte proliferation and differentiation, fatty acid uptake, and fatty acid storage but not in hepatocyte or skeletal muscle proliferation. TZDs possess the ability to shunt and preserve energy substrates, thus promoting the storage of fat in adipose tissue rather than in the liver or muscle. This results in decreased intramyocellular FFA content and decreased liver fat content and hepatic steatosis. Consequently, TZDs improve insulin sensitivity in the liver, skeletal muscle, and the adipose tissue.[2-4]

CLASSIFICATION OF TZDS

There are several subtypes or ligands of TZDs; however, the main classes are the γ, α, and δ ligands.[2-4] In this regard, the metabolic effects in patients with T2D depend on the subtype of PPAR. In this context, the γ class has the predominant effect on glucose and carbohydrate metabolism because of an increase in insulin sensitivity in the liver, skeletal muscle, and adipose tissue. Nevertheless, the mechanisms of insulin sensitization in the insulin-sensitive tissues remain unknown. In this regard, patients treated with TZDs increase peripheral glucose disposal during euglycemic hyperinsulinemic clamp as assessed by total glucose disposal (M) value or M/I insulin (M/I) and minimal model method by twofold[12,13] and reduce homeostasis model assessment (HOMA-IR) by 50%.[12,13] In addition, TZDs increase hepatic insulin sensitivity as evidenced by effective insulin-mediated suppression of basal hepatic glucose production (HGP).[2-4]

In general, serum insulin levels decrease during treatment with TZDs. The direct effects of TZDs on β-cell secretion and functionality in humans remain debatable, however. Recently, it was demonstrated that TZDs preserve the β-cell secretion as assessed by HOMA-B% and frequently sampled intravenous glucose tolerance test (FSIVGT).[12-15] The direct mechanism of TZDs on β-cell secretion in humans, however, has not been proven. In general, the fasting and postglucose serum insulin responses decrease during TZD treatment of patients with T2D. This has been attributed predominantly to improved hepatic and peripheral insulin sensitivity but not to TZDs' mediated suppression of β-cell secretion. Recently, Osei et al.[16] examined the mechanism of the lower peripheral insulin levels. The study measured insulin clearance (IC) or hepatic insulin extraction (HIE) using C-peptide/insulin molar ratio during the use of rosiglitazone for 3 months in African Americans with prediabetes and impaired glucose tolerance.[17] The study demonstrated that rosiglitazone increased insulin clearance and HIE in patients with prediabetes, IGT, and diabetes.[17] Although, the mechanism of this intriguing result remains uncertain, it is possible that changes in hepatic insulin receptors or metabolism by rosiglitazone could be partly responsible. Thus, clearly, other potential molecular mechanisms of TZDs on insulin metabolism (e.g., hepatic CEACAM 1) could play a role, but this remains to be investigated.[18] Whether this is a class effect of TZDs or it is specific to rosiglitazone remains to be elucidated in patients with and without T2D and in other racial and ethnic populations.

FFAs have a significant impact on hepatic glucose metabolism and peripheral insulin action. One of the mechanisms of TZDs is to increase hepatic insulin action and decrease hepatic glucose production by reducing serum FFA levels. Several previous studies have suggested that elevated FFA is associated with both hepatic and skeletal muscle insulin resistance. Because TZD treatment reduces serum FFA levels, this could be one of the mechanisms for improving insulin sensitivity in vivo in the liver and skeletal muscles. Finally, the reduction in circulating FFA by TZDs also can contribute to the reduced hepatic triglyceride synthesis.[20]

TZDS AND ADIPOCYTOKINES

bioactive product from adipose tissue

Adipose tissue is the largest endocrine organ in the body. There has been increasing interest in the role of adipocytokines in the development of T2D and cardiovascular diseases (CVDs).[2-4] These adipocytokines include adiponectin, interleukin (IL)-6 and IL-8, and tumor necrosis factor–alpha (TNF-α). Further-

adipocytokines
{
- *inflammatory mediator – IL-6, IL-8*
- *angiogenic protein – VEGF*
- *metabolic regulator – adiponectin, leptin*
}

more, these adipocytokines have variable effects on glucose metabolism and insulin sensitivity.

Adiponectin is a 244aa protein synthesized, produced, and secreted solely by adipose tissue. TZDs increase adiponectin levels while they suppress TNF-α and IL-6.[19] Physiologically, adiponectin is an endogenous insulin sensitizer in the peripheral muscle tissues and the liver. Previous studies have shown direct relationships between adiponectin, insulin sensitivity, and metabolic syndrome. Low serum adiponectin has been associated with T2D and coronary artery disease. In this regard, several previous studies have reported increased adiponectin levels during TZD treatment of patients with T2D and prediabetes.[19] Indeed, TZD-induced increases in adiponectin levels could play a mechanistic role in the increases in the hepatic and skeletal muscle insulin sensitivity. Paradoxically, although diet-induced and surgically induced weight loss increases adiponectin levels, TZD treatment often is associated with weight gain and increased adiponectin levels. This paradoxical relationship remains to be elucidated. In contrast to adiponectin, IL-6 and TNF-α cause insulin resistance and β-cell dysfunction. These peptides have been partly responsible for the subclinical inflammatory properties as assessed by hsCRP in obese patients with T2D. T2D is regarded as a subclinical inflammatory state with increased hsCRP. Therefore, the effects of TZDs in reducing inflammation (i.e., anti-inflammatory property) are important in patients with T2D and perhaps CVD and metabolic syndrome. The mechanism of these anti-inflammatory properties of TZDs, however, remains unknown. In this context, it is well established that inflammation worsens insulin resistance and β-cell function. In this regard, several previous studies have shown that hsCRP, as a marker of subclinical inflammation, has been associated with increased prevalence and incidence of metabolic syndrome and coronary artery diseases. Indeed, cardiovascular outcome studies using statins have reported that reduction in cardiac events and morbidity and mortality is associated with reduction in hsCRP.

TZDS AND PREVENTION OF TYPE 2 DIABETES

The pleotropic actions of TZDs make these agents suitable candidates not only for the treatment of established patients with T2D, but also for the prevention of T2D in patients with prediabetes and IGT.[7,12-15] In this regard, several clinical trials support these concepts in the prevention of diabetes in patients with prediabetes.[2-5] Buchman et al.[12] reported that troglitazone prevented incident T2D in Latino women with a history of gestational diabetes mellitus (GDM). This study, referred to as TRIPOD, showed that troglitazone reduced the incidence of T2D by ~58%.[12] The extension of the study with pioglitazone (PIPOD) showed that pioglitazone (similar to troglitazone) was associated with reduced incidence of T2D in Latino women with former GDM.[13] In these studies, the investigators demonstrated that TZD preserved insulin secretion and insulin sensitivity and both significantly reduced progression of T2D. Furthermore, troglitazone was studied in the Diabetes Prevention Program (DPP), a National Institutes of Health (NIH)-sponsored multicenter, multiethnic study in patients with prediabetes and IGT.[7] Patients were randomized into lifestyle intervention, metformin, troglitazone, or placebo. The troglitazone arm was discontinued after a major adverse event, however; the limited use of troglitazone also was associated with reduced incident T2D.[8] During the mean 0.9 year (range 0.5–1.5 years) of intervention, troglitazone reduced the incidence of T2D by 75% when compared with the placebo group.[8] This effect of troglitazone was in part due to improved insulin sensitivity with maintenance of insulin secretion. During the 3-year follow-up of troglitazone, the rate of incidence of T2D was similar to that of placebo. Thus, TZDs prevented or reduced the incidence of T2D, but this was not sustained after withdrawal. No long-term postintervention studies, however, were performed in the DREAM and ACT NOW studies to address this question. In the DPP, the metformin group lost the glycemic benefits within 16 weeks after completion of the study, while the lifestyle arm sustained the lower incident T2D for at least 10 years. In a short-term study, DeFronzo et al.[14] studied the effects of pioglitazone in reversing IGT in the ACT NOW study. The study revealed that pioglitazone can reverse IGT back to normal by improving insulin sensitivity in the liver and peripheral muscles.[14]

Given the potential benefits of TZDs on glucose metabolism, it was important to demonstrate the long-term benefits of TZDs on these parameters in patients with IGT randomized into rosiglitazone or placebo in the DREAM study. This study showed a reduction in incident T2D in patients with prediabetes. The DREAM study was associated with 62% reduction in incident T2D. This was associated with significant improvement in β-cell (HOMA-B%) and insulin sensitivity (HOMA-IR) as the potential mechanism for delaying or preventing the development of T2D.

TZDS AS MONOTHERAPY OR COMBINATION THERAPY ON METABOLIC CONTROL IN TYPE 2 DIABETES

TZDs have become one of the mainstays and backbones in the treatment of patients with T2D.[1,5] TZDs have a general appeal to primary care providers and diabetologists because they are well tolerated, easy to administer orally, and require no renal-dosing adjustments in patients with chronic kidney disease (CKD), when used as monotherapy. TZDs are not associated with hypoglycemia. Because of their mechanism of action, however, the lowering of serum glucose is delayed for 4–6 weeks with a peak action at 10–14 weeks. In general, TZDs given as monotherapy, reduce the fasting glucose by an average of 40–50 mg/dl, postprandial serum glucose by 50–60 mg/dl, and A1C by 1–1.5%. TZDs reduce serum triglycerides by 15–20% and low-density lipoprotein cholesterol (LDL-C) by 10% with minimal effect on high-density lipoprotein cholesterol (HDL-C), but these effects vary depending on the TZD.

In general, TZDs can be prescribed as monotherapy in patients with T2D. The initiating dose of rosiglitazone is 2 mg/day with a maximum dose of 8 mg/day. Similarly, the initiating dose of pioglitazone is 15 mg/day and can be titrated to a maximum dose of 45 mg/day. Because of the complexity of T2D, however, most patients tend to receive the combination of TZDs and other oral antidiabetic medications (i.e., metformin, sulfonylurea), glucagon-like peptide-1(GLP-1) agonists, and insulin. This approach is based on the concept of maximizing the effects of these drugs on the pathophysiology of T2D. In addition, the combination therapy provides flexibility for primary care providers in selection of antidiabetic regimen and in achieving the American Diabetes Association or the American Association of Clinical Endocrinologists–recommended A1C goals of <7% and <6.5%, respectively.

Finally, the clinical application of TZDs in patients with T2D has synergistic effects when combined with other antidiabetic agents. Most of the previous clinical trials consisted of short- and intermediate-term studies randomized to TZD or placebo in patients receiving background antidiabetic medications. Most of the studies lasted 26–52 weeks with an open-label extension period (1–2 years). These studies, however, showed that during the active phase, TZDs reduced A1C by at least 1%, which persisted during the open-label extension studies. This metabolic benefit of TZD, however, was associated with weight gain of 2–3 kg.

A major disadvantage of the oral agents, such as sulfonylureas, is the high rate of primary and secondary failures. Thus, to examine the durability of the glycemic benefits of TZDs on glucose regulation, β-cell function, and insulin sensitivity, the ADOPT study randomized patients with T2D into three arms—namely, metformin, glyburide, and rosiglitazone—for 5 years.[21,22] The study revealed that rosiglitazone sustained the glucose control as assessed by fasting glucose and A1C longer than did glyburide and metformin. The study confirmed that glucose control assessed by A1C and fasting plasma glucose was more durable in patients treated with TZDs (i.e., rosiglitazone when compared with metformin and glyburide).[21,22]

TZDS AND CARDIOVASCULAR DISEASES IN TYPE 2 DIABETES

TZDs have pleotropic effects, which theoretically have beneficial effects in reducing cardiovascular risk factors in some patients. These effects include improvement not only in glucose and A1C but also lipids and lipoproteins. Indeed, the lipids–lipoprotein benefit tends to be more favorable with pioglitazone than rosiglitazone in the head-to-head comparative studies in patients with T2D. Recent studies tested the theoretical benefits of TZDs improving CVD outcomes in patients with T2D.[23–25] The primary composite CVD outcomes in most of these studies were cardiovascular mortality (deaths) and cardiac endpoints such as congestive heart failure and acute myocardial infarctions. The studies failed to show significant benefit of TZDs on overall mortality and composite primary endpoints. Parenthetically, there were some significant beneficial secondary endpoints, but these have been inconclusive and difficult to explain. Whether there is increased incidence of ischemic heart disease associated with TZDs in patients with T2D remain uncertain, however. In the PROACTIVE study, the use of pioglitazone did not reveal significant improvement in the primary composite cardiac outcomes.[23,24] Furthermore, in the subgroup of patients adequately treated with statins, pioglitazone conferred no CVD benefit despite similar glycemic control. Rosiglitazone showed potential negative CVD outcomes, but this remains controversial.[22] Furthermore, in the RECORD study, no significant reduction in composite CVD endpoints was found in patients with T2D assigned to rosiglitazone when compared with controls. The study was considered underpowered with inadequate sample size for detailed statistical analysis. Recently, an independent meta-analysis indicated that TZDs as a class could have worse CVD outcomes in patients with

T2D than the non-TZD treated control group on oral medications, such as metformin. There is, however, persistent evidence that rosiglitazone is associated with more cardiovascular outcomes relative to pioglitazone.[26]

ADVERSE EFFECTS OF TZDS IN TYPE 2 DIABETES

TZDs generally are well tolerated with minimum side or adverse effects. The major adverse effects of TZDs are weight gain, edema, and congestive heart failure.[14-18] In addition, there are recent reports of atypical bone fractures in the hands and feet.[14,15] The etiology of the atypical fractures associated with TZDs remain unknown.

TZDS AND INCIDENT CANCER

A recent report that PPAR agonist could be associated with increased incident cancers has raised serious concern in the medical community. PPAR-γ agonists have been shown to induce apoptosis in several malignant cell lines and to inhibit the invasive activity of colon and breast cancer cells. In contrast, animal toxicity studies have suggested a possible increased cancer risk in multiple organs in association with a wide variety of PPAR-γ and dual PPAR-α/-γ agonists. Indeed, recent findings suggest that synthetic PPAR-γ ligands may affect cell growth independent of its glucose metabolism. Recent reports that pioglitazone is associated with increased incidence of bladder cancer have raised major concerns; however, this observation remains inconclusive and debatable.[27] Furthermore, it is uncertain whether there is an association of rosiglitazone treatment and incident bladder cancer.

FUTURE OF TZDS IN TYPE 2 DIABETES

The controversies surrounding the use of TZDs raise questions on the use of these agents in the future. Metabolically, however, these agents have proven to be important and effective in patients with T2D either as monotherapy or in combination therapy. One of the downsides for the use of TZDs is the high retail cost. The introduction of generic TZDs on the market globally could provide an opportunity for more patients to receive TZDs. Such patients, however, ought to be selected carefully based on U.S. Food and Drug Administration (FDA)-approved indications and contraindications and should be monitored carefully by experienced providers.

CONCLUSION

TZDs have been on the market for two decades for patients with T2D. Although TZDs have added important metabolic benefits on glucose and lipid metabolism, the recent reports of increasing congestive heart failure, weight gain, and edema; atypical fractures of the hands and feet bones; and the potential incident bladder cancer have raised concerns on the continued use of these agents in patients with T2D. Given the lack of significant CVD outcomes benefit, therefore, the long-term use of TZDs in clinical patients with T2D needs to be reevaluated carefully.

ACKNOWLEDGMENT

The authors thank the staff at the CCTS NIH# UL1TRR000090 and the patient volunteers for their participation and American Diabetes Association Clinical Research Award.

REFERENCES

1. Nathan DM, Buse JB, Davidson MB, et al., American Diabetes Association, European Association for Study of Diabetes. Medical management of hyperglycemia in type 2 diabetes: a consensus algorithm for the initiation and adjustment of therapy: a consensus statement of the American Diabetes Association and the European Association for the Study of Diabetes. *Diabetes Care* 2009;32:193–203.

2. Yki-Järvinen H. Thiazolidinediones. *N Engl J Med* 2004;351;1106–1118.

3. Grey A, et al. The peroxisome proliferator-activated receptor-gamma agonist rosiglitazone decreases bone formation and bone mineral density in healthy postmenopausal women: a randomized, controlled trial. *J Clin Endocrinol Metab* 2007;92:1305–1310.

4. Nathan DM. Thiazolidinediones for initial treatment of type 2 diabetes? *N Engl J Med* 2006;355:2477–2480.

5. Miyazaki Y, De Filippis E, Bajaj M, et al. Predictors of improved glycemic control with rosiglitazone therapy in type 2 diabetic patients: a practical approach for the primary care physician. *Br J Diabetes Vasc Dis* 2005;5:28–35.

6. Buchanan TA. (How) can we prevent type 2 diabetes? *Diabetes* 2007;56:1502–1507.

7. Knowler WC, Barrett-Connor E, Fowler SE, et al. Reduction in the incidence of type 2 diabetes with lifestyle intervention or metformin. *N Engl J Med* 2002;346:393–403.

8 The Diabetes Prevention Program Research Group. Prevention of type 2 diabetes with troglitazone in the Diabetes Prevention Program. *Diabetes* 2005;54(4):1150–1156.

9. Aubert RE, Herrera V, Chen W, Haffner SM, Pendergrass M. Rosiglitazone and pioglitazone increase fracture risk in women and men with type 2 diabetes. *Diabetes Obes Metab* 2010;12(8):716–721.

10. Murphy CE. Effects of thiazolidinediones on bone loss and fracture. *Ann Pharmacother* 2007;41(12):2014–2018.

11. Meymeh RH, Wooltorton E. Diabetes drug pioglitazone (Actos): risk of fracture. *CMAJ* 2007;177(7):723–724.

12. Buchanan TA, Xiang AH, Peters RK, Kjos SL, Marroquin A, Goico J, Ochoa C, Tan S, Berkowitz K, Hodis HN, Azen S. Preservation of pancreatic beta cell function and prevention of type 2 diabetes by pharmacological treatment of insulin resistance in high-risk Hispanic women. *Diabetes* 2002;51:2796–2803.

13. Xiang AH, Peters RK, Siri L, Kjos S, Marroquin A, Goico J, Ochoa C, Miwa Kawakubo M, Buchanan TA. Effect of pioglitazone on pancreatic β-cell function and diabetes risk in Hispanic women with prior gestational diabetes. *Diabetes* 2006;55(2):517–522.

14. DeFronzo RA, Tripathy D, Schwenke DC, Banerji M, Bray GA, Buchanan TA, Clement SC, Henry RR, Hodis HN, Kitabchi AE, Mack WJ, Mudaliar S, Ratner RE, Williams K, Stentz FB, Musi N, Reaven PD. Pioglitazone for diabetes prevention in impaired glucose tolerance; ACT NOW Study. *N Engl J Med* 2011;24;364(12):1104–1115.

15. Scheen AJ. DREAM study: prevention of type 2 diabetes with ramipril and/or rosiglitazone in persons with dysglycaemia but no cardiovascular disease. *Rev Med Liege* 2006;61(10):728–732.

15. Hanefeld M, Schaper F. Pioglitazone for diabetes prevention in impaired glucose tolerance drug therapy for the prevention of type 2 diabetes. Is there a medical rationale? *Brit J Diabetes Vascular Disease* 2011;11(4):168–174.

16. Kahn SK, Haffner SM, Heise MA, Herman WH, Holman RR, Jones NP, Kravitz BG, John M, et al. for the ADOPT Study Group. Glycemic durability of rosiglitazone, metformin, or glyburide monotherapy. *N Engl J Med* 2006;355:2427–2443.

17. Osei K, Gaillard TE, Schuster D. Thiazolidinediones increase hepatic insulin extraction in African Americans with impaired glucose tolerance and type 2 diabetes mellitus. A pilot study of rosiglitazone. *Metabolism* 2007;56(1):24–29.

18. Poy MN, Yang Y, Rezaei K, Fernström MA, Lee AD, Kido Y, Erickson SK, Najjar SM. CEACAM1 regulates insulin clearance in liver. *Nat Genet* 2002;30(3):270–276.

19. Osei K, Gaillard T, Kaplow J, Bullock M, Schuster D. Effects of rosiglitazone on plasma adiponectin, insulin sensitivity, and insulin secretion in high-risk African Americans with impaired glucose tolerance test and type 2 diabetes. *Metabolism* 2004;53(12):1552–1557.

20. Roberts TB, Price G, Perseghin KF, Petersen DL, Rothman GW, Cline GI. Shulman mechanism of free fatty acid-induced insulin resistance in humans. *J Clin Invest* 1996;97(12):2859–2865.

21. Viberti G, Kahn SE, Greene DA, Herman WH, Zinman B, Holman RR, Haffner SM, Levy D, et al. A Diabetes Outcome Progression Trial (ADOPT).

An international multicenter study of the comparative efficacy of rosiglitazone, glyburide, and metformin in recently diagnosed type 2 diabetes. *Diabetes Care* 2002;25(10):1737–1743.

22. Scheen AJ. ADOPT study: which first-line glucose-lowering oral medication in type 2 diabetes? *Rev Med Liege* 2007;62(1):48–52.

23. Dormandy JA, Charbonnel B, Eckland DJ, et al. Secondary prevention of macrovascular events in patients with type 2 diabetes in the PROACTIVE Study (Prospective Pioglitazone Clinical Trial in Macrovascular Events): a randomised controlled trial. *Lancet* 2005;366:1279–1289.

24. Erdmann E, Dormandy JR, Massi-Benedetti M, Charbonnel B. PROactive 07: Pioglitazone in the treatment of type 2 diabetes: results of the PROactive study. *Vasc Health Risk Manag* 2007; 3(4):355–370.

25. Home PD, Jones NP, Pocock SJ, Beck-Nielsen H, Gomis R, Hanefeld M, Komajda M, Curtis P; for the RECORD Study Group. Rosiglitazone RECORD study: glucose control outcomes at 18 months. *Diabet Med* 2007;24(6):626–634.

26. Loke YK, Kwok CS, Singh S. Comparative cardiovascular effects of thiazolidinediones: Systematic review and meta-analysis of observational studies. *BMJ* 2011:342:d1309. doi;10.1136/bmj.d1309.

27. Ferrara A, Lewis JD, Quesenberry CP Jr, Peng T, Strom BL, Van Den Eeden SK, Ehrlich SF, Habel LA. Cohort study of pioglitazone and cancer incidence in patients with diabetes. *Diabetes Care* 2011;34(4):923–929.

Chapter 24

Dipeptidyl-Peptidase 4 Inhibitors

Pablo Aschner, MD, MSc

Sitagliptin

INTRODUCTION

The incretin effect of hormones secreted by intestinal cells to enhance insulin secretion in response to meals is well known.[1] The effect of the main incretin hormone glucagon-like peptide-1 (GLP-1) in lowering blood glucose was demonstrated >20 years ago.[2] Native GLP-1 is rapidly degraded (within minutes) by the enzyme dipeptidyl-peptidase 4 (DPP-4), which also hydrolyzes other peptides, including the glucose-dependent insulinotropic polypeptide (GIP).[3] Thus, it became clear that to turn the incretin effect into a pharmacological tool, the enzymatic degradation needed to be avoided. This initially was achieved by exendin-4, a natural occurring GLP-1 receptor agonist found in the saliva of the Gila monster, which proved to be resistant to DPP-4.[4] Shortly after this finding, a synthetic version of exendin-4, exenatide, became an effective glucose-lowering drug.[5] Many GLP-1 receptor agonists have been produced in recent years. All of them need to be injected subcutaneously, and their advantage in glucose control and weight reduction is somewhat counterbalanced by their gastrointestinal side effects. In addition, several oral DPP-4 inhibitors have been developed and are effective and well-tolerated pharmacological agents for the management of patients with type 2 diabetes (T2D). This chapter reviews the mechanism of action, efficacy, and safety of DPP-4 inhibitors in the treatment of people with T2D.

MECHANISM OF ACTION OF DPP-4 INHIBITORS

DPP-4 is a membrane-associated peptidase widely distributed in many tissues and found in a soluble form. At the molecular level, it cleaves two amino acids from the N-terminus of the intact forms of both GLP-1 and GIP, resulting in truncated metabolites that are largely inactive.[6] DPP-4 inhibitors have been designed as low-molecular-weight, orally active agents with high affinity and specificity for the enzyme. Approximately 80% of the DPP-4 enzyme inhibition is needed to increase by two- to threefold the levels of the biologically active form of GLP-1. Most DPP-4 inhibitors remain active in pharmacologic range up to 24 hours after a single-dose administration. Because the incretin action of GLP-1 as an insulin secretagogue is glucose dependent, and its effect ceases when the plasma glucose level is within the normal range, it is expected that DPP-4 inhibitors will control high glucose levels both in the postprandial and fasting period without causing hypoglycemia. Additionally, GLP-1 inhibits glucagon secretion in a glucose-

DOI: 10.2337/9781580405096.24

dependent manner; therefore, DPP-4 inhibitors also will control the hyperglucagonemia observed in patients with diabetes.[7] The first successful DPP-4 inhibitor developed for clinical use was vildagliptin,[8] and sitagliptin was the first DPP-4 inhibitor approved by the U.S. Food and Drug Administration (FDA) in 2006 for the treatment of people with T2D. After that approval, many other DPP-4 inhibitors were approved by the FDA, including saxagliptin, linagliptin, and alogliptin.

The glucose-lowering action is a class effect shared by all the DPP-4 inhibitors; however, these agents differ in their pharmacokinetic (PK) and pharmacodynamic (PD) properties, which influence their safety profile and drug interactions (Table 24.1).[9] In general, all DPP-4 inhibitors are safe and can be used in the majority of patients with T2D; however, vildagliptin is not recommended in patients with impaired hepatic function and only saxagliptin and linagliptin are approved for use in patients with severe hepatic failure. All DPP-4 inhibitors with the exception of linagliptin need dose adjustment when used in patients with impaired renal function, although this recommendation is based on their PK (levels rise) and not on safety issues (safe up to eight times their therapeutic dose).

EFFICACY OF DPP-4 INHIBITORS

Early randomized clinical trials (RCTs) comparing DPP-4 inhibitors and placebo as monotherapy in patients with T2D showed a reduction in A1C around –0.6% to –0.8%, which was considered lower than with other antidiabetic drugs, such as metformin, sulphonylureas, and thiazolidinediones.[10,11] The mean baseline A1C in

Table 24.1 Pharmacokinetics and Pharmacodynamics of DPP-4 Inhibitors

Generic name	Chemical structure	Metabolism	Excretion	DPP-4 inhibition
Vildagliptin	Cyanopyrrolidine Peptidomimetic	Hydrolyzed to inactive metabolite	Renal (22% as parent, 55% as inactive metabolite)	>80%, 12 hours postdose
Sitagliptin	β-amino acid-based Peptidomimetic	Not appreciably metabolized	Renal (~80% unchanged)	>80%, 24 hours postdose
Saxagliptin	Cyanopyrrolidine Peptidomimetic	Hepatic to active metabolite	Renal (12–29% as parent, 21–52% as active metabolite)	~70%, 24 hours postdose
Linagliptin	Xanthine-based Nonpeptidomimetic	Not appreciably metabolized	Biliary (>70% unchanged as parent)	~70%, 24 hours postdose
Alogliptin	Modified pyrimidinedione Nonpeptidomimetic	Not appreciably metabolized	Renal (>70% unchanged)	~75%, 24 hours postdose

the early studies with DPP-4 inhibitors was ~8%; however, when the efficacy was explored in subgroups with different baseline A1C levels, those with higher values (≥9%) had greater mean reduction (–1.5%). Thus, as reported in a recent metaregression analysis, the change in A1C with DPP-4 inhibitors and other glucose-lowering drugs is dependent on the baseline A1C levels.[12] When the initial trials with sitagliptin and vildagliptin were included in the metaregression analysis, it was concluded that the smaller decreases in the A1C levels could be explained by lower baseline values than those reported with other glucose-lowering drugs.[13] Later, head-to-head RCTs and meta-analyses reported noninferiority between DPP-4 inhibitors and other classes of antidiabetic drugs. The most recent meta-analysis reported that sulfonylureas are slightly superior to DPP-4 inhibitors in reducing A1C from baseline (mean A1C difference –0.07%, 95% confidence interval [CI] –0.03 to –0.11%), but they are equally effective in achieving an A1C <7% (risk ratio 1.06, 95% CI 0.98–1.14). Metformin was also more effective than DPP-4 inhibitors as monotherapy (mean A1C difference –0.2%, 95% CI –0.08 to –0.32%) but a difference of <0.4% is not considered clinically meaningful. DPP-4 inhibitors are as effective as thiazolidinediones (mean A1C difference –0.09%, 95% CI –0.07 to 0.24). The A1C reduction achieved with GLP-1 receptor agonists is greater than with DPP-4 inhibitors (mean A1C difference –0.49%, 95% CI –0.31 to –0.67).[14] In addition, basal insulin also has been found to be more effective than DPP-4 inhibitors when added to metformin (mean A1C difference –0.59%, 95% CI –0.77 to –0.42).[15] Adding DPP-4 inhibitors to metformin, sulfonylureas, or thiazolidinediones has been proven effective in reducing A1C by –0.7 to –1% compared with placebo.

The synergistic effect of combining metformin with DPP-4 inhibitors is of particular interest, as metformin enhances the biological effect of GLP-1 by increasing GLP-1 secretion, suppressing activity of DPP-4, and upregulating the expression of GLP-1 receptors in pancreatic β-cells.[16] The combination of metformin with a DPP-4 inhibitor has synergistic effects in reducing fasting and postmeal plasma glucose, increasing GLP-1 secretion, and β-cell function, decreasing plasma glucagon, and inhibiting endogenous glucose production.[17]

All of the DPP-4 inhibitors have been studied in combination with metformin in drug-naive patients with T2D. The combination of a DPP-4 inhibitor and 2,000 mg of metformin results in a mean A1C reduction ≥1.7% and with 51–66% of patients achieving a target A1C <7% after 24–108 weeks of therapy (Table 24.2). In patients staring with a baseline A1C >11%, the mean A1C reduction was ≥3%.[18-24] In a recent meta-analysis, the difference in the mean A1C reduction between initial combination therapy with metformin plus DPP-4 inhibitors and metformin alone was –0.49% (95% CI –0.57 to –0.40) in favor of the combination.[25-29] Similar results have been reported with the initial combination of a DPP-4 inhibitor and pioglitazone.[30-32]

DPP-4 inhibitors also have been studied in triple combination therapy with insulin and other oral agents (Table 24.3). When sitagliptin was added to metformin and glimepiride, there was a mean A1C reduction of 0.9% from a baseline of 8.3%, with 23% of the patients achieving an A1C <7%.[33-37] DPP-4 inhibitors also have been tested as add-on therapy to insulin in patients with T2D,[38-43] resulting in a reduction in A1C by –0.5 to –0.7% during a median follow-up of 24 weeks.[44]

Table 24.2 Efficacy of Initial Combination of DPP-4 Inhibitors and Metformin or Pioglitazone Therapy

DPP-4 inhibitor, daily dose	Combined with	Follow-up (weeks)	Mean baseline A1C (%)	Mean A1C (%) reduction	Patients achieving goal A1C <7% (%)		
					Combination therapy	Monotherapy*	NNT to achieve goal
Sitagliptin 100 mg	Metformin 2,000 mg	24	8.8	-2.1	66	38	5
		108		-1.7	60	45	7
		24	11.2	-2.9			
Vildagliptin 100 mg		24	~8.6	-1.8	65	43	8
		24	12.2	-3.2			
Saxagliptin 10 mg		24	~9.5	-2.5	60	41	5
		76		-2.3	51	35	6
Linagliptin 5 mg		24	8.7	-1.7	59	48	9
		24	11.8	-3.7			
Sitagliptin 100 mg	Pioglitazone 45 mg	56	9.4	-2.4	61	36	4
Vildagliptin 100 mg +	Pioglitazone 30 mg	24	8.7	-1.9	65	43	5
Linagliptin 5 mg		24	8.6	-1.06	43	31	8
Alogliptin 25 mg		26	8.8	-1.7	63	34	3

Note: NNT = number needed to treat.

TOLERABILITY AND SAFETY

DPP-4 inhibitors are generally well tolerated. The pooled incidence of adverse events from Phase 2 and 3 RCTs comparing DPP-4 inhibitors to placebo have not shown clinically significant differences in patients treated up to 2 years.[45]

RCTs comparing DPP-4 inhibitors to sulfonylureas have shown significant lower incidence of hypoglycemia with the use of DPP-4 inhibitors. Additionally, these studies showed a difference in weight of ~2 kg because of the weight increase in patients treated with sulfonylureas and a slight decrease in those taking DPP-4 inhibitors, particularly in patients receiving combination therapy with metformin. Similar results were found when DPP-4 inhibitors were compared with basal insulin as an add-on to metformin. As expected, the risk of hypoglycemia increases when a DPP-4 inhibitor is added to therapy with sulfonylurea or to insulin, and the rate is proportional to the improvement of glucose control.

In RCTs comparing DPP-4 inhibitors and thiazolidinediones, the risk of hypoglycemia is about the same, but there is a significant weight difference of ~3 kg because of the weight increase with thiazolidinediones.

When metformin is compared with DPP-4 inhibitors, there is an increased risk of gastrointestinal side effects (~70%), including diarrhea, nausea, and vomiting, in patients taking the biguanide, which is not seen with DPP-4 inhibitors. On the other hand, there is a weight difference ~1.5 kg in favor of metformin.

As with all the new glucose-lowering drugs, there is concern about the cardiovascular safety of DPP-4 inhibitors. Pooled analyses of Phase 3 RCTs and meta-analysis have reported no increased signal in cardiovascular adverse events; however, in most Phase 3 studies, the cardiovascular events were not included as preestablished outcomes. Recently, the regulatory agencies and particularly the FDA have recommended that long-term cardiovascular-endpoint RCTs should be started as soon as a new glucose-lowering drug is filed for approval. This has been done with all the DPP-4 inhibitors and two of these trials already have been reported. The recent Saxagliptin Assessment of Vascular Outcomes in Patients with Diabetes Mellitus (SAVOR)–Thrombolysis in Myocardial Infarction (TIMI) 53 trial randomly assigned 16,492 patients with T2D with a history of, or at risk for, cardiovascular events to receive saxagliptin or placebo in addition to standard care and followed them for a median of 2.1 years. No difference was found in the incidence of the primary endpoint, which was a composite of cardiovascular death, myocardial infarction, or ischemic stroke (hazard ratio 1.00; 95% CI 0.89–1.12; $P = 0.99$). There was also no difference in the incidence of the major secondary endpoint of a composite of cardiovascular death, myocardial infarction, stroke, hospitalization for unstable angina, coronary revascularization, or heart failure, but more patients in the saxagliptin group than in the placebo group were hospitalized for heart failure (3.5 vs. 2.8%; hazard ratio 1.27; 95% CI 1.07–1.51; $P = 0.007$).[46]

The Examination of Cardiovascular Outcomes with Alogliptin versus Standard of Care (EXAMINE) trial randomly assigned 5,380 patients with T2D and either an acute myocardial infarction or unstable angina requiring hospitalization within the previous 15–90 days to receive alogliptin or placebo in addition to existing antihyperglycemic and cardiovascular drug therapy and were followed for up to 40 months (median, 18 months). The incidence of the primary endpoint of

Table 24.3 Efficacy of Triple Oral Combination Therapy with DPP-4 Inhibitors

Add-on	Baseline treatment	Comparator	Follow-up (weeks)	Mean baseline A1C (%)	Mean A1C (%) reduction with triple combination	Patients achieving goal A1C <7% with triple combination (%)	NNT to achieve goal
Sitagliptin	Metformin + Glimepiride	PBO	24	8.3	−0.89 vs. PBO	23 vs. 1	5
Linagliptin	Metformin + sulfonylurea	PBO	24	8.1	−0.62 vs. PBO	29 vs. 8	5
Sitagliptin	Metformin + Pioglitazone	PBO	54	8.8	−0.8 vs. PBO	26 vs. 14	8
Alogliptin + Pioglitazone	Metformin	Pioglitazone	26	8.5	−1.4 with −0.9 without Alogliptin	56 vs. 31 (A1C ≤7%)	4
Sitagliptin	Metformin + Pioglitazone	Glimepiride	54	7.2	−0.7 Sitagliptin −1.1 Glimepiride	NA	NA

Note: PBO = placebo; NNT = number needed to treat.

a composite of death from cardiovascular causes, nonfatal myocardial infarction, or nonfatal stroke was not increased with alogliptin therapy (hazard ratio 0.96; upper boundary of the one-sided repeated confidence interval, 1.16; $P < 0.001$ for noninferiority).[47] In both studies, A1C levels were significantly lower with the DPP-4 inhibitor compared with placebo (mean difference −0.36% with alogliptin and −0.3% after 2 years with saxagliptin, $P < 0.001$ for both). Additional studies with other DPP-4 inhibitors will be reported during the next few years.[48]

A concern with incretin-based therapies is their pancreatic safety, as some rodent studies reported an increased β-cell neogenesis and reduced β-cell apoptosis resulting in increased β-cell mass. To date, no evidence of such effects has been observed in humans with the exception of a recent controversial study that reported increased exocrine cell proliferation and increased pancreatic intraepithelial neoplasia in organ donors treated with incretin-based therapy compared with controls.[49] These findings could be attributed to differences in age and sex between cases and controls.[49] Because GLP-1 receptors are found in pancreatic ducts, however, it has been suggested that exocrine pancreatic cells could be affected, leading to acinar and duct cell metaplasia, which are potentially premalignant changes present in patients with chronic pancreatitis. Although some studies in rodents with GLP-1 receptor agonists and with DPP-4 inhibitors have shown increased turnover and proliferation of ductal cells as well as increased lipase and pancreatitis score, the majority have not observed these changes, and others have found some protection against experimentally induced pancreatitis. In humans, the pooled analysis of Phase 2 and 3 RCTs as well as a recent meta-analysis[50] demonstrated no increase in the incidence of pancreatitis and pancreatic cancer, although there have been several case reports of pancreatitis linked to the postmarketing use of these drugs. Pharmacoepidemiological studies using administrative databases do not confirm this association with the exception of two studies: one based on the analysis of the FDA Adverse Event Reporting System (FAERS), which may have a reporting bias and should not be used for incidence calculations, and another study based on hospitalizations in which the role of potential risk-modifying factors could not be completely ruled out. The association of incretin therapy and pancreatitis and pancreatic tumors is a matter of debate,[51,52] and long-term Phase 4 cardiovascular safety trials, which are adjudicating pancreatic events, may solve this controversy. The SAVOR trial found no difference in the incidence of adjudicated cases of pancreatitis (acute pancreatitis, 0.2% in the saxagliptin group and 0.1% in the placebo group, $P = 0.17$, and chronic pancreatitis, <0.1 and 0.1% in the two groups, respectively, $P = 0.18$). There were five cases of pancreatic cancer in the saxagliptin group and 12 cases in the placebo group ($P = 0.095$).[46] Similarly, in the EXAMINE trial, no difference was found in the incidence of acute pancreatitis (0.4% in the alogliptin group and 0.3% in the placebo group, $P = 0.5$) or chronic pancreatitis (0.2 and 0.1%, respectively, $P = 1.0$). Recently, the FDA and EMA, after an extensive evaluation of experimental and clinical evidence regarding incretin-based therapy and risk of pancreatic cancer, reported that there is no conclusive evidence in support of this association. It should be noted, however, that pancreatitis is considered a potential risk associated with these drugs and that both agencies continue to investigate this safety signal.[53]

DPP-4 INHIBITORS IN CLINICAL PRACTICE

All the DPP-4 inhibitors with the exception of vildagliptin are prescribed as a once-daily pill given at any time of the day and with no restriction regarding meals. Some DPP-4 inhibitors are also available as fixed-dose combination with metformin in an attempt to increase compliance, and in those cases, the dose of the DPP-4 inhibitor is divided to match with the twice-daily administration of high doses of metformin. Fixed-dose combination with metformin XR has a 24-hour duration of action and is better tolerated than regular metformin, but it has to be given twice daily when the total daily dose of metformin is >1,000 mg.

The most recent position statement of the American Diabetes Association (ADA) and the European Association for the Study of Diabetes (EASD) include DPP-4 inhibitors for combination therapy when initial monotherapy with metformin fails to achieve the desired glucose control. Although the algorithm does not show any preference among sulfonylureas, thiazolidinediones, DPP-4 inhibitors, GLP-1 receptor agonists, or insulin therapy, it points out that incretin-based therapies are the best alternative when avoiding hypoglycemia and weight gain.[54] The American Association of Clinical Endocrinologists (AACE) recently published their treatment algorithm placing incretin-based therapies as a top choice when dual therapy is indicated.[55] These guidelines also recommended the use of incretin agents in combination with metformin when entry A1C is ≥7.5%. Similarly, the Global Partnership for Effective Diabetes Management considered initiating combination therapy of metformin and a DPP-4 inhibitor for the management of patients with A1C ≥9%.[56] Based on the safety and efficacy data, the Latin American Diabetes Association (ALAD) recently proposed DPP-4 inhibitors as the best choice to initiate in combination with metformin in patients with A1C >8%. When A1C is below that value, monotherapy with metformin is the best choice, but a DPP-4 inhibitor could be added if the A1C target is not achieved. DPP-4 inhibitors can be used as first-line monotherapy when metformin is contraindicated or not tolerated. RCTs have shown that these agents are effective and safe in people with T2D and renal failure. DPP-4 inhibitors, except linagliptin, are excreted primarily by the kidneys either as the parent molecule or as metabolites. Therefore, the dose needs to be adjusted in the presence of kidney failure (Table 24.4). They are also useful in elderly patients who are vulnerable to hypoglycemia and gastrointestinal side effects and who may not need to lose weight. RCTs have shown that they have the same efficacy and safety profile as in younger patients.[57]

DPP-4 inhibitors have not been approved for use in pregnancy and in patients with type 1 diabetes (T1D), but recent reports in patients with T1D have reported a benefit in improving glucose control in combination with insulin therapy, probably because of the effect on glucagon secretion.

CONCLUSION

DPP-4 inhibitors are glucose-dependent insulin secretagogues as well as glucose-dependent inhibitors of glucagon secretion. They are effective in reducing A1C equal to other oral glucose-lowering drugs but with a better safety profile because

Table 24.4 Prescribing Information for DPP-4 Inhibitors

DPP-4 inhibitor	Daily dose (mg)				
	Normal renal function	Renal insufficiency		Mild/ moderate	
		Moderate	Severe/ ESRD		
	CrCl > 50 ml/min	CrCl 50-30 ml/min	CrCl <30 ml/in	hepatic insufficiency	Drug interactions
Sitagliptin	100 mg QD	50 mg QD	25 mg QD	No dose adjustment	
Vildagliptin	50 mg bid	50 mg QD	50 mg QD	Not recommended	
Saxagliptin	2.5–5 mg QD	2.5 mg QD	2.5 mg QD	No dose adjustment	Limit to 2.5 mg QD with CYP3A4/5 inhibitors
Alogliptin	25 mg QD	12.5 mg QD	6.25 mg QD	Use with caution	
Linagliptin	5 QD	5 QD	5 QD	No dose adjustment	Efficacy is reduced with strong P-gp or CYP3A4 inducer

Note: CrCl = creatinine clearance; QD = once daily; BID = twice daily; ESRD = end-stage renal disease; P-gp = P-glycoprotein.

their use is not associated with hypoglycemia or weight gain. They can be used as monotherapy when metformin is contraindicated and in dual or triple combination with other oral agents or insulin. Recent trials have demonstrated their cardiovascular safety, and thus far, there is no hard evidence of increased risk of pancreatic damage with the use of DPP-4 inhibitors in patients with diabetes.

REFERENCES

1. Creutzfeldt W. The incretin concept today. *Diabetologia* 1979;16:75–85.

2. Gutniak M, Orskov C, Holst JJ, Ahren B, Efendic S. Antidiabetogenic effect of glucagon-like peptide-1 (7-36) amide in normal subjects and patients with diabetes mellitus. *N Engl J Med* 1992;326:1316–1322.

3. Mentlein R, Gallwitz B, Schmidt WE. Dipeptidyl-peptidase IV hydrolyses gastric inhibitory polypeptide, glucagon-like peptide-1(7-36)amide, peptide histidine methionine and is responsible for their degradation in human serum. *Eur J Biochem* 1993;214:829–835.

4. Goke R, Fehmann HC, Linn T, Schmidt H, Krause M, Eng J, Goke B. Exendin-4 is a high potency agonist and truncated exendin-(9-39)-amide an

antagonist at the glucagon-like peptide 1-(7-36)-amide receptor of insulin-secreting beta-cells. *J Biol Chem* 1993;268:19650–19655.

5. Kolterman OG, Buse JB, Fineman MS, Gaines E, Heintz S, Bicsak TA, Taylor K, Kim D, Aisporna M, Wang Y, Baron AD. Synthetic exendin-4 (exenatide) significantly reduces postprandial and fasting plasma glucose in subjects with type 2 diabetes. *J Clin Endocrinol Metab* 2003;88:3082–3089.

6. Holst JJ, Deacon CF. Inhibition of the activity of dipeptidyl-peptidase IV as a treatment for type 2 diabetes. *Diabetes* 1998;47:1663–1670.

7. Deacon CF, Ahrén B, Holst JJ. Inhibitors of dipeptidyl peptidase IV: a novel approach for the prevention and treatment of type 2 diabetes? *Expert Opin Investig Drugs* 2004;13:1091–1102.

8. Villhauer EB, Brinkman JA, Naderi GB, Burkey BF, Dunning BE, Prasad K, Mangold BL, Russell ME, Hughes TE. 1-[[(3-hydroxy-1-adamantyl)amino] acetyl]-2-cyano-(S)-pyrrolidine: a potent, selective, and orally bioavailable dipeptidyl peptidase IV inhibitor with antihyperglycemic properties. *J Med Chem* 2003;46(13):2774–2789.

9. Deacon CF. Dipeptidyl peptidase-4 inhibitors in the treatment of type 2 diabetes: a comparative review. *Diabetes Obes Metab* 2011;13:7–18.

10. Pratley RE, Jauffret-Kamel S, Galbreath E, Holmes D. Twelve-week monotherapy with the DPP-4 inhibitor vildagliptin improves glycemic control in subjects with type 2 diabetes. *Horm Metab Res* 2006;38:423–428.

11. Aschner P, Kipnes MS, Lunceford JK, Sanchez M, Mickel C, Williams-Herman DE; for the Sitagliptin Study 021 Group. Effect of the dipeptidyl dipeptidase-4 inhibitor sitagliptin as monotherapy on glycemic control in patients with type 2 diabetes. *Diabetes Care* 2006;29:2632–2637.

12. Bloomgarden ZT, Dodis R, Viscoli CM, Holmboe ES, Inzucchi SE. Lower baseline glycemia reduces apparent oral agent glucose-lowering efficacy: a meta-regression analysis. *Diabetes Care* 2006;29:2137–2139.

13. Bloomgarden ZT, Inzucchi SE. New treatments for diabetes. *N Engl J Med* 2007;356:2219–2220.

14. Karagiannis T, Paschos P, Konstantinos Paletas K, David R, Matthews DR, Tsapas A. Dipeptidyl peptidase-4 inhibitors for treatment of type 2 diabetes mellitus in the clinical setting: systematic review and meta-analysis. *BMJ* 2012;344:e1369.

15. Aschner P, Chan J, Owens DR, Picard S, Wang E, Dain MP, Pilorget V, Echtay A, Fonseca V; EASIE Investigators. Insulin glargine versulfonylureas sitagliptin in insulin-naive patients with type 2 diabetes mellitus uncontrolled on metformin (EASIE): a multicentre, randomised open-label trial. *Lancet* 2012;379:2262–2269.

16. Liu Y, Hong T. Combination therapy of dipeptidyl peptidase-4 inhibitors and metformin in type 2 diabetes: rationale and evidence. *Diabetes Obes Metab* 2013 May 13. doi: 10.1111/dom.12128. [Epub ahead of print].

17. Solis-Herrera C, Triplitt C, Garduno-Garcia J, Adams J, Defronzo RA, Cersosimo E. Mechanisms of glucose lowering of dipeptidyl peptidase-4 inhibitor sitagliptin when used alone or with metformin in type 2 diabetes: a double-tracer study. *Diabetes Care* 2013;36:2756–2762.

18. Goldstein BJ, Feinglos MN, Lunceford JK, Johnson J, Williams-Herman D; for the Sitagliptin 036 Study Group. Effect of initial combination therapy with sitagliptin, a dipeptidyl peptidase-4 inhibitor, and metformin on glycemic control in patients with type 2 diabetes. *Diabetes Care* 2007;30:1979–1987.

19. Williams-Herman D, Johnson J, Teng R, Golm G, Kaufman KD, Goldstein BJ, Amatruda JM. Efficacy and safety of sitagliptin and metformin as initial combination therapy and as monotherapy over 2 years in patients with type 2 diabetes. *Diabetes Obes Metab* 2010;12: 442–451.

20. Bosi E, Dotta F, Jia Y, Goodman M. Vildagliptin plus metformin combination therapy provides superior glycaemic control to individual monotherapy in treatment-naive patients with type 2 diabetes mellitus. *Diabetes Obes Metab* 2009;11:506–515.

21. Jadzinsky M, Pfützner A, Paz-Pacheco E, Xu Z, Allen E, Chen R; for the CV181-039 Investigators. Saxagliptin given in combination with metformin as initial therapy improves glycaemic control in patients with type 2 diabetes compared with either monotherapy: a randomized controlled trial. *Diabetes Obes Metab* 2009;11:611–622.

22. Pfützner A, Paz-Pacheco E, Allen E, Frederich R, Chen R; for the CV181039 Investigators. Initial combination therapy with saxagliptin and metformin provides sustained glycaemic control and is well tolerated for up to 76 weeks. *Diabetes Obes Metab* 2011;13:567–576.

23. Haak T, Meinicke T, Jones R, Weber S, von Eynatten M, Woerle HJ. Initial combination of linagliptin and metformin improves glycaemic control in type 2 diabetes: a randomized, double-blind, placebo-controlled study. *Diabetes Obes Metab* 2012;14:565–574.

24. Rosenstock J, Inzucchi SE, Seufert J, Fleck PR, Wilson CA, Mekki Q. Initial combination therapy with alogliptin and pioglitazone in drug-naïve patients with type 2 diabetes. *Diabetes Care* 2010;33:2406–2408.

25. Wu D, Li L, Liu C. Efficacy and safety of dipeptidyl peptidase-4 inhibitors and metformin as initial combination therapy and as monotherapy in patients with type 2 diabetes mellitus: a meta-analysis. *Diabetes Obes Metab* 2014;16:30–37.

26. Yoon KH, Steinberg H, Teng R, Golm GT, Lee M, O'Neill EA, Kaufman KD, Goldstein BJ. Efficacy and safety of initial combination therapy with sitagliptin and pioglitazone in patients with type 2 diabetes: a 54-week study. *Diabetes Obes Metab* 2012;14:745–752.

27. Rosenstock J, Kim SW, Baron A, Camisasca R-P, Cressier F, Couturier A, Dejager S. Efficacy and tolerability of initial combination therapy with vilda-

gliptin and pioglitazone compared with component monotherapy in patients with type 2 diabetes. *Diabetes Obes Metab* 2007;9:175–185.

28. Gomis R, Espadero R-M, Jones R, Woerle HJ, Dugi KA. Efficacy and safety of initial combination therapy with linagliptin and pioglitazone in patients with inadequately controlled type 2 diabetes: a randomized, double-blind, placebo-controlled study. *Diabetes Obes Metab* 2011;13:653–661.

29. Rosenstock J, Inzucchi SE, Seufert J, Fleck PR, Wilson CA, Mekki Q. Initial combination therapy with alogliptin and pioglitazone in drug-naïve patients with type 2 diabetes. *Diabetes Care* 2010;33:2406–2408.

30. Rosenstock J, Brazg R, Andryuk PJ, Lu K, Stein P; for the Sitagliptin Study 019 Group. Efficacy and safety of the dipeptidyl peptidase-4 inhibitor sitagliptin added to ongoing pioglitazone therapy in patients with type 2 diabetes: a 24-week, multicenter, randomized, double-blind, placebo-controlled, parallel-group study. *Clin Ther* 2006;28:1556–1568.

31. Garber AJ, Schweitzer A, Baron A, Rochotte E, Dejager S. Vildagliptin in combination with pioglitazone improves glycaemic control in patients with type 2 diabetes failing thiazolidinedione monotherapy: a randomized, placebo-controlled study. *Diabetes Obes Metab* 2007;9:166–174.

32. Hollander P, Li J, Frederich R, Allen E, Chen R; for the CV181013 Investigators. Safety and efficacy of saxagliptin added to thiazolidinedione over 76 weeks in patients with type 2 diabetes mellitus. *Diabetes Vasc Dis Res* 2011;8:125–135.

33. Hermansen K, Kipnes M, Luo E, Fanurik D, Khatami H, Stein P for the Sitagliptin Study 035 Group. Efficacy and safety of the dipeptidyl peptidase-4 inhibitor, sitagliptin, in patients with type 2 diabetes mellitus inadequately controlled on glimepiride alone or on glimepiride and metformin. *Diabetes Obes Metab* 2007;9:733–745.

34. Owens DR, Swallow R, Dugi KA, Woerle HJ. Efficacy and safety of linagliptin in persons with type 2 diabetes inadequately controlled by a combination of metformin and sulphonylurea: a 24-week randomized study. *Diabet Med* 2011;28:1352–1361.

35. Dobs AS, Goldstein BJ, Aschner P, Horton ES, Umpierrez GE, Duran L, Hill JS, Chen Y, Golm GT, Langdon RB, Williams-Herman DE, Kaufman KD, Amatruda JM, Ferreira JC. Efficacy and safety of sitagliptin added to ongoing metformin and rosiglitazone combination therapy in a randomized placebo-controlled 54-week trial in patients with type 2 diabetes. *J Diabetes* 2013;5:68–79.

36. Derosa G, Cicero AFG, Franzetti IG, Querci F, Carbone A, Piccinni MN, D'Angelo A, Fogari E, Maffioli P. A comparison between sitagliptin or glibenclamide in addition to metformin + pioglitazone on glycaemic control and b-cell function: the triple oral therapy. *Diabetes Med* 2013;30:846–854.

37. DeFronzo R, Burant CF, Fleck P, Wilson C, Mekki Q, Pratley RE. Efficacy and tolerability of the dpp-4 inhibitor alogliptin combined with pioglitazone,

in metformin-treated patients with type 2 diabetes. *J Clin Endocrinol Metab* 2012;97:1615–1622.

38. Vilsbøll T, Rosenstock J, Yki-Jarvinen H, Cefalu WT, Chen Y, Luo E, Musser B, Andryuk PJ, Ling Y, Kaufman KD, Amatruda JM, Engel SS, Katz L. Efficacy and safety of sitagliptin when added to insulin therapy in patients with type 2 diabetes. *Diabetes Obes Metab* 2010;12:167–177.

39. Fonseca V, Schweizer A, Albrecht D, Baron MA, Chang I, Dejager S. Addition of vildagliptin to insulin improves glycaemic control in type 2 diabetes. *Diabetologia* 2007;50:1148–1155.

40. Kothny W, Foley J, Kozlovski P, Shao Q, Gallwitz B, Lukashevich V. Improved glycaemic control with vildagliptin added to insulin, with or without metformin, in patients with type 2 diabetes mellitus. *Diabetes Obes Metab* 2013;15:252–257.

41. Yki-Järvinen H, Rosenstock J, Durán-Garcia S, Pinnetti S, Bhattacharya S, Thiemann S, Patel S, Woerle HJ. Effects of adding linagliptin to basal insulin regimen for inadequately controlled type 2 diabetes: a ≥52-week randomized, double-blind study. *Diabetes Care* 2013;36:3875–3881.

42. Rosenstock J, Rendell MS, Gross JL, Fleck PR, Wilson CA, Mekki Q. Alogliptin added to insulin therapy in patients with type 2 diabetes reduces HbA1c without causing weight gain or increased hypoglycaemia. *Diabetes Obes Metab* 2009;11:1145–1152.

43. Barnett AH, Charbonnel B, Donovan M, Fleming D, Chen R. Effect of saxagliptin as add-on therapy in patients with poorly controlled type 2 diabetes on insulin alone or insulin combined with metformin. *Curr Med Res Opin* 2012;28:513–523.

44. Rizos EC, Ntzani EE, Papanas N, Tsimihodimos V, Mitrogianni Z, Maltezos E, Elisaf MS. Combination therapies of DPP4 inhibitors and GLP1 analogues with insulin in type 2 diabetic patients: a systematic review. *Curr Vasc Pharmacol* 2012 [Epub ahead of print].

45. Goossen K, Gräber S. Longer term safety of dipeptidyl peptidase-4 inhibitors in patients with type 2 diabetes mellitus: systematic review and meta-analysis. *Diabetes Obes Metab* 2012;14:1061–1072.

46. Scirica BM, Bhatt DL, Braunwald E, Steg G, Davidson J, Hirshberg B, Ohman P, Frederich R, Wiviott SD, Hoffman EB, Cavender MA, Udell JA, Desai NR, Mozenson O, McGuire DK, Ray KK, Leiter LA, Raz I; for the SAVOR-TIMI 53 Steering Committee and Investigators. Saxagliptin and cardiovascular outcomes in patients with type 2 diabetes mellitus. *N Engl J Med* 2013;369:1317–1326.

47. White WB, Cannon CP, Heller SR, Nissen SE, Bergenstal RM, Bakris GL, Perez AT, Fleck PR, Mehta CR, Kupfer S, Wilson C, Cushman WC, Zannad F; for the EXAMINE Investigators. Alogliptin after acute coronary syndrome in patients with type 2 diabetes. *N Engl J Med* 2013;369:1327–1335.

48. Scheen AJ. Cardiovascular effects of dipeptidyl peptidase-4 inhibitors: from risk factors to clinical outcomes. *Postgrad Med* 2013;125:7–20.

49. Butler AE, Campbell-Thompson M, Gurlo T, Dawson DW, Atkinson M, Butler PC. Marked expansion of exocrine and endocrine pancreas with incretin therapy in humans with increased exocrine pancreas dysplasia and the potential for glucagon-producing neuroendocrine tumors. *Diabetes* 2013;62:2595–2604.

50. Monami M, Dicembrini I, Mannucci E. Dipeptidyl peptidase-4 inhibitors and pancreatitis risk: a meta-analysis of randomized clinical trials. *Diabetes Obes Metab* 2013 [Epub ahead of print].

51. Butler PC, Elashoff M, Elashoff R, Gale EA. A critical analysis of the clinical use of incretin-based therapies: are the GLP-1 therapies safe? *Diabetes Care* 2013;36:2118–2125.

52. Nauck MA. A critical analysis of the clinical use of incretin-based therapies: the benefits by far outweigh the potential risks. *Diabetes Care* 2013;36:2126–2132.

53. Egan AG, Blind E, Dunder K, de Graeff PA, Hummer T, Bourcier T, Rosebraugh C. Pancreatic safety of incretin-based drugs — FDA and EMA assessment. *N Engl J Med* 2014;370:794–797.

54. Inzucchi SE, Bergenstal RM, Buse JB, Diamant M, Ferrannini E, Nauck M, Peters AL, Tsapas A, Wender R, Matthews DR; American Diabetes Association (ADA); European Association for the Study of Diabetes (EASD). Management of hyperglycemia in type 2 diabetes: a patient-centered approach: Position statement of the American Diabetes Association (ADA) and the European Association for the Study of Diabetes (EASD). *Diabetes Care* 2012;35:1364–1379.

55. Garber AJ, Abrahamson MJ, Barzilay JI, Blonde L, Bloomgarden ZT, Bush MA, Dagogo-Jack S, Davidson MB, Einhorn D, Garvey WT, Grunberger G, Handelsman Y, Hirsch IB, Jellinger PS, McGill JB, Mechanick JI, Rosenblit PD, Umpierrez G, Davidson MH. AACE comprehensive diabetes management algorithm 2013. *Endocr Pract* 2013;19:327–336.

56. Bailey CJ, Aschner P, Del Prato S, Lasalle J, Ji L, Matthaei S; on behalf of the Global Partnership for Effective Diabetes Management. Individualized glycaemic targets and pharmacotherapy in type 2 diabetes. *Diab Vasc Dis Res* 2013 [Epub ahead of print].

57. Schwartz SL. Treatment of elderly patients with type 2 diabetes mellitus: a systematic review of the benefits and risks of dipeptidyl peptidase-4 inhibitors. *Am J Geriatr Pharmacother* 2010;8:405–418.

Chapter 25

Glucagon-Like Peptide-1 Receptor Agonist Therapy for Type 2 Diabetes

Dima L. Diab, MD
David A. D'Alessio, MD

exenitid

INTRODUCTION

Glucagon-like peptide-1 (GLP-1) is a regulatory peptide that is essential for normal glucose homeostasis. GLP-1 acts in great part by augmenting insulin secretion after meal ingestion in a glucose-dependent manner, but it also has other actions that tend to lower blood glucose.[1] GLP-1 is produced from the proglucagon gene in the L-cells that are distributed mainly in the distal small intestine and colon. The primary impetus for GLP-1 release is the presence of nutrients in the gut, and L-cells are stimulated by a variety of substrates, including carbohydrates, fats, and proteins.[2-7] In addition, it is now known that other factors also stimulate the release of GLP-1, including interleukin-6 (IL-6)[8] and bile acids.[9] Although the mechanism by which nutrients stimulate the L-cells to secrete GLP-1 is not known, both neural and hormonal mechanisms have been invoked, because serum GLP-1 concentrations increase as early as 5–10 minutes following meal ingestion, which is well before the nutrients pass into the lower gut where most L-cells are located.[10]

GLP-1 receptors (GLP-1Rs) were first discovered on islet β-cells, but it is now clear that this member of the family B G-protein coupled receptors also is expressed by other cells, including central and peripheral neurons, cardiac myocytes, endothelial cells, and subpopulations of immune cells and pneumocytes; the GLP-1R also is expressed in the intestine and kidneys.[1] The major effects of GLP-1 include enhancing glucose-stimulated insulin biosynthesis and secretion, suppressing postprandial glucagon release, decreasing appetite and food intake, reducing hepatic glucose production, and delaying gastric emptying.[1,11-13] Once released from L-cells, GLP-1 is rapidly metabolized by a serine protease, dipeptidyl peptidase 4 (DPP-4), which is expressed ubiquitously on the surface of vascular endothelial cells, but in especially high amounts in the kidney, intestinal brush-border membranes, hepatocytes, and pulmonary vasculature. The N-terminal cleavage of GLP-1 by DPP-4 is rapid, resulting in a half-life of 1–2 minutes for GLP-1 in the circulation.[13] Elimination of bioactive and truncated GLP-1 from the circulation also occurs via renal clearance.

HISTORY OF DEVELOPMENT AND KEY CHARACTERISTICS OF GLP-1 MIMETICS

It has long been known that peptides expressed in the gastrointestinal tract stimulate insulin secretion and that these account for the two to three times greater insulin

DOI: 10.2337/9781580405096.25

secretion resulting from oral glucose ingestion as compared with isoglycemic intravenous glucose (i.e., the incretin effect).[14] Of the range of gut peptides known to stimulate insulin secretion in vitro or in healthy humans, however, only GLP-1 retains significant insulinotropic activity in people with type 2 diabetes (T2D).[15] Research indicates that the incretin effect is impaired in T2D and that people with T2D have a decreased β-cell responsiveness to GLP-1.[16] Supraphysiologic doses of GLP-1, however, retain the capability to enhance glucose-induced insulin secretion in diabetic patients.[17] Furthermore, infusions of GLP-1 have been found to suppress α-cell secretion of glucagon in diabetic subjects.[7,18] The combination of these effects on islet cell secretion causes a significant reduction in fasting[19] and postprandial hyperglycemia.[20] The major barrier to successful therapeutic use of GLP-1 as an antidiabetic agent is the rapid inactivation by DPP-4. Strategies designed to circumvent the rapid metabolism of GLP-1 have resulted in the development of GLP-1 mimetics (GLP-1 receptor agonists [GLP-1 RAs]) that are resistant to DPP-4 and thus have longer half-lives than natural GLP-1. The discovery of exendin-4, a naturally DPP-4-resistant GLP-1 analog, originally purified from the saliva of the Gila monster (*Heloderma suspectum*), had a great impact to advance this area of therapeutics.[7]

GLP-1 RAs have become an active area of drug development. These agents vary in their chemical structures and pharmacokinetics. They are highly specific for the GLP-1R, however, and thus mimic the actions established for native GLP-1. Three GLP-1 RAs are currently available for the management of hyperglycemia in patients with T2D. Exenatide (Byetta), a synthetic replica of exendin-4, has been available clinically since 2005 and is administered twice daily. Liraglutide (Victoza), a GLP-1 analog modified to include a fatty acid side chain to facilitate albumin binding, has a longer half-life and is suitable for once-daily injection; this agent received approval in 2010. An extended-release form of exenatide, exenatide ER (Bydureon), is administered weekly and has been available since 2012. Because they are peptides, these agents are administered subcutaneously. The key pharmacologic characteristics of the commercially available GLP-1 RAs are summarized in Table 25.1.[21–24] Exenatide BID and exenatide ER are eliminated predominantly through glomerular filtration, whereas liraglutide is not cleared renally but rather is metabolized endogenously.

CLINICAL USE

GLP-1 RAs have multiple physiologic effects that lead to improved clinical outcomes in T2D. They increase insulin secretion in response to elevated glucose, and they decrease glucagon release, improving fasting and postprandial glucose levels as well as reducing glycated hemoglobin (A1C).[25–27] Because these effects are glucose dependent, these agents pose a relatively low risk of hypoglycemia. In clinical trials, GLP-1 RAs increased the risk of hypoglycemia only when combined with sulfonylureas.[28] Moreover, despite the effect of GLP-1R signaling to reduce plasma glucagon, GLP-1 RAs do not interfere with hypoglycemic counterregulation.[29,30]

Preclinical human studies demonstrated potent effects of GLP-1 to reduce food intake.[31] Studies in animals indicate that GLP-1 activates satiety pathways in

Table 25.1 Key Pharmacologic Characteristics of Commercially Available GLP-1 RAs

Characteristic	Exenatide BID (Byetta)	Liraglutide (Victoza)	Exenatide ER (Bydureon)
Description	Synthetic exendin-4	Human GLP-1 modified with amino acid substitution and acyl chain addition	Exenatide contained in hydrolysable polymer microspheres
Administration	Subcutaneous injection twice daily before meals	Subcutaneous injection once daily, any time	Subcutaneous injection, once weekly, any time but immediately after suspension
Half-life	2.4 hours	13 hours	~2 weeks
Time to peak concentration	2.1 hours	8–12 hours	6–7 weeks

Sources: Neumiller JJ. Differential chemistry (structure), mechanism of action, and pharmacology of GLP-1 receptor agonists and DPP-4 inhibitors. *J Am Pharm Assoc* 2009;49(Suppl 1):S16–29; *package inserts:* Byetta: http://documents.byetta.com/Byetta_PI.pdf. Accessed 15 August 2013; Bydureon: http://documents.bydureon.com/Bydureon_PI.pdf. Accessed 15 August 2013; Victoza: www.novo-pi.com/victoza.pdf. Accessed 15 August 2013.

the brain and interacts with other systems regulating energy balance.[32] These effects extend to the use of GLP-1 RAs in clinical practice, where most patients receiving these drugs lose weight; subjects in clinical trials lose an average of 3 kg over 6–12 months of treatment.[33] Liraglutide currently is under investigation as therapy for weight loss in people without diabetes.[34] Use of GLP-1 RAs also is associated with a reduction of common markers of cardiovascular risk, including blood pressure, total cholesterol, triglycerides, and C-reactive protein.[35] It is not clear whether these effects are independent of weight loss, although the effect of GLP-1 RAs to lower blood pressure seems likely to be related to a direct effect on natriuresis.[36] Both exenatide and liraglutide have been noted to increase heart rate by 3–5 beats/minute.

One of the earliest actions observed with the infusion of GLP-1 into humans was delayed gastric emptying,[37] an effect that occurs most prominently with supraphysiologic amounts of peptide. Because GLP-1 RAs are given in supraphysiologic amounts, and mimic precisely the actions of native GLP-1, it is not surprising that these drugs also have a significant impact on gastric motility.[38] The delayed passage of meal carbohydrate from the stomach results in a slower rise in postprandial glycemia and contributes to the effect of GLP-1 RAs on glycemic control in T2D.[39] Evidence suggests that short-acting GLP-1 RAs like exenatide may have a larger effect on gastric emptying than longer-acting agents.[40] On the basis of animal studies, the effect of GLP-1 to delay gastric emptying is neurally mediated,[1] but it is not clear whether the nausea and other adverse effects of GLP-1 RAs are associated with the effects of these drugs to cause satiety and delay gastric emptying.

GLP-1 RAs are approved by the U.S. Food and Drug Administration (FDA) as an adjunct to diet and exercise in adult patients with T2D, although liraglutide and exenatide ER are not recommended as first-line monotherapy. Exenatide and liraglutide are approved in combination with basal insulin, whereas exenatide ER is not. These agents may provide benefits in prediabetes although evidence is insufficient from amply powered clinical trials to support this indication, and they are not FDA-approved for the treatment of this condition.[41,42]

A position statement of the American Diabetes Association (ADA) and the European Association for the Study of Diabetes (EASD) proposes that initial treatment with a GLP-1 RA might be useful in occasional cases in which weight loss is seen as an essential aspect of therapy.[43] The current American Association of Clinical Endocrinologists (AACE) treatment algorithm suggests that GLP-1 RAs are second in hierarchy after metformin for monotherapy in patients with A1C <7.5% and first in hierarchy for intensification of therapy (dual or triple therapy).[44]

GLP-1 RAs IN CLINICAL TRIALS

Numerous clinical trials have illustrated the efficacy of GLP-1 RAs as monotherapy as well as in combination with increasingly complex diabetes therapy regimens.[26,45–48] Specifically, GLP-1 RAs have demonstrated improved glycemic control when added to one agent or a combination of two or three agents, including metformin, sulfonylureas, and thiazolidinediones. GLP-1 RAs used with DPP-4 inhibitors have not been well studied, and in fact, they are not approved by the FDA for use in combination with DPP-4 inhibitors.

Post hoc analyses of pooled data from 16 exenatide randomized controlled trials showed significant A1C reductions from baseline.[49] Furthermore, these patients had significant reductions in fasting plasma glucose levels and body weight regardless of duration of diabetes. A similar post hoc analysis of seven trials evaluating the effectiveness of exenatide ER also revealed significant improvements in glycemic control and body weight regardless of diabetes duration.[50] In both studies, hypoglycemia was more common overall in patients who were taking a concomitant sulfonylurea than in patients who were not. Studies looking at efficacy according to background therapy showed similar findings, with significant reductions in A1C from baseline in patients on 0, 1, or 2–3 background agents.[51,52] Results of analyses of liraglutide effect on glycemic control by diabetes stage were consistent with the observations from exenatide studies.[53]

The use of short-acting exenatide and liraglutide in combination with basal insulin also has been associated with improved overall glycemic control.[54–56] Exenatide with insulin glargine, and the addition of insulin detemir to regimens including once-daily liraglutide, are associated with significant reductions in A1C levels compared with either basal insulin or GLP-1 RA alone. It is worth noting that there was significant weight loss when exenatide was added to insulin glargine and that there was no weight gain when insulin detemir was added to a regimen that included liraglutide. With both of these combinations, hypoglycemia rates were very low.

Head-to-head trials with the available GLP-1 RAs reveal greater reduction in fasting glucose, glucagon, and glycated hemoglobin levels with the longer-acting GLP-1 RAs (see Table 25.2), but greater reductions in postprandial glucose levels with the shorter-acting exenatide.[40,57–59] More than 75% of patients lost weight in these clinical trials, with similar weight changes reported among the different GLP-1 RAs, ranging generally between 2 and 4 kg, with the exception of greater weight loss with liraglutide compared with weekly exenatide in the Diabetes Therapy Utilization: Researching Changes in A1C, Weight and Other Factors Through Intervention with Exenatide Once Weekly (DURATION-6) trial (Table 25.2). A meta-analysis of published studies revealed that the highest maintenance doses of the GLP-1 RAs were associated with changes from baseline in mean A1C

Table 25.2 Glycemic Control with the Currently Available GLP-1 RAs: Head-to-Head Trial Results

Study	GLP-1 RA	ΔA1C (%)	ΔFPG (mg/dl)	ΔWeight (kg)
DURATION-1 (N = 295, 30 weeks)	Exenatide BID	−1.5	−25	−3.6
	Exenatide ER	−1.9*	−41*	−3.7
DURATION-5 (N = 252, 24 weeks)	Exenatide BID	−0.9	−12	−1.4
	Exenatide ER	−1.6*	−35*	−2.3
LEAD-6 (N = 464, 26 weeks)	Exenatide BID	−0.8	−11	−2.9
	Liraglutide	−1.1*	−29*	−3.2
DURATION-6 (N = 911, 26 weeks)	Exenatide ER	−1.3	−32	−2.7
	Liraglutide	−1.5*	−38*	−3.6*

Note: DURATION = Diabetes Therapy Utilization: Researching Changes in A1C, Weight and Other Factors Through Intervention with Exenatide Once Weekly; FPG = fasting plasma glucose; GLP-1 RA = GLP-1 receptor agonists; LEAD = Liraglutide Effect and Action in Diabetes.

* P <0.05 vs. GLP-1 RA.

Sources: DURATION-1: Drucker DJ, Buse JB, Taylor K, et al. Exenatide once weekly versus twice daily for the treatment of type 2 diabetes: a randomised, open-label, non-inferiority study. *Lancet* 2008;372:1240–1250; DURATION-5: Blevins T, Pullman J, Malloy J, et al. DURATION-5: exenatide once weekly resulted in greater improvements in glycemic control compared with exenatide twice daily in patients with type 2 diabetes. *J Clin Endocrinol Metab* 2011;96:1301–1310; LEAD-6: Buse JB, Rosenstock J, Sesti G, et al. Liraglutide once a day versus exenatide twice a day for type 2 diabetes: a 26-week randomised, parallel-group, multinational, open-label trial (LEAD-6). *Lancet* 2009;374:39–47; DURATION-6: Buse JB, Nauck M, Forst T, et al. Exenatide once weekly versus liraglutide once daily in patients with type 2 diabetes (DURATION-6): a randomised, open-label study. *Lancet* 2013;381:117–124.

of –1.1 to –1.6% and confirmed that the mean reductions in fasting glucose levels with exenatide once weekly or liraglutide once daily were apparently greater than those with exenatide twice daily.[60] Beyond the traditional clinical measures of diabetes therapy, studies assessing treatment satisfaction showed improvements in satisfaction scores that were overall greater with the long-acting GLP-1 RAs as compared with short-acting exenatide.[61,62]

ADVERSE EVENTS AND SAFETY CONCERNS

Adverse events of GLP-1 RAs are predominantly gastrointestinal. Nausea is a common adverse effect but can be reduced with dose titration; it is generally mild to moderate in intensity and wanes with duration of therapy. It also has been reported less frequently with the long-acting agents.[40] In clinical trials, these agents have not been shown to pose an increased risk of hypoglycemia overall.[63]

Prescribing information for all three GLP-1 RAs includes precautions regarding the potential risk of pancreatitis; however, no causal link to incretin mimetics has been identified at this time. Thirty-six postmarketing reports of acute pancreatitis, including cases of necrotizing or hemorrhagic pancreatitis and fatalities, in patients taking exenatide were submitted via the Medwatch system soon after its introduction; many of these cases were associated only tangentially with exenatide use, but there were three episodes of recurrent pancreatitis in patients restarted after their initial event.[64] Although retrospective cohort studies have not identified an increased risk,[65] a recent case-control study showed that current use of GLP-1-based therapies within 30 days and recent use past 30 days and <2 years were associated with significantly increased odds of acute pancreatitis compared with nonusers (adjusted odds ratio, 2.24; 95% confidence interval [CI], 1.36–3.68] and 2.01; 95% CI, 1.37–3.18, respectively).[66] In response to this study, the AACE and ADA published a press release stating that this does not provide the basis for changing treatment in people with diabetes.[67] Pancreatitis should be considered in patients with persistent severe abdominal pain, and GLP-1 RAs should be discontinued in such patients. Although the use of GLP-1 RAs in people with a history of pancreatitis is not strictly contraindicated, it may not be prudent.

There have also been reports of an increased risk of subclinical pancreatic inflammation and pancreatic cancer in exenatide users,[68] although no causal relationship has been established. After a review of currently available data, the FDA stated that there was insufficient evidence to confirm an increased risk of pancreatic cancer with the use of GLP-1-based therapies, but the FDA is continuing to evaluate all available data to further understand this potential safety issue.[69] Several large randomized clinical trials are ongoing to evaluate the cardiovascular safety of GLP-1 RAs; it is expected that these studies will provide increased information on which to assess the risk of the drugs on pancreatic disease.

Prescribing information for all three agents also includes precautions regarding renal failure. There have been 78 reported cases of acute renal failure or renal insufficiency in patients using exenatide.[70] The relationship between these findings and exenatide could not be determined, and common characteristics of these cases included dehydration and concomitant use of nephrotoxic agents. The recently discovered natriuretic actions of GLP-1 RAs provide a direct mechanism that may contribute as well. Nevertheless, it currently is recommended that both short-acting exenatide and exenatide ER should be used cautiously in patients with moderate kidney impairment and should not be used at all in patients with severe impairment in renal function (creatinine clearance <30 ml/minute). In contrast, because the kidneys are not a major route of clearance for liraglutide, there are no recommendations against the use of this agent in patients with kidney disease. Clinicians should follow the guidelines in Table 25.3 for the use of GLP-1 RAs in patients with impaired kidney function.

Prescribing information for liraglutide and exenatide ER also includes precautions regarding a potential risk of medullary thyroid cancer. Observations in rodents prompted these label statements,[71] and although any potential risk in humans is unknown,[72,73] these agents should not be prescribed to patients with personal or family history of medullary thyroid cancer or multiple endocrine neoplasia 2. To date, results of randomized trials do not suggest any detrimental effect of GLP-1 RAs on cardiovascular events.[74,75]

FUTURE DEVELOPMENTS

Several GLP-1 RAs currently are in clinical development. Lixisenatide, a synthetic analog of exendin-4, which is injected once daily, has demonstrated efficacy in phase 3 trials as monotherapy as well as in combination with oral antidiabetic drugs and insulin.[76-81] Albiglutide, an albumin-GLP-1 fusion protein, is also currently in phase 3 trials for the treatment of T2D as a once-weekly injection.[82-85] Semaglutide is another promising GLP-1 analog administered as a once-weekly injection and currently is in phase 3 clinical development for T2D.[86] Finally, dulaglutide and langlenatide are GLP-1 RAs linked to the constant region of immu-

Table 25.3 Use of GLP-1 RAs in Chronic Kidney Disease

Renal status	Exenatide BID and Exenatide ER	Liraglutide
Mild impairment (CrCl >50 ml/minute)	No adjustment	No adjustment Use with caution when initiating or escalating doses
Moderate impairment (CrCl 30–50 ml/minute)	Use with caution	
Severe impairment (CrCl <30 ml/minute) or ESRD	Should not be used	
Renal transplant	Use with caution	

Note: CrCl = creatinine clearance; ESRD = end-stage renal disease.

Sources: Available at http://documents.byetta.com/Byetta_PI.pdf. Accessed 15 August 2013; Available at http://documents.bydureon.com/Bydureon_PI.pdf. Accessed 15 August 2013; Available at http://www.novo-pi.com/victoza.pdf. Accessed 15 August 2013.

noglobulin G, the Fc region. Dulaglutide has demonstrated efficacy in terms of glycemic control when given as a once-weekly injection in a large phase 3 trial.[87,88] Langlenatide holds promise to show even longer duration of action and currently is being investigated in phase 2 trials for the treatment of T2D as once-weekly and once-monthly applications.[89] Upcoming phase 3 data from the next generation of long-acting GLP-1 RAs will reveal whether the efficacy within this class of drugs can be improved without affecting safety. Evidence is increasing that GLP-1 RAs may be beneficial as adjunct therapies in type 1 diabetes, and ongoing trials are assessing the efficacy of such agents in the setting of islet transplantation. As mentioned, liraglutide is also under investigation as a therapy for weight loss in people without diabetes.

CONCLUSION

At this time, three GLP-1 RAs are widely available for clinical use. These provide significant improvement in glycemic control across the progression of T2D, but only exenatide and liraglutide are FDA approved for use with basal insulin. In clinical trials, long-acting agents—including once-daily liraglutide and once-weekly exenatide—improve fasting plasma glucose and A1C levels to a greater extent than twice-daily exenatide, although short-acting exenatide may be more advantageous for patients who primarily require improvement in their postprandial glucose levels. In addition, adherence to long-acting agents may be greater than that for twice-daily administration, providing another rationale for the use of such agents. Despite the need for administration by injection and the potential for gastrointestinal side effects, other characteristics of incretin mimetics, including glycemic control efficacy, weight loss, and low risk of hypoglycemia, make these agents compare favorably with other treatment options for T2D. The major adverse effects of GLP-1 RAs are nausea, vomiting, and other gastrointestinal symptoms. Safety concerns currently under investigation include acute pancreatitis and renal failure.

REFERENCES

1. Campbell JE, Drucker DJ. Pharmacology, physiology, and mechanisms of incretin hormone action. *Cell Metab* 2013;17:819–837.

2. Diakogiannaki E, Gribble FM, Reimann F. Nutrient detection by incretin hormone secreting cells. *Physiol Behav* 2012;106:387–393.

3. Tolhurst G, Heffron H, Lam YS, et al. Short-chain fatty acids stimulate glucagon-like peptide-1 secretion via the G-protein-coupled receptor FFAR2. *Diabetes* 2012;61:364–371.

4. Oya M, Kitaguchi T, Pais R, Reimann F, Gribble F, Tsuboi T. The G protein-coupled receptor family C group 6 subtype A (GPRC6A) receptor is involved in amino acid-induced glucagon-like peptide-1 secretion from GLUTag cells. *J Biol Chem* 2013;288:4513–4521.

5. Reimann F, Tolhurst G, Gribble FM. G-protein-coupled receptors in intestinal chemosensation. *Cell Metab* 2012;15:421–431.

6. Tolhurst G, Reimann F, Gribble FM. Intestinal sensing of nutrients. *Handb Exp Pharmacol* 2012:309–335.

7. Diab DL, D'Alessio DA. The contribution of enteroinsular hormones to the pathogenesis of type 2 diabetes mellitus. *Curr Diab Rep* 2010;10:192–198.

8. Ellingsgaard H, Hauselmann I, Schuler B, et al. Interleukin-6 enhances insulin secretion by increasing glucagon-like peptide-1 secretion from L cells and alpha cells. *Nat Med* 2011;17:1481–1489.

9. Parker HE, Wallis K, le Roux CW, Wong KY, Reimann F, Gribble FM. Molecular mechanisms underlying bile acid-stimulated glucagon-like peptide-1 secretion. *Br J Pharmacol* 2012;165:414–423.

10. Salehi M, D'Alessio DA. New therapies for type 2 diabetes based on glucagon-like peptide 1. *Cleve Clin J Med* 2006;73:382–389.

11. Nicolaus M, Brodl J, Linke R, Woerle HJ, Goke B, Schirra J. Endogenous GLP-1 regulates postprandial glycemia in humans: relative contributions of insulin, glucagon, and gastric emptying. *J Clin Endocrinol Metab* 2011;96:229–236.

12. Witte AB, Gryback P, Jacobsson H, et al. Involvement of endogenous glucagon-like peptide-1 in regulation of gastric motility and pancreatic endocrine secretion. *Scand J Gastroenterol* 2011;46:428–435.

13. Drucker DJ. The biology of incretin hormones. *Cell Metab* 2006;3:153–165.

14. Creutzfeldt W, Nauck M. Gut hormones and diabetes mellitus. *Diabetes Metab Rev* 1992;8:149–177.

15. Nauck MA, Heimesaat MM, Orskov C, Holst JJ, Ebert R, Creutzfeldt W. Preserved incretin activity of glucagon-like peptide 1 [7-36 amide] but not of synthetic human gastric inhibitory polypeptide in patients with type-2 diabetes mellitus. *J Clin Invest* 1993;91:301–307.

16. Kjems LL, Holst JJ, Volund A, Madsbad S. The influence of GLP-1 on glucose-stimulated insulin secretion: effects on beta-cell sensitivity in type 2 and nondiabetic subjects. *Diabetes* 2003;52:380–386.

17. Hojberg PV, Zander M, Vilsboll T, et al. Near normalisation of blood glucose improves the potentiating effect of GLP-1 on glucose-induced insulin secretion in patients with type 2 diabetes. *Diabetologia* 2008;51:632–640.

18. Hare KJ, Knop FK, Asmar M, et al. Preserved inhibitory potency of GLP-1 on glucagon secretion in type 2 diabetes mellitus. *J Clin Endocrinol Metab* 2009;94:4679–4687.

19. Nauck MA, Kleine N, Orskov C, Holst JJ, Willms B, Creutzfeldt W. Normalization of fasting hyperglycaemia by exogenous glucagon-like peptide 1 (7-36 amide) in type 2 (non-insulin-dependent) diabetic patients. *Diabetologia* 1993;36:741–744.

20. Rachman J, Barrow BA, Levy JC, Turner RC. Near-normalisation of diurnal glucose concentrations by continuous administration of glucagon-like peptide-1 (GLP-1) in subjects with NIDDM. *Diabetologia* 1997;40:205–211.

21. Neumiller JJ. Differential chemistry (structure), mechanism of action, and pharmacology of GLP-1 receptor agonists and DPP-4 inhibitors. *J Am Pharm Assoc* 2009;49(Suppl 1):S16–S29.

22. Byetta package insert. Available at http://documents.byetta.com/Byetta_PI.pdf. Accessed 15 August 2013.

23. Bydureon package insert. Available at http://documents.bydureon.com/Bydureon_PI.pdf. Accessed 15 August 2013.

24. Victoza package insert. Available at www.novo-pi.com/victoza.pdf. Accessed 15 August 2013.

25. Blonde L, Russell-Jones D. The safety and efficacy of liraglutide with or without oral antidiabetic drug therapy in type 2 diabetes: an overview of the LEAD 1-5 studies. *Diabetes Obes Metab* 2009;11(Suppl 3):26–34.

26. Russell-Jones D, Cuddihy RM, Hanefeld M, et al. Efficacy and safety of exenatide once weekly versus metformin, pioglitazone, and sitagliptin used as monotherapy in drug-naive patients with type 2 diabetes (DURA-TION-4): a 26-week double-blind study. *Diabetes Care* 2012;35:252–258.

27. DeFronzo RA, Okerson T, Viswanathan P, Guan X, Holcombe JH, MacConell L. Effects of exenatide versus sitagliptin on postprandial glucose, insulin and glucagon secretion, gastric emptying, and caloric intake: a randomized, cross-over study. *Curr Med Res Opin* 2008;24:2943–2952.

28. Monami M, Marchionni N, Mannucci E. Glucagon-like peptide-1 receptor agonists in type 2 diabetes: a meta-analysis of randomized clinical trials. *Eur J Endocrinol* 2009;160:909–917.

29. Nauck MA, Heimesaat MM, Behle K, et al. Effects of glucagon-like peptide 1 on counterregulatory hormone responses, cognitive functions, and insulin secretion during hyperinsulinemic, stepped hypoglycemic clamp experiments in healthy volunteers. *J Clin Endocrinol Metab* 2002;87:1239–1246.

30. Degn KB, Brock B, Juhl CB, et al. Effect of intravenous infusion of exenatide (synthetic exendin-4) on glucose-dependent insulin secretion and counter-regulation during hypoglycemia. *Diabetes* 2004;53:2397–2403.

31. Verdich C, Flint A, Gutzwiller JP, et al. A meta-analysis of the effect of glucagon-like peptide-1 (7-36) amide on ad libitum energy intake in humans. *J Clin Endocrinol Metab* 2001;86:4382–4389.

32. Barrera JG, Sandoval DA, D'Alessio DA, Seeley RJ. GLP-1 and energy balance: an integrated model of short-term and long-term control. *Nat Rev Endocrinol* 2011;7:507–516.

33. Vilsboll T, Christensen M, Junker AE, Knop FK, Gluud LL. Effects of glucagon-like peptide-1 receptor agonists on weight loss: systematic review and meta-analyses of randomised controlled trials. *BMJ* 2012;344:d7771.

34. Astrup A, Rossner S, Van Gaal L, et al. Effects of liraglutide in the treatment of obesity: a randomised, double-blind, placebo-controlled study. *Lancet* 2009;374:1606–1616.

35. Mundil D, Cameron-Vendrig A, Husain M. GLP-1 receptor agonists: a clinical perspective on cardiovascular effects. *Diab Vasc Dis Res* 2012;9:95–108.

36. Skov J, Dejgaard A, Frokiaer J, et al. Glucagon-like peptide-1 (GLP-1): effect on kidney hemodynamics and renin-angiotensin-aldosterone system in healthy men. *J Clin Endocrinol Metab* 2013;98:E664–E671.

37. Nauck MA, Niedereichholz U, Ettler R, et al. Glucagon-like peptide 1 inhibition of gastric emptying outweighs its insulinotropic effects in healthy humans. *Am J Physiol* 1997;273:E981–E988.

38. Drucker DJ, Nauck MA. The incretin system: glucagon-like peptide-1 receptor agonists and dipeptidyl peptidase-4 inhibitors in type 2 diabetes. *Lancet* 2006;368:1696–1705.

39. Linnebjerg H, Park S, Kothare PA, et al. Effect of exenatide on gastric emptying and relationship to postprandial glycemia in type 2 diabetes. *Regul Pept* 2008;151:123–129.

40. Drucker DJ, Buse JB, Taylor K, et al. Exenatide once weekly versus twice daily for the treatment of type 2 diabetes: a randomised, open-label, non-inferiority study. *Lancet* 2008;372:1240–1250.

41. Rosenstock J, Klaff LJ, Schwartz S, et al. Effects of exenatide and lifestyle modification on body weight and glucose tolerance in obese subjects with and without pre-diabetes. *Diabetes Care* 2010;33:1173–1175.

42. Astrup A, Carraro R, Finer N, et al. Safety, tolerability and sustained weight loss over 2 years with the once-daily human GLP-1 analog, liraglutide. *Int J Obes (Lond)* 2012;36:843–854.

43. Inzucchi SE, Bergenstal RM, Buse JB, et al. Management of hyperglycemia in type 2 diabetes: a patient-centered approach: position statement of the American Diabetes Association (ADA) and the European Association for the Study of Diabetes (EASD). *Diabetes Care* 2012;35:1364–1379.

44. Garber AJ, Abrahamson MJ, Barzilay JI, et al. AACE comprehensive diabetes management algorithm 2013. *Endocr Pract* 2013;19:327–336.

45. Moretto TJ, Milton DR, Ridge TD, et al. Efficacy and tolerability of exenatide monotherapy over 24 weeks in antidiabetic drug-naive patients with type 2 diabetes: a randomized, double-blind, placebo-controlled, parallel-group study. *Clin Ther* 2008;30:1448–1460.

46. Bergenstal RM, Wysham C, Macconell L, et al. Efficacy and safety of exenatide once weekly versus sitagliptin or pioglitazone as an adjunct to metfor-

min for treatment of type 2 diabetes (DURATION-2): a randomised trial. *Lancet* 2010;376:431–439.

47. Russell-Jones D, Vaag A, Schmitz O, et al. Liraglutide vs insulin glargine and placebo in combination with metformin and sulfonylurea therapy in type 2 diabetes mellitus (LEAD-5 met+SU): a randomised controlled trial. *Diabetologia* 2009;52:2046–2055.

48. Pratley RE, Nauck M, Bailey T, et al. Liraglutide versus sitagliptin for patients with type 2 diabetes who did not have adequate glycaemic control with metformin: a 26-week, randomised, parallel-group, open-label trial. *Lancet* 2010;375:1447–1456.

49. Pencek R, Blickensderfer A, Li Y, Brunell SC, Anderson PW. Exenatide twice daily: analysis of effectiveness and safety data stratified by age, sex, race, duration of diabetes, and body mass index. *Postgrad Med* 2012;124:21–32.

50. Pencek R, Blickensderfer A, Li Y, Brunell SC, Chen S. Exenatide once weekly for the treatment of type 2 diabetes: effectiveness and tolerability in patient subpopulations. *Int J Clin Pract* 2012;66:1021–1032.

51. Pencek R, Brunell SC, Li Y, Hoogwerf BJ, Malone J. Exenatide once weekly for the treatment of type 2 diabetes mellitus: clinical results in subgroups of patients using different concomitant medications. *Postgrad Med* 2012;124:33–40.

52. Pencek R, Brunell SC, Li Y, Hoogwerf BJ, Malone J. Use of concomitant glucose-lowering therapies and associated treatment results observed in clinical trials of twice-daily exenatide. *Endocr Pract* 2012;18:227–237.

53. Garber AJ. Liraglutide in oral antidiabetic drug combination therapy. *Diabetes Obes Metab* 2012;14(Suppl 2):13–19.

54. Buse JB, Bergenstal RM, Glass LC, et al. Use of twice-daily exenatide in basal insulin-treated patients with type 2 diabetes: a randomized, controlled trial. *Ann Intern Med* 2011;154:103–112.

55. DeVries JH, Bain SC, Rodbard HW, et al. Sequential intensification of metformin treatment in type 2 diabetes with liraglutide followed by randomized addition of basal insulin prompted by A1C targets. *Diabetes Care* 2012;35:1446–1454.

56. Rosenstock J, Rodbard HW, Bain SC, et al. One-year sustained glycemic control and weight reduction in type 2 diabetes after addition of liraglutide to metformin followed by insulin detemir according to HbA1c target. *J Diabetes Complications* 2013 Sep-Oct;27(5):492–500.

57. Blevins T, Pullman J, Malloy J, et al. DURATION-5: exenatide once weekly resulted in greater improvements in glycemic control compared with exenatide twice daily in patients with type 2 diabetes. *J Clin Endocrinol Metab* 2011;96:1301–1310.

58. Buse JB, Rosenstock J, Sesti G, et al. Liraglutide once a day versus exenatide twice a day for type 2 diabetes: a 26-week randomised, parallel-group, multinational, open-label trial (LEAD-6). *Lancet* 2009;374:39–47.

59. Buse JB, Nauck M, Forst T, et al. Exenatide once weekly versus liraglutide once daily in patients with type 2 diabetes (DURATION-6): a randomised, open-label study. *Lancet* 2013;381:117–124.

60. Aroda VR, Henry RR, Han J, et al. Efficacy of GLP-1 receptor agonists and DPP-4 inhibitors: meta-analysis and systematic review. *Clin Ther* 2012;34:1247–1258, e22.

61. Best JH, Boye KS, Rubin RR, Cao D, Kim TH, Peyrot M. Improved treatment satisfaction and weight-related quality of life with exenatide once weekly or twice daily. *Diabet Med* 2009;26:722–728.

62. Schmidt WE, Christiansen JS, Hammer M, Zychma MJ, Buse JB. Patient-reported outcomes are superior in patients with type 2 diabetes treated with liraglutide as compared with exenatide, when added to metformin, sulphonylurea or both: results from a randomized, open-label study. *Diabet Med* 2011;28:715–723.

63. Liu SC, Tu YK, Chien MN, Chien KL. Effect of antidiabetic agents added to metformin on glycaemic control, hypoglycaemia and weight change in patients with type 2 diabetes: a network meta-analysis. *Diabetes Obes Metab* 2012;14:810–820.

64. U.S. Food and Drug Administration. Byetta safety update for healthcare professionals. Available at www.fda.gov/Drugs/DrugSafety/PostmarketDrugSafetyInformationforPatientsandProviders/DrugSafetyInformationforHeathcareProfessionals/ucm190406.htm. Accessed 1 August 2013.

65. Dore DD, Bloomgren GL, Wenten M, et al. A cohort study of acute pancreatitis in relation to exenatide use. *Diabetes Obes Metab* 2011;13:559–566.

66. Singh S, Chang HY, Richards TM, Weiner JP, Clark JM, Segal JB. Glucagonlike peptide 1-based therapies and risk of hospitalization for acute pancreatitis in type 2 diabetes mellitus: a population-based matched case-control study. *JAMA Intern Med* 2013;173:534–539.

67. American Association of Clinical Endocrinologists. Correcting and replacing: American Association of Clinical Endocrinologists, American Diabetes Association issue joint response to published JAMA article. Available at http://media.aace.com/press-release/correcting-and-replacing-american-association-clinical-endocrinologists-american-diabe. Accessed 1 August 2013.

68. Butler PC, Elashoff M, Elashoff R, Gale EA. A critical analysis of the clinical use of incretin-based therapies: are the GLP 1 therapies safe? *Diabetes Care* 2013;36:2118–2125.

69. U.S. Food and Drug Administration. FDA drug safety communication: FDA investigating reports of possible increased risk of pancreatitis and pre-can-

cerous findings of the pancreas from incretin mimetic drugs for type 2 diabetes. Available at www.fda.gov/Drugs/DrugSafety/ucm343187. htm?source=govdelivery. Accessed 1 August 2013.

70. U.S. Food and Drug Administration. Byetta (exenatide) - renal failure. Available at www.fda.gov/safety/MedWatch/SafetyInformation/SafetyAlerts-forHumanMedicalProducts/ucm188703.htm. Accessed 1 August 2013.

71. Bjerre Knudsen L, Madsen LW, Andersen S, et al. Glucagon-like peptide-1 receptor agonists activate rodent thyroid C-cells causing calcitonin release and C-cell proliferation. *Endocrinology* 2010;151:1473–1486.

72. Boess F, Bertinetti-Lapatki C, Zoffmann S, et al. Effect of GLP1R agonists taspoglutide and liraglutide on primary thyroid C-cells from rodent and man. *J Mol Endocrinol* 2013;50:325–336.

73. Gier B, Butler PC, Lai CK, Kirakossian D, DeNicola MM, Yeh MW. Glucagon like peptide-1 receptor expression in the human thyroid gland. *J Clin Endocrinol Metab* 2012;97:121–131.

74. Monami M, Cremasco F, Lamanna C, et al. Glucagon-like peptide-1 receptor agonists and cardiovascular events: a meta-analysis of randomized clinical trials. *Exp Diabetes Res* 2011;2011:215764.

75. Monami M, Dicembrini I, Nardini C, Fiordelli I, Mannucci E. Effects of glucagon-like peptide-1 receptor agonists on cardiovascular risk: a meta-analysis of randomized clinical trials. *Diabetes Obes Metab* 2014 Jan;16(1):38–47.

76. Ratner RE, Rosenstock J, Boka G. Dose-dependent effects of the once-daily GLP-1 receptor agonist lixisenatide in patients with type 2 diabetes inadequately controlled with metformin: a randomized, double-blind, placebo-controlled trial. *Diabet Med* 2010;27:1024–1032.

77. Hramiak I, Raccah D, Ceriello A, et al. Meta-analysis of GLP-1 receptor agonist lixisenatide use in patients insufficiently controlled with oral antihyperglycemic agents. *Can J Diabetes* 2013;37(Suppl 4):S37–S38.

78. Riddle MC, Aronson R, Home P, et al. Adding once-daily lixisenatide for type 2 diabetes inadequately controlled by established basal insulin: a 24-week, randomized, placebo-controlled comparison (GetGoal-L). *Diabetes Care* 2013;36:2489–2496.

79. Riddle MC, Forst T, Aronson R, et al. Adding once-daily lixisenatide for type 2 diabetes inadequately controlled with newly initiated and continuously titrated basal insulin glargine: a 24-week, randomized, placebo-controlled study (GetGoal-Duo 1). *Diabetes Care* 2013;36:2497–2503.

80. Rosenstock J, Raccah D, Koranyi L, et al. Efficacy and safety of lixisenatide once daily versus exenatide twice daily in type 2 diabetes inadequately controlled on metformin: a 24-week, randomized, open-label, active-controlled study (GetGoal-X). *Diabetes Care* 2013;36:2945–2951.

81. Sigalas J, Bonadonna R, Puig-Domingo M, et al. Lixisenatide significantly increases the probability of a a1c response in patients not adequately controlled on oral antihyperglycemic agents. *Can J Diabetes* 2013;37(Suppl 4): S43.

82. Bush MA, Matthews JE, De Boever EH, et al. Safety, tolerability, pharmacodynamics and pharmacokinetics of albiglutide, a long-acting glucagon-like peptide-1 mimetic, in healthy subjects. *Diabetes Obes Metab* 2009;11:498–505.

83. Matthews JE, Stewart MW, De Boever EH, et al. Pharmacodynamics, pharmacokinetics, safety, and tolerability of albiglutide, a long-acting glucagon-like peptide-1 mimetic, in patients with type 2 diabetes. *J Clin Endocrinol Metab* 2008;93:4810–4817.

84. St Onge EL, Miller SA. Albiglutide: a new GLP-1 analog for the treatment of type 2 diabetes. *Expert Opin Biol Ther* 2010;10:801–806.

85. Rosenstock J, Reusch J, Bush M, Yang F, Stewart M. Potential of albiglutide, a long-acting GLP-1 receptor agonist, in type 2 diabetes: a randomized controlled trial exploring weekly, biweekly, and monthly dosing. *Diabetes Care* 2009;32:1880–1886.

86. Nauck MA, Petrie JR, Sesti G, et al. Abstracts of the 48th EASD (European Association for the Study of Diabetes) Annual Meeting of the European Association for the Study of Diabetes. October 1–5, 2012. Berlin, Germany. The once-weekly human GLP-1 analogue semaglutide provides significant reductions in HbA1c and body weight in patients with type 2 diabetes. *Diabetologia* 2012;55(Suppl 1):S7.

87. Grunberger G, Chang A, Garcia Soria G, Botros FT, Bsharat R, Milicevic Z. Monotherapy with the once-weekly GLP-1 analogue dulaglutide for 12 weeks in patients with type 2 diabetes: dose-dependent effects on glycaemic control in a randomized, double-blind, placebo-controlled study. *Diabet Med* 2012;29:1260–1267.

88. Guerci B, Weinstock R, Umpierrez G, et al. Safety and efficacy of dulaglutide versus sitagliptin after 104 weeks in type 2 diabetes (AWARD-5). *Can J Diabetes* 2013;37(Suppl 4):S44–S45.

89. Lorenz M, Evers A, Wagner M. Recent progress and future options in the development of GLP-1 receptor agonists for the treatment of diabesity. *Bioorg Med Chem Lett* 2013;23:4011–4018.

Chapter 26

α-Glucosidase Inhibitors

Josée Leroux-Stewart, MD
Rémi Rabasa-Lhoret, MD, PhD
Jean-Louis Chiasson, MD

INTRODUCTION

Lifestyle intervention including diet and exercise remains the cornerstone of treatment strategies for patients with type 2 diabetes (T2D). If the A1C is high from the beginning or remains above target after 2–3 months of lifestyle modifications, and if there are no contraindications, it is recommended to start with metformin.[1] Metformin is effective in reducing hepatic glucose production and thus in decreasing fasting plasma glucose (FPG). In many patients, however, postprandial hyperglycemia persists, accounting in part for the sustained increase in A1C.[2] It has been suggested that postprandial glycemic excursions contribute to the development of diabetes-specific complications and could be involved in the development of macrovascular complications.[3-7] We now have a number of oral antidiabetic medications that specifically target postprandial hyperglycemia: the meglitinides, the dipeptidyl peptidase-4 (DPP-4) inhibitors, and the α-glucosidase inhibitors (AGIs).

The AGIs delay the digestion of complex carbohydrates, therefore decreasing the postprandial rise in plasma glucose and the rise in plasma insulin, reproducing the effect of a low–glycemic-index high-fiber diet. AGIs show a moderate but constant and sustained reduction of A1C whether they are used as monotherapy or in combination, in patients with both type 1 diabetes (T1D) and T2D. They have an excellent safety profile but often are associated with gastrointestinal symptoms. These side effects can be minimized greatly by the "start low and go slow" policy (e.g., starting at the lower available dose for a single meal and based on tolerance titrating upward slowly).

MECHANISM OF ACTION

AGIs competitively block small intestine brush border α-glucosidases, which are essential to hydrolyze di-, oligo-, and polysaccharides to monosaccharides for absorption.[8] Normally, carbohydrates are primarily and rapidly absorbed in the first part of the small intestine. With the use of AGIs, carbohydrate absorption is prolonged throughout the small intestine, resulting in a slower absorption rate and a reduction in the postprandial plasma glucose rise.[9]

Three AGIs have been developed (acarbose, miglitol, and voglibose) and all have similar pharmacological profiles.[10,11] Acarbose, the agent most studied, is a pseudotetrasaccharide of microbial origin, structurally analogous to an oligosac-

 DOI: 10.2337/9781580405096.26

charide derived from starch digestion. It has a high affinity for the carbohydrate-binding site of various α-glucosidases, exceeding the affinity (10- to 100,000-fold) of regular oligosaccharides from nutritional carbohydrates. Because of its structure, acarbose cannot be cleaved and, therefore, enzymatic hydrolysis is blocked. It also is absorbed poorly, therefore displaying its inhibitory activity throughout the small intestine up to the ileum. Binding, however, is reversible. Acarbose is then cleaved in the large intestine by bacterial enzymes into several metabolizable intermediates and four methylpyrogallol derivatives. Thus, even though acarbose itself is poorly absorbed, 35% of an oral dose appears as metabolites in the urine.[12] Because of their specificity for α-glucosidases, β-glucosidases (e.g., lactases) are not inhibited and so the digestion of lactose is not affected.[8]

PHARMACOLOGICAL CHARACTERISTICS

Because of their mechanism of action, certain important aspects of AGI must be known by treating physicians and patients when initiating them to maximize their efficacy and tolerability.

AGIs must be present at the site of enzymatic action at the same time as the polysaccharides, oligosaccharides, or disaccharides. Therefore, AGIs must be taken within the first 15 minutes of each meal to be efficient.[13]

By blocking small intestine α-glucosidases, AGIs cause a considerable amount of undigested carbohydrates to spill into the colon. This gives way to intracolonic fermentation and consequent gas production. Therefore, abdominal distention, flatulence, and diarrhea are frequent side effects of AGIs. With time, however, treatment will induce α-glucosidase synthesis in the distal part of the small intestine, thus minimizing the carbohydrate load reaching the colon. This explains the necessity of initiating treatment at a low dose and increasing it slowly to give the small intestine time to adapt and increase its α-glucosidase content. Therefore, it is recommended to start low (i.e., 25 or 50 mg each day for 1 week) and then increase gradually by 25–50 mg each subsequent week.[12,14–16]

The dose-response relationship of acarbose has been studied in large multicenter trials at doses ranging from 25 to 300 mg three times daily (TID). Despite slight differences, these trials indicate that the 100 mg TID dose evokes a near-maximal response.[14,17] To decrease the risk of side effects, however, the maximum recommended dose of acarbose is 50 mg TID for patients <60 kg and 100 mg TID for patients >60 kg.[18] Interestingly, it has been shown that a low dose of 25 mg TID of acarbose already can significantly reduce FPG, postprandial plasma glucose (PPG), and A1C.[14] Concurrent administration of antacids, bile acid resins, intestinal absorbents, or digestive enzyme preparations may reduce the effect of AGIs and so may necessitate an increase in dosage.

CLINICAL EFFICACY OF α GLUCOSIDASE INHIBITORS

The benefit of adding AGIs to the diet alone or in combination with other agents in patients with T1D or T2D has been investigated in several randomized, double-blind, placebo-controlled trials, as well as in open-labeled controlled studies and postmarketing surveillance trials. Regardless of the concurrent treatment, the glucose-lowering effect of AGIs is seen from the first week of therapy, and is maintained even after 5 years, independent of sex or ethnicity.[19–23]

EFFICACY OF α-GLUCOSIDASE INHIBITORS VERSUS PLACEBO

In a Cochrane systematic review of 28 studies comparing the effect of acarbose versus placebo in patients with T2D, acarbose showed a significant reduction in PPG of –2.32 mmol/l and in FBG of –1.09 mmol/l. Furthermore, through their effects on FBG and PPG, AGIs significantly affected A1C with a decline of 0.77%.[24]

EFFICACY OF α-GLUCOSIDASE INHIBITORS IN COMPARISON TO OTHER HYPOGLYCEMIC AGENTS

Many studies have compared AGIs head to head with other agents in patients with T2D. Ten studies comparing AGIs to sulfonylureas showed a mean adjusted A1C reduction of 0.74% versus 1.18%, respectively.[17,25–33] Fewer studies have compared AGIs to metformin. In one study, acarbose (300 mg/day) had the same efficacy as metformin (1,700 mg/day), with a mean A1C reduction of 1%.[34] Another study showed that miglitol (300 mg/day) had a lower efficacy than metformin (1,500 mg/day), but the combination of both drugs had a synergistic effect (A1C –1.8%).[35] Compared to thiazolidinediones, two studies showed a slightly better performance on A1C in the pioglitazone groups. Weight, however, was either unchanged or increased with the use of pioglitazone, as opposed to a significant weight reduction in the AGI-treated groups.[36,37] Finally, DPP-4 inhibitors have been compared to AGIs in five double-blind randomized trials. Overall, the mean adjusted A1C reduction was of 0.54% in the AGI groups versus 0.9% in the DPP-4 inhibitor groups.[38–42]

EFFICACY OF α-GLUCOSIDASE INHIBITORS IN ASSOCIATION WITH OTHER HYPOGLYCEMIC AGENTS

Because the mechanism of action of AGI is different from that of other oral hypoglycemic agents, an additive benefit can be expected when given in combination with other agents. This has been confirmed in several different trials. The benefit of adding acarbose to sulfonylurea therapy seemed comparable to the addition of metformin for lowering A1C with a mean decrease of 0.81%.[17,28,43–47] In patients with T2D who are suboptimally controlled with metformin, the addition of acarbose similarly produced a reduction of 0.85% in A1C.[21,22,48–51] Finally, when combined sulfonylurea and biguanide therapy failed to achieve adequate glycemic control, the addition of acarbose resulted in a reduction of 0.81% in A1C.[21,36,52–55]

EFFICACY OF α-GLUCOSIDASE INHIBITORS IN COMPARISON TO INSULIN IN PATIENTS WITH T2D

The addition of acarbose has been compared to the introduction of bedtime neutral protamine Hagedorn (NPH) insulin in patients with T2D insufficiently controlled with combined sulfonylurea and metformin treatment. Although adding acarbose resulted in improvement of metabolic control compared to placebo (A1C –0.8% versus –0.2%), it was less effective than insulin (A1C –2.3%).[56] Therefore, this strategy could be considered as a compromise for patients who refuse insulin injections.

EFFICACY OF α-GLUCOSIDASE INHIBITORS IN ASSOCIATION WITH INSULIN IN PATIENTS WITH T2D

Combining AGIs with insulin therapy resulted in significant metabolic improvement in several studies, with a mean adjusted reduction in A1C of 0.5%. There was no significant effect on insulin dosages, but also no weight gain.[17,57–61]

EFFICACY OF α-GLUCOSIDASE INHIBITORS IN PATIENTS WITH T1D

AGIs were added to insulin treatment in eight studies in patients with T1D resulting in a mean-adjusted A1C decrease of 0.54%.[62–69] Although acute studies have shown an insulin-sparing effect of AGI,[63,70–72] the largest placebo-controlled trial in patients with T1D could not confirm that observation.[66] Interestingly, studies have shown that when AGIs were added to regular insulin, there was a decrease in the risk of nocturnal and daytime hypoglycemia as well as during postprandial exercise.[73–76]

EFFICACY OF α-GLUCOSIDASE INHIBITORS IN PATIENTS WITH IMPAIRED GLUCOSE TOLERANCE

In the Study to Prevent Non-Insulin-Dependent Diabetes Mellitus (STOP-NIDDM) trial, subjects with impaired glucose tolerance (IGT) were randomized to either placebo or acarbose to investigate the potential of AGIs to prevent or delay the development of T2D. On the basis of two consecutive positive oral glucose tolerance tests, acarbose reduced the risk of developing T2D by 36.4%.[77] The trial also showed that acarbose treatment was associated with a significant increase in the conversion of IGT to normal glucose tolerance (hazard ratio [HR] = 1.42, 95% confidence interval [CI] 1.24–1.62; P <0.0001). Overall, the study indicated that 11 patients should be treated for 3.3 years to prevent or delay one case of T2D. Moreover, in patients with the metabolic syndrome, only 5.8 patients had to be treated to prevent one case of diabetes, an efficacy similar to that of lifestyle modification.[78] Similarly, another multicenter randomized, double-blind trial was performed in patients with IGT, randomly assigned to receive either voglibose or placebo.[79] Voglibose treatment was associated with a highly significant reduction of 40.5% in the risk of developing T2D compared to placebo. It also significantly increased the conversion of IGT to normal glucose tolerance. Therefore, AGIs are effective in decreasing the risk of diabetes in subjects with IGT.

OTHER EFFECTS OF α-GLUCOSIDASE INHIBITORS

CARDIOVASCULAR RISK FACTORS

AGIs have been shown to lower the postprandial triglyceride rise[80,81] and most studies have reported a small but significant reduction of fasting triglyceride levels.[48,80,82–84] The effects on fasting total cholesterol and high-density lipoprotein cholesterol appear to be minor or marginally significant.[19,82,83,85] Furthermore, AGIs have been shown to decrease insulin resistance in most[77,86–90] but not all studies.[91–93] The negative results in the latter studies may be related to the very poor glycemic control. A meta-analysis of seven randomized, double-blind, placebo-controlled trials with patients with T2D measuring the effects of acarbose on metabolic parameters revealed that systolic blood pressure was significantly lowered by 2.7 mmHg with acarbose treatment.[94] Data from the STOP-NIDDM trial indicated that acarbose could delay the appearance of new cases of high blood pressure in IGT patients.[95] Finally, AGIs have been shown to have a neutral effect on weight in many studies.[21,96] In fact, the use of AGIs does not seem to affect energy intake, nutrient intake, or dietary patterns.[97,98] Carbohydrates that reach the colon are metabolized by bacteria into short chain fatty acids, which then are absorbed, resulting in no or minimal caloric loss.[99] AGIs, however, also have produced weight loss (~1 kg) in several other studies.[10,19,38,48,52,77,97] Overall, AGIs exert neutral or slightly favorable effects on cardiovascular risk factors.

POTENTIAL EFFECTS ON THE PREVENTION OF MACROVASCULAR DIABETIC COMPLICATIONS

Accumulating evidence suggests that AGIs could reduce macrovascular complications associated with diabetes. Carotid artery intima-media thickness (IMT) is recognized as an independent predictor of coronary heart disease and stroke.[100–102] Because postprandial hyperglycemia has been associated with increased common carotid IMT,[103,104] much interest has emerged regarding the potential effect of AGIs on that parameter. Five randomized controlled trials studied the progression of carotid IMT with or without AGIs in patients with IGT or T2D.[82,83,85,105,106] All studies were associated with a significant decrease in the annual progression of carotid IMT when treated with AGIs, suggesting an anti-atherosclerotic effect. Likewise, a meta-analysis of seven randomized placebo-controlled trials in patients with T2D showed a highly significant relative risk reduction of 35% for any cardiovascular event in the acarbose-treated groups.[94] This was further supported by the STOP-NIDDM trial in which acarbose treatment in subjects with IGT was associated with a 49% reduction in cardiovascular events.[95]

INDICATIONS FOR α-GLUCOSIDASE INHIBITOR THERAPY

When diet and exercise fail to maintain optimal blood glucose control, prescription of AGIs should be considered in patients with T2D in the following situations:

- As primary therapy for the following:
  - *Patients with normal or slightly elevated fasting blood glucose but with postprandial hyperglycemia.* This population includes most recently diagnosed patients for whom postprandial hyperglycemia contributes significantly to increased A1C.[2] When diet and exercise fail to normalize blood glucose, AGIs can bring glycemic control into the desirable range for an important portion of these patients.
  - *Elderly patients with diabetes.* This patient population can highly benefit from AGI treatment because of its excellent safety profile and its low hypoglycemic and drug interaction risks.[9,15,28,86] Beside its impact on postprandial blood glucose, AGIs could address a rare but important clinical problem in the elderly population: postprandial hypotension.[107,108] Patient symptoms can be confused with hypoglycemia and although exact pathophysiology is unclear, reducing postprandial hyperglycemia can contribute to reduced postprandial hypotension in patients with T1D or T2D.[109–111]
  - *As an alternative to other oral hypoglycemic agents when they are contraindicated.*
- As an adjunct therapy for the following:
  - Patients with inadequate glycemic control under other hypoglycemic agents, because the combination of AGIs with all other treatments has demonstrated a moderate but significant and sustained glycemic improvement.

TOLERABILITY

AGIs are particularly safe drugs. As monotherapy, they do not cause hypoglycemia.[21] They, however, may potentiate the hypoglycemic action of sulfonylureas or insulin and so a reduction in dosage of concomitant hypoglycemic agents may be necessary when AGIs are introduced.[23] If patients taking AGIs experience hypoglycemia, they should be treated with glucose because the absorption of sucrose (but not lactose) and complex carbohydrates is delayed by the drug, particularly if it occurs early after meal. Patients should be educated on this aspect.

As mentioned earlier, the main side effects of AGIs are gastrointestinal symptoms, such as abdominal distention, flatulence, and diarrhea in ~50% of patients. These symptoms are dose dependent and tend to decrease with continued treatment. Therefore, the best strategy to minimize these side effects is to use a "start low and go slow" dosage policy.[13,77] The importance of this was confirmed by the positive relationship between higher initial doses and higher discontinuation rates.[16] In fact, the discontinuation rate, close to 25% in most large trials, is mostly related to these gastrointestinal side effects due to high initial doses.[22,34,77] Although some studies including the U.K. Prospective Diabetes Study have reported higher discontinuation rates of up to 40%,[16,21,23] many others have found a much lower rate of patients unable to tolerate AGIs, which is comparable to that observed with biguanides (i.e., 5–7%).[14,20,44,112] No clear explanations are available for such discrepancies, but false evaluation of the gastrointestinal side effects can lead to unnecessary gastroenterologist consultations.[16] Despite these frequent gastrointestinal symptoms, the quality of life of patients on AGIs has been shown to be as good, if not better, than with sulfonylurea or insulin therapy.[15,113]

Pneumatosis cystoides intestinalis (also known as pseudolipomatosis, pneumatosis coli, or intestinal emphysema) is a rare condition in which gas is abnormally found in the submucosa or subserosa of the bowel wall. Its relevance must be interpreted within the clinical context as it can be suggestive of a severe underlying condition, such as bowel infarction, but can also be a benign incidental discovery. Interestingly, all three AGIs have been associated with this finding, perhaps because of abnormally raised intracolonic pressure from fermentation of nonabsorbed carbohydrates. We have found 18 case reports of such associations: 10 cases with voglibose, 7 with acarbose, and 1 with miglitol.[114–131] The onset occurred from 1 week to 11 years after starting treatment, when patients complained of abdominal pain, distension, or rectal bleeding. Three patients were asymptomatic and this was an incidental finding. Conservative treatment was employed in all but one case, where surgery was judged appropriate. Treatment consists of immediate discontinuation of the drug with, in some cases, the use of antibiotics or the administration of oxygen, as oxygen is toxic to the anaerobic intestinal bacteria. All 18 cases reported complete clinical and radiological healing usually within the month following the discontinuation of the drug.

In ~3 million patient-years of international postmarketing experience with acarbose, 62 cases of serum transaminase elevations >500 international units per liter have been reported.[18] For 55 of the 59 cases for which follow-up was recorded, hepatic abnormalities improved or resolved upon discontinuation. Moreover, two cases of severe hepatotoxic reaction categorized as probable idiosyncratic reaction related to acarbose have been reported.[132,133] Thus, hepatic reactions are rare and unpredictable.

Rare interactions with digoxin have been reported, resulting in either lowered or increased digoxin plasma levels. Thus, monitoring probably should be done when AGI therapy is initiated or the dose is modified.[134]

Formal contraindications to AGIs include intestinal malabsorption syndromes, inflammatory bowel disease, colonic ulceration, partial intestinal obstruction, and cirrhosis. They also are contraindicated in cases of severe renal impairment (creatinine clearance <25 ml/minute), in children <12 years of age, and in pregnant or lactating women because of a lack of data in these groups. Interestingly, studies have been performed in rabbits at doses up to 32 times those given to humans and have revealed no evidence of teratogenicity.[18]

Because trials in diabetic cirrhotic patients have demonstrated a positive action of acarbose on glycemic control without adverse effects on liver function, restrictions related to cirrhosis probably could be withdrawn.[135,136] It has been mentioned that acarbose even could be used to treat hepatic encephalopathy, but this has yet to be approved for that indication.[137]

CONCLUSION

By delaying the digestion of complex carbohydrates, AGIs significantly decrease the postprandial rise in plasma glucose, resulting in a modest but constant reduction of A1C, regardless of the therapeutic regimen already in place. In subjects with IGT, these drugs can prevent or delay the onset of T2D and hypertension and also have been associated with a reduction in cardiovascular events. Additional benefits of AGIs are the lack of hypoglycemia with monotherapy, no weight gain, and an excellent safety profile. Although gastrointestinal symptoms are frequent, they can be minimized greatly by initiating treatment at a low dose and titrating upward slowly.

REFERENCES

1. American Diabetes Association. Standards of medical care in diabetes—2014. *Diabetes Care* 2014;37(Suppl 1):S14–S80.

2. Monnier L, Lapinski H, Colette C. Contributions of fasting and postprandial plasma glucose increments to the overall diurnal hyperglycemia of type 2 diabetic patients: variations with increasing levels of HbA(1c). *Diabetes Care* 2003;26(3):881–885.

3. American Diabetes Association. Postprandial blood glucose. *Diabetes Care* 2001;24(4):775–778.

4. Bonora E, Muggeo M. Postprandial blood glucose as a risk factor for cardiovascular disease in Type II diabetes: the epidemiological evidence. *Diabetologia* 2001;44(12):2107–2114.

5. The DECODE Study Group. Glucose tolerance and cardiovascular mortality: comparison of fasting and 2-hour diagnostic criteria. *Arch Intern Med* 2001;161(3):397–405.

6. Davidson J. Should postprandial glucose be measured and treated to a particular target? Yes. *Diabetes Care* 2003;26(6):1919–1921.

7. American Diabetes Association. Standards of medical care in diabetes—2013. *Diabetes Care* 2013;36(Suppl 1):S11–S66.

8. Bischoff H. The mechanism of alpha-glucosidase inhibition in the management of diabetes. *Clin Investig Med* 1995;18(4):303–311.

9. Rabasa-Lhoret R, Chiasson JL. Potential of alpha-glucosidase inhibitors in elderly patients with diabetes mellitus and impaired glucose tolerance. *Drugs & Aging* 1998;13(2):131–143.

10. Vichayanrat A, Ploybutr S, Tunlakit M, Watanakejorn P. Efficacy and safety of voglibose in comparison with acarbose in type 2 diabetic patients. *Diabetes Res Clin Prac* 2002;55(2):99–103.

11. Kageyama S, Nakamichi N, Sekino H, Nakano S. Comparison of the effects of acarbose and voglibose in healthy subjects. *Clin Therap* 1997;19(4):720–729.

12. Lebovitz HE. alpha Glucosidase inhibitors as agents in the treatment of diabetes. *Diabetes Rev* 1998;6(2):132–145.

13. Rosak C, Nitzsche G, Konig P, Hofmann U. The effect of the timing and the administration of acarbose on postprandial hyperglycaemia. *Diabet Med* 1995;12(11):979–984.

14. Fischer S, Hanefeld M, Spengler M, Boehme K, Temelkova-Kurktschiev T. European study on dose-response relationship of acarbose as a first-line drug in non-insulin-dependent diabetes mellitus: efficacy and safety of low and high doses. *Acta Diabetol* 1998;35(1):34–40.

15. Josse RG, Chiasson JL, Ryan EA, Lau DC, Ross SA, Yale JF, et al. Acarbose in the treatment of elderly patients with type 2 diabetes. *Diabetes Res Clin Prac* 2003;59(1):37–42.

16. Catalan VS, Couture JA, LeLorier J. Predictors of persistence of use of the novel antidiabetic agent acarbose. *Arch Intern Med* 2001;161(8):1106–1112.

17. Coniff RF, Shapiro JA, Seaton TB, Hoogwerf BJ, Hunt JA. A double-blind placebo-controlled trial evaluating the safety and efficacy of acarbose for the treatment of patients with insulin-requiring type II diabetes. *Diabetes Care* 1995;18(7):928–932.

18. Bayer HealthCare Pharmaceuticals Inc. Precose (acarbose) prescribing information 2013. Available at www.accessdata.fda.gov/drugsatfda_docs/label/2012/020482s025lbl.pdf. Accessed 4 March 2014.

19. Mertes G. Safety and efficacy of acarbose in the treatment of type 2 diabetes: data from a 5-year surveillance study. *Diabetes Res Clin Prac* 2001;52(3):193–204.

20. Li C, Hung YJ, Qamruddin K, Aziz MF, Stein H, Schmidt B. International noninterventional study of acarbose treatment in patients with type 2 diabetes mellitus. *Diabetes Res Clin Prac* 2011;92(1):57–64.

21. Holman RR, Cull CA, Turner RC. A randomized double-blind trial of acarbose in type 2 diabetes shows improved glycemic control over 3 years (U.K. Prospective Diabetes Study 44). *Diabetes Care* 1999;22(6):960–964.

22. Chiasson JL, Josse RG, Hunt JA, Palmason C, Rodger NW, Ross SA, et al. The efficacy of acarbose in the treatment of patients with non-insulin-dependent diabetes mellitus. A multicenter controlled clinical trial. *Ann Intern Med* 1994;121(12):928–935.

23. Buse J, Hart K, Minasi L. The PROTECT Study: final results of a large multicenter postmarketing study in patients with type 2 diabetes. Precose Resolution of Optimal Titration to Enhance Current Therapies. *Clin Ther* 1998;20(2):257–269.

24. Van de Laar FA, Lucassen PL, Akkermans RP, Van de Lisdonk EH, Rutten GE, Van Weel C. Alpha-glucosidase inhibitors for type 2 diabetes mellitus. *Cochrane Database Syst Rev* 2005(2):Cd003639.

25. Hoffmann J, Spengler M. Efficacy of 24-week monotherapy with acarbose, glibenclamide, or placebo in NIDDM patients. The Essen Study. *Diabetes Care* 1994;17(6):561-566.

26. Segal P, Feig PU, Schernthaner G, Ratzmann KP, Rybka J, Petzinna D, et al. The efficacy and safety of miglitol therapy compared with glibenclamide in patients with NIDDM inadequately controlled by diet alone. *Diabetes Care* 1997;20(5):687–691.

27. Salman S, Salman F, Satman I, Yilmaz Y, Ozer E, Sengul A, et al. Comparison of acarbose and gliclazide as first-line agents in patients with type 2 diabetes. *Curr Med Res Opin* 2001;16(4):296–306.

28. Johnston PS, Lebovitz HE, Coniff RF, Simonson DC, Raskin P, Munera CL. Advantages of alpha-glucosidase inhibition as monotherapy in elderly type 2 diabetic patients. *J Clin Endocrinol Metab* 1998;83(5):1515–1522.

29. van de Laar FA, Lucassen PL, Kemp J, van de Lisdonk EH, van Weel C, Rutten GE. Is acarbose equivalent to tolbutamide as first treatment for newly diagnosed type 2 diabetes in general practice? A randomised controlled trial. *Diabetes Res Clin Prac* 2004;63(1):57–65.

30. Fischer S, Patzak A, Rietzsch H, Schwanebeck U, Kohler C, Wildbrett J, et al. Influence of treatment with acarbose or glibenclamide on insulin sensitivity in type 2 diabetic patients. *Diabetes Obes Metab* 2003;5(1):38–44.

31. Pagano G, Marena S, Corgiat-Mansin L, Cravero F, Giorda C, Bozza M, et al. Comparison of miglitol and glibenclamide in diet-treated type 2 diabetic patients. *Diabet Med* 1995;21(3):162–167.

32. Rosenthal JH, Mauersberger H. Effects on blood pressure of the alpha-glucosidase inhibitor acarbose compared with the insulin enhancer glibenclamide in patients with hypertension and type 2 diabetes mellitus. *Clin Drug Invest* 2002;22(10):695–701.

33. Kovacevic I, Profozic V, Skrabalo Z, Cabrijan T, Zjacic-Rotkvic V, Goldoni V, et al. Multicentric clinical trial to assess efficacy and tolerability of acarbose (BAY G 5421) in comparison to glibenclamide and placebo. *Diabetol Croat* 1997;26:83–89.

34. Hoffmann J, Spengler M. Efficacy of 24-week monotherapy with acarbose, metformin, or placebo in dietary-treated NIDDM patients: the Essen-II Study. *Am J Med* 1997;103(6):483–490.

35. Chiasson JL, Naditch L. The synergistic effect of miglitol plus metformin combination therapy in the treatment of type 2 diabetes. *Diabetes Care* 2001;24(6):989–994.

36. Derosa G, Mereu R, D'Angelo A, Salvadeo SA, Ferrari I, Fogari E, et al. Effect of pioglitazone and acarbose on endothelial inflammation biomarkers

during oral glucose tolerance test in diabetic patients treated with sulphonylureas and metformin. *J Clin Pharm Ther* 2010;35(5):565–579.

37. Fujitaka K, Otani H, Jo F, Jo H, Nomura E, Iwasaki M, et al. Comparison of metabolic profile and adiponectin level with pioglitazone versus voglibose in patients with type-2 diabetes mellitus associated with metabolic syndrome. *Endocr J* 2011;58(6):425–432.

38. Pan C, Yang W, Barona JP, Wang Y, Niggli M, Mohideen P, et al. Comparison of vildagliptin and acarbose monotherapy in patients with type 2 diabetes: a 24-week, double-blind, randomized trial. *Diabet Med* 2008; 25(4):435–441.

39. Iwamoto Y, Kashiwagi A, Yamada N, Terao S, Mimori N, Suzuki M, et al. Efficacy and safety of vildagliptin and voglibose in Japanese patients with type 2 diabetes: a 12-week, randomized, double-blind, active-controlled study. *Diabetes Obes Metab* 2010;12(8):700–708.

40. Seino Y, Fujita T, Hiroi S, Hirayama M, Kaku K. Efficacy and safety of alogliptin in Japanese patients with type 2 diabetes mellitus: a randomized, double-blind, dose-ranging comparison with placebo, followed by a long-term extension study. *Curr Med Res Opin* 2011;27(9):1781–1792.

41. Iwamoto Y, Tajima N, Kadowaki T, Nonaka K, Taniguchi T, Nishii M, et al. Efficacy and safety of sitagliptin monotherapy compared with voglibose in Japanese patients with type 2 diabetes: a randomized, double-blind trial. *Diabetes Obes Metab* 2010;12(7):613–622.

42. Kawamori R, Inagaki N, Araki E, Watada H, Hayashi N, Horie Y, et al. Linagliptin monotherapy provides superior glycaemic control versus placebo or voglibose with comparable safety in Japanese patients with type 2 diabetes: a randomized, placebo and active comparator-controlled, double-blind study. *Diabetes Obes Metab* 2012;14(4):348–357.

43. Hsieh SH, Shih KC, Chou CW, Chu CH. Evaluation of the efficacy and tolerability of miglitol in Chinese patients with type 2 diabetes mellitus inadequately controlled by diet and sulfonylureas. *Acta Diabetol* 2011;48(1):71–77.

44. Willms B, Ruge D. Comparison of acarbose and metformin in patients with type 2 diabetes mellitus insufficiently controlled with diet and sulphonylureas: a randomized, placebo-controlled study. *Diabet Med* 1999;16(9):755–761.

45. Calle-Pascual AL, Garcia-Honduvilla J, Martin-Alvarez PJ, Vara E, Calle JR, Munguira ME, et al. Comparison between acarbose, metformin, and insulin treatment in type 2 diabetic patients with secondary failure to sulfonylurea treatment. *Diabet Med* 1995;21(4):256–260.

46. Bayraktar M, Van Thiel DH, Adalar N. A comparison of acarbose versus metformin as an adjuvant therapy in sulfonylurea-treated NIDDM patients. *Diabetes Care* 1996;19(3):252–254.

47. May C. Efficacy and tolerability of stepwise increasing dosage of acarbose in patients with non-insulin-dependent diabetes mellitus (NIDDM), treated with sulfonylureas. [German] Wirksamkeit Und Vertraglichkeit Von Einschleichend Dosierter Acarbose Bei Patienten Mit Nichtinsulinpflichtigem Diabetes Mellitus (Typ-II-Diabetes) Unter Sulfonylharnstofftherapie. *Diabetes und Stoffwechsel* 1995;4(1):3–8.

48. Wang JS, Lin SD, Lee WJ, Su SL, Lee IT, Tu ST, et al. Effects of acarbose versus glibenclamide on glycemic excursion and oxidative stress in type 2 diabetic patients inadequately controlled by metformin: a 24-week, randomized, open-label, parallel-group comparison. *Clin Ther* 2011;33(12):1932–1942.

49. Rosenstock J, Brown A, Fischer J, Jain A, Littlejohn T, Nadeau D, et al. Efficacy and safety of acarbose in metformin-treated patients with type 2 diabetes. *Diabetes Care* 1998;21(12):2050–2055.

50. Phillips P, Karrasch J, Scott R, Wilson D, Moses R. Acarbose improves glycemic control in overweight type 2 diabetic patients insufficiently treated with metformin. *Diabetes Care* 2003;26(2):269–273.

51. Halimi S, Le Berre MA, Grange V. Efficacy and safety of acarbose add-on therapy in the treatment of overweight patients with type 2 diabetes inadequately controlled with metformin: a double-blind, placebo-controlled study. *Diabetes Res Clin Prac* 2000;50(1):49–56.

52. Derosa G, Salvadeo SA, D'Angelo A, Ferrari I, Mereu R, Palumbo I, et al. Metabolic effect of repaglinide or acarbose when added to a double oral antidiabetic treatment with sulphonylureas and metformin: a double-blind, cross-over, clinical trial. *Curr Med Res Opin* 2009;25(3):607–615.

53. Lam KS, Tiu SC, Tsang MW, Ip TP, Tam SC. Acarbose in NIDDM patients with poor control on conventional oral agents. A 24-week placebo-controlled study. *Diabetes Care* 1998;21(7):1154–1158.

54. Soonthornpun S, Rattarasarn C, Thamprasit A, Leetanaporn K. Effect of acarbose in treatment of type II diabetes mellitus: a double-blind, crossover, placebo-controlled trial. *J Med Assoc Thailand* 1998;81(3):195–200.

55. Kaye TB. Triple oral antidiabetic therapy. *J Diabetes Comp* 1998;12(6):311–313.

56. Lopez-Alvarenga JC, Aguilar-Salinas CA, Velasco-Perez ML, Arita-Melzer O, Guillen LE, Wong B, et al. Acarbose vs. bedtime NPH insulin in the treatment of secondary failures to sulphonylurea-metformin therapy in type 2 diabetes mellitus. *Diabetes Obes Metab* 1999;1(1):29–35.

57. Yilmaz H, Gursoy A, Sahin M, Guvener Demirag N. Comparison of insulin monotherapy and combination therapy with insulin and metformin or insulin and rosiglitazone or insulin and acarbose in type 2 diabetes. *Acta Diabetol* 2007;44(4):187–192.

58. Nemoto M, Tajima N, Kawamori R. Efficacy of combined use of miglitol in type 2 diabetes patients receiving insulin therapy: placebo-controlled double-blind comparative study. *Acta Diabetol* 2011;48(1):15–20.

59. Standl E, Baumgartl HJ, Fuchtenbusch M, Stemplinger J. Effect of acarbose on additional insulin therapy in type 2 diabetic patients with late failure of sulphonylurea therapy. *Diabetes Obes Metab* 1999;1(4):215–220.

60. Guvener N, Gedik O. Effects of combination of insulin and acarbose compared with insulin and gliclazide in type 2 diabetic patients. *Acta Diabetol* 1999;36(1–2):93–97.

61. Schnell O, Mertes G, Standl E. Acarbose and metabolic control in patients with type 2 diabetes with newly initiated insulin therapy. *Diabetes Obes Metab* 2007;9(6):853–858.

62. Gerard J, Luyckx AS, Lefebvre PJ. Improvement of metabolic control in insulin dependent diabetics treated with the alpha-glucosidase inhibitor acarbose for two months. *Diabetologia* 1981;21(5):446–451.

63. Marena S, Tagliaferro V, Cavallero G, Pagani A, Montegrosso G, Bianchi W, et al. Double-blind crossover study of acarbose in type 1 diabetic patients. *Diabet Med* 1991;8(7):674–678.

64. Sels JP, Verdonk HE, Wolffenbuttel BH. Effects of acarbose (Glucobay) in persons with type 1 diabetes: a multicentre study. *Diabetes Res Clin Prac* 1998;41(2):139–145.

65. Riccardi G, Giacco R, Parillo M, Turco S, Rivellese AA, Ventura MR, et al. Efficacy and safety of acarbose in the treatment of type 1 diabetes mellitus: a placebo-controlled, double-blind, multicentre study. *Diabet Med* 1999;16(3):228–232.

66. Hollander P, Pi-Sunyer X, Coniff RF. Acarbose in the treatment of type I diabetes. *Diabetes Care* 1997;20(3):248–253.

67. Escobar-Jimenez F, de Leiva A, Pinon F, Soler J, Tebar J, Sancho MA, et al. [Clinical effectiveness and tolerance of acarbose in the treatment of insulin-dependent diabetic patients (type I)]. *Med Clin* 1993;100(13):488–491.

68. Viviani GL, Camogliano L, Borgoglio MG. Acarbose treatment in insulin-dependent diabetics. A double-blind crossover study. *Curr Ther Res Clin E* 1987;42(1):1–11.

69. Austenat E. Recent therapy studies with acarbose in type I diabetics. *Endokrinologie und Stoffwechsel* 1991;12:19–24.

70. Dimitriadis G, Hatziagellaki E, Alexopoulos E, Kordonouri O, Komesidou V, Ganotakis M, et al. Effects of alpha-glucosidase inhibition on meal glucose tolerance and timing of insulin administration in patients with type I diabetes mellitus. *Diabetes Care* 1991;14(5):393–398.

71. Juntti-Berggren L, Pigon J, Hellstrom P, Holst JJ, Efendic S. Influence of acarbose on post-prandial insulin requirements in patients with type 1 diabetes. *Diabetes Nutr Metab* 2000;13(1):7–12.

72. Lecavalier L, Hamet P, Chiasson JL. The effects of sucrose meal on insulin requirement in IDDM and its modulation by acarbose. *Diabet Med* 1986;12(3):156–161.

73. Rabasa-Lhoret R, Burelle Y, Ducros F, Bourque J, Lavoie C, Massicotte D, et al. Use of an alpha-glucosidase inhibitor to maintain glucose homoeostasis during postprandial exercise in intensively treated type 1 diabetic subjects. *Diabet Med* 2001;18(9):739–744.

74. McCulloch DK, Kurtz AB, Tattersall RB. A new approach to the treatment of nocturnal hypoglycemia using alpha-glucosidase inhibition. *Diabetes Care* 1983;6(5):483–487.

75. Nagai E, Katsuno T, Miyagawa J, Konishi K, Miuchi M, Ochi F, et al. Effects of miglitol in combination with intensive insulin therapy on blood glucose control with special reference to incretin responses in type 1 diabetes mellitus. *Endocr J* 2011;58(10):869–877.

76. Jandrain B, Pirnay F, Scheen A, Lacroix M, Mosora F, Lefèbvre PJ. Comparative metabolic availability of glucose and sucrose and the effect of acarbose on sucrose utilization during exercise in type I diabetic patients. In *Acarbose for the Treatment of Diabetes Mellitus.* Creutzfeldt W, Ed. Berlin, Springer, 1988, p. 180–181.

77. Chiasson JL, Josse RG, Gomis R, Hanefeld M, Karasik A, Laakso M. Acarbose for prevention of type 2 diabetes mellitus: the STOP-NIDDM randomised trial. *Lancet* 2002;359(9323):2072–2077.

78. Hanefeld M, Karasik A, Koehler C, Westermeier T, Chiasson JL. Metabolic syndrome and its single traits as risk factors for diabetes in people with impaired glucose tolerance: the STOP-NIDDM trial. *Diabetes Vasc Dis Res* 2009;6(1):32–37.

79. Kawamori R, Tajima N, Iwamoto Y, Kashiwagi A, Shimamoto K, Kaku K. Voglibose for prevention of type 2 diabetes mellitus: a randomised, double-blind trial in Japanese individuals with impaired glucose tolerance. *Lancet* 2009;373(9675):1607–1614.

80. Ogawa S, Takeuchi K, Ito S. Acarbose lowers serum triglyceride and postprandial chylomicron levels in type 2 diabetes. *Diabetes Obes Metab* 2004;6(5):384–390.

81. Kado S, Murakami T, Aoki A, Nagase T, Katsura Y, Noritake M, et al. Effect of acarbose on postprandial lipid metabolism in type 2 diabetes mellitus. *Diabetes Res Clin Prac* 1998;41(1):49–55.

82. Oyama T, Saiki A, Endoh K, Ban N, Nagayama D, Ohhira M, et al. Effect of acarbose, an alpha-glucosidase inhibitor, on serum lipoprotein lipase mass

levels and common carotid artery intima-media thickness in type 2 diabetes mellitus treated by sulfonylurea. *J Atheroscler Thromb* 2008;15(3):154–159.

83. Koyasu M, Ishii H, Watarai M, Takemoto K, Inden Y, Takeshita K, et al. Impact of acarbose on carotid intima-media thickness in patients with newly diagnosed impaired glucose tolerance or mild type 2 diabetes mellitus: a one-year, prospective, randomized, open-label, parallel-group study in Japanese adults with established coronary artery disease. *Clin Ther* 2010;32(9):1610–1617.

84. Mughal MA, Memon MY, Zardari MK, Tanwani RK, Ali M. Effect of acarbose on glycemic control, serum lipids and lipoproteins in type 2 diabetes. *J Pakistan Med Assoc* 2000;50(5):152–156.

85. Yamasaki Y, Katakami N, Hayaishi-Okano R, Matsuhisa M, Kajimoto Y, Kosugi K, et al. Alpha-glucosidase inhibitor reduces the progression of carotid intima-media thickness. *Diabetes Res Clin Prac* 2005;67(3):204–210.

86. Meneilly GS, Ryan EA, Radziuk J, Lau DC, Yale JF, Morais J, et al. Effect of acarbose on insulin sensitivity in elderly patients with diabetes. *Diabetes Care* 2000;23(8):1162–1167.

87. Chiasson JL, Josse RG, Leiter LA, Mihic M, Nathan DM, Palmason C, et al. The effect of acarbose on insulin sensitivity in subjects with impaired glucose tolerance. *Diabetes Care* 1996;19(11):1190–1193.

88. Shinozaki K, Suzuki M, Ikebuchi M, Hirose J, Hara Y, Harano Y. Improvement of insulin sensitivity and dyslipidemia with a new alpha-glucosidase inhibitor, voglibose, in nondiabetic hyperinsulinemic subjects. *Metab Clin Exp* 1996;45(6):731–737.

89. Laube H, Linn T, Heyen P. The effect of acarbose on insulin sensitivity and proinsulin in overweight subjects with impaired glucose tolerance. *Exp Clin Endocrinol Diabetes* 1998;106(3):231–233.

90. Delgado H, Lehmann T, Bobbioni-Harsch E, Ybarra J, Golay A. Acarbose improves indirectly both insulin resistance and secretion in obese type 2 diabetic patients. *Diabetes Metab* 2002;28(3):195–200.

91. Reaven GM, Lardinois CK, Greenfield MS, Schwartz HC, Vreman HJ. Effect of acarbose on carbohydrate and lipid metabolism in NIDDM patients poorly controlled by sulfonylureas. *Diabetes Care* 1990;13 (Suppl 3):32–36.

92. Jenney A, Proietto J, O'Dea K, Nankervis A, Traianedes K, D'Embden H. Low-dose acarbose improves glycemic control in NIDDM patients without changes in insulin sensitivity. *Diabetes Care* 1993;16(2):499–502.

93. Johnson AB, Taylor R. Does suppression of postprandial blood glucose excursions by the alpha-glucosidase inhibitor miglitol improve insulin sensitivity in diet-treated type II diabetic patients? *Diabetes Care* 1996;19(6):559–563.

94. Hanefeld M, Cagatay M, Petrowitsch T, Neuser D, Petzinna D, Rupp M. Acarbose reduces the risk for myocardial infarction in type 2 diabetic patients: meta-analysis of seven long-term studies. *Eur Heart J* 2004;25(1):10–16.

95. Chiasson JL, Josse RG, Gomis R, Hanefeld M, Karasik A, Laakso M. Acarbose treatment and the risk of cardiovascular disease and hypertension in patients with impaired glucose tolerance: the STOP-NIDDM trial. *JAMA* 2003;290(4):486–494.

96. Coniff RF, Shapiro JA, Seaton TB. Long-term efficacy and safety of acarbose in the treatment of obese subjects with non-insulin-dependent diabetes mellitus. *Arch Intern Med* 1994;154(21):2442–2448.

97. Wolever TM, Chiasson JL, Josse RG, Hunt JA, Palmason C, Rodger NW, et al. Small weight loss on long-term acarbose therapy with no change in dietary pattern or nutrient intake of individuals with non-insulin-dependent diabetes. *Inter J Obes Relat Metab Disord* 1997;21(9):756–763.

98. Lindstrom J, Tuomilehto J, Spengler M. Acarbose treatment does not change the habitual diet of patients with type 2 diabetes mellitus. The Finnish Acarbos Study Group. *Diabet Med* 2000;17(1):20–25.

99. Santeusanio F, Compagnucci P. A risk-benefit appraisal of acarbose in the management of non-insulin-dependent diabetes mellitus. *Drug Saf* 1994;11(6):432–444.

100. O'Leary DH, Polak JF, Kronmal RA, Manolio TA, Burke GL, Wolfson SK Jr. Carotid-artery intima and media thickness as a risk factor for myocardial infarction and stroke in older adults. Cardiovascular Health Study Collaborative Research Group. *N Engl J Med* 1999;340(1):14–22.

101. Bots ML, Hoes AW, Koudstaal PJ, Hofman A, Grobbee DE. Common carotid intima-media thickness and risk of stroke and myocardial infarction: the Rotterdam Study. *Circulation* 1997;96(5):1432–1437.

102. Lorenz MW, Markus HS, Bots ML, Rosvall M, Sitzer M. Prediction of clinical cardiovascular events with carotid intima-media thickness: a systematic review and meta-analysis. *Circulation* 2007;115(4):459–467.

103. Hanefeld M, Koehler C, Schaper F, Fuecker K, Henkel E, Temelkova-Kurktschiev T. Postprandial plasma glucose is an independent risk factor for increased carotid intima-media thickness in non-diabetic individuals. *Atherosclerosis* 1999;144(1):229–235.

104. Bonora E, Kiechl S, Oberhollenzer F, Egger G, Bonadonna RC, Muggeo M, et al. Impaired glucose tolerance, type II diabetes mellitus and carotid atherosclerosis: prospective results from the Bruneck Study. *Diabetologia* 2000;43(2):156–164.

105. Hanefeld M, Chiasson JL, Koehler C, Henkel E, Schaper F, Temelkova-Kurktschiev T. Acarbose slows progression of intima-media thickness of the

carotid arteries in subjects with impaired glucose tolerance. *Stroke* 2004;35(5):1073–1078.

106. Nakamura T, Matsuda T, Kawagoe Y, Ogawa H, Takahashi Y, Sekizuka K, et al. Effect of pioglitazone on carotid intima-media thickness and arterial stiffness in type 2 diabetic nephropathy patients. *Metab: Clin Exp* 2004; 53(10):1382–1386.

107. Jansen RW, Lipsitz LA. Postprandial hypotension: epidemiology, pathophysiology, and clinical management. *Ann Intern Med* 1995;122(4):286–295.

108. Puisieux F, Bulckaen H, Fauchais AL, Drumez S, Salomez-Granier F, Dewailly P. Ambulatory blood pressure monitoring and postprandial hypotension in elderly persons with falls or syncopes. *J Gerontol A Biol Sci Med Sci* 2000;55(9):M535–540.

109. Yamamoto N, Sasaki E, Arishima T, Ito M, Tanaka H, Terasaki J, et al. Combination therapy for postprandial and orthostatic hypotension in an elderly patient with type 2 diabetes mellitus. *J Am Geriatr Soc* 2006;54(4):727–728.

110. Sasaki E, Goda K, Nagata K, Kitaoka H, Ohsawa N, Hanafusa T. Acarbose improved severe postprandial hypotension in a patient with diabetes mellitus. *J Diabetes Comp* 2001;15(3):158–161.

111. Maule S, Tredici M, Dematteis A, Matteoda C, Chiandussi L. Postprandial hypotension treated with acarbose in a patient with type 1 diabetes mellitus. *Clin Auton Res* 2004;14(6):405–407.

112. Krentz AJ, Ferner RE, Bailey CJ. Comparative tolerability profiles of oral antidiabetic agents. *Drug Saf* 1994;11(4):223–241.

113. Deutschmann R, Moser M, Mertes G, Eds. Favourable quality of life for acarbose-treated patients with type II diabetes when compared with other treatments. *Diabetes* 1997;46(Suppl 1):292A.

114. Hayakawa T, Yoneshima M, Abe T, Nomura G. Pneumatosis cystoides intestinalis after treatment with an alpha-glucosidase inhibitor. *Diabetes Care* 1999;22(2):366–367.

115. Azami Y. Paralytic ileus accompanied by pneumatosis cystoides intestinalis after acarbose treatment in an elderly diabetic patient with a history of heavy intake of maltitol. *Internal Med* 2000;39(10):826–829.

116. Maeda A, Yokoi S, Kunou T, Murata T. [A case of pneumatosis cystoides intestinalis assumed to be induced by acarbose administration for diabetes mellitus and pemphigus vulgaris]. *Nihon Shokakibyo Gakkai zasshi* 2002;99(11):1345–1349.

117. Yanaru R, Hizawa K, Nakamura S, Yoshimura R, Watanabe K, Nakamura U, et al. Regression of pneumatosis cystoides intestinalis after discontinuing of alpha-glucosidase inhibitor administration. *J Clin Gastroenterol* 2002;35(2):204–205.

118. Hisamoto A, Mizushima T, Sato K, Haruta Y, Tanimoto Y, Tanimoto M, et al. Pneumatosis cystoides intestinalis after alpha-glucosidase inhibitor treatment in a patient with interstitial pneumonitis. *Intern Med* 2006;45(2):73–76.

119. Furio L, Vergura M, Russo A, Bisceglia N, Talarico S, Gatta R, et al. Pneumatosis coli induced by acarbose administration for diabetes mellitus. Case report and literature review. *Minerva Gastroenterologica e Dietologica* 2006;52(3):339–346.

120. Maeda Y, Inaba N, Aoyagi M, Kanda E, Shiigai T. Fulminant pneumatosis intestinalis in a patient with diabetes mellitus and minimal change nephrotic syndrome. *Intern Med* 2007;46(1):41–44.

121. Saito M, Tanikawa A, Nakasute K, Tanaka M, Nishikawa T. Additive contribution of multiple factors in the development of pneumatosis intestinalis: a case report and review of the literature. *Clin Rheumatol* 2007;26(4):601–603.

122. Tsujimoto T, Shioyama E, Moriya K, Kawaratani H, Shirai Y, Toyohara M, et al. Pneumatosis cystoides intestinalis following alpha-glucosidase inhibitor treatment: a case report and review of the literature. *World J Gastroenterol* 2008;14(39):6087–6092.

123. Vogel Y, Buchner NJ, Szpakowski M, Tannapfel A, Henning BF. Pneumatosis cystoides intestinalis of the ascending colon related to acarbose treatment: a case report. *J Med Case Reports* 2009;3:9216.

124. Kojima K, Tsujimoto T, Fujii H, Morimoto T, Yoshioka S, Kato S, et al. Pneumatosis cystoides intestinalis induced by the alpha-glucosidase inhibitor miglitol. *Intern Med* 2010;49(15):1545–1548.

125. Wu SS, Yen HH. Images in clinical medicine. Pneumatosis cystoides intestinalis. *N Engl J Med* 2011;365(8):e16.

126. Shimojima Y, Ishii W, Matsuda M, Tojo K, Watanabe R, Ikeda S. Pneumatosis cystoides intestinalis in neuropsychiatric systemic lupus erythematosus with diabetes mellitus: case report and literature review. *Mod Rheumatol* 2011;21(4):415–419.

127. Miyagawa M, Kanemasa H, Nakagawa S, Nitan T, Matsumoto M, Tokita K, et al. A case of pneumatosis cystoides intestinalis after treatment with an alpha-glucosidase inhibitor. [Japanese]. *Gastroenterol Endosc* 2006;48(3):329–333.

128. Tachibana Y, Band H, Asai J, Notsumata K, Toya D, Tanaka N, et al. A case of pneumatosis cystoides intestinalis with abdominal free air. *Nihon Arukoru Yakubutsu Igakkai Zasshi* 2002;22:1103–1106.

129. Matsuda Y, Yoshida H, Sugimoto H, Tanaka K. A case of pneumatosis cystoides intestinalis with intraperitoneal free air in palliative care. *J Jpn Surg Assoc* 2004;65:3288–3292.

130. Yasuoka R, Sonoyama Y, Fujiki H, Morita S, Mitsuo M, Kadotani Y. A case of intestinal emphysema with pneumoperitoneum in which a-glucosidase inhibitor participated. *J Jpn Surg Assoc* 2007;68(8):2014–2018.

131. Nagahara Y, Hakoda T, Imada T, Kurose H, Okuno T, Yoshida T. Pneumatosis cystoides intestinalis after treatment with an alpha-glucosidase inhibitor. *Diabetes J* 2006;34:104–107.

132. Andrade RJ, Lucena MI, Rodriguez-Mendizabal M. Hepatic injury caused by acarbose. *Ann Intern Med* 1996;124(10):931.

133. Carrascosa M, Pascual F, Aresti S. Acarbose-induced acute severe hepatotoxicity. *Lancet* 1997;349(9053):698–699.

134. Magner J, Amatruda J. Alpha-glucosidase inhibitors in the treatment of diabetes. In *Diabetes Mellitus: A Fundamental and Clinical Text*. Philadelphia, Lippincott Williams & Wilkins, 2000, p. 797–803.

135. Gentile S, Turco S, Guarino G, Sasso FC, Torella R. Aminotransferase activity and acarbose treatment in patients with type 2 diabetes. *Diabetes Care* 1999;22(7):1217–1218.

136. Gentile S, Turco S, Guarino G, Oliviero B, Annunziata S, Cozzolino D, et al. Effect of treatment with acarbose and insulin in patients with non-insulin-dependent diabetes mellitus associated with non-alcoholic liver cirrhosis. *Diabetes Obes Metab* 2001;3(1):33–40.

137. Gentile S, Guarino G, Romano M, Alagia IA, Fierro M, Annunziata S, et al. A randomized controlled trial of acarbose in hepatic encephalopathy. *Clin Gastroenterol Hepatol* 2005;3(2):184–191.

Chapter 27

[handwritten: Work in the brain — can't use for T1D or ketoacidosis]

Cycloset: A Sympatholytic, D2-Dopamine Agonist for the Treatment of Type 2 Diabetes

Ralph A. DeFronzo, MD

[handwritten: pramipexole (Mirapex) ropinirole (Requip)]

INTRODUCTION

[handwritten: Parlodel]

Bromocriptine is a sympatholytic D2-dopamine agonist approved for the treatment of type 2 diabetes (T2D). A recent review has examined its efficacy and safety in the treatment of patients with T2D.[1] On the basis of animal and human studies, timed bromocriptine administration within 2 hours of awakening is believed to augment low hypothalamic dopamine levels. It also inhibits excessive sympathetic tone within the central nervous system (CNS), resulting in a reduction in postmeal plasma glucose levels due to enhanced suppression of hepatic glucose production (Figure 27.1).

PHARMACOKINETICS

Cycloset (bromocriptine mesylate) tablets are rapidly absorbed within 30 minutes[2] and reach the maximum plasma concentration in 60 minutes. Absorption is delayed by food. There is extensive hepatic first-pass extraction and metabolism, and only 5–10% of the ingested dose reaches the systemic circulation.[3,4] Ninety-eight percent of ingested bromocriptine is excreted via the biliary route with an elimination half-life of ~6 hours. Within the liver, bromocriptine is extensively metabolized by the cytochrome P450 system, specifically CYP3A4. Cycloset differs from traditional bromocriptine formulations, such as Parlodel, in its quick release that provides peak concentrations within 60 minutes. There is no AB-rated equivalent for Cycloset.

DOSING

Cycloset comes as 0.8 mg tablets. The starting dose is 0.8 mg/day and can be titrated to a maximum of 4.8 mg/day. Cycloset is administered as a once daily dose within 2 hours of awakening. Individuals with T2D are believed to have an early morning dip in dopaminergic tone, which leads to increased sympathetic activity.[5] Circadian plasma prolactin levels closely parallel changes in hypothalamic dopamine levels and insulin sensitivity.[6,7] In lean, normal glucose-tolerant, insulin-sensitive humans, plasma prolactin concentrations peak at night during sleep. In contrast, obese insulin-resistant individuals have elevated (twofold) daytime plasma prolactin levels,[2] consistent with reduced dopaminergic tone.[8] Administration of Cycloset within 2 hours of awakening reduces the elevated prolactin levels[2,9,10] and is thought to restore dopaminergic activity, thereby reducing postprandial plasma

DOI: 10.2337/9781580405096.27

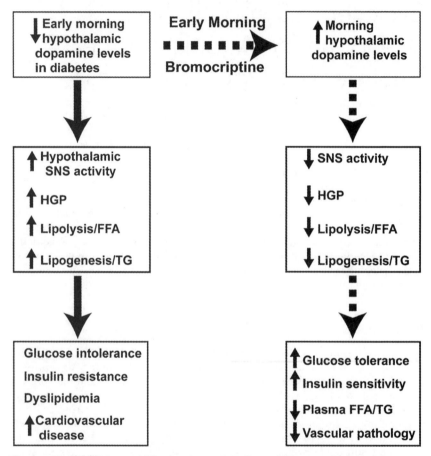

Figure 27.1 — Proposed Mechanism of Action of Bromocriptine to Improve Glucose Homeostasis and Insulin Sensitivity

Note: HGP = hepatic glucose production; TG = triglyceride; FFA = free fatty acids.

glucose, triglyceride, and free-fatty-acid (FFA) concentrations without increasing plasma insulin levels (see discussion in the section Mechanism of Action).

MECHANISM OF ACTION

The mechanism of action of Cycloset remains unknown. In nondiabetic obese hyperinsulinemic subjects,[10] bromocriptine reduced fasting and postprandial (standardized meals) glucose levels without change in body weight and with a decrease in fasting and postprandial plasma insulin concentrations without change in muscle insulin sensitivity. In an 8-week study, timed bromocriptine reduced day-long plasma glucose, triglyceride, and FFA levels without a change in body weight and a decrease in plasma insulin concentration in nondiabetic obese women.[11] Insulin-stimulated glucose disposal, measured with the insulin suppression test, was not altered. Because the insulin suppression test primarily reflects insulin-mediated glucose disposal in muscle, the improvement in postprandial plasma glucose levels[11] most likely reflects enhanced suppression of hepatic glucose production by insulin, similar to what has been described in animals.[12] No study, however, has examined hepatic glucose production following glucose ingestion or in response to a physiologic increase in plasma insulin concentration in humans.

In a 16-week double-blind, placebo-controlled study in 22 obese subjects with T2D, Cycloset reduced A1C by 1.2%, fasting plasma glucose by 54 mg/dl, and mean plasma glucose during oral glucose tolerance test by 46 mg/dl without change in plasma insulin concentration or body weight.[13] During a two-step euglycemic-hyperinsulinemic clamp, there was no improvement in insulin sensitivity during the first, physiologic insulin clamp step (plasma insulin concentration ~80 μU/ml).[13] These results are consistent with the insulin suppression test[11] and demonstrate that within the physiologic range of hyperinsulinemia, Cycloset does not improve insulin action in muscle.

In a 12-week study[14] in insulin-treated subjects with T2D, Cycloset reduced A1C by 0.7% and mean plasma glucose concentration (7 A.M. to 7 P.M.) by 8% without change in body weight. These results are consistent with an improvement in insulin sensitivity, although the site (i.e., liver versus muscle) remains to be defined.

PHASE 3 EFFICACY TRIALS

Four phase 3 trials have evaluated the efficacy of Cycloset versus placebo in the treatment of patients with T2D.[2,15,16] The four trials included a 24-week monotherapy trial ($n = 159$)[2]; two 24-week add-on to sulfonylurea trials ($n = 494$)[2]; and a 52-week add-on to various oral antidiabetic agents trial (see Table 27.1).[16] Results of these four studies consistently demonstrated a placebo-subtracted

Table 27.1 Phase 3 Cycloset Efficacy Trials

	N	Duration (months)	Baseline A1C (%)	Placebo-subtracted change in A1C (%)	P value
Monotherapy	159	6	8.7	−0.56	<0.02
Add-on to SU	494	6	9.4	−0.55	<0.0001
Add-on to various OHAs	3,095	12	8.3	−0.6 to −0.9	<0.01–0.001

Note: SU = sulfonylurea; OHA = oral hypoglycemic agent.

decline in A1C of 0.5–0.7%. Subjects with T2D in the monotherapy and add-on to sulfonylurea studies[2] were admitted to the clinical research center (CRC) for 12 hours (7 A.M. to 7 P.M.) and received standardized meals for breakfast, lunch, and dinner (5 P.M.). Relative to placebo, Cycloset significantly reduced fasting, post-breakfast, postlunch, and postdinner glucose, FFA, and triglyceride concentrations without change in serum insulin level or body weight.

In the monotherapy and add-on to sulfonylurea studies, a prespecified analysis was performed on Cycloset responders (minimum A1C decrease from baseline = 0.3% at week 8) versus the entire Cycloset-treated group (Figure 27.2). In the mono-therapy and add-on to sulfonylurea trials, the decrements in A1C from baseline were –0.65 and –0.63, respectively, and responders represented 63 and 65% of the total Cycloset-treated group.[2] The placebo-subtracted difference in A1C in responders was 1% in both monotherapy and add-on to sulfonylurea trials (Figure 27.2).

In a large 52-week randomized, double-blind, placebo-controlled trial, Cyclo-set was added to therapy in patients with poorly controlled (A1C >8.3%) T2D who were taking one to two oral hypoglycemic agents (OHAs).[14–16] The placebo-subtracted decrease in A1C ranged from 0.6 to 0.9% and was consistent in sub-jects failing any OHA, failing metformin ± OHA, failing metformin + sulfonylurea, and failing thiazolidinedione ± OHA (Figure 27.3).[16–18]

SAFETY AND TOLERABILITY

In the Cycloset monotherapy and add-on to sulfonylurea trials,[2] side effects that occurred more commonly in Cycloset versus placebo were nausea (32 vs. 8%), asthenia (12 vs. 6%), constipation (11 vs. 4%), dizziness (12 vs. 8%), head-ache (13 vs. 9%), somnolence (4.3 vs. 1.3%), and rhinitis (13 vs. 4%). In general, these side effects were mild and transient. In the pooled Cycloset phase 3 trials, adverse events leading to discontinuation occurred in 24% of Cycloset-treated subjects compared with 9% of placebo-treated subjects. This difference was driven by gastrointestinal events, primarily nausea. There was no increase in serious adverse events in the Cycloset group compared with the placebo group. There was no difference in the incidence of hypoglycemia between the Cycloset and pla-cebo-treated groups in any trial.

ALL-CAUSE SAFETY TRIAL

A large ($n = 3,070$) 52-week, randomized, placebo-controlled,[1,2] double-blind trial evaluated overall and cardiovascular safety of Cycloset in patients with T2D treated with diet alone, one to two OHAs, or insulin alone or with one OHA.[16] There were 8.6% serious adverse events in the Cycloset group versus 9.6% in the placebo group (hazard ratio [HR] 0.89, P = NS). Thirty-two diabetic patients (3.2%) in the Cycloset group versus 37 patients (1.8%) in the placebo group experienced a prespecified cardiovascular event (myocardial infarction, stroke, hospitalization for angina, hospitalization for congestive heart failure [CHF], coronary revasculariza-tion, and death) (HR 0.60, two-sided 95% confidence internal [CI] 0.37–0.96, P = 0.036) (Figure 27.3). Using the major adverse cardiac events endpoint (myocardial infarction, stroke, and death), the HR was reduced in Cycloset versus placebo-treated subjects (HR 0.45, two-sided 95% CI 0.205–0.996, $P < 0.05$) (Figure 27.3).

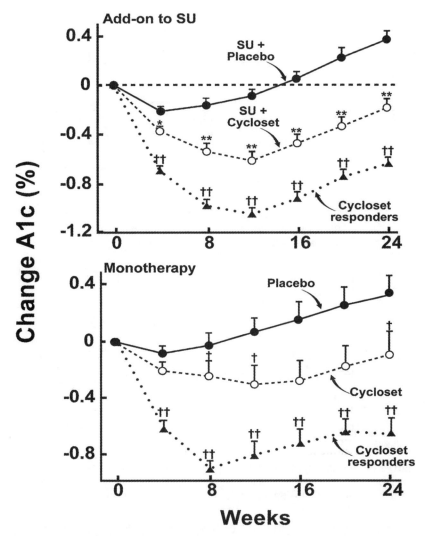

Figure 27.2—Change in A1C in Cycloset-Diabetes Subjects (Total Group) and Placebo-Treated Subjects

Note: Cycloset responders (defined as a ≥0.3% decrease in A1C at week 8) had a significantly greater decline in A1C (placebo-subtracted ΔA1C = 1.0%) than the total group.[1] SU = sulfonylurea. $^*P < 0.01$; $^{**}P < 0.001$; $^\dagger P < 0.04$ for Cycloset responders vs. total Cycloset group; $^{\dagger\dagger}P < 0.0001$ for Cycloset responders vs. placebo.

On the basis of the composite cardiovascular outcome, 79 patients with diabetes needed to be treated for 1 year to avoid one cardiovascular event.

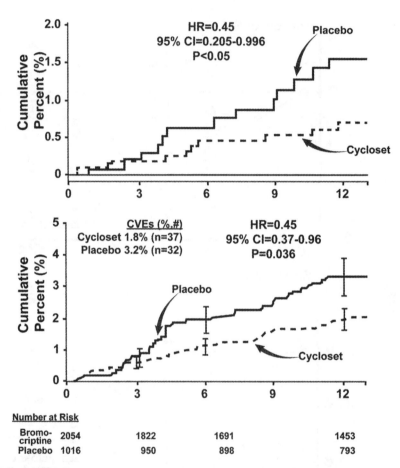

Figure 27.3—Kaplan–Meier Plots in Patients with T2D

Top: Kaplan–Meier plot of time to first cardiovascular event (myocardial infarction, stroke, and death) in subjects with T2D treated with Cycloset or placebo for 52 weeks.[14]

Bottom: Kaplan–Meier plot of time to first cardiovascular event (myocardial infarction, stroke, hospitalization for angina or CHF, coronary revascularization, and death) in 3,070 subjects with T2D treated with Cycloset or placebo for 52 weeks.[15]

Note: CVEs = cardiovascular events.

The mechanisms by which timed bromocriptine reduced cardiovascular events remains undefined. In the cardiovascular safety trial,[16] bromocriptine reduced A1C by 0.6% ($P < 0.0001$), systolic/diastolic blood pressure by 2/1 mmHg ($P < 0.02$), heart rate by 1 beat/minute ($P = 0.02$), and plasma triglyceride by 0.08

mmol/l (P = 0.02). These changes were modest, however, and seem unlikely to explain the 40% decrease in composite cardiovascular outcome. In animal studies, bromocriptine attenuates the effect of CNS sympathetic overactivity on the vasculature,[19,20] and a direct inhibitory effect of bromocriptine on mitogen-stimulated proliferation of rat vascular muscle cells and human aortic smooth muscle cells has been demonstrated in vitro.[21] In the high fat–fed, spontaneously hypertensive rat, bromocriptine reduced pathologically elevated endothelial nitric oxide synthase (eNOS) and inducible NOS (iNOS) levels.[22] At present, it is unclear whether the salutatory effect of bromocriptine to reduce cardiovascular events[16] is related to the drug's beneficial effect on any of these pathologic processes or atherosclerotic risk factors.

WARNINGS

Although uncommon, orthostatic hypotension can occur, particularly upon initiation of Cycloset therapy, and assessment of orthostatic vital signs is recommended before starting therapy. Hallucinations, confusion, and psychiatric disorders have been reported with bromocriptine, but none were observed in the Cycloset trials.

DRUG–DRUG INTERACTIONS

Cycloset is a dopamine receptor agonist and concomitant use with dopamine receptor antagonists (clozapine, olanzapine, ziprasidone) or metoclopramide may reduce its effectiveness. If used in combination with ergot-related drugs, Cycloset may increase the occurrence of ergot-related side effects (nausea, vomiting) or reduce the effectiveness of the ergot therapy when used to treat migraines. Concurrent use of ergot agents within 6 hours of Cycloset dosing is not recommended. Cycloset undergoes extensive hepatic metabolism by CYP3A4, and potent inhibitors or inducers of CYP3A4 may increase or decrease plasma Cycloset levels. Therefore, caution should be used when using Cycloset with such medications (e.g., HIV protease inhibitors, azole antimycotics). Dopamine receptor agonists are indicated for the treatment of Parkinson's disease, hyperprolactinemia, and acromegaly. Since the effectiveness and safety of Cycloset in patients taking such medications is not known, the use of Cycloset is not recommended. Because the active ingredient (bromocriptine mesylate) in Cycloset is highly bound, it may increase the unbound fraction of other highly protein-bound medications (salicylates, sulfonamides, chloramphenicol, probenecid) and alter their effectiveness and risk for side effects.

USE IN PREGNANCY, NURSING MOTHERS, AND PEDIATRIC POPULATION

Because Cycloset has not been studied in pregnant women or in pediatric patients, it is contraindicated in these populations. Bromocriptine inhibits lactation and Cycloset is contraindicated in nursing mothers.

CONCLUSION

Both as monotherapy and in combination with other OHAs, timed bromocriptine (Cycloset) causes a 0.6–0.7% reduction in A1C and reduces plasma triglyceride and FFA concentrations in patients with T2D. In a 52-week safety study, Cycloset decreased the cardiovascular composite endpoint by 40%. Other advantages of Cycloset include the absence of hypoglycemia because insulin secretion is not stimulated, weight neutrality, no need for dose adjustment in patients with moderate renal insufficiency, lack of edema and CHF, and good side-effect profile.

ACKNOWLEDGMENTS

Ralph A. DeFronzo has received grants from Takeda, Bristol-Myers Squibb, Boehringer Ingelheim, and Amylin Pharmaceuticals and has been a board member of and consulted for Takeda, Amylin Pharmaceuticals, Bristol-Myers Squibb, Janssen, Novo Nordisk, Lexicon, and Boehringer Ingelheim. He is a member of the speakers' bureau for Bristol-Myers Squibb, Janssen, and Novo Nordisk. No other potential conflicts of interest relevant to this article were reported.

Lorrie Albarado and Amy Richardson (University of Texas Health Science Center, San Antonio, TX) provided expert secretarial assistance in preparation of the manuscript.

REFERENCES

1. DeFronzo RA. Bromocriptine: a sympathoylytic, D2-dopamine agonist for the treatment of type 2 diabetes. *Diabetes Care* 2011;34:789–794.

2. Cincotta AH, Meier AH, Cincotta M Jr. Bromocriptine improves glycaemic control and serum lipid profile in obese type 2 diabetic subjects: a new approach in the treatment of diabetes. *Expert Opin Investig Drugs* 1999;8:1683–1707.

3. Maurer G, Schreier E, Delaborde S, Loosli HR, Nufer R, Shukla AP. Fate and disposition of bromocriptine in animals and man. I: structure elucidation of the metabolites. *Eur J Drug Metab Pharmacokinet* 1982;7:281–292.

4. Maurer G, Schreier E, Delaborde S, Nufer R, Shukla AP. Fate and disposition of bromocriptine in animals and man. II: Absorption, elimination and metabolism. *Eur J Drug Metab Pharmacokinet* 1983;8:51–62.

5. Luo S, Luo J, Cincotta AH. Chronic ventromedial hypothalamic infusion of norepinephrine and serotonin promotes insulin resistance and glucose intolerance. *Neuroendocrinology* 1999;70:460–465.

6. Cincotta AH. Hypothalamic role in the insulin resistance syndrome. In *Insulin Resistance Syndrome*. Hansen B, Shaffrir E, Eds. London, Taylor and Francis, 2002, p. 271–312.

7. Meier AHCA. Circadian rhythms regulate the expression of the thrifty genotype/phenotype. *Diabetes Reviews* 1996;4:464–487.

8. Wang GJ, Volkow ND, Logan J, et al. Braindopamine and obesity. *Lancet* 2001;357:354–357.

9. Pijl H. Reduced dopaminergic tone in hypothalamic neural circuits: expression of a thrifty genotype underlying the metabolic syndrome? *Eur J Pharmacol* 2003;480:125–131.

10. Cincotta AH, Meier AH. Bromocriptine (Ergoset) reduces body weight and improves glucose tolerance in obese subjects. *Diabetes Care* 1996;19:667–670.

11. Kamath V, Jones CN, Yip JC, et al. Effects of a quick-release form of bromocriptine (Ergoset) on fasting and postprandial plasma glucose, insulin, lipid, and lipoprotein concentrations in obese nondiabetic hyperinsulinemic women. *Diabetes Care* 1997;20:1697–1701.

12. Cincotta AH, Meier AH. Bromocriptine inhibits in vivo free fatty acid oxidation and hepatic glucose output in seasonally obese hamsters (Mesocricetus auratus). *Metabolism* 1995;44:1349–1355.

13. Pijl H, Ohashi S, Matsuda M, Miyazaki Y, Mahankali A, Kumar V, Pipek R, Iozzo P, Lancaster JL, Cincotta AH, DeFronzo RA. Bromocriptine: a novel approach to the treatment of type 2 diabetes. *Diabetes Care* 23:1154-1161, 2000.

14. Schwartz S. Bromocriptine (Ergoset) improves glycemic control in type 2 diabetes on insulin. *Diabetes* 1999;48(Suppl 1):A99.

15. Scranton R, Cincotta A. Bromocriptine unique formulation of adopamine agonist for the treatment of type 2 diabetes. *Expert Opin Pharmacother* 2010;11:269–279.

16. Gaziano JM, Cincotta AH, Connor CM, et al. Randomized clinical trial of quick release bromocriptine among patients with type 2 diabetes on overall safety and cardiovascular outcomes. *Diabetes Care* 2010;33:1503–1508.

17. Scranton REFW, Ezrokhi M, Gaziano JM, Cincotta AH. Quick release bromocriptine (Cycloset TM) improves glycaemic control in patients with diabetes failing metformin/sulfonylurea combination therapy. *Diabetologia* 2008;51:S372–S373.

18. Cincotta AHGJ, Ezrokhi M, Scranton R. Cycloset (Quick-Release Bromocriptine Mesylate), a novel centrally acting treatment for type 2 diabetes (Abstract). *Diabetologia* 2008;51:S22.

19. Franchi F, Lazzeri C, Barletta G, Ianni L, Mannelli M. Centrally mediated effects of bromocriptine on cardiac sympathovagal balance. *Hypertension* 2001;38:123–129.

20. Liang Y, Cincotta AH. Increased responsiveness to the hyperglycemic, hyperglucagonemic and hyperinsulinemic effects of circulating norepinephrine in ob/ob mice. *Int J Obes Relat Metab Disord* 2001;25:698–704.

21. Zhang Y, Cincotta AH. Inhibitory effects of bromocriptine on vascular smooth muscle cell proliferation. *Atherosclerosis* 1997;133:37–44.

22. Ezrokhi MTY, Luo S, Cincotta AH. Timed dopamine agonist treatment ameliorates both vascular nitrosative/oxidative stress pathology and aortic stiffness in arteriosclerotic, hypertensive SHR rats. *Diabetes* 2010;59(Suppl 1):252–OR.

Chapter 28

Sodium-Glucose Cotransporter-2 Inhibitors and Type 2 Diabetes

MUHAMMAD A. ABDUL-GHANI, MD, PhD
LUKE NORTON, PhD
RALPH A. DEFRONZO, MD

INTRODUCTION

Hyperglycemia is the major factor responsible for the development of microvascular complications and plays an important role in the pathogenesis of type 2 diabetes (T2D) by means of glucotoxicity. Effective glycemic control not only reduces the incidence of microvascular complications, but also corrects the metabolic abnormalities that contribute to the progression of the disease. Progressive β-cell failure and side effects, including hypoglycemia and weight gain, associated with many current therapies present obstacles to the achievement of optimal and durable glycemic control in T2D. Inhibitors of the renal sodium-glucose cotransporter 2 (SGLT-2) have been developed to reduce the plasma glucose concentration by inducing glucosuria. Because the mechanism of action is independent of β-cell function and tissue sensitivity to insulin, the SGLT-2 inhibitors improve glycemic control while avoiding hypoglycemia and they promote weight loss. We have written two recent reviews[1,2] on the SGLT-2 inhibitors, and many of the concepts and some of the wording overlap with these prior publications. This chapter reviews the renal handling of glucose and summarizes the available data concerning the mechanism of action, efficacy, and safety of this novel class of antidiabetic agents.

GLUCOSE FILTRATION AND REABSORPTION

With a glomerular filtration rate of 180 liters/day and a mean day-long plasma glucose concentration of ~100 mg/dl, the kidney filters ~180 grams of glucose per day.[1,2] In subjects with normal glucose tolerance, all of the filtered glucose is reabsorbed in the proximal tubule. The maximum glucose transport capacity (Tm) of the proximal tubule is approximately 375 mg/minute. Renal glucose reabsorption occurs in the proximal tubule primarily in the S1 and S3 segments (Figure 28.1) by SGLTs, which couple glucose to sodium reabsorption. The electrochemical gradient generated by active sodium transport provides the energy for glucose transport. SGLT-2 has low affinity–high capacity for glucose transport, mediates glucose transport in the S1 segment, and reabsorbs about 80–90% of filtered glucose. SGLT 1 has high affinity–low capacity for glucose transport, mediates glucose transport in the S3 segment, and reabsorbs the remaining 10–20% of filtered glucose. In normal individuals, the filtered glucose load is <375 mg/minute, and all filtered glucose is reabsorbed and returned to the circulation. If the filtered glucose load exceeds 375 mg/minute, as often occurs in subjects with poorly con-

DOI: 10.2337/9781580405096.28

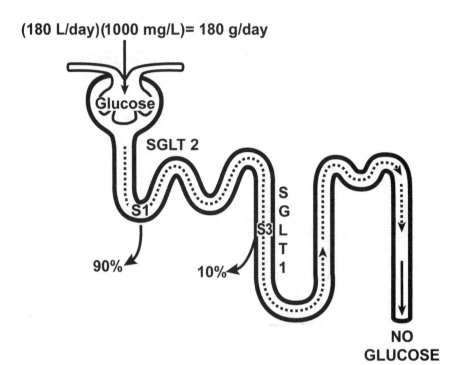

(180 L/day)(1000 mg/L)= 180 g/day

Figure 28.1—Renal handling of glucose.

trolled T2D, the maximum renal tubular reabsorptive capacity is exceeded and all glucose in excess of the Tm is excreted in the urine. The plasma glucose concentration at which the filtered glucose load reaches 375 mg/minute is called the threshold and is ~180 mg/dl in normal glucose-tolerant subjects (Figure 28.2). When the threshold is exceeded, the glucose excretion rate increases linearly and parallels the filtered glucose load. The reabsorption and excretion curves display a nonlinear transition as the Tm for glucose is approached. This "rounding" of the curves is termed splay and has been explained by heterogeneity in the Tm of individual nephrons or glomerulotubular imbalance.[1,2]

In type 1 diabetes (T1D)[3] and T2D,[4,5] the renal Tm and threshold for glucose are paradoxically increased[4,5] (Figure 28.3). The increased glucose reabsorption observed in diabetic patients is explained by an increase in the expression, as well as in the activity of the SGLT-2 transporter, in the proximal tubule.[6] In diabetic patients, it would be desirable for the kidney to excrete the excess filtered glucose load and restore normoglycemia. In contrast, the increased Tm and threshold for glucose minimizes glucosuria and exacerbates the hyperglycemia.

On the basis of these pathophysiologic considerations, it follows that development of specific inhibitors of the renal SGLT-2 transporter provides a rational approach for the treatment of diabetic patients. This approach not only decreases

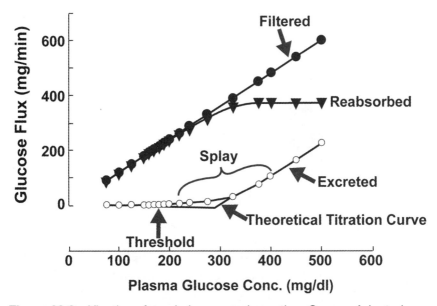

Figure 28.2—Kinetics of renal glucose reabsorption. *Source:* Adapted with permission from Abdul-Ghani MA, Norton L, DeFronzo RA. Role of sodium-glucose cotransporter 2 (SGLT-2) inhibitors in the treatment of type 2 diabetes. *Endocr Rev* 2011;32:515–531.

the plasma glucose concentration but also can be expected to have additional metabolic benefits effects on blood pressure (due to mild negative sodium balance) and weight loss (due to loss of calories in the urine).[1] The specificity of drugs that inhibit SGLT-2 over SGLT-1 (which is present in both the gut and kidney) avoids impaired intestinal glucose absorption and diarrhea. Persistent glucosuria potentially could cause an increase in urinary tract infections. Subjects with familial renal glucosuria, however, are asymptomatic and maintain normal renal function throughout their lives.[7]

PHARMACOLOGICAL INHIBITORS OF RENAL GLUCOSE UPTAKE

Phlorizin, isolated from the bark of apple trees, was the first SGLT inhibitor to be identified.[8] It competitively inhibits both SGLT-1 and SGLT-2 in the proximal tubule, producing glucosuria in normal glucose-tolerant subjects, but it was not developed because of low bioavailability following oral administration and inhibition of SGLT-1 in the gastrointestinal tract. On the basis of the structure of phlorizin, several other compounds with greater bioavailability following oral administration and higher selectivity for SGLT-2 compared with SGLT-1 have been developed and are in varying stages of development for clinical use.[1]

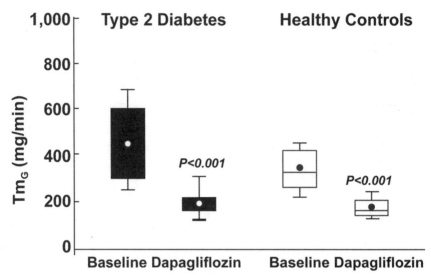

Figure 28.3—Effect of dapagliflozin on the renal maximal reabsorptive capacity for glucose Tm_G in type 2 diabetic and normal glucose-tolerant healthy control subjects. *Source:* DeFronzo RA, Hompesch M, Kasichayanula S, Liu X, Hong Y, Pfister M, Morrow LA, Leslie BR, Bouton DW, Ching A, Lacreta FP, Griffen SC. Characterization of renal glucose reabsorption in response to dapagliflozin in healthy subjects and subjects with type 2 diabetes. *Diabetes Care* 2013;36:3169–3176.

INHIBITION OF RENAL GLUCOSE TRANSPORT CORRECTS HYPERGLYCEMIA: PROOF OF CONCEPT

Studies performed with phlorizin in 90% pancreatectomized diabetic rats have provided proof of concept for the efficacy of SGLT-2 inhibition in the treatment of hyperglycemia. Chronic phlorizin administration induced glucosuria and normalized both the fasting and fed plasma glucose levels in these diabetic rodents.[1] Phlorizin also completely reversed insulin resistance and corrected the defects in both first- and second-phase insulin secretion.[9–11] Recent studies in T2D humans treated with dapagliflozin for only 14 days have demonstrated significant reductions in fasting and postprandial plasma glucose concentration, improved muscle glucose uptake (by 26%), and enhanced β-cell function (by 89%),[12] thus reproducing the findings in diabetic animals.

Familial renal glucosuria, a benign condition, has provided assurance for the safety of pharmacological inhibition of SGLT-2.[7] Affected individuals with loss-of-function mutations in the gene encoding for the SGLT-2 transporter[13] manifest varying degrees of glucosuria (20–200 grams/day). Despite the glucosuria, these subjects are asymptomatic and do not experience hypoglycemia.[7] These observations provide proof of concept that pharmacological inhibition of SGLT-2 is a safe and effective strategy for reducing the plasma glucose concentration in diabetic subjects.[1]

SGLT-2 INHIBITORS IN T2D SUBJECTS

Canagliflozin (Invokana)

Canagliflozin is the first SGLT-2 inhibitor approved for the treatment of T2D in the U.S.[14] In humans, the half-life is ~16 hours, making it suitable for once-daily administration.[15] Canagliflozin is absorbed rapidly after oral administration, achieving maximal plasma concentration within 2 hours. Canagliflozin is highly protein bound (~99%) and renal excretion is low (~1%).[15] An inert glucuronoside conjugate is the major metabolite. Although canagliflozin possesses some inhibitory action on SGLT-1, this effect is of little clinical significance with respect to further augmenting renal glucose excretion or inhibiting glucose absorption by the gastrointestinal tract.

Dosing. The starting dose of canagliflozin is 100 mg/day, given before breakfast.[14] If additional glycemic control is required, the dose can be increased to 300 mg/day. The time interval for titrating from 100 to 300 mg/day is up to the discretion of the physician. In patients with an estimated glomerular filtration rate (eGFR) <60 ml/minute, the efficacy decreases,[16] and there is an increased incidence of volume/osmotic-related side effects.[14] Therefore, the dose is restricted to 100 mg/day in patients with an eGFR 45–60 ml/minute. Canagliflozin should not be used in patients with an eGFR <45 ml/minute because of lack of efficacy.[14] If after instituting therapy the eGFR declines to <45 ml/minute on two consecutive determinations, it is recommended that the drug be discontinued.

Glycemic Efficacy. Canagliflozin is approved: (1) for use in patients with T2D treated with diet and exercise; (2) as add-on therapy in diabetic patients treated with monotherapy, including metformin, sulfonylureas, pioglitazone, or dipeptidyl peptidase-4 (DPP-4) inhibitors; (3) as add-on therapy in patients with diabetes treated with any two of the previous two oral antidiabetic agents; (4) as combination therapy with insulin or a glucagon-like peptide-1 (GLP-1) receptor agonist.[14,17–23] As with other oral antidiabetic agents, the decline in A1C is related to the starting A1C. In T2D patients with a starting A1C of ~8%, one can expect an A1C decrement of ~0.8–1% irrespective of the accompanying antidiabetic regimen. In a head-to-head study in inadequately controlled patients with T2D on metformin, the reduction in A1C with canagliflozin ($\Delta = -1.03\%$) was significantly greater ($P < 0.0001$) than with sitagliptin ($\Delta = -0.66\%$)[18] (Figure 28.4). In a head-to-head study with glimiperide added to a background of metformin, canagliflozin (300 mg/day) was slightly more effective in reducing the A1C ($\Delta = -0.12\%$, $P < 0.01$) after 1 year and was associated with a weight loss of 4.0 kg compared to weight gain of 0.7 kg.[24] Hypoglycemia was common with glimiperide and uncommon with canagliflozin (5 vs. 34% of patients per year). When used as monotherapy or add-on to metformin, sulfonylurea, or metformin/sulfonylurea, the reduction in A1C was maintained after 2 years.[25]

Nonglycemic Benefits. Canagliflozin also improves two important cardiovascular risk factors: obesity and blood pressure. Because canagliflozin works on the kidney to promote glucosuria, diabetic patients lose ~80–90 grams/day of glucose

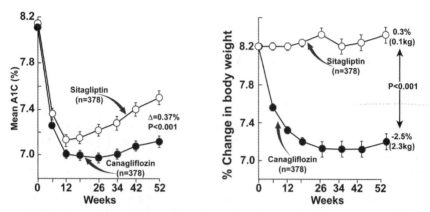

Figure 28.4—Effect of canagliflozin and sitagliptin on the time course of change in A1c and body weight in type 2 diabetic patients. *Source:* Schernthaner G, Gross JL, Rosenstock J, Guarisco M, Fu M, Yee J, Kawaguchi M, Canovatchel W, Meininger G. Canagliflozin compared with sitagliptin for patients with type 2 diabetes who do not have adequate glycemic control with metformin plus sulfonylurea: a 52 week randomized trial. *Diabetes Care* 2013;36:2508–2515.

in the urine. This amounts to the loss of ~320–360 calories/day and weight loss of 2–3 kg during the first year of treatment is a consistent finding in all studies[14] (Figure 28.4). The weight loss is most rapid during the first 3 months, begins to slow during months 3–6, and reaches a plateau during months 6–12. Importantly, weight regain is uncommon.

Canagliflozin also produces consistent reductions of systolic/diastolic blood pressure of 4–6/1–2 mmHg across all studies.[14,26,27] The reduction in blood pressure occurs within the initial 2–4 weeks after the initiation of therapy, is greatest in individuals with an elevated blood pressure at baseline, and persists for up to 1–2 years, or for the duration of therapy. The reduction in blood pressure most likely is explained by the negative salt and water balance that occurs during the first 3–4 days of initiating therapy, and this is reflected by a 1–2% increase in hematocrit. Another plausible explanation for the drop in blood pressure is local inhibition of the renin angiotensin system secondary to enhanced sodium delivery to the juxtaglomerular apparatus. The decrease in blood pressure correlates poorly with the reduction in body weight, which is more gradual in onset. It is likely, however, that the decrease in body weight contributes to the long-term maintenance of blood pressure reduction.

Side Effects. Potential side effects with canagliflozin, as well as with all SGLT-2 inhibitors under development, include hypoglycemia, dyslipidemia, altered renal function, electrolyte disturbances, urinary tract infection, genital mycotic infections, and volume- and osmotic-related events.[14]

Hypoglycemia is a potential side effect of all hypoglycemic agents. However, because canagliflozin and other SGLT-2 inhibitors decrease the plasma glucose concentration without augmenting insulin secretion or inhibiting the counter-regulatory response, hypoglycemia is uncommon (2–4%) when this class of drugs is used as monotherapy or in combination with pioglitazone, metformin, or a DPP-4 inhibitor and, most important, severe hypoglycemia is extremely rare. When used in combination with a sulfonylurea or insulin,[14,21,22] the reported incidence of hypoglycemia is similar to that observed with the sulfonylureas alone or insulin alone.

A small reduction in eGFR of ~4-5 ml/minute/1.73 m² has been observed during the first month of therapy with canagliflozin.[14] This most likely results from the mild intravascular volume depletion, and the eGFR returns to normal when the drug is discontinued. Disturbances in the serum sodium concentration have not been observed. Rare cases of hyperkalemia have been observed with the 300 mg/day dose of canagliflozin in patients with an eGFR = 45–60 ml/minute/1.73 m² (the 300 mg/day dose is contraindicated with eGFR <60) and who were taking an angiotensin-converting enzyme (ACE) or angiotensin-receptor blocker (ARB) or a potassium-sparing diuretic.[14] No clinically significant changes in serum calcium, parathyroid hormone (PTH), vitamin D, or bone mineral density have been observed with canagliflozin, and a dedicated bone study is under way. Consistent with the inhibition of sodium-coupled uric acid reabsorption in the proximal tubule and the human glucose transporter 9 (GLUT-9) that exchanges luminal glucose for uric acid in the distal tubule, a modest drop in serum uric acid of ~1.0 mg/dl is observed. Small, clinically insignificant changes in serum magnesium (–0.6%) and phosphate (+1.5%) have been reported.[14]

The serum low-density lipoprotein (LDL) cholesterol concentration has been shown to increase by 4.4 and 8.8 mg/dl with the 100 and 300 mg/day dose of canagliflozin in association with a small increase in apolipoprotein (apo) B100.[14] Plasma triglyceride concentration decreased by 7.7–10.2% and high-density lipoprotein (HDL) cholesterol increased by 5–6.3%.[24] The mechanism(s) responsible for the rise in LDL cholesterol is (are) unknown but could result from hemoconcentration or transfer of cholesterol from triglyceride to apo B100.

Because canagliflozin, and all SGLT-2 inhibitors, promote glucosuria, they pose a risk for urinary tract infections (UTIs) and genital infections. Diabetic subjects treated with canagliflozin, 100 mg/day, had a small increase in the incidence of UTIs compared with the comparator (5.9 vs. 4%).[14,28,29] The incidence of UTIs (4.3%), however, in the group treated with canagliflozin, 300 mg/day, was similar to that in the comparator group. All UTIs involved the lower urinary tract and responded well to usual antibiotic therapy.

The incidence of vulvovaginitis is increased significantly in women treated with canagliflozin versus comparator (~10 vs. ~3%).[14,30,31] Most infections are mild and respond well to local therapy. Women who experience a mycotic infection are more likely to have a recurrent infection. Men who are treated with canagliflozin also experience an increased incidence of balanitis compared with the comparator (~5 vs. ~1%). The incidence is not as high as in females, however, and primarily affects uncircumcised males.

Drug-Drug Interactions. Canagliflozin is metabolized by UDP-glucuronosyl transferase (UGT) enzyme. Therefore, when used in combination with drugs such as rifampin, phenytoin, phenobarbital, ritonavir, it is advisable to use the 300 mg/day canagliflozin tablet. In diabetic patients treated with digoxin, canagliflozin increased the mean plasma digoxin area under the curve by 20% and the peak level by 36%. Therefore, it is advisable to check the serum digoxin level after initiating canagliflozin.

Contraindications. Canagliflozin has not been studied in pregnancy and nursing mothers or in children <18 years old and should not be used in these populations.[14] Canagliflozin has not been studied in patients with diabetes who have severe liver disease and is contraindicated in this population.[14]

Dapagliflozin (Farxiga)[1,2]

Dapagliflozin was approved for the treatment of patients with T2D in Europe in 2013. Phase 3 trials in the U.S. have been completed, and dapagliflozin was approved in 2014 by the U.S. Food and Drug Administration (FDA). Dapagliflozin has a half-life of 17–18 hours and is administered once daily producing sustained glucosuria over 24 hours.[32] Dapagliflozin is absorbed rapidly, achieving a maximal plasma concentration at ~2 hours. Dapagliflozin is highly protein bound (97–98%) and renal excretion is low (2–4%). An inert glucuronide conjugate is the major metabolite.

Dosing. Dapagliflozin comes in two strengths, 5 and 10 mg. The recommended starting dose is 5 mg/day, with escalation to 10 mg/day if additional A1C reduction is needed. The efficacy of dapagliflozin is reduced in patients with diabetes with an eGFR between 45 and 60 ml/minute/1.73 m², and dapagliflozin is largely ineffective at eGFRs <45 ml/minute/1.73 m². In the U.S. and in Europe, dapagliflozin is not recommended in patients with diabetes who have an eGRF <60 ml/minute/1.73 m².

Efficacy. Treatment with dapagliflozin for 12 weeks reduced the A1C by about 0.7% without any apparent dose dependency in 389 subjects with T2D with a baseline A1C of 7.8–8%.[32] The reduction in A1C was similar to that observed with metformin, and the reductions in fasting and postprandial plasma glucose concentrations accounted approximately equally for the decline in A1C.[33]

In five Phase 3 trials,[34] treatment with dapagliflozin (N = 6,798 randomized to dapagliflozin and placebo in a 2:1 ratio; 5 and 10 mg/day) consistently caused a significant decrease in A1C of 0.6–0.7 (baseline A1C ~8–8.2%) compared with placebo, independent of the background therapy. A similar decrease in A1C was observed when dapagliflozin was given as monotherapy or added to metformin, sulfonylurea, thiazolidinedione, or insulin. The 10 mg/day dapagliflozin dose produced an ~25 and 55 mg/dl decrease in the fasting and 2-hour plasma glucose concentrations, respectively. The decrease in A1C caused by dapagliflozin was independent of gender, ethnicity, race, BMI, or duration of T2D. As expected, dapagliflozin produced a greater reduction in A1C in patients with higher baseline A1C. In a 24-week study, dapagliflozin reduced the A1C by 2.88% (5 mg/day) and 2.66% (10 mg/day) in a subgroup (n = 78) of subjects with baseline A1C 10.1–12%.[35]

Because the mechanism of action of dapagliflozin is independent of insulin secretion and insulin action, the efficacy of dapagliflozin is independent of β-cell function, severity of insulin resistance, or diabetes duration. Wilding et al.[36] randomized 71 insulin-treated (≥50 units/day) patients with T2D who also were receiving an insulin sensitizer (metformin and/or thiazolidinedione) to add-on therapy with dapagliflozin (5 and 10 mg/day) or placebo. The insulin dose was reduced by 50% at the start of therapy, while the insulin sensitizer dose was unchanged. After 12 weeks, the placebo-subtracted declines in A1C were 0.70 and 0.78%, respectively (P <0.01 vs. placebo), despite the 50% reduction in insulin dose. In another study, 151 subjects with new-onset diabetes (<1 year) and 58 subjects with longstanding (11 years) T2D were randomly assigned to 10 or 20 mg/day of dapagliflozin for 12 weeks.[37] Subjects with longstanding diabetes were in poor glycemic control (A1C = 8.4%), despite large doses of insulin (>50 units/day) plus metformin and a thiazolidinedione. Dapagliflozin caused a comparable decline in A1C in both groups.

In a head-to-head comparison of dapagliflozin with sulfonylurea as add-on therapy in individuals with poorly controlled T2D on metformin therapy,[38] both groups exhibited the same decline in mean A1C (-0.52%). In this study, subjects had a relatively low initial A1C, and 25% of participants had a baseline A1C <7%.

Two-year follow-up results with dapagliflozin treatment have been reported in two trials.[39,40] In subjects treated with metformin, the decrease from baseline in A1C was -0.54% at 1 year and -0.80% at 2 years. Similarly, in a head-to-head study of dapagliflozin versus glipizide, an additional -0.34% decrease in A1C was observed in the second year in subjects treated with dapagliflozin compared with a -0.12% decrease in subjects treated with glipizide.[39] About 70 and 90% of subjects in the two studies,[39,40] respectively, entered the second-year extension study. Thus, it is difficult to determine whether the decrease in A1C during the second year was due to dapagliflozin or selection bias in the subjects entering the second-year extension study. Nevertheless, the results of both studies demonstrate that the glucose-lowering effect of dapagliflozin does not wane with time up to a 2-year period.

Nonglycemic Benefits. Dapagliflozin treatment promoted between 2.2 and 3.1 kg of weight loss and a modest reduction in both systolic and diastolic blood pressure. The amount of glucosuria observed with dapagliflozin (50–60 grams/day) is equivalent to a daily caloric loss of about 200 to 240 calories/day, which over the course of 12 weeks could explain the 2–3 kg weight loss. In the study by Wilding et al.,[36] the placebo-subtracted reduction in body weight in insulin-treated subjects with T2D was 2.4–2.6 kg, reflecting both the loss of glucose in the urine and reduction (50%) in insulin dose.

Side Effects. Compared with patients treated with metformin or placebo, dapagliflozin therapy was associated with small increases in 24-hour urine volume, blood urea nitrogen/creatinine ratio, and hematocrit consistent with a modest reduction in intravascular volume. Serum uric acid declined by ~1.0%, while serum magnesium increased slightly by 0.10–0.15 mg/dl. No clinically significant changes in serum sodium, calcium, or phosphate have been observed. Genital infections (12 vs. 3%) and UTIs (11 vs. 6%) were increased, more so in females than in males. Hypoglycemia has not been observed in the absence of concomitant sulfonylurea or insulin therapy. Dapagliflozin causes a small increase in serum HDL cholesterol (3–4%) and modest decrease (~6%) in serum triglyceride; LDL cholesterol did not change significantly.

In Phase 3 studies of dapagliflozin, an increased incidence of bladder and breast cancer was observed. The total number of cases, however, was small (10 for each cancer). This finding was surprising, because neither breast nor bladder tissue express SGLT-2. In addition, rigorous 2-year carcinogenic studies in animals failed to demonstrate any preneoplastic or neoplastic changes. Because breast and especially bladder cancer take many years to develop, whereas the exposure to dapagliflozin was short (generally <1 year), the significance of the increased incidence of these two tumors remains to be determined. Of note, 8 of the 9 dapagliflozin-treated patients with bladder cancer had hematuria at the time of entry into the study. Moreover, detection bias for bladder cancer may have been due to the frequent testing for UTIs, which could have led to the discovery of microscopic hematuria. Nonetheless, because of this potential carcinogenic signal, the FDA has asked for post-approval follow-up safety data regarding cancer risk with dapagliflozin.[1]

Empagliflozin

Empagliflozin[1,2] is a highly selective SGLT-2 inhibitor that is absorbed rapidly, reaching maximal plasma concentrations in 1.5 hours.[41,42] The drug is highly protein bound, with a long terminal half-life, making it suitable for once-daily administration. Approximately 18% of the drug is excreted in the urine following single-dose administration.

Similar to other SGLT-2 inhibitors, empagliflozin produces a dose-dependent glucosuria in both normal subjects and those with T2D.[43-45] In a placebo-controlled 12-week study in 495 subjects with diabetes with poor glycemic control on metformin, empagliflozin caused a dose-dependent decrease in both the fasting plasma glucose (FPG) concentration and A1C with placebo-subtracted decreases in FPG and A1C of 27 mg/dl and 0.7%, respectively, with a dose of 25 mg/day.[46] Empagliflozin was scheduled to be reviewed by the U.S. FDA in March 2014.

Ipragliflozin

In a 12-week double-blind study, 361 Japanese subjects with T2D treated with ipragliflozin[1,2] at doses ranging from 12.5 to 100 mg/day experienced a 0.9% reduction in A1C at the two highest doses (50 and 100 mg/day).[47] Body weight also was dose-dependently reduced by up to 2 kg in the 100 mg/day dose. In a 16-week study, ipragliflozin monotherapy (50 mg/day) caused a 1.2% decrease from baseline (8.3%) in A1C in 62 individuals with T2D.[48]

LX4211

In a Phase 2A study, LX4211, which inhibits SGLT-2 and to a lesser extent SGLT-1, at doses of 150 and 300 mg/day reduced the A1C by 1.2%, but the starting A1C (8.2–8.5%) was higher than in most other studies, and the placebo decreased the A1C by 0.5%.[49,50] In a 12-week study, LX4211 at doses of 75, 200, and 400 mg reduced A1C by –0.43, –0.79, and –0.95, respectively, in association with significant reductions in body weight, blood pressure, and serum triglycerides.[51] Because LX2411 possesses significant activity against the SGLT-1 transporter, gut glucose absorption is inhibited and may provide greater A1C lowering than specific SGLT-2 inhibitors. Furthermore, the glucose that is delivered to the distal small bowel and large bowel is converted to fatty acid derivatives, which stimulate GLP-1 and peptide YY (PYY) release from L-cells.[52] The increase in GLP-1 has the potential to augment insulin and inhibit glucagon secretion, resulting in a further enhancement of glucose tolerance. Consistent with this, preliminary studies in patients with T2D demonstrate that combination therapy with a DPP-4 inhibitor plus LX4211 produces a synergistic increase in active GLP-1 after a meal challenge.[52]

CONCLUSION

Current data in humans indicate that inhibition of the SGLT-2 transporter is an effective and novel strategy to reduce the plasma glucose concentration in subjects with T2D.[1,2] Canagliflozin and dapagliflozin have demonstrated a good safety profile, modest weight loss, a decrease in blood pressure, and A1C reduction of ~0.8% with a starting A1C of ~8%. Because the SGLT-2 inhibitors have a mechanism of action that is independent of insulin secretion or the presence of insulin resistance, the efficacy of this class of drugs is not anticipated to decline with progressive β-cell failure or in the presence of severe insulin resistance, although it will decrease with declining renal function at eGFR of <60 ml/minute. This class of drugs can be used in combination with all other antidiabetic medications with anticipated additive efficacy on glycemic control. The SGLT-2 inhibitors also are effective as monotherapy in newly diagnosed patients with diabetes. To the extent that glucotoxicity contributes to the demise in β-cell function in subjects with impaired glucose tolerance or impaired fasting glucose, these drugs also may prove useful in the treatment of prediabetes. Currently available data indicate that the SGLT-2 inhibitors have a good safety profile. In addition, the asymptomatic clinical presentation of subjects with familial renal glucosuria, despite multiple generations of the disease, supports the likely long-term safety of pharmacological inhibition of SGLT-2.

DISCLOSURE

Conflicts of interest: M.A. Abdul-Ghani: none; L. Norton: none; R.A. DeFronzo is a member of the advisory board of Amylin, Takeda, Boehringer Ingelheim, Novo Nordisk, Janssen, Lexicon, AstraZeneca, and Bristol-Myers Squibb; RAD has received grant support from Amylin, Bristol-Myers Squibb, Takeda, and Boehringer-Ingelheim, and he is a member of the speakers bureau of Bristol-Myers Squibb, AstraZeneca, Janssen, and Novo Nordisk.

REFERENCES

1. Abdul-Ghani MA, Norton L, DeFronzo RA. Efficacy and safety of SGLT-2 inhibitors in the treatment of type 2 diabetes mellitus. *Curr Diab Rep* 2012;12(3):230–238.

2. Abdul-Ghani MA, Norton L, DeFronzo RA. Role of sodium-glucose cotransporter 2 (SGLT 2) inhibitors in the treatment of type 2 diabetes. *Endocr Rev* 2011;32:515–531.

3. Mogensen CE. Urinary albumin excretion in early and long-term juvenile diabetes. *Scand J Clin Lab Invest* 1971;28:183–193.

4. Farber SJ, Berger EY, Earle DP. Effect of diabetes and insulin of the maximum capacity of the renal tubules to reabsorb glucose. *J Clin Invest* 1951;30:125–129.

5. DeFronzo RA, Hompesch M, Kasichayanula S, Liu X, Hong Y, Pfister M, Morrow LA, Leslie BR, Boulton DW, Ching A, Lacreta FP, Griffen SC. Characterization of renal glucose reabsorption in response to dapagliflozin in healthy subjects and subjects with type 2 diabetes. *Diabetes Care* 2013;36:3169–3176.

6. Rahmoune H, Thompson PW, Ward JM, Smith CD, Hong G, Brown J. Glucose transporters in human renal proximal tubular cells isolated from the urine of patients with non-insulin-dependent diabetes. *Diabetes* 2005;54:3427–434.

7. Santer R, Calado J. Familial renal glucosuria and SGLT-2: from a Mendelian trait to a therapeutic target. *Clin J Am Soc Nephrol* 2010;5:133–141.

8. Chassis H, Jolliffe N, Smith H. The action of phlorizin on the excretion of glucose, xylose, sucrose, creatinine, and urea by man. *J Clin Invest* 1933;12:1083–1089.

9. Rossetti L, Smith D, Shulman GI, Papachristou D, DeFronzo RA. Correction of hyperglycemia with phlorizin normalizes tissue sensitivity to insulin in diabetic rats. *J Clin Invest* 1987;79:1510–1515.

10. Rossetti L, Shulman GI, Zawalich W, DeFronzo RA. Effect of chronic hyperglycemia on in vivo insulin secretion in partially pancreatectomized rats. *J Clin Invest* 1987;80:1037–1044.

11. Kahn BB, DeFronzo RA, Cushman SW, Rossetti L. Normalization of blood glucose in diabetic rats with phlorizin treatment reverses insulin-resistant glucose transport in adipose cells without restoring glucose transporter gene expression. *J Clin Invest* 1999;87:561–570.

12. Merovci A, Solis-Herrera C, Daniele G, Eldor R, Fiorentino TV, Tripathy D, Xiong J, Perez Z, Norton L, Abdul-Ghani MA, DeFronzo R. Dapagliflozin improves muscle insulin sensitivity but enhances glucose production. *J Clin Invest* 2014;124:509–514.

13. Santer R, Kinner M, Lassen CL, Schneppenheim R, Eggert P, Bald M, Brodehl J, Daschner M, Ehrich JH, Kemper M, Li Volti S, Neuhaus T, Skovby F, Swift PG, Schaub J, Klaerke D. Molecular analysis of the SGLT-2 gene in patients with renal glucosuria. *J Am Soc Nephrol* 2003;14:2873–2882.

14. Canagliflozin package insert. Available at www.invokanahcp.com/prescribing-information.pdf. Accessed 28 February 2014.

15. Devineni D, Curtin CR, Polidori D, Gutierrez MJ, Murphy J, Rusch S, Rothenberg PL. Pharmacokinetics and pharmacodynamics of canagliflozin,

a sodium glucose co-transporter 2 inhibitor, in subjects with type 2 diabetes mellitus. *J Clin Pharmacol* 2013;53:601–610.

16. Yale JF, Bakris G, Cariou B, Yue D, David-Neto E, Xi L, Figueroa K, Wajs E, Usiskin K, Meininger G. Efficacy and safety of canagliflozin in subjects with type 2 diabetes and chronic kidney disease. *Diabetes Obes Metab* 2013;15:463–473.

17. Clar C, Gill JA, Court R, Waugh N. Systemic review of SGLT2 receptor inhibitors in dual or triple therapy in type 2 diabetes. *BMJ* 2:e001007, 2012. Doi:10.136/bmjopen-2012-001007.

18. Schernthaner G, Gross JL, Rosenstock J, Guarisco M, Fu M, Yee J, Kawaguchi M, Canovatchel W, Meininger G. Canagliflozin compared with sitagliptin for patients with type 2 diabetes who do not have adequate glycemic control with metformin plus sulfonylurea: a 52-week randomized trial. *Diabetes Care* 2013;36:2508–2515..

19. Devineni D, Morrow L, Hompesch M, Skee D, Vandebosch A, Murphy J, Ways K, Schwartz S. Canagliflozin improves glycaemic control over 28 days in subjects with type 2 diabetes not optimally controlled on insulin. *Diabetes Obes Metab* 2012;14:539–545.

20. Stenlof K, Cefalu WT, Kim K-A, Jodar E, Alba M, Edwards R, Tong C, Canovatchel W, Meininger G. Efficacy and safety of canagliflozin (CANA) monotherapy in subjects with type 2 diabetes mellitus (T2DM) over 52 weeks. *Diabetes* 2013;62(Suppl 1):A303.

21. Fulcher G, Matthews D, Perkovic V, Mahaffrey KW, Weiss R, Rosenstock J, Capuano G, Desai M, Shaw W, Vercruysse F, Meinringer G, Neal B. Canagliflozin (CANA) in subjects with type 2 diabetes mellitus (T2DM) inadequately controlled on sulfonylurea (SU) monotherapy: a CANVAS substudy. *Diabetes* 2013;62(Suppl 1):A292.

22. Rosenstock J, Davies M, Dumas R, Dessai M, Alba M, Capuano G, Meininger G. Effects of canagliflozin added on to basal insulin +/- other antihyperglycemic agents in type 2 diabetes. *Diabetes* 2013;62(Suppl 1):A280.

23. Wysham C, Woo V, Mathieu C, Desai M, Alba M, Capuano G, Meininger G. Canagliflozin (CANA) added on to dipeptidyl peptidase-4 inhibitors (DPP-4i) or glucagon-like peptide-1 (GLP-1) agonists with or without other antihyperglycemic agents (AHAs) in type 2 diabetes mellitus (T2DM). *Diabetes* 2013;62(Suppl 1):A279.

24. Cefalu WT, Leiter LA, Yoon K-H, Arias P, Niskanen L, Xie J, Balis DA, Canovatchel W, Meininger G. Efficacy and safety of canagliflozin versus glimepiride in patients with type 2 diabetes inadequately controlled with metformin (CANTATA-SU): 52 week results from a randomised, double-blind, phase 3 non-inferiority trial. *Lancet* 2013;382:941–950.

25. Cefalu WT, Leiter LA, Yoon K-H, Langslet G, Arias P, Xie J, Balis DA, Millington D, Vercruysse F, Canovatchel W, Meininger G. Canagliflozin (CANA) demonstrates durable glycemic improvements over 104 weeks ver-

sus glimepiride (GLIM) in subjects with type 2 diabetes mellitus (T2DM) on metformin (MET). American Diabetes Association Scientific Sessions, Chicago, 2013 (late breaker abstract).

26. Weir M, Janusezewicz A, Gilbert R, Lavalle Gonzales F, Meininger G. Lower blood pressure (BP) with canagliflozin (CANA) in subjects with type 2 diabetes mellitus (T2DM). *Diabetes* 2013;62(Suppl 1):A278.

27. Blonde L, Wilding J, Chiasson J-L, Polidori D, Meininger G, Stein P. Canagliflozin (CANA) lowers A1c and blood pressure (BP) through weight loss-independent (WL-I) and weight loss-associated (WL-A) mechanisms. *Diabetes* 2013;62(Suppl 1):A288.

28. Nicolle LE, Capuano G, Fung A, Usiskin K. Urinary tract infection (UTI) with canagliflozin (CANA) in subjects with type 2 diabetes mellitus (T2DM). *Diabetes* 2013;62(Suppl 1):A296.

29. Nicolle LE, Capuano G, Ways K, Usiskin K. Effect of canagliflozin, a sodium glucose co-transporter 2 (SGLT-2) inhibitor, on bacteriuria and urinary tract infection in subjects with type 2 diabetes enrolled in a 12-week, phase 2 study. *Curr Med Res Opin* 2012;28:1167–1171.

30. Nyirjesy P, Sobel J, Fung A, Gassmann-Mayer C, Ways K, Usiskin K. Genital mycotic infections with canagliflozin (CANA) in subjects with type 2 diabetes mellitus (T2DM). *Diabetes* 2013;62(Suppl 1):A276.

31. Nyirjesy P, Zhao Y, Ways K, Usiskin K. Evaluation of vulvovaginal symptoms and Candida colonization in women with type 2 diabetes mellitus treated with canagliflozin, a sodium glucose co-transporter 2 inhibitor. *Curr Med Res Opin* 2012;28:1173–1178.

32. Meng W, Ellsworth BA, Nirschl AA, McCann PJ, Patel M, Girotra RN, Wu G, Sher PM, Morrison EP, Biller SA, Zahler R, Deshpande PP, Pullockaran A, Hagan DL, Morgan N, Taylor JR, Obermeier MT, Humphreys WG, Khanna A, Discenza L, Robertson JG, Wang A, Han S, Wetterau JR, Janovitz EB, Flint OP, Whaley JM, Washburn WN. Discovery of dapagliflozin: a potent, selective renal sodium-dependent glucose cotransporter 2 (SGLT-2) inhibitor for the treatment of type 2 diabetes. *J Med Chem* 2008;51:1145–1149.

33. List JF, Woo V, Morales E, Tang W, Fiedorek FT: Sodium-glucose cotransport inhibition with dapagliflozin in type 2 diabetes. *Diabetes Care* 2009;32:650–657.

34. U.S. Food and Drug Administration. Background document: dapagliflozin. Available at www.fda.gov/downloads/advisorycommittees/committeesmeetingmaterials/drugs/endocrinologicandmetabolicdrugsadvisorycommittee/ucm262996.pdf. Accessed 9 April 2014.

35. Ferrannini E, Ramos SJ, Salsali A, Tang W, List JF. Dapagliflozin monotherapy in type 2 diabetic patients with inadequate glycemic control by diet and exercise: a randomized, double-blind, placebo-controlled, phase 3 trial. *Diabetes Care* 2010;33:2217–2224.

36. Wilding JP, Norwood P, T'Joen C, Bastien A, List JF, Fiedorek FT. A study of dapagliflozin in patients with type 2 diabetes receiving high doses of insulin plus insulin sensitizers: applicability of a novel insulin-independent treatment. *Diabetes Care* 2009;32:1656–1662.

37. Zhang L, Feng Y, List J, Kasichayanula S, Pfister M. Dapagliflozin treatment in patients with different stages of type 2 diabetes mellitus: effects on glycaemic control and body weight. *Diabetes Obes Metab* 2010;12:510–516.

38. Nauck MA, Del Prato S, Meier JJ, Duran-Garcia S, Rohwedder K, Elze M, Parikh SJ. Dapagliflozin versus glipizide as add-on therapy in patients with type 2 diabetes who have inadequate glycemic control with metformin: a randomized, 52-week, double-blind, active-controlled noninferiority trial. *Diabetes Care* 2011;34:2015–2022.

39. Baily CJ, Gross JL, Yadav M, Iqbal N, Mansfield Ta, List JF. Sustained efficacy of dapagliflozin when added to metformin in type 2 diabetes inadequately controlled by metformin monotherapy. *Diabetologia* 2011;54(Suppl 1): A146.

40. Del Prato S, Nauck M, Rohwedder K, Thouerkuuf A, Longkilde AM, Parikh S. Long term efficacy and safety of add-on dapagliflozin vs add-on glipizide in patients with type 2 diabetes mellitus inadequately controlled with metformin: 2 year results. *Diabetologia* 2011;54(Suppl 1):A852.

41. Macha S, Dieterich S, Mattheus M, Seman LJ, Broedl UC, Woerle HJ. Pharmacokinetics of empagliflozin, a sodium glucose cotransporter-2 (SGLT-2) inhibitor, and metformin following co-administration in healthy volunteers. *Int J Clin Pharmacol Ther* 2013;51:132–140.

42. Grempler R, Thomas L, Eckhardt M, Himmelsbach F, Sauer A, Sharp DE, Bakker RA, Mark M, Klein T, Eickelmann P. Empagliflozin, a novel selective sodium glucose cotransporter-2 (SGLT-2) inhibitor: characterisation and comparison with other SGLT-2 inhibitors. *Diabetes Obes Metab* 2012;14:83–90.

43. Heise T, Seewaldt-Becker E, Macha S, Hantel S, Huber K, Pinnetri S, Seman L, Hans-Juergen W. BI 10773, a sodium glucose co-transporter inhibitor (SGLT-2), is safe and efficacious following 4-week treatment in patients with type 2 diabetes. *Diabetes* 2010;59(Suppl 1):A172.

44. Koiwai K, Seman L, Yamamura N, Macha S, Taniguchi A, Negishi T, Sosoko S, Dugi KA. Safety, tolerability, pharmacokinetics and pharmacoydnamics of single doses of BI 10773. A sodium-glucose co-transporter inhibitor (SGLT-2), in Japanese healthy volunteers. *Diabetes* 2010;59(Suppl 1):A571.

45. Hanesen KB, Knop FK, Andersen NW, Diep TA, Rosenkilde MM, Holst JJ, Hansen HH. A naturally occurring ligand activates the GLP-1 in vivo. *Diabetes* 2010;59(Suppl 1):A174.

46. Rosenstock J, Jelaska A, Seman L, Pinnetri S, Hantel S, Woerle HJ. Efficacy and safety of BI 10773, a new sodium glucose cotransporter-2 (SGLT-2)

inhibitor, in type 2 diabetes inadequately controlled on metformin. *Diabetes* 2011;60(Suppl 1):A271.

47. Kashiwagi A, Ursuno A, Kazura K, Yoshida S, Kageyama S. ASP1941, a novel selective SGLT-2 inhibitor, was effective and safe in Japanese healthy volunteers and patients with type 2 diabetes mellitus. *Diabetes* 2010;59(Suppl 1): A21.

48. Takinami A, Tukinami Y, Kuzuta K, Yoshida S, Utsuno A, Nagase I, Kashiwagi A. Ipragliflozin improved glycemic control with additional benefit of reduction of body weight and blood pressure in Japanese patients with type 2 diabetes mellitus: BRIGHTEN Study. *Diabetologia* 2011;54(Suppl):A149.

49. Zambrowicz B, Freiman J, Brown PM, Frazier KS, Turnage A, Bronner J, Ruff D, Shadoan M, Banks P, Mseeh F, Rawlins DB, Goodwin NC, Mabon R, Harrison BA, Wilson A, Sands A, Powell DR. LX 4211, a dual SGLT1/ SGLT2 inhibitor, improved glycemic control in patients with type 2 diabetes in a randomized, placebo-controlled trial. *Clin Pharmacol Therap* 2012; 92:158–169.

50. Zambrowicz B, Freiman J, Brown PM, Frazier KS, Turnage A, Bronner J, Ruff D, Shadoan M, Banks P, Mseeh F, Rawlins DB, Goodwin NC, Mabon R, Harrison BA, Wilson A, Sands A, Powell DR. LX4211, a dual SGLT-1/ SGLT-2 inhibitor, improved glycemic control in patients with type 2 diabetes in a randomized, placebo-controlled trial. *Clin Pharmacol Ther* 2012;92:158–169.

51. Powell DR, Smith M, Greer J, Harris A, Zhao S, DaCosta C, Mseeh F, Shadoan MK, Sands A, Zambrowicz B, Ding ZM. LX4211 increases serum glucagon-like peptide 1 and peptide YY levels by reducing sodium/glucose cotransporter 1 (SGLT-1)-mediated absorption of intestinal glucose. *J Pharmacol Exp Ther* 2013;345:250–259.

52. Zambrowicz B, Ding ZM, Ogbaa I, Frazier K, Banks P, Turnage A, Freiman J, Smith M, Ruff D, Sands A, Powell D. Effects of LX4211, a dual SGLT-1/ SGLT-2 inhibitor, plus sitagliptin on postprandial active GLP-1 and glycemic control in type 2 diabetes. *Clin Ther* 2013;35:273–285, e277.

Chapter 29

Insulin Therapy in Type 2 Diabetes

Darin E. Olson, MD, PhD
Mary Rhee, MD, MS
Lawrence S. Phillips, MD

INTRODUCTION

In the natural history of type 2 diabetes (T2D), most patients exhibit progressive β-cell dysfunction and loss of insulin secretion over time. As β-cell function decreases, most oral medications typically used in T2D, which act by facilitating β-cell secretion of insulin or decreasing insulin resistance, become insufficient to control glucose levels, leading to the need for insulin treatment. Although the pharmacology of insulin in T2D is similar to that in type 1 diabetes (T1D), the absence of absolute insulin deficiency for most patients with T2D allows for more options for implementing insulin therapy. Clinical decision making will be influenced not only by glucose levels but also by patient preference and understanding, the stage of the disease, and the presence or absence of comorbidities. The goals of insulin therapy to establish metabolic control, achieve glycemic goals, and prevent long-term complications in T2D must be balanced against the risk of hypoglycemia. This chapter discusses insulin treatment in T2D, with particular focus on the indications and methods of using insulin.

HISTORY OF INSULIN DEVELOPMENT AND USE

The development of insulin and its various formulations is reviewed briefly here (for a discussion about its use in regard to the treatment of T1D, see Chapter 9). Early in the history of insulin therapy, only animal insulins were available, but both recombinant human insulin and insulin analogs now are used routinely. Different insulin formulations have been developed to achieve various pharmacodynamic profiles. The action of the insulin preparations typically is described in terms of the time to onset, time to peak effect, and duration. Currently available formulations and their characteristic pharmacodynamic profiles are listed in Chapter 31, Table 31.3. Recombinant human insulin in the form of regular human insulin has a relatively rapid absorption, and when mixed with protamine (neutral protamine Hagedorn, NPH), it has a slower absorption and onset of action. These types of insulin can be administered separately or mixed together in the same syringe, either mixed manually or in premixed formulations (e.g., 70/30 NPH/regular insulin). Insulin analogs, developed nearly two decades after the first recombinant human insulin, have more rapid (insulin aspart, insulin lispro, insulin glulisine) or slower and more consistent (insulin glargine, insulin detemir) phar-

DOI: 10.2337/9781580405096.29

461

macodynamic characteristics. The key difference in the various insulin formulations is the time course of action after subcutaneous injection.

INSULIN ANALOGS [more expensive / mimic normal physiology]

A major advance in the past 20 years has been the development of human insulin analogs. Insulin analogs have been modified with amino acid changes and the addition of fatty acid moieties to alter absorption characteristics or half-life in the circulation and to mimic important aspects of normal physiology. The analogs have either a more rapid time course that allows for better matching to meals with a quick onset and shorter duration of action, or a longer time course that allows for more consistent action over a prolonged time period for basal insulin coverage and minimal peaking effects. The new preparations of insulin allow for more flexible and convenient timing of insulin administration, but they often require more frequent injections.

Beyond the trade-off between convenience and frequency of administration, one major established benefit of the new analogs is a moderate reduction in hypoglycemia,[1,2] but a clear benefit on overall glycemic control or prevention of diabetic complications has been difficult to establish when compared with human insulin preparations.[3,4] The currently available insulin analogs are more expensive than the NPH and regular human insulin preparations, and varying experience among providers may affect the choice of the insulin preparation prescribed.

Rapid-Acting Analogs

Rapid-acting analogs currently include insulin lispro, insulin aspart, and insulin glulisine. They each have similar time courses of action, with more rapid onset and shorter duration than regular insulin, more closely mimicking the normal physiologic response of insulin to a meal. As such, they primarily are used before meals to match the metabolic requirements of the meal, and ideally they should be matched to the timing, size, and carbohydrate content of a meal, as well as the insulin sensitivity of the patient. Rapid-acting analogs also can be used as a supplement to "correct" elevated glucose levels back toward the target range.

Given their pharmacodynamic profile, both the rapid-acting insulin analogs and regular insulin can provide flexibility with regard to meal frequency, timing, and size, which is not possible with premixed insulin preparations.[5] Moreover, adding rapid-acting analogs before the largest meal in T2D consistently has been shown to reduce late-postprandial hypoglycemia.[6,7] Consistent reduction in overall glycemia in T2D, however, has not been observed when compared with other insulin formulations.[2] When considering short-acting insulin and rapid-acting insulin, at the higher doses of insulin often seen with T2D, the relative difference in the rapidity of action of the rapid-acting analogs compared with regular insulin is not as different as that observed at lower insulin doses.[8]

Relatively Peakless Long-Acting Analogs

Long-acting insulin analogs currently available in the U.S. include insulin glargine and insulin detemir (a newer long-acting analog recently available in some other countries is not discussed here). These long-acting analogs have less prominent "peaking" than NPH and other mixed preparations, and they provide greater likelihood of once-a-day basal coverage for many patients. They also have been found to produce less hypoglycemia while achieving similar or improved overall glycemic control compared with NPH,[9] with convenient once-daily dosing, but at a higher cost.

INSULIN PREPARATIONS AND DEVICES

The standard insulin concentration is 100 units/milliliter (U/ml) of insulin (U-100) packaged in 10 ml vials, which can be drawn into calibrated syringes that typically hold up to 50 or 100 units of insulin. (A more concentrated form, U-500, is discussed later as an option for a subset of patients with extremely high insulin needs.) All of the human insulins and insulin analogs are available in either vials or insulin pen devices for more convenient administration. The insulin pens hold 300 units of insulin and can deliver doses up to 60 or 80 units at a time, depending on the source. These devices have been shown to be more readily accepted by patients in clinical trials because of the relative ease of use but at a relatively higher cost. Despite the ease of use and patient acceptability, there have not been proven glycemic benefits over injecting insulin with syringes.[10]

INSULIN USE IN TYPE 2 DIABETES

INDICATIONS FOR INSULIN USE

A wide range of patients with T2D may benefit from insulin therapy.[11,12] The most common indications for the initiation of insulin therapy in T2D include the following:

1. Progressive β-cell dysfunction with insufficient insulin secretion relative to the degree of insulin resistance despite maximal treatment with oral or noninsulin therapies
2. Severe hyperglycemia with associated glucose toxicity
3. Hospitalization for an acute illness or surgery
4. Side effects with or contraindication to use of oral or noninsulin therapies
5. Pregnancy
6. Patient preference

Insulin initiation earlier in the natural history of T2D may be considered as well and will be discussed later in this chapter. Given all of these considerations, the choices and role of insulin therapy in T2D must be individualized.

Stage of Disease

Most patients early in the natural history of T2D may not require insulin to achieve standard glycemic goals. Advanced stages of T2D, however, in which β-cell function has deteriorated significantly, often require the initiation of insulin treatment as prior oral or noninsulin injectable therapy becomes less effective. In these later stages, when patients are no longer able or likely to achieve glycemic goals with the addition or intensification of another noninsulin agent, then the addition of insulin is necessary and typical.

Severe Hyperglycemia

Regardless of where the patient may be in the natural history of diabetes, when glucose levels become severely elevated—often in association with infection, medication noncompliance, initial presentation of undiagnosed diabetes, or other significant metabolic stress or medical decompensation—β-cell function can become severely impaired as a consequence of glucose toxicity and lipotoxicity. Patients may present with hyperosmolar nonketotic hyperglycemia, and a subset of the population with T2D may develop diabetic ketoacidosis. In these circumstances, oral and noninsulin injectable medications typically used for T2D are not sufficient to correct metabolic derangements or reduce glucose levels to the target range, and exogenous insulin is needed for management. Depending on the stage of disease, and therefore the degree of loss of β-cell function, some patients eventually may be able to transition off insulin and on to oral or other noninsulin injectable diabetes therapies once the glucose levels improve sufficiently and remain relatively stable.

Hospitalization

In most cases, insulin is the preferred treatment option in patients who are hospitalized for acute illness or surgery. Insulin treatment in the hospital setting will be addressed briefly in this section (for a detailed discussions, see Chapters 33 and 34). Because glucose levels tend to rise during hospitalization because of metabolic stress, and because most, if not all, oral and noninsulin medications should be discontinued upon admission to reduce potential adverse effects, insulin is often the first-line treatment during hospitalization in place of prior outpatient treatment regimens. Management with insulin in the hospital generally should mirror the outpatient approach to a basal-bolus insulin regimen with a focus on administering scheduled subcutaneous doses of insulin (as basal alone or as a basal-bolus regimen), or even intravenous insulin when needed. Additional "correction" or "supplemental" doses of rapid-acting insulin to acutely reduce high glucose levels may be beneficial, but it generally is not recommended to rely only on a traditional sliding-scale approach, which provides only correction dosing in the absence of a plan for scheduled insulin. Inpatient management may require extra caution to avoid hypoglycemia and account for frequent metabolic fluctuations. In patients who start insulin during hospitalization, diabetes education and discharge planning should begin as early as possible and should include reevaluation of the final diabetes management plan before discharge with regard to either restarting previously effective oral or noninsulin agents without insulin, or continuing insulin treatment with or without previous noninsulin medications.

Side Effects with or Contraindication to Alternative Therapies

If patients cannot take the available oral or injected noninsulin medications because of side effects, allergies, or contraindications to use, then insulin may be initiated earlier in the disease course.

Pregnancy

All of the oral and injected noninsulin medications used in diabetes management have been assigned to pregnancy categories B or C by the U.S. Food and

Drug Administration. Therefore, insulin remains the mainstay of treatment in women with diabetes who become pregnant and in pregnant women who develop gestational diabetes mellitus that cannot be controlled sufficiently with lifestyle changes. Further discussion of diabetes treatment in pregnancy can be found in Chapters 14 and 15.

Patient Preferences

In addition to the various metabolic and pharmacologic factors considered for insulin use, the decision to initiate insulin treatment and the insulin regimen chosen should take into consideration the preferences and capabilities of the patient. Particular considerations with regard to insulin treatment include the patient's ability to self-administer insulin; willingness to administer insulin at the necessary frequency and schedule; ability to adjust insulin dosages according to differences in diet, physical activity, and glucose levels; and ability to monitor glucose levels as needed. Issues that influence the patient's preference often involve daily schedules and mental or physical limitations.

INSULIN USAGE IN TYPE 2 DIABETES

Basal Insulin

Patients who can improve their glycemic control by using basal insulin include those with persistently elevated prebreakfast glucose or A1C levels above goal despite oral or injected noninsulin therapy, and those who are unable or unwilling to add other agents. Some patients may choose insulin over other options either because of its ability to effectively achieve glycemic goals or β-cell preservation or its benefits in reducing long-term complications, despite the known risks of hypoglycemia and weight gain.

Types of Insulin. The insulin formulations currently used for basal insulin treatment include intermediate-acting insulin (NPH) and long-acting insulin analogs (insulin glargine, insulin detemir).

Methods of Dosing and Titration. NPH, insulin glargine, or insulin detemir typically are recommended to be given in the evening with the goal of achieving near-normal glucose levels in the morning, although different dosing times (e.g., morning) and frequencies (e.g., twice daily) may be indicated in select patients. Dosing in the evening is somewhat less likely to be associated with hypoglycemia than dosing at other times of the day. The dose usually can be titrated according to prebreakfast glucose levels, and starting the day with normal or near-normal glucose levels makes it easier to control glucose levels during the day. Although most patients will not get 24-hour coverage with a single dose of NPH at bedtime, they often can achieve significant reductions in prebreakfast glucose levels, which improves how other oral or noninsulin injectable medications control glucose for the remainder of the day.[13] Insulin detemir has been effective when given once daily, but it may not provide 24-hour coverage in all patients, especially at lower doses; it is more likely to cover a 24-hour period as the dose increases.[14] Insulin glargine is the most likely to have 24-hour coverage, although clinical experience has shown that many patients may require insulin glargine more than once a day to optimize control.

Comparisons among the different basal insulin options have shown similar glycemic control, but slightly more hypoglycemia with NPH compared with detemir and glargine.[3] Initial trials with insulin detemir suggested that there was less weight gain with this agent,[15,16] but that has not been consistent in later studies, and current consensus does not include that as a reason to choose it over the other options.

Starting doses can be weight based (e.g., 0.1–0.2 units/kilogram [U/kg]) or empirical (e.g., 10–20 units), and the patient usually will have to advance the dose to achieve prebreakfast goals. There are several methods for titrating up the dose. First, a target blood glucose range should be chosen that is appropriate for the patient's symptoms, hypoglycemia risk, and overall glycemic goals. Glucose goals within the typical target ranges advocated by different guidelines, which generally fall between 70 and 130 mg/dl, are appropriate for most patients. Prebreakfast glucose levels of 75–100 or even 75–95 mg/dl have been targeted successfully in some research studies. Patients at risk for hypoglycemia, including those with hypoglycemic unawareness or with hypoglycemic symptoms at glucose values above the expected normal range, should be given higher target goals, such as 100–150 mg/dl before meals, to be more certain that very low glucose levels can be avoided. Titration can occur as frequently as every day when advancing the dose slowly to achieve fasting goals, or as infrequently as every 3 months to evaluate and target A1C goals. Most diabetes specialists favor more rapid titration using blood glucose target goals. Examples of titration schemes include increasing every day by 1–5 units until reaching glucose targets (smaller increases for patients using lower doses or closer to goals, larger increases for patients at higher dose or further from goals), increasing by 10% for patients near to target goals, or by 20% for those further from target goals, or according to tabulated titration schedules that have been effective in treating to target studies.[13,17-23]

Example 29.1 — Basal Insulin

A 45-year-old man with T2D on metformin and a sulfonylurea has an A1C level of 8.4% and feels "bad" if his sugar level is ~100 mg/dl, but he has newly elevated urinary albumin levels >30 mg/24 hours and he wishes to prevent long-term renal failure. He weighs 120 kg. Multiple options are discussed, and he and his health care provider choose to start basal insulin glargine at a dose of 20 units at bedtime. He is given an initial fasting glucose goal of 100–150 mg/dl and advised to advance the dose by 2 additional units every 2–3 days until his prebreakfast glucose is at goal. He calls back a week later and has advanced the dose to 32 units, and his prebreakfast glucose levels have decreased from 220 to 140 mg/dl without any reported hypoglycemia. After confirming that he is not consuming extra calories in the evening after dinner, he is advised to continue that dose. He calls back a week later saying that his prebreakfast glucose has risen again to 180 mg/dl. The dose is increased to 35 units, and he is instructed to increase by +5 units at a time every 2–3 days with a new prebreakfast glucose goal of 80–120 mg/dl. He increases the dose two times in the next week, and calls with reported prebreakfast glucose levels of 96, 114, and 124 over the past 3 days. He is advised to continue the current dose of insulin, record glucose levels at other times of the day, and to contact the provider if there are any hypoglycemic episodes.

Multidose Insulin: Basal-Bolus and Split-Mixed

Many patients require both basal and prandial insulin, including patients with advanced T2D, severe hyperglycemia, or other specific circumstances that preclude other oral or noninsulin injected therapies (e.g., pregnancy, side effects, or contraindications to oral and noninsulin injected therapies). Patients who cannot achieve optimal glycemic targets despite adequate titration of a basal insulin with or without other noninsulin injected medications, also would benefit from the addition of prandial insulin to basal insulin treatment.

A multidose insulin regimen can be prescribed in many ways. It is important to work with the patient to match the plan of therapy to his or her ability and willingness to adhere to the regimen. In general, using fewer injections requires the patient to adapt meals and physical activity to the insulin schedule, while using more injections can provide greater flexibility for the patient, allowing the patient to adapt the insulin schedule to the patient's lifestyle and schedule.

Types of Insulin

We will describe two main types of multidose insulin treatment: 1) basal-bolus insulin (basal insulin + prandial insulin) and 2) split-mixed insulin (NPH insulin + regular insulin twice daily; NPH + regular insulin in the morning, regular insulin before supper, and NPH at bedtime). Premixed formulations of 70/30 NPH/ regular or insulin aspart or 75/25 insulin lispro also may be used. In the basal-bolus regimen, a long-acting insulin (typically glargine or detemir, but less commonly NPH) provides basal insulin coverage, and a rapid-acting insulin (typically insulin lispro, insulin aspart, or insulin glulisine, but less commonly regular insulin) is added before meals to provide prandial coverage.

Despite the patient's initial preference, a chosen insulin plan may not be effective, and other options should be offered if there is excessive hypoglycemia or inadequate glycemic control, or if the patient's preferences, schedule, lifestyle, or comorbidities change.

Methods of Dosing and Titration

The dosing and titration of multidose insulin regimens are similar to those in patients with T1D (see Chapter 9). Some differences expected in patients with T2D typically include a requirement for higher doses, less dependence on 24-hour insulin coverage or precise mealtime doses (as patients have remaining β-cell function), continued benefit from concomitant oral agents, and less risk of hypoglycemia with less marked glycemic excursions.

Basal-Bolus Insulin Regimen. For the basal-bolus insulin regimen, long-acting insulins (e.g., glargine, detemir) provide basal coverage, usually starting once daily, and usually at bedtime, or sometimes twice a day to ensure 24-hour coverage. To minimize the risk of nocturnal hypoglycemia, it may be better to emphasize use of glargine at suppertime rather than at bedtime, but detemir usually is given at bedtime. A rapid-acting insulin analog or short-acting regular insulin is added before every meal to provide prandial coverage. When initiating a multidose regimen with long-acting basal insulin and rapid-acting analogs for bolus treatment, the usual starting total daily insulin dose is ≥0.5 U/kg, where ~50% (0.25 U/kg) is

[handwritten annotations at top of page:]

Basal regimens

80 kg. (0.1–0.2 U/kg)   8 U/d   glargine 8 U qhs. or NPH 8 U qhs

Basal Bolus Regimen

80 kg
40 U/d (0.5 U/kg)
20 U basal + 20 U bolus
20 U glargine qhs + 7 U lispro AC TID

6 Y

80 kg
40 U/d (0.5 U/kg)
10 U NPH + 30 U RI
10 U NPH qhs + 10 U RI AC TID

goal: 80–120 FBG   <180 AC

given as a daily dose of the basal insulin, and the remaining 50% is given in divided doses at mealtimes of the prandial, or bolus, insulin.

Example 29.2—Basal-Bolus Insulin Regimen

An 80-kg individual who is no longer adequately controlled with noninsulin agents for T2D is given the recommendation to start insulin. He prefers the flexibility of a basal-bolus regimen because he eats at different times of the day depending on his work schedule. The initial total daily dose is calculated as 40 units (0.5 U/kg), and distributed as 20 units (50% of the total daily dose) of basal insulin per day and 7 units (50% of the total daily dose, divided in three doses) before each meal. Basal insulin detemir is started at bedtime. He starts the insulin and is told to titrate the basal insulin to prebreakfast glucose goals of 80–120 mg/dl and the mealtime doses to keep postprandial glucose <180 mg/dl. He meets with a certified diabetes educator in the following week and has prebreakfast glucose levels in the 180–230 range. The basal insulin is increased to 24 units, and he is instructed to make further increases on his own until the prebreakfast glucose is at goal, increasing by 2 units at a time if the fasting glucose is above goal. Two weeks later, he has increased the basal insulin to 30 units, and mealtime insulin to 8 units to achieve the stated goals.

[handwritten: NPH]

A multidose regimen may use NPH insulin and regular insulin. The usual starting total daily insulin dose is the same as the regimens with long-acting insulin plus rapid-acting insulin analogs, but the distribution of the insulin doses may be different. Starting with a total daily insulin dose of ≥0.5 U/kg, the initial insulin doses commonly are divided equally across the four injections: one-quarter given as NPH insulin at bedtime, and one-quarter given as regular insulin before each of three meals. NPH insulin must be administered in the evening or at bedtime to provide overnight basal insulin coverage and cannot provide full 24-hour basal coverage unless also given at other times of day. Because of the extended duration of action of regular insulin compared with the rapid-acting analogs, regular insulin given before each of three meals not only provides prandial coverage but also provides some basal coverage between meals during the day. Giving NPH insulin at suppertime can increase the risk of hypoglycemia in the middle of the night, which coincides with a peak effect of NPH; this risk can be minimized by moving the NPH dose to bedtime.

Although multidose insulin regimens involve more frequent insulin injections, they also allow greater flexibility in the timing and number of meals. Patients are not required to eat three meals per day at regular times each day (if they skip a meal, they simply do not take rapid-acting analog insulin at that time), as opposed to the split-mixed regimen or use of premixed insulins discussed in the following section. Flexibility is somewhat limited using an NPH plus regular insulin regimen. Because the NPH insulin will not provide true 24-hour basal coverage, skipping a meal and the associated premeal bolus of regular insulin can create a period without insulin coverage.

The distribution of basal and bolus insulin doses varies depending on multiple factors, such as insulin resistance, meal size and carbohydrate proportions, and use of exogenous glucocorticoids. Recognizing that patients have different insulin sensitivities and meal patterns is important when choosing and titrating prandial insulin doses.

Split-Mixed Insulin Regimen. Some patients prefer fewer injections than required with basal-bolus regimens. This can be achieved by mixing an intermediate insulin (NPH) and a short- or rapid-acting insulin together in one injection (e.g., NPH insulin + regular insulin) before breakfast and before supper. By allowing the patients to mix two insulins with different pharmacodynamic profiles, the patient benefits from the combined effects of each insulin in a single injection. The mixed insulin regimen thus approximates both basal and prandial insulin coverage throughout the day while limiting injections to only two per day, split up typically before morning and evening meals.

This requires that patients conform their meal schedules to the time-action profiles of the insulin regimen: they must eat on a regular schedule every day, and match the mealtimes to the expected peak effects of the mixed insulin. Patients who are not able to maintain a consistent meal schedule to match mealtimes to the pharmacodynamics of the split-mixed regimen should consider the greater flexibility and adaptability of a basal-bolus regimen. Some patients who are new to insulin initially may benefit from the limited number of injections as they learn about and get used to using insulin.

The primary role of the health care provider is to match the doses of the split-mixed insulin regimen to the patient's schedule and insulin needs. Longer-acting analogs cannot be mixed with other insulins in the same syringe, and the rapid-acting analogs are approved only for mixing together in preformulated packaging. NPH and regular can be mixed together by the patient at independent doses.

Commonly, NPH and regular insulin are mixed and administered in the morning before breakfast and again before the evening meal. The regular insulin dose in the morning provides prandial coverage for breakfast, and the delayed peak and intermediate duration of the NPH insulin provides both daytime basal coverage and prandial coverage for a midday meal. In the second dose administered before supper, the regular insulin provides prandial coverage for the evening meal, and the NPH is intended to provide overnight basal coverage. As noted earlier, giving NPH insulin with the evening meal may—either as split-mixed or premixed insulin—increase the risk of hypoglycemia around 3:00 A.M. (because of the ~8-hour peak of NPH action). If this is a problem, the risk of nocturnal hypoglycemia can be reduced by giving the NPH insulin at bedtime. Premixed insulin, however, should not be given at bedtime except in individual cases in which patients eat late at night, requiring additional insulin.

The starting total daily insulin dose is the same as for the multidose insulin regimen (≥ 0.5 U/kg), which then traditionally is distributed as two-thirds given before breakfast and one-third given before supper; at each of these times, the dosage is divided two-thirds as NPH and one-third as regular insulin. This traditional approach, however, may not match the needs of the patient if supper is the much larger meal. If this is a problem, the distribution of the total daily insulin dose can be adjusted so that a relatively greater dose of regular insulin is given before the evening meal. Another consideration is that even though the breakfast meal tends to be smaller than the evening meal, patients may need more insulin in the morning because they are more insulin resistant at that time because of the dawn phenomenon, demanding a greater dose of both NPH and regular insulin in the morning.

As a first approximation, independent titration of the different doses can be done by taking into account the expected time course of the different doses of regular insulin and NPH, such that prebreakfast glucose measurements can be used to titrate the evening dose of NPH, late morning or prelunch glucose can be used to titrate the morning dose of regular insulin, afternoon or predinner glucose can be used to titrate the morning dose of NPH, and late night or bedtime blood glucose can be used to titrate the evening dose of regular insulin.

Patients must understand how to properly mix NPH and regular insulin. To avoid accidentally introducing any protamine from the NPH into the regular insulin vial, the best practice is to draw up regular insulin into the syringe first, followed by NPH insulin.

Example 29.3 — Split-Mixed Insulin Regimen

An 80-kg patient with T2D has suboptimal glycemic control on three oral agents, and now requires insulin treatment. He prefers to try just two shots of insulin a day to try to match three consistent meals a day. He is started with a total daily insulin dose of 40 units (0.5 U/kg). An initial dose might be 27 units before breakfast (two-thirds of the total daily dose) and 13 units before supper (one-third of the total daily dose). Of the 27 units given before breakfast, 18 units (two-thirds of the breakfast dose) of NPH would be mixed with 9 units (one-third of the breakfast dose) of regular insulin. Of the 13 units given before supper, 9 units (two-thirds of the supper dose) of NPH would be mixed with 4 units (one-third of the supper dose) of regular insulin. The patient sees a pharmacist and is instructed to draw the regular insulin into the syringe first before drawing the NPH into the same syringe, and injecting 30 minutes before breakfast and supper. The patient is instructed to record glucose levels four times a day and returns in a week to report average glucose levels. The prebreakfast glucose is 160 mg/dl, midday is 200 mg/dl, presupper is 200 mg/dl, and bedtime is 240 mg/dl. His largest meal is supper, and he has reduced the portions at lunch in an attempt to lose weight. He is advised to change the morning doses of NPH to 20 units, the morning dose of regular insulin to 10 units, the evening dose of regular insulin to 8 units, and the evening dose of NPH to 10 units.

OTHER OPTIONS

Premixed Formulations

The premixed insulin formulations have intermediate- and either rapid- or short-acting insulin premixed in a vial or pen. These formulations essentially allow patients to administer a split-mixed insulin regimen without having to manually mix the two insulin doses. The currently available premixed formulations include NPH insulin plus regular insulin (70/30 NPH/regular, 50/50 NPH/regular), aspart protamine plus aspart (70/30 Novolog), and lispro protamine plus lispro (75/25 Humalog, 50/50 Humalog). The 70/30, 75/25, and 50/50 insulin formulations provide a mixture of 70% of the intermediate-acting insulin with 30% of the short-acting insulin, 75% intermediate-acting insulin with 25% short-acting insulin, and 50% intermediate-acting insulin with 50% short-acting insulin, respectively.

As with the split-mixed insulin regimen discussed previously, the premixed insulins, in theory, provide a biphasic insulin profile in which the initial peak corresponds to the timing of the rapid- or short-acting insulin, and the peak of the intermediate-acting insulin is expected 6–8 hours later, with an overall period of coverage typically expected to be ~12–14 hours. Premixed insulin formulations typically are administered twice per day and work best in patients who have consistent schedules, do not need precise dose adjustments, are not able to mix doses of insulin on their own, are not able to perform multiple daily injections, or have higher glucose goals. Because of problems with hypoglycemia, it is more difficult to achieve A1C levels <7 or <6.5% with premixed insulins.[24] A common approach to initiating the premixed insulins is to use a slightly larger dose in the morning and a lower dose in the evening (e.g., two-thirds in the morning and one-third in the evening, as with the split-mixed regimen). Ideally the doses should be chosen to match the timing and size of the patients' meals. For example, more equivalent doses might be used twice a day in patients who eat just two reasonably small meals a day or who have a pattern of eating multiple small meals spread out consistently through the day.

The 50/50 premixed insulin formulations are not used as commonly as the 70/30 or 75/25 premixed formulations. The 50/50 premixed insulin is effective mainly for patients who eat relatively large meals or eat only two meals a day.

One limitation of the premixed formulations of insulin is the inability to adjust the doses differentially to match basal and prandial needs. Consequently, an increase in the dose will increase both the intermediate-acting and rapid- or short-acting insulin doses. For example, it would be difficult to optimally adjust the dose of a premixed formulation given in the morning in a patient who has near-normal prelunch glucose but elevated pre-supper glucose. In this example, increasing the morning insulin dose to achieve pre-supper glucose goals puts the patient at risk for pre-lunch hypoglycemia, but making no dose changes allows persistent pre-supper hyperglycemia with overall suboptimal glycemic control.

High-Concentration Insulin U-500

Some patients with T2D have very high insulin needs requiring large doses of insulin. Once the injection doses become larger than the volume capacity of typical insulin syringes, or the subcutaneous insulin depots become uncomfortably large for the patient, it may be preferable to use a more concentrated form of insulin. Currently, regular human insulin is available in a concentrated formulation, called U-500 (5 times the concentration of the standard U-100 formulations, or 500 U/ml). Use of concentrated insulin has been advocated in some patients who require >200 U/day of insulin, or in any patient who cannot comfortably inject enough insulin using the standard preparations. Typical dosing schedules are two to three times a day before the main meals, and doses should be titrated by matching daily eating habits to conform to insulin action and checking premeal glucose levels to avoid hypoglycemia. The pharmacodynamic profile of U-500 regular insulin is between that of regular and NPH insulin,[25,26] and patients may have to adjust their meals to match the times when it is most active a few hours after injecting.

Insulin Pumps

Insulin pumps typically are used in patients with T1D, but they can be effective and used under the same guiding principles in patients with T2D. Higher doses of insulin may be required. Insulin pumps are discussed in greater detail in Chapter 11.

ADVERSE EFFECTS OF INSULIN

HYPOGLYCEMIA IN PATIENTS WITH T2D TREATED WITH INSULIN

Hypoglycemia is the main risk factor when using insulin. Patients, or their caregivers, should be educated about typical symptoms of hypoglycemia and appropriate urgent treatment, which is discussed in detail in Chapter 40. Hypoglycemia in the setting of insulin therapy may be reduced with long-acting relatively peakless analogs instead of NPH as basal insulin. Likewise, rapid-acting analogs are associated with less hypoglycemia compared with regular insulin as mealtime insulin. Although there is debate regarding the utility of self-monitoring of blood glucose in patients with T2D on oral agents,[27,28] consensus is clear that it is necessary to ensure safety and safely titrate therapy when using insulin. In addition to short-term adverse effects of hypoglycemia, recognition is emerging that tight glycemic goals in patients at high risk for cardiovascular disease may increase the risk of hypoglycemia, and these tight goals are associated with worse outcomes when hypoglycemia is encountered.[29,30] Therefore, it is appropriate to reduce intensification in patients with cardiovascular risk and recurrent hypoglycemia.

WEIGHT GAIN IN PATIENTS WITH T2D TREATED WITH INSULIN

Because insulin promotes glucose uptake in insulin-dependent tissues, and thereby reduces energy lost through glucosuria, any excess carbohydrate consumption beyond metabolic needs is likely to be stored predominantly as fat. Therefore, patients may expect that effective insulin therapy in the absence of eating less is likely to lead to weight gain. There is newly evolving understanding of the neurological and psychological regulation of eating that is affected by insulin and insulin resistance that likely contributes as well.

INSULIN ALLERGY

All formulations of insulin are generally well tolerated, particularly because currently available recombinant human insulins and insulin analogs have effectively replaced the previous animal-insulin formulations. Clinically significant allergies to the newer formulations of insulin may still occur, however, although at a frequency far less than previously experienced with the animal-based insulin formulations. Case reports of reactions to the protamine in NPH or the new analogs continue, but they occur at a low enough frequency as to greatly reduce the prior concern for insulin allergies, which was more prominent in past recommendations of using insulin in T2D.

LIPOHYPERTROPHY AND LIPOATROPHY

Nonallergic injection site reactions may occur, especially if injections are given repeatedly at the same site. Fatty tissue in the subcutaneous space may have an atrophic, fibrotic, or hypertrophic response, which can be detected on physical examination and is associated with inconsistent insulin absorption and action. Patients should be advised to rotate injection sites to avoid this problem and to avoid any sites at which visible or palpable abnormalities have developed.

IMPORTANT CONSIDERATIONS

INSULIN INITIATION EARLIER IN THE NATURAL HISTORY

Although most patients and many clinicians view insulin as a treatment of "last resort" for T2D, there are important reasons for considering insulin earlier in the disease. In addition to improving glycemic control, insulin is one of the few agents with documented benefit in reducing long-term complications of T2D. Moreover, exogenous insulin is an effective method of providing rest to the β-cells with subsequent preservation of β-cell function, which has been associated with better long-term glycemic control.[31] One randomized controlled trial investigated the effect of short-term intensive glycemic control, comparing insulin and oral hypoglycemic agents in patients newly diagnosed with diabetes.[32] After rapid correction of hyperglycemia followed by a 2-week maintenance period of normoglycemia, study medications were discontinued, and patients were monitored for remission or relapse of diabetes based on fasting and 2-hour postchallenge glucose levels. Intensive insulin treatment was associated with a 31–44% relative risk reduction for relapse at 1 year compared with treatment with oral agents, with improved acute insulin responses after 1 year. These findings were confirmed in another study which investigated similar outcomes but with a longer treatment period with basal insulin.[33] Patients with T2D treated with metformin were given additional glargine insulin for 8 weeks. Both first- and second-phase insulin secretion increased significantly, demonstrating improved β-cell function with early insulin treatment. The ORIGIN study of insulin glargine in patients with prediabetes also demonstrated a 30–35% reduction in progression to diabetes, presumably because of preservation of β-cell function.[34] Given this potential benefit of insulin therapy in these studies of early T2D, safe use of insulin in patients with a low risk of hypoglycemia earlier in the natural history of the disease can begin with a dosage of 0.1–0.15 units of glargine or detemir insulin given once a day in the evening, titrated to achieve normal glucose levels (75–100 mg/dl) before breakfast.

"ATYPICAL" TIME COURSES OF INSULIN ACTION

The pharmacodynamic profiles for each insulin formulation generally remain similar from patient to patient. Significant variability in the action of some of the insulin formulations can occur, however, which affect the peak and duration of action. Understanding the common variations in the action of the available insulin formulations is important when using insulin.

NPH Insulin

Although the frequently quoted average peak of action for NPH insulin is 6–8 hours with a duration of 12–20 hours, in some patients, the peak occurs as soon as 3–4 hours after injection. In these patients, the earlier peak can be associated with pre-lunch hypoglycemia when NPH is given as part of a split-mixed or premixed regimen before breakfast and with bedtime or early nocturnal hypoglycemia at 1:00–2:00 a.m. when NPH is given before supper. In such cases, switching to basal-bolus regimens with other insulin analogs may be needed.

Insulin Glargine

For most patients, insulin glargine provides relatively peakless action that lasts for nearly 24 hours.[35] Particularly at lower doses, however, the action of glargine insulin may not extend for the entire 24-hour period, but rather may fall short at 18–20 hours, or may have modest dose-dependent peaking effects several hours after administration.[36]

If the duration of glargine insulin action is shorter than usual, patients may report that when glargine is administered before the evening meal, glucose levels are consistently high the following afternoon (as the insulin levels wane). Further proof of short duration of action can be obtained if there is a rise in glucose levels from post-lunch to pre-supper. In such cases, better control can be obtained if the basal insulin is split into two doses, one given in the morning and the other at night.

Some patients may benefit from taking insulin glargine before the evening meal instead of bedtime, because they experience an early peak of insulin action. Such an early peak can present as hypoglycemia during the night when glargine is given at bedtime, and can prevent increasing the dose to achieve pre-breakfast glycemic goals. This problem can be alleviated by moving the insulin glargine from bedtime dosing to pre-supper or by switching from insulin glargine to insulin detemir. Dosing insulin glargine at earlier times of the day, including before breakfast, has been similarly effective in clinical trials with some reduction in nocturnal hypoglycemia.[37,38]

In addition, some patients taking glargine before supper and titrating dosage according to the pre-breakfast glucose levels may experience problems with hypoglycemia before supper. This may be due to a combination of diet, physical activity, and waning of morning insulin resistance (due to the dawn phenomenon, which is rare in T2D).[39] In such patients, control can be improved by replacing the glargine with other basal insulins, such as insulin detemir, that can be given twice a day.

Insulin Detemir

Although insulin detemir was developed as a once-daily basal insulin, the duration of action, especially at lower doses, is often shorter than 24 hours.[40] Therefore, twice-daily dosing of insulin detemir may be needed.

CONCLUSION

Even with the many new pharmacologic developments of oral and noninsulin injectable medications for the treatment of T2D, insulin therapy remains a standard and effective treatment for achieving glycemic control. The indications for insulin therapy are varied and range from β-cell failure late in T2D, to severe hyperglycemia at the first clinical presentation and disease diagnosis, or even preservation of β-cell function early in the disease. Insulin therapy consistently achieves glycemic goals and may delay the progression of the course of the disease, while preventing microvascular complications. With the newer insulin analogs, the benefits of insulin treatment usually should be more attainable with minimal risk of hypoglycemia when prescribed appropriately, according to the pharmacodynamics of the insulin formulation and tailored individually to the patient's needs.

REFERENCES

1. Bazzano LA, Lee LJ, Shi L, Reynolds K, Jackson JA, Fonseca V. Safety and efficacy of glargine compared with NPH insulin for the treatment of type 2 diabetes: a meta-analysis of randomized controlled trials. *Diabet Med* 2008;25:924–932.

2. Mannucci E, Monami M, Marchionni N. Short-acting insulin analogues vs. regular human insulin in type 2 diabetes: a meta-analysis. *Diabetes Obes Metab* 2009;11:53–59.

3. Monami M, Marchionni N, Mannucci E. Long-acting insulin analogues versus NPH human insulin in type 2 diabetes: a meta-analysis. *Diabetes Res Clin Pract* 2008;81:184–189.

4. Rosenstock J, Fonseca V, McGill JB, Riddle M, Halle JP, Hramiak I, Johnston P, Davis M. Similar progression of diabetic retinopathy with insulin glargine and neutral protamine Hagedorn (NPH) insulin in patients with type 2 diabetes: a long-term, randomised, open-label study. *Diabetologia* 2009;52:1778–1788.

5. Rys P, Pankiewicz O, Lach K, Kwaskowski A, Skrzekowska-Baran I, Malecki MT. Efficacy and safety comparison of rapid-acting insulin aspart and regular human insulin in the treatment of type 1 and type 2 diabetes mellitus: a systematic review. *Diabetes Metab* 2011;37:190–200.

6. Lankisch MR, Ferlinz KC, Leahy JL, Scherbaum WA. Introducing a simplified approach to insulin therapy in type 2 diabetes: A comparison of two single-dose regimens of insulin glulisine plus insulin glargine and oral antidiabetic drugs. *Diabetes Obes Metab* 2008;10:1178–1185.

7. Owens DR, Luzio SD, Sert-Langeron C, Riddle MC. Effects of initiation and titration of a single pre-prandial dose of insulin glulisine while continuing titrated insulin glargine in type 2 diabetes: a 6-month 'proof-of-concept' study. *Diabetes Obes Metab* 2011;13:1020–1027.

8. Evans M, Schumm-Draeger PM, Vora J, King AB. A review of modern insulin analogue pharmacokinetic and pharmacodynamic profiles in type 2 diabetes: improvements and limitations. *Diabetes Obes Metab* 2011;13:677–684.

9. Home PD, Fritsche A, Schinzel S, Massi-Benedetti M. Meta-analysis of individual patient data to assess the risk of hypoglycaemia in people with type 2 diabetes using NPH insulin or insulin glargine. *Diabetes Obes Metab* 2010;12:772–779.

10. Korytkowski M, Bell D, Jacobsen C, Suwannasari R. A multicenter, randomized, open-label, comparative, two-period crossover trial of preference, efficacy, and safety profiles of a prefilled, disposable pen and conventional vial/syringe for insulin injection in patients with type 1 or 2 diabetes mellitus. *Clin Ther* 2003;25:2836–2848.

11. Inzucchi SE, Bergenstal RM, Buse JB, Diamant M, Ferrannini E, Nauck M, Peters AL, Tsapas A, Wender R, Matthews DR. Management of hyperglycaemia in type 2 diabetes: a patient-centered approach. Position statement of the American Diabetes Association (ADA) and the European Association for the Study of Diabetes (EASD). *Diabetologia* 2012;55:1577–1596.

12. Inzucchi SE, Bergenstal RM, Buse JB, Diamant M, Ferrannini E, Nauck M, Peters AL, Tsapas A, Wender R, Matthews DR, American Diabetes Association, European Association for the Study of Diabetes. Management of hyperglycemia in type 2 diabetes: a patient-centered approach: position statement of the American Diabetes Association (ADA) and the European Association for the Study of Diabetes (EASD). *Diabetes Care* 2012;35:1364–1379.

13. Riddle MC, Rosenstock J, Gerich J, Insulin Glargine Study. The treat-to-target trial: randomized addition of glargine or human NPH insulin to oral therapy of type 2 diabetic patients. *Diabetes Care* 2003;26:3080–3086.

14. Swinnen SG, Simon AC, Holleman F, Hoekstra JB, Devries JH. Insulin detemir versus insulin glargine for type 2 diabetes mellitus. *The Cochrane Database of Systematic Reviews* 2011:CD006383.

15. Hollander P, Cooper J, Bregnhoj J, Pedersen CB. A 52-week, multinational, open-label, parallel-group, noninferiority, treat-to-target trial comparing insulin detemir with insulin glargine in a basal-bolus regimen with mealtime insulin aspart in patients with type 2 diabetes. *Clin Ther* 2008;30:1976–1987.

16. Rosenstock J, Davies M, Home PD, Larsen J, Koenen C, Schernthaner G. A randomised, 52-week, treat-to-target trial comparing insulin detemir with insulin glargine when administered as add-on to glucose-lowering drugs in insulin-naive people with type 2 diabetes. *Diabetologia* 2008;51:408–416.

17. Blonde L, Merilainen M, Karwe V, Raskin P, TITRATE Study Group. Patient-directed titration for achieving glycaemic goals using a once-daily basal insulin analogue: an assessment of two different fasting plasma glucose targets—the TITRATE study. *Diabetes Obes Metab* 2009;11:623–631.

18. Davies M, Storms F, Shutler S, Bianchi-Biscay M, Gomis R. Improvement of glycemic control in subjects with poorly controlled type 2 diabetes: compari-

son of two treatment algorithms using insulin glargine. *Diabetes Care* 2005;28:1282–1288.

19. Gerstein HC, Yale JF, Harris SB, Issa M, Stewart JA, Dempsey E. A randomized trial of adding insulin glargine vs. avoidance of insulin in people with type 2 diabetes on either no oral glucose-lowering agents or submaximal doses of metformin and/or sulphonylureas. The Canadian INSIGHT (Implementing New Strategies with Insulin Glargine for Hyperglycaemia Treatment) Study. *Diabet Med* 2006;23:736–742.

20. Hermansen K, Davies M, Derezinski T, Martinez Ravn G, Clauson P, Home P. A 26-week, randomized, parallel, treat-to-target trial comparing insulin detemir with NPH insulin as add-on therapy to oral glucose-lowering drugs in insulin-naive people with type 2 diabetes. *Diabetes Care* 2006;29:1269–1274.

21. Kennedy L, Herman WH, Strange P, Harris A, Team GA. Impact of active versus usual algorithmic titration of basal insulin and point-of-care versus laboratory measurement of HbA1c on glycemic control in patients with type 2 diabetes: the Glycemic Optimization with Algorithms and Labs at Point of Care (GOAL A1C) trial. *Diabetes Care* 2006;29:1–8.

22. Meneghini LF, Rosenberg KH, Koenen C, Merilainen MJ, Luddeke HJ. Insulin detemir improves glycaemic control with less hypoglycaemia and no weight gain in patients with type 2 diabetes who were insulin naive or treated with NPH or insulin glargine: clinical practice experience from a German subgroup of the PREDICTIVE study. *Diabetes Obes Metab* 2007;9:418–427.

23. Yki-Jarvinen H, Juurinen L, Alvarsson M, Bystedt T, Caldwell I, Davies M, Lahdenpera S, Nijpels G, Vahatalo M. Initiate Insulin by Aggressive Titration and Education (INITIATE): a randomized study to compare initiation of insulin combination therapy in type 2 diabetic patients individually and in groups. *Diabetes Care* 2007;30:1364–1369.

24. Rosenstock J, Ahmann AJ, Colon G, Scism-Bacon J, Jiang H, Martin S. Advancing insulin therapy in type 2 diabetes previously treated with glargine plus oral agents: prandial premixed (insulin lispro protamine suspension/lispro) versus basal/bolus (glargine/lispro) therapy. *Diabetes Care* 2008;31:20–25.

25. de la Pena A, Riddle M, Morrow LA, Jiang HH, Linnebjerg H, Scott A, Win KM, Hompesch M, Mace KF, Jacobson JG, Jackson JA. Pharmacokinetics and pharmacodynamics of high-dose human regular U-500 insulin versus human regular U-100 insulin in healthy obese subjects. *Diabetes Care* 2011;34:2496–2501.

26. Davidson MB, Navar MD, Echeverry D, Duran P. U-500 regular insulin: clinical experience and pharmacokinetics in obese, severely insulin-resistant type 2 diabetic patients. *Diabetes Care* 2010;33:281–283.

27. Malanda UL, Bot SD, Nijpels G. Self-Monitoring of blood glucose in noninsulin-using type 2 diabetic patients: it is time to face the evidence. *Diabetes Care* 2013;36:176–178.

28. Polonsky WH, Fisher L. Self-monitoring of blood glucose in noninsulin-using type 2 diabetic patients: right answer, but wrong question: self-monitoring of blood glucose can be clinically valuable for noninsulin users. *Diabetes Care* 2013;36:179–182.

29. Bonds DE, Miller ME, Bergenstal RM, Buse JB, Byington RP, Cutler JA, Dudl RJ, Ismail-Beigi F, Kimel AR, Hoogwerf B, Horowitz KR, Savage PJ, Seaquist ER, Simmons DL, Sivitz WI, Speril-Hillen JM, Sweeney ME. The association between symptomatic, severe hypoglycaemia and mortality in type 2 diabetes: retrospective epidemiological analysis of the ACCORD study. *BMJ* 2010;340:b4909. Accessed on 29 January 2014.

30. Duckworth W, Abraira C, Moritz T, Reda D, Emanuele N, Reaven PD, Zieve FJ, Marks J, Davis SN, Hayward R, Warren SR, Goldman S, McCarren M, Vitek ME, Henderson WG, Huang GD. Glucose control and vascular complications in veterans with type 2 diabetes. *N Engl J Med* 2009;360:129–139.

31. Retnakaran R, Zinman B. Short-term intensified insulin treatment in type 2 diabetes: long-term effects on β-cell function. *Diabetes Obes Metab* 2012;14(Suppl 3):161–166.

32. Weng J, Li Y, Xu W, Shi L, Zhang Q, Zhu D, Hu Y, Zhou Z, Yan X, Tian H, Ran X, Luo Z, Xian J, Yan L, Li F, Zeng L, Chen Y, Yang L, Yan S, Liu J, Li M, Fu Z, Cheng H. Effect of intensive insulin therapy on beta-cell function and glycaemic control in patients with newly diagnosed type 2 diabetes: a multicentre randomised parallel-group trial. *Lancet* 2008;371:1753–1760.

33. Pennartz C, Schenker N, Menge BA, Schmidt WE, Nauck MA, Meier JJ. Chronic reduction of fasting glycemia with insulin glargine improves first- and second-phase insulin secretion in patients with type 2 diabetes. *Diabetes Care* 2011;34:2048–2053.

34. Gerstein HC, Bosch J, Dagenais GR, Diaz R, Jung H, Maggioni AP, Pogue J, Probstfield J, Ramachandran A, Riddle MC, Ryden LE, Yusuf S. Basal insulin and cardiovascular and other outcomes in dysglycemia. *N Engl J Med* 2012;367:319–328.

35. Lepore M, Pampanelli S, Fanelli C, Porcellati F, Bartocci L, Di Vincenzo A, Cordoni C, Costa E, Brunetti P, Bolli GB. Pharmacokinetics and pharmacodynamics of subcutaneous injection of long-acting human insulin analog glargine, NPH insulin, and ultralente human insulin and continuous subcutaneous infusion of insulin lispro. *Diabetes* 2000;49:2142–2148.

36. Wang Z, Hedrington MS, Gogitidze N, Briscoe VJ, Richardson MA, Younk L, Nicholson W, Tate DB, Davis SN. Dose-response effects of insulin glargine in type 2 diabetes. *Diabetes Care* 2010;33:1555–1560.

37. Fritsche A, Schweitzer MA, Haring HU, Study G. Glimepiride combined with morning insulin glargine, bedtime neutral protamine Hagedorn insulin, or bedtime insulin glargine in patients with type 2 diabetes. A randomized, controlled trial. *Ann Intern Med* 2003;138:952–959.

38. Standl E, Maxeiner S, Raptis S. Once-daily insulin glargine administration in the morning compared to bedtime in combination with morning glimepiride in patients with type 2 diabetes: an assessment of treatment flexibility. *Horm Metab Res* 2006;38:172–177.

39. Carroll MF, Hardy KJ, Burge MR, Schade DS. Frequency of the dawn phenomenon in type 2 diabetes: implications for diabetes therapy. *Diabetes Technol Ther* 2002;4:595–605.

40. Plank J, Bodenlenz M, Sinner F, Magnes C, Gorzer E, Regittnig W, Endahl LA, Draeger E, Zdravkovic M, Pieber TR. A double-blind, randomized, dose-response study investigating the pharmacodynamic and pharmacokinetic properties of the long-acting insulin analog detemir. *Diabetes Care* 2005;28:1107–1112.

Chapter 30

Current and New Long-Acting Insulin Analogs in Development: The Quest for a Better Basal Insulin

David R. Owens, CBE, MD, FRCP
Julio Rosenstock, MD

Insulin remains the most effective and consistent means of controlling blood glucose levels in diabetes, limited only by hypoglycemia. Following the epoch-making discovery by Banting and Best in 1922,[1] rapid progress was made to escalate production and purification of insulin together with the development of various pharmaceutical formulations and modes of delivery in an attempt to mimic the pattern of endogenous insulin secretion, which has continued up to the present day.[2] The primary aim of exogenous insulin administration is to attempt to simulate the body's physiological insulin secretion, but most current advances fall short of mimicking physiologic delivery to the liver. Endogenous insulin secretion essentially is divided into two phases: a low-level "basal" component, when insulin is secreted continuously (~40% of total secretion over a 24-hour period); and a stimulated or "bolus" component, where additional insulin is secreted in response to nutrient intake.[3] Basal insulin secretion functions primarily to inhibit hepatic glucose production in the fasting state (especially overnight), whereas prandial-bolus insulin secretion combats the meal-related glycemic excursions. Depending on their duration of action, subcutaneously administered insulin can be classified as short-acting (prandial or bolus), intermediate-acting, long-acting (basal), or pre-mixed preparations. This chapter focuses on the evolution of basal insulin and basal insulin analog preparations, including those at an advanced stage of development (Table 30.1).

THE HISTORY OF INSULIN DEVELOPMENT

A simplified historic overview of the evolution of insulin preparations is represented in Figure 30.1. Soon after the availability of crude short-acting insulin, the first attempts were made to develop products with prolonged absorption to reduce the burden involved with the number of daily injections. Several substances, including gum arabic solutions and epinephrine, were added to insulin with the aim of delaying its absorption from the subcutis, but all were unsuccessful.[4] In the 1930s, insulin initially was complexed with protein (protamine) and zinc in an attempt to retard the absorption of insulin from the subcutaneous tissue. As a consequence, neutral protamine Hagedorn (NPH) was introduced in 1946, a formulation of insulin and protamine in "isophane" proportions (i.e., no excess of either protamine or insulin), which possessed an "intermediate" duration of action.[5] NPH insulin, considered to be a "breakthrough" at that time, quickly

DOI: 10.2337/9781580405096.30

Table 30.1 — Pharmacological Profile of Different Basal Insulins

Basal insulin classifica-tion	Insulin prep-aration	Onset (hours)*	Peak (hours)	Duration (hours)†	Within subject variability (CV%)‡	Timing of administration	References
Intermedi-ate or long-acting	NPH	1–3	4–6	12–16	68	Usually taken once- or twice-daily	[14, 15, 23, 56]
Long-acting analog	Glargine	0.5–2	Flat, no peak	~24	32–82	Usually taken once-daily at the same time every day	[14, 23, 53, 57, 74, 108]
	Detemir	0.5–2	Flat, no peak	~20	27	Usually taken once- or twice-daily	[15, 23, 53, 57]
	Degludec¶	NR	Flat, no peak	>42	20	Once-daily, any time of the day	[75, 79, 80]
	LY2605541	NR	Flat, no peak	>36	<18§	Once-daily	[106–108]
	U300	NR	Flat, no peak	>36	NR	Once-daily	[112–114]

Source: Table adapted from Rossetti et al.[64] Where possible, pharmacokinetic and phar-macodynamic data are based on subjects with T1D.

Note: CV = coefficient of variation; NPH = neutral protamine Hagedorn; NR = not reported.

*Onset of action based on definitions used in glucose clamp studies. Definition can vary between studies.

†Duration of action based on glucose clamp studies.

‡Within-subject (or intrasubject) variability (day-to-day variability) is expressed as the coef-ficient of variation (CV%) of the AUC-GIR study period from clamp studies.

¶Not available for clinical use in the U.S. Degludec is approved for use in some other countries.

§In healthy subjects.

became established as the main basal insulin during the twentieth century and was administered twice-daily in conjunction with short-acting insulin preparations in people with type 1 diabetes (T1D) and once- or twice-daily in those with type 2 diabetes (T2D) usually in addition to oral antidiabetic agents (OADs). A premixed formulation of NPH with soluble insulin also became available, almost retaining the properties of the individual components, and obviating the need to mix the

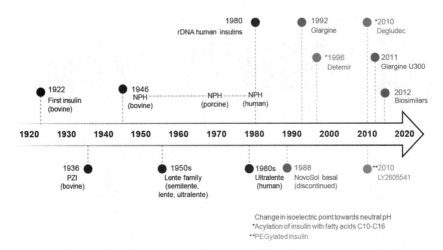

Figure 30.1—Start of timelines for the development of insulin formulations.

Notes: Species preparation, where relevant, is shown in parentheses. NPH = neutral protamine Hagedorn; PZI = protamine zinc insulin; rDNA = recombinant DNA.

short- and intermediate-acting insulins before administration. Shortly afterward, early in the 1950s, a series of protein-free insulin zinc suspensions were introduced, referred to as the lente family, i.e., semilente, lente, and ultralente insulins, possessing a short, intermediate, or long duration of action, respectively.[6]

For both NPH and the lente insulins, the initial source of extracted insulin was bovine pancreas. This later was superseded by porcine pancreas, which had reduced antigenicity and a shorter duration of action. Bovine ultralente had a large crystal structure (25 microns) that contributed to its prolonged duration of action and therefore was the first long-acting basal insulin suitable for a once-daily administration. As bovine ultralente was substantially antigenic, however, the insulin antibodies obtunded the action of the mealtime short-acting insulin. Considerable efforts continued to be made to improve the purity of the extracted insulin utilizing methods including recrystallization and gel filtration, and culminating in the emergence of monocomponent insulins in the 1970s.[7]

A further perceived "breakthrough" was the development of human insulin in the early 1980s, initially derived semisynthetically from porcine insulin.[8,9] Later, human insulin was produced biosynthetically by recombinant DNA (rDNA) technology, using either *Escherichia coli* or Saccharomyces vectors.[10–12] Subsequently, all insulin preparations were reformulated using human insulin, which possesses a shorter duration of action than the animal equivalent.[2] The need for resuspension of the turbid insulin suspensions before injection was a major limitation to the predictability and time-action characteristics of these preparations.[13] Human NPH has a gradual onset of action (within 1–3 hours), a peak effect at 4–6 hours, and a highly variable duration of action of 12–16 hours, which is influenced further by the dose and site of subcutaneous administration.[9,14,15] Its peak effect therefore can compound the action of the short-acting analogs and confer a propensity for hypoglycemia especially between meals and at nighttime. Consequently, to provide basal coverage over a 24-hour period, human NPH often is given twice-daily in people with T1D and once (pre-evening meal or before bedtime) or twice-daily in T2D. Despite these limitations, human NPH remains widely used in clinical practice, in part because of widespread availability and lower cost. Although human ultralente had a longer duration of action than NPH, it also was associated with larger day-to-day variability, erratic peaks, and consequently frequent episodes of hypoglycemia, resulting in discontinuation of this product.[9,14,16] These various limitations provided the stimulus to continue the search for soluble and longer-acting insulin preparations to better represent normal physiological basal insulin secretion (Box 30.1).[2,9]

The advent of rDNA technology in the 1980s allowed for the modification of the amino-acid sequence of human insulin to alter its time-action characteristics.[8,9] This led to the development of insulin analogs with pharmacokinetic and pharmacodynamic properties with additional benefits to that of previous human insulin preparations.[2]

CURRENT LONG-ACTING INSULIN ANALOGS

INSULIN GLARGINE

Initial efforts were focused on adjusting the isoelectric point of insulin toward a neutral pH, which resulted in precipitation of the insulin in the subcutaneous tissue, thereby delaying its absorption.[2] Eventually after a number of unsuccessful attempts, soluble insulin glargine (glargine) was developed and approved for commercial use, with a rate of absorption from the subcutaneous tissue much slower and flatter than that of NPH and negligibly influenced by the site of injection.[17]

Glargine is modified from human insulin in two ways: There is elongation of the C-terminal of the β-chain with retention of two di-arginyl molecules at position B30, and a substitution of asparagine with glycine at A21 (Figure 30.2). These changes alter the isoelectric point and improve the stability of this product.[18] Glargine remains soluble in the acidic pH (~4.5) of its pharmaceutical formulation, precipitating after injection into the neutral pH environment of the subcutaneous tissue, leading to a delay in absorption and thereby prolonging its duration of action.[2,17,19] In the subcutaneous tissue, glargine undergoes rapid transformation to two main active metabolites, M1 (Gly^{A21}) and M2 (Gly^{A21}, des-Thr^{B30}), with

---

Box 30.1—Ideal Features for a Basal Insulin
- A prolonged pharmacodynamic profile with at least 24-hour duration of action and without a discernible peak effect
- Simplicity of dose adjustments to achieve FPG <100 mg/dl
- Predictable action without intra- and interindividual variability
- Low risk of hypoglycemia
- Limited weight gain or some weight loss
- No undesirable cardiovascular or carcinogenic side effects
- Well tolerated in both T1D and T2D

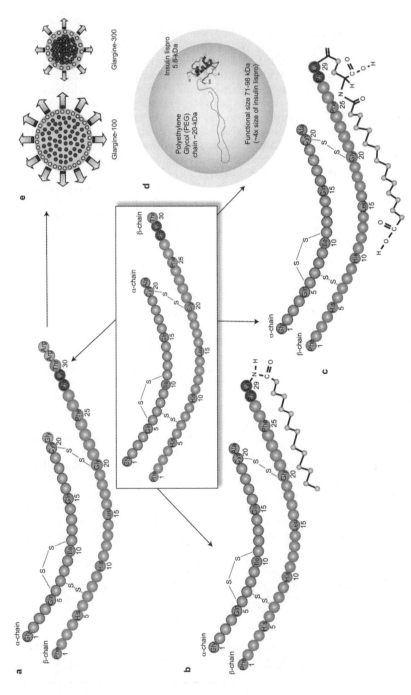

Figure 30.2—Strategies employed to develop long-acting basal insulins with prolonged in vivo half-lives. The primary, secondary, and ribbon structures of insulin with α- and β-chains that are held together by three disulphide bonds is indicated in the central panel. The surrounding panels show strategies employed to develop **a** | glargine; **b** | detemir; **c** | degludec; **d** | PEGylated Lispro (LY2605541) and **e** | glargine U300.

in vitro activity similar to that of human insulin.[20] These metabolites of glargine possess a very low affinity for the human insulin-like growth factor-1 receptor (IGF-1R) and a low mitogenic–metabolic potency ratio. The M1 metabolite predominates and accounts for ~90% of the daily plasma insulin absorbed into the systemic circulation.[21,22]

Glucose clamp studies have been used as the standard approach to study the pharmacokinetic and pharmacodynamic characteristics of insulin preparations (Table 30.1). In such studies, soluble glargine was shown to have a duration of action of up to 24 hours, a flatter time-action profile, and reduced variability, especially at the lower dose range, when compared with NPH,[14,23,24] thus enabling once-daily administration.

Many studies have demonstrated both in patients with T1D and T2D that glargine is as effective as NPH in lowering glycated hemoglobin (A1C) levels,[25,26] with a consistent reduced risk of symptomatic and nocturnal hypoglycemia.[27,28] The lower risk of hypoglycemia and the once-daily administration have facilitated the implementation of more intensive or systematic insulin dose titrations, resulting in greater proportions of patients achieving and maintaining target A1C levels.[2] Indeed, in people with T2D who are insufficiently controlled on OADs, the addition of basal glargine systematically titrated to target fasting plasma glucose (FPG) of <100 mg/dl (<5.5 mmol/l) often results in a significantly higher proportion of subjects achieving target A1C levels of <7% without hypoglycemia.[25,29] Perhaps one of the major contributions of glargine was the introduction of the concept of treat-to-target applied to FPG levels, which translated to a simple message of "fix fasting first" that facilitated the early initiation of insulin in T2D by general physicians. The majority of patients with T2D can be controlled adequately by once-daily injection if adequately titrated.[30,31] The added flexible timing of injection (morning, pre-dinner, or pre-bedtime),[32,33] and no need to eat at defined times,[34] provides convenience and treatment satisfaction.[35] Further long-term observational studies have demonstrated that glargine added to OADs can attain and sustain target A1C levels in T2D.[2,36] Also, the early introduction of glargine after the failure of diet and metformin has resulted in good control with a low risk of hypoglycemia and minimal weight gain.[37] Adequate dose titration to target FPG achieved and sustained good control in the majority of patients who failed on OADs from 3 months onward.[38] Increased cost compared with NPH, however, remains a barrier to more widespread use.

The long-term safety of glargine has been investigated in two trials. In a randomized controlled trial, there was no difference between NPH and glargine in the development or progression of microvascular disease (diabetic retinopathy) over 5 years.[39] The cardiovascular safety of glargine was evaluated in the recently reported ORIGIN trial, which involved 12,537 persons at high cardiovascular disease risk with either early T2D or prediabetes, randomized to treatment with glargine or standard care.[40] Following a median follow-up period of 6.2 years, glargine demonstrated a neutral effect with no adverse effect on cardiovascular outcomes (hazard ratio [HR] 1.02; 95% confidence interval [CI], 0.94–1.11; $P = 0.63$) despite a relatively low but still a threefold higher risk of hypoglycemia. Over the course of the study, 28% of those individuals with prediabetes were less likely to convert to diabetes ($P = 0.006$) if treated with glargine.

In 2009, four international studies highlighted a potential association between glargine and cancer, especially breast cancer.[41-44] Subsequent follow-up of larger epidemiologic studies, however, specifically designed to properly explore databases and a meta-analysis of randomized controlled trials, did not support such a link.[45-47] In addition, there was no excess risk of cancer on exposure to glargine in the ORIGIN trial (HR 1.00; $P = 0.97$).[40,48]

INSULIN DETEMIR

Insulin detemir (detemir) was the second basal analog developed using rDNA technology.[49] This is a first-generation acylated insulin derivative that differs from human insulin in two ways: deletion of amino acid threonine at position 30 of the β-chain and addition of 14-carbon aliphatic fatty acid to the ε amino group of lysine in position B29 (Figure 30.2). These changes enable detemir to slowly bind to and dissociate from the subcutaneous tissue and circulating albumin, resulting in a "floating depot" of multimeric complexes that prolong the duration of action.[50] The appended fatty acid chain is hypothesized to interfere with binding to the insulin receptor (IR), thereby lowering the potency of detemir and requiring detemir to be reformulated at a fourfold higher insulin concentration per unit relative to other insulin preparations (24 vs. 6 nmol/unit).[51,52]

Glucose clamp studies show that detemir has a flat, protracted time-action profile with a duration of action of ~20 hours depending how end-of-insulin action is defined (Table 30.2).[15,53,54] Several studies also indicate reduced day-to-day glucose variability, as measured by a smaller coefficient of variation of pharmacodynamic endpoints, compared with NPH and glargine, but the clinical relevance has been difficult to substantiate.[23,55,57] Clinical studies also show reduced day-to-day variability in self-measured FPG levels with detemir compared with NPH.[58-61] Other than a reduced propensity for hypoglycemia, particularly nocturnal hypoglycemia, and slightly less weight gain compared with NPH,[62] the clinical implications of the latter small effect on diabetes management are uncertain. In a study in subjects with T1D, the time-action profile for detemir at steady state was significantly shorter than that for glargine, 23.3 and 27.1 hours, respectively,[57] which is in keeping with evidence that a proportion of patients require two doses of detemir per day for optimal basal coverage. Not all clamp studies are infallible, however, and results may vary depending on the study population, methodology, and predefined definitions for start and end of insulin action.[63,64]

The efficacy and safety of detemir and glargine have been compared in many studies involving people with T1D and T2D.[65-71] In T1D, it has been demonstrated clearly that once- or twice-daily detemir achieves a similar improvement in glycemic control and risk of hypoglycemia to once-daily glargine.[2,65,66] In the first head-to-head study comparing detemir and glargine in insulin-naive subjects with T2D uncontrolled with OAD treatments, both preparations were commenced once-daily in the evening, although those on detemir were allowed to add a second dose in the morning if the pre-dinner glucose level was elevated once the FPG was controlled adequately.[2,67] At study end, both insulins achieved similar meaningful improvements in A1C but with detemir at the expense of ~30% higher insulin doses and 55% of the subjects necessitating twice-daily injections, whereas glargine remained on once-daily injection at bedtime as per study design. A sub-

Table 30.2 Comparative Pharmacology and Safety of Long-Acting Basal Insulin Analogs

	Glargine	Detemir	Degludec	LY2605541	U300 glargine
Structure	Retention of two, and substitution of one amino acid	Addition of acylated fatty acid chain at B29	Lack of B30; addition glutamic acid spacer and diacylated fatty acid chain at B29	Insulin lispro covalently bound, via a urethane bond at lysine B28, to a 20-kDa PEG chain	Not known
Mechanism of protraction of action	Precipitation at acidic pH in subcutis	Binding to albumin in subcutis and system circulation	Multi-hexamer chain formation in subcutis and albumin binding in systemic circulation	Increasing the hydrodynamic size of the insulin-PEG complex	Compact subcutis depot with a smaller surface area than glargine
Risk of hypoglycemia	Low	Low	Low	Low	Low
Risk of nocturnal hypoglycemia	Low	Low	Lowest	Low	Low
Risk of severe hypoglycemia	Low	Low	Low	Low	Low
Miscibility with short-acting insulin	No	Yes	Yes	Not known	Not known
Miscibility with GLP-1 receptor agonists	Yes	Yes	Yes	Not known	Not known
CV risk	No risk	Not known	Not known*	Not known	Not known
Cancer risk	No risk	Not known	Not known	Not known	Not known

Note: GLP-1 = glucagon-like peptide; CV = cardiovascular; PEG = polyethylene glycol.

*Approved in the EU and other countries but did not meet U.S. FDA requirements for cardiovascular safety.

sequent study comparing detemir twice-daily versus glargine once-daily from the time of randomization confirmed comparable efficacy with higher doses with detemir.[68] A more recent study, however, demonstrated that glycemic control was inferior with detemir when both basal insulins were randomized to a once-daily administration, as shown by significantly different final A1C levels with detemir and glargine (7.5 and 7.1%, respectively) and 38 and 53% of the patients, respectively, reaching target A1C ≤7%.[69] Weight decreased with detemir and increased with glargine (–0.5 kg and +1.0 kg, respectively) and hypoglycemia was slightly less with detemir, probably reflecting higher glucose control. When given together with short-acting insulin analogs in T2D (basal-bolus therapy), detemir (once- or twice-daily) and glargine (once-daily) were similar in terms of improving glycemic control and safety.[2,70,71] The evidence from trials shows that most patients require a higher dose of detemir than glargine[65–68,70]; indeed, in several trials twice-daily detemir dosing was used in a high proportion of such patients.[66,67,70] Weight gain is less, around –0.8 kg, with detemir than glargine when both are given once-daily; however, when detemir is administered twice-daily for equivalent efficacy, weight gain is similar to that seen with once-daily glargine.[2,69,71]

INSULIN DEGLUDEC

Insulin degludec (degludec), a second-generation acylated-soluble insulin analog, is the newest basal insulin analog to enter clinical practice following an extensive clinical development program that deserves expanded coverage. Currently, degludec is approved for use in Europe, Japan, and Mexico, but it is not yet approved in the U.S. (2014) for the reasons that will be discussed in the following paragraphs. Degludec is prepared by deletion of threonine at position B30 of human insulin and the attachment of a 16-carbon fatty diacyl chain to the B29 lysine residue with a glutamic acid as a spacer (Figure 30.2).[2,72] Degludec has a low affinity for the human IGF-1R, comparable with human insulin, and a low mitogenic–metabolic potency ratio.[73]

In its pharmaceutical formulation, degludec is a di-hexamer in the presence of zinc and phenol. Following subcutaneous injection, there is a rapid loss of phenol in the subcutis, which changes the configuration of degludec into soluble multi-hexamer chains. Then the zinc slowly diffuses from this complex, with these multi-hexamers breaking down into dimers and monomers before entering the systemic circulation.[2,72] The microprecipitation of the multi-hexamers in the sub-cutaneous tissue results in delayed absorption, which is the predominant mechanism underlying its prolonged duration of action profile. Reversible binding to circulating albumin also contributes, but to a lesser extent, to the prolongation of action.[74,75]

Degludec was developed at the standard concentration of 100 U/ml (600 nmol/ml) but also is available at a higher concentration of 200 U/ml (1200 nmol/ml) to accommodate the need of larger doses (up to 160 U) in a single insulin pen device. Degludec preparations should be titrated at 6 nmol/unit, equivalent to that for glargine. Significantly higher circulating insulin concentrations are bound to the albumin because of the long-chain fatty acid on the β-chain of degludec compared with glargine (6,000 vs. 50 pmol/l) although the free insulin component has not been determined.[76] Degludec also has been developed in combination with a rapid insulin analog (insulin aspart) in a soluble premixed formulation in a 70:30 ratio. It appears that this premixed formulation is not associated with the formation of hybrid hexamers that otherwise may lead to unpredictable and suboptimal pharmacokinetic profiles.[2,77]

Glucose clamp studies show that steady state is achieved after 2–3 days of multiple doses of once-daily degludec, with a stable flat pharmacokinetic–pharmacodynamic profile (Table 30.2).[74,75,78] It has been estimated that degludec has a half-life of ~25 hours, with an apparent residual action exceeding 42 hours, and it is measurable in the circulation for at least 120 hours (5 days) following subcutaneous administration.[75,79,80] The intra-subject variability appears to be lower compared with glargine in subjects with T1D.[74]

A large number of randomized, open-label, multicenter, treat-to-target trials (active control over 6–12 months) have evaluated the efficacy and safety of degludec in both T1D[81–83] and T2D,[84–90] mainly versus glargine. The primary efficacy endpoint in all these trials was A1C. Insulin doses were adjusted once-weekly according to self-monitored pre-breakfast blood glucose to achieve aggressive fasting glucose target values of 70–90 mg/dl (4–5 mmol/l), which are lower than previous treat-to-target trials conducted with glargine.[2] Whereas degludec was administered consistently at dinnertime, the time of administration of glargine, although not recorded, was presumed to be at bedtime.[2] In addition, two trials have compared degludec versus detemir (initially given in the evening with a second dose at breakfast if needed) [NCT00978627] or versus the dipeptidyl peptidase-4 inhibitor sitagliptin.[90]

All the comparative trials confirmed degludec as non-inferior to glargine for the change from baseline in A1C.[2] In T1D, the mean reduction in A1C at endpoint (6–12 months) generally was smaller (<1%) than in T2D (>1%), in part because of the lower baseline values for the former group.[91] The FPG was lowered more with degludec than glargine, detemir, or sitagliptin at the end of the active treatment period,[91] although this did not reach statistical significance in 6 of the 11 trials.[2]

In addition, 2 trials (one each in T1D and T2D) utilized flexible dosing intervals of ~8–40 hours by alternating doses of degludec given in the morning or evening on successive days, and compared with consistent once-daily dosing with degludec or glargine.[2,83,87] In both trials, the flexible dosing regimen did not compromise glycemic control (A1C and FPG) or safety (similar hypoglycemia) versus either comparator, and therefore offered the possibility of dosing flexibility, which may or may not improve patient adherence. In contrast, a three-times-weekly regimen for degludec (either in the morning or evening) was less effective in lowering blood glucose and was accompanied by higher rates of hypoglycemia when compared with once-daily glargine,[91] leading to discontinuation of the development of this regimen program.

Although weight gain tended to be slightly greater with degludec than glargine or detemir in most trials, this did not reach statistical significance at the end of treatment.[2] The mean total daily insulin dose was slightly lower with degludec than comparator treatments in all except two of the trials in T2D.[85,87] Whereas smaller insulin doses normally are associated with lesser reductions in A1C and fewer hypoglycemic episodes,[91] these relationships did not occur in a consistent manner across the trials.

The definition of "confirmed" hypoglycemia across all the trials was a plasma glucose of <56 mg/dl (3.1 mmol/l), irrespective of symptoms, as well as severe events requiring assistance from another person.[2,92] This definition differs from that advocated by the American Diabetes Association, which requires both the presence of clinical symptoms of hypoglycemia and documented evidence of a low plasma glucose, albeit at a higher threshold of ≤70 mg/dl (3.9 mmol/l).[92,93] Also, "confirmed" nocturnal hypoglycemia was defined as events occurring between 00:01 and 05:59 (a 6-hour time period).

A small but statistically significant reduction in the rate of confirmed hypoglycemia events (number of events per patient-year of exposure), mainly nocturnal hypoglycemia, was seen with degludec versus comparators in several trials.[2] However, the rates of overall, nocturnal, and severe confirmed hypoglycemia were inconsistent between trials and the magnitude of the absolute differences were relatively small. In T2D on basal insulin only, rates of overall confirmed hypoglycemia were similar for degludec and glargine.[84,86–88,90] There were no obvious differences in the rates of overall confirmed hypoglycemia episodes observed between degludec (fixed or flexible dosing) or degludec–aspart and the comparator insulins.[2]

Across trials, there was a numerically smaller rate of nocturnal confirmed hypoglycemic episodes recorded with degludec versus comparator, which reached statistical significance in several trials.[2] There was some inconsistency in rates of nocturnal confirmed hypoglycemia between individual trials, however. It also has been suggested that this difference may be artifactual, reflecting differences in the timing of administration of the comparator insulins.[2,91] Degludec was administered consistently with the evening meal in all trials with peak glucose lowering as expected 12 hours later. In contrast, glargine was most likely given predominantly at bedtime with maximal levels achieved ~4–12 hours later (i.e., during the time period for measuring nocturnal events). Other proposed explanations include familiarity with the comparator product, overaggressive FBG targets, or missing data.[2,91]

A meta-analysis of seven Phase III trials indicated that the relative risk of confirmed hypoglycemia, overall (risk ratio [RR] 0.91; 95% CI 0.83–0.99) and nocturnal (RR 0.74; 95% CI 0.65–0.85), was lower with degludec than glargine in the combined patient population of T1D and T2D, but the differences in absolute numbers were small.[2,94] Subsequent subgroup analyses of the data indicated clear geographic differences.[84] In the U.S. subgroup of whom 64% had T1D, no differences in the rate of overall confirmed hypoglycemia were observed between degludec and glargine.[91] Differences in overall hypoglycemia were seen clearly in patients with T2D but not in those with T1D. Similarly, the rate of nocturnal confirmed hypoglycemia was lower with degludec compared with glargine only in T2D (RR 0.68; 95% CI 0.57–0.82) and equivalent in T1D (RR 0.83; 95% CI 0.69–1.00).[94] Importantly, there was no difference in the percentage of patients achieving an A1C target <7% without hypoglycemia.[95]

The degludec Phase III program included a premixed formulation of degludec-aspart. These trials compared premixed degludec-aspart with once- or twice-daily detemir in T1D,[96] and twice-daily premixed insulin (biphasic-aspart 30/70)[97,98] or once-daily glargine[82,99] in people with T2D.[2] The degludec-aspart preparation was administered once- or twice-daily with dinner or before the largest meal of the day. In subjects with T1D, aspart also was given before the remaining meals and compared with standard basal-bolus therapy using detemir and aspart.[96] The fixed combination of degludec-aspart was found to be non-inferior to the insulin comparators (detemir, glargine, or premixed 70/30) in all trials,[2] although in one trial in Japanese subjects with T1D, A1C was significantly lower with degludec-aspart than with once-daily glargine.[99]

As part of the U.S. Federal Drug Administration (FDA) regulatory approval process, a prespecified meta-analysis of trial data was performed. Degludec (either alone or in combination with aspart) initially was associated with a possible 10% increase in the risk of major adverse cardiovascular events, including nonfatal myocardial infarction, nonfatal stroke, and cardiovascular death (MACE) plus unstable angina (MACE+) (HR 1.10; 95% CI 0.68–1.77; incidence rate 1.48 vs. 1.44 events per 100 patient-years of exposure) relative to active comparators.[2,82] This estimate was based on only 80 cases over 5,444 patient-years of exposure and included events up to 7 days after drug discontinuation. Further updated analyses, including additional ongoing long-term extension data from these trials capturing more cardiovascular events (132 cases over 7,716 patient-years of exposure), showed further worsening of the HRs with all 95% upper-bound CI crossing the 1.8 limit necessary for FDA drug approval with varying results, depending on the definition of MACE (inclusion or exclusion of unstable angina).[2,82,91] On the basis of these findings, the FDA requested additional cardiovascular data from a dedicated cardiovascular outcomes trial before degludec could be approved in the U.S.[2,100] In contrast, the Japanese and European regulatory agencies concluded from the data presented by the sponsor, without separate statistical analyses, that there was no indication of increased cardiovascular risk with degludec and approved its use.[95] Debate continues about the potential cardiovascular risk of degludec.[101] This is only likely to be resolved when results of a randomized, double-blind, cardiovascular outcome trial (DEVOTE; NCT01959529) versus glargine in ~7,500 patients with T2D become available. Data from an interim analysis are anticipated within 2–3 years presumably for registration purposes.

POTENTIAL FUTURE BASAL INSULIN ANALOGS

PEGYLATED LISPRO (LY2605541)

LY2605541 is a long-acting insulin that comprises insulin lispro covalently bound, via a urethane bond at lysine B28, to a 20-kDa polyethylene glycol (PEG) chain, thereby increasing the hydrodynamic size of the insulin-PEG complex (Figure 30.2).[2,102] This large size delays insulin absorption from the site of subcutaneous injection and also reduces renal clearance, which collectively results in a prolongation of action. LY2605541 has a lower binding affinity for the IR and IGF-1R than lispro, and a lower mitogenic potency than human insulin.[103] A labeled-clamp study in dogs suggests that LY2605541 may have a hepatoselective action on glucose metabolism,[104] similar to that seen with endogenous insulin and in contrast to other exogenous insulins that have a preference for action in peripheral tissues.[105] It has been suggested that because of its much larger size, this insulin may have greater liver access through the fenestrated hepatic sinusoidal endothelium and lesser transport through the peripheral endothelium, resulting in higher insulin action and exposure to the liver than to the muscle and adipose tissues.

Glucose clamp studies in patients with T2D show that steady-state is achieved in 7–10 days after multiple doses of once-daily LY2605541 with low peak-to-trough fluctuation, resulting in a flat glucose infusion rate (GIR) profile and duration of action longer than 24 hours.[106,107] The estimated half-life was ~2–3 days (45–75 hours) depending on dose, with low intra-patient variability. In healthy individuals, a single dose of LY2605541 showed a relatively flat GIR profile that was sustained for >36 hours.[108]

In Phase II clinical trials in T1D and T2D (12–16 weeks treatment duration),[109,110] LY2605541 achieved glycemic control relatively comparable to glargine with some minor differences but mostly similar rates of overall hypoglycemia. Rates of intraday blood glucose variability, nocturnal hypoglycemia, and weight loss, however, were significantly better with LY2605541 than with glargine. More specifically, in the T1D short-term crossover trial, mean glucose levels, fasting blood glucose variability, and A1C were slightly but significantly reduced with LY2605541 compared with insulin glargine, but total hypoglycemia rate was higher for LY2605541 and the nocturnal hypoglycemia rate was lower compared with glargine.[103] Data from a subset of patients with T2D who underwent continuous glucose monitoring suggested that LY2605541 is associated with reduced blood glucose variability versus glargine.[111] An interesting finding with LY2605541 is the modest weight loss noted previously that contrasts with the small weight gain usually seen with glargine. The 8-week Phase II crossover study in T1D also demonstrated a small but significant reduction in prandial insulin doses, probably reflecting longer and better basal insulin coverage during daytime.[110]

Modest elevations in liver enzymes, triglyceride, and LDL-cholesterol levels, although still within the normal range, were observed with LY2605541, but the clinical significance of these changes is uncertain. Ongoing Phase III trials in T1D and T2D will include additional hepatic function monitoring and careful characterization of lipid changes.

An extensive Phase III trial program involving eight pivotal studies in T1D and T2D (IMAGINE trials I to VII and one trial in Asia, involving ~6,000 patients) is underway with first results expected in 2014. Several of the trials are powered for assessment of the risk of hypoglycemia. For the first time in an insulin development program, several of the IMAGINE trials are being conducted in a double-blind fashion that will generate valuable comparative data, especially for the analyses of differences in hypoglycemia.

GLARGINE U300

Glargine U300 (U300) is a new higher-strength formulation of glargine at 300 U/ml rather than the usual 100 U/ml, which alters its pharmacokinetic and pharmacodynamic properties (Figure 30.2).[2] Following subcutaneous injection, U300 forms a compact subcutaneous depot with a smaller surface area, which results in more gradual and prolonged release from the subcutaneous depot when compared with glargine.[2]

Glucose clamp studies in patients with T1D show that U300 has a flat pharmacokinetic and pharmacodynamic profile (low peak-to-trough ratio)[112–114] with
apparently a smoother starting profile than glargine U100. The GIR profile of
U300 was dose dependent and glucose lowering was evident up to 36 hours after
injection (end of study) (Table 30.2).[112–114] Metabolic degradation to M1 and M2
metabolites is the same as for glargine.[115]

In Phase III trials in insulin-treated T2D patients with high insulin requirements (EDITION I on basal-bolus and EDITION II on basal insulin plus OADs)
and in EDITION III on insulin-naïve T2D patients on OADs, glycemic control
was comparable with once-daily U300 versus glargine U100 over 6 months.[116–118]
Two of these trials (EDITION I and II) showed that U300 was associated with a
small but significant reduction in the incidence (percentage of patients with at
least one event) of confirmed nocturnal hypoglycemia (≤70 mg/ml) combined
with severe hypoglycemia, during the final 3 months of treatment and with a
lower occurrence of any nocturnal hypoglycemic event during the total 6-month
study period.[2] As with degludec, however, the reporting of the results emphasize
relative percentages of hypoglycemia reduction rather than absolute numbers of
hypoglycemic events, which are low in magnitude and of uncertain clinical relevance. In contrast to the results of the EDITION I and II studies, the rates of
severe and nocturnal confirmed hypoglycemia in EDITION III during the final
3 months were not statistically significant and only numerically lower with U300
but the full hypoglycemia analyses have not yet been reported. Initial evidence
indicates that to achieve equivalent efficacy, a 10% higher dose of U300 was
required.

An additional two studies (EDITION IV and JP1) compared U300 with
glargine in patients with T1D treated with basal-bolus insulin.[118] Similar reductions from baseline in A1C between U300 and glargine were seen at 6 months;
data on the rates of hypoglycemia are pending.

BIOSIMILAR BASAL INSULINS

The next few years will see the emergence of biosimilar versions of glargine in
view of the expiration of patent protection of the commercial form of this insulin in
late 2014. Biosimilars are copies of licensed biological products that are produced
to ensure that their physiochemical characteristics, immunogenicity, efficacy, and
safety are similar to the brand-name therapies.[119] Biosimilars are not generics and
are new biological products similar but not identical to the biological reference
medicine. The regulatory process for approval is far more rigorous in view of the
multiple factors involved in production of biosimilars from genetic engineering to
fermentation, extraction, purification, and formulation processes. They therefore
are deemed to eventually be acceptable forms of the original biological therapy by
regulatory agencies if they meet all the requirements to demonstrate similar immunogenicity, equivalent pharmacokinetic–pharmacodynamic data, comparability in
efficacy, and safety. In addition, evidence of interchangeability may need to be dem
onstrated, which will be a major challenge. The leading contender is LY2963016,
developed by Lilly and Boehringer Ingelheim, which has been studied in Phase III
trials in >1,000 patients with T1D and T2D (ELEMENT1 [NCT01421147] and
ELEMENT 2 [NCT01421459], respectively), using the marketed glargine as the

active comparator. No trial results have been reported to date. It is unclear, however, whether LY2963016 is a true biosimilar of glargine. Although both have the same amino acid sequence, further differences in formulation are not known. LY2963016 was filed and was undergoing review by the European Medicines Agency in July 2013. Other companies, including Merck, are also reported to be developing biosimilar versions of glargine. Several copies currently are available in countries such as India and China but no published data are available. There are concerns, however, about the potential hazards of these drugs and the relative paucity of adequate regulatory mechanisms in their approval and pharmacovigilance processes in those countries.[119] This area of development will probably expand as a result of global economic constraints considered by regulatory agencies.

ALTERNATIVE APPROACHES TO PROVIDE BASAL INSULIN

Although insulin pumps have been used for several decades using short- or rapid-acting insulin for continuous subcutaneous insulin infusion, particularly in patients with T1D, the practicalities and expense of traditional pump technology have limited their use.[120] Recent developments to simplify these delivery systems have resulted in "patch pumps," a new generation of pumps that are smaller than existing pumps. These integrate an insulin reservoir, delivery system, and cannula into a small, wearable, disposable, or semidisposable device that is attached to the skin by an adhesive patch.[121,122] Some are controlled by handheld remote devices. Thus, patch pumps offer a simple means to deliver basal-bolus insulin therapy over several days or a 1-week period. The small size and relative simplicity makes these pumps more suitable than conventional pumps for use in T2D. The lack of long-term data demonstrating sustained efficacy and compliance, however, is a concern and cost remains an issue. Table 30.3 lists currently available patch pumps for insulin delivery.

Table 30.3 Patch Pumps for Insulin Delivery

Name	Manufacturer	Availability	Duration of use
V-Go	Valeritas, Bridgewater, NJ, U.S.	U.S.	Disposable, 1-day use
PaQ	CeQur SA, Horw, Switzerland	Europe*	3-day use
Solo	Roche Diabetes Care, Mannheim, Germany	Europe, U.S.†	90-day use
Finesse	Johnson & Johnson, New Brunswick, NJ, U.S.	FDA	3-day use
Cellnovo	Swansea, Wales, U.K.	Not available	
JewelPUMP	Debiotech S.A., Lausanne, Switzerland	Not available	

Note: *CE Mark approval, due to be launched in 2014.

†Approved but not yet launched.

FIXED-RATIO BASAL INSULIN PLUS GLP-1 RECEPTOR AGONIST COMBINATION TREATMENT

In addition to the development of new basal insulins, the combination of a basal insulin analog with a glucagon-like peptide (GLP)-1 receptor agonist offers new therapeutic options for patients with T2D, reducing reliance on prandial insulin to optimize daytime and postprandial glucose control. Completed trials indicate that adding GLP-1 receptor agonists to insulin or vice-versa is associated with beneficial effects on glycemic control and body weight, with a low incidence of hypoglycemia.[123]

Degludec and glargine are both undergoing evaluation using fixed-ratio concentrations with the GLP-1 analogs liraglutide and lixisenatide, respectively. A single once-daily dose combination of degludec and the GLP-1 analog liraglutide (IDegLira) has been developed. In Phase III trials (DUAL I and II) in both insulin-naïve patients and patients with T2D who were uncontrolled on basal insulin, IDegLira achieved greater A1C reductions compared with degludec and liraglutide alone after 6 months' treatment.[124,125] IDegLira also was associated with significant weight loss when compared with degludec alone, without increased risk of hypoglycemia. This agent was submitted for review by the European Medicines Agency in May 2013.

LixiLan is a once-daily fixed-ratio formulation combining glargine with lixisenatide, a once-daily short-acting GLP-1 receptor agonist. A Phase II proof-of-concept study in patients with T2D showed that treatment with LixiLan resulted in substantial A1C reductions with associated weight loss and without an increased risk of hypoglycemia compared with glargine in metformin-treated T2D.[126] LixiLan currently is being studied in two multicenter, 30-week, Phase III randomized clinical trials, LixiLan-O (NCT02058147) and LixiLan-L (NCT02058160), in subjects with T2D not at glycemic target despite OADs in the former study or on basal glargine with or without metformin in the latter study.

CONCLUSION

The two soluble long-acting analogs—glargine and detemir—represent a significant advance in basal insulin supplementation since the introduction of the intermediate-acting insulin suspensions NPH, lente and ultralente.[2] In contrast to NPH, both analogs reduce the risk for hypoglycemia and especially nocturnal hypoglycemia, achieve a lower FPG, and reduce day-to-day glucose variability, with no requirement for resuspension. Glargine predominantly is administered once-daily, whereas detemir may need to be given twice-daily and at higher insulin doses to achieve equivalent efficacy according to individual requirements.[2]

In recent years, several new insulin analog preparations have been developed, which are aimed at extending the duration of action of insulin to >24 hours. The next generation of basal insulins, degludec, LY2605541, and glargine U300, use different pharmacological mechanisms to achieve a flatter and more extended pharmacokinetic–pharmacodynamic profile compared with existing therapies. To date, findings indicate similar glycemic control compared with the existing therapies but with slightly lower rates of hypoglycemia. The absolute difference in the rates of hypoglycemia with these new insulins, especially during the day when most events occur, is relatively small. Thus, the clinical relevance of these new long-acting basal insulins remains uncertain given the lack of a significant improvement in glycemic control. Therefore, these new insulin agents do not seem to represent a greater therapeutic advance compared with that of glargine and detemir over NPH except perhaps for modest weight loss, rather than just less weight gain induced by LY2605541, which needs to be confirmed in Phase III studies, as well as its liver and lipid safety.

Each of the new formulations, however, offers potential practical benefits to patients in terms of greater flexibility in dose timing and reduced injection volumes. The value of such potential benefits also remains to be established. In addition, extensive clinical trials with the newer insulin formulations need to provide reassurance relating to their short and empirically long-term safety in addition to clarifying their place and role in the management paradigm of T1D or the insulin-requiring person with T2D. The future undoubtedly will offer a number of choices in providing basal insulin supplementation, ranging from conventional insulins, insulin analogs, biosimilar insulins, and insulins delivered by a range of devices and pumps. The strength of the clinical evidence and economic considerations will contribute to determining the utility of the different options available and their impact on the recipient and society.

REFERENCES

1. Banting FG, Best CH, Collip JB, Campbell WR, Fletcher AA. Pancreatic extracts in the treatment of diabetes mellitus. *Can Med Assoc J* 1922;12(3):141–146.

2. Owens DR, Matfin G, Monnier L. Basal insulin analogues in the management of diabetes mellitus: what progress have we made? *Diabetes Metab Res Rev* 2014;30(2):104–119.

3. Owens DR, Bolli GB. Beyond the era of NPH insulin—long-acting insulin analogs: chemistry, comparative pharmacology, and clinical application. *Diabetes Technol Ther* 2008;10(5):333–349.

4. Best CH. The prolongation of insulin action. *Ohio J Sci* 1937;37:362–377.

5. Krayenbuhl C, Rosenberg T. Crystalline protamine insulin. *Rep Steno Mem Hosp Nord Insulinlab* 1946;1:60–73.

6. Hallas-Møller K. The lente insulins. *Diabetes* 1956;5(1):7–14.

7. Schlichtkrull J, Brange J, Christiansen AH, Hallund D, Heding LG, Jørgensen KH, Munkgaard Rasmussen S, Sørensen E, Vølund A. Monocomponent insulin and its clinical implications. *Horm Metab Res* 1974;5(Suppl 1): 134–143.

8. Brange J, Ribel U, Hansen JF, Dodson G, Hansen MT, Havelund S, Melberg SG, Norris F, Norris K, Snel L, Sørensen AR, Voigt HO. Monomeric insulins obtained by protein engineering and their medical implications. *Nature* 1988;333(6174):679–682.

9. Hirsch IB. Insulin analogues. *N Engl J Med* 2005;352(2):174–183.

10. Goeddel DV, Kleid DG, Bolivar F, Heyneker HL, Yansura DG, Crea R, Hirose T, Kraszewski A, Itakura K, Riggs AD. Expression in *Escherichia coli* of chemically synthesized genes for human insulin. *Proc Natl Acad Sci U S A* 1979;76(1):106–110.

11. Chance RE, Kroeff EP, Hoffmann JA, Frank BH. Chemical, physical, and biologic properties of biosynthetic human insulin. *Diabetes Care* 1981;4(2):147–154.

12. Markussen J, Damgaard U, Jørgensen KH, Sorensen E, Thim L. Human monocomponent insulin. Chemistry and characteristics. *Acta Med Scand* 1983;671(Suppl):99–105.

13. Binder C. Absorption of injected insulin. A clinical-pharmacological study. *Acta Pharmacol Toxicol* 1969;27(Suppl 2):1–84.

14. Lepore M, Pampanelli S, Fanelli C, Porcellati F, Bartocci L, Di Vincenzo A, Cordoni C, Costa E, Brunetti P, Bolli GB. Pharmacokinetics and pharmacodynamics of subcutaneous injection of long-acting human insulin analog glargine, NPH insulin, and ultralente human insulin and continuous subcutaneous infusion of insulin lispro. *Diabetes* 2000;49(12):2142–2148.

15. Plank J, Bodenlenz M, Sinner F, Magnes C, Gorzer E, Regittnig W, Endahl LA, Draeger E, Zdravkovic M, Pieber TR. A double-blind, randomized, dose-response study investigating the pharmacodynamic and pharmacokinetic properties of the long-acting insulin analog detemir. *Diabetes Care* 2005;28(5):1107–1112.

16. Scholtz HE, Pretorius SG, Wessels DH, Becker RH. Pharmacokinetic and glucodynamic variability: assessment of insulin glargine, NPH insulin and insulin ultralente in healthy volunteers using a euglycaemic clamp technique. *Diabetologia* 2005;48(10):1988–1995.

17. Owens DR, Coates PA, Luzio SD, Tinbergen JP, Kurzhals R. Pharmacokinetics of ^{125}I-labeled insulin glargine (HOE 901) in healthy men: comparison with NPH insulin and the influence of different subcutaneous injection sites. *Diabetes Care* 2000;23(6):813–819.

18. Bolli GB, Owens DR. Insulin glargine. *Lancet* 2000;356(9228):443–445.

19. Heinemann L, Linkeschova R, Rave K, Hompesch B, Sedlak M, Heise T. Time-action profile of the long-acting insulin analog insulin glargine (HOE901) in comparison with those of NPH insulin and placebo. *Diabetes Care* 2000;23(5):644–649.

20. Kuerzel GU, Shukla U, Scholtz HE, Pretorius SG, Wessels DH, Venter C, Potgieter MA, Lang AM, Koose T, Bernhardt E. Biotransformation of insulin glargine after subcutaneous injection in healthy subjects. *Curr Med Res Opin* 2003;19(1):34–40.

21. Bolli GB, Hahn AD, Schmidt R, Eisenblaetter T, Dahmen R, Heise T, Becker RH. Plasma exposure to insulin glargine and its metabolites M1 and M2 after

subcutaneous injection of therapeutic and supratherapeutic doses of glargine in subjects with type 1 diabetes. *Diabetes Care* 2012;35(12):2626–2630.

22. Lucidi P, Porcellati F, Rossetti P, Candeloro P, Andreoli AM, Cioli P, Hahn A, Schmidt R, Bolli GB, Fanelli CG. Metabolism of insulin glargine after repeated daily subcutaneous injections in subjects with type 2 diabetes. *Diabetes Care* 2012;35(12):2647–2649.

23. Heise T, Nosek L, Ronn BB, Endahl L, Heinemann L, Kapitza C, Draeger E. Lower within-subject variability of insulin detemir in comparison to NPH insulin and insulin glargine in people with type 1 diabetes. *Diabetes* 2004;53(6):1614–1620.

24. Porcellati F, Rossetti P, Ricci NB, Pampanelli S, Torlone E, Campos SH, Andreoli AM, Bolli GB, Fanelli CG. Pharmacokinetics and pharmacodynamics of the long-acting insulin analog glargine after 1 week of use compared with its first administration in subjects with type 1 diabetes. *Diabetes Care* 2007;30(5):1261–1263.

25. Rosenstock J, Dailey G, Massi-Benedetti M, Fritsche A, Lin Z, Salzman A. Reduced hypoglycemia risk with insulin glargine: a meta-analysis comparing insulin glargine with human NPH insulin in type 2 diabetes. *Diabetes Care* 2005;28(4):950–955.

26. Horvath K, Jeitler K, Berghold A, Ebrahim SH, Gratzer TW, Plank J, Kaiser T, Pieber TR, Siebenhofer A. Long-acting insulin analogues versus NPH insulin (human isophane insulin) for type 2 diabetes mellitus. *Cochrane Database Syst Rev* 2007;(2):CD005613.

27. Mullins P, Sharplin P, Yki-Jarvinen H, Riddle MC, Haring HU. Negative binomial meta-regression analysis of combined glycosylated hemoglobin and hypoglycemia outcomes across eleven Phase III and IV studies of insulin glargine compared with neutral protamine Hagedorn insulin in type 1 and type 2 diabetes mellitus. *Clin Ther* 2007;29(8):1607–1619.

28. Home PD, Fritsche A, Schinzel S, Massi-Benedetti M. Meta-analysis of individual patient data to assess the risk of hypoglycaemia in people with type 2 diabetes using NPH insulin or insulin glargine. *Diabetes Obes Metab* 2010;12(9):772–779.

29. Riddle MC, Rosenstock J, Gerich J. The treat-to-target trial: randomized addition of glargine or human NPH insulin to oral therapy of type 2 diabetic patients. *Diabetes Care* 2003;26(11):3080–3086.

30. Wang F, Carabino JM, Vergara CM. Insulin glargine: a systematic review of a long-acting insulin analogue. *Clin Ther* 2003;25(6):1541–1577.

31. Pieber TR, Eugene-Jolchine I, Derobert E. Efficacy and safety of HOE 901 versus NPH insulin in patients with type 1 diabetes. The European Study Group of HOE 901 in type 1 diabetes. *Diabetes Care* 2000;23(2):157–162.

32. Ashwell SG, Gebbie J, Home PD. Optimal timing of injection of once-daily insulin glargine in people with type 1 diabetes using insulin lispro at mealtimes. *Diabet Med* 2006;23(1):46–52.

33. DeVries JH, Nattrass M, Pieber TR. Refining basal insulin therapy: what have we learned in the age of analogues? *Diabetes Metab Res Rev* 2007;23(6):441–454.

34. Mucha GT, Merkel S, Thomas W, Bantle JP. Fasting and insulin glargine in individuals with type 1 diabetes. *Diabetes Care* 2004;27(5):1209–1210.

35. Witthaus E, Stewart J, Bradley C. Treatment satisfaction and psychological well-being with insulin glargine compared with NPH in patients with type 1 diabetes. *Diabet Med* 2001;18(8):619–625.

36. Schreiber SA, Ferlinz K, Haak T. The long-term efficacy of insulin glargine plus oral antidiabetic agents in a 32-month observational study of everyday clinical practice. *Diabetes Technol Ther* 2008;10(2):121–127.

37. Fonseca V, Gill J, Zhou R, Leahy J. An analysis of early insulin glargine added to metformin with or without sulfonylurea: impact on glycaemic control and hypoglycaemia. *Diabetes Obes Metab* 2011;13(9):814–822.

38. Owens DR, Dain M-P, Traylor L, Landgraf W. Early onset of glycaemic improvements after insulin initiation with insulin glargine in patients with type 2-diabetes mellitus uncontrolled with OADS: pooled analysis from clinical trials (abstract P-170). *Diabetes Technol Ther* 2013;15(S1):A88.

39. Rosenstock J, Fonseca V, McGill JB, Riddle M, Halle JP, Hramiak I, Johnston P, Davis M. Similar progression of diabetic retinopathy with insulin glargine and neutral protamine Hagedorn (NPH) insulin in patients with type 2 diabetes: a long-term, randomised, open-label study. *Diabetologia* 2009;52(9):1778–1788.

40. Gerstein HC, Bosch J, Dagenais GR, Diaz R, Jung H, Maggioni AP, Pogue J, Probstfield J, Ramachandran A, Riddle MC, Rydén LE, Yusuf S; ORIGIN Trial Investigators. Basal insulin and cardiovascular and other outcomes in dysglycemia. *N Engl J Med* 2012;367(4):319–328.

41. Hemkens LG, Grouven U, Bender R, Gunster C, Gutschmidt S, Selke GW, Sawicki PT. Risk of malignancies in patients with diabetes treated with human insulin or insulin analogues: a cohort study. *Diabetologia* 2009;52(9):1732–1744.

42. Currie CJ, Poole CD, Gale EA. The influence of glucose-lowering therapies on cancer risk in type 2 diabetes. *Diabetologia* 2009;52(9):1766–1777.

43. Jonasson JM, Ljung R, Talbäck M, Haglund B, Gudbjörnsdòttir S, Steineck G. Insulin glargine use and short-term incidence of malignancies: a population-based follow-up study in Sweden. *Diabetologia* 2009;52(9):1745–1754.

44. Colhoun HM. Use of insulin glargine and cancer incidence in Scotland: a study from the Scottish Diabetes Research Network Epidemiology Group. *Diabetologia* 2009;52(9):1755–1765.

45. Boyle P, Koechlin A, Boniol M, Robertson C, Bolli G, Rosenstock J. Updated meta-analysis of cancer risk among users of insulin glargine (abstract). *Diabetes* 2012;61(Suppl 1):A345.

46. Habel LA, Danforth KN, Quesenberry CP, Capra A, Van Den Eeden SK, Weiss NS, Ferrara A. Cohort study of insulin glargine and risk of breast, prostate, and colorectal cancer among patients with diabetes. *Diabetes Care* 2013;36(12):3953–3960.

47. Stürmer T, Marquis MA, Zhou H, Meigs JB, Lim S, Blonde L, Macdonald E, Wang R, Lavange LM, Pate V, Buse JB. Cancer incidence among those initiating insulin therapy with glargine versus human NPH insulin. *Diabetes Care* 2013;36(11):3517–3525.

48. Bordeleau L, Yakubovich N, Dagenais GR, Rosenstock J, Probstfield J, Chang YP, Ryden LE, Pirags V, Spinas GA, Birkeland KI, Ratner RE, Marin-Neto JA, Keltai M, Riddle MC, Bosch J, Yusuf S, Gerstein HC. The association of basal insulin glargine and/or n-3 fatty acids with incident cancers in patients with dysglycemia. *Diabetes Care* 2014;Feb 26. [Epub ahead of print].

49. Barlocco D. Insulin detemir. Novo Nordisk. *Curr Opin Investig Drugs* 2003;4(4):449–454.

50. Havelund S, Plum A, Ribel U, Jonassen I, Volund A, Markussen J, Kurtzhals P. The mechanism of protraction of insulin detemir, a long-acting, acylated analog of human insulin. *Pharm Res* 2004;21(8):1498–1504.

51. European Medicines Agency. European Medicines Agency. Levemir. European Public Assessment Report Scientific Discussion, 15 August 2006. Available at www.ema.europa.eu/docs/en_GB/document_library/EPAR_-_Scientific_Discussion/human/000528/WC500036658.pdf. Accessed 30 March 2014.

52. Vigneri R, Squatrito S, Sciacca L. Insulin and its analogs: actions via insulin and IGF receptors. *Acta Diabetol* 2010;47(4):271–278.

53. Porcellati F, Rossetti P, Busciantella NR, Marzotti S, Lucidi P, Luzio S, Owens DR, Bolli GB, Fanelli CG. Comparison of pharmacokinetics and dynamics of the long-acting insulin analogs glargine and detemir at steady state in type 1 diabetes: a double-blind, randomized, crossover study. *Diabetes Care* 2007;30(10):2447–2452.

54. Luzio SD, Dunseath GJ, Atkinson MD, Owens DR. A comparison of the pharmacodynamic profiles of insulin detemir and insulin glargine: a single dose clamp study in people with type 2 diabetes. *Diabetes Metab* 2013;39(6):537–542.

55. Klein O, Lynge J, Endahl L, Damholt B, Nosek L, Heise T. Albumin-bound basal insulin analogues (insulin detemir and NN344): comparable time-action profiles but less variability than insulin glargine in type 2 diabetes. *Diabetes Obes Metab* 2007;9(3):290–299.

56. Wutte A, Plank J, Bodenlenz M, Magnes C, Regittnig W, Sinner F, Ronn B, Zdravkovic M, Pieber TR. Proportional dose-response relationship and lower within-patient variability of insulin detemir and NPH insulin in subjects with type 1 diabetes mellitus. *Exp Clin Endocrinol Diabetes* 2007;115(7):461–467.

57. Koehler G, Treiber G, Wutte A, Korsatko S, Mader JK, Semlitsch B, Pieber TR. Pharmacodynamics of the long-acting insulin analogues detemir and glargine following single-doses and under steady-state conditions in patients with type 1 diabetes. *Diabetes Obes Metab* 2014;16(1):57–62.

58. Vague P, Selam JL, Skeie S, De Leeuw I, Elte JWF, Haahr H, Kristensen A, Draeger E. Insulin detemir is associated with more predictable glycemic control and reduced risk of hypoglycemia than NPH insulin in patients with type 1 diabetes on a basal-bolus regimen with premeal insulin aspart. *Diabetes Care* 2003;26(3):590–596.

59. Home P, Bartley P, Russell-Jones D, Hanaire-Broutin H, Heeg JE, Abrams P, Landin-Olsson M, Hylleberg B, Lang H, Draeger E. Insulin detemir offers improved glycemic control compared with NPH insulin in people with type 1 diabetes: a randomized clinical trial. *Diabetes Care* 2004;27(5):1081–1087.

60. Russell-Jones D, Simpson R, Hylleberg B, Draeger E, Bolinder J. Effects of QD insulin detemir or neutral protamine Hagedorn on blood glucose control in patients with type I diabetes mellitus using a basal-bolus regimen. *Clin Ther* 2004;26(5):724–736.

61. Pieber TR, Draeger E, Kristensen A, Grill V. Comparison of three multiple injection regimens for type 1 diabetes: morning plus dinner or bedtime administration of insulin detemir vs. morning plus bedtime NPH insulin. *Diabet Med* 2005;22(7):850–857.

62. Frier BM, Russell-Jones D, Heise T. A comparison of insulin detemir and neutral protamine Hagedorn (isophane) insulin in the treatment of diabetes: a systematic review. *Diabetes Obes Metab* 2013;15(11):978–986.

63. Heise T, Pieber TR. Towards peakless, reproducible and long-acting insulins. An assessment of the basal analogues based on isoglycaemic clamp studies. *Diabetes Obes Metab* 2007;9(5):648–659.

64. Rossetti P, Ampudia-Blasco FJ, Ascaso JF. Old and new basal insulin formulations: understanding pharmacodynamics is still relevant in clinical practice. *Diabetes Obes Metab* 2014;Jan 8. [Epub ahead of print].

65. Pieber TR, Treichel HC, Hompesch B, Philotheou A, Mordhorst L, Gall MA, Robertson LI. Comparison of insulin detemir and insulin glargine in subjects with type 1 diabetes using intensive insulin therapy. *Diabet Med* 2007;24(6):635–642.

66. Heller S, Koenen C, Bode B. Comparison of insulin detemir and insulin glargine in a basal-bolus regimen, with insulin aspart as the mealtime insulin, in patients with type 1 diabetes: a 52-week, multinational, randomized, open-

label, parallel-group, treat-to-target noninferiority trial. *Clin Ther* 2009;31(10):2086–2097.

67. Rosenstock J, Davies M, Home PD, Larsen J, Koenen C, Schernthaner G. A randomised, 52-week, treat-to-target trial comparing insulin detemir with insulin glargine when administered as add-on to glucose-lowering drugs in insulin-naive people with type 2 diabetes. *Diabetologia* 2008;51(3):408–416.

68. Swinnen SG, Dain MP, Aronson R, Davies M, Gerstein HC, Pfeiffer AF, Snoek FJ, DeVries JH, Hoekstra JB, Holleman F. A 24-week, randomized, treat-to-target trial comparing initiation of insulin glargine once-daily with insulin detemir twice-daily in patients with type 2 diabetes inadequately controlled on oral glucose-lowering drugs. *Diabetes Care* 2010;33(6):1176–1178.

69. Meneghini L, Kesavadev J, Demissie M, Nazeri A, Hollander P. Once-daily initiation of basal insulin as add-on to metformin: a 26-week, randomized, treat-to-target trial comparing insulin detemir with insulin glargine in patients with type 2 diabetes. *Diabetes Obes Metab* 2013;15(8):729–736.

70. Hollander P, Cooper J, Bregnhoj J, Pedersen CB. A 52-week, multinational, open-label, parallel-group, noninferiority, treat-to-target trial comparing insulin detemir with insulin glargine in a basal-bolus regimen with mealtime insulin aspart in patients with type 2 diabetes. *Clin Ther* 2008;30(11):1976–1987.

71. Raskin P, Gylvin T, Weng W, Chaykin L. Comparison of insulin detemir and insulin glargine using a basal-bolus regimen in a randomized, controlled clinical study in patients with type 2 diabetes. *Diabetes Metab Res Rev* 2009;25(6):542–548.

72. Jonassen I, Havelund S, Hoeg-Jensen T, Steensgaard DB, Wahlund PO, Ribel U. Design of the novel protraction mechanism of insulin degludec, an ultra-long-acting basal insulin. *Pharm Res* 2012;29(8):2104–2114.

73. Nishimura E, Sørensen AR, Hansen BF, Stidsen CE, Olsen GS, Schaffer L, Bonnesen C, Hegelund AC, Lundby A, Jonassen I. Insulin degludec: a new ultra-long, basal insulin designed to maintain full metabolic effect while minimizing mitogenic potential (abstract 974). *Diabetologia* 2010;53(Suppl 1):S388–S389.

74. Heise T, Hermanski L, Nosek L, Feldman A, Rasmussen S, Haahr H. Insulin degludec: four times lower pharmacodynamic variability than insulin glargine under steady-state conditions in type 1 diabetes. *Diabetes Obes Metab* 2012;14(9):859–864.

75. Heise T, Nosek L, Bottcher SG, Hastrup H, Haahr H. Ultra-long-acting insulin degludec has a flat and stable glucose-lowering effect in type 2 diabetes. *Diabetes Obes Metab* 2012;14(10):944–950.

76. Monnier L, Colette C, Owens D. Basal insulin analogs: from pathophysiology to therapy. What we see, know, and try to comprehend? *Diabetes Metab* 2013;39(6):468–476.

77. Jonassen I, Hoeg-Jensen T, Havelund S, Ribel U. Ultra-long acting insulin degludec can be combined with rapid-acting insulin aspart in a soluble co-formulation (abstract 380). *J Pept Sci* 2010;16(Suppl 1):32.

78. Heise T, Nosek L, Coester H-V, Roepstorff C, Segel S, Lassota N, Haahr HL. Steady state is reached within two to three days of once-daily administration of ultra-long-acting insulin degludec (abstract 1013-P). *Diabetes* 2012;61(Suppl 1):A259.

79. Kurtzhals P, Heise T, Strauss HM, Bottcher SG, Granhall C, Haahr H, Jonassen I. Multi-hexamer formation is the underlying basis for the ultra-long glucose-lowering effect of insulin degludec (abstract). *Diabetologia* 2011;54(Suppl 1):S426.

80. Heise T, Hovelmann U, Nosek L, Bottcher SG, Granhall C, Haahr H. Insulin degludec: two-fold longer half-life and a more consistent pharmacokinetic profile than insulin glargine (abstract 1046). *Diabetologia* 2011;54(Suppl 1):S425.

81. Heller S, Buse J, Fisher M, Garg S, Marre M, Merker L, Renard E, Russell-Jones D, Philotheou A, Francisco AM, Pei H, Bode B. Insulin degludec, an ultra-longacting basal insulin, versus insulin glargine in basal-bolus treatment with mealtime insulin aspart in type 1 diabetes (BEGIN Basal-Bolus Type 1): a phase 3, randomised, open-label, treat-to-target non-inferiority trial. *Lancet* 2012;379(9825):1489–1497.

82. Novo Nordisk. Insulin degludec and insulin degludec/insulin aspart treatment to improve glycemic control in patients with diabetes mellitus. Briefing information for the November 8, 2012, meeting of the Endocrinologic and Metabolic Drugs Advisory Committee. Available at www.fda.gov/downloads/AdvisoryCommittees/CommitteesMeetingMaterials/Drugs/EndocrinologicandMetabolicDrugsAdvisoryCommittee/UCM327017.pdf. Accessed 30 March 2014.

83. Mathieu C, Hollander P, Miranda-Palma B, Cooper J, Franek E, Russell-Jones D, Larsen J, Tamer SC, Bain SC. Efficacy and safety of insulin degludec in a flexible dosing regimen vs insulin glargine in patients with type 1 diabetes (BEGIN: Flex T1): a 26-week randomized, treat-to-target trial with a 26-week extension. *J Clin Endocrinol Metab* 2013;98(3):1154–1162.

84. Zinman B, Philis-Tsimikas A, Cariou B, Handelsman Y, Rodbard HW, Johansen T, Endahl L, Mathieu C. Insulin degludec versus insulin glargine in insulin-naive patients with type 2 diabetes: a 1-year, randomized, treat-to-target trial (BEGIN Once Long). *Diabetes Care* 2012;35(12):2464–2471.

85. Garber AJ, King AB, Del Prato S, Sreenan S, Balci MK, Munoz-Torres M, Rosenstock J, Endahl LA, Francisco AM, Hollander P. Insulin degludec, an ultra-longacting basal insulin, versus insulin glargine in basal-bolus treatment with mealtime insulin aspart in type 2 diabetes (BEGIN Basal-Bolus Type 2): a phase 3, randomised, open-label, treat-to-target non-inferiority trial. *Lancet* 2012;379(9825):1498–1507.

86. Onishi Y, Iwamoto Y, Yoo SJ, Clauson P, Tamer SC, Park S. Insulin degludec compared with insulin glargine in insulin-naïve patients with type 2 diabetes: a 26-week, randomized, controlled, pan-Asian, treat-to-target trial. *J Diabetes Invest* 2013;4(6):605–612.

87. Meneghini L, Atkin SL, Gough SC, Raz I, Blonde L, Shestakova M, Bain S, Johansen T, Begtrup K, Birkeland KI. The efficacy and safety of insulin degludec given in variable once-daily dosing intervals compared with insulin glargine and insulin degludec dosed at the same time daily: a 26-week, randomized, open-label, parallel-group, treat-to-target trial in individuals with type 2 diabetes. *Diabetes Care* 2013;36(4):858–864.

88. Gough SC, Bhargava A, Jain R, Mersebach H, Rasmussen S, Bergenstal RM. Low-volume insulin degludec 200 units/mL once daily improves glycemic control similar to insulin glargine with a low risk of hypoglycemia in insulin-naive patients with type 2 diabetes: a 26-week, randomized, controlled, multinational, treat-to-target trial: the BEGIN LOW VOLUME trial. *Diabetes Care* 2013;36(9):2536–2542.

89. Zinman B, DeVries JH, Bode B, Russell-Jones D, Leiter LA, Moses A, Johansen T, Ratner R. Efficacy and safety of insulin degludec three times a week versus insulin glargine once a day in insulin-naive patients with type 2 diabetes: results of two phase 3, 26 week, randomised, open-label, treat-to-target, non-inferiority trials. *Lancet Diabetes Endocrinol* 2013;1(2):123–131.

90. Philis-Tsimikas A, Del Prato S, Satman I, Bhargava A, Dharmalingam M, Skjoth TV, Rasmussen S, Garber AJ. Effect of insulin degludec versus sitagliptin in patients with type 2 diabetes uncontrolled on oral antidiabetic agents. *Diabetes Obes Metab* 2013;15(8):760–766.

91. FDA. U.S. Food and Drug Administration—FDA Briefing Information, insulin degludec and insulin degludec/aspart, for the November 8, 2012 Meeting of the Endocrinologic and Metabolic Drugs Advisory Committee. Available at www.fda.gov/downloads/AdvisoryCommittees/Committees-MeetingMaterials/Drugs/EndocrinologicandMetabolicDrugsAdvisory-Committee/UCM327015.pdf. Accessed 30 March 2014.

92. American Diabetes Association Workgroup on Hypoglycemia. Defining and reporting hypoglycemia in diabetes. *Diabetes Care* 2005;28(5):1245–1249.

93. Seaquist ER, Anderson J, Childs B, Cryer P, Dagogo-Jack S, Fish L, Heller SR, Rodriguez H, Rosenzweig J, Vigersky R. Hypoglycemia and diabetes: a report of a workgroup of the American Diabetes Association and The Endocrine Society. *Diabetes Care* 2013;36(5):1384-1395.

94. Ratner RE, Gough SC, Mathieu C, Del Prato S, Bode B, Mersebach H, Endahl L, Zinman B. Hypoglycaemia risk with insulin degludec compared with insulin glargine in type 2 and type 1 diabetes: a pre-planned meta-analysis of phase 3 trials. *Diabetes Obes Metab* 2013;15(2):175–184.

95. European Medicines Agency. Committee for Medicinal Products for Human Use (CHMP) Assessment Report for tresiba (insulin degludec). 20 Septem-

ber 2012. Available at www.ema.europa.eu/docs/en_GB/document_library/ EPAR_-_Public_assessment_report/human/002498/WC500139010.pdf. Accessed 30 March 2014.

96. Hirsch IB, Bode B, Courreges JP, Dykiel P, Franek E, Hermansen K, King A, Mersebach H, Davies M. Insulin degludec/insulin aspart administered once daily at any meal, with insulin aspart at other meals versus a standard basal-bolus regimen in patients with type 1 diabetes: a 26-week, phase 3, randomized, open-label, treat-to-target trial. *Diabetes Care* 2012;35(11):2174–2181.

97. Fulcher G, Bantwal G, Christiansen JS, Andersen T, Mersebach H, Niskanen LK. Superior FPG control and reduced hypoglycaemia with IDegAsp vs BIAsp 30 in adults with type 2 diabetes mellitus inadequately controlled on pre/self-mixed insulin: a randomised phase 3 trial (abstract 1044). *Diabetologia* 2013;56(Suppl 1):S419.

98. Christiansen JS, Chow FCC, Choi DS, Taneda S, Hirao K, Park Y, Andersen T, Gall M-A, Kaneko S. Superior FPG control and less nocturnal hypoglycaemia with IDegAsp vs BIAsp 30 in Asian subjects poorly controlled on basal or pre/self-mixed insulin: randomised phase 3 trial (abstract 1045). *Diabetologia* 2013;56(Suppl 1):S420.

99. Onishi Y, Ono Y, Rabol R, Endahl L, Nakamura S. Superior glycaemic control with once-daily insulin degludec/insulin aspart versus insulin glargine in Japanese adults with type 2 diabetes inadequately controlled with oral drugs: a randomized, controlled phase 3 trial. *Diabetes Obes Metab* 2013;15(9):826–832.

100. Novo Nordisk. Company announcement, 10 February 2013. Available at www.novonordisk.com/include/asp/exe_news_attachment.asp?s AttachmentGUID=83700060-0ce3-4577-a35a-f3e57801637d. Accessed 30 March 2014.

101. Schmidt TA, Rosen CJ, Yudkin JS. European Medicines Agency must take account of cardiovascular harm associated with degludec insulin. *BMJ* 2013;346:f3731. doi: 10.1136/bmj.f3731.

102. Hansen RJ, Cutler Jr GB, Vick A, Koester A, Li S, Siesky AM, Beals JM. LY2605541: leveraging hydrodynamic size to develop a novel basal insulin (abstract 896-P). *Diabetes* 2012;61(Suppl 1):A228.

103. Owens RA, Lockwood JF, Dunbar JD, Zhang C, Ruan X, Kahl SD, Beals JM. In vitro characterization of novel basal insulin LY2605541: reduced mitogenicity and IGF-IR binding (abstract 1643-P). *Diabetes* 2012;61(Suppl 1):A425.

104. Moore MC, Smith MS, Sinha VP, Beals JM, Michael MD, Jacober SJ, Cherrington AD. Novel PEGylated basal insulin LY2605541 has a preferential hepatic effect on glucose metabolism. *Diabetes* 2014;63(2):494–504.

105. Shojaee-Moradie F, Powrie JK, Sundermann E, Spring MW, Schuttler A, Sonksen PH, Brandenburg D, Jones RH. Novel hepatoselective insulin analog: studies with a covalently linked thyroxyl-insulin complex in humans. *Diabetes Care* 2000;23(8):1124–1129.

106. Morrow LA, Hompesch M, Jacober SJ, Choi SL, Qu Y, Sinha VP. LY2605541 (LY) exhibits a flatter glucodynamic profile than insulin glargine (GL) at steady state in subjects with type 1 diabetes (T1D) (abstract 917-P). *Diabetes* 2013;62(Suppl 1):A233.

107. Sinha VP, Howey DC, Choi SL, Mace KF, Heise T. Steady-state pharmacokinetics and glucodynamics of the novel, long-acting basal insulin LY2605541 dosed once-daily in patients with type 2 diabetes mellitus. *Diabetes Obes Metab* 2014;16(4):344–350.

108. Sinha VP, Choi SL, Soon DK, Mace KF, Yeo KP, Lim ST, Howey DC. Single-dose pharmacokinetics and glucodynamics of the novel, long-acting basal insulin LY2605541 in healthy subjects. *J Clin Pharmacol* 2014;Feb 6. [Epub ahead of print].

109. Bergenstal RM, Rosenstock J, Arakaki RF, Prince MJ, Qu Y, Sinha VP, Howey DC, Jacober SJ. A randomized, controlled study of once-daily LY2605541, a novel long-acting basal insulin, versus insulin glargine in basal insulin-treated patients with type 2 diabetes. *Diabetes Care* 2012;35(11):2140–2147.

110. Rosenstock J, Bergenstal RM, Blevins TC, Morrow LA, Prince MJ, Qu Y, Sinha VP, Howey DC, Jacober SJ. Better glycemic control and weight loss with the novel long-acting basal insulin LY2605541 compared with insulin glargine in type 1 diabetes: a randomized, crossover study. *Diabetes Care* 2013;36(3):522–528.

111. Bergenstal RM, Rosenstock J, Bastyr EJ III, Prince MJ, Qu Y, Jacober SJ. Lower glucose variability and hypoglycemia measured by continuous glucose monitoring with novel long-acting insulin LY2605541 versus insulin glargine. *Diabetes Care* 2014;37(3):659–665.

112. Tillner J, Bergmann K, Teichert L, Dahmen R, Heise T, Becker RHA. Euglycemic clamp profile of new insulin glargine U300 formulation in patients with type 1 diabetes (T1DM) is different from glargine U100 (abstract 920-P). *Diabetes* 2013;62(Suppl 1):A234.

113. Dahmen R, Bergmann K, Lehmann A, Tillner J, Thomas J, Heise T, Becker RHA. New insulin glargine U300 formulation evens and prolongs steady state PK and PD profiles during euglycemic clamp in patients with type 1 diabetes (T1DM) (abstract 113-OR). *Diabetes* 2013;62(Suppl 1):A29.

114. Shiramoto M, Eto T, Watanabe A, Irie S, Fukuzaki A, Bergmann K, Takahashi Y, Dahmen R, Koyama M, Becker RHA. Single dose of new insulin glargine Gla-300 formulation has a flatter and prolonged PK/PD profile than Gla-100 in Japanese subjects with type 1 diabetes (abstract 1031). *Diabetologia* 2013;56(Suppl 1):S414.

115. Steinstraesser A, Schmidt R, Bergmann K, Dahmen R, Becker RHA. Metabolism of insulin glargine in humans is the same regardless of formulation, Gla-100 or Gla-300 (abstract 1032). *Diabetologia* 2013;56(Suppl 1):S415.

116. Riddle MC, Bolli GB, Ziemen M, Muehlen-Bartmer I, Bizet F, Home PD. New insulin glargine formulation: glucose control and hypoglycemia in

people with type 2 diabetes using basal and mealtime insulin (EDITION I) (abstract 43-LB). *Diabetes* 2013;62(Suppl 1A):LB12.

117. Yki-Järvinen H, Bergenstal RM, Ziemen M, Wardecki M, Muehlen-Bartmer I, Boelle E, Riddle M. An investigational new insulin U300: glucose control and hypoglycemia in people with type 2 diabetes on basal insulin and OADs (EDITION II) (abstract: OP-0075), Oral Presentation, World Diabetes Congress, Melbourne, Australia, 2–6 December 2013.

118. Press Release. Sanofi announces new Phase 3 results for investigational new insulin U300. 3 December 2013. Available at http://en.sanofi.com/Images/35096_20131203_U300_ED_II_III_IV_JPI_en.pdf. Accessed 30 March 2014.

119. Owens DR, Landgraf W, Schmidt A, Bretzel RG, Kuhlmann MK. The emergence of biosimilar insulin preparations: a cause for concern? *Diabetes Technol Ther* 2012;14(11):989–996.

120. Owens DR. Insulin preparations with prolonged effect. *Diabetes Technol Ther* 2011;13(Suppl 1):S5–S14.

121. Anhalt H, Bohannon NJ. Insulin patch pumps: their development and future in closed-loop systems. *Diabetes Technol Ther* 2010;12(Suppl 1):S51–S58.

122. Fry A. Insulin delivery device technology 2012: where are we after 90 years? *J Diabetes Sci Technol* 2012;6(4):947–953.

123. Holst JJ, Vilsboll T. Combining GLP-1 receptor agonists with insulin: therapeutic rationales and clinical findings. *Diabetes Obes Metab* 2013;15(1):3–14.

124. Buse JB, Gough SC, Woo VC, Rodbard HW, Linjawi S, Poulsen P, Damgaard LH, Bode BW. IDegLira, a novel fixed ratio combination of insulin degludec and liraglutide, is efficacious and safe in subjects with type 2 diabetes: a large, randomized Phase 3 trial (abstract). *Diabetes* 2013;62(Suppl 1):65–OR.

125. Buse JB, Vilsbøll T, Thurman J, Blevins T, Langbakke IH, Damgaard LH, Rodbard HW. Liraglutide contributes significantly to glycaemic control achieved in IDegLira: a double-blind Phase 3 trial in type 2 diabetes. Oral presentation (OP-0082) at the World Diabetes Congress for the International Diabetes Federation (IDF), Melbourne, Australia, 2–6 December 2013.

126. Rosenstock J, Diamant M, Silvestre L, Souhami E, Zhou T, Fonseca V. Efficacy and safety of insulin glargine/lixisenatide fixed combination versus insulin glargine alone on top of metformin in type 2 diabetic patients (abstract). *Diabetes* 2014;63(Suppl 1):OR033.

Chapter 31
Combination Therapy in Type 2 Diabetes

Matthew C. Riddle, MD
Kevin C. J. Yuen, MD, FRCP (UK)

INTRODUCTION

Type 2 diabetes (T2D) is a chronic metabolic disorder characterized by relative insulin deficiency and multiple other metabolic and endocrine abnormalities. A progressive decline of the β-cell response of insulin secretion to metabolic needs is the central pathogenic feature, but in most cases, peripheral and hepatic resistance to the actions of insulin are also major contributing factors. Abnormalities of gastrointestinal function, satiety, and weight control contribute to the clinical syndrome as well as the dysregulation of fat, salt, and water metabolism. Together these abnormalities lead to hyperglycemia, obesity, dyslipidemia, hypertension, and the cardiovascular and microvascular complications of diabetes. Because of this multifactorial pathogenesis, metabolic control is difficult to attain and understandably requires combinations of therapies that have different mechanisms of action to produce additive effects. The inability of treatment with a single drug to maintain glycemic control over time has been well demonstrated in the United Kingdom Prospective Diabetes Study (UKPDS). At the same time, long-term follow-up of treatment in the UKPDS and other studies has shown that intervention early in the course of T2D can reduce later risks of microvascular complications, and although the evidence is less convincing, perhaps also cardiovascular complications. Recent guidance from several professional societies therefore emphasizes the need for systematic and progressive use of combinations of antihyperglycemic agents. Metformin is the preferred first-line therapy, but with disease progression, its combination with additional agents becomes necessary. When oral combination therapy is not fully effective, adding one or more injections of insulin has been recommended. Recently, several new classes of drugs have added to the choices available. The importance of combination regimens is further illustrated by the availability of many fixed-ratio coformulations, allowing for simplified dosing of commonly used agents.

AVAILABLE AGENTS

Information regarding currently available classes of antihyperglycemic agents, with some of their properties, is shown in Tables 31.1–31.4. The ability of each agent to lower A1C is usually greatest when the agent is used as monotherapy and somewhat lower when added as a second or third agent in combination regimens, later in the course of diabetes. Clinical studies have shown that agents from differ-

DOI: 10.2337/9781580405096.31

Table 31.1 Currently Available Classes of Antihyperglycemic Agents

Class and drug	Mode of action					Glycemic effects		Other effects	
	Decrease hepatic glucose output	Increase plasma insulin	Slow CHO absorption	Increase peripheral glucose uptake	Increase glycosuria	Decrease fasting plasma glucose	Decrease post-prandial increments	Weight	Blood pressure
Biguanide Metformin	+++			+		+++	+	↓	
Sulfonylurea Gliclazide	+++	++				+++	+	↑	
Glimepiride	+++	++				+++	+	↑	
Glipizide	+++	++				+++	+	↑	
Glyburide	+++	++				+++	+	↑	
Nonsulfonylurea secretatogue Nateglinide	++	+++		+		+	++	↑	
Repaglinide	++	+++		+		++	++	↑	
Thiazolidinedione Pioglitazone	++			+++		++	+	↑	↓
Rosiglitazone	++			+++		++	+	↑	↓
DPP-4 inhibitor Alogliptin	++	+				++	+		
Linagliptin	++	+				++	+		
Saxagliptin	++	+				++	+		
Sitagliptin	++	+				++	+		
Vildagliptin	++	+				++	+		
α-Glucosidase inhibitor Acarbose	+		+++			+	++		
Miglitol	+		+++			+	++		
SGLT-2 blocker Canagliflozin					+++	++	+	↓	↓
Dapaglifozin[a]					+++	++	+	↓	↓
Bile acid sequestrant Colesevelam	++					++	++		
Dopamine R agonist Bromocriptine	++					++	++	↓	
Long-acting insulin Human NPH	+++	++		+		+++		↑	
Degludec[a]	+++	++		+		+++		↑	
Detemir	+++	++		+		+++		↑	
Glargine	+++	+++		+		+++		↑	

(continued)

Table 31.1 Currently Available Classes of Antihyperglycemic Agents *(continued)*

Class and drug	Mode of action					Glycemic effects		Other effects	
	Decrease hepatic glucose output	Increase plasma insulin	Slow CHO absorption	Increase peripheral glucose uptake	Increase glycosuria	Decrease fasting plasma glucose	Decrease post-prandial increments	Weight	Blood pressure
Short-acting insulin									
Human regular	+++	+++		+++		+	++	↑	
Aspart	+++	+++		+++		+	++	↑	
Glulisine	+++	+++		+++		+	++	↑	
Lispro	+++	+++		+++		+	++	↑	
Long-acting GLP-1R agonist									
Exenatide (once weekly)	+++	+	+			+++	+	↓	↓
Liraglutide	+++	+	+			+++	+	↓	↓
Short-acting GLP-1R agonist									
Exenatide (twice-daily)	+	+	+++			+	+++	↓	↓
Lixisenatide[a]	+	+	+++			++	++	↓	↓
Amylin R agonist									
Pramlintide			+++				+++	↓	

Note: CHO = carbohydrate; DPP-4 = dipeptidyl peptidase-4; GLP-1 = glucagon-like polypeptide 1; NPH = neutral protamine Hagedorn; SGLT-2 = sodium-dependent glucose transporter two.
[a]Dapagliflozin, degludec, and lixisenatide are not currently available in the United States but are approved in other countries.

ent classes in most cases can be effectively and safely combined. Characteristics of individual agents are described in greater detail in other chapters of this book. At present, evidence regarding long-term comparative effectiveness of different drug combinations is limited, and thus no evidence-based recommendations regarding the combination regimens preferred in different settings are available. Ultimately, the choice of combination therapy undertaken should take into account multiple factors, such as disease duration; concurrent comorbidities; life expectancy; expected complications, including the risk of hypoglycemia; and the patient's personal preferences, capacity for self-care, availability of social support, and financial resources.

Table 31.2 Clinical Features of Oral Medications

Medications (commercial name)	Drug class	Common side effects	Contraindications	Percent A1C lowering as monotherapy
Metformin (Glucophage, Glucophage XR), and generics	Biguanide	GI (nausea, vomiting, diarrhea, abdominal pain), vitamin B12 deficiency	T1D, DKA, renal impairment (Cr > 1.5 men, > 1.4 women), liver impairment	1–2%
Glipizide (Glucotrol), glimepiride (Amaryl), glyburide (Micronase, DiaBeta, Glynase, Pres Tab), and generics	Sulfonylurea	Hypoglycemia, weight gain	T1D, DKA	1–2%
Pioglitazone (Actos)*, rosiglitazone (Avandia)**, and generics	TZD	Edema, weight gain, bone fractures	T1D, DKA, symptomatic CHF	0.75–1.5%
Repaglinide (Prandin), netaglinide (Starlix), and generics	Meglitinide	Hypoglycemia, weight gain	T1D, DKA	0.75–1.5%
Acarbose (Precose), miglitol (Glyset), and generics	α-Glucosidase inhibitor	GI (flatulence, diarrhea, abdominal discomfort)	T1D, DKA, liver impairment, chronic intestinal disease	0.5–1%
Sitagliptin (Januvia), saxagliptin (Onglyza), linagliptin (Tradjenta)	DPP-4 inhibitor	Hypersensitivity	T1D, pancreatitis, hypersensitivity	0.5–1%
Bromocriptine mesylate (Cycloset)	Dopamine receptor agonist	GI, orthostatic hypotension, somnolence, psychosis, dizziness	T1D, DKA, syncope, migraines	0.5–1%
Canaglifozin (Invokana), dapaglifozin (Forxiga)†	SGLT-2 blocker	Genito-urinary infections, constipation, diarrhea, nausea, urinary frequency	T1D, chronic urinary tract infections, severe renal impairment, end-stage renal disease	0.7–1%
Colesevelam (Welchol)	Bile acid sequestrant	Constipation, hypertriglyceridemia, decreased absorption of drugs	T1D, DKA, chronic intestinal disease, hypertriglyceridemia, pancreatitis	0.5–1%

Note. CHF = congestive heart failure; DKA = diabetic ketoacidosis; DPP-4 = dipeptidyl peptidase-4; GI = gastrointestinal; SGLT-2 = sodium-dependent glucose transporter two; T1D = type 1 diabetes; TZD = thiazolidinedione.
*Possible association with bladder cancer.
**Use restricted, possible association with myocardial infarction.
†Dapagliflozin is not currently available in the U.S. but is approved in other countries.

Table 31.3 Clinical Features of Insulin

Type	Product (commercial name)	Onset of action	Time to peak	Duration	Administration
Rapid-acting	Lispro (Humalog) Aspart (Novolog) Glulisine (Apidra)	15–20 minutes	1–2 hours	3–5 hours	15 minutes before or just after meals in patients with gastroparesis
Short-acting	Regular (Humulin R, Novolin R)	30–40 minutes	2–4 hours	4–6 hours	30–45 minutes before meals
Intermediate-acting	NPH (Humulin N, Novolin N)	1–2 hours	4–8 hours	8–12 hours	Once or twice daily
Long-acting basal	Glargine (Lantus), Detemir (Levemir)	1–2 hours	No pronounced peak	20–24 hours	Not dependent on meals Usually once daily
Ultralong-acting	Degludec (Tresiba)†	1–2 hours	No pronounced peak	24–72 hours	Not dependent on meals Usually once daily
Premixed	70/30 NPH/R 75/25 Protamine-lispro/Lispro 70/30 Protamine-aspart/Aspart 50/50 Protamine-lispro/Lispro	1–2 hours	4–8 hours	8–12 hours	30–60 minutes before meals
Concentrated	U-500 (Humulin U-500, U-500R)	30–40 minutes	2–4 hours	6–10 hours	30 minutes before meals

Note: NPH = neutral protamine Hagedorn.
†Degludec is not currently available in the U.S. but is approved in other countries.

PHYSIOLOGIC RATIONALE

INSULIN DEFICIENCY AND INSULIN RESISTANCE

The most obvious need for combination therapy stems from the presence of both insulin deficiency and insulin resistance in most patients with T2D. Moreover, progressive decline of insulin secretory capacity from the time of diagnosis ensures that single-drug therapy will remain effective for no more than 3 years in most cases. Thus, early use of the combination of an agent that enhances insulin availability (a sulfonlyurea or insulin) with one that improves the sensitivity of target tissues to insulin (metformin or pioglitazone) commonly is recommended. Metformin and pioglitazone act by different mechanisms and at different sites. Metformin primarily improves the sensitivity of the liver to effects of insulin, whereas pioglitazone acts mainly through improved responsiveness of the peripheral tissues (adipose tissue and muscle) to insulin, with some additional effects at the liver. Hence, these insulin-sensitizing agents have additive effects when used

Table 31.4 Clinical Features of Injectable Medications Other Than Insulins

Medications (commercial name)	Drug class	Common side effects	Contra-indications	Percent A1C lowering as monotherapy
Exenatide (Byetta)	Short-acting GLP-1 agonist	Nausea, vomiting, diarrhea, abdominal pain, pancreatitis (rare)	T1D, ketoacidosis, pancreatitis	0.5–1%
Lixisenatide (Lyxumia)†	Intermediate-acting GLP-1 agonist	Nausea, vomiting, headache, diarrhea, abdominal pain, pancreatitis (rare)	T1D, ketoacidosis, pancreatitis	0.7–1%
Liraglutide (Victoza)	Intermediate-acting GLP-1 agonist	Nausea, vomiting, diarrhea, abdominal pain, pancreatitis (rare)	T1D, ketoacidosis, pancreatitis, personal or family history of medullary carcinoma of thyroid or multiple endocrine neoplasia 2	1–2%
Exenatide extended-release (Bydureon)	Long-acting GLP-1 agonist	GI (nausea, vomiting, diarrhea, abdominal pain), pancreatitis (rare)	T1D, ketoacidosis, pancreatitis, personal or family history of medullary carcinoma of thyroid or multiple endocrine neoplasia 2	1–2%
Pramlintide (Symlin)	Amylin mimetic	GI (nausea, vomiting)	Confirmed gastroparesis	0.5–1%

Note: GI = gastrointestinal; GLP-1 = glucagon-like polypeptide 1; T1D = type 1 diabetes.
†Lixisenatide is not currently available in the U.S. but is approved other countries.

together. In contrast, sulfonylureas and the nonsulfonlylurea secretagogues have similar mechanisms of action and do not provide additive effects.

MINIMIZATION OF SIDE EFFECTS

Combination therapy can improve glycemic control while limiting side effects. The maximal dosage of many therapeutic agents is determined by their undesired symptomatic effects. At the same time, half-maximal dosage can provide more than half the desired therapeutic effect with much lower risk of side effects. For example, the usual maximal dosage of metformin (2,000 mg/day) causes significant gastrointestinal side effects in 25–30% of people. Limiting the dosage of metformin to 1,000 mg/day allows up to 70% of the total therapeutic effect but with less risk of nausea and diarrhea. Therefore, use of submaximal dosage of two agents can achieve both a greater glycemic effect and fewer undesired effects than full dosage of either agent alone. The same principle applies to the combination of oral agents with insulin. Continuing metformin when starting basal insulin is desirable because metformin enhances the buffering effects of endogenous insulin secretion and can reduce the risk of hypoglycemia that might accompany higher doses of basal insulin when used alone. In addition, concurrent use of metformin can limit the gain of weight frequently accompanying progressive increases of insulin dosage.

BASAL VERSUS POSTPRANDIAL CONTROL

In the absence of diabetes, basal glucose is controlled by less complex mechanisms than those limiting mealtime increments of glucose. Basal glucose levels mainly are determined by the rate of hepatic glucose production, and this is controlled most strongly by modulation of the levels of insulin and glucagon in the portal vein. In contrast, increases of plasma glucose after meals normally are limited by an array of responses, including a rapid increase of insulin and suppression of glucagon secretion, increased plasma levels of amylin and glucagon-like peptide-1 (GLP-1) and declining levels of ghrelin, and neurally mediated alteration of glucose production by the liver and uptake by peripheral tissues. In addition, gastric emptying decreases and satiety increases after eating. Many of these intricate mechanisms are impaired in T2D, and correcting postprandial glycemic patterns can be challenging.

Both overnight and between-meal glucose levels (fasting or basal) and the increments above premeal levels (postprandial) are increased in most people with diabetes, and both components of hyperglycemia typically worsen with increasing duration of diabetes. In the absence of pharmacotherapy, basal hyperglycemia contributes more to the overall glycemic exposure of tissues than do the further increments after meals, but with treatment, this relationship changes. At present, the most widely used treatments for T2D, including metformin, sulfonylureas, pioglitazone, dipeptidyl peptidase-4 (DPP-4) inhibitors, basal insulin, and long-acting GLP-1 receptor agonists, act mainly on fasting and between-meal hyperglycemia. Use of these agents early in the course of T2D reduces fasting glucose levels, but increments after meals may persist. When these agents do not maintain adequate control of overall hyperglycemia, as measured by A1C levels, the remaining defect is mainly postprandial. In this setting, agents that mainly affect mealtime increments of glucose can be added. Use of rapid-acting insulin together with long-acting insulin to improve postprandial control is a form of combination therapy. In some cases, adding an injection of rapid-acting insulin with one or more meals can improve glycemic control with less risk of hypoglycemia than might occur with a continued increase of dosage of basal insulin alone. Other agents with important mealtime glycemic effects include nateglinide and repaglinide, acarbose, and miglitol, as well as the short-acting GLP-1 receptor agonists exenatide and lixisenatide.

DESIRABLE NONGLYCEMIC EFFECTS

Beyond improving glycemic control, use of combination therapy can assist with the management of other metabolic risk factors. The ability of metformin to limit weight gain and sometimes promote modest weight loss is an important example of this kind of benefit. In the UKPDS, treatment with metformin alone led to slower gain of weight over time than was observed with treatment with lifestyle, sulfonylurea, or basal insulin. Other studies confirm that this weight-limiting effect persists when metformin is combined with other agents. A similar beneficial effect on weight accompanies the use of GLP-1 receptor agonists and sodium-dependent glucose cotransporter 2 (SGLT-2) blockers, and both of these classes of agents have beneficial effects on blood pressure. When the control of these risk factors becomes increasingly important, combination regimens including these agents may be helpful.

WELL-TESTED VERSUS NEWER THERAPIES

Any discussion of combination therapy requires consideration of how agents that have been in use for many years may differ from newer ones. Objective evidence for medical benefit relative to risks from treatments is highly desirable, and because of the extended course of time over which the complications of diabetes develop, this cannot be obtained in the first few years of use of newer agents. Strong evidence for the limitation of microvascular complications (and some evidence for the reduction of cardiovascular complications) is available for metformin, sulfonylureas, and insulins mainly because of the extensive experience with the use of these agents, which have been available for a long time. Suggestive evidence for medical benefits of acarbose and pioglitazone exists, but side effects and safety concerns have constrained the use of these agents to some degree. At present, therefore, combinations of metformin, sulfonylureas, and insulin lie at the center of most guidelines for standard treatment of T2D.

The newer classes of drugs—DPP-4 inhibitors, GLP-1 receptor agonists, SGLT-2 blockers, and the amylin receptor agonist pramlintide—have proven abilities to improve metabolic control and treat specific defects, but the long-term balance of benefit versus risk for these agents remains to be clarified by upcoming studies with long-term follow-up. Accordingly, they generally are recommended to be used in special circumstances rather than as a routine. In the case of the GLP-1-related therapies, an active debate on benefits versus risks (notably the possible risk of pancreatitis and certain cancers) is in progress. In addition, significant differences in the costs of older versus newer classes of agents cannot be ignored. Nevertheless, the need to individualize treatment for patients who are not successful with the more common combinations of agents supports the use of a wide variety of combinations in varying circumstances.

COMMON REGIMENS USED SOON AFTER DIAGNOSIS

LIFESTYLE WITH METFORMIN OR SULFONYLUREA

Combining intensification of lifestyle intervention with initial oral pharmacotherapy is justified at the time of diagnosis of diabetes. In most cases, metformin is the first choice, but ~5% of people cannot tolerate even the lowest doses of this drug, and in this situation, a low initial dosage of a sulfonylurea (such as 0.5–1 mg of glimepiride or 2.5 mg of long-acting glipizide) may be effective. Glyburide, a sulfonylurea that has been used widely in the past, is less suitable for early treatment and has now fallen out of favor due to its propensity to cause hypoglycemia and weight gain. Either metformin or a sulfonylurea used together with lifestyle modifications as an initial treatment can reliably improve glycemic control, with A1C reductions of 1.5–2% common when the starting level is ≥9%.

METFORMIN WITH SULFONYLUREA, PIOGLITAZONE, OR DPP-4 INHIBITORS

The combination of metformin with a sulfonylurea is the typical regimen to follow lifestyle modifications with either agent alone. These agents have additive effects on glycemic control, and together often maintain A1C levels near the target range for several years after initiation. When one of them presents difficulties, such as nausea or diarrhea with metformin or hypoglycemia with a sulfonylurea, alternatives are available. Pioglitazone, currently the only thiazolidinedione widely available, and the DPP-4 inhibitors (linagliptin, saxagliptin, sitagliptin, and vildagliptin) similarly are able to provide moderate improvement of glycemic control (usually A1C reductions of 0.5–1%) when added to prior monotherapy, while adding little additional risk of hypoglycemia or other symptoms. Whereas pioglitazone often causes weight gain and fluid retention, the DPP-4 inhibitors are weight neutral and can be used in patients with renal impairment. Several new oral glucose-lowering agents are now available for use without inducing weight gain, although experience with them is limited. One such agent is canagliflozin, the first of the SGLT-2 blockers to be approved for use in the U.S., which has been reported to reduce A1C by 0.5–1%. This class of agents works by decreasing renal glucose and sodium reabsorption and thereby reducing blood glucose levels; however, experience is still too limited to assess how problematic the genito-urinary symptoms, which are the leading side effect, may prove to be. Colesevelam, a bile acid sequestrant that appears to act by a hepatic mechanism, has been shown to reduce A1C levels by ~0.5% when used in combination with other agents. Finally, sustained-release bromocriptine appears to exert a neurally mediated effect on gluconeogenesis leading to a ~0.5% decrement in A1C. Canagliflozin also reduces weight and blood pressure, while colesevelam and bromocriptine can have desirable effects on plasma lipids.

ORAL AGENTS WITH BASAL INSULIN OR A GLP-1 RECEPTOR AGONIST

When two oral agents do not provide adequate glycemic control, a third oral agent may be added, but the glycemic benefit may be modest due to declining insulin secretory reserve. A more effective approach at this stage of disease progression is the addition of a long-acting insulin or a GLP-1 receptor agonist to the previously used oral agents. Long experience and proven medical benefit make adding basal insulin the leading choice for most patients. Systematic titration of glargine, detemir, degludec, or NPH insulin with continuation of oral agents can restore A1C to ≤7% for >50% of patients, and when the A1C level is <8% at the time insulin is started, 75% of patients can attain this level of success. The main undesired effects are weight gain (typically 1–2 kg), a ~50% likelihood of at least one symptomatic hypoglycemic event, and a 1–2% risk of hypoglycemia needing assistance. Because of the potential for weight gain and hypoglycemia associated with the use of insulin, consideration of a GLP-1 receptor agonist as the initial injected therapy is an attractive alternative. The long-acting agents of this class, once-daily liraglutide and once-weekly exenatide, are about as effective as basal insulin in restoring glycemic control to the A1C target in most cases. The main advantages of this approach are loss of weight (typically at least 2 kg), lower risk of hypoglycemia, and less frequent need for self-testing of glucose to guide dosing. The main disadvantage of the GLP-1 receptor agonists, aside from uncertainty about long-term safety, is the relatively high rate of nausea and other gastrointestinal symptoms. Up to 25–30% of patients have some symptoms of this kind when starting therapy and ~5% discontinue for this reason.

INDIVIDUALIZED REGIMENS USED LATER IN THE NATURAL HISTORY OF DIABETES

BASAL INSULIN WITH MEALTIME INSULIN

The most common prior regimen at the time when it becomes necessary to add an agent specifically targeting postprandial hyperglycemia is basal insulin with one or more oral agents. Even when fasting glucose levels are controlled to the 100–140 mg/dl range, prominent elevations of glucose after meals can lead to A1C levels between 7 and 8.5%. The traditional next step has been to add injections of rapid-acting insulin with meals to control daytime as well as overnight glucose levels, while continuing one or more oral agents. At this time, it is common practice to stop a sulfonylurea or thiazolidinedione, if either is being used, but continuation of these agents at reduced dosage may be helpful for some patients. The transition from basal insulin without mealtime insulin to the combination of basal with prandial insulins can be made most effective in a stepwise fashion, beginning with a single injection of prandial insulin (4–6 units is a common starting dose) given before the most problematic meal, usually breakfast or dinner. Injections of rapid-acting insulin with other meals can be added later if necessary. Twice-daily injections of premixed formulations of long-acting with rapid-acting insulins also can be used effectively, but they have limited dosing flexibility and greater risk of hypoglycemia. Many patients with T2D are successful with basal and mealtime insulin in combination with oral therapies, but this regimen also presents some practical difficulties. Risks of hypoglycemia and weight gain may be greater than with basal insulin alone and have been postulated to cause further cardiovascular risks. The need to increase the frequency of glucose testing to guide insulin dosing adds to the patient's burden of treatment. Also, despite the theoretically unlimited ability of insulin to control hyperglycemia, some people continue to have A1C levels above the target range. As a result, other combination-therapy approaches to management of postprandial hyperglycemia now are receiving renewed attention.

BASAL INSULIN WITH A GLP-1 RECEPTOR AGONIST

Insulins and GLP-1 receptor agonists have complementary effects. Basal insulin is the most effective treatment available for the control of basal hyperglycemia, but it may induce hypoglycemia and weight gain. Treatment with a GLP-1 receptor agonist favors weight loss and does not increase the risk of hypoglycemia when used alone and does not necessarily require more glucose testing. Thus, combining either long-acting or short-acting GLP-1 receptor agonists with basal insulin is an attractive option to improve glycemic control while limiting weight gain, with the short-acting GLP-1 receptor agonists (exenatide, lixisenatide) being more effective in reducing postprandial hyperglycemia. More experience is needed to identify which groups of patients are best suited to this combination, but if long-term safety can be demonstrated, this method of managing postprandial hyperglycemia has advantages for some patients, especially older or frail individuals for whom hypoglycemia poses significant risk. In addition, the amylin receptor agonist pramlintide has favorable effects on postprandial hyperglycemia and weight that resemble those of shorter-acting GLP-1 receptor agonists. It is approved for use only when both basal and mealtime insulin are needed, must be given just before meals with careful dose titration to limit nausea, and at present is used infrequently for T2D. α-Glucosidase inhibitors can be effective in limiting after-meal hyperglycemia when used in combination with basal insulin and can have desirable effects on weight. They require careful dose titration, however, to minimize gastrointestinal side effects.

GOALS AND OBJECTIVES OF THERAPY

To attain the goal of minimizing the development and progression of complications of diabetes, several objectives for glycemic management should be considered. Diagnosis of diabetes ideally is made soon after the first appearance of hyperglycemia, and treatment should be started promptly. The effectiveness of treatment can be optimized and side effects can be minimized by combination therapy using submaximal dosage of individual agents with the timely addition of other agents as needed. The ability of this approach to maintain good glycemic control for at least 5 years in early T2D was demonstrated in the ORIGIN trial, either with oral combination therapy or by adding basal insulin to a previous oral regimen. A significant challenge in this process lies in identifying patients whose response to therapy is below expectation and in individualizing treatment by selecting a combination of therapies with properties best suited to the patient's physiologic needs, personal preferences, and financial resources. This approach to combination therapy allows for the initial use of well-tested agents followed, when necessary, by judicious introduction of newer agents with especially desirable features for specific clinical situations. Ongoing studies of several newer classes of glucose-lowering agents offer the potential to improve the individualization of drug combinations and to identify subgroups for which specific drug combinations have high ratios of benefit to risk.

BIBLIOGRAPHY

RATIONALE FOR COMBINATION THERAPY

Bennett WL, Maruther NM, Singh S, Segal JB, Wilson LM, Chatterjee R, Marinopoulos SS, Puhan MA, Ranasinghe P, Block L, Nicholson WK, Hutfless S, Bass EB, Bolen S. Comparative effectiveness and safety of medications for type 2 diabetes: an update including new drugs and 2-drug combinations. *Ann Intern Med* 2011;154:602–613.

Inzucchi SE. Oral antihyperglycemic therapy for type 2 diabetes: scientific review. *JAMA* 2002;287;360–373.

The ORIGIN Trial Investigators. Characteristics associated with maintenance of mean A1C <6.5% in people with dysglycemia in the ORIGIN trial. *Diabetes Care* 2013;36:2915–2922.

Phung OJ, Scholle JM, Talwar M, Coleman CI. Effect of noninsulin antidiabetic drugs added to metformin therapy on glycemic control, weight gain, and hypoglycemia in type 2 diabetes. *JAMA* 2010;303:1410–1418.

Riddle M. Combining sulfonylureas and other oral agents. *Am J Med* 2000;108(Suppl 6A):15S–22S.

Riddle MC. Glycemic management of type 2 diabetes: an emerging strategy with oral agents, insulins, and combinations. *Endocrinol Metab Clin North Am* 2005;34:77–98.

U.K. Prospective Diabetes Study Group. U.K. Prospective Diabetes Study 16: overview of 6 years' of therapy of type II diabetes: a progressive disease. *Diabetes* 1995;44:1249–1258.

Yki-Jarvinen H. Combination therapies with insulin in type 2 diabetes. *Diabetes Care* 2001;24:758–767.

ORAL AGENT COMBINATIONS

Dobs AS, Goldstein BJ, Aschner P, Horton ES, Umpierrez GE, Duran L, Hill JS, Chen Y, Golm GT, Langdon RB, Williams-Herman ED, Kaufman KD, Amatruda JM, Arjona-Ferreira JC. Efficacy and safety of sitagliptin added to ongoing metformin and rosiglitazone combination therapy in a randomized placebo-controlled 54-week trial in patients with type 2 diabetes. *J Diab* 2012;5:68–79.

Scheen AJ, Charpentier G, Ostgren CJ, Hellqvist A, Gause-Nilsson I. Efficacy and safety of saxagliptin in combination with metformin compared with sitagliptin in combination with metformin in adult patients with type 2 diabetes mellitus. *Diabetes Metab Res Rev* 2010;26:540–549.

Schernthaner G, Gross JL, Rosenstock J, Guarisco M, Fu M, Yee J, Kawaguchi M, Canovatchel W, Meininger G. Canagliflozin compared with sitagliptin for patients with type 2 diabetes who do not have adequate glycemic control with metformin plus sulfonylurea: a 52-week randomized trial. *Diabetes Care* 2013;36:2508–2515.

Umpierrez G, Issa M, Vlajnic A. Glimepiride versus pioglitazone combination therapy in subjects with type 2 diabetes inadequately controlled on metformin monotherapy: results of a randomized trial. *Curr Med Res Opin* 2006;22:751–759.

INSULINS AND ORAL AGENTS

Davidson MB, Raskin P, Tanenberg RJ, Vlajnic A, Hollander P. A stepwise approach to insulin therapy in patients with type 2 diabetes and basal insulin treatment failure. *Endocr Pract* 2011;17:395–403.

Riddle MC, Vlajnic A, Zhou R, Rosenstock J: Baseline HbA1c predicts attainment of 7.0% HbA1c target with structured titration of insulin glargine in type 2 diabetes: a patient-level analysis of 12 studies. *Diab Obes Metab.* Accessed 5 April 2013.

Wulffele MG, Kooy A, Lehert P, Bets D, Ogterop JC, van der Berg BB, Donker AJM, Stehouwer DCA. Combination insulin and metformin in the treatment of type 2 diabetes. *Diabetes Care* 2002;25:2133–2140.

GLP-1R AGONISTS WITH ORAL AGENTS OR INSULIN

Buse JB, Bergenstal RM, Glass LC, Heilmann CR, Lewis MS, Kwan AYM, Hoogwerf BJ, Rosenstock J. Use of twice-daily exenatide in basal insulin-treated patients with type 2 diabetes: a randomized, controlled trial. *Ann Intern Med* 2011;154:103–111.

Drucker DJ, Buse JB, Taylor K, Kendall DM, Trautmann M, Zhuang D, Porter L, for the DURATION-1-Study Group. Exenatide once weekly versus twice daily for the treatment of type 2 diabetes: a randomized, open-label, non-inferiority study. *Lancet* 2008;372:1240–1250.

Nauck M, Frid A, Hermansen K, Shay NS, Tankova T, Mitha IH, Zdrackovic M, During M, Matthews DR, for the LEAD-2 Study Group. Efficacy and safety comparison on liraglutide, glimepiride, and placebo, all in combination with metformin, in type 2 diabetes: the LEAD (Liraglutide Effect and Action in Diabetes)-2 study. *Diabetes Care* 2009;32:84–90.

Riddle MC, Forst T, Aronson R, Sauque-Reyna L, Souhami E, Silvestre L, Ping Lin, Rosenstock J. Adding one-daily lixisenatide for type 2 diabetes inadequately controlled with newly initiated and continuously titrated basal insulin glargine: a 24-week randomized placebo-controlled study (GetTGoal-Duo1). *Diabetes Care* 2013;36:2497–2503.

Russell-Jones D, Vaag A, Schmitz O, Sethi BK, Lalic N, Antic S, Zdravkovic M, Ravn GM, Simo R, on behalf of the Liraglutide Effect and Action in Diabetes 5 (LEAD-5) met+SU Study Group. Liraglutide vs insulin glargine and placebo in combination with metformin and sulfonylurea therapy is type 2 diabetes mellitus (LEAD-5 met+SU): a randomized controlled trial. *Diabetologia* 2009;52:2046–2055.

CLINICAL GUIDELINES

Garber AJ, Abrahamson MJ, Barzilay JI, Blonde L, Bloomgarden ZT, Bush MA, Dagogo-Jack S, Davidson MB, Einhorn D, Garvey WT, Grunberger G, Handelsman Y, Hirsch IB, Jellinger PS, McGill JB, Mechanick JI, Rosenbllit PD, Umpierrez GI, Davidson MH. American Association of Clinical Endocrinologists' comprehensive diabetes management algorithm 2013 consensus statement: executive summary. *Endocr Pract* 2013;19:536–547.

Inzucchi SE, Bergenstal RM, Buse JB, Diamant M, Ferrannini E, Nauck M, Peters AL, Tsapas A, Wender R, Matthews DR. Management of hyperglycemia in type 2 diabetes: a patient-centered approach. Position statement of the American Diabetes Association (ADA) and the European Association for the Study of Diabetes (EASD). *Diabetes Care* 2012;35:1364–1379.

Nathan DM, Buse JB, Davidson MB, Ferrannini E, Holman RR, Sherwin R, Zinman B. Medical management of hyperglycemia in type 2 diabetes: a consensus algorithm for the initiation and adjustment of therapy. *Diabetes Care* 2009;32:193–203.

Chapter 32

Role of Bariatric Surgery in the Treatment of Type 2 Diabetes

Steven K. Malin, PhD
Sangeeta R. Kashyap, MD

OVERVIEW OF OBESITY PROMOTING TYPE 2 DIABETES

Obesity is a worldwide problem associated with increased rates of morbidity and mortality and decreased quality of life. In 2008, the World Health Organization estimated that there were 1.4 billion overweight adults (>20 years of age) and at least 500 million obese adults worldwide.[1] The definition of overweight according to the World Health Organization is a BMI of 25 kg/m² or more, and obesity as a BMI of >30 kg/m². However, obese patients are further characterized into class I (BMI 30–34.9 kg/m²), class II (BMI 35–39.9 kg/m²), class III (BMI >40 kg/m²), and class IV (>50 BMI kg/m²), because disease prevalence increases progressively from a BMI >20 kg/m² and exponentially from a BMI >35 kg/m².[1]

In the U.S., the Centers for Disease Control and Prevention conducted the National Health and Nutrition Examination Surveys that suggested nearly 75 million adults are obese. Although the prevalence of obesity has more than doubled over the past 40 years (13.4% in 1960–1962 vs. 35.1% in 2005–2006) in adults ages 20–74 years, obesity rates appear to have plateaued as of late.[2] Unfortunately, the subcategories of obesity have undergone a distribution shift, such that the prevalence of superobesity (>50 BMI kg/m²) in 1960–1962 of 0.9% had risen to 6.2% in 2005–2006.[3,4]

Obesity is responsible for >2.8 million deaths worldwide per year, owing to an increased prevalence of related comorbidities, including hypertension, heart disease, stroke, back and lower extremity weight-bearing degenerative problems, cancer, and type 2 diabetes (T2D).[4] Moreover, obesity is an independent risk factor for death and some reports indicate that there is a 20–40% increase in mortality in those who are overweight and upward of 300% among those who are obese.[5] Although numerous weight-loss interventions show initial promising results, the long-term success is highly variable. In 1991, the National Institutes of Health established surgical therapy guidelines for morbid obesity (BMI >40 kg/m² or BMI >35 kg/m²) in the presence of substantial complications.[6] Since then, the number of bariatric procedures has increased radically to >200,000 procedures performed in the U.S. in 2007, according to the American Society of Bariatric Surgery, with 170,000 patients undergoing Roux-en-Y gastric bypass operation. The patients electing to have these procedures have been primarily young women (~80%) of Caucasian descent with private insurance (~80%) and severe obesity (BMI >47 kg/m²).[7] Although most adults have attempted to lose weight at some point in their lives,[8] bariatric surgery is the only effective long-term weight-loss

DOI: 10.2337/9781580405096.32

therapy for severely obese individuals. Given the prevalence of obesity in the U.S., particularly class III obesity, there are almost 10,000 potential surgical candidates for every bariatric surgery.[9] Thus, it is likely that the use of bariatric surgery for weight loss and metabolic health will continue to rise over the next several years.

This chapter examines the impact of bariatric surgery on glucose and insulin metabolism. There is increasing evidence for the use of bariatric surgery to treat T2D in patients whose BMI is >35 kg/m². Central to improvements in glycemic control is enhanced sensitivity of bodily tissues to insulin as well as a stark increase in β-cell function. Special attention is given to weight-loss–dependent and –independent mechanisms that have been proposed to be altered by bariatric surgery and explain diabetes remission. The chapter also discusses the efficacy of using bariatric surgery as a therapeutic modality to improve cardiometabolic health in relation to surgery risk.

OBESITY AS A CULPRIT IN THE PATHOGENESIS OF TYPE 2 DIABETES

Insulin resistance and progressive pancreatic β-cell dysfunction are hallmark characteristics of T2D.[10] Obesity is a chief risk factor for the development of hyperglycemia, as excess body fat contributes to elevations in circulating free fatty acids and adipocyte-derived cytokines that mediate insulin resistance via inflammatory pathways.[11,12] The U.S. Diabetes Prevention Program demonstrated that modest weight loss (5–10% of initial body weight) through low-fat diet and increased physical activity (150 minutes/week of moderate intensity) reduced the incidence of T2D in adults with impaired glucose tolerance.[13] Moreover, in the Action for Health in Diabetes (Look AHEAD) study of the National Institutes of Health, lifestyle modification greatly improved glucose homeostasis after 1 year, although reductions in cardiovascular events were not seen.[14] In any event, these observations support the use of lifestyle modification as a medical treatment for T2D.[15] It is worth considering, however, that adherence to lifestyle changes is difficult, and oftentimes requires the addition of medications to restore glycemic control by reducing insulin resistance (biguanides, glitazones) and/or improving insulin secretion (incretin mimetics and sulfonylureas). Unfortunately, evidence reporting that these medications guarantee diabetes control is limited, and almost half of all patients fail to achieve the American Diabetes Association goal for glycemic control (i.e., A1C levels <7%).[16]

TYPES OF BARIATRIC SURGERY

Bariatric procedures are an effective means for inducing weight loss and improving glycemic control. Bariatric surgery tends to promote upward of 25% of the patient's total body weight. In addition, of those with T2D, nearly 85% achieve at least better glycemic control and need fewer antidiabetic medications, whereas an average of 78% achieve normal glycemic control without taking any antidiabetic medications.[17] Interestingly, not all bariatric surgeries cause the same effect on body weight, diabetes remission, and cardiometabolic resolution (Table 32.1).

Table 32.1 Metabolic Effects of Conventional Bariatric Techniques

	Rates of improvement (%) after surgery		
Improvement	LAGB	RYGB	BPD
Excess weight loss	46.2	59.5	63.3
Resolution of type 2 diabetes	56.7	80.3	95.1
Remission of dyslipidemia	59	97	99
Resolution of hypertension	43	68	83
Operative mortality	0.1	0.5	1.1

Note: LAGB = laparoscopic adjustable gastric banding; RYGB = Roux-en-Y gastric bypass; BPD = biliopancreatic diversion.
Source: Adapted from Buchwald H, Avidor Y, Braunwald E, Jensen MD, Pories W, Fahrbach K, Schoelles K. Bariatric surgery: a systematic review and meta-analysis. *JAMA* 2004;292(14):1724–1737.

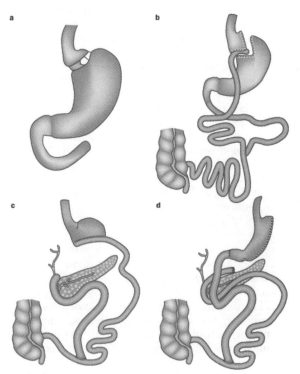

Figure 32.1—Conventional Bariatric Operations

Source: Adapted from Rubino et al.[40]

Bariatric procedures are classified as restrictive or malabsorptive (Figure 32.1) based on the presumed mechanism of weight loss.[18]

Gastric restrictive procedures limit gastric volume and, hence, restrict the intake of calories by inducing satiety. This procedure does not exclude or redirect food in the gastrointestinal tract. These medical therapies often include some "band" (i.e., laparoscopic adjustable gastric banding [LAGB]) or surgical resizing of the stomach with a stapler to create a small pouch (i.e., sleeve gastrostomy [SG] or vertical gastroplasty [VBG]) that limits food intake.[4] Afterward, patients lose ~46.2% of their excess body weight, while roughly 56.7% have T2D remission.

The LAGB surgical procedure is the second most common bariatric approach to weight loss. The procedure involves an adjustable plastic and silicone ring placed around the proximal stomach just beneath the gastresopageal junction.[4] A subcutaneous access port allows the degree of band constriction to be adjusted by the injection or withdrawal of saline.[20] Although the risk of death and morbidity is low following LAGB surgery, the amount of weight loss obtained is small compared with malabsorptive procedures.[4]

SG is a relatively new surgical procedure for the management of obesity. This procedure involves stapling the stomach over a sizing tube (11–20 mm) after resection of the greater curvature.[21] Interestingly, SG was originally developed as part of the biliopancreatic diversion with duodenal switch (BPD-DS), as the first-line treatment for superobesity.[22] Now, it is used more often as a stand-alone procedure (SG accounted for 7.8% of primary bariatric operations in 2010).[23] The effectiveness of SG on weight loss and resolution of comorbidities is less than that of Roux-en-Y gastric bypass (RYGB) but greater than that of LAGB. These results suggest that, at least, in the short term, SG is an efficacious method for weight loss.[4]

Malabsorptive procedures are designed to reduce the area of intestinal mucosa available for nutrient absorption and to restrict caloric intake similar to the way of LAGB. But, because the small intestine is shortened, these surgical approaches have an added component of malabsorption of fat and nutrients. Afterward, more patients experience remission of T2D (82–99%) than after gastric restrictive operations, even in patients with longer duration of disease, including those treated with insulin (Table 32.2). BPD consists of a partial gastrectomy, resulting in a 200–500 ml proximal gastric pouch and creation of a distal Roux and proximal biliary limb by division of the small bowel 200 cm proximal to the terminal ileum.[4] The gastric pouch then is anastomosed to the end of the Roux limb, and the biliary limb is attached 50 cm proximal to the iliocecal valve.[19] This procedure was later modified by creating a gastric sleeve with a maximum reservoir (150–200 ml). The small bowel then is divided at two points: 4–5 cm distal to the pylorus and 250 cm proximal to the terminal ileum.[4] The proximal duodenal end is reconnected to the last 250 cm of the small intestine and the biliary limb is anastomosed 100 cm proximal to the terminal ileum.[4] This protocol effectively created the BPD-DS and maintains the integrity of the antrum, pylorus, and short segment of the duodenum, and vagal nerve integrity. In theory, this protocol provides an advantage at maintaining a more physiologic digestive behavior than other surgical techniques.[24] The BPD-DS, however, is complex and not used as often as RYGB surgery. RYGB is considered the gold standard for bariatric surgery,[18,24] and the procedure involves creating a gastric pouch, Roux limb, and biliary limb.

Table 32.2 Antidiabetic Effects of Bariatric Surgery

	LAGB	RYGB	BPD
Rate of diabetes remission	Slow	Rapid	Rapid
Insulin sensitivity	Improved	Improved	Supernormal
Insulin secretion	Reduced	Increased	Reduced
GLP-1	No change	Increased	Increased
GIP	No change	Increased	Increased
PYY	No change	No change or increase	Reduced

Note: GLP = glucagon-like polypeptide; PYY = polypeptide tyrosine-tyrosine; GIP = glucose-dependent insulinotropic peptide; LAGB = laparoscopic adjustable gastric banding; RYGB = Roux-en-Y gastric bypass; BPD = biliopancreatic diversion.

Surgical staplers are used to create a small, vertically oriented gastric pouch with a volume of <30 cm^3. The Roux and biliary limbs are created by dividing the small bowel 30–40 cm from the ligament of Trietz. Restoration of continuity occurs by connecting the distal end of the divided bowel (Roux limb) to the pouch, creating a gastrojejunostomy, and anastomosing the biliary limb ~100–150 cm distal to the gastrojejunostomy.[4] The final size of the pouch is ~95% of the original stomach, and the entire duodenum and a portion of the jejunum are effectively bypassed, thereby restricting the volume of food ingested.[18,24]

Taken together, the efficacy of bariatric surgery on diabetes remission or metabolic health will differ depending on the surgery. The speed at which T2D goes into remission differs with restrictive vs. malabsorptive procedures (Table 32.2). After RYGB and BPD, diabetes remits within days, even before the patient has lost much weight. This does not happen after restrictive procedures.[25]

EFFECTS OF BARIATRIC SURGERY ON WEIGHT LOSS

The largest, prospective intervention-based trial that examined the effects of bariatric surgery (i.e., LAGB vs. VBG vs. RYGB) on 4,047 obese patients with healthy matched treated controls was the Swedish Obesity Study.[26] The results demonstrated that the surgical groups lost on average 23%, 17%, and 18% body weight at 2, 10, and 20 years, respectively.[27] The control group, however, gained weight at each respective time point. Buchwald et al. conducted a meta-analysis on the effects of bariatric surgery–induced weight loss and obesity-related comorbidities. It was reported that at 2 years postsurgery the overall excess weight loss for 10,172 patients was 61.2%.[17]

EFFECTS OF BARIATRIC SURGERY ON GLYCEMIA

The notion that bariatric surgery "cures" diabetes, or at the very least causes remission, has been recognized for >20 years. A classic study by Pories et al.[28]

demonstrated in 141 patients with T2D or impaired glucose tolerance that all but two individuals had normalized glucose tolerance within 10 days after RYGB. At 7.6 years after surgery, 83% of the diabetic patients were off their antidiabetic drugs, and 99% of those with impaired glucose tolerance were normoglycemic with a normal fasting glucose and hemoglobin A1C.[29] In the Swedish Obesity Study, at 2 years postsurgery with an average weight loss of nearly 28 kg, 72% of patients had complete resolution of T2D compared with 21% of controls.[26] Many of these patients had been able to stop taking oral hypoglycemic drugs or insulin, which is in contrast to the control group who had an increased need for these agents. Moreover, the proportion of patients treated with diet alone rose from 59 to 73% in the surgical group compared with a decline from 55 to 34% in the nonsurgical group. These results are similar to those of Schauer et al.[30] who observed marked improvements in morbidly obese patients with T2D based on A1C or impaired fasting glucose. After RYGB, fasting glucose and A1C had returned to normal levels in 83% of cases. In addition, nearly 80% of patients needed less oral antidiabetic agents or insulin. Scopinaro et al.[31,32] reported long-term follow-up data on 312 patients with T2D who underwent BPD and indicated that 99% of patients achieved normal glucose concentrations by 1 year after surgery. At 10 years after surgery, 98% of the patients were still in complete remission of diabetes (defined as normal glucose levels without the use of antidiabetic medications). Together, these studies demonstrate significant benefit for reducing the progression to T2D in adults with impaired glucose tolerance (or prediabetes). The risk of developing T2D in the study by Pories et al. was 30 times lower,[29] whereas in the Swedish Obesity Study,[26] the frequency of diabetes was 30 times lower at 2 years and 5 times lower at 8 years after surgery. This latter observation highlights that remission of diabetes is complex, and further research is needed to understand whether weight regain or a genetic predisposition toward diabetes affects the relapse of diabetes over time.

The magnitude of glycemic control benefit is specific to the medical therapy or surgical technique used (Figure 32.2). Complete resolution of T2D was observed in ~98% of patients who underwent BPD (with or without DS), 84% who underwent RYGB, 72% who underwent VBG, and 48% who underwent adjustable gastric band.[17] Other factors that appear to predict diabetes remission include the mildest severity of diabetes (diet controlled or duration <5 years), lower central obesity as measured by waist circumference, and the greatest weight loss after surgery.[33] Conversely, patients who do not resolve diabetes postsurgery were usually older or had a more prolonged pre-surgical disease course.[28,34,35]

EFFECT OF BARIATRIC SURGERY ON GLYCEMIC CONTROL: RANDOMIZED CONTROL TRIALS

Although much of the literature seems encouraging with respect to the effect of surgery on diabetes remission, the major limitation with this work is the lack of randomized control trials (RCTs). In the past few years, however, large randomized trials have evaluated the effects of various bariatric procedures in obese cohorts with T2D.

Dixon et al.[36] had conducted one of the early RCTs in patients with T2D. Patients were randomized to a medical treatment group utilizing strategies rec-

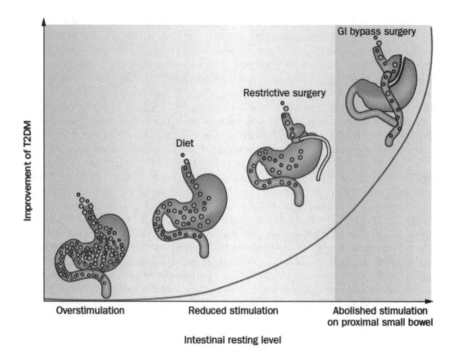

Figure 32.2—Hypothetical Model of Nutrient-Stimulated Gastrointestinal Dysfunction in Type 2 Diabetes

Source: Adapted from Rubino et al.[40]

ommended by the American Diabetes Association guidelines or to a surgery group to undergo laparoscopic adjustable gastric banding. Two years following surgery, diabetes remission (A1C <6.2% and a normal fasting glucose level) was 73% in the surgery group compared with only 13% in the medical treatment group. Individuals undergoing bariatric surgery lost 20.7% compared with 1.7% of body weight in the medical treatment arm.[36] A possible limitation of the work, however, was that vigorous medical weight-loss strategies such as those used in the Diabetes Prevention Study and the Look AHEAD trial[14] were not employed.

The Surgical Treatment and Medications Potentially Eradicate Diabetes Efficiently (STAMPEDE) trial was recently conducted to determine the effects of bariatric surgery on controlling glycemia in obese individuals with T2D. In the STAMPEDE trial, Schauer et al.[37] compared the effects of RYGB and SG vs. intensive medical therapy at 1 year post-operation in 150 obese patients with uncontrolled T2D. Individuals were randomized to surgical or medical therapy groups, and the primary end point was an A1C <6.0% (the most stringent criteria to date; Figure 32.3). The results indicated that RYGB and SG each produced significant improvements in A1C with 42 and 37% of patients in RYGB and SG,

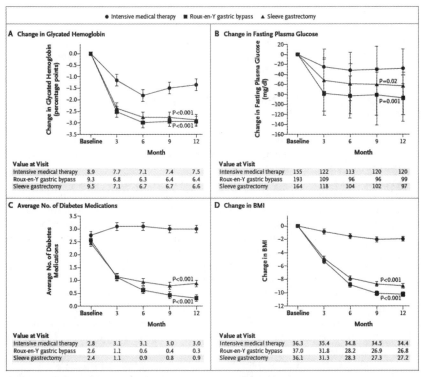

Figure 32.3—Effect of Bariatric Surgery on Metabolic Outcomes

Source: Adapted from Schauer PR, Kashyap SR, Wolski K, Brethauer SA, Kirwan JP, Pothier CE, Thomas S, Abood B, Nissen SE, Bhatt DL. Bariatric surgery versus intensive medical therapy in obese patients with diabetes. *N Engl J Med* 2012;366(17):1567–1576.

respectively, meeting glycemic control criteria. Consistent with these results, were those of the Diabetes Surgery Study whereby Ikramuddin et al.[38] compared the effects of RYGB with intensive medical therapy in 120 patients with T2D. A unique aspect of this study was that the end-point goal was the composite of the triple end-point goal: A1C <7.0%, a low-density lipoprotein (LDL) cholesterol of <100 mg/dl, and systolic blood pressure <130 mmHg. The results highlight RYGB as the more effective therapy for improving glycemic control, as 46% of RYGB patients improved glucose status compared with 11% with medical therapy. In a similar study, Mingrone et al.[39] included 60 patients between the ages of 30 and 60 years with a BMI >35 kg/m² with T2D (duration at least 5 years). Individuals were assigned randomly to either conventional medical therapy or gastric bypass (i.e., RYGB) or BPD. The primary end-point was the rate of diabetes remission at 2 years, which was defined as a fasting glucose <100 mg/dl and an A1C level of <6.5% in the absence of pharmacotherapy. The results demonstrate that conventional medical therapy was not able to normalize glucose status in any patient, whereas RYGB and BPD promoted diabetes remission in 75 and 95% of patients, respectively. Taken together, bariatric surgery appears to result in dramatic improvements in glycemic control and weight loss in obese patients with T2D. Further studies are required to assess the durability of this improved glycemic control and weight loss with the propensity to develop T2D.

MECHANISMS OF IMPROVEMENT IN T2D WITH BARIATRIC SURGERY

Three major mechanisms for the improvement in glucose homeostasis following bariatric surgery have been proposed, and these include: weight loss, nutrient malabsorption, and gut hormonal changes.

Weight loss may play a role in the resolution of T2D in obese patients since negative energy balance (or caloric deficit) improves insulin sensitivity.[40] This, in turn, would contribute to β-cell rest and improve pancreatic function. Indeed, the rate of diabetes resolution at 2 years post-surgery, compared with year one, was significantly correlated with the improvement in weight loss.[41] Moreover, postsurgery, patients have changes in food frequency (e.g., snack numbers, portion size) and food preference. Interestingly, these patients typically have reduced preference for sweet and fat-tasting foods.[42] Although less food intake clearly contributes to weight loss, the normalization of blood glucose and insulin levels following RYGB or BPD occurs well before any significant weight loss.[43] In fact, restrictive-malabsorptive procedures (LAGB) produce fewer cases of diabetes remission than mixed procedures (RYGB or BPD) despite comparable weight loss.[44] Therefore, diabetes resolution is not the result of weight loss alone.

Another theory is that bariatric surgery ameliorates insulin resistance and β-cell dysfunction by reducing the intestinal absorption of glucose and lipids. Because these nutrients in excess are known to promote reactive oxygen species and inflammation,[45] reducing glucose and lipid absorption would reduce the accumulation of intermediate lipid byproducts in multiple tissues (e.g., skeletal muscle, liver, and adipose) and directly or indirectly reduce the secretion of hormones secreted from adipocytes that impair insulin signaling. Although nutrient malabsorption is clinically evident after BPD, it does not occur after standard RYGB,[46] suggesting that additional factors may drive improvements in glycemic control.[47]

An alternative theory for explaining the anti-diabetic effects of bariatric surgery is linked to the rerouting of nutrient flow through the gastrointestinal tract. Rubino et al. have hypothesized that overstimulation of the gastrointestinal tract by overeating could lead to metabolic disturbances that promote hyperglycemia, whereas restricting food contact with the gastrointestinal tract could improve these conditions.[40] A possible mechanism for improving insulin sensitivity or β-cell function is related to the secretion of various hormones (see Gut Hormones as a Candidate for Diabetes Remission and Weight Loss for more details) released by the gut in response to the rerouting of food intake (Figure 32.4).[48] RYGB procedure excludes the duodenum, while BPD excludes both the duodenum and jejunum and results in altered distributions of carbohydrate and fat absorption.[48] Subsequently, this altered nutrient delivery is linked to higher anorectic hormones that induce satiety (e.g., glucagon-like polypeptide 1 [GLP-1] and polypeptide tyrosine-tyrosine [PYY]) and lower levels of the orexigeneic hormone ghrelin.[48]

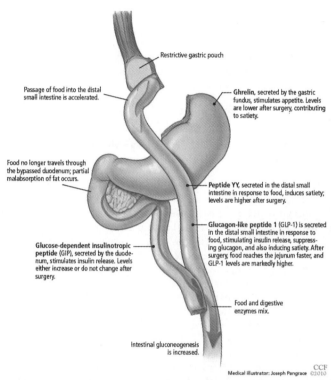

Figure 32.4—Role of Gut Hormones in Possibly Explaining the Remission of Type 2 Diabetes Following Roux-en-Y Surgery

Source: Adapted from Kashyap SR, Gatmaitan P, Brethauer S, Schauer PR. Bariatric surgery for type 2 diabetes: weighing the impact for obese patients. *Cleve Clin J Med* 2010;77(7):468–476. Reprinted with permission from the publisher.

On the basis of these observations, the "hindgut" and "foregut" hypotheses have been raised. The hindgut hypothesis (also referred to as the lower intestinal or distal hypothesis) proposed by Cummings et al.[49] suggests that diabetes control is due to accelerated delivery of nutrients to the distal intestine, which augments an insulinotropic signal (e.g., GLP-1) that improves glucose homeostasis via enhanced insulin action. Indeed, augmented GLP-1 secretion increases the insulin response to nutrient intake, and at least in animal models, induces β-cell proliferation,[50] which together reduce blood glucose levels. In contrast, the foregut hypothesis (also referred to as upper intestinal or proximal hypothesis), raised by Rubino et al.,[51] suggests that nutrient interactions in the duodenum and proximal jejunum are diabetogenic and, hence, bypassing the duodenum would alleviate this intestinal factor that induces insulin resistance and β-cell dysfunction.[52] Although the hindgut and foregut hypotheses often are explained in terms of hormonal changes, they are exclusive of altered nutrient flow that affects neural signaling. In addition, the hindgut and foregut hypotheses often are presented as mutually exclusive theories. Although this approach is convenient for didactic purposes, no data actually exist excluding portions of the upper or lower intestine. In addition, the molecular mechanism by which gastric bypass surgery, or other surgical techniques, improves glucose metabolism is unclear, but alterations in gastrointestinal hormones and neural signals linked to the gastrointestinal tract likely are key.[40]

GUT HORMONES AS A CANDIDATE FOR DIABETES REMISSION AND WEIGHT LOSS

Gastrointestinal hormones that increase insulin secretion following meal intake are known as incretins. Of interest, they have this effect only when glucose is orally consumed, not when it is infused intravenously.[53] GLP-1 and glucose-dependent insulinotropic peptide (GIP) account for ~60% of the nutrient-related insulin secretion. In addition, GLP-1 has been shown to suppress glucagon and ghrelin, as well as delay gastric emptying, which delays digestion and reduces postprandial hyperglycemia.[54] GLP-1 also acts on the brain to induce satiety, although the mechanisms remain largely unknown. Laferrere et al.[55] and others reported increased postprandial levels of GLP-1 within 4 weeks following RYGB, whereas levels of GLP-1 did not rise with comparable weight loss induced by diet. These findings are consistent with data in patients with T2D at 1 and 2 years following RYGB in which elevated GLP-1 was associated significantly with insulin action.[56] Moreover, in the STAMPEDE trial, RYGB was shown to augment GLP-1 and β-cell function to a greater extent than either SG or intensive medical therapy 2 years postsurgery.[57] In general, RYGB is reported to enhance insulin secretion, whereas gastric-restrictive procedures reduce the need to secrete insulin.[58] On the other hand, GIP is secreted in the K-cells located mainly in the duodenum and proximal jejunum and released in response to nutrients (mainly lipid). Unlike, GLP-1, GIP is more involved in lipid metabolism (storage) and thus is thought to play a more direct role in the pathogenesis of obesity. The effect of bariatric surgery on GIP is more controversial than the findings of GLP-1, such that the role of GIP is less clear on the regulation of lower fat mass or weight maintenance.[42]

Noninsulinotropic gut hormones are altered after RYGB and include PYY and ghrelin. Like GLP-1, PYY is secreted by the L-cells of the distal small intestine and is responsible for increasing satiety and delaying gastric emptying after meals. Several studies consistently have documented increases in postprandial PYY and GLP-1 after gastric bypass.[59–61] Ghrelin is a gastric hormone produced primarily in the stomach with secondary secretion emanating from the proximal small intestine. Ghrelin is best known as an appetite-stimulating hormone, but it also has additional effects on impairing insulin sensitivity and reducing glucose-stimulated insulin secretion.[62] Ghrelin suppression usually is improved post-RYGB or SG, suggesting that suppression of hunger signals helps sustain weight loss. In contrast, ghrelin levels typically rise following diet-induced weight loss.[63] The efficacy of bariatric surgery on ghrelin, however, is controversial.[56,64]

EFFECTS OF BARIATRIC SURGERY ON DYSLIPIDEMIA AND HYPERTENSION

In addition to substantially reducing hyperglycemia, bariatric surgery also reduces cardiometabolic risk by lowering dyslipidemia and hypertension. Atherogenic dyslipidemia is strongly associated with insulin resistance, inflammation–thrombotic states, and visceral fat, and is defined as low high-density lipoprotein (HDL) cholesterol and elevated triglycerides, apolipoprotein B, and small LDL particles. Results of a meta-analysis showed marked decreases in levels of total cholesterol, LDL, and triglycerides after bariatric procedures.[65] In fact, ~70% of patients experience an improvement in hyperlipidemia and maximum improvements typically are derived from BPD and RYGB groups.[17] In the Swedish Obesity Study, significant improvements were observed in triglyceride and HDL concentrations at 2 and 10 years in the surgical versus the control group.[26] In recent randomized controlled trials, including the Diabetes Surgery Study and STAMPEDE, bariatric surgery has been shown to decrease triglycerides and increase HDL concentrations to a greater extent than medical therapy alone.[37-39] Collectively, these data demonstrate that bariatric surgery is not only effective at regulating blood glucose levels and sustaining weight loss, but also an effective treatment option for improving blood lipid profiles in obese individuals. These findings are likely to contribute to the overall reduction in cardiovascular disease events seen 20 years postsurgery.[27]

Hypertension is highly associated with obesity, and there is good evidence that weight loss reduces blood pressure.[66] In general, a decrease of 1% body weight leads to a 1 mmHg decrease in systolic blood pressure and a 2 mmHg decrease in diastolic blood pressure.[67,68] Similar to effects on dyslipidemia, hyperglycemia, and weight loss, bariatric surgery across all procedures has good effects on reducing blood pressure. In particular, ~61 and 79% of the total population with hypertension had it either resolved or improved up to 2 years postsurgery.[17] The Swedish Obesity Study examined the effect of obesity on hypertension by investigating the 8-year incidence of hypertension in obese patients treated with bariatric surgery (VGB, GB, and RYGB) versus obese matched controls.[69] The results indicated no overall difference in systolic blood pressure and an increase in diastolic blood pressure at 8 years compared with the control group. RYGB, however, did appear to be the more favorable surgical procedure for decreasing systolic and diastolic blood pressure at 10 years (by 4.7 and 10.4%, respectively, $P < 0.10$).[26] Nevertheless, to understand why systolic blood pressure did not improve, an examination of weight loss and age were analyzed.[69] It was reported that despite rapid improvements in body weight and blood pressure by 1 year, the slight increase in systolic and diastolic blood pressure over subsequent years was linked to the rate of weight gain and age. In fact, in the surgical group, the effect on blood pressure of 1 year (time between baseline and last observation in the study) was up to 4 times greater than the effect of 1 kg regained. Together, these results suggest that blood pressure is linked more closely to the direction of weight change than to the initial weight loss, but age is an important factor. Bariatric surgery did not decrease diastolic blood pressure, but rather diastolic blood pressure was increased postsurgery. Given that pulse pressure is associated with increased risk for coronary artery disease,[70] Sjostrom et al. examined whether surgery could lower pulse pressure compared with a control group.[69] The results indicated that the weight reduction postsurgery lowered the rate of increase in pulse pressure seen in obese patients. Taken together, the results of bariatric surgery on blood pressure are not a simple relationship, but there do seem to be some protective effects on the risk for future coronary heart disease.

RISKS OF BARIATRIC SURGERY

A common concern raised about bariatric surgery is that it is associated with a markedly elevated risk of postsurgical complications and mortality. A meta-analysis of 361 studies that included 85,048 patients, however, showed an overall mortality of 0.28% within 30 days of surgery, and a mortality of 0.35% between 30 days and 2 years after surgery.[71] In addition, a prospective observational study known as the Longitudinal Assessment of Bariatric Surgery was conducted at multiple sites within the U.S.[72] The major finding was that the 30-day death rate among individuals undergoing RYGB or LAGB was 0.3%.[72] Buchwald et al.[71] performed a meta-analysis of 136 bariatric studies that included 22,094 patients. The 30-day operative death rates were 1.1% with BPD, 0.5% with RYGB, and 0.1% with restrictive procedures. Importantly, although several complications from bariatric surgery may increase the 30-day in-hospital mortality, older age, BMI >50 kg/m^2, male gender, hypertension, diabetes, and pulmonary embolus risk appear to account for the majority of deaths.[71,72] Nevertheless, death rates after bariatric surgery must be weighed against the long-term cardiovascular risk of continued obesity and T2D.[48] In fact, bariatric surgery has been shown to increase life expectancy[5,73] in part because of reductions in cardiovascular risk factors and diabetes. Interestingly, patients undergoing bariatric surgery have a 32–73% lower long-term death rate than matched controls who do not undergo surgery.[5,73]

LAGB is considered to be the safest of the current bariatric procedures. It does not involve bowel anastomosis, and the risk of major hemorrhage, gastric perforation, and pulmonary embolism is <1%. Late complications requiring reoperation include band slippage or prolapse (5–10%) and band erosion (1–3%). The entire intestinal tract is left intact, so subsequent nutritional deficiencies are rare.[74] RYGB, on the other hand, carries an overall risk of major complication of 10–15%. Anastomotic leak (1–5%), pulmonary embolism (<1%), and hemorrhage (1–4%) can be life threatening but are rare if the staff are experienced. Late complications, such as ulcer or stricture formation at the gastrojejunostomy site, occur in 5–10% of cases and are managed nonoperatively.[48]

In 30–70% of patients, nutritional deficiencies occur and require some nutritional support. The patients at highest risk of developing severe nutritional deficiencies include those who have lost >10% of their body weight by 1 month, have anastomotic stenosis, have undergone surgical revision, and have persistent vomiting.[48,75] Protein calorie malnutrition is also a concern and can be recognized by signs such as edema, hypoalbuminemia, anemia, and hair loss. To minimize these effects, it generally is recommended that patients consume between 60–80 g of protein and ~800 kcal/day. Vitamin deficiencies are common and can lead to peripheral neuropathy (B$_{12}$), Wernicke encephalopathy (B$_1$), metabolic bone disease (vitamin D, calcium), and iron-deficient anemia. Subsequently, monitoring iron stores, nutrient levels, and vitamin levels before bariatric surgery is recommended as well as every 6 months after surgery.[75–77] Bone density screening is included in these recommendations at baseline and at follow-up every 2–3 years.

In some cases, severe hypoglycemia has been documented after RYGB and is associated with prandial hyperinsulinemia due to elevated GLP-1 levels.[78] Neuroglycopenia and seizures have been reported in severe cases. Initial treatment of hypoglycemia involves dietary modification targeting carbohydrate restriction and management by an endocrinologist.[79] In addition to carbohydrate restriction, pharmacotherapy targeting carbohydrate absorption with acarbose may be indicated as well as the use of agents that inhibit insulin secretion (diazoxide, octreotide).

Relapse of diabetes control has been documented in 20–40% of cases,[80] especially in those that undergo restrictive (lap banding, sleeve gastrectomy) procedures. Relapse may be associated with poor residual pancreatic β-cell function indicated by severity and duration of diabetes, insulin use, and weight regain that occurs from 18–24 months post procedure.

IMPLICATIONS FOR BARIATRIC SURGERY IN PATIENTS WITH TYPE 2 DIABETES

The National Institutes of Health current guidelines for physicians considering bariatric surgery in their patients include people with a BMI of 40 kg/m^2 or higher, or a BMI >35 kg/m^2 with at least two obesity-related comorbidities (e.g., hyperglycemia, dyslipidemia, hypertension). The metabolic health risk of mortality from diabetes justifies the risk of surgery. Bariatric surgery appears to be a viable treatment option for all obese patients (BMI >35 kg/m^2) with T2D who have struggled to lose weight through conventional lifestyle approaches.[48] In addition, although recent evidence suggests that patients with a BMI 30–35 kg/m^2 experience greater weight loss and better immediate glucose outcomes when compared with nonsurgical treatments, the evidence for recommending bariatric surgery in class I obesity is insufficient at this point until more long-term outcomes and complications from surgery are studied.[81] This chapter has focused on the effects of bariatric surgery on glucose and cardiometabolic health in obese adults. Recent work has suggested that adolescents have favorable improvements in weight reduction, glycemic control, and cardiovascular risk factors.[82,83] As with recommending bariatric surgery for individuals with a BMI between 30 and 35 kg/m^2, there is limited long-term follow-up data on reproductive physiology and complications in the pediatric populations to determine the usefulness of bariatric surgery as a medical approach for improving short-term and lifelong metabolic health.

Whether obesity in itself is a medical disease or a chief risk factor for the development of insulin resistance and pancreatic β-cell dysfunction, obesity is an important causal factor in the development of T2D.[84] Lifestyle modification and weight loss are considered first-line therapeutic strategies for alleviating insulin resistance and poor insulin secretion capacity. Based on current evidence, bariatric surgery appears to be a reasonable medical intervention to promote weight loss and improve glycemic control, if lifestyle and pharmacological attempts fail. In addition, bariatric surgery has protective effects on dyslipidemia and blood pressure, suggesting that bariatric surgery may lower the risk of future heart disease. Thus, when the individual risk factors for obesity-related diabetes and coronary heart disease are taken into consideration, the results presented herein highlight bariatric surgery as a potentially effective therapy for lowering metabolic disease risk and overall mortality. Given that bariatric surgery also poses low risk in itself, surgery appears to be a credible treatment strategy to accelerate the reversal of obesity-induced metabolic disease. Follow-up for monitoring of comorbidity status, nutrient deficiencies, and weight regain–related issues are essential for optimizing patient care.

REFERENCES

1. Obesity and overweight. Fact sheet no 311. Geneva, World Health Organization, 2013.

2. Flegal KM, Carroll MD, Kit BK, Ogden CL. Prevalence of obesity and trends in the distribution of body mass index among US adults, 1999-2010. *JAMA* 2012;307(5):491–497.

3. Ogden CL, Carroll MD, Curtin LR, McDowell MA, Tabak CJ, Flegal KM. Prevalence of overweight and obesity in the United States, 1999-2004 *JAMA* 2006;295(13):1549–1555.

4. Noria SF, Grantcharov T. Biological effects of bariatric surgery on obesity-related comorbidities. *Can J Surg* 2013;56(1):47–57.

5. Adams KF, Schatzkin A, Harris TB, Kipnis V, Mouw T, Ballard Barbash R, Hollenbeck A, Leitzmann MF. Overweight, obesity, and mortality in a large prospective cohort of persons 50 to 71 years old. *N Engl J Med* 2006;355(8):763–778.

6. NIH conference. Gastrointestinal surgery for severe obesity. Consensus development conference panel. *Ann Intern Med* 1991;115(12):956–961.

7. Santry HP, Gillen DL, Lauderdale DS. Trends in bariatric surgical procedures. *JAMA* 2005;294(15):1909–1917.

8. Serdula MK, Mokdad AH, Williamson DF, Galuska DA, Mendlein JM, Heath GW. Prevalence of attempting weight loss and strategies for controlling weight. *JAMA* 1999;282(14):1353–1358.

9. Alt SJ. Bariatric surgery programs growing quickly nationwide. *Health Care Strateg Manage* 2001;19(9):1, 7–23.

10. DeFronzo RA, Abdul Ghani MA. Preservation of ß-cell function: the key to diabetes prevention. *J Clin Endocrinol Metab* 2011;96(8):2354–2366.

11. Despres JP, Lemieux I, Prud'homme D. Treatment of obesity: need to focus on high risk abdominally obese patients. *BMJ* 2001;322(7288):716–720.

12. Samuel VT, Shulman GI. Mechanisms for insulin resistance: common threads and missing links. *Cell* 2012;148(5):852–871.

13. Knowler WC, Barrett-Connor E, Fowler SE, Hamman RF, Lachin JM, Walker EA, Nathan DM, Diabetes Prevention Program Research Group. Reduction in the incidence of type 2 diabetes with lifestyle intervention or metformin. *N Engl J Med* 2002 Feb 7;346(6):393–403.

14. Wing RR, Bolin P, Brancati FL, Bray GA, Clark JM, Coday M, Crow RS, Curtis JM, Egan CM, Espeland MA, Evans M, Foreyt JP, Ghazarian S, Gregg EW, Harrison B, Hazuda HP, Hill JO, Horton ES, Hubbard VS, Jakicic J, Jeffery RW, Johnson KC, Kahn SE, Kitabchi A, Knowler WC, Lewis CE, Maschak-Carey BJ, Montez MG, Murillo A, Nathan DM, Patricio J, Peters A, Pi-Sunyer X, Pownall H, Reboussin D, Regensteiner JG, Rickman AD, Ryan DH, Safford M, Wadden TA, Wagenknecht L, West DS, Williamson DF, Yanovski SZ. Cardiovascular effects of intensive lifestyle intervention in type 2 diabetes. *New Engl J Med* 2013;369(2):145–154.

15. Church TS, Blair SN, Cocreham S, Johannsen N, Johnson W, Kramer K, Mikus CR, Myers V, Nauta M, Rodarte RQ, Sparks L, Thompson A, Earnest C. Effects of aerobic and resistance training on hemoglobin A1c levels in patients with type 2 diabetes: a randomized controlled trial. *JAMA* 2010;304(20):2253–2262.

16. Diagnosis and classification of diabetes mellitus. *Diabetes Care* 2009;32(Suppl 1): S62–S67.

17. Buchwald H, Avidor Y, Braunwald E, Jensen MD, Pories W, Fahrbach K, Schoelles K. Bariatric surgery: a systematic review and meta-analysis. *JAMA* 2004;292(14):1724–1737.

18. Steinbrook R. Surgery for severe obesity. *N Engl J Med* 2004;350(11):1075–1079.

19. Colquitt JL, Picot J, Loveman E, Clegg AJ. Surgery for obesity. *Cochrane Database of Systematic Reviews* 2009(2):CD003641–CD003641.

20. Parikh MS, Fielding GA, Ren CJ. U.S. experience with 749 laparoscopic adjustable gastric bands: intermediate outcomes. *Surg Endosc* 2005;19(12):1631–1635.

21. Gagner M, Deitel M, Kalberer TL, Erickson AL, Crosby RD. The second international consensus summit for sleeve gastrectomy. *Surg Obes Relat Dis* 2009;5(4):476–485.

22. Hess DS. Biliopancreatic diversion with a duodenal switch. *Obesity Surg* 1998;8(3).267–202.

23. Hutter MM, Schirmer BD, Jones DB, Ko CY, Cohen ME, Merkow RP, Nguyen NT. First report from the American College of Surgeons Bariatric Surgery Center Network: laparoscopic sleeve gastrectomy has morbidity and

effectiveness positioned between the band and the bypass. *Ann Surg* 2011;254(3):410–420.

24. Rubino F. Bariatric surgery: effects on glucose homeostasis. *Curr Opin Clin Nutr Metab Care* 2006;9(4):497–507.

25. Buchwald H, Estok R, Fahrbach K, Banel D, Jensen MD, Pories WJ, Bantle JP, Sledge I. Weight and type 2 diabetes after bariatric surgery: systematic review and meta-analysis. *Am J Med* 2009;122(3):248–256.e5.

26. Sjöström L. Lindroos AK, Peltonen M, Torgerson J, Bouchard C, Carlsson B, Dahlgren S, Larsson B, Narbro K, Sjöström CD, Sullivan M, Wedel H; Swedish Obese Subjects Study Scientific Group. Lifestyle, diabetes, and cardiovascular risk factors 10 years after bariatric surgery. *N Engl J Med* 2004; 351(26):2683–2693.

27. Sjöström L, Peltonen M, Jacobson P, Sjöström CD, Karason K, Wedel H, Ahlin S, Anveden Å, Bengtsson C, Bergmark G, Bouchard C, Carlsson B, Dahlgren S, Karlsson J, Lindroos AK, Lönroth H, Narbro K, Näslund I, Olbers T, Svensson PA, Carlsson LM. Bariatric surgery and long-term cardiovascular events. *JAMA* 2012;307(1):56–65.

28. Pories WJ, Caro JF, Flickinger EG, Meelheim HD, Swanson MS. The control of diabetes mellitus (NIDDM) in the morbidly obese with the Greenville gastric bypass. *Ann Surg* 1987;206(3):316–323.

29. Pories WJ, Swanson MS, MacDonald KG, Long SB, Morris PG, Brown BM, Barakat HA, deRamon RA, Israel G, Dolezal JM. Who would have thought it? An operation proves to be the most effective therapy for adult-onset diabetes mellitus. *Ann Surg* 1995;222(3):339–350.

30. Schauer PR, Burguera B, Ikramuddin S, Cottam D, Gourash W, Hamad G, Eid G, Mattar S, Ramanathan R, Barinas Mitchel E, Rao RH, Kuller L, Kelley D. Effect of laparoscopic roux-en Y gastric bypass on type 2 diabetes mellitus. *Ann Surg* 2003;238(4):467–484.

31. Scopinaro N, Papadia F, Marinari G, Camerini G, Adami G. Long-term control of type 2 diabetes mellitus and the other major components of the metabolic syndrome after biliopancreatic diversion in patients with BMI <35 kg/m². *Obesity Surg* 2007;17(2):185–192.

32. Scopinaro N, Marinari GM, Camerini GB, Papadia FS, Adami GF. Specific effects of biliopancreatic diversion on the major components of metabolic syndrome: a long-term follow-up study. *Diabetes Care* 2005;28(10):2406–2411.

33. Torquati A, Lutfi R, Abumrad N, Richards WO. Is roux-en-Y gastric bypass surgery the most effective treatment for type 2 diabetes mellitus in morbidly obese patients? *J Gastrointest Surg* 2005;9(8):1112–1116.

34. Pories WJ, MacDonald KG, Flickinger EG, Dohm GL, Sinha MK, Barakat HA, May HJ, Khazanie P, Swanson MS, Morgan E. Is type II diabetes mellitus (NIDDM) a surgical disease? *Ann Surg* 1992;215(6):633–642.

35. Sugerman HJ, Wolfe LG, Sica DA, Clore JN. Diabetes and hypertension in severe obesity and effects of gastric bypass-induced weight loss. *Ann Surg* 2003;237(6):751–756.

36. Dixon JB, O'Brien PE, Playfair J, Chapman L, Schachter LM, Skinner S, Proietto J, Bailey M, Anderson M. Adjustable gastric banding and conventional therapy for type 2 diabetes: a randomized controlled trial. *JAMA* 2008; 299(3):316–323.

37. Schauer PR, Kashyap SR, Wolski K, Brethauer SA, Kirwan JP, Pothier CE, Thomas S, Abood B, Nissen SE, Bhatt DL. Bariatric surgery versus intensive medical therapy in obese patients with diabetes. *N Engl J Med* 2012;366(17):1567–1576.

38. Ikramuddin S, Korner J, Lee WL, Connett JE, Inabnet WB, Billington CJ, Thomas AJ, Leslie DB, Chong K, Jeffery RW, Ahmed L, Vella A, Chuang LM, Bessler M, Sarr MG, Swain JM, Laqua P, Jensen M, Bantle J. Roux-en-Y gastric bypass vs intensive medical management for the control of type 2 diabetes, hypertension, and hyperlipidemia: the Diabetes Surgery Study randomized clinical trial. *JAMA* 2013;309(21):2240–2249.

39. Mingrone G, Panunzi S, De Gaetano A, Guidone C, Iaconelli A, Leccesi L, Nanni G, Pomp A, Castagneto M, Ghirlanda G, Rubino F. Bariatric surgery versus conventional medical therapy for type 2 diabetes. *N Engl J Med* 2012;366(17):1577–1585.

40. Rubino F, R'bibo SL, del Genio F, Mazumdar M, McGraw T. Metabolic surgery: the role of the gastrointestinal tract in diabetes mellitus. *Nat Rev Endocrinol* 2010;6(2):102–109.

41. Ponce J, Haynes B, Paynter S, Fromm R, Lindsey B, Shafer A, Manahan E, Sutterfield C. Effect of lap-band-induced weight loss on type 2 diabetes mellitus and hypertension. *Obesity Surg* 2004;14(10):1335–1342.

42. Ionut V, Bergman R. Mechanisms responsible for excess weight loss after bariatric surgery. *J Diabetes Sci Technol* 2011;5(5):1263–1282.

43. Isbell JM, Tamboli RA, Hansen EN, Saliba J, Dunn JP, Phillips SE, Marks Shulman PA, Abumrad NN. The importance of caloric restriction in the early improvements in insulin sensitivity after roux-en-Y gastric bypass surgery. *Diabetes Care* 2010;33(7):1438–1442.

44. Buchwald H, Oien DM. Metabolic/bariatric surgery worldwide 2008. *Obesity Surg* 2009;19(12):1605–1611.

45. Evans JL, Goldfine ID, Maddux BA, Grodsky GM. Are oxidative stress-activated signaling pathways mediators of insulin resistance and beta-cell dysfunction? *Diabetes* 2003;52(1):1–8.

46. Marceau P, Hould FS, Simard S, Lebel S, Bourque RA, Potvin M, Biron S. Biliopancreatic diversion with duodenal switch. *World J Surg* 1998;22(9):947–954.

47. Brolin RE, LaMarca LB, Kenler HA, Cody RP. Malabsorptive gastric bypass in patients with superobesity. *J Gastrointest Surg* 2002;6(2):195–203.

48. Kashyap SR, Gatmaitan P, Brethauer S, Schauer PR. Bariatric surgery for type 2 diabetes: weighing the impact for obese patients. *Cleve Clin J Med* 2010;77(7):468–476.

49. Cummings DE. Endocrine mechanisms mediating remission of diabetes after gastric bypass surgery. *Int J Obes* 2009;33(Suppl 1):S33–S40.

50. Pournaras DJ, le Roux CW. Obesity, gut hormones, and bariatric surgery. *World J Surg* 2009;33(10):1983–1988.

51. Rubino F. The early effect of the Roux-en-Y gastric bypass on hormones involved in body weight regulation and glucose metabolism. *Ann Surg* 2004;240(2):236–242.

52. Salinari S, Debard C, Bertuzzi A, Durand C, Zimmet P, Vidal H, Mingrone G. Jejunal proteins secreted by db/db mice or insulin-resistant humans impair the insulin signaling and determine insulin resistance. *PLoS ONE* 2013;8(2):e56258.

53. Vollmer K, Holst JJ, Baller B, Ellrichmann M, Nauck MA, Schmidt WE, Meier JJ. Predictors of incretin concentrations in subjects with normal, impaired, and diabetic glucose tolerance. *Diabetes* 2008;57(3):678–687.

54. Holst JJ, Vilsbll T, Deacon CF. The incretin system and its role in type 2 diabetes mellitus. *Mol Cell Endocrinol* 2009;297(1–2):127–136.

55. Laferrère B, Teixeira J, McGinty J, Tran H, Egger JR, Colarusso A, Kovack B, Bawa B, Koshy N, Lee H, Yapp K, Olivan B. Effect of weight loss by gastric bypass surgery versus hypocaloric diet on glucose and incretin levels in patients with type 2 diabetes. *J Clin Endocrinol Metab* 2008;93(7):2479–2485.

56. Malin SK, Samat A, Wolski K, Abood B, Pothier CE, Bhatt DL, Nissen S, Brethauer SA, Schauer PR, Kirwan JP, Kashyap SR. Improved acylated ghrelin suppression at 2 years in obese patients with type 2 diabetes: effects of bariatric surgery vs. standard medical therapy. *Int J Obes (Lond)*; 2013 Oct 29. doi: 10.1038/ijo.2013.196. [Epub ahead of print.]

57. Kashayp SR, Bhatt DL, Wolski K, Wantanabe RM, Abdul-Ghani MA, Abood B, Pothier CE, Brethauer S, Nissen SE, Gupta M, Kirwan JP, Schauer PR. Metabolic effects of bariatric surgery in patients with moderate obesity and type 2 diabetes: analysis of a randomized control trial comparing surgery vs. intensive medical treatment. *Diabetes Care* 2013 36(8):2175–2182.

58. Kashyap SR, Daud S, Kelly KR, Gastaldelli A, Win H, Brethauer S, Kirwan JP, Schauer PR. Acute effects of gastric bypass versus gastric restrictive surgery on beta-cell function and insulinotropic hormones in severely obese patients with type 2 diabetes. *Int J Obes* 2010;34(3):462–471.

59. Korner J, Bessler M, Inabnet W, Taveras C, Holst JJ. Exaggerated glucagon-like peptide-1 and blunted glucose-dependent insulinotropic peptide secre-

tion are associated with Roux-en-Y gastric bypass but not adjustable gastric banding. *Surg Obes Relat Dis* 2007;3(6):597–601.

60. Hanusch Enserer U, Ghatei MA, Cauza E, Bloom SR, Prager R, Roden M. Relation of fasting plasma peptide YY to glucose metabolism and cardiovascular risk factors after restrictive bariatric surgery. *Wien Klin Wochenschr* 2007;119(9–10):291–296.

61. le Roux CW, Aylwin SJ, Batterham RL, Borg CM, Coyle F, Prasad V, Shurey S, Ghatei MA, Patel AG, Bloom SR. Gut hormone profiles following bariatric surgery favor an anorectic state, facilitate weight loss, and improve metabolic parameters. *Ann Surg* 2006;243(1):108–114.

62. Tong J, Prigeon RL, Davis HW, Bidlingmaier M, Kahn SE, Cummings DE, Tschop MH, D'Alessio D. Ghrelin suppresses glucose-stimulated insulin secretion and deteriorates glucose tolerance in healthy humans. *Diabetes* 2010;59(9):2145–2151.

63. Cummings DE, Weigle DS, Frayo RS, Breen PA, Ma MK, Dellinger EP, Purnell JQ. Plasma ghrelin levels after diet-induced weight loss or gastric bypass surgery. *N Engl J Med* 2002;346(21):1623–1630.

64. Falken Y, Hellstrom PM, Holst JJ, Naslund E. Changes in glucose homeostasis after Roux-en-Y gastric bypass surgery for obesity at day three, two months, and one year after surgery: role of gut peptides. *J Clin Endocrinol Metab* 2011;96(7):2227–2235.

65. Bouldin MJ, Ross LA, Sumrall CD, Loustalot FV, Low AK, Land KK. The effect of obesity surgery on obesity comorbidity. *Am J Med Sci* 2006;331(4):183–193.

66. Neter JE, Stam BE, Kok FJ, Grobbee DE, Geleijnse JM. Influence of weight reduction on blood pressure: a meta-analysis of randomized controlled trials. *Hypertension* 2003;42(5):878–884.

67. Dornfeld LP, Maxwell MH, Waks AU, Schroth P, Tuck ML. Obesity and hypertension: long-term effects of weight reduction on blood pressure. *Int J Obes* 1985;9(6):381–389.

68. Hypertension Prevention Trial Research Group. The Hypertension Prevention Trial: three-year effects of dietary changes on blood pressure. hypertension prevention trial research group. *Arch Intern Med* 1990;150(1):153–162.

69. Sjöström CD, Peltonen M, Sjöström L. Blood pressure and pulse pressure during long-term weight loss in the obese: the Swedish Obese Subjects (SOS) intervention study. *Obes Res* 2001;9(3):188–195.

70. Benetos A, Rudnichi A, Safar M, Guize L. Pulse pressure and cardiovascular mortality in normotensive and hypertensive subjects. *Hypertension* 1998;32(3):560–564.

71. Buchwald H, Estok R, Fahrbach K, Banel D, Sledge I. Trends in mortality in bariatric surgery: a systematic review and meta-analysis. *Surgery* 2007;142(4):621–632.

72. Flum DR, Belle SH, King WC, Wahed AS, Berk P, Chapman W, Pories W, Courcoulas A, McCloskey C, Mitchell J, Patterson E, Pomp A, Staten MA, Yanovski SZ, Thirlby R, Wolfe B. Perioperative safety in the longitudinal assessment of bariatric surgery. *N Engl J Med* 2009;361(5):445–454.

73. Sjöström L, Narbro K, Sjöström CD, Karason K, Larsson B, Wedel H, Lystig T, Sullivan M, Bouchard C, Carlsson B, Bengtsson C, Dahlgren S, Gummesson A, Jacobson P, Karlsson J, Lindroos AK, Lönroth H, Näslund I, Olbers T, Stenlöf K, Torgerson J, Agren G, Carlsson LM; Swedish Obese Subjects Study. Effects of bariatric surgery on mortality in Swedish obese subjects. *N Engl J Med* 2007;357(8):741–752.

74. Tucker ON, Szomstein S, Rosenthal RJ. Nutritional consequences of weight-loss surgery. *Med Clin North Am* 2007;91(3):499–514.

75. Davies DJ, Baxter JM. Nutritional deficiencies after bariatric surgery. *Obesity Surg* 2007;17(9):1150–1158.

76. Ritz P, Becouarn G, Douay O, Salle A, Topart P, Rohmer V. Gastric bypass is not associated with protein malnutrition in morbidly obese patients. *Obesity Surg* 2009;19(7):840–844.

77. Angstadt JD, Bodziner RA. Peripheral polyneuropathy from thiamine deficiency following laparoscopic Roux-en-Y gastric bypass. *Obesity Surg* 2005;15(6):890–892.

78. Service GJ, Thompson GB, Service FJ, Andrews JC, Collazo Clavell ML, Lloyd RV. Hyperinsulinemic hypoglycemia with nesidioblastosis after gastric-bypass surgery. *N Engl J Med* 2005;353(3):249–254.

79. Goldfine AB, Mun EC, Devine E, Bernier R, Baz Hecht M, Jones DB, Schneider BE, Holst JJ, Patti ME. Patients with neuroglycopenia after gastric bypass surgery have exaggerated incretin and insulin secretory responses to a mixed meal. *J Clin Endocrinol Metab* 2007;92(12):4678–4685.

80. Arterburn DE, Bogart A, Sherwood NE, Sidney S, Coleman KJ, Haneuse S, O'Connor PJ, Theis MK, Campos GM, McCulloch D, Selby J. A multisite study of long-term remission and relapse of type 2 diabetes mellitus following gastric bypass. *Obesity Surg* 2013;23(1):93–102.

81. Maggard-Gibbons M, Maglione M, Livhits M, Ewing B, Maher AR, Hu J, Li Z, Shekelle PG. Bariatric surgery for weight loss and glycemic control in non-morbidly obese adults with diabetes: a systematic review. *JAMA* 2013; 309(21):2250–2261.

82. Inge TH, Miyano G, Bean J, Helmrath M, Courcoulas A, Harmon CM, Chen MK, Wilson K, Daniels SR, Garcia VF, Brandt ML, Dolan LM. Reversal of type 2 diabetes mellitus and improvements in cardiovascular risk factors after surgical weight loss in adolescents. *Pediatrics* 2009;123(1):214–222.

83. Inge TH, Zeller MH, Jenkins TM, Helmrath M, Brandt ML, Michalsky MP, Harmon CM, Courcoulas A, Horlick M, Zanthakos SA, Dolan L, Mitsnefes M, Barnett SJ, Buncher R; for the Teen-Labs Consortium. Perioperative out-

comes of adolescents undergoing bariatric surgery: the Teen-Longitudinal Assessment of Bariatric Surgery (Tee-LABS) Study. *JAMA Pediatr* 2013; 168(1):47–53.

84. Beal E. The pros and cons of designating obesity a disease: the new AMA designation stirs debate. *Am J Nurs* 2013;113(11):18–19.

Chapter 33
Diabetes in the Elderly

MEDHA N. MUNSHI, MD

INTRODUCTION

In the U.S., one in four people ≥65 years has diabetes. The number of elderly people with diabetes is projected to increase over the next few decades since the fastest growing segment of the population is that >85 years of age. This population of older patients with diabetes has one of the highest impacts on the health care system, both in terms of economic expenditure and in terms of population health. There are unique challenges in managing diabetes in the elderly population. There is scant evidence-based data available to guide better management of this growing segment. When the same strategies used in young adults are used in elderly patients with diabetes, there is an increased risk of noncompliance, lack of benefits, and higher risk of treatment-related complications, especially hypoglycemia. This chapter discusses the unique features in pathophysiology, clinical presentations, comorbid conditions, goal setting, and treatment strategies for older adults with diabetes.

SCOPE OF THE PROBLEM

In 2011, among U.S. residents >65 years of age, 10.9 million, or 26.9%, had diabetes compared with 11.3% in the younger population.[1] Anticipated growth in the total U.S. population between 2002 and 2020 is ~17%, while the estimated increase in people with diabetes during this period is ~44%. This increase is largely due to the increase in the size of the elderly population,[2] which is projected to reach 70 million by 2030.[3] The socioeconomic cost of the diabetes epidemic among older adults is also significant. Older adults with diabetes have high prevalence of diabetes-related complications with the highest rate of myocardial infarction, end-stage renal disease, visual impairment, lower extremity amputations, and diabetes-related hospitalizations, of any age-group (www.cdc.gov/diabetes/statistics, accessed 8/1/13). The percentage of adults ≥75 years with diabetes who need assistance with day-to-day activities is more than twice that of younger adults with diabetes (www.cdc.gov/diabetes/statistics, accessed 8/1/13). In addition, elderly patients with diabetes have higher all-cause mortality and morbidity when compared with elderly people without diabetes.[4] The economic impact of these conditions is enormous. In 2012, out of the estimated $245 billion in health care expenditure attributable to diabetes, $144.5 billion (59%) was for services provided to elderly patients, including hospitalizations, nursing facility resources, physician office visits, and prescription medications.[5]

DOI: 10.2337/9781580405096.33

PATHOPHYSIOLOGY

The differences between older patients compared with younger patients with diabetes primarily stem from the pathophysiology of aging combined with alteration in glucose metabolism.[6] In addition, conditions associated with aging such as coexisting illnesses, increased adiposity, decreased muscle mass, decreased physical activity, and effect of medications used to treat comorbidities further affect abnormal glucose metabolism in the elderly.[7]

Metabolic Alteration

Abnormal insulin secretion and resistance to insulin action are pathophysiological factors in the development of type 2 diabetes (T2D). The metabolic profile in older adults with diabetes is distinct when compared with younger and middle-aged patients.[8] The older adults with diabetes show normal fasting hepatic glucose production compared with elevated hepatic glucose production in younger patients.[8] The abnormality in insulin secretions is related to alterations in insulin release, loss of pulsatility, loss of first-phase insulin secretion, and decreased response to incretin hormones with aging.[9] Abnormal insulin sensitivity commonly is seen with aging and is exacerbated by confounding factors, such as higher body fat content and loss of fat-free mass.[10] Compared with young adults, obese older people with diabetes have relatively normal insulin secretion but marked resistance to insulin-mediated glucose disposal. On the other hand, lean older people with diabetes have profound impairment in glucose-induced insulin secretion but minimal resistance to insulin action.[8,11]

Environmental Impact

A diet high in simple sugars, saturated fat, and total energy—and low in fiber and complex carbohydrates—is linked to higher risk of diabetes at all ages. Dietary modification and exercise improve diabetes in both young and old patients with diabetes. In addition, however, aging causes structural and functional changes in skeletal muscles, which form the basis of changes in body composition and metabolic abnormalities such as insulin resistance.[12] Higher fat-to-muscle ratio with a central distribution of fat, and lack of physical activity, are common with aging and contribute to higher risk of diabetes. The role of nutritional deficiency in the development or prevention of diabetes in older adults is not completely clear.

Genetic Predisposition

Age-related changes in glucose metabolism are exacerbated by genetic predisposition in older adults. The specific genes responsible have not been identified, however. Family history of diabetes and certain ethnic groups, such as African American, Asian American, American Indian, and Hispanic descent, confers higher risk of developing diabetes with aging, supporting the hypothesis of genetic predisposition.

Other Factors

A variety of aging-related changes have been shown to add to the risk of abnormal glucose metabolism. The presence of inflammation as measured by pro-inflammatory cytokines, such as tumor necrosis factor-α[13] and C-reactive protein[14], have been associated with higher risk of diabetes in elderly patients. On the other hand, an adipocytokine known to increase insulin sensitivity (adiponectin) has been found to be associated with lower risk of diabetes in older men and women.[15] Age-associated reductions in mitochondrial oxidative and phosphorylation activity also have been shown to contribute to insulin resistance in the elderly.[16] Autoimmunity has been shown to play a role in the impairment of glucose-induced insulin secretion in lean older people with diabetes.[6] Levels of sex steroids also affect the development of diabetes in elderly. Low levels of testosterone in men and higher levels of testosterone in women are associated with higher risk of insulin resistance and diabetes in this age-group.[17]

OVERALL APPROACH AND PRINCIPLES OF CARE

Successful management of diabetes in older adults warrants a better understanding of the unique presentation and course of the disease in this population. As in younger adults, the primary goal of diabetes management in older adults is to prevent or slow the onset and progression of acute and chronic complications associated with this disease. An additional goal in the older population is to prevent treatment-related complications, especially hypoglycemia, which can be more harmful than the disease itself. Finally, maintaining an acceptable quality of life is usually an overarching goal in caring for older adults with diabetes. Unfortunately, the older adults are underrepresented in diabetes research studies, and the evidence-based guidelines specifically targeted toward elderly persons are difficult to formulate. The American Diabetes Association (ADA) and the American Geriatrics Society have published recommendations for optimal care for older adults largely based on expert consensus.[18] The key to developing an optimal management strategy is to consider clinical (comorbidities such as cognitive dysfunction, depressions), functional (e.g., hearing and vision loss, physical disabilities), and psychosocial (financial and social adversities) barriers before formulating treatment plans. With this approach, the treatment plans would be appropriate for older patients' coping abilities and self-care capacity. Table 33.1 shows unique considerations and management strategies in older adults with diabetes.

CLINICAL CHARACTERISTICS AND PRESENTATION OF OLDER ADULTS WITH DIABETES

Clinical characteristics of older adults with diabetes depend on their clinical, functional, and psychosocial status. There is a considerable heterogeneity in clinical presentation based on a patient's functional status (healthy versus fragile elderly), presence of comorbidities (diabetes related or not), duration of disease (long vs. short), treatment regimen (insulin regimen vs. oral medications), living situation (alone vs. with caregivers), and economic status (adequacy of resources). Patients' ability to care for themselves depends significantly on all of these factors and characteristics. Table 33.2 shows characteristics of older adults with diabetes living in the community, in assisted-living facilities, and in nursing homes.

Table 33.1 Unique Considerations and Management Strategies in the Care of Older Adults with Diabetes

Important considerations	Unique issues in older adults	Management strategies
Hypoglycemia	■ Even mild episode combined with other medical conditions may result in catastrophic falls, fractures, and poor quality of life	■ Avoid medications with high risk of hypoglycemia
	■ High risk of hypoglycemia unawareness and missed reporting	■ Carefully look for hidden/subtle symptoms of hypoglycemia ■ Consider continuous glucose monitoring if hypoglycemia suspected but not reported
Geriatric syndromes	■ Suspect unrecognized self-care barriers if 　—recent unexpected deterioration in control 　—frequent errors in medications/judgment 　—fails to achieve glycemic goal after reasonable attempts 　—seems overwhelmed with self-care issues	■ Screen for cognitive dysfunction, depression, physical disabilities, polypharmacy, chronic pain ■ Improve barriers such as depression, polypharmacy ■ Simplify regimen to fit barriers that are not reversible, such as cognitive dysfunction, physical disability
Goal setting	■ Avoiding hypoglycemia is as important as achieving target A1C goal ■ Individuals with multiple chronic conditions may have difficulty achieving individual disease goals for all conditions ■ Goals may change if overall health changes	■ Weigh risk of hypoglycemia before setting A1C goal ■ Balance glycemic goal and other chronic disease goals with overall life goals and patient preferences ■ Assess and adjust goals periodically
Treatment strategies	■ Patients' ability to learn new information might be limited, causing stress and errors ■ Barriers to self-care, such as cognitive dysfunction or physical disability, are not reversible ■ Changes in dietary habits are more difficult ■ Many older adults feel discouraged with other health issues and avoid exercise due to pain	■ Assess patients' ability to perform self-care before developing strategy for disease management ■ Simpler regimen may help compliance and avoid large excursions ■ Simple dietary plans to avoid large carbohydrate load through the day ■ Provide detailed prescription for individualized physical activity and constant encouragement

Table 33.2 Characteristics of Older Adults with Diabetes in Different Settings

Living status	Patient characteristics	Issues pertaining to diabetes management
Community-dwelling	■ High functioning ■ Perform self-care independently with/without caregiver support	■ Consider comorbidities that interfere with ability to perform self-care ■ Avoid complex regimen and medications that increase risk of hypoglycemia
Assisted care facilities	■ Needs some support with IADL ■ Higher caregiver needs	■ Frail population, more comorbidities ■ May/may not have control over meal content ■ Need some assistance with medication management ■ Cannot get help with insulin injection—may become an issue if acutely ill or confused and unable to follow complex regimen
Nursing homes	■ Low functioning ■ Assistance with ADL and IADL ■ Total dependence for self-care ■ Limited life expectancy ■ High burden of comorbidities	■ Little control over timing or content of diet ■ Higher risk of side effects with oral medications ■ Higher risk of acute illness, anorexia, dementia/delirium interfering with BG ■ Self-care performed by NH staff

In addition, the unique pathophysiology of diabetes manifests as unique clinical presentation of the disease in this population. As the renal threshold for glucose increases with age, glycosuria may not be detected at usual levels,[19] masking the symptoms of polyuria. The polydipsia also may be absent because of impaired thirst mechanisms in this population. The absence of classic symptoms of hyperglycemia puts patients at a higher risk of dehydration and nonketotic hyperosmolar state.[20] Thus, in some of the older patients, infections, neuropathic pain, and weight loss may manifest as initial presentation of diabetes. The clinical presentation also alters in this population on the basis of coexisting medical condition, especially geriatric syndrome described in the next section.

GERIATRIC SYNDROME

The older population with diabetes is at higher risk for many coexisting medical conditions. Some of these conditions, such as macrovascular and microvascular complications of diabetes, are well recognized by medical providers. A group of conditions termed geriatric syndrome also occur at a higher frequency in older adults and typically are not associated with diabetes. These conditions include cognitive impairment, depression, functional decline, chronic pain, polypharmacy, and urinary incontinence.[21] The importance of recognizing these conditions with sometimes subtle presentations lies in the fact that they interfere with the patient's ability to perform self-care.[22,23] Although geriatric assessment and screening for these conditions are recommended in all older adults with diabetes, time constraints are major barriers in the current medical environment. If, however, older patients with diabetes start making errors in managing diabetes and develop coping difficulties, they should be screened for geriatric syndrome.

Cognitive Dysfunction

Cognitive impairment in older adults with diabetes may manifest as deficits in psychomotor efficiency, global cognition, episodic memory, semantic memory, and working memory.[24] Executive dysfunction mediated by the frontal lobe commonly is found in older adults with diabetes and affects behaviors, such as problem solving, planning, organization, insight, reasoning, and attention.[25] In a study evaluating adults >70 years in a geriatric diabetes clinic, one-third of the study population had cognitive dysfunction, which was associated with poor diabetes control.[23] In a large randomized study, however, tighter control of both blood glucose and blood pressure failed to prevent the progression of cognitive decline.[26] In older patients, it is important to identify cognitive dysfunction early so that simpler treatment plans are formulated to avoid such complications as hypoglycemia from missing a meal or incorrect dosing or timing of insulin. Some of the short-screening tools to screen for cognitive function include clock drawing test and Montreal Cognitive Assessment.[27,28]

Depression

Depression in older adults with diabetes is common and is associated with poor glycemic control, decreased adherence to treatment strategies, increased functional disability, and mortality.[29-31] Untreated depression can interfere with patients' ability to perform self-care, while treatment of depression leads to improved mood and quality of life.[32] A large randomized study showed lower mortality in elderly depressed patients treated with comprehensive care management at their primary care practice compared with those treated with usual care.[33] Depression can remain undiagnosed in older adults and screening with short clinical tools, such as the geriatric diabetes scale, is recommended in elderly patients.[34]

Functional Dysfunction and Falls

In the past, the significant health burden in older patients with diabetes was attributed primarily to vascular complications. Recently, clinical researchers conducted a large community-based case control study that examined in detail the nature of functional impairment in older patients with diabetes.[35] They found that compared with age-matched control subjects living in the same community, older patients with diabetes have a reduction in physical function and health status. Those patients with diabetes also were more likely to use a mobility aid, such as a cane or a walker, and are dependent on caregivers for day-to-day activities. This population is at higher risk for falls due to lower-limb dysfunction, cardiovascular disease, polypharmacy, and impaired balance, among other factors.[36]

Polypharmacy

Prevention and management of multiple chronic diseases in older adults require the use of multiple medications. In addition, older patients need symptomatic medications for a variety of ailments, and supplements in the form of vitamins. In fact, the elderly population is the highest consumer of the over-the-counter medications.[37] Thus, older adults in general, and those with diabetes in particular, often take six to eight medications daily.[38] Many phamacokinetics (decreased renal and hepatic blood flow and metabolism, slowed peristalsis), and pharmacodynamics changes occur with aging that affect metabolism and clearance of the drug and promote drug-drug interactions, putting older patients at high risk of adverse drug reactions.[39] Polypharmacy increases the probability of nonadherence because of many of these factors. It is extremely important to keep the medication list current and review it at each medical visit.

Other Commonly Occurring Medical Conditions

Chronic pain, urinary incontinence, and hearing and vision impairment are some of the other conditions with high prevalence in older adults with diabetes.[18] These conditions are thought to be the natural process with aging; however, they interfere with patients' ability to perform self-care and they lower quality of life. Efforts should be made to assess for these commonly occurring symptoms and their management should be part of overall diabetes management.

GOAL SETTING

Goal setting for glycemia in older adults demands careful weighing of risks and benefits of the disease and its treatment. It is imperative that treatment of diabetes and its complications (especially hypoglycemia) should not be worse than the disease. Recently, several studies have elucidated a "J-shaped" relationship between chronic disease goals and mortality. A large retrospective study showed that both very low and very high A1C levels were associated with higher all-cause mortality and cardiac events.[40] The lowest hazard ratio for mortality in this study was found at an A1C of 7.5%. Another prospective cohort study found a "U-shaped" relationship between blood pressure control and risk of coronary heart disease in patients with diabetes.[41] The "U-shaped" relationship converted into an inverse relationship in older patients (>60 years) in this study, suggesting that low blood pressure was more dangerous to this population than uncontrolled blood pressures. These results, when combined with results of the large prospective studies (ADVANCE, ACCORD, VADT),[42–44] reveal no cardiovascular outcome risk reduction of tight glycemic control and no possible harm, especially in the older population, suggesting no role for intensive management in this population.

The recommendations from the expert consensus published with support of the ADA suggest that the goals of glucose, blood pressure, and lipid control should be based on overall health status, particularly comorbidity burden, cognitive function, and ability to perform day-to-day activities,[18] without excessive stress on chronological age. In addition, it is also important to consider the medications required to achieve the glycemic goal. The medications that have high risk of hypoglycemia (insulin, secretagogues) should be used cautiously, and the glycemic goal in patients using them should be less stringent. On the other hand, medications with low risk of hypoglycemia (metformin, dipeptidyl peptidase [DPP]-4 inhibitors, glucagon-like polypeptide 1 [GLP-1] agonists, α-glucosidase inhibitors) can be used safely to achieve better glycemic goal. Figure 33.1 shows the

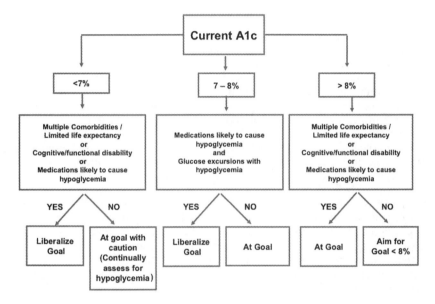

Figure 33.1—Framework for Goal Adjustment in Older Adults with Diabetes.

general approach to goal setting in older adults with diabetes. The overall approach should be to get the best glycemic control without exposing the patient to the risks of hypoglycemia and its consequences. Figure 33.1 also shows the suggested framework for glycemic goals in older adults based on their comorbidities, functional and cognitive status, and the treatment modality.

HYPOGLYCEMIA

Hypoglycemia in older adults needs special focus for several reasons. Older patients with diabetes are at higher risk of hypoglycemia compared with the younger population.[18,45] Although hypoglycemia is the limiting factor in achieving tight glycemic control in all adults with diabetes, it has grave consequences in the older population. Even a mild-to-moderate episode of hypoglycemia may result in falls, fractures, hospitalizations, and aggravation of existing medical conditions, such as cognitive dysfunction and coronary artery disease.[46] Many factors, such as decreased renal clearance, polypharmacy, drug-drug interactions, and coexisting comorbidities, contribute to the higher risk of hypoglycemia in the elderly. In older adults with diabetes, there is a bidirectional association between hypoglycemia and cognitive dysfunction.[47] In a cross-sectional database analysis of older veterans with diabetes, cognitive dysfunction was found in 13.1% of patients between 65 and 75 years and in 24.2% in those ≥75 years,[48] and it was associated independently with hypoglycemia. In addition, older patients have hypoglycemia unawareness and prolongation of hypoglycemia-induced reaction time, both of which put this population at high risk of severe hypoglycemic episodes.[49] Finally, hypoglycemia is associated with lower health-related quality of life.[22]

Another important difference in symptoms of hypoglycemia between younger and older patients with diabetes is the lack of the autonomic warning symptoms. In older adults, such symptoms as confusion, delirium, weakness, dizziness, and falls are common and may suggest neuroglycopenic manifestations of hypoglycemia. This is in contrast to typical adrenergic symptoms of hypoglycemia seen in younger adults (e.g., tremors, palpitation, sweating). In addition, symptoms of hypoglycemia may occur at lower blood glucose levels and may be harder to recognize in older adults.[50] Neuroglycopenic symptoms in older adults frequently can be misconstrued to be secondary to other medical conditions, such as a transient ischemic attack, dementia, or orthostatic hypotension, and can remain unrecognized by both older patients and providers. Unrecognized and untreated hypoglycemia may lead to unintended consequences, such as injurious falls and fear of falls, limiting activity in older adults and resulting in noncompliance with medications. The first step in avoiding this vicious cycle is to educate patients and their caregivers regarding different presentations of hypoglycemia with aging. Patients' ability to recognize and treat hypoglycemia should be assessed periodically during the clinic visits along with reinforcement of education regarding precipitating factors and prevention of hypoglycemia.

TREATMENT STRATEGIES

LIFESTYLE MODIFICATIONS

Exercise

Regular exercise for older patients with diabetes is as important as in their younger counterparts. Diabetes is associated with lower skeletal muscle strength and quality in the aging population.[51] Exercise can improve muscle strength, gait, and balance and can reduce the risk of falls with improvement in overall quality of life in older adults. Even low-intensity exercise can yield benefits in this population and is associated with better self-rated physical health and feeling of well-being.[52] Older people can safely start exercise at low intensity and gradually increase as tolerated. Resistance training in this age-group has been associated with improvement in glycemic control.[53] In fact, patients with multiple chronic conditions, such as hypertension, hypercholesteremia, osteoarthritis, and cardiovascular diseases, can have higher benefits, as all of these conditions may improve with exercise.

Diet

Dietary habits affect glycemic control in all patients with diabetes, including older adults.[54,55] Dietary modification, however, may have a limited role in older adults compared with the younger population. Lifelong eating habits, difficulty changing basic structure of the diet, dependence on other people for shopping and preparing food, inconsistent appetite, demands of other health issues, and financial concerns are some of the factors that make it difficult to change dietary habits.

Simple teaching methods to distribute carbohydrates throughout the day to avoid large load in a single meal can improve glucose excursions in many older individuals. Decreased food intake and weight loss are bigger concerns in many elderly patients with diabetes and are associated with nutritional deficiency, increased morbidity, and mortality.[56-58] In a cohort of >3,300 patients with T2D followed over a 10-year period, higher body weight was associated with lower mortality in patients >65 years of age compared with younger population.[59]

PHARMACOLOGICAL MANAGEMENT OF DIABETES IN OLDER ADULTS

Basic principles of pharmacological management of diabetes in older adults are similar to the younger population. The first line of therapy after lifestyle modifications remains metformin in all patients with diabetes. The second and the third line of therapeutic agents should be chosen based on the risk of hypoglycemia, efficacy, major side effects, cost, and total treatment burden in an individual patient.[60] For older patients, "start low and go slow" is an important principle. Some of the unique considerations to keep in mind in older individuals are as follows.

Oral and Noninsulin Hypoglycemic Agents

Metformin remains the drug of choice as the first-line therapy for all patients. Recent meta-analysis is reassuring in its finding that metformin can be used safely in lower doses up to a glomerular filtration rate of 30 mg/minute. This is an attractive agent to use because of its low risk of hypoglycemia. Renal insufficiency, gastrointestinal side effects, and weight loss are common limiting factors in older adults taking metformin.

The longer-acting insulin secretagogues, such as the sulfonylureas (glipizide, glimepiride), are commonly used medications. They are inexpensive and most medical providers are familiar with this group of drugs. These medications, however, pose a significant risk of hypoglycemia. Glyburide in particular increases the risk of hypoglycemia in elderly and should be avoided.[61] The shorter-acting secretagogues, such as repaglinide and nateglinide, act similarly to the sulfonylureas but with more focused action just after meals. The advantage of these medications is that they are taken just before a meal, and if a meal is skipped or added, the dose of the medication can be skipped or added, respectively. The dose also may be adjusted if a person has a variable appetite. This approach is especially useful in frail elderly nursing home patients with variable food intake.

α-Glucosidase inhibitors (acarbose and miglitol) are fairly safe in older adults and can be used to control small postprandial elevations in blood glucose. The main side effects that limit their use are flatulence and diarrhea, which are common, and can be problematic for older people.

The incretin-mimetic agents include DPP-4 inhibitors (sitagliptin, saxagliptin) and GLP-1 analogs (exenatide, liraglutide). Both of these groups have low risk of hypoglycemia, making them attractive for use in older adults. The DPP-4 inhibitors are well tolerated in elderly people without weight loss and can be used with renal dosing in patients with renal insufficiency. Their efficacy is lower, however, when compared with other agents. GLP-1 analogs induce weight loss and should be avoided in frail elderly with weight loss. It is available only in an injectable format and requires the ability to self-inject, which might be problematic in some older adults. Extended-release formulations that can be used once a week are also attractive for patients needing caregiver support for injections. Pramlintide, a synthetic analog of amylin, requires multiple subcutaneous injections, and its role in the management of diabetes in the elderly is limited.

Insulin

Insulin sometimes is underutilized in the elderly because of fear (by the physician, patient, or family) that it is too complicated or dangerous. In many older patients, however, glycemic control improves substantially when insulin treatment is individualized and monitored carefully with regular follow-up. The benefits of insulin should be weighed against its risk of hypoglycemia, which is higher with insulin compared with oral medications. Careful assessment of risk factors for hypoglycemia should be carried out before deciding on insulin therapy. An older adult's ability to manage a complex insulin regimen may change with increasing age or worsening overall health. A recent analysis of pooled data from randomized studies has shown that the relative contribution of basal hyperglycemia is lower, whereas that of postprandial hyperglycemia is greater in older compared with younger patients at all A1C levels.[62] Thus, with better understanding of unique glucose patterns in the elderly and with the availability of various types of insulin with different time-action curves, individualization of regimen is possible. Adding a once-a-day dose of basal insulin can be a safe and effective method of initiating insulin therapy in those who demonstrate suboptimal glycemic control on oral hypoglycemia agents.[63,64]

CONCLUSION

Older patients with diabetes are a heterogeneous group characterized by unique challenges and barriers to optimal diabetes care. Providing diabetes treatment to older adults is more than just replicating the same adult care in an aging population. Many aspects of the disease, including pathophysiology, clinical presentation, doses and side effects of medications, dietary consideration, exercise strategies, and impact of disease on quality of life are different and require special consideration in an older adult with diabetes when compared with younger adults. A multidisciplinary approach, by a team of caregivers, needs to apply strategies that look beyond just glycemic control to include screening for and treating complications, as well as considering concomitant conditions like depression, cognitive dysfunction, and physical limitations. Treatment plans should be safe with low risk of hypoglycemia, and flexible, so that they can incorporate new challenges or considerations associated with declining overall health, level of function, and the patient's wishes with acceptable quality of life.

REFERENCES

1. Centers for Disease Control and Prevention. National diabetes fact sheet: general information and national estimates on diabetes in United States.

Atlanta, U.S. Department of Health and Human Services, 2011. http://www.cdc.gov/diabetes/pubs/pdf/ndfs_2011.pdf.

2. Hogan P, Dall T, Nikolov P. Economic costs of diabetes in the US in 2002. *Diabetes Care* 2003;26(3):917–932.

3. Narayan KM, et al. Impact of recent increase in incidence on future diabetes burden: U.S., 2005-2050. *Diabetes Care* 2006;29(9):2114–2116.

4. Bertoni AG, et al. Excess mortality related to diabetes mellitus in elderly Medicare beneficiaries. *Ann Epidemiol* 2004;14(5):362–367.

5. American Diabetes Association. Economic costs of diabetes in the U.S. in 2012. *Diabetes Care* 2013;36(4):1033–1046.

6. Meneilly GS, Tessier D. Diabetes in elderly adults. *J Gerontol A Biol Sci Med Sci* 2001;56(1):M5–M13.

7. Sinclair AJ, Meneilly GS. Re-thinking metabolic strategies for older people with type 2 diabetes mellitus: implications of the UK Prospective Diabetes Study and other recent studies. *Age Ageing* 2000;29(5):393–397.

8. Meneilly GS, Elahi D. Metabolic alterations in middle-aged and elderly lean patients with type 2 diabetes. *Diabetes Care* 2005;28(6):1498–1499.

9. Meneilly GS, Elliott T. Metabolic alterations in middle-aged and elderly obese patients with type 2 diabetes. *Diabetes Care* 1999;22(1):112–118.

10. Elahi D, et al. Glucose tolerance, glucose utilization and insulin secretion in ageing. *Novartis Found Symp* 2002;242:222–242; discussion 242–246.

11. Meneilly GS, et al. NIDDM in the elderly. *Diabetes Care* 1996;19(12):1320–1325.

12. Nair KS. Aging muscle. *Am J Clin Nutr* 2005;81(5):953–963.

13. Lechleitner M, et al. Tumour necrosis factor-alpha plasma levels in elderly patients with type 2 diabetes mellitus—observations over 2 years. *Diabet Med* 2002;19(11):949–953.

14. Barzilay JI, et al. The relation of markers of inflammation to the development of glucose disorders in the elderly: the Cardiovascular Health Study. *Diabetes* 2001;50(10):2384–2389.

15. Kanaya AM, et al. Adipocytokines attenuate the association between visceral adiposity and diabetes in older adults. *Diabetes Care* 2004;27(6):1375–1380.

16. Petersen KF, et al. Mitochondrial dysfunction in the elderly: possible role in insulin resistance. *Science* 2003;300(5622):1140–1142.

17. Oh JY, et al. Endogenous sex hormones and the development of type 2 diabetes in older men and women: the Rancho Bernardo study. *Diabetes Care* 2002;25(1):55–60.

18. Kirkman MS, et al. Diabetes in older adults. *Diabetes Care* 2012;35(12):2650–2664.

19. Meneilly GS. The pathophysiology of diabetes in the elderly. In *Geriatric Diabetes*. Munshi, M, Eds. New York, Informa Healthcare, 2007, p. 29–36.

20. Munshi MN, Blair E, Coopan R. Diabetes in the older adult. In *Joslin's Diabetes Deskbook: A Guide for Primary Care Providers*. Richard S. Beaser, MD and the Staff of Joslin Diabetes Center, Eds. Boston, Joslin Publications Department, 2007, p. 623–639.

21. Munshi M. Managing the "geriatric syndrome" in patients with type 2 diabetes. *Consult Pharm* 2008;23(Suppl B):12–16.

22. Laiteerapong N, et al. Correlates of quality of life in older adults with diabetes: the Diabetes and Aging Study. *Diabetes Care* 2011;34(8):1749–1753.

23. Munshi M, et al. Cognitive dysfunction is associated with poor diabetes control in older adults. *Diabetes Care* 2006;29(8):1794–1799.

24. Iwata I, Munshi MN. Cognitive and psychosocial aspects of caring for elderly patients with diabetes. *Curr Diab Rep* 2009;9(2):140–146.

25. Munshi MN, et al. Which aspects of executive dysfunction influence ability to manage diabetes in older adults? *Diabet Med* 2012;29(9):1171–1177.

26. Launer LJ, et al. Effects of intensive glucose lowering on brain structure and function in people with type 2 diabetes (ACCORD MIND): a randomised open-label substudy. *Lancet Neurol* 2011;10(11):969–977.

27. Nishiwaki Y, et al. Validity of the clock-drawing test as a screening tool for cognitive impairment in the elderly. *Am J Epidemiol* 2004;160(8):797–807.

28. Smith T, Gildeh N, Holmes C. The Montreal Cognitive Assessment: validity and utility in a memory clinic setting. *Can J Psychiatry* 2007;52(5):329–332.

29. Nouwen A, et al. Type 2 diabetes mellitus as a risk factor for the onset of depression: a systematic review and meta-analysis. *Diabetologia* 2010;53(12):2480–2486.

30. Lustman PJ, et al. Depression and poor glycemic control: a meta-analytic review of the literature. *Diabetes Care* 2000;23(7):934–942.

31. Lin EH, et al. Relationship of depression and diabetes self-care, medication adherence, and preventive care. *Diabetes Care* 2004;27(9):2154–2160.

32. Lustman PJ, Clouse RE. Depression in diabetic patients: the relationship between mood and glycemic control. *J Diabetes Complications* 2005;19(2):113–122.

33. Bogner HR, et al. Diabetes, depression, and death: A randomized controlled trial of a depression treatment program for older adults based in primary care (PROSPECT). *Diabetes Care* 2007;30(12):3005–3010.

34. Montorio I, Izal M. The geriatric depression scale: a review of its development and utility. *Int Psychogeriatr* 1996;8(1):103–112.

35. Sinclair AJ, Conroy SP, Bayer AJ. Impact of diabetes on physical function in older people. *Diabetes Care* 2008;31(2):233–235.

36. Wallace C, et al. Incidence of falls, risk factors for falls, and fall-related fractures in individuals with diabetes and a prior foot ulcer. *Diabetes Care* 2002;25(11):1983–1986.

37. Bruno JJ, Ellis JJ. Herbal use among US elderly: 2002 National Health Interview Survey. *Ann Pharmacother* 2005;39(4):643–648.

38. Orwig D, Brandt N, Gruber-Baldini AL. Medication management assessment for older adults in the community. *Gerontologist* 2006;46(5):661–668.

39. Bressler R, Bahl JJ. Principles of drug therapy for the elderly patient. *Mayo Clin Proc* 2003;78(12):1564–1577.

40. Currie CJ, et al. Survival as a function of HbA(1c) in people with type 2 diabetes: a retrospective cohort study. *Lancet* 2010; Feb 6; 375(9713):481–489.

41. Zhao W, et al. Aggressive blood pressure control increases coronary heart disease risk among diabetic patients. *Diabetes Care* 2013; Oct; 36(10):3287–3296.

42. Patel A, et al. Intensive blood glucose control and vascular outcomes in patients with type 2 diabetes. *N Engl J Med* 2008;358(24):2560–2572.

43. Gerstein HC, et al. Effects of intensive glucose lowering in type 2 diabetes. *N Engl J Med* 2008;358(24):2545–2559.

44. Duckworth W, et al. Glucose control and vascular complications in veterans with type 2 diabetes. *N Engl J Med* 2009;360(2):129–139.

45. Leese GP, et al. Frequency of severe hypoglycemia requiring emergency treatment in type 1 and type 2 diabetes: a population-based study of health service resource use. *Diabetes Care* 2003;26(4):1176–1180.

46. Johnston SS, et al. Association between hypoglycaemic events and fall-related fractures in Medicare-covered patients with type 2 diabetes. *Diabetes Obes Metab* 2012;14(7):634–643.

47. Yaffe K, et al. Association between hypoglycemia and dementia in a biracial cohort of older adults with diabetes mellitus. *JAMA* 2013;173(14):1300–1306.

48. Feil DG, et al. Risk of hypoglycemia in older veterans with dementia and cognitive impairment: implications for practice and policy. *J Am Geriatr Soc* 2011;59(12):2263–2272.

49. Bremer JP, et al. Hypoglycemia unawareness in older compared with middle-aged patients with type 2 diabetes. *Diabetes Care* 2009;32(8):1513–1517.

50. Matyka K, et al. Altered hierarchy of protective responses against severe hypoglycemia in normal aging in healthy men. *Diabetes Care* 1997;20(2):135–141.

51. Park SW, et al. Decreased muscle strength and quality in older adults with type 2 diabetes: the Health, Aging, and Body Composition study. *Diabetes* 2006;55(6):1813–1818.

52. Buman MP, et al. Objective light-intensity physical activity associations with rated health in older adults. *Am J Epidemiol* 2010;172(10):1155–1165.

53. Castaneda C, et al. A randomized controlled trial of resistance exercise training to improve glycemic control in older adults with type 2 diabetes. *Diabetes Care* 2002;25(12):2335–2341.

54. Miller CK, et al. Nutrition education improves metabolic outcomes among older adults with diabetes mellitus: results from a randomized controlled trial. *Prev Med* 2002;34(2):252–259.

55. Redmond EH, et al. Improvement in A1C levels and diabetes self-management activities following a nutrition and diabetes education program in older adults. *J Nutr Elder* 2006;26(1–2):83–102.

56. Wedick NM, et al. The relationship between weight loss and all-cause mortality in older men and women with and without diabetes mellitus: the Rancho Bernardo study. *J Am Geriatr Soc* 2002;50(11):1810–1815.

57. Knudtson MD, et al. Associations with weight loss and subsequent mortality risk. *Ann Epidemiol* 2005;15(7):483–491.

58. Newman AB, et al. Weight change in old age and its association with mortality. *J Am Geriatr Soc* 2001;49(10):1309–1318.

59. Zoppini G, et al. Body mass index and the risk of mortality in type II diabetic patients from Verona. *Int J Obes Relat Metab Disord* 2003;27(2):281–285.

60. Inzucchi SE, et al. Management of hyperglycemia in type 2 diabetes: a patient-centered approach: position statement of the American Diabetes Association (ADA) and the European Association for the Study of Diabetes (EASD). *Diabetes Care* 2012;35(6):1364–1379.

61. American Geriatrics Society 2012 Beers Criteria Update Expert Panel. Updated Beers criteria for potentially inappropriate medication use in older adults. *J Am Geriatr Soc* 2012;60(4):616–631.

62. Munshi MN, et al. Contributions of basal and prandial hyperglycemia to total hyperglycemia in older and younger adults with type 2 diabetes mellitus. *J Am Geriatr Soc* 2013;61(4):535–541.

63. Karnieli E, et al. Observational study of once-daily insulin detemir in people with type 2 diabetes aged 75 years or older: a sub-analysis of data from the Study of Once daily LeVEmir (SOLVE). *Drugs Aging* 2013;30(3):167–175.

64. Pandya N, et al. Efficacy and safety of insulin glargine compared to other interventions in younger and older adults: a pooled analysis of nine open-label, randomized controlled trials in patients with type 2 diabetes. *Drugs Aging* 2013;30(6):429–438.

Chapter 34

Diabetes in Intensive Care Units and Non-ICU Settings

Kara Hawkins, MD
Amy C. Donihi, PharmD, BCPS
Mary T. Korytkowski, MD

INTRODUCTION

More than 20% of hospitalized patients in the U.S. have diabetes as an associated diagnosis. Cardiovascular disorders are listed as the most common reasons for admission, whereas short-term complications, such as severe hyperglycemia and hypoglycemia, are listed as the second most common reasons. Approximately 50% of these hospitalizations represent readmissions and many are potentially preventable.[1-3]

When people with diabetes are hospitalized, they experience longer and more costly hospital stays than those without diabetes.[3] Some of this burden is related to inadequate care in the outpatient setting with a failure to achieve metabolic goals as recommended by the American Diabetes Association (ADA), and others are due to inadequate attention to the glycemic management in the hospital.[4-9] Many providers feel inadequately prepared to address the complexity of care required of a multidose and multicomponent insulin regimen.[10,11]

Although it would be advantageous to sequester diabetes patients on nursing units where dedicated attention to their glycemic management could be maintained, this is not feasible given the large numbers of patients and the diverse reasons for hospitalization. It is therefore important for hospitals to develop systems of care that promote patient safety and ensure optimal outcomes by providing a rational approach to inpatient diabetes management. This chapter will address the components of inpatient diabetes care that can help hospital systems achieve these goals.

COMPONENTS OF A HOSPITAL-BASED GLYCEMIC MANAGEMENT PROGRAM

The most important component of any inpatient diabetes management program (IDMP) is the establishment of accepted blood glucose (BG) targets that guide the use of diabetes medications. There are published guidelines for BG targets in both noncritically and critically ill patients.[12-15] In patients who are not critically ill, the recommendations are to maintain fasting and premeal BG targets between 100 and 140 mg with maximal random BG <180 mg/dl.[12-14] These goals can be modified for patients with multiple comorbidities or limited life expectancy, but even in this group of patients, maintaining BG ≤200 mg/dl avoids symptomatic glucosuria with associated polyuria and polydipsia, while also minimizing risk for associated electrolyte abnormalities and hospital-acquired infections.[16]

DOI: 10.2337/9781580405096.34

Modification of a diabetes treatment regimen is recommended when BG declines to <100 mg/dl as a way of reducing risk for hypoglycemia.[12-14]

Glycemic goals in critically ill patients are similar to what has been recommended for noncritically ill patients.[12-14] It generally is recommended that BG levels be maintained between 140 and 180 mg/dl with consideration of lower targets of 110–180 mg/dl in critically ill surgical patients provided that this can be achieved and maintained with low risk for moderate hypoglycemia (MH), defined as BG <70 mg/dl, or severe hypoglycemia (SH).[12-14] Other glycemic goal ranges that have been recommended generally fall within these ranges.[15-17]

An integrated IDMP can provide a framework for guiding goal-directed management in the hospital.[10,18] An interdisciplinary team approach contributes to the coordination of care among physicians, nurses, pharmacists, and nutrition services, as well as laboratory, risk management, quality improvement, and patient safety personnel.[19-21]

NUTRITION

An often overlooked but essential component of an IDMP is nutrition, which requires coordination with the administration of diabetes medications.[22,23] For patients who are eating regular meals, little data provide support for one dietary approach over another. Current recommendations suggest that providing meals with a consistent number of carbohydrate calories at each specified meal may allow for better coordination of insulin doses with a reduction in risk for hypoglycemia.[12-14,24]

When coordinating insulin therapy with meals, the use of rapid-acting analogs before meals is preferred. Unlike regular insulin, which requires dosing in advance of a meal, the rapid-acting analogs allow dosing when the meal is in front of the patient.[25] These agents also may provide more effective glycemic control with less hypoglycemia than regular insulin.[26] To facilitate the appropriate timing of insulin administration with meals, some hospitals have developed interventions that provide patients with a sign on their meal tray that prompts a call to the nurse for the premeal insulin.[22]

HOSPITAL ADMISSION

All patients with diabetes require documentation of an A1C at the time of hospital admission, unless there is a measurement available from the preceding 2–3 months.[12-14] The A1C provides information regarding the adequacy of the home diabetes regimen before admission, the need for intensification of the current regimen while in the hospital, and what to anticipate at time of hospital discharge.

DIABETES MANAGEMENT IN NONCRITICALLY ILL PATIENTS

Insulin is the preferred therapy for the management of diabetes and hyperglycemia in the hospital setting.[12-14] There is no single recommendation for how to adjust insulin therapy at the time of hospital admission for patients taking insulin before admission (Table 34.1). Some patients require modification of their home regimen because of current clinical status, illness severity, antici-

Table 34.1 Suggested Approach for Insulin Therapy in the Hospital in Patients with Diabetes

Patients who take insulin before admission	■ Assess home glucose control and factors that may influence glycemic control in the hospital. ■ If home glucose control is adequate and the patient is eating a similar amount of food compared with at home, continue the current insulin regimen in combination with correction (supplemental) insulin. If the patient is eating less than at home, then reduce insulin dose. ■ Hold mealtime insulin if the patient will be taking nothing by mouth. ■ For patients with A1C >8%, consider increasing current insulin doses or modifying current insulin regimen.
Patients not taking insulin before admission who have a sustained requirement for correction insulin (i.e., ≥2 doses/day) or an A1C of ≥6.5%	■ Start weight-based basal-plus or basal-bolus insulin regimen (Table 34.2).
Patients with well-controlled diabetes who are at risk for hyperglycemia while in the hospital	■ Start correction insulin for 24–48 hours. ■ If there is a consistent requirement for correction doses of insulin, convert to weight-based basal-plus or basal-bolus insulin regimen (Table 34.2).

pated caloric intake and physical activity, and use of medications that affect glycemic control, whereas others may safely continue their usual outpatient doses.

Sliding-scale insulin (SSI) is never appropriate for use as the sole method of glycemic management in any patient with type 1 diabetes (T1D) or insulin-requiring type 2 diabetes (T2D).[12–14,27] By definition, patients with T1D have absolute insulin deficiency that puts them at high risk for severe hyperglycemia and even diabetic ketoacidosis (DKA) when insulin is withheld. SSI monotherapy places these patients at high risk for uncontrolled hyperglycemia and hypoglycemia, hospital-acquired infections, and prolonged length of stay (LOS).[28] The terms "correction" or "supplemental insulin," rather than SSI, are a more accurate way of describing doses of rapid or short-acting insulin preparations administered at specified intervals (premeal in patients who are eating; every 4–6 hours in patients who are not eating) according to results of bedside BG monitoring. Patients with sustained hyperglycemia, a persistent requirement for correction insulin (i.e., ≥2 doses per day), or an A1C ≥6.5% usually will require scheduled insulin therapy (Table 34.2).

TYPE 1 DIABETES

All patients with T1D will require continuation of insulin when they are hospitalized. Those who will be eating regular meals usually can continue their

Table 34.2 Recommendations for Initiating Insulin in the Hospitalized Patient

For patients with lean body type or renal insufficiency or age >70 years	Option 1: Calculate 0.2–0.3 units/kg as total daily dose (TDD) Option 2: Calculate 0.15 units/kg as basal insulin dose Use either option in combination with correction insulin
For patients who are obese or insulin resistant	Option 1: Calculate 0.4 units/kg as TDD for BG 140–200* Calculate 0.5 units/kg as TDD for BG >200* Option 2: Calculate 0.2 units/kg as basal insulin dose for BG 140–200 Calculate 0.25 units/kg as basal insulin dose for BG >200 Use either option in combination with correction insulin

*Prescribe 50–60% of TDD as basal and 40–50% of TDD as mealtime insulin

Suggested insulin regimens for basal-bolus insulin:

- Basal: glargine or detemir q 12–24 hours
- Nutritional: rapid-acting insulin before each meal (Note: hold dose if meal is missed)
- Correction: use same rapid-acting insulin before each meal

Suggested insulin regimens for basal-plus (correction) insulin:

- Basal: glargine or detemir q 12–24 hours
- Correction: rapid-acting insulin QAC if ordered with meals, otherwise every 6 hours

Correction insulin scales (to be used with basal insulin or as monotherapy for no more than 48 hours)

	Low dose (use for lean patients, type 1, or eGFR <30)	Moderate dose (usual starting scale)	High dose (use only if TDD >100 units/day)
<70 mg/dl	Begin hypoglycemia protocol	Begin hypoglycemia protocol	Begin hypoglycemia protocol
70–140 mg/dl	0 units	0 units	0 units
141–180 mg/dl	1 units	2 units	3 units
181–220 mg/dl	2 units	4 units	6 units
221–260 mg/dl	3 units	6 units	9 units
261–300 mg/dl	4 units	8 units	12 units
301–340 mg/dl	5 units	10 units	15 units
>340 mg/dl	6 units and call doctor	12 units and call doctor	18 units and call doctor

Note: eGFR = estimated glomerular filtration rate.

home insulin regimen when the A1C is at goal (Table 34.1). Patients who will not be eating for a specified period of time can continue to receive their long- or intermediate-acting insulin in combination with correction insulin for BG above goal range.

TYPE 2 DIABETES

Patients with T2D do not have the same absolute insulin requirement as those with T1D, but they are at high risk for severe hyperglycemia, hyperosmolar hyperglycemic nonketotic syndrome, and even DKA in the setting of acute illness. The majority of patients with insulin-requiring T2D before admission will require continuation of insulin when they are hospitalized. Patients treated with lifestyle interventions or oral diabetes medications (ODM) before admission should have bedside BG monitoring to determine whether they will need scheduled insulin. Patients who maintain BG <140 mg/dl while off all diabetes medications may not require continuation of bedside BG monitoring. Correction insulin alone may be appropriate for short-term use in patients with previously well-controlled T2D or for those for whom it is not known whether there will be an ongoing insulin requirement. When BG levels consistently exceed 140 mg/dl, patients may require scheduled insulin. These patients can be transitioned safely to basal-bolus or basal-plus-insulin regimens using weight-based calculations (Table 34.2).[29-31] The use of basal-plus-insulin regimens, defined as use of long-acting insulin in combination with correction insulin, is preferred for patients who are fasted in preparation for procedures or surgery. One study demonstrated that the use of basal-plus-insulin therapy was as effective as basal-bolus insulin therapy with less hypoglycemia in patients with T2D.[32] In this study, 375 patients with T2D treated with diet, ODM, or low-dose insulin before admission (≤0.4 units/kg/day) were randomized to basal-bolus, basal plus, or correction insulin monotherapy. Glycemic control was similar between the basal-bolus and basal-plus-insulin groups (*P* = 0.16) when compared with the SSI monotherapy (*P* = 0.04). The incidence of MH (16 and 13%, respectively) was higher than the correction insulin–only group (3%) (*P* = 0.02).

FREQUENCY OF BG MONITORING

Bedside BG monitoring is an essential component of inpatient diabetes management. Patients who are eating can have this done before meals and bedtime, whereas those who are not eating or who are receiving continuous enteral or parenteral nutrition can have this done every 4–6 hours. All patients with diabetes as well as all those with persistent BG >140 mg/dl or who receive therapies associated with hyperglycemia such as corticosteroids will require continuation of BG monitoring for the duration of their hospitalization.

Many factors can affect the accuracy of point-of-care glucose meters in the hospital setting, including variation in user experience, hematocrit, pH, and blood oxygen or carbon dioxide level.[33] The reader is referred to several excellent reviews on meter accuracy and safety in the inpatient setting.[33,34]

CONTINUOUS SUBCUTANEOUS INSULIN INFUSIONS IN HOSPITALIZED PATIENTS

Many patients with T1D and insulin-treated T2D use continuous subcutaneous insulin infusion (CSII) therapy with an insulin pump in the outpatient setting. Several studies have demonstrated that selected patients can continue CSII therapy in the hospital setting using principles of diabetes self-management.[35-37] Some hospitals have formalized insulin pump protocols that require patient attestation that they have the proper supplies and knowledge for continued CSII use and that they agree to document infusion rates, bolus doses, and BG values with nursing personnel. The availability of hospital personnel who are knowledgeable in CSII therapy allows for ongoing assessment of the continued safety of CSII use by an individual patient and can guide transition to scheduled subcutaneous (SQ) insulin therapy when patients are no longer capable of self-management, or they have a diagnostic study, such as magnetic resonance imaging, that requires temporary discontinuation of the pump.[35-37]

Patients with altered mental status, high suicide risk, or severe illness require transition to scheduled insulin therapy. When transitioning patients from CSII to multiple daily insulin doses, the total daily dose of basal insulin delivered with the pump device can be used to guide dosing for long- or intermediate-acting insulin. The dose of prandial insulin can be based on the usual premeal doses a patient was taking at home as either a fixed dose or as an insulin-to-carbohydrate ratio. In situations in which a patient is unable to provide this information, a weight-based calculation for insulin therapy can be made (Table 34.2).

CONTINUOUS INTRAVENOUS INSULIN THERAPY IN NONCRITICAL CARE AREAS

Some hospitals allow the administration of continuous intravenous insulin infusions (CII) for noncritically ill patients with more severe degrees of hyperglycemia who are not able to achieve desired glycemic targets with SQ insulin.[38] Patients who eat meals during CII therapy have more hyperglycemia and hypoglycemia when compared with those who are not eating.[39] This suggests the need for prandial SQ insulin in those who are eating to control postprandial hyperglycemia. CII is recommended for use by nurses who have been trained to use these protocols in a safe and effective manner.

USE OF ORAL DIABETES OR NONINSULIN INJECTABLE AGENTS IN THE HOSPITAL

Very few data are available investigating the use of noninsulin therapies in the hospital. The majority of patients will have or will develop contraindications to the use of ODM or noninsulin injectable therapies when hospitalized.[12-14] A minority of patients with well-controlled T2D who are clinically stable and eating regular meals may be able to continue these agents as long as there are no contraindications. Metformin, the most commonly used ODM, must be discontinued in patients with risk factors for lactic acidosis (i.e., decompensated congestive heart failure, renal insufficiency, hypoperfusion, chronic pulmonary disease), and those who have received intravenous (IV) contrast dye.[40] Sulfonylureas (SU) can cause severe and prolonged hypoglycemia, especially in patients >65 years old, with stage IV chronic kidney disease (CKD) (glomerular filtration rate [GFR] <30 ml/minute/1.73m²), and when used concurrently with intermediate- or long-acting insulin preparations.[38]

There has been much interest in using dipeptidyl peptidase-IV (DPP-IV) inhibitors agents or glucagon-like peptide-1 (GLP-1) analogs for management of patients with T2D because of their general tolerability and low incidence of hypoglycemia.[42] When used in place of IV insulin in critically ill patients, these agents have the potential to reduce nurse time for monitoring of BG levels and adjustments of CII. These benefits, however, have not yet been demonstrated. To date, the studies done using these agents have been performed in small numbers of patients where almost 50% of subjects required rescue therapy with insulin to achieve and maintain glycemic control. In addition, there have been no observed reductions in the frequency of hypoglycemia, frequency of BG monitoring, or nurse time.[42] Although these remain promising therapies in the outpatient setting or in stable hospitalized patients with T2D, it is important to wait for results from well-conducted, adequately powered studies that demonstrate efficacy and safety of their inpatient use.

GLYCEMIC MANAGEMENT DURING PARENTERAL AND ENTERAL NUTRITION

Patients with and without diabetes who receive parenteral or enteral nutrition are at risk for hyperglycemia.[43,44] At a minimum, patients started on this therapy should have BG monitoring at regular intervals with initiation or modification of scheduled insulin therapy to maintain glycemic control. Patients receiving enteral nutrition usually will require basal insulin to achieve and maintain adequate glycemic control.[43] Use of correction insulin alone may be an acceptable initial therapy; however, scheduled basal or basal-bolus insulin is required once a consistent insulin requirement is demonstrated. Long-acting basal insulin preparations have been demonstrated to be safe and effective in patients receiving enteral nutrition; however, they pose a risk for hypoglycemia in the event of abrupt discontinuation of nutritional supplementation if an alternate source of glucose is not provided immediately.[29,43] Use of 70/30 biphasic insulin or intermediate-acting insulin (neutral protamine Hagedorn [NPH]) administered at intervals of 2–3 times a day may result in less hypoglycemia during continuous or cyclic enteral feedings.[45] For patients receiving enteral nutrition over 12–18 hours, NPH in combination with short-acting (regular) insulin can be given at the initiation of the feedings followed by additional doses of scheduled regular insulin at 6-hour intervals for the duration of the feedings.

Patients receiving total parenteral nutrition (TPN) are treated optimally by having insulin added to their daily TPN bag based on their BG monitoring results and dose of correction (SQ) insulin administered during the previous day. Sole use of SQ insulin may result in unacceptable BG control and a higher risk of hypoglycemia, especially if the TPN is unexpectedly held or stopped after SQ doses of insulin are administered.

A common cause of hypoglycemia in the hospital is the unexpected interruption of parenteral or enteral nutrition after a patient has received their SQ long- or intermediate-acting insulin. Protocols for preventing hypoglycemia in these patients incorporate standing orders for initiation of an alternate glucose source, such as dextrose 10%, administered IV at the same rate of enteral or parenteral nutrition administration as a way of minimizing risk for hypoglycemia.[43]

STEROID THERAPY

Systemic glucocorticoids are used to treat acute exacerbations of chronic obstructive pulmonary disease, as part of chemotherapeutic or antirejection protocols; to prevent postoperative nausea; and in patients with relative adrenal insufficiency of acute illness. Intra-articular glucocorticoids also are associated with elevations in glucose levels for up to 48 hours following administration.[46] These agents are used frequently in the inpatient setting and represent a major contributor to the frequency and severity of hyperglycemia in patients with and without a prior history of diabetes.[47] In high doses, steroids not only increase insulin resistance but also have effects on β-cell function.[48]

The fact that not all patients develop hyperglycemia in the setting of glucocorticoid therapy suggests the need for a measured and deliberate approach to the detection, prevention, and management of glycemic excursions that occur with the various glucocorticoid protocols used in the hospital setting. All patients with diabetes require close glycemic monitoring with initiation of glucocorticoid therapy. Patients who have a history of steroid-associated hyperglycemia can have their insulin doses preemptively increased with initiation of steroid therapy. Those who are new to steroid therapy can have their doses increased once it becomes apparent that they experience deteriorations in glycemic control.

There are several suggested approaches to the management of steroid-associated hyperglycemia. One method involves increasing doses of basal and bolus insulin by up to 40–50% depending on the dose of steroid used. Another approach that can be effective in the management of regimens using prednisone or prednisolone is to administer NPH insulin using a weight-based calculation of 0.1 unit/kg for each 10 mg dose of prednisone or prednisolone up to a maximal dose of 0.4 units/kg for doses of 40 mg or greater.[49,50] These dosing regimens are meant to be used as a guide to therapy because there can be significant variability in insulin requirements among patients. In some cases, it is reasonable to use CII over a period of 12 hours to determine the dose of SQ insulin required to maintain desired levels of glycemic control with prolonged or intermittent steroid therapy. One benefit of using NPH-based regimens is that the dose can be administered at the time of steroid administration. If steroids are discontinued abruptly, then the dose of NPH also is discontinued, minimizing risk for hypoglycemia.

DIABETES AND HYPERGLYCEMIA IN THE INTENSIVE CARE UNIT

Hyperglycemia is common in critically ill patients with and without diabetes.[8] Following publication of a landmark study demonstrating significant improvements in patient outcomes using CII protocols targeting near euglycemia (e.g., 80–110 mg/dl) in surgical intensive care unit (ICU) patients, many hospitals introduced protocols with similar glycemic targets to improve outcomes in their patient populations.[51-53] Several studies, however, performed in different patient populations with protocols targeting BG 80–110 mg/dl, were unable to reproduce the favorable results of the surgical study (Table 34.3).[54-57] In fact, protocols targeting near euglycemia were observed to be associated with a higher risk for both MH and SH, which was related to higher mortality.[58,59]

The Normoglycemia in Intensive Care Evaluation-Survival Using Glucose Algorithm Regulation (NICE-SUGAR) study provided a turning point in recommendations for the glycemic management of critically ill patients.[56] Surgical and nonsurgical patients with or without a history of diabetes who received intensive insulin therapy (IIT) experienced more all-cause and cardiovascular mortality at 90 days (odds ratio [OR] 1.14). No differences were observed for ICU or hospital LOS, days of mechanical ventilation, or renal replacement therapy.[56] In response to this evidence of harm without clear benefit from protocols targeting near euglycemia, recommendations for glycemic targets in critically ill patients were mod-

Table 34.3 Selected ICU Studies with Intensive Insulin Therapy

Study	n	BG goal (mg/dl)	Patient type	Rate of hypoglyce-mia*	Conclusion
Leuven 1 2001	1,548	IIT 80–110 vs. 180–200	Single-center surgical ICU	IIT 2.5% Usual care 0.39%	Decreased ICU mortality (ARR 3.4%) Decreased in-hospital mortality (ARR 3.7%)
Leuven II 2006	1,200	IIT 90–110 vs. 180–200	Single-center medical ICU	IIT 18.7% Usual care 3.1%	No difference in in-hospital mortality Decreased morbidity in IIT group
VISEP 2008	537	IIT 80–110 vs. 180–200	Multicenter ICU sepsis/septic shock	IIT 12.1% Usual care 2.1%	Stopped early due to high rates of hypoglycemia in IIT group
Glucon-trol 2009	1,101	IIT 80–110 vs. 140–180	Multicenter mixed ICU	IIT 8.7% Conventional 2.7%	Stopped early due to hypoglycemia rates and thus underpowered to show any difference in mortality
NICE-SUGAR 2009	6,104	IIT 81–108 vs. <180	Multicenter mixed ICU	IIT 6.8% Conventional 0.5%	Increased mortality in the IIT group

Note: ARR = absolute risk reduction; BG = blood glucose; ICU = intensive care unit; IIT = intensive insulin therapy.
*Hypoglycemia defined as BG ≤40 mg/dl in Leuven I, Leuven II, and VISEP. Hypoglycemia defined as BG <40 mg/dl in Glucontrol.

ified to BG of 140–180 mg/dl for the majority of patients, with consideration for lower targets (110–140 mg/dl) in surgical ICU patients.[12,13] These more lenient protocols have been demonstrated to have low risk for both MH and SH, while still avoiding severe hyperglycemia.[17,60] The Society for Critical Care Medicine recommends maintaining BG levels of <150 mg/dl with CII.[15]

CONTINUOUS IV INSULIN INFUSION PROTOCOLS

CII is the most effective way to treat hyperglycemia in critically ill patients who can have ongoing variability in insulin sensitivity requiring frequent adjustments in insulin dose.[12,13,17,60,61] Of the many CII protocols published, those that effectively achieve and maintain desired BG targets with low risk for hypoglycemia using algorithms for insulin dose adjustments according to changes in BG are considered optimal.[53,60,61] For the most part, computer-based protocols result in a higher percentage of BG in the target range with lower rates of SH than paper-based protocols.[62,63] Selected features of several CII protocol studies can be seen in Table 34.3. A sample protocol can be found in Figure 34.1.

TRANSITION FROM IV TO SUBCUTANEOUS INSULIN

CII is labor intensive and, at most institutions, are done only in an ICU because of the amount of nursing care that is required. Too often, in an attempt to quickly move a patient out of the ICU, CII is stopped and SSI is started with subsequent deterioration in glycemic control. All patients with diabetes require the administration of SQ insulin before discontinuation of CII to maintain desired BG.[64,65] The majority of published transition protocols estimate transition doses of basal insulin by averaging the last 6–8 hours of the insulin infusion rate and multiplying by 20, which gives ~80% of previous insulin requirement over the preceding 24 hours. This strategy has been demonstrated to be both safe and effective.[66,67] The dose of basal insulin at time of transition can vary from 40 to 80% of the prior total daily insulin requirement.[67]

Variables associated with difficult transitions from IV to SQ insulin include age ≥72 years, high insulin infusion rates, and glucose variability in the 24 hours before transition.[68] The timing of the transition is another key factor in maintaining BG control. In one study, patients transitioned to SQ insulin ≤1 day after cardiac surgery had only 35% of BG in the target range.[69] Daily adjustments to insulin doses are required as patients begin to resume regular meals with gradual reductions in physiological stress and insulin doses.[70]

When transitioning from IV to SQ insulin, the dose of long- or intermediate-acting insulin typically is administered at least 2 hours before CII is stopped, allowing time for sufficient absorption of SQ insulin. If short- or rapid-acting insulin is administered with the basal insulin, the time period can sometimes be reduced to 1–2 hours. To prevent rebound hyperglycemia, some protocols administer SQ glargine in combination with CII.[64] In one study comparing glargine 0.25 units/kg in combination with CII with CII alone, those receiving basal insulin had a significant reduction (94 vs. 33%) in the percentage of patients experiencing hyperglycemia (BG >180 mg/dl) in the 12-hour period following CII discontinuation.[64] There were three MH events in the CII alone group and none in the group receiving basal insulin. These results suggest that administration of low-dose glargine insulin during CII may reduce the risk for rebound hyperglycemia following transition from IV to SQ insulin.[64]

In general, it is prudent to delay transition from CII until infusion rates are relatively stable and patients are ready to eat. Patients who will resume usual meals can receive 50% of the calculated transition dose as glargine with the remaining insulin administered as rapid-acting insulin in divided doses before meals.[68] Patients with poor appetites can receive more of the transition dose as basal insulin in combination with correction or supplemental insulin administered 3–4 times daily.[67] In older patients or those with renal insufficiency or rapidly changing clinical status, more conservative transition doses are appropriate.[68,70]

HYPOGLYCEMIA

The avoidance of hypoglycemia is a major challenge with any IDMP and remains a major barrier to achieving glycemic targets in the hospital setting. The fact that many hospitalized patients often are unable to sense or report symptoms of hypoglycemia due to use of sedating medications or factors related to their underlying illness increases risk for unrecognized or untreated hypoglycemia with potential for adverse sequelae.[71,72] Similar to what occurs with hyperglycemia, hypoglycemia also results in release of proinflammatory cytokines with an increase in reactive oxygen species.[73] Severe or prolonged hypoglycemia can result in seizures, cardiac arrhythmias, irreversible brain damage, and death.[74]

An association between SH mortality risk in critically ill patients has been demonstrated in several studies using protocols targeting euglycemia.[54,55] The NICE-SUGAR study demonstrated a nearly twofold increase in the hazard ratio for mortality with both MH and SH in critically ill patients.[58] A recent analysis of data from two large observational cohorts and one prospective study that included patients with varying severity of illness and ICU LOS also demonstrated independent associations for mortality in patients experiencing MH or SH when compared with those without hypoglycemia.[72]

An association between hypoglycemia and mortality has also been reported in noncritically ill patients.[71] In a retrospective cohort study of >4,000 admissions for patients with known diabetes hospitalized on general medical wards, BG ≤50 mg/dl occurred in 7.7% of all admissions and 3% of all patients. Both early and late mortality was higher among patients who had at least one hypoglycemic episode (inpatient mortality: 2.96 vs. 0.82%; mortality at 1 year after discharge: 27.8 vs. 14.1%). Both inpatient mortality and hospital LOS increased according to the severity and frequency of hypoglycemic episodes.[71]

There are several identified risk factors for hypoglycemia in hospitalized patients. These include poor coordination of insulin administration and food delivery, abrupt changes in nutritional intake or renal function, tapering steroid doses without appropriate reductions in insulin, and inappropriate insulin dosing.[75] In one study of hospitalized patients taking SU, 19% of patients experienced at least one episode of hypoglycemia.[41] A low estimated GFR (eGFR), age >65 years, and use of SU in combination with basal insulin were all identified as risk factors for hypoglycemia in this study.

Figure 34.1—Example continuous IV insulin infusion protocol targeting a goal blood glucose of 140–180 mg/dl designed and used at the University of Pittsburgh Medical Center.

☒ Start IV insulin infusion (1 unit/mL). Waste 15 mL of infusion through new tubing and every time tubing is changed.

INITIAL BG (mg/dL):

181–200   Start IV insulin infusion at 1 units/hour
201–250   Start IV insulin infusion at 2 units/hour
251–300   Give 2 units insulin IV push and start IV insulin infusion at 2 units/hour
>300   Give 4 units insulin IV push and start IV insulin infusion at 4 units/hour

☒ Check blood glucose (BG) 1 hour after each rate change (or q1h) until stable (at least 2 values between 140–180). BG checks can then be reduced to q2h. Once BGs are within desired range for 12 hours, reduce BG checks to q4h.

☒ Restart q1h checking if any change in insulin infusion rate occurs OR if there is significant change in clinical condition, vasopressor therapy, CVVHD, nutritional support, or glucocorticoid therapy.

☒ The site for BG checks should remain consistent. It is preferred to use either an arterial line or "VAMP" on a central line.

☒ Confirm BG via lab STAT if BG>500, HCT <25, or if clinical judgment indicates.

☒ Confirm BG with meter if BG<70 or if BG changes more than 100 mg/dL on a stable IV infusion.

☒ Notify MD when insulin infusion rate exceeds 10 units/hr or if 4 consecutive BGs are >250 mg/dL.

SUBSEQUENT INSULIN ADJUSTMENT:

BG (mg/dL)	Current rate 0.1–3.9 units/hour	Current rate 4–6.9 units/hour	Current rate 7–10 units/hour	Current rate >10 units/hour*
<70	**(1) D/C insulin. Give 50mL (1 amp) D50 IV. Recheck BG in 15 min.** Repeat as necessary. (Do not restart insulin until at least 1 hr after D50.) Notify MD. If no continuous glucose, start IV fluid as per page 1. Restart insulin at 50% (half) previous rate when BG >140 AND it is at least 1 hr after D50. Recheck BG in 1 hr.			
70–99	**(2) D/C insulin.** Recheck BG in 1 hr and then hourly. When BG >140, restart insulin but decrease rate by 50% (half) and recheck BG in 1 hr.			

continued

BG (mg/dL)	Current rate 0.1–3.9 units/hour	Current rate 4–6.9 units/hour	Current rate 7–10 units/hour	Current rate >10 units/hour*
100–139	**(3.1)** If BG drop >25 mg/dl from last check, **D/C insulin.** Recheck BG in 1 hr and then hourly. When BG >140, restart insulin but decrease rate by 50% (half) and recheck BG in 1 hr. **(3.2)** Otherwise, **decrease** by 0.5 units/hr (if current rate <0.5 units/hr, then D/C) and recheck BG in 1 hr.	**(4.1)** If BG drop >25 mg/dl from last check, **D/C insulin.** Recheck BG in 1 hr and then hourly. When BG >140, restart insulin but decrease rate by 2 units/hr and recheck BG in 1 hr. **(4.2)** Otherwise, **decrease** rate by 1 unit and recheck BG in 1 hr.	**(5.1)** If BG drop >25 mg/dl from last check, **D/C insulin.** Recheck BG in 1 hr and then hourly. When BG >140, restart insulin but decrease rate by 3 units/hr and recheck BG in 1 hr. **(5.2)** Otherwise, **decrease** rate by 1.5 units and recheck BG in 1 hr.	**(6.1)** If BG drop >25 mg/dl from last check, **D/C insulin.** Recheck BG in 1 hr and then hourly. When BG >140, restart insulin but decrease rate by 4 units/hr and recheck BG in 1 hr. **(6.2)** Otherwise, **decrease** rate by 2 units and recheck BG in 1 hr.
140–180	**(7.1)** If BG drop >50 mg/dl from last check, **D/C insulin.** Recheck BG in 1 hr and then hourly. Restart insulin (as long as BG>140), but decrease rate by 50% (half) and recheck BG in 1 hr. **(7.2)** If BG drop 25–50 mg/dl from last check, **decrease** rate by 50% (half) and recheck BG in 1 hr. **(7.3)** Otherwise, **make no changes.** If BGs 140–180 for 2 consecutive hours, recheck q2h.	**(8.1)** If BG drop >50 mg/dl from last check, **D/C insulin.** Recheck BG in 1 hr and then hourly. Restart insulin (as long as BG>140), but decrease rate by 2 units/hr and recheck BG in 1 hr. **(8.2)** If BG drop 25–50 mg/dl from last check, **decrease** by 2 units/hr and recheck BG in 1 hr. **(8.3)** Otherwise, **make no changes.** If BGs 140–180 for 2 consecutive hours, recheck q2h.	**(9.1)** If BG drop >50 mg/dl from last check, **D/C insulin.** Recheck BG in 1 hr and then hourly. Restart insulin (as long as BG>140), but decrease rate by 3 units/hr and recheck BG in 1 hr. **(9.2)** If BG drop 25–50 mg/dl from last check, **decrease** by 3 units/hr and recheck BG in 1 hr. **(9.3)** Otherwise, **make no changes.** If BGs 140–180 for 2 consecutive hours, recheck q2h.	**(10.1)** If BG drop >50 mg/dl from last check, **D/C insulin.** Recheck BG in 1 hr and then hourly. Restart insulin (as long as BG>140), but decrease rate by 4 units/hr and recheck BG in 1 hr. **(10.2)** If BG drop 25–50 mg/dl from last check, **decrease** by 4 units/hr and recheck BG in 1 hr. **(10.3)** Otherwise, **make no changes.** If BGs 140–180 for 2 consecutive hours, recheck q2h.

continued

Figure 34.1 — Example continuous IV insulin infusion protocol targeting a goal blood glucose of 140–180 mg/dl designed and used at the University of Pittsburgh Medical Center. (*continued*)

BG (mg/dL)	Current rate 0.1–3.9 units/hour	Current rate 4–6.9 units/hour	Current rate 7–10 units/hour	Current rate >10 units/hour*
181–250	**(11.1)** If BG drop >50 mg/dl, **decrease** rate by 50% (half) and recheck BG in 1 hr.	**(12.1)** If BG drop >50 mg/dl, **decrease** rate by 2 units/hr and recheck BG in 1 hr.	**(13.1)** If BG drop >50 mg/dl, **decrease** rate by 3 units/hr and recheck BG in 1 hr.	**(14.1)** If BG drop >50 mg/dl, **decrease** rate by 4 units/hr and recheck BG in 1 hr.
	(11.2) If BG drop 25-50 mg/dl from last check, make **no change** and recheck BG in 1 hr.	**(12.2)** If BG drop 25-50 mg/dl from last check, make **no change** and recheck BG in 1 hr.	**(13.2)** If BG drop 25-50 mg/dl from last check, make **no change** and recheck BG in 1 hr.	**(14.2)** If BG drop 25-50 mg/dl from last check, make **no change** and recheck BG in 1 hr.
	(11.3) Otherwise, **increase** rate by 1 unit/hr and recheck BG in 1 hr.	**(12.3)** Otherwise, **increase** rate by 1.5 units/hr and recheck BG in 1 hr.	**(13.3)** Otherwise, **increase** rate by 2 units/hr and recheck BG in 1 hr.	**(14.3)** Otherwise, **increase** rate by 3 units/hr and recheck BG in 1 hr.
>250	**(15.1)** If BG drop ≥25 mg/dl from last check, make **no change** and recheck BG in 1 hr.	**(16.1)** If BG drop ≥25 mg/dl from last check, make **no change** and recheck BG in 1 hr.	**(17.1)** If BG drop ≥25 mg/dl from last check, make **no change** and recheck BG in 1 hr.	**(18.1)** If BG drop ≥25 mg/dl from last check, make **no change** and recheck BG in 1 hr.
	(15.2) Otherwise, **give** 2 units insulin IV push AND **increase** rate by 1 unit/hr. Recheck BG in 1 hr.	**(16.2)** Otherwise, **give** 2 units insulin IV push AND **increase** rate by 1.5 units/hr. Recheck BG in 1 hr.	**(17.2)** Otherwise, **give** 2 units insulin IV push AND **increase** rate by 2 units/hr. Recheck BG in 1 hr.	**(18.2)** Otherwise, **give** 2 units insulin IV push AND **increase** rate by 3 units/hr. Recheck BG in 1 hr.

The contribution of renal insufficiency to risk for hypoglycemia was demonstrated in one trial of hospitalized patients with T2D and eGFR <45 ml/minute randomized to once-daily glargine and three-times daily glulisine using weight-based dose calculation of 0.25 or 0.5 units/kg/day.[76] Both groups had a similar percentage of BG values in the target range (100–180 mg/dl), but the group receiving the lower doses had less hypoglycemia (30 vs. 15.8%; *P* = 0.08).[76] What is notable about this study is the frequency of hypoglycemia with the lower dosing regimen, again demonstrating a need for a higher level of caution with insulin dosing in patients with renal insufficiency.

Although no studies establish direct causation between hypoglycemia and mortality, prompt recognition and treatment for any BG <70 mg/dl certainly is warranted as a way to prevent progression to SH. The use of nurse-directed hypoglycemia treatment protocols (HTP) has helped alleviate the frequency and SH events in some hospitals (Table 34.4).[21,77,78] Standard recommendations for hypoglycemia treatment suggest administration of 15–20 grams of oral carbohydrates or glucose followed by a repeat BG 15 minutes later.[79] Few studies are investigating the optimal dose of oral glucose needed to treat hypoglycemia that also mini-

Table 34.4 Example of a Hypoglycemia Treatment Protocol

	Blood glucose 50–69 mg/dl	Blood glucose <50 mg/dl
For patients who are alert	Give one of the following: ■ 1 tube (15 grams) glucose gel ■ 3 graham crackers ■ 4 oz. apple juice ■ 6 oz. clear nondiet soft drink	Give one of the following: ■ 2 tubes (30 grams) glucose gel ■ 4 oz. apple juice and 3 graham crackers ■ 6 oz. clear nondiet soft drink and 3 graham crackers
For NPO patients or patients unable to swallow (alert)	Give one of the following: ■ Dextrose 50% 30 ml = 15 grams of dextrose ■ Dextrose 20% 75 ml = 15 grams of dextrose ■ Dextrose 10% 150 ml = 15 grams of dextrose ■ Glucagon 1 mg IM/SQ followed by dextrose 10% (D10W) at 50ml/hour Communicate event to doctor after treatment initiated to obtain orders for adjustment of dextrose infusions, if needed.	
For patients on IV insulin infusion	Stop the IV insulin infusion and use one of the following: ■ Dextrose 50% 30 ml = 15 grams of dextrose ■ Dextrose 20% 75 ml = 15 grams of dextrose ■ Dextrose 10% 150 ml = 15 grams of dextrose	
For patients with a decreased level of consciousness	Call the medical emergency team and use one of the following: ■ Dextrose 50% IV push (1 amp) = 25 grams of dextrose ■ Dextrose 20% 125 ml = 25 grams of dextrose ■ Dextrose 10% 250 ml = 25 grams of dextrose If D50 is not available, or there will be a delay in obtaining dextrose solutions, give glucagon 1 mg IM/SQ followed by a continuous infusion of D10W or D20W.	

Note: IM = intramuscular; IV = intravenous; SQ = subcutaneous.

mize rebound hyperglycemia in the inpatient setting. In one study of 51 unresponsive patients with BG <72 mg/dl who were attended by paramedics before transfer to the hospital found no difference in the time to resolution of mental status changes (~8 minutes) in those randomized to dextrose 10% delivered in 5-gram aliquots every minute (median total dose 10 grams) or to 25 grams of dextrose 50% ($P = 0.001$).[80] The median post-treatment BG, however, was significantly lower in the patients receiving aliquots of dextrose 10% (112 vs. 169 mg/dl, $P = 0.003$).

Many hypoglycemic events can be prevented by using appropriately dosed insulin that is adjusted according to bedside BG results on at least a daily basis. Avoiding the use of SU medications in patients >65 years old or those who have renal insufficiency can reduce the risk for both MH and prolonged SH. In patients with diabetes who receive insulin in the hospital for glycemic management, it is best to discontinue the SU. Finally, use of nurse-directed HTP promotes early recognition and treatment of mild hypoglycemia to MH, avoiding progression to more severe episodes.

CONCLUSION

Studies investigating short- and long-term clinical outcomes in patients with diabetes according to treatment strategies and glycemic measures have led to the development of guidelines and consensus statements that specify target BG levels and methods of achieving these targets.[12-15] Several important principles can guide the management of these patients in the hospital:

- Patients who are treated with insulin before admission will almost always require insulin therapy in the hospital setting.
- Discontinuation of scheduled insulin therapy in patients previously treated with insulin can result in severe hyperglycemia with the risk for DKA and hyperosmolar syndromes.
- Very little data guide the management of patients with T2D treated with ODM or noninsulin injectable therapies in the hospital. It generally is recommended that these agents be used cautiously or not at all in this setting.
- Weight-based algorithms adjusted for age, renal function, and a general assessment of insulin sensitivity can be safely used to determine doses of basal and prandial insulin therapy.
- SSI is inappropriate for use as monotherapy in patients with T1D or any previously insulin-treated diabetes.
- Correction insulin in conjunction with regular BG monitoring can be used for short periods of time in patients with newly diagnosed T2D, or T2D previously treated with ODM for whom the need for scheduled insulin is uncertain.
- Determination of an A1C at time of admission for all hospitalized patients with diabetes allows for assessment of the adequacy of the home regimen and modification of the regimen at the time of hospital discharge.

REFERENCES

1. Kim H, Helmer DA, Zhao Z, Boockvar K. Potentially preventable hospitalizations among older adults with diabetes. *Am J Managed Care* 2011;17:e419–e426.

2. Kim H, Ross JS, Melkus GD, Zhao Z, Boockvar K. Scheduled and unscheduled hospital readmissions among patients with diabetes. *Am J Managed Care* 2010;16:760–767.

3. Jiang HJ, Stryer D, Friedman B, Andrews R. Multiple hospitalizations for patients with diabetes. *Diabetes Care* 2003;26:1421–1426.

4. Kim S. Burden of hospitalizations primarily due to uncontrolled diabetes: implications of inadequate primary health care in the United States. *Diabetes Care* 2007;30:1281–1282.

5. Umpierrez G, Maynard G. Glycemic chaos (not glycemic control) still the rule for inpatient care: how do we stop the insanity? *J Hosp Med* 2006;1:141–144.

6. Cook CB, Jameson KA, Hartsell ZC, Boyle ME, Leonhardi BJ, Farquhar-Snow M, Beer KA. Beliefs about hospital diabetes and perceived barriers to glucose management among inpatient midlevel practitioners. *Diabetes Educ* 2008;34:75–83.

7. Cook CB, Kongable GL, Potter DJ, Abad VJ, Leija DE, Anderson M. Inpatient glucose control: a glycemic survey of 126 U.S. hospitals. *J Hosp Med* (Online) 2009;4:E7–E14.

8. Swanson CM, Potter DJ, Kongable GL, Cook CB. Update on inpatient glycemic control in hospitals in the United States. *Endocr Pract* 2011;17:853–861.

9. Smith WD, Winterstein AG, Johns T, Rosenberg E, Sauer BC. Causes of hyperglycemia and hypoglycemia in adult inpatients. *Am J Health Syst Pharm* 2005;62:714–719.

10. Desimone ME, Blank GE, Virji M, Donihi A, DiNardo M, Simak DM, Buranosky R, Korytkowski MT. Effect of an educational inpatient diabetes management program on medical resident knowledge and measures of glycemic control: a randomized controlled trial. *Endocr Pract* 2012;18:238–243.

11. Rubin DJ, Moshang J, Jabbour SA. Diabetes knowledge: are resident physicians and nurses adequately prepared to manage diabetes? *Endocr Pract* 2007;13:17–21.

12. Moghissi ES, Korytkowski MT, DiNardo M, Einhorn D, Hellman R, Hirsch IB, Inzucchi SE, Ismail-Beigi F, Kirkman MS, Umpierrez GE, American Association of Clinical Endocrinologists, American Diabetes Association. American Association of Clinical Endocrinologists and American Diabetes Association consensus statement on inpatient glycemic control. *Endocr Pract* 2009;15:353–369.

13. Moghissi ES, Korytkowski MT, DiNardo MM, Einhorn D, Hellman R, Hirsch IB, Inzucchi SE, Ismail-Beigi F, Kirkman MS, Umpierrez GE. American Association of Clinical Endocrinologists and American Diabetes Association consensus statement on inpatient glycemic control. *Diabetes Care* 2009;32:1119–1131.

14. Umpierrez GE, Hellman R, Korytkowski MT, Kosiborod M, Maynard GA, Montori VM, Seley JJ, Van den Berghe G. Management of hyperglycemia in hospitalized patients in noncritical care setting: an Endocrine Society clinical practice guideline. *J Clin Endocrinol Metab* 2012;97:16–38.

15. Jacobi J, Bircher N, Krinsley J, Agus M, Braithwaite SS, Deutschman C, Freire AX, Geehan D, Kohl B, Nasraway SA, Rigby M, Sands K, Schallom L, Taylor B, Umpierrez G, Mazuski J, Schunemann H. Guidelines for the use of an insulin infusion for the management of hyperglycemia in critically ill patients. *Crit Care Med* 2012;40:3251–3276.

16. Korytkowski M, Moghissi E, Umpierrez G. Intensive insulin therapy in hospitalized patients. *Ann Intern Med* 2011;154:846–847; author reply 847–848.

17. Marvin MR, Inzucchi SE, Besterman BJ. Computerization of the Yale insulin infusion protocol and potential insights into causes of hypoglycemia with intravenous insulin. *Diabetes Technol Ther* 2013;15:1–7.

18. Donihi AC, Gibson JM, Noschese ML, DiNardo MM, Koerbel GL, Curll M, Korytkowski MT. Effect of a targeted glycemic management program on provider response to inpatient hyperglycemia. *Endocr Pract* 2011;17:552–557.

19. Hermayer KL, Cawley P, Arnold P, Sutton A, Crudup J, Kozlowski L, Hushion TV, Sheakley ML, Epps JA, Weil RP, Carter RE. Impact of improvement efforts on glycemic control and hypoglycemia at a university medical center. *J Hosp Med* 2009;4:331–339.

20. Thompson R, Schreuder AB, Wisse B, Jarman K, Givan K, Suhr L, Corl D, Pierce B, Knopp R, Goss JR. Improving insulin ordering safely: the development of an inpatient glycemic control program. *J Hosp Med* 2009;4:E30–35.

21. Korytkowski M, Dinardo M, Donihi AC, Bigi L, Devita M. Evolution of a diabetes inpatient safety committee. *Endocr Pract* 2006;12(Suppl 3):91–99.

22. Donihi AC, Abriola C, Hall R, Korytkowski MT. Getting the timing right in the hospital: synching insulin administration with meal tray arrival. *Diabetes* 2010;59:1028–P.

23. Freeland B, Penprase BB, Anthony M. Nursing practice patterns: timing of insulin administration and glucose monitoring in the hospital. *Diabetes Educ* 2011;37:357–362.

24. Curll M, DiNardo M, Noschese M, Korytkowski MT. Menu selection, glycaemic control, and satisfaction with standard and patient-controlled consistent carbohydrate diet meal plans in hospitalised patients with diabetes. *Qual Saf Health Care* 2010;19:355–359.

25. Guerra YS, Lacuesta EA, Yrastorza R, Miernik J, Shakya N, Fogelfeld L. Insulin injections in relation to meals in the hospital medicine ward: comparison of 2 protocols. *Endocr Pract* 2011;17:737–746.

26. Meyer C, Boron A, Plummer E, Voltchenok M, Vedda R. Glulisine versus human regular insulin in combination with glargine in noncritically ill hospitalized patients with type 2 diabetes: a randomized double-blind study. *Diabetes Care* 2010;33:2496–2501.

27. Hirsch IB. Sliding scale insulin: time to stop sliding. *JAMA* 2009;301:213–214.

28. Hawkins K, Korytkowski M. Inpatient management and specific procedures. In *American Diabetes Association/JDRF Type 1 Diabetes Sourcebook*. Peters A, Laffel L, Eds. Alexandria, VA, American Diabetes Association, 2013, p. 531–541.

29. Umpierrez GE. Basal versus sliding-scale regular insulin in hospitalized patients with hyperglycemia during enteral nutrition therapy. *Diabetes Care* 2009;32:751–753.

30. Umpierrez GE, Smiley D, Jacobs S, Peng L, Temponi A, Mulligan P, Umpierrez D, Newton C, Olson D, Rizzo M. Randomized study of basal-bolus insulin therapy in the inpatient management of patients with type 2 diabetes undergoing general surgery (RABBIT 2 surgery). *Diabetes Care* 2011;34:256–261.

31. Umpierrez GE, Smiley D, Zisman A, Prieto LM, Palacio A, Ceron M, Puig A, Mejia R. Randomized study of basal-bolus insulin therapy in the inpatient management of patients with type 2 diabetes (RABBIT 2 trial). *Diabetes Care* 2007;30:2181–2186.

32. Umpierrez GE, Smiley D, Hermayer K, Khan A, Olson DE, Newton C, Jacobs S, Rizzo M, Peng L, Reyes D, Pinzon I, Fereira ME, Hunt V, Gore A, Toyoshima MT, Fonseca VA. Randomized study comparing a basal bolus with a basal plus correction insulin regimen for the hospital management of medical and surgical patients with type 2 diabetes: Basal Plus trial. *Diabetes Care* 2013;36:2169–2174.

33. Rebel A, Rice MA, Fahy BG. Accuracy of point-of-care glucose measurements. *J Diabetes Science Technol* 2012;6:396–411.

34. Hellman R. Glucose meter inaccuracy and the impact on the care of patients. *Diabetes Metab Res Rev* 2012;28:207–209.

35. Noschese ML, DiNardo MM, Donihi AC, Gibson JM, Koerbel GL, Saul M, Stefanovic-Racic M, Korytkowski MT. Patient outcomes after implementation of a protocol for inpatient insulin pump therapy. *Endocr Pract* 2009;15:415–424.

36. Cook CB, Beer KA, Seifert KM, Boyle ME, Mackey PA, Castro JC. Transitioning insulin pump therapy from the outpatient to the inpatient setting: a review of 6 years' experience with 253 cases. *J Diabetes Sci Technol* 2012;6:995–1002.

37. Bailon RM PB, Miller-Cage V, Boyle ME, Castro JC, Bourgeois PB, Cook CB. Continuous subcutaneous insulin infusion (insulin pump) therapy can be safely used in the hospital in select patients. *Endocr Pract* 2009;15:24–29.

38. Kelly JL, Hirsch IB, Furnary AP. Implementing an intravenous insulin protocol in your practice: practical advice to overcome clinical, administrative, and financial barriers. *Semin Thorac Cardiovasc Surg* 2006;18:346–358.

39. Smiley D, Rhee M, Peng L, Roediger L, Mulligan P, Satterwhite L, Bowen P, Umpierrez GE. Safety and efficacy of continuous insulin infusion in noncritical care settings. *J Hosp Med* 2010;5:212–217.

40. Calabrese AT, Coley KC, DaPos SV, Swanson D, Rao RH. Evaluation of prescribing practices: risk of lactic acidosis with metformin therapy. *Arch Intern Med* 2002;162:434–437.

41. Deusenberry CM, Coley KC, Korytkowski MT, Donihi AC. Hypoglycemia in hospitalized patients treated with sulfonylureas. *Pharmacotherapy* 2012;32:613–617.

42. Umpierrez GE, Korytkowski M. Is incretin-based therapy ready for the care of hospitalized patients with type 2 diabetes? Insulin therapy has proven itself and is considered the mainstay of treatment. *Diabetes Care* 2013;36:2112–2117.

43. Korytkowski MT, Salata RJ, Koerbel GL, Selzer F, Karslioglu E, Idriss AM, Lee KKW, Moser AJ, Toledo FGS. Insulin therapy and glycemic control in hospitalized patients with diabetes during enteral nutrition therapy: a randomized controlled clinical trial. *Diabetes Care* 2009;32:594–596.

44. Cheung NW, Napier B, Zaccaria C, Fletcher JP. Hyperglycemia is associated with adverse outcomes in patients receiving total parenteral nutrition. *Diabetes Care* 2005;28:2367–2371.

45. Hsia E, Seggelke SA, Gibbs J, Rasouli N, Draznin B. Comparison of 70/30 biphasic insulin with glargine/lispro regimen in non-critically ill diabetic patients on continuous enteral nutrition therapy. *Nutr Clin Pract* 2011;26:714–717.

46. Even JL, Crosby CG, Song Y, McGirt MJ, Devin CJ. Effects of epidural steroid injections on blood glucose levels in patients with diabetes mellitus. *Spine* 2012;37:E46–E50.

47. Donihi AC, Raval D, Saul M, Korytkowski MT, DeVita MA. Prevalence and predictors of corticosteroid-related hyperglycemia in hospitalized patients. *Endocr Pract* 2006;12:358–362.

48. van Raalte DH, van Genugten RE, Linssen MM, Ouwens DM, Diamant M. Glucagon-like peptide-1 receptor agonist treatment prevents glucocorticoid-induced glucose intolerance and islet-cell dysfunction in humans. *Diabetes Care* 2001;34:412–417.

49. Clore JN, Thurby-Hay L. Glucocorticoid-induced hyperglycemia *Endocr Pract* 2009;15:469–474.

50. Seggelke SA, Gibbs J, Draznin B. Pilot study of using neutral protamine Hagedorn insulin to counteract the effect of methylprednisolone in hospitalized patients with diabetes. *J Hosp Med* 2011;6:175–176.

51. Van den Berghe G, Wouters P, Weekers F, Verwaest C, Bruyninckx F, Schetz M, Vlasselaers D, Ferdinande P, Lauwers P, Bouillon R. Intensive insulin therapy in the critically ill patients. *N Engl J Med* 2001;345:1359–1367.

52. Krinsley JS. Effect of an intensive glucose management protocol on the mortality of critically ill adult patients. *Mayo Clin Proc* 2004;79:992–1000.

53. Rea RS, Donihi AC, Bobeck M, Herout P, McKaveney TP, Kane-Gill SL, Korytkowski MT. Implementing an intravenous insulin infusion protocol in the intensive care unit. *Am J Health Syst Pharm* 2007;64:385–395.

54. Brunkhorst FM, Engel C, Bloos F, Meier-Hellmann A, Ragaller M, Weiler N, Moerer O, Gruendling M, Oppert M, Grond S, Olthoff D, Jaschinski U, John S, Rossaint R, Welte T, Schaefer M, Kern P, Kuhnt E, Kiehntopf M, Hartog C, Natanson C, Loeffler M, Reinhart K, German Competence Network Study; Intensive insulin therapy and pentastarch resuscitation in severe sepsis. *N Engl J Med* 2008;358:125–139.

55. Van den Berghe G, Wilmer A, Hermans G, Meersseman W, Wouters PJ, Milants I, Van Wijngaerden E, Bobbaers H, Bouillon R. Intensive insulin therapy in the medical ICU. *N Engl J Med* 2006;354:449–461.

56. Finfer S, Chittock DR, Su SY-S, Blair D, Foster D, Dhingra V, Bellomo R, Cook D, Dodek P, Henderson WR, Hebert PC, Heritier S, Heyland DK, McArthur C, McDonald E, Mitchell I, Myburgh JA, Norton R, Potter J, Robinson BG, Ronco JJ (Investigators N-SS). Intensive versus conventional glucose control in critically ill patients. *N Engl J Med* 2009;360:1283–1297.

57. Preiser JC, Devos P, Ruiz-Santana S, Melot C, Annane D, Groeneveld J, Iapichino G, Leverve X, Nitenberg G, Singer P, Wernerman J, Joannidis M, Stecher A, Chiolero R. A prospective randomised multi-centre controlled trial on tight glucose control by intensive insulin therapy in adult intensive care units: the Glucontrol Study. *Intensive Care Med* 2009;35:1738–1748.

58. Finfer S, Liu B, Chittock DR, Norton R, Myburgh JA, McArthur C, Mitchell I, Foster D, Dhingra V, Henderson WR, Ronco JJ, Bellomo R, Cook D, McDonald E, Dodek P, Hebert PC, Heyland DK, Robinson BG. Hypoglycemia and risk of death in critically ill patients. *N Engl J Med* 2012;367:1108–1118.

59. Griesdale DEG, de Souza RJ, van Dam RM, Heyland DK, Cook DJ, Malhotra A, Dhaliwal R, Henderson WR, Chittock DR, Finfer S, Talmor D. Intensive insulin therapy and mortality among critically ill patients: a meta-analysis including NICE-SUGAR study data. *Can Med Assoc J* 2009;180:821–827.

60. Magaji V, Nayak S, Donihi AC, Willard L, Jampana S, Nivedita P, Eder R, Johnston J, Korytkowski MT. Comparison of insulin infusion protocols targeting 110-140 mg/dl in patients after cardiac surgery. *Diabetes Technol Ther* 2012;14:1013–1017.

61. Goldberg PA, Siegel MD, Sherwin RS, Halickman JI, Lee M, Bailey VA, Lee SL, Dziura JD, Inzucchi SE. Implementation of a safe and effective insulin infusion protocol in a medical intensive care unit. *Diabetes Care* 2004;27:461–467.

62. Krikorian A, Ismail-Beigi F, Moghissi ES. Comparisons of different insulin infusion protocols: a review of recent literature. *Curr Opin Clin Nutr Metab Care* 2010;13:198–204.

63. Boord JB, Sharifi M, Greevy RA, Griffin MR, Lee VK, Webb TA, May ME, Waitman LR, May AK, Miller RA. Computer-based insulin infusion protocol improves glycemia control over manual protocol. *J Am Med Inform Assoc* 2007;14:278–287.

64. Hsia E, Seggelke S, Gibbs J, Hawkins RM, Cohlmia E, Rasouli N, Wang C, Kam I, Draznin B. Subcutaneous administration of glargine to diabetic patients receiving insulin infusion prevents rebound hyperglycemia. *J Clin Endocrinol Metab* 2012;97:3132–3137.

65. Bode BW, Braithwaite SS, Steed RD, Davidson PC. Intravenous insulin infusion therapy: indications, methods, and transition to subcutaneous insulin therapy. *Endocr Pract* 2004;10(Suppl 2):71–80.

66. DeSantis AJ, Schmeltz LR, Schmidt K, O'Shea-Mahler E, Rhee C, Wells A, Brandt S, Peterson S, Molitch ME. Inpatient management of hyperglycemia: the Northwestern experience. *Endocr Pract* 2006;12:491–505.

67. Schmeltz LR, DeSantis AJ, Schmidt K, O'Shea-Mahler E, Rhee C, Brandt S, Peterson S, Molitch ME. Conversion of intravenous insulin infusions to subcutaneously administered insulin glargine in patients with hyperglycemia. *Endocr Pract* 2006;12:641–650.

68. Avanzini F, Marelli G, Donzelli W, Busi G, Carbone S, Bellato L, Colombo EL, Foschi R, Riva E, Roncaglioni MC, De Martini M, Desio Diabetes Diagram Study G. Transition from intravenous to subcutaneous insulin: effectiveness and safety of a standardized protocol and predictors of outcome in patients with acute coronary syndrome. *Diabetes Care* 2011;34:1445–1450.

69. Shomali ME, Herr DL, Hill PC, Pehlivanova M, Sharretts JM, Magee MF. Conversion from intravenous insulin to subcutaneous insulin after cardiovascular surgery: transition to target study. *Diabetes Technol Ther* 2011;13:121–126.

70. Furnary AP, Braithwaite SS. Effects of outcome on in-hospital transition from intravenous insulin infusion to subcutaneous therapy. *Am J Cardiol* 2006;98:557–564.

71. Turchin A, Matheny ME, Shubina M, Scanlon JV, Greenwood B, Pendergrass ML. Hypoglycemia and clinical outcomes in patients with diabetes hospitalized in the general ward. *Diabetes Care* 2009;32:1153–1157.

72. Krinsley JS, Schultz MJ, Spronk PE, Harmsen RE, van Braam Houckgeest F, van der Sluijs JP, Melot C, Preiser JC. Mild hypoglycemia is independently associated with increased mortality in the critically ill. *Crit Care* 2011;15:R173.

73. Razavi Nematollahi L, Kitabchi AE, Stentz FB, Wan JY, Larijani BA, Tehrani MM, Gozashti MH, Omidfar K, Taheri E. Proinflammatory cytokines in response to insulin-induced hypoglycemic stress in healthy subjects. *Metab Clin Exp* 2009;58:443–448.

74. Egi MMD, Bellomo RMD, Stachowski EMD, French CJMD, Hart GKMD, Taori GMD, Hegarty CB, Bailey MP. Hypoglycemia and outcome in critically ill patients. *Mayo Clinic Proc* 2010;85:217–224.

75. Elliott MB, Schafers SJ, McGill JB, Tobin GS. Prediction and prevention of treatment-related inpatient hypoglycemia. *J Diabetes Science Technol* 2012;6:302–309.

76. Baldwin D, Zander J, Munoz C, Raghu P, DeLange-Hudec S, Lee H, Emanuele MA, Glossop V, Smallwood K, Molitch M. A randomized trial of two weight-based doses of insulin glargine and glulisine in hospitalized subjects with type 2 diabetes and renal insufficiency. *Diabetes Care* 2012;35:1970–1974.

77. DiNardo M, Donihi A, DeVita M, Siminerio L, Rao H, Korytkowski M. A nurse-directed protocol for recognition and treatment of hypoglycemia in hospitalized patients. *Practical Diabetol* 2005;24:37–44.

78. DiNardo M, Noschese M, Korytkowski M, Freeman S. The medical emergency team and rapid response system: finding, treating, and preventing hypoglycemia. *Jt Comm J Qual Patient Saf* 2006;32:591–595.

79. American Diabetes Association. Standards of medical care for patients with diabetes mellitus. *Diabetes Care* 2013;36:S11–S166.

80. Moore C, Woollard M. Dextrose 10% or 50% in the treatment of hypoglycaemia out of hospital? A randomised controlled trial. *Emerg Med J* 2005;22:512–515.

Chapter 35

Perioperative Hyperglycemia Management

Dawn Smiley, MD, MSCR

INTRODUCTION

Over the past 10 years, the number of surgeries in the U.S. has increased. Although nearly two-thirds of all surgeries are performed in the outpatient setting,[1] a report from the National Institutes of Health (NIH) revealed that there were as many as 51.4 million inpatient surgeries in the U.S. in 2010 and this number is expected to rise.[2] It also is known that patients with diabetes are more likely to undergo surgery than people without diabetes, with nearly 25% of people with diabetes requiring surgery over time.[3-5] Many of these surgeries are related directly to the macrovascular and microvascular complications as evidenced by the fact that cardiothoracic procedures, limb amputations, and eye surgeries are common in patients with diabetes. Surgery in patients with diabetes is associated with longer hospital stay, greater perioperative morbidity and mortality, and higher health care resource utilization compared with subjects without diabetes.[6-8] Thus, it is imperative that health care providers are knowledgeable about the appropriate management of diabetes and hyperglycemia in the perioperative period for patients in the inpatient and outpatient setting.

Diabetes is one of the most common diagnoses in hospitalized patients,[9] and it represents up to 20% of the total surgical population in the U.S.[6] and >10% in the U.K.,[10] with more recent reports showing 26.2% in England alone.[11] The reported prevalence of hyperglycemia in the surgical setting varies greatly depending on patient populations, types of surgeries performed, and regions. For instance, one large U.S. retrospective study found that 40% of patients undergoing noncardiac surgery had mean blood glucose (BG) >140 mg/dl; however, other studies have found that up to 80% of patients experience hyperglycemia after cardiac surgery[12,13] and 12% of patients without a history of diabetes will experience significant hyperglycemia (BG >200 mg/dl) on the day following surgery.[13] Those patients with new-onset hyperglycemia (no previous history of diabetes) will experience a worse clinical outcome as determined by longer length of stay, increased rate of infection complications, and higher mortality rate compared with those subjects with normoglycemia and a previous history of diabetes. Furthermore, observational studies show that up to 40% of patients admitted to the hospital have fasting glucose levels exceeding 126 mg/dl (7 mmol/l) or two or more random glucose levels >200 mg/dl (11.1 mmol/l) and that one-third of patients with hyperglycemia have stress hyperglycemia without a preceding history of diabetes.[9,14] In addition to this physiologic stress of surgery, hospitalized patients may develop perioperative hyperglycemia related to

DOI: 10.2337/9781580405096.35

the stress of concomitant illness or infection, treatment with corticosteroids, anesthetics and other medications, and densely caloric enteral and parenteral nutritional supplements.[5,15]

In addition to significantly more complications, several studies have shown that hospital costs are higher in patients with diabetes and hyperglycemia who undergo surgery compared with those without diabetes, and most of this can be attributed to a higher number of postoperative complications and greater length of stay (LOS) in the hospital.[16–18] Studies have shown that medical expenditures are 2.3-fold higher in patients with diabetes compared with those without diabetes, and inpatient costs are higher because of the increased LOS, resource utilization, and complication rates.[19,20]

This chapter reviews the evidence that hyperglycemia is associated with poor outcomes in surgical patients, the pathophysiology of hyperglycemia during trauma and surgical stress, the current published guidelines, and common postoperative complications in patients with diabetes. The chapter also provides practical recommendations for the preoperative, intraoperative, and postoperative management of hyperglycemia in patients with and without diabetes.

BACKGROUND

Hyperglycemia can cause myriad complications in patients who undergo surgical procedures, and the degree of risk depends on age, diabetes treatment, length of time with diabetes, preceding level of control, existing comorbidities, malnutrition, and general physical fitness.[4] Furthermore, perioperative mortality for some surgical procedures can be up to 50% higher in patients with diabetes compared with those without diabetes,[6] and a large case-control study showed that the odds ratio for perioperative mortality in noncardiac surgery is 1.19 (95% confidence interval [CI] 1.1–1.3) per mmol/l increase of glucose level.[8] BG levels >180 mg/dl can lead to dehydration because of the resultant osmotic diuresis. This osmotic diuresis in the face of hyperglycemia and relative hypoinsulinemia can result in the development of hyperglycemic-hyperosmolar syndrome (HHS) and diabetic ketoacidosis (DKA).[21,22] These hyperglycemic crises are associated with increased morbidity and mortality, particularly in such procedures as cardiac bypass where it is associated with up to 42% mortality.[23] BG levels >180 mg/dl also are associated with impaired wound healing and increased risk of infection. A study from Furnary et al. found that patients with diabetes have a 1.5- to 3-fold higher chance of developing deep sternal wound infections after coronary artery bypass graft (CABG) surgery.[24] Infections like these account for 66% of postoperative complications and cause up to one-fourth of perioperative deaths in patients with diabetes. The increased risk of infection and sepsis has been linked to altered chemotaxis and decreased phagocytic burst activity of the leukocytes,[25] and one study showed that insulin treatment compared with conventional treatment improves neutrophil function in patients with diabetes undergoing cardiac surgery.[26] Wound healing also can be hindered by any underlying circulation problems, nerve damage, and weakened immune systems that may exist in a state of poorly controlled diabetes.[27] Finally, stress-induced hyperglycemia can contribute to increased osmolality, endothelial dysfunction, and thrombosis because of the activation of the coagulation cascade; in turn, this can lead to ischemia and frank infarction.[4] Furthermore, patients with diabetes who have underlying cardiovascular (CV) and renal disease, autonomic neuropathy, and mobility issues will be more susceptible to develop intraoperative arrhythmias and ischemia, postoperative renal failure, hypotension, and postoperative pressure ulcers, respectively.[28]

Increasing evidence suggests that in hospitalized patients, with and without diabetes, the presence of hyperglycemia is a marker of poor outcome and can acutely trigger dehydration, impair immunologic response to infection, and promote inflammation and endothelial dysfunction.[29-34] Hyperglycemia also is associated with increased infections, length of hospital stay, resource utilization, and perioperative mortality compared with normoglycemic patients without diabetes.[4,9,13,35-40] This risk is heightened in the face of surgical intervention. Pomposelli et al. showed that general surgery patients had a 5.7-fold relative risk for serious postoperative infections (sepsis, pneumonia, and wound infection) when any postoperative BG was >220 mg/dl,[7] and the sentinel study by Van den Berghe et al. showed that critical care surgery patients with hyperglycemia had 34% higher mortality compared with patients with BG <110 mg/dl.[13] More important, having a preceding diagnosis of diabetes can increase perioperative mortality up to 50% compared with those without diabetes. [6,14,41]

Despite this convincing evidence and several published insulin protocols, intensive glycemic control is not aggressively pursued because of the fear of hypoglycemia in the face of nothing by mouth (NPO) status and its association with increased risk of poor outcomes.[42-44] Additionally the pivotal Normoglycemia in Intensive Care Evaluation-Survival Using Glucose Algorithm Regulation (NICE-SUGAR) study in surgical and medical patients with hyperglycemia in the intensive care unit (ICU) setting showed that patients who were being treated more aggressively (81–108 vs.144–180 mg/dl) had significantly higher mortality and hypoglycemia.[45] A subsequent meta-analysis by Griesdale, however, found that surgical patients, especially those undergoing cardiothoracic surgery, had a significant mortality benefit from tighter glycemic control.[46] Recently, Buchleitner et al. reviewed 12 randomized trials in patients with diabetes undergoing surgery to compare outcomes between intensive versus conventional glycemic control groups (694 vs. 709 patients, respectively) and found higher rates of hypoglycemia in the intensive group and no differences in mortality or outcomes.[47] This review underscores the fact that further evidence is needed before more aggressive targets can be recommended for patients undergoing general surgery. Furthermore, surgeons and anesthesiologists desire easy, straightforward protocols that are quick to implement. The lack of institutionally accepted protocols, inconsistent use of guidelines, and patient refusal of scheduled insulin serve as further barriers to treating patients in the perioperative setting with an insulin regimen other than sliding-scale insulin (SSI). Guidelines on the inpatient management of diabetes based on evidence and expert opinion have helped to mold the standard of care in medical centers and have increased adoption of written protocols. This practice of following guidelines can result in improved glycemic control and lower rates of hypoglycemia.

PROCESSES UNDERLYING THE DEVELOPMENT OF
HYPERGLYCEMIA IN THE PERIOPERATIVE SETTING

A surgical patient has multifactorial reasons to develop hyperglycemia that are independent of any background of preceding diabetes or prediabetes. Surgical stress is characterized by increased levels of counterregulatory hormones (catecholamines, cortisol, glucagon, and growth hormone) and inflammatory cytokines, such as tumor necrosis factor-α, interleukin-6, and interleukin-1β.[5,48–51] The magnitude of the counterregulatory response is related directly to the baseline glycemic control, severity of surgery, and the type of anesthesia used during the procedure.[52,53] The counterregulatory response results in insulin resistance, increased hepatic glucose output, impaired peripheral glucose utilization, and relative insulin deficiency (Table 35.1).[5,54,55] In addition to alterations in insulin sensitivity, poor β-cell responsiveness also can occur during surgery, although the mechanism underlying this effect is unclear. The additional insult of absolute or relative insulin deficiency as can be seen with uncontrolled diabetes can beget further increases in catecholamines and glucagon levels, leading to increased gluconeogenesis and glycogenolysis and inhibition of glucose uptake from the peripheral tissues.[5,15,56,57]

Surgery also can activate mediators of inflammation such as tumor necrosis factor-alpha (TNF-α), interleukins, nuclear factor kappa-B (NF-κB), and intercellular adhesion molecule (ICAM) that can lead to increased hepatic and skeletal muscle

Table 35.1 Counterregulatory Hormones and Mediators of Inflammation Associated with Surgery and Stress Hyperglycemia

Hormones	Effect
Cortisol	↑ skeletal muscle IR, ↑ lipolysis → substrate for↑ gluconeogenesis
Epinephrine	↑ skeletal muscle IR, ↑ gluconeogenesis and glycogenolysis, ↑ lipolysis, ↓ insulin secretion
Norepinephrine	↑ gluconeogenesis (at high levels), ↑ lipolysis
Glucagon	↑ gluconeogenesis and glycogenolysis
Growth hormone	↑ skeletal muscle IR, ↑ gluconeogenesis, ↑ lipolysis
Inflammation mediators	**Effect**
Tumor necrosis factor Nuclear factor-κB Interleukins 1 & 6	↑ skeletal and hepatic IR

Note: IR = insulin resistance; TNF = tumor necrosis factor.
Source: Adapted from McCowen KC, Malhotra A, Bistrian BR. Stress-induced hyperglycemia. *Crit Care Clinics* 2001;17:107–124; Smiley D, Umpierrez GE. Management of hyperglycemia in hospitalized patients. *Ann NY Acad Sci* 2010;1212:1–11.

insulin resistance.[58] These molecules also can alter the immune system[59] and in turn cause disruption in wound healing. TNF-α, in particular, activates c-Jun NH$_2$-terminal kinase (JNK), a signaling protein molecule that phosphorylates insulin receptor substrate-1 (IRS-1) and prevents insulin-mediated activation of phosphatidylinositol 3-kinase (PI 3-kinase) involved in tissue glucose uptake.[60]

The type of anesthesia may contribute to the development or degree of hyperglycemia during surgery. General anesthesia, compared with local or epidural anesthesia, is associated with higher rates of hyperglycemia and higher catecholamine, cortisol, and glucagon levels.[53,61,62] Volatile anesthetic agents, such as halothane and isoflurane, can cause hyperglycemia via inhibition of insulin secretion[63,64] and can increase hepatic glucose production.[65] Epidural analgesia, however, has been found to abolish the hyperglycemic response to surgery[66] and has minimal effects on carbohydrate metabolism or counterregulatory hormonal response in the intraoperative period.[67] Finally, some older studies suggest that the type of surgery and not just the type of anesthesia affect glycemia in the perioperative setting.[68] For instance, Weddell and Gale reported that the average BG excursion during intraperitoneal surgery is 93 mg/dl versus only 52 mg/dl in superficial surgeries.[69]

Many patients experience nausea after surgery due to pain and the residual effects of anesthesia, a delay in the return to bowel function, or being too ill to eat (i.e., sedated and ventilated). A medical nutrition therapy (MNT) consult is important in the postoperative setting, and in the U.S. the standard approach is for enteral or parenteral feeds to be initiated if it is anticipated that a surgical patient will eat <60% of their recommended caloric intake over 5–7 days or if they need gastrointestinal (GI) rest; however, in Europe, it is usual that patients are started on *total parenteral nutrition* (TPN) shortly after surgery.[70] One large, U.S. database that included surgical patients showed that nutritional support is associated with lower costs, lower rate of infection, and shorter LOS.[71] Medical nutrition therapy using these modalities, however, can cause or exacerbate hyperglycemia because of excess carbohydrate delivery or elevated free fatty acid levels, and intervention is needed to decrease the chance of poor outcomes.

INPATIENT GLYCEMIC MANAGEMENT IN SURGICAL PATIENTS: TREATMENT OPTIONS AND SPECIAL CONSIDERATIONS

As mentioned, a large body of evidence suggests that hyperglycemia in surgical patients, with and without diabetes, is associated with an increased risk of complications and death,[4,7,35,36,38] and thus, it would follow that focused management of glycemic levels would beget better outcomes. Glycemic management with insulin therapy in surgical patients with critical illness has been shown to reduce the risk of multiorgan failure, infections, postoperative arrhythmias, and LOS in the intensive care setting and mortality.[13,24,72,73] Additionally, glucose control also has been associated with decreased postoperative complications in noncritically ill patients admitted to general surgery.[74] This study by Umpierrez et al. found that significantly more patients reached glycemic targets with a scheduled basal-bolus insulin regimen compared with the use of SSI alone (53 vs. 31%, respectively), and the composite complication, which included wound infection, pneumonia, respiratory failure, acute renal failure, and bacteremia, was significantly lower. The landmark NICE-SUGAR trial, along with the Efficacy of Volume Substitution and Insulin Therapy in Severe Sepsis (VISEP) and Glucontrol trials, challenged "tight" glycemic control for patients in the ICU due to significant hypoglycemia, yet found no harm in maintaining BG levels <180 mg/dl.[45,75,76]

On the basis of these findings in observational and interventional studies, targeted BG management is recommended in surgical patients with and without diabetes or hyperglycemia in the perioperative period. Several guidelines have since been published to guide the management of hyperglycemia in the ICU and non-ICU setting (Table 35.2). Perhaps the most followed position statements are from the American Association of Clinical Endocrinologists/American Diabetes Association (AACE/ADA),[77] the Endocrine Society,[78] and the National Health Services

Table 35.2 Recommended Glycemic Goals Based on the Surgical Setting

Organization	Setting	Target BG range (md/dl)	Preprandial	Random
ADA/AACE, 2009	ICU	140–180 or 110–140*	—	≤180
	Non-ICU	100–140	100–140	≤180
NHS, 2011	ICU	108–180 but 72–216 is acceptable	—	<180
Endocrine Society, 2012	Non-ICU	100–140; <200 for special cases†	100–140	<180
CDA, 2013	ICU	144–180; 90–180 for minor and - moderate surgeries	—	<180
	Non-ICU	90–180	90–144	<180
ACP, 2013	ICU	140–200	—	<200

Note: ACP = American College of Physicians; ADA/AACE = American Diabetes Association and American Association for Clinical Endocrinologists; BG = blood glucose; CDA = Canadian Diabetes Association; ICU = intensive care unit; NHS = U.K. National Health Services.
*Surgical ICU, healthier patients, cardiovascular insults, total parenteral nutrition use, significant hyperglycemia in the first 24 hours of admission.
†Terminal illness, limited life expectancy, or recurrent hypoglycemia.
Sources: Moghissi ES, Korytkowski MT, DiNardo M, et al. American Association of Clinical Endocrinologists and American Diabetes Association consensus statement on inpatient glycemic control. *Diabetes Care* 2009;32:1119–1131; Dhatariya K, Levy N, Kilvert A, et al. NHS diabetes guideline for the perioperative management of the adult patient with diabetes. *Diabet Med* 2012;29:420–433; Umpierrez GE, Hellman R, Korytkowski MT, et al. Management of hyperglycemia in hospitalized patients in non-critical care setting: an Endocrine Society clinical practice guideline. *J Clin Endocrinol Metab* 2012;97:16–38; Houlden R, Capes S, Clement M, Miller D. Canadian Diabetes Association 2013 clinical practice guidelines for the prevention and management of diabetes in Canada: in-hospital diabetes management. *Can J Diabetes* 2013;37:S77–S81; Qaseem A, Chou R, Humphrey LL, Shekelle P; for the Clinical Guidelines Committee of the American College of Physicians. Inpatient glycemic control: best practice advice from the Clinical Guidelines Committee of the American College of Physicians. *Am J Med Qual* 2013. [Epub ahead of print http://ajm.sagepub.com/content/early/2013/06/06/1062860613489339]

(NHS).[79] Additionally, several recent guidelines have been published by the ADA,[80,81] Joint British Diabetes Societies (NHS),[10] and Canadian Diabetes Association[82] that specifically make recommendations for the perioperative management of patients with diabetes. Although each authoritative organization may have slightly different ranges or key recommendations particular to the patient population, they are similar and based on data from landmark studies and expert opinion. These clinical guidelines are useful because they allow medical staff and institutions to formalize treatment plans for patients with diabetes or hyperglycemia, define the process for point-of-care BG testing, outline monitoring for potential inpatient complications, stress the need for diabetes education, and help with the transition to the outpatient arena. The Planning Research in Inpatient Diabetes (PRIDE) consortium has been formed to fill in gaps of evidence for inpatient glucose management, and it is anticipated that the knowledge gained from this movement will shape future guidelines for perioperative diabetes management.[83]

Because diabetes, in addition to malnutrition, is a significant risk factor for surgical site infections and worse outcomes,[84] it is important to assess glycemic control and CV risk factors before admitting the patient for elective surgery. There are no randomized controlled trials or ample data to determine what the optimal A1C or BG level should be before surgery; however, NHS guidelines recommend that patients be referred to a diabetes specialist preoperatively if the A1C is >8.5% to optimize glycemic control before surgery.[10] Comorbidities that could affect outcomes, such as uncontrolled hypertension and malnutrition, should be addressed before surgery if possible. Before inpatient surgery, the Endocrine Society recommends the discontinuation of oral and noninsulin injectable antidiabetic agents and the initiation of scheduled insulin for patients with diabetes who develop hyperglycemia in the perioperative period.[78]

Despite controversy about just how aggressive glycemic control should be in the inpatient setting, it is widely accepted that a measure of BG control needs to be taken to improve perioperative outcomes for patients with diabetes and stress hyperglycemia.[13,85,86] The most recent joint position statement from the AACE/ADA[77] recommends intervention for any patient with a BG >180 mg/dl in the ICU and to maintain target glucose levels at 140–180 mg/dl. The guidelines further recommend tighter control of 110–140 mg/dl for patients who are younger, are healthier, have undergone surgery, or have had a CV procedure. The Society of Critical Care Medicine, however, recommends that insulin be initiated in the postoperative period when BG levels are ≥150 mg/dl, and in cases of trauma and CV surgery, the BG levels optimally should be maintained at <150 mg/dl.[87]

In the ICU setting, continuous insulin infusion (CII) is the preferred method for controlling hyperglycemia,[77] although guidelines from the Society for Critical Care Medicine outline that subcutaneous (SQ) insulin may be an alternative treatment for select ICU patients who do not have type 1 diabetes (T1D), hemodynamic instability, or wavering clinical status (hypothermia, edema, frequent interruption of dextrose intake).[87] Thus, for the surgical ICU population where altered PO status, volume shifts, and blood pressure fluctuations are common, the use of a CII would be preferred over SQ insulin for hyperglycemia management in this setting. Several CII protocols have been published, including the dynamic, static, and columnar algorithms or computer-guided algorithms, such as Glucommander, Glytec, or EndoTool that can be used to attain glycemic goals.[13,86,88]

There are no randomized controlled trials to determine which protocol may be best for surgical patients; however, institutionally accepted protocols that are followed are more effective and associated with fewer episodes of hypoglycemia.[89] When the patient is ready to have CII discontinued or transitioned to a hospital unit, SQ insulin should be administered 2–4 hours before discontinuation of the drip to avoid rebound hyperglycemia. The insulin rate during the last 4–6 hours of CII can be used to extrapolate the total daily insulin that will be given as SQ insulin. Although several authors have described how to calculate the total dose of insulin needed, it is customary that 75–80% of the daily CII dose be given as a basal and prandial insulin (rapid-acting vs. regular) doses, divided proportionally, based on the patient's insulin sensitivity, renal function, and ability to eat.[10,77] For patients without a previous history of diabetes who require >2 units/hour of CII, it is recommended that these individuals also be transitioned to a scheduled SQ regimen rather than SSI alone.[78]

In the non-ICU setting, it is recommended that preprandial BG levels be maintained at 100–140 mg/dl and random BG levels <180 mg/dl. A scheduled SQ insulin regimen is the preferred method for treatment of hyperglycemia in the non-ICU setting,[80,81] and oral antidiabetic agents should be discontinued in most cases, as they currently have limited roles in the inpatient setting mostly because of a lack of substantial data in this area, inability to titrate oral agents in response to glycemic excursions, potential postoperative nausea and appetite changes, unpredictable timing of meal delivery, variable diet status (e.g., NPO), and potential toxicities associated with oral agents (e.g., metformin and intravenous [IV] contrast). A recent pilot study, however, investigating the use of sitagliptin in general medicine and surgery patients with type 2 diabetes (T2D) was promising when it showed that treatment with sitagliptin alone or in combination with basal insulin is safe and effective for the management of hyperglycemia.[90]

A series of studies from Umpierrez et al. repeatedly has shown that a basal ± bolus regimen is superior to SSI alone,[74,91,92] and the ADA does not recommend the sole use of SSI based on these studies and several other supporting trials.[81] The recent Basal Plus trial, which included general surgical and medicine patients with T2D, evaluated the efficacy and safety of using insulin glargine plus rapid-acting, correctional dose insulin if needed for BG >140 mg/dl. The regimen proved to be just as effective as a true basal-bolus regimen without the advent of more hypoglycemia and the need for fewer injections.[92] The treatment algorithm outlined in Figure 35.1 from this randomized controlled trial can be used for non-ICU surgical patients in the inpatient setting and is predicated on whether or not the patient is able to eat. As long as BG levels are not low, the basal insulin can be increased by 10% for fasting blood glucose (FBG) levels 140–180 mg/dl and 20% if the FBG levels are >200 mg/dl. On the basis of the A1C, patients in this study were discharged to home on either their home regimen (A1C <7%), oral antidiabetic drugs (OADs) and basal insulin (A1C 7–9%), or basal-bolus insulin (>9%). This type of algorithmic approach may have long-term benefits, as a study by Wexler et al. found that inpatient diabetes management significantly improved glycemic control 1 year from time of discharge in patients who were newly placed on insulin.[93]

Perhaps one of the main factors limiting more proactive glycemic control in the hospital setting would be the association with an increased risk of hypoglycemia.[86,94] Previous studies have shown that the rate of severe hypoglycemia (<40

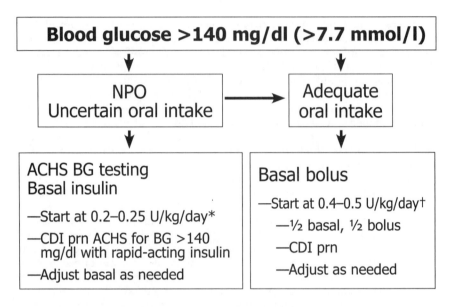

Figure 35.1— Basal plus insulin regimen approach in the non-ICU setting.
Note: ACHS = preprandial and bedtime; BG = blood glucose; CDI = correctional dose insulin; kg = kilogram; NPO = nothing by mouth; U = units.
*Reduce to 0.15 U/kg/day if age ≥70 years or creatinine ≥2.0 mg/dl
†Reduce to 0.3 U/kg/day if age ≥70 years or creatinine ≥2.0 mg/dl

mg/dl) in the ICU is 5–19%.[13,37,45,75,76] In the non-ICU setting, however, where hypoglycemia is defined as <70 or <60 mg/dl, the rates range from 5 to 33%.[74,91,95,96] Although most hypoglycemic events are mild and without significant clinical consequences,[97] in the cardiothoracic patient, hypoglycemia may result in excess catecholamine release that may aggravate myocardial ischemia or cause arrhythmias.[98,99] Additionally, it has been well documented that hypoglycemia can increase inflammation just as hyperglycemia does.[100] Risk assessment for more aggressive glycemic control in surgical patients must take into account the negative implications of hypoglycemic events and the potential benefits of wound healing and decreased postoperative complications. Continued staff education and the use of frequent BG monitoring facilitate early detection and treatment of hypoglycemic events.[5,86] Increased mortality has been identified with the development of spontaneous hypoglycemia and not with insulin-induced hypoglycemia.[101,102]

Most of the special considerations in the following section are reviewed in other chapters. The following provides an overview and options for the management of hyperglycemia in the surgical setting for certain clinical cases.

TYPE 1 DIABETES

The same ICU, non-ICU, and same-day surgery guidelines can be employed for the management of patients with T1D,[77,78,80] but some precautions should be taken in this patient population. Regardless of the type or length of surgery, insulin should never be stopped in patients with T1D as this could lead to severe hyperglycemia or diabetic ketoacidosis (DKA). The patient's home regimen and degree of adherence should be documented, and it should be recognized that insulin requirements can increase in cases of prolonged surgery (>60 minutes), infection, and glucocorticoid treatment. The NHS guidelines suggest that a CII and IV fluids be initiated in patients with T1D if the omission of more than one meal is expected.[10] As with any insulin drip, it is important to concomitantly infuse 5% glucose to avoid the risk of hypoglycemia or catabolism. Additionally, patients with T1D should be monitored closely for the development of ketosis and DKA and treated accordingly. Once the patient is ready to be transitioned from CII, the clinician should plan to provide overlap with long-acting SQ insulin at least 2–3 hours before discontinuing the insulin drip. If the patient is eating, they can receive prandial insulin, and the CII can be discontinued 1–2 hours afterward.[10,82] It should be stressed to the nursing and medical staff that basal insulin should never be stopped in patients with T1D, as this could lead to a glycemic crisis and worsen outcomes.

There are very few data on the use of continuous subcutaneous insulin infusions (CSII) in the management of people with diabetes undergoing surgery. Clinical scenarios in which a hemodynamically stable, surgical patient could remain on their basal CSII would be in the instance of a limited NPO period, knowledgeable medical staff, and adequate pump supplies (i.e., insertion needle, tubing). If more than one meal is to be missed, the insulin pump should be removed and CII should be used. For those postoperative patients who qualify to be on CSII and who are cleared to eat and are not cognitively impaired, prandial boluses should be resumed once the patient is eating and drinking normally and correctional dose insulin can be used as needed.[10]

STRESS HYPERGLYCEMIA

Stress hyperglycemia (defined as a BG >140 mg/dl) is common in the postsurgical setting and its prevalence depends on the type of surgery, length and complexity of the procedure, underlying comorbidities, and age of the patient.[29] For instance, the reported prevalence has been up to 34% in pancreatic surgery cases[103] and >80% in cardiothoracic surgery patients.[12] Furthermore, some studies have shown that patients who undergo laparoscopic procedures have fewer postoperative BG excursions compared with open surgeries.[104,105]

Similar to patients with diabetes, there have been extensive observational and prospective randomized controlled trials in critically ill patients without diabetes that indicate a strong association between hyperglycemia and poor clinical outcomes.[106] A large retrospective study in a community teaching hospital of >2,000 consecutively admitted patients found that subjects with newly diagnosed or stress hyperglycemia had increased hospital mortality (16 vs. 3%) and longer LOS (9.0 vs. 5.5 days) compared with patients with known diabetes. Additionally, these patients were more likely to require transitional or nursing home care.[9] In a meta-analysis of 32 studies, investigators found that patients with stress hyperglycemia in the setting of stroke had higher rates of mortality (unadjusted RR 3.07 vs. 1.30, respectively) and worse rates of functional recovery than those with known diabetes.[39] Another study found that patients who underwent CV procedures with BG values >200 mg/dl, irrespective of diabetes status, had higher mortality, more wound infections, and longer hospital stays.[35] Furthermore, a large retrospective analysis by Falciglia et al. including nearly 260,000 patients admitted to ICUs showed that the mortality risk was significantly greater at each quartile range of BG for patients without a history of diabetes.[107] The landmark Leuven studies[13,37] showed significant benefit for mortality and complication rates in surgical ICU and medical ICU populations consisting mostly of patients with stress hyperglycemia rather than preexisting diabetes. Thus, the management of hyperglycemia is also important in surgical patients without diabetes with stress hyperglycemia and the same published guidelines should be used.[77,78] In addition to initiating glycemic management in the inpatient setting, identifying patients with stress hyperglycemia and educating them is essential because it is estimated that one-third to two-thirds of these individuals will develop prediabetes or diabetes over time, with one study finding that 60% develop diabetes at 1 year of hospitalization.[108,109] An A1C should be done for all patients with stress hyperglycemia, especially because statistics show that up to one-third of patients, particularly in the U.S., actually will have undiagnosed diabetes (A1C ≥6.5%).[110] In fact, one study found that 24% of orthopedic patients in the hospital had unrecognized diabetes or impaired fasting glucose (IFG) and 64% with a FBG >100 mg/dl still had elevated BG levels at the time of outpatient follow-up. Perhaps more disconcerting is the fact that this study found that none of the patients with newly diagnosed diabetes or IFG had point-of-care testing or mention of hyperglycemia in the discharge summary.[111] Although the best time to reassess glycemic status is not well defined, authoritative organizations generally recommend that a hemoglobin A1C, FBG, or oral glucose tolerance test be done at 4–6 weeks following discharge from the hospital to determine whether the patient has prediabetes or diabetes.[10,77,78]

TOTAL PARENTERAL NUTRITION

It is estimated that >50% of patients who receive TPN and up to 30% who receive enteral feeds will experience hyperglycemia.[112] There are no randomized controlled trials to guide specific management of hyperglycemia in these populations; however, the AACE/ADA guidelines call for insulin treatment if the BG levels are >180 mg/dl for patients in the ICU setting and in the non-ICU setting. Furthermore, the Endocrine Society guidelines recommend that a scheduled SQ insulin regimen be given to any patient on TPN or tube feeds who has a persistent BG of >140 mg/dl. Several publications exist to guide the initiation of insulin for patients receiving specialized MNT,[113–116] and a straightforward, stepwise approach can be used as outlined in Figure 35.2.

BARIATRIC SURGERY

With the growing prevalence of obesity and limited responses to pharmaceutical agents and lifestyle intervention, bariatric surgery increasingly is considered as a treatment for patients with diabetes and significant obesity-related morbidity. Bariatric surgeries, particularly the Roux-en-Y and biliopancreatic diversion pro-

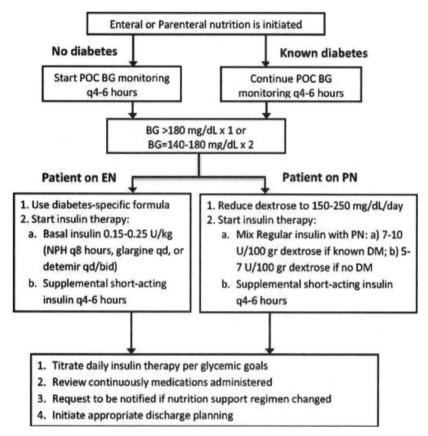

Figure 35.2—Algorithm for treating hyperglycemia in patients receiving enteral or parenteral nutrition.

Note: BG = blood glucose; DM = diabetes mellitus; EN = enternal nutrition; PN = parenteral nutrition; POC = point-of-care; U = units.

Source: Gosmanov AR, Umpierrez GE. Management of hyperglycemia during enteral and parenteral nutrition therapy. *Curr Diabetes Rep* 2013;13:155–162. Reprinted with permission from the publisher.

cedures, are unique from other surgeries in that glycemic control significantly improves immediately after surgery in the vast majority of patients and 75–95% of patients remain in near-normoglycemic remission for 2 years following the surgery.[117,118] Because of strict limitations of oral intake and calories and the immediate enhancement of incretin and adipokine pathways, the majority of gastric bypass patients with T2D require little to no insulin in the postoperative period.

Outside of the updated 2013 published practice guidelines,[119] there are no randomized controlled trials or consensus statements to specify the management of BG levels in the postoperative setting following bariatric procedures. Until more formal guidelines are released, clinicians can follow the current ICU and non-ICU diabetes guidelines (as mentioned), specify MNT, and reconcile the patient's preoperative diabetes regimen before discharge.[120]

OUTPATIENT SURGERY: TREATMENT OPTIONS AND CONCERNS

In the U.S., >60% of elective surgeries are performed in the outpatient setting, and it is estimated that this number will increase by another 15% over the next few years.[121] There are not well-defined, evidence-based guidelines for management of diabetes for patients undergoing outpatient or day surgery. The NHS guidelines, however, outline the following steps to ensure that diabetes is assessed and is part of the comprehensive care plan.[10]

1. Have a system in place to preoperatively identify patients with suboptimal diabetes control.
2. Have protocols in place for day surgeries to avoid unnecessary admissions.
3. Prioritize patients with diabetes on the procedure log.
4. Identify patients who will require an extended period of being NPO and provide them with written information on diabetes management at time of discharge.
5. Avoid evening procedures for patients with diabetes to minimize the period of being NPO, the use of a CSII, and unnecessary admission for observation.

The Society for Ambulatory Anesthesia (SAA) also published a consensus statement for patients with diabetes undergoing outpatient surgery.[122] Using the Cochrane Library database (January 1980–November 2009), the expert panel used the GRADE system (Grading of Recommendations, Assessment, Development, and Evaluation) to address particular clinical considerations. The society underscores the fact that evidence is insufficient regarding preoperative management of oral antidiabetic agents and insulin. The SAA has recommended that oral antidiabetics and noninsulin injectables should not be taken on the day of surgery until normal food intake is resumed. This is in contrast to the U.K. NHS guidelines, which give specific recommendations on adjustments for antidiabetic medications (Tables 35.3 and 35.4) and state that oral antidiabetic agents can be taken if only one meal will be missed on the day of surgery. In general, patients who are on insulin before surgery should continue to take their prescribed doses on the day before surgery; however, some experts suggest that basal insulin should be reduced by a third if the patient with diabetes tends to eat throughout the day or reports that the BG decreases >36 mg/dl overnight *and* is scheduled for an early morning surgery. This practice of reducing the basal dose of insulin is controversial, and only one retrospective study has shown that the usual basal insulin dose is well tolerated.[123] Adjustments can be made as suggested in Table 35.4 for patients who are on premixed or prandial insulins.[10] Until more data are published to guide the direction of perioperative hyperglycemia management in the outpatient setting, maintain BG levels at <180 with a goal of 140–180 mg/dl during the immediate perioperative period and resume the ADA outpatient guidelines

Table 35.3 Guideline for Perioperative Adjustment of Insulin (no more than *one* missed meal)

Insulin	Day prior to admission	Day of surgery Patient for AM surgery	Patient for PM surgery
Once daily evening (e.g., insulin glargine, insulin detemir, insulin degludec, NPH)	No dose change*	Check BG on admission	Check BG on admission
Once daily morning (e.g., insulin glargine, insulin detemir, insulin degludec, NPH)	No dose change	No dose change* Check BG on admission	No dose change* Check BG on admission
Twice daily (e.g., premixed insulin 70/30, 75/25, or 50/50, twice daily glargine, detemir or NPH)	No dose change	Halve the usual AM dose Check BG on admission Leave the evening meal dose unchanged	Halve the usual AM dose Check BG on admission Leave the evening meal dose unchanged
Twice daily–separate injections of short-acting (e.g., insulin lispro, insulin aspart, insulin glulisine, regular insulin) **and intermediate-acting** (e.g., NPH or insulin iso-phane)	No dose change	Calculate the total dose of both AM insulins and give half as intermedi-ate-acting only in the AM Check BG on admission Leave the evening meal dose unchanged	Calculate the total dose of both AM insu-lins and give half as intermediate-acting only in the AM Check BG on admission Leave the evening meal dose unchanged
3, 4, or 5 injections daily	No dose change	**Basal bolus regimens:** Omit the AM and lunch-time short-acting insu-lins Keep the basal unchanged* **Premixed AM insulin:** Halve the AM dose and omit lunchtime dose Check BG on admission	Take usual AM insulin dose(s) Omit lunchtime dose Check BG on admission

Note: BG = blood glucose; NPH = neutral protamine Hagedorn; AM = morning; PM = afternoon.
*Can consider reducing the usual dose of long-acting analog by a third. This reduction should be considered for any patient who eats throughout the day.

Source: Modified from Dhatariya K, Levy N, Kilvert A, et al. NHS diabetes guideline for the perioperative management of the adult patient with diabetes. *Diabet Med* 2012;29: 420–433.

Table 35.4 Guideline for Perioperative Adjustment of Oral Antidiabetic Agents and Noninsulin Injectables (no more than *one* missed meal)

Medication class	Day prior to admission	Day of surgery	
		Patient for AM surgery	Patient for PM surgery
Biguanide*	Take as normal	Take as normal	Take as normal
Sulfonylurea	Take as normal	Once daily AM, omit twice daily, omit AM	Once daily AM, omit twice daily, omit AM and PM
Meglitinide	Take as normal	Omit AM dose if NPO	Give AM dose if eating
DPP-IV inhibitor	Take as normal	Omit on day of surgery	Omit on day of surgery
Thiazolidinedione	Take as normal	Take as normal	Take as normal
α-Glucosidase inhibitor	Take as normal	Omit AM dose if NPO	Give AM dose if eating
SGLT-2 inhibitor	Take as normal	Omit on day of surgery	Omit on day of surgery
GLP-1 analog	Take as normal	Omit on day of surgery	Omit on day of surgery

Note: AM = morning; DPP-IV = dipeptidyl peptidase-IV; GLP-1 = glucagon-like peptide-1; NPO = nothing by mouth; PM = afternoon; SGLT-2 = sodium-glucose cotransporter-2.
*If contrast medium is to be used and glomerular filtration rate is <50 ml/minute/1.73m^2, metformin should be omitted on the day of the procedure and for the following 48 hours.

Source: Modified from Dhatariya K, Levy N, Kilvert A, et al. NHS diabetes guideline for the perioperative management of the adult patient with diabetes. *Diabet Med* 2012;29:420–433.

(premeal BG 70–130 mg/dl, postprandial <180 mg/dl) within 1 week of surgery, per the current AACE/ADA guidelines.[77,80,81] Although no evidence indicates the best insulin formulation for hyperglycemia management in ambulatory surgical patients with diabetes, SQ SSI continues to be the mainstay for most patients. For surgeries that require >1 hour of anesthesia or where more than one meal will be missed, the medical team may want to consider using an intraoperative insulin drip to maintain glycemic control and a CII in the postoperative period, if needed (BG >180 mg/dl). Patients with T1D will require basal insulin or a CII during the procedure and requirements may vary significantly from those for patients with T2D. Omission or underdosing of insulin in this population can lead quickly to severe glycemic crises and poor outcomes.

Based on the type of surgery, preceding glycemic control (A1C), degree of insulin needs in the postoperative period, and patient's ability to eat, a good outpatient regimen and follow-up plan can be formulated before discharge from the surgical center. Note, however, that 1–11% of ambulatory surgical patients have to be admitted to the hospital following procedures,[124] with one study indicating that surgery duration of ≥60 minutes is the most important predictor of unanticipated admission.[125] In the case of admission, the inpatient guidelines as previously outlined should be followed.

CONCLUSION

Studies have provided evidence that inpatient hyperglycemia in surgical patients is associated with worsened outcomes and that improved glycemic control can result in better clinical outcomes and reduce mortality in certain clinical scenarios. It is not clear, however, what the absolute glucose target cutoffs should be to achieve the maximal clinical benefit and at the same time avoid increased risk of hypoglycemia. CII is the preferred regimen for critically ill patients in the ICU and scheduled SQ administration with a basal-bolus regimen with correctional insulin is the preferred method for achieving glycemic control in the non-ICU setting.[126] Oral antidiabetic agents typically are not appropriate for most hospitalized surgical patients; however, more data will be forthcoming to address the potential role of these treatments. In addition to adequate control of glucose in the hospital or in the outpatient surgical suite, it is imperative that a discharge plan is formulated early during the hospital course that includes patient education and postoperative expectations, medication reconciliation, glycemic goals, and adequate follow-up.

Several guidelines and position statements offer medical institutions evidence-based guidelines for the management of inpatient hyperglycemia in both the ICU and non-ICU settings.[126] More research is needed, however, to further delineate the patient populations that would benefit most from more aggressive control, which treatment regimens are the safest and most effective, and what the optimal treatment would be for patients undergoing outpatient procedures. Additionally, current research projects will address whether supplementation with glutamine will enhance the metabolic response to glucose control and whether there is benefit for using an artificial pancreas intraoperatively.

REFERENCES

1. Cullen KA, Hall MJ, Golosinskiy A. Ambulatory surgery in the United States, 2006. *National Health Statistics Reports* 2009:1–25.

2. Centers for Disease Control and Prevention. National Hospital Discharge Survey, 2010. Available at http://www.cdc.gov/nchs/fastats/insurg.htm. Accessed October 2013.

3. Hirsch IB, McGill JB, Cryer PE, White PF. Perioperative management of surgical patients with diabetes mellitus. *Anesthesiology* 1991;74:346–359.

4. Clement S, Braithwaite SS, Magee MF, et al. Management of diabetes and hyperglycemia in hospitals. *Diabetes Care* 2004;27:553–591.

5. Smiley D, Umpierrez GE. Perioperative glucose control in the diabetic or nondiabetic patient. *South Med J* 2006;99:580–589; quiz 90–91.

6. Frisch A, Chandra P, Smiley D, et al. Prevalence and clinical outcome of hyperglycemia in the perioperative period in noncardiac surgery. *Diabetes Care* 2010;33:1783–1788.

7. Pomposelli JJ, Baxter JK 3rd, Babineau TJ, et al. Early postoperative glucose control predicts nosocomial infection rate in diabetic patients. *JPEN* 1998;22:77–81.

8. Noordzij PG, Boersma E, Schreiner F, et al. Increased preoperative glucose levels are associated with perioperative mortality in patients undergoing noncardiac, nonvascular surgery. *Eur J Endocrinol* 2007;156:137–142.

9. Umpierrez GE, Isaacs SD, Bazargan N, You X, Thaler LM, Kitabchi AE. Hyperglycemia: an independent marker of in-hospital mortality in patients with undiagnosed diabetes. *J Clin Endocrinol Metab* 2002;87:978–982.

10. Dhatariya K, Levy N, Kilvert A, et al. NHS diabetes guideline for the perioperative management of the adult patient with diabetes. *Diabet Med* 2012;29:420–433.

11. Health and Social Care Information Centre. National Diabetes Inpatient Audit 2012. Available at http://www.hscic.gov.uk/catalogue/PUB10506. Accessed November 2013.

12. Schmeltz LR, DeSantis AJ, Thiyagarajan V, et al. Reduction of surgical mortality and morbidity in diabetic patients undergoing cardiac surgery with a combined intravenous and subcutaneous insulin glucose management strategy. *Diabetes Care* 2007;30:823–828.

13. Van den Berghe G, Wouters P, Weekers F, et al. Intensive insulin therapy in critically ill patients. *N Engl J Med* 2001;345:1359–1367.

14. Levetan CS, Passaro M, Jablonski K, Kass M, Ratner RE. Unrecognized diabetes among hospitalized patients. *Diabetes Care* 1998;21:246–249.

15. Dagogo-Jack S, Alberti KG. Management of diabetes mellitus in surgical patients. *Diabetes Spectrum* 2002;15:44–48.

16. Sadhu AR, Ang AC, Ingram-Drake LA, Martinez DS, Hsueh WA, Ettner SL. Economic benefits of intensive insulin therapy in critically Ill patients: the Targeted Insulin Therapy to Improve Hospital Outcomes (TRIUMPH) project. *Diabetes Care* 2008;31:1556–1561.

17. Krinsley JS, Jones RL. Cost analysis of intensive glycemic control in critically ill adult patients. *Chest* 2006;129:644–650.

18. Van den Berghe G, Wouters PJ, Kesteloot K, Hilleman DE. Analysis of healthcare resource utilization with intensive insulin therapy in critically ill patients. *Crit Care Med* 2006;34:612–616.

19. American Diabetes Association. Economic costs of diabetes in the U.S. in 2012. *Diabetes Care* 2013;36:1033–1046.

20. Carral F, Olveira G, Salas J, Garcia L, Sillero A, Aguilar M. Care resource utilization and direct costs incurred by people with diabetes in a Spanish hospital. *Diabetes Res Clin Pract* 2002;56:27–34.

21. Walker M, Marshall SM, Alberti KG. Clinical aspects of diabetic ketoacidosis. *Diabetes Metab Rev* 1989;5:651–663.

22. Brenner WI, Lansky Z, Engelman RM, Stahl WM. Hyperosomolar coma in surgical patients: an iatrogenic disease of increasing incidence. *Ann Surg* 1973;178:651–654.

23. Seki S. Clinical features of hyperosmolar hyperglycemic nonketotic diabetic coma associated with cardiac operations. *J Thorac Cardiovasc Surg* 1986; 91:867–873.

24. Furnary AP, Zerr KJ, Grunkemeier GL, Starr A. Continuous intravenous insulin infusion reduces the incidence of deep sternal wound infection in diabetic patients after cardiac surgical procedures. *Ann Thorac Surg* 1999;67:352–360; discussion 60-62.

25. Alexiewicz JM, Kumar D, Smogorzewski M, Klin M, Massry SG. Polymorphonuclear leukocytes in non-insulin-dependent diabetes mellitus: abnormalities in metabolism and function. *Ann Intern Med* 1995;123:919–24.

26. Rassias AJ, Marrin CA, Arruda J, Whalen PK, Beach M, Yeager MP. Insulin infusion improves neutrophil function in diabetic cardiac surgery patients. *Anesth Analg* 1999;88:1011–1016.

27. Geerlings SE, Hoepelman AI. Immune dysfunction in patients with diabetes mellitus (DM). *FEMS Immunol Med Microbiol* 1999;26:259–265.

28. Tamai D, Awad AA, Chaudhry HJ, Shelley KH. Optimizing the medical management of diabetic patients undergoing surgery. *Conn Med* 2006;70:621–630.

29. McCowen KC, Malhotra A, Bistrian BR. Stress-induced hyperglycemia. *Crit Care Clin* 2001;17:107–124.

30. Rayfield EJ, Ault MJ, Keusch GT, Brothers MJ, Nechemias C, Smith H. Infection and diabetes: the case for glucose control. *Am J Med* 1982;72:439–450.

31. Giugliano D, Marfella R, Coppola L, et al. Vascular effects of acute hyperglycemia in humans are reversed by L-arginine. Evidence for reduced availability of nitric oxide during hyperglycemia. *Circulation* 1997;95:1783–1790.

32. Montori VM, Bistrian BR, McMahon MM. Hyperglycemia in acutely ill patients. *JAMA* 2002;288:2167–2169.

33. Dandona P. Endothelium, inflammation, and diabetes. *Curr Diabetes Rep* 2002;2:311–315.

34. Booth G, Stalker TJ, Lefer AM, Scalia R. Elevated ambient glucose induces acute inflammatory events in the microvasculature: effects of insulin. *Am J Physiol Endocrinol Metab* 2001;280:E848–E856.

35. Van den Berghe G, Wouters PJ, Bouillon R, et al. Outcome benefit of intensive insulin therapy in the critically ill: Insulin dose versus glycemic control. *Crit Care Med* 2003;31:359–366.

36. Finney SJ, Zekveld C, Elia A, Evans TW. Glucose control and mortality in critically ill patients. *JAMA* 2003;290:2041–2047.

37. Van den Berghe G, Wilmer A, Hermans G, et al. Intensive insulin therapy in the medical ICU. *N Engl J Med* 2006;354:449–461.

38. Malmberg K, Ryden L, Efendic S, et al. Randomized trial of insulin-glucose infusion followed by subcutaneous insulin treatment in diabetic patients with acute myocardial infarction (DIGAMI study): effects on mortality at 1 year. *J Am Coll Cardiol* 1995;26:57–65.

39. Capes SE, Hunt D, Malmberg K, Pathak P, Gerstein HC. Stress hyperglycemia and prognosis of stroke in nondiabetic and diabetic patients: a systematic overview. *Stroke* 2001;32:2426–2432.

40. Edelson GW, Fachnie JD, Whitehouse FW. Perioperative management of diabetes. *Henry Ford Hosp Med J* 1990;38:262–265.

41. Rayman G. Inpatient audit. *Diabetes Update* 2010:18.

42. Malouf R, Brust JC. Hypoglycemia: causes, neurological manifestations, and outcome. *Ann Neurol* 1985;17:421–430.

43. Unger RH. Nocturnal hypoglycemia in aggressively controlled diabetes. *N Engl J Med* 1982;306:1294.

44. Ben-Ami H, Nagachandran P, Mendelson A, Edoute Y. Drug-induced hypoglycemic coma in 102 diabetic patients. *Arch Intern Med* 1999;159:281–284.

45. Investigators N-SS, Finfer S, Chittock DR, et al. Intensive versus conventional glucose control in critically ill patients. *N Engl J Med* 2009;360:1283–1297.

46. Griesdale DE, de Souza RJ, van Dam RM, et al. Intensive insulin therapy and mortality among critically ill patients: a meta-analysis including NICE-SUGAR study data. *CMAJ* 2009;180:821–827.

47. Buchleitner AM, Martinez-Alonso M, Hernandez M, Sola I, Mauricio D. Perioperative glycaemic control for diabetic patients undergoing surgery. *Cochrane Reviews* 2012;9:CD007315.

48. Madsen SN, Engguist A, Badawi I, Kehlet H. Cyclic AMP, glucose and cortisol in plasma during surgery. *Horm Metab Res* 1976;8:483–485.

49. Lang CH, Dobrescu C, Bagby GJ. Tumor necrosis factor impairs insulin action on peripheral glucose disposal and hepatic glucose output. *Endocrinology* 1992;130:43–52.

50. Hotamisligil GS, Murray DL, Choy LN, Spiegelman BM. Tumor necrosis factor alpha inhibits signaling from the insulin receptor. *Proc Natl Acad Sci U S A* 1994;91:4854–4858.

51. Coursin DB, Connery LE, Ketzler JT. Perioperative diabetic and hyperglycemic management issues. *Crit Care Med* 2004;32:S116–S125.

52. Hirsch IB, McGill JB. Role of insulin in management of surgical patients with diabetes mellitus. *Diabetes Care* 1990;13:980–991.

53. Rehman HU, Mohammed K. Perioperative management of diabetic patients. *Curr Surg* 2003;60:607–611.

54. Umpierrez GE, Kitabchi AE. ICU care for patients with diabetes. *Curr Opinions Endocrinol* 2004;11:75–81.

55. Halter JB, Pflug AE. Relationship of impaired insulin secretion during surgical stress to anesthesia and catecholamine release. *J Clin Endocrinol Metab* 1980;51:1093–1098.

56. Clutter WE, Rizza RA, Gerich JE, Cryer PE. Regulation of glucose metabolism by sympathochromaffin catecholamines. *Diabetes Metab Rev* 1988;4:1–15.

57. McMahon M, Gerich J, Rizza R. Effects of glucocorticoids on carbohydrate metabolism. *Diabetes Metab Rev* 1988;4:17–30.

58. Metchick LN, Petit WA, Jr., Inzucchi SE. Inpatient management of diabetes mellitus. *Am J Med* 2002;113:317–323.

59. Stentz FB, Umpierrez GE, Cuervo R, Kitabchi AE. Proinflammatory cytokines, markers of cardiovascular risks, oxidative stress, and lipid peroxidation in patients with hyperglycemic crises. *Diabetes* 2004;53:2079–2086.

60. del Aguila LF, Claffey KP, Kirwan JP. TNF-alpha impairs insulin signaling and insulin stimulation of glucose uptake in C2C12 muscle cells. *Am J Physiol* 1999;276:E849–E855.

61. Scherpereel PA, Tavernier B. Perioperative care of diabetic patients. *Eur J Anaesthesiol* 2001;18:277–294.

62. Pflug AE, Halter JB. Effect of spinal anesthesia on adrenergic tone and the neuroendocrine responses to surgical stress in humans. *Anesthesiology* 1981;55:120–126.

63. Hikasa Y, Kawanabe H, Takase K, Ogasawara S. Comparisons of sevoflurane, isoflurane, and halothane anesthesia in spontaneously breathing cats. *Vet Surg* 1996;25:234–243.

64. Desborough JP, Jones PM, Persaud SJ, Landon MJ, Howell SL. Isoflurane inhibits insulin secretion from isolated rat pancreatic islets of Langerhans. *Br J Anaesth* 1993;71:873–876.

65. Lattermann R, Schricker T, Wachter U, Georgieff M, Goertz A. Understanding the mechanisms by which isoflurane modifies the hyperglycemic response to surgery. *Anesth Analg* 2001;93:121–127.

66. Brandt MR, Kehlet H, Faber O, Binder C. C-peptide and insulin during blockade of the hyperglycaemic response to surgery by epidural analgesia. *Clin Endocrinol* 1977;6:167–170.

67. Wolf AR, Eyres RL, Laussen PC, et al. Effect of extradural analgesia on stress responses to abdominal surgery in infants. *Br J Anaesth* 1993;70:654–660.

68. Clarke RS. The hyperglycaemic response to different types of surgery and anaesthesia. *Br J Anaesth* 1970;42:45–53.

69. Weddell AG, Gale HED. Changes in the blood-sugar level associated with surgical operations. *Br J Surg* 1934;22:80–87.

70. Cresci G. Targeting the use of specialized nutritional formulas in surgery and critical care. *JPEN* 2005;29:S92–S95.

71. Heyland DK, Montalvo M, MacDonald S, Keefe L, Su XY, Drover JW. Total parenteral nutrition in the surgical patient: a meta-analysis. *Can J Surg* 2001;44:102–111.

72. Furnary AP, Gao G, Grunkemeier GL, et al. Continuous insulin infusion reduces mortality in patients with diabetes undergoing coronary artery bypass grafting. *J Thorac Cardiovasc Surg* 2003;125:1007–1021.

73. Lazar HL, Chipkin SR, Fitzgerald CA, Bao Y, Cabral H, Apstein CS. Tight glycemic control in diabetic coronary artery bypass graft patients improves perioperative outcomes and decreases recurrent ischemic events. *Circulation* 2004;109:1497–1502.

74. Umpierrez GE, Smiley D, Jacobs S, et al. Randomized study of basal-bolus insulin therapy in the inpatient management of patients with type 2 diabetes undergoing general surgery (RABBIT 2 surgery). *Diabetes Care* 2011;34:256–261.

75. Brunkhorst FM, Engel C, Bloos F, et al. Intensive insulin therapy and pentastarch resuscitation in severe sepsis. *N Engl J Med* 2008;358:125–139.

76. Preiser JC, Devos P, Ruiz-Santana S, et al. A prospective randomised multicentre controlled trial on tight glucose control by intensive insulin therapy in adult intensive care units: the Glucontrol study. *Intensive Care Med* 2009;35:1738–1748.

77. Moghissi ES, Korytkowski MT, DiNardo M, et al. American Association of Clinical Endocrinologists and American Diabetes Association consensus statement on inpatient glycemic control. *Diabetes Care* 2009;32:1119–1131.

78. Umpierrez GE, Hellman R, Korytkowski MT, et al. Management of hyperglycemia in hospitalized patients in non-critical care setting: an Endocrine Society clinical practice guideline. *J Clin Endocrinol Metab* 2012;97:16–38.

79. Diabetes UK. Inpatient care for people with diabetes. Macleod House, June 2013. Available at http://www.diabetes.org.uk/Documents/Position%20 statements/diabetes-uk-position-statement-inpatient-care-0613.pdf. Accessed September 2013.

80. American Diabetes Association. Standards of medical care in diabetes—2013. *Diabetes Care* 2013;36(Suppl 1):S11–S66.

81. American Diabetes Association. Standards of medical care in diabetes—2014. *Diabetes Care* 2014;37(Suppl 1):S14-S80.

82. Canadian Diabetes Association Clinical Practice Guidelines Expert Committee of the Canadian Diabetes Advisory Board. Canadian Diabetes Association 2013 clinical practice guidelines for the prevention and management of diabetes in Canada. *Can J Diabetes* 2013;37:S1–S212.

83. Draznin B, Gilden J, Golden SH, et al. Pathways to quality inpatient management of hyperglycemia and diabetes: a call to action. *Diabetes Care* 2013;36:1807–1814.

84. Malone DL, Genuit T, Tracy JK, Gannon C, Napolitano LM. Surgical site infections: reanalysis of risk factors. *J Surg Res* 2002;103:89–95.

85. Trence DL, Kelly JL, Hirsch IB. The rationale and management of hyperglycemia for in-patients with cardiovascular disease: time for change. *J Clin Endocrinol Metab* 2003;88:2430–2437.

86. Goldberg PA, Siegel MD, Sherwin RS, et al. Implementation of a safe and effective insulin infusion protocol in a medical intensive care unit. *Diabetes Care* 2004;27:461–467.

87. Jacobi J, Bircher N, Krinsley J, et al. Guidelines for the use of an insulin infusion for the management of hyperglycemia in critically ill patients. *Crit Care Med* 2012;40:3251–3276.

88. Davidson PC, Steed RD, Bode BW. Glucommander: a computer-directed intravenous insulin system shown to be safe, simple, and effective in 120,618 h of operation. *Diabetes Care* 2005;28:2418–2423.

89. Cobaugh DJ, Maynard G, Cooper L, et al. Enhancing insulin-use safety in hospitals: practical recommendations from an ASHP Foundation expert consensus panel. *AJHP* 2013;70:1404–1413.

90. Umpierrez GE, Gianchandani R, Smiley D, et al. Safety and efficacy of sitagliptin therapy for the inpatient management of general medicine and surgery patients with type 2 diabetes: a pilot, randomized, controlled study. *Diabetes Care* 2013;36:3430–3435.

91. Umpierrez GE, Smiley D, Zisman A, et al. Randomized study of basal-bolus insulin therapy in the inpatient management of patients with type 2 diabetes (RABBIT 2 trial). *Diabetes Care* 2007;30:2181–2186.

92. Umpierrez GE, Smiley D, Hermayer K, et al. Randomized study comparing a basal-bolus with a basal plus correction insulin regimen for the hospital management of medical and surgical patients with type 2 diabetes: Basal Plus trial. *Diabetes Care* 2013;36:2169–2174.

93. Wexler DJ, Beauharnais CC, Regan S, Nathan DM, Cagliero E, Larkin ME. Impact of inpatient diabetes management, education, and improved discharge transition on glycemic control 12 months after discharge. *Diabetes Res Clin Pract* 2012;98:249–256.

94. Kagansky N, Levy S, Rimon E, et al. Hypoglycemia as a predictor of mortality in hospitalized elderly patients. *Arch Intern Med* 2003;163:1825–1829.

95. Umpierrez GE, Hor T, Smiley D, et al. Comparison of inpatient insulin regimens with detemir plus aspart versus neutral protamine hagedorn plus regular in medical patients with type 2 diabetes. *J Clin Endocrinol Metab* 2009;94:564–569.

96. Queale WS, Seidler AJ, Brancati FL. Glycemic control and sliding scale insulin use in medical inpatients with diabetes mellitus. *Arch Intern Med* 1997;157:545–552.

97. Bode BW, Braithwaite SS, Steed RD, Davidson PC. Intravenous insulin infusion therapy: indications, methods, and transition to subcutaneous insulin therapy. *Endocrine Pract* 2004;10(Suppl 2):71–80.

98. Desouza C, Salazar H, Cheong B, Murgo J, Fonseca V. Association of hypoglycemia and cardiac ischemia: a study based on continuous monitoring. *Diabetes Care* 2003;26:1485–1489.

99. Robinson RT, Harris ND, Ireland RH, Lindholm A, Heller SR. Comparative effect of human soluble insulin and insulin aspart upon hypoglycaemia-induced alterations in cardiac repolarization. *Br J Clin Pharmacol* 2003;55:246–251.

100. Razavi Nematollahi L, Kitabchi AE, Stentz FB, et al. Proinflammatory cytokines in response to insulin-induced hypoglycemic stress in healthy subjects. *Metabolism* 2009;58:443–448.

101. Boucai L, Southern WN, Zonszein J. Hypoglycemia-associated mortality is not drug-associated but linked to comorbidities. *Am J Med* 2011;124:1028–1035.

102. Kosiborod M, Inzucchi SE, Goyal A, et al. Relationship between spontaneous and iatrogenic hypoglycemia and mortality in patients hospitalized with acute myocardial infarction. *JAMA* 2009;301:1556–1564.

103. Shi Z, Tang S, Chen Y, et al. Prevalence of stress hyperglycemia among hepatopancreatobiliary postoperative patients. *Int J Clin Exp Med* 2013;6:799–803.

104. Engin A, Bozkurt BS, Ersoy E, Oguz M, Gokcora N. Stress hyperglycemia in minimally invasive surgery. *Surg Laparosc Endosc* 1998;8:435–437.

105. Nguyen NT, Goldman CD, Ho HS, Gosselin RC, Singh A, Wolfe BM. Systemic stress response after laparoscopic and open gastric bypass. *J Am Coll Surg* 2002;194:557–566; discussion 66–67.

106. McDonnell ME, Umpierrez GE. Insulin therapy for the management of hyperglycemia in hospitalized patients. *Endocrinol Metab Clin* 2012;41:175–201.

107. Falciglia M, Freyberg RW, Almenoff PL, D'Alessio DA, Render ML. Hyperglycemia-related mortality in critically ill patients varies with admission diagnosis. *Crit Care Med* 2009;37:3001–3009.

108. Greci LS, Kailasam M, Malkani S, et al. Utility of HbA(1c) levels for diabetes case finding in hospitalized patients with hyperglycemia. *Diabetes Care* 2003;26:1064–1068.

109. Dungan KM, Braithwaite SS, Preiser JC. Stress hyperglycaemia. *Lancet* 2009;373:1798–1807.

110. Centers for Disease Control and Prevention. National Diabetes Fact Sheet: General Information and National Estimates on Diabetes in the United States, 2011. Atlanta, Department of Health and Human Services, Centers for Disease Control and Prevention, 2011.

111. Sheehy AM, Benca J, Glinberg SL, et al. Preoperative "NPO" as an opportunity for diabetes screening. *J Hosp Med* 2012;7:611–616.

112. Gosmanov AR, Umpierrez GE. Medical nutrition therapy in hospitalized patients with diabetes. *Curr Diabetes Rep* 2012;12:93–100.

113. McClave SA, Martindale RG, Vanek VW, et al. Guidelines for the provision and assessment of nutrition support therapy in the adult critically ill patient: Society of Critical Care Medicine (SCCM) and American Society for Parenteral and Enteral Nutrition (A.S.P.E.N.). *JPEN* 2009;33:277–316.

114. Singer P, Berger MM, Van den Berghe G, et al. ESPEN guidelines on parenteral nutrition: intensive care. *Clin Nutr* 2009;28:387–400.

115. Bankhead R, Boullata J, Brantley S, et al. Enteral nutrition practice recommendations. *JPEN* 2009;33:122–167.

116. Gosmanov AR, Umpierrez GE. Management of hyperglycemia during enteral and parenteral nutrition therapy. *Curr Diabetes Rep* 2013;13:155–162.

117. Mingrone G, Panunzi S, De Gaetano A, et al. Bariatric surgery versus conventional medical therapy for type 2 diabetes. *N Engl J Med* 2012;366:1577–1585.

118. Buchwald H, Estok R, Fahrbach K, et al. Weight and type 2 diabetes after bariatric surgery: systematic review and meta-analysis. *Am J Med* 2009;122:248–256 e5.

119. Mechanick JI, Youdim A, Jones DB, et al. Clinical practice guidelines for the perioperative nutritional, metabolic, and nonsurgical support of the bariatric surgery patient—2013 update: cosponsored by American Association of Clinical Endocrinologists, the Obesity Society, and American Society for Metabolic and Bariatric Surgery. *Obesity* 2013;21(Suppl 1):S1–S27.

120. Schlienger JL, Pradignac A, Luca F, Meyer L, Rohr S. Medical management of diabetes after bariatric surgery. *Diabetes Metab* 2009;35:558–561.

121. Peng L, Norris E. Outpatient surgery. Available at http://www.emedicinehealth.com/outpatient_surgery/page13_em.htm. Accessed October 2013.

122. Joshi GP, Chung F, Vann MA, et al. Society for Ambulatory Anesthesia consensus statement on perioperative blood glucose management in diabetic patients undergoing ambulatory surgery. *Anesth Analg* 2010;111:1378–1387.

123. Modi A, Lipp A, Dhatariya K. An audit of a new diabetic management regime suitable for day and short stay surgery. *Journal of One-Day Surgery* 2009;19:A2.

124. Morales R, Esteve N, Casas I, Blanco C. Why are ambulatory surgical patients admitted to hospital?: Prospective study. *Ambulatory Surgery* 2002;9:197–205.

125. Mingus ML, Bodian CA, Bradford CN, Eisenkraft JB. Prolonged surgery increases the likelihood of admission of scheduled ambulatory surgery patients. *J Clin Anesth* 1997;9:446–450.

126. Smiley D, Umpierrez GE. Management of hyperglycemia in hospitalized patients. *Ann N Y Acad Sci* 2010;1212:1–11.

ACKNOWLEDGMENTS

Dr. Dawn Smiley is supported in part by research grants from the NIH-NIDDK (K08-DK-083036-01A1), Merck, Sanofi Aventis, and Abbott Nutrition.

Chapter 36

Post-Transplant Diabetes: Diagnosis, Consequences, and Management

Brian Boerner, MD
Vijay Shivaswamy, MD
Jennifer Larsen, MD

INTRODUCTION

Improved graft and patient survival has led to an increasing number of transplant recipients who require long-term care. Preexisting diabetes can contribute to the need for transplant, such as kidney, heart, or pancreas. In others, diabetes can develop after transplant. This type of diabetes has been called new-onset diabetes after transplantation (NODAT) but is now designated as post-transplant diabetes (PTDM) by the International Consensus panel as well as many U.S. transplant groups. Many transplant candidates do not receive optimal screening for diabetes. Thus, diabetes diagnosed after transplant may not be new-onset, but represents previously unrecognized or undiagnosed diabetes in some. This chapter reviews the criteria for diagnosis, contributing causes, and the impact of PTDM on other transplant outcomes. It also describes how the transplant setting affects the management of diabetes, whether preexisting or PTDM, inside and outside the hospital.

DIAGNOSIS

An international consensus panel established the first and only diagnostic criteria for diabetes after transplant in 2003, patterned after the American Diabetes Association (ADA) criteria at the time (Table 36.1).[1] This remains the primary guideline for diagnosis for all transplant groups. This first guideline, unlike the ADA diagnostic criteria, did not exclude the first acute hospitalization for transplantation, which commonly includes the administration of high-dose corticosteroids. A follow-up International Consensus panel has concluded that the diagnosis should be reserved for persistent significant hyperglycemia, consistent with current ADA guidelines, after discharge from the hospital and once the recipient is on stable, maintenance immunosuppression. The ADA has since added hemoglobin A1C ($\geq 6.5\%$) as a diagnostic criterion for diabetes in nontransplant patients.[2] A1C, however, has not been adopted as a diagnostic criterion for PTDM. In fact, A1C may underestimate risk in transplant patients, who frequently have anemia and reduced red cell survival, because of chronic kidney or liver disease. Although a normal A1C does not exclude PTDM, an elevated A1C does suggest the diagnosis and is used with glucose values to monitor long-term management. Importantly, even diabetes diagnosed 10 years after transplant, whether in an adult or pediatric recipient, still is considered PTDM, although the consequences are likely to be different than those diagnosed early after transplant, largely summarized in this chapter.

There are three criteria for diagnosis of new diabetes after transplant:[1] *1)* fasting plasma glucose ≥126 mg/dl (or 7 mmol/l) after no caloric intake for at least 8 hours; *2)* random plasma glucose ≥200 mg/dl or 11.1 mmol/l with symptoms of diabetes; or *3)* 2-hour plasma glucose in a 75-gram oral glucose tolerance test (OGTT) ≥200 mg/dl or 11.1 mmol/l. Because fasting glucose is lower in patients with chronic kidney or liver disease, OGTT or postprandial glucose testing are more sensitive measures for diagnosis. A1C can underestimate risk in many transplant patients so should not be used alone for diagnosis. If, however, A1C is significantly elevated (>6.5%), diabetes is strongly suggested.

EPIDEMIOLOGY AND PATHOPHYSIOLOGY

Risk factors for PTDM are similar to those described for type 2 diabetes (T2D),[3-10,15-18] and include age (over 45 years), family history of T2D, race and ethnicity (African American or Hispanic), preexisting glucose intolerance, elevated BMI, hepatitis C or cytomegalovirus (CMV) infection, hypertriglyceridemia, or other features of metabolic syndrome.[3,4] Most if not all of the major candidate genes for T2D also have been implicated as risk factors for PTDM, including TCF7L2, KCNJ11, SLC30A8, HHEX, CDKAL1, CDKN2A/B, and KCNQ1 polymorphisms.[5-8] Type 1 diabetes (T1D) candidate genes also have been implicated, such as interleukins IL-7R, IL-17E, IL-17R, and IL-17RB.[9] Polymorphism of the NFATc4 gene also may contribute to PTDM.[10] Like T2D, PTDM is linked to both insulin resistance and reduced insulin secretion, based on insulin clamp and oral glucose tolerance tests.[11-14]

Specific immunosuppression medications predict and contribute to risk, particularly corticosteroids and the calcineurin inhibitor tacrolimus.[3,15,16] But cyclosporine and mTOR inhibitors, such as sirolimus, have also been associated with PTDM.[16-18] The calcineurin inhibitors largely reduce insulin secretion, while sirolimus has a greater impact on insulin sensitivity, and both are associated with islet apoptosis.[19-23]

Additional factors that have been associated with PTDM after kidney transplant include number of rejection episodes, deceased over living donor graft, polycystic kidney disease, and hypertensive vascular disease.[63-65] Although hepatitis C infection is strongly associated with PTDM, all causes of cirrhosis are associated with greater risk of PTDM following liver transplant.[35]

Prevalence of PTDM varies with the type of transplant (e.g., kidney, heart, liver) and the specific transplant center, as their candidate populations also vary with respect to diabetes risk factors such as prevalence of obesity and/or race and ethnicity. Table 36.1 summarizes the prevalence of PTDM, concentrating on estimates published after 2003, when more consistent criteria for diagnosis of PTDM have been used.

Table 36.1 Prevalence of PTDM

Type of graft	Prevalence estimate	References
Kidney	14–74%	(Vincenti et al., 2007; Sulanc et al., 2005; Kamar et al., 2007; Valderhaug et al., 2009)
Liver	7–30%	(Pageaux et al., 2009)
Heart	11–38%	(Ye et al., 2010)

Note: These estimates are based on criteria for PTDM prior to revised guidelines for adults, as there are no consensus guidelines for screening or diagnosis in children, which included diagnosis in the hospital setting. Pancreas and islet transplant are excluded as diabetes diagnosis after these transplants are more likely to be due to graft failure.

Sources: Vincenti F, Friman S, Scheuermann E, Rostaing L, Jenssen T, Campistol JM, et al. Results of an international, randomized trial comparing glucose metabolism disorders and outcome with cyclosporine versus tacrolimus. *Am J Transplant* 2007;7(6):1506–1514; Sulanc E, Lane JT, Puumala SE, Groggel GC, Wrenshall LE, Stevens RB. New-onset diabetes after kidney transplantation: an application of 2003 International Guidelines. *Transplantation* 2005;80(7):945–952; Kamar N, Mariat C, Delahousse M, Dantal J, Al Najjar A, Cassuto E, et al. Diabetes mellitus after kidney transplantation: a French multicentre observational study. *Nephrol Dialysis Transplant* 2007;22(7):1986–1993; Valderhaug TG, Jenssen T, Hartmann A, Midtvedt K, Holdaas H, Reisaeter AV, et al. Fasting plasma glucose and glycosylated hemoglobin in the screening for diabetes mellitus after renal transplantation. *Transplantation* 2009;88(3):429–434; Pageaux GP, Faure S, Bouyabrine H, Bismuth M, Assenat E. Long-term outcomes of liver transplantation: diabetes mellitus. *Liver Transplant* 2009;15(Suppl 2):S79–82; Ye X, Kuo HT, Sampaio MS, Jiang Y, Reddy P, Bunnapradist S. Risk factors for development of new-onset diabetes mellitus in adult heart transplant recipients. *Transplantation* 2010;89(12):1526–1532.

CONSEQUENCES OF PTDM

PTDM affects patient and graft survival, infections, and cardiovascular events in different transplant groups. After kidney transplant, PTDM decreases patient survival largely attributed to cardiovascular disease (CVD).[24–27] In fact, PTDM is an independent risk factor for CVD.[28–30] PTDM also decreases graft survival after kidney transplant compared with nondiabetic recipients in most studies,[26,31–34] but not all,[24,35] largely due to increased mortality. Postoperative hyperglycemia is itself positively associated with graft rejection compared with controls, whether or not diabetes was diagnosed.[36–38]

After liver transplant, PTDM and postoperative hyperglycemia (glucose >200 mg/dl) is also associated with increased acute allograft rejection and graft failure.[39–42] PTDM is associated with reduced short-term but does not consistently affect long-term survival after liver transplant.[40–45] After heart transplant, PTDM is not associated with increased rejection episodes, transplant vasculopathy, or reduced patient or graft survival.[46]

PTDM also can increase post-transplant infections. Those with PTDM are more likely to have CMV in kidney and lung transplants, sepsis after kidney transplant, and minor bacterial and fungal infections after liver transplant.[41,42,44,47–50] In fact, perioperative hyperglycemia alone is associated with greater infections immediately after liver and kidney transplant.[38,51,52]

GLUCOSE MANAGEMENT AFTER TRANSPLANT

Hyperglycemia, whether identified before or after transplant, warrants glucose management, inside and outside of the hospital. The diagnosis of PTDM, like pretransplant diabetes, should precipitate the management of other factors that affect future diabetes complications, such as lipids or blood pressure, with consideration for the specific transplant setting.

INPATIENT MANAGEMENT OF GLUCOSE IN THE TRANSPLANT PATIENT

Glucose control in the hospital improves length of stay, infections, wound healing, and mortality in non-transplant populations.[53-57] However, the one prospective study of glucose control in kidney transplant patients demonstrated no value of more intensive glucose management (70–110 mg/dl) compared to usual control (<180 mg/dl) as there were no benefits and they experienced greater graft rejection.[58] As a result, current recommendations for glucose management after transplant follows current ADA guidelines, which are based largely on the Normoglycemia in Intensive Care Evaluation-Survival Using Glucose Algorithm Regulation (NICE-SUGAR) trial (Table 36.2).[2]

Table 36.2 Proposed Inpatient Blood Glucose Goals and Glycemic Regimens for Transplant Recipients

Goal blood glucose level	
Critically ill patients	140–180 mg/dl
Noncritically ill patients	Premeal <140 mg/dl Random <180 mg/dl
Recommended treatment strategies	
IV insulin infusion	Critically ill, severe insulin resistance, high-dose steroids, enteral or parenteral nutrition
Subcutaneous insulin	Stable patient, predictable nutrition, steroids tapering, IV insulin not available
Oral diabetes medication	Generally not recommended in the inpatient setting

Note: Supplemental scale insulin should be ordered in most patients in addition to fixed insulin doses for those transitioning to or on oral diabetes medications.

Sources: These criteria are based on ADA guidelines for inpatient management of hyperglycemia. American Diabetes Association. Standards of medical care in diabetes—2013. *Diabetes Care* 2013;36(Suppl 1):S11–66; Therasse A, Wallia A, Molitch ME. Management of post-transplant diabetes. *Curr Diab Rep* 2013;13(1):121–129.

Glucose tolerance can change dramatically after transplant with changes in corticosteroid dose, infection, pain, nutritional intake and source (intravenous vs. enteral), and overall clinical status. Thus, hospital management often requires daily adjustments of insulin. Initially, a tightly regulated intravenous insulin infusion protocol is generally required, transitioning to subcutaneous insulin when stable as recently described.[59] Many immunosuppression protocols and treatment of rejection include intermittent corticosteroid administration. To reduce or prevent episodic hyperglycemia, or overshoot hypoglycemia from supplemental insulin once the effect of the corticosteroids wanes, intermediate-acting insulin (NPH) is often prescribed to be given at the same time as the corticosteroid dose. Before hospital discharge, all patients, or their designated caregiver, should be taught to perform self–glucose monitoring and insulin administration as many will require intermittent or long-term insulin therapy. Oral diabetes medications can be initiated or restarted close to planned discharge if overall insulin requirements are relatively low, and there are no contraindications. After hospital discharge, insulin or other oral medications will likely require frequent adjustments based on glucose records.

LONG-TERM OUTPATIENT MANAGEMENT OF DIABETES AFTER TRANSPLANT

Overall A1C goal <7% is reasonable for most,[2] but a higher A1C goal may be safer in those with recurrent, severe hypoglycemia; advanced complications; or limited life expectancy. The Kidney Disease: Improving Global Outcomes (KDIGO) guidelines have suggested a target A1C of 7–7.5%, preferring the use of agents with less risk of hypoglycemia.[60] Dietary changes and regular exercise also can improve glucose after kidney transplant.[61] Many transplant recipients will require insulin, which should be tailored to their lifestyle, meal pattern, kidney function, and immunosuppression. Considerations for use of diabetes agents after transplant are summarized in Table 36.3. The transplant setting can affect management of other factors important to the prevention of diabetes complications as outlined in Table 36.4. Bone loss and fracture are also more common in diabetes patients after transplant so bone density surveillance should be a routine part of post-transplant care.[62]

Table 36.3 Considerations for the Use of Diabetes Agents for Diabetes Treatment After Transplantation

Agent	Considerations after transplant	References
Biguanides (metformin)	Effective in stable KTX patients but contraindicated for many other TX groups, including during acute hospitalizations.	(Hecking et al., 2013; Therasse et al., 2012)
Sulfonylureas	Not recommended with GFR <30 ml/minute due to risk of hypoglycemia. Often ineffective as monotherapy after TX.	(Hecking et al., 2013; Therasse et al., 2012)

(continued)

Table 36.3 Considerations for the Use of Diabetes Agents for Diabetes Treatment After Transplantation *(continued)*

Agent	Considerations after transplant	References
TZDs	Can aggravate weight gain, edema, and bone loss, which may already be concerns. Safe and efficacious in short term after KTX, sometimes preferred with steatohepatitis after liver TX but not studied after cardiac TX. Relative risk of bladder cancer with this agent in TX patients unknown.	(Hecking et al., 2013; Therasse et al., 2012)
Megli-tinides	Preferred over sulfonylureas as less risk of hypoglycemia due to shorter half-life with low GFR.	(Hecking et al., 2013; Therasse et al., 2012)
α-Glucosidase inhibitors (acarbose)	Often inadequate to achieve glucose goals.	No available studies
GLP-1 agonists	Nausea and reduced intestinal motility has potential to impact immunosuppressant levels.	No available studies
DPP-4 inhibitors	No dose reduction required unless GFR <30 ml/minute. No significant risk of hypoglycemia.	(Gueler et al., 2013; Lane et al., 2011; Werzowa et al., 2013)
Insulin	Must be tailored to meals and corticosteroid dosing schedule. NPH dose can cover intermittent corticosteroid administration independent of other diabetes treatment. Total dose requirements will change with GFR.	(Hecking et al., 2013)
Sodium glucose cotransporter-2 (SGLT-2) inhibitors	The safety of this class of agents in transplant patients is unknown. Because they can cause dehydration, which could compromise their kidney graft, as well as increase their risk for genitourinary infections, a risk that might be further magnified by immunosuppression, their use in this population should be restricted to a research protocol until safety has been assured.	

Note: KTX = kidney transplant; GFR = glomerular filtration rate; TX = transplant; TZD = thiazolidinedione; GLP-1 = glucagon-like peptide-1; DPP-4 = dipeptidyl peptidase-4 inhibitor.
Sources: Hecking M, Werzowa J, Haidinger M, Horl WH, Pascual J, Budde K, et al. Novel views on new-onset diabetes after transplantation: development, prevention and treatment. *Nephrol Dial Transplant* 2013;28(3):550–566; Therasse A, Wallia A, Molitch ME. Management of post-transplant diabetes. *Curr Diab Rep* 2012;13(1):121–129; Gueler I, Mueller S, Helmschrott M, Oeing CU, Erbel C, Frankenstein L, et al. Effects of vildagliptin (Galvus(R)) therapy in patients with type 2 diabetes mellitus after heart transplantation. *Drug Des Devel Ther* 2013;7:297–303; Lane JT, Odegaard DE, Haire CE, Collier DS, Wrenshall LE, Stevens RB. Sitagliptin therapy in kidney transplant recipients with new-onset diabetes after transplantation. *Transplantation* 2011;92(10):e56–57; Werzowa J, Hecking M, Haidinger M, Lechner F, Doller D, Pacini G, et al. Vildagliptin and pioglitazone in patients with impaired glucose tolerance after kidney transplantation: a randomized, placebo-controlled clinical trial. *Transplantation* 2013;95(3):456–462.

Table 36.4 Impact of Transplant on Other ADA Recommended Diabetes Care Guidelines

Measure	ADA guidelines	KDIGO guidelines	Transplant considerations	References
Aspirin	75–162 mg/day	65–100 mg/day	■ Restart after immediate postoperative period. ■ Improves graft survival and prevents CVD events. ■ Increases GI bleeds.	(American Diabetes Association, 2013; Kasiske et al., 2009)
Blood pressure	Goal <140/80 mmHg; ACE inhibitor or ARB with elevated blood pressure or proteinuria	Goal <130/80 mmHg; ACE inhibitor or ARB with elevated blood pressure or proteinuria	■ Restart ACE/ARB 1–3 months after transplant. ■ Continue unless serum creatinine increases >25–30%. ■ CCBs can change immune suppressant metabolism.	(American Diabetes Association, 2013; Kasiske et al., 2009)
Urine albumin/creatinine	Goal: <30 mg/grams Measure annually	Urine protein/creatinine 1st month after KTX, then every 3 months for 1 year, and then annually	■ Sirolimus can increase and CNIs can reduce urine protein independent of other factors. ■ Urine albumin/creatinine used over protein in non-KTX patients.	(American Diabetes Association, 2013; Kasiske et al., 2009)
Fasting lipids	Goal: LDL <100 mg/dl or <70 mg/dl or start statin with CVD or significant CVD risk	Goal <100 mg/dl, and lower if it can be achieved safely but no data to support goal <70 mg/dl after KTX	■ Statins, ezetimibe, and fibrates have been used singly or with fish oil ■ Statins, fenofibrates, and niacin can all singly cause drug–drug interactions with immunosuppressants so statin plus fibrates should be avoided altogether.	(American Diabetes Association, 2013; Kasiske et al., 2009; KDOQI, 2012)
Eye exam	Annually	No recommendations	■ Greater risk of infections and cataracts due to immunosuppression and corticosteroids. ■ At risk for diabetic retinal disease.	(American Diabetes Association, 2013)
Foot exam	Annual	No recommendations	■ Slow resolution of neuropathy and immunosuppression increases risk for injury and infection. ■ Early diabetic foot education strongly recommended.	(American Diabetes Association, 2013)

Note: CVD = cardiovascular disease; GI = gastrointestinal; ACE = angiotensin-converting enzyme; ARB = angiotensin receptor blocker; CCB = calcium channel blocker; KTX = kidney transplant; CNI = calcineurin inhibitor (cyclosporine or tacrolimus); LDL = low-density lipoprotein. *Sources:* American Diabetes Association. Standards of medical care in diabetes—2013. *Diabetes Care* 2013;36(Suppl 1):S11–S66; Kasiske BL, Zeier MG, Chapman JR, Craig JC, Ekberg H, Garvey CA, et al. KDIGO clinical practice guideline for the care of kidney transplant recipients: a summary. *Kidney Int* 2009;77(4):299–311; KDOQI clinical practice guideline for diabetes and CKD: 2012 Update. *Am J Kidney Dis* 2012;60(5):850–886.

CONCLUSION

PTDM affects transplant outcomes, including graft and patient survival, as well as risk of infections and CVD. Management of diabetes after transplant, including measures to prevent diabetic complications, must take into consideration drug–drug interactions that can occur between immunosuppression medications and the medications used to treat hypertension and lipid disorders in diabetes patients.

REFERENCES

1. Davidson J, Wilkinson A, Dantal J, Dotta F, Haller H, Hernandez D, et al. New-onset diabetes after transplantation: 2003 International consensus guidelines. Proceedings of an international expert panel meeting. Barcelona, Spain, 19 February 2003. *Transplantation* 2003;75(10 Suppl):SS3–S24.

2. American Diabetes Association. Standards of medical care in diabetes—2013. *Diabetes Care* 2013;36(Suppl 1):S11–66.

3. Hecking M, Werzowa J, Haidinger M, Horl WH, Pascual J, Budde K, et al. Novel views on new-onset diabetes after transplantation: development, prevention and treatment. *Nephrol Dial Transplant* 2013;28(3):550–566.

4. Therasse A, Wallia A, Molitch ME. Management of post-transplant diabetes. *Curr Diab Rep* 2012;13(1):121–129.

5. Ghisdal L, Baron C, Le Meur Y, Lionet A, Halimi JM, Rerolle JP, et al. TCF7L2 polymorphism associates with new-onset diabetes after transplantation. *J Am Soc Nephrol* 2009;20(11):2459–2467.

6. Kang ES, Kim MS, Kim CH, Nam CM, Han SJ, Hur KY, et al. Association of common type 2 diabetes risk gene variants and posttransplantation diabetes mellitus in renal allograft recipients in Korea. *Transplantation* 2009;88(5):693–698.

7. Kurzawski M, Dziewanowski K, Kedzierska K, Wajda A, Lapczuk J, Drozdzik M. Association of transcription factor 7-like 2 (TCF7L2) gene polymorphism with posttransplant diabetes mellitus in kidney transplant patients medicated with tacrolimus. *Pharmacol Rep* 2011;63(3):826–833.

8. Tavira B, Coto E, Torres A, Diaz-Corte C, Diaz-Molina B, Ortega F, et al. Association between a common KCNJ11 polymorphism (rs5219) and new-onset posttransplant diabetes in patients treated with tacrolimus. *Mol Genet Metab* 2012;105(3):525–527.

9. Kim YG, Ihm CG, Lee TW, Lee SH, Jeong KH, Moon JY, et al. Association of genetic polymorphisms of interleukins with new-onset diabetes after transplantation in renal transplantation. *Transplantation* 2012;93(9):900–907.

10. Chen Y, Sampaio MS, Yang JW, Min D, Hutchinson IV. Genetic polymorphisms of the transcription factor NFATc4 and development of new-onset

diabetes after transplantation in Hispanic kidney transplant recipients. *Transplantation* 2012;93(3):325–330.

11. Ekstrand AV, Eriksson JG, Gronhagen-Riska C, Ahonen PJ, Groop LC. Insulin resistance and insulin deficiency in the pathogenesis of posttransplantation diabetes in man. *Transplantation* 1992;53(3):563–569.

12. Midtvedt K, Hartmann A, Hjelmesaeth J, Lund K, Bjerkely BL. Insulin resistance is a common denominator of post-transplant diabetes mellitus and impaired glucose tolerance in renal transplant recipients. *Nephrol Dial Transplant* 1998;13(2):427–431.

13. Nam JH, Mun JI, Kim SI, Kang SW, Choi KH, Park K, et al. Beta-cell dysfunction rather than insulin resistance is the main contributing factor for the development of postrenal transplantation diabetes mellitus. *Transplantation* 2001;71(10):1417–1423.

14. Hagen M, Hjelmesaeth J, Jenssen T, Morkrid L, Hartmann A. A 6-year prospective study on new onset diabetes mellitus, insulin release and insulin sensitivity in renal transplant recipients. *Nephrol Dial Transplant* 2003;18(10):2154–2159.

15. Porrini E, Moreno JM, Osuna A, Benitez R, Lampreabe I, Diaz JM, et al. Prediabetes in patients receiving tacrolimus in the first year after kidney transplantation: a prospective and multicenter study. *Transplantation* 2008;85(8):1133–1138.

16. Vincenti F, Friman S, Scheuermann E, Rostaing L, Jenssen T, Campistol JM, et al. Results of an international, randomized trial comparing glucose metabolism disorders and outcome with cyclosporine versus tacrolimus. *Am J Transplant* 2007;7(6):1506–1514.

17. Johnston O, Rose CL, Webster AC, Gill JS. Sirolimus is associated with new-onset diabetes in kidney transplant recipients. *J Am Soc Nephrol* 2008;19(7):1411–1418.

18. Sulanc E, Lane JT, Puumala SE, Groggel GC, Wrenshall LE, Stevens RB. New-onset diabetes after kidney transplantation: an application of 2003 International Guidelines. *Transplantation* 2005;80(7):945–952.

19. Bell E, Cao X, Moibi JA, Greene SR, Young R, Trucco M, et al. Rapamycin has a deleterious effect on MIN-6 cells and rat and human islets. *Diabetes* 2003;52(11):2731–2739.

20. Fraenkel M, Ketzinel-Gilad M, Ariav Y, Pappo O, Karaca M, Castel J, et al. mTOR inhibition by rapamycin prevents beta-cell adaptation to hyperglycemia and exacerbates the metabolic state in type 2 diabetes. *Diabetes* 2008;57(4):945–957.

21. Johnson JD, Ao Z, Ao P, Li H, Dai LJ, He Z, et al. Different effects of FK506, rapamycin, and mycophenolate mofetil on glucose-stimulated insulin release and apoptosis in human islets. *Cell Transplant* 2009;18(8):833–845.

22. Larsen JL, Bennett RG, Burkman T, Ramirez AL, Yamamoto S, Gulizia J, et al. Tacrolimus and sirolimus cause insulin resistance in normal Sprague Dawley rats. *Transplantation* 2006;82(4):466–470.

23. Shivaswamy V, McClure M, Passer J, Frahm C, Ochsner L, Erickson J, et al. Hyperglycemia induced by tacrolimus and sirolimus is reversible in normal Sprague-Dawley rats. *Endocrine* 2010;37(3):489–496.

24. Revanur VK, Jardine AG, Kingsmore DB, Jaques BC, Hamilton DH, Jindal RM. Influence of diabetes mellitus on patient and graft survival in recipients of kidney transplantation. *Clin Transplant* 2001;15(2):89–94.

25. Cosio FG, Pesavento TE, Kim S, Osei K, Henry M, Ferguson RM. Patient survival after renal transplantation: IV. Impact of post-transplant diabetes. *Kidney Int* 2002;62(4):1440–1446.

26. Kasiske BL, Snyder JJ, Gilbertson D, Matas AJ. Diabetes mellitus after kidney transplantation in the United States. *Am J Transplant* 2003;3(2):178–185.

27. Joss N, Staatz CE, Thomson AH, Jardine AG. Predictors of new onset diabetes after renal transplantation. *Clin Transplant* 2007;21(1):136–143.

28. Wauters RP, Cosio FG, Suarez Fernandez ML, Kudva Y, Shah P, Torres VE. Cardiovascular consequences of new-onset hyperglycemia after kidney transplantation. *Transplantation* 2012;94(4):377–382.

29. Lentine KL, Brennan DC, Schnitzler MA. Incidence and predictors of myocardial infarction after kidney transplantation. *J Am Soc Nephrol* 2005;16(2):496–506.

30. Hjelmesaeth J, Hartmann A, Leivestad T, Holdaas H, Sagedal S, Olstad M, et al. The impact of early-diagnosed new-onset post-transplantation diabetes mellitus on survival and major cardiac events. *Kidney Int* 2006;69(3):588–595.

31. Roth D, Milgrom M, Esquenazi V, Fuller L, Burke G, Miller J. Posttransplant hyperglycemia. Increased incidence in cyclosporine-treated renal allograft recipients. *Transplantation* 1989;47(2):278–281.

32. Miles AM, Sumrani N, Horowitz R, Homel P, Maursky V, Markell MS, et al. Diabetes mellitus after renal transplantation: as deleterious as non-transplant-associated diabetes? *Transplantation* 1998;65(3):380–384.

33. Cole EH, Johnston O, Rose CL, Gill JS. Impact of acute rejection and new-onset diabetes on long-term transplant graft and patient survival. *Clin J Am Soc Nephrol* 2008;3(3):814–821.

34. Matas AJ, Gillingham KJ, Humar A, Ibrahim HN, Payne WD, Gruessner RW, et al. Posttransplant diabetes mellitus and acute rejection: Impact on kidney transplant outcome. *Transplantation* 2008;85(3):338–343.

35. Kuo HT, Sampaio MS, Vincenti F, Bunnapradist S. Associations of pretransplant diabetes mellitus, new-onset diabetes after transplant, and acute rejection with transplant outcomes: an analysis of the Organ Procurement and

Transplant Network/United Network for Organ Sharing (OPTN/UNOS) database. *Am J Kidney Dis* 2010;56(6):1127–1139.

36. Ganji MR, Charkhchian M, Hakemi M, Nederi GH, Solymanian T, Saddadi F, et al. Association of hyperglycemia on allograft function in the early period after renal transplantation. *Tranplant Proc* 2007;39(4):852–854.

37. Valderhaug, TG, Helmesaeth J, . Jenssen T, Roislien J, Leivestad T, Hartmann A. Early posttransplantation hyperglycemia in kidney transplant recipients is associated with overall long-term graft losses *Transplantation* 2012;94(7):714–720.

38. Thomas MC, Mathew TH, Russ GR, Rao MM, Moran J. Early peri-operative glycaemic control and allograft rejection in patients with diabetes mellitus: a pilot study. *Transplantation* 2001;72(7):1321–1324.

39. Wallia A, Parikh ND, Molitch ME, Mahler E, Tian L, Huang JJ, et al. Posttransplant hyperglycemia is associated with increased risk of liver allograft rejection. *Transplantation* 2010;89(2):222–226.

40. Navasa M, Bustamante J, Marroni C, Gonzalez E, Andreu H, Esmatjes E, et al. Diabetes mellitus after liver transplantation: prevalence and predictive factors. *J Hepatol* 1996;25(1):64–71.

41. John PR, Thuluvath PJ. Outcome of patients with new-onset diabetes mellitus after liver transplantation compared with those without diabetes mellitus. *Liver Transplant* 2002;8(8):708–713.

42. Moon JI, Barbeito R, Faradji RN, Gaynor JJ, Tzakis AG. Negative impact of new-onset diabetes mellitus on patient and graft survival after liver transplantation: long-term follow up. *Transplantation* 2006;82(12):1625–1628.

43. Trail KC, McCashland TM, Larsen JL, Heffron TG, Stratta RJ, Langnas AN, et al. Morbidity in patients with posttransplant diabetes mellitus following orthotopic liver transplantation. *Liver Transplant Surg* 1996;2(4):276–283.

44. Trail KC, Stratta RJ, Larsen JL, Ruby EI, Patil KD, Langnas AN, et al. Results of liver transplantation in diabetic recipients. *Surgery* 1993;114(4):650–656; discussion 656–658.

45. Baid S, Cosimi AB, Farrell ML, Schoenfeld DA, Feng S, Chung RT, et al. Posttransplant diabetes mellitus in liver transplant recipients: risk factors, temporal relationship with hepatitis C virus allograft hepatitis, and impact on mortality. *Transplantation* 2001;72(6):1066–1072.

46. Klingenberg R, Gleissner C, Koch A, Schnabel PA, Sack FU, Zimmermann R, et al. Impact of pre-operative diabetes mellitus upon early and late survival after heart transplantation: a possible era effect. *J Heart Lung Transplant* 2005;24(9):1239–1246.

47. von Kiparski A, Frei D, Uhlschmid G, Largiader F, Binswanger U. Posttransplant diabetes mellitus in renal allograft recipients: a matched-pair control study. *Nephrol Dialysis Transplant* 1990;5(3):220–225.

48. Sumrani NB, Delaney V, Ding ZK, Davis R, Daskalakis P, Friedman EA, et al. Diabetes mellitus after renal transplantation in the cyclosporine era: an analysis of risk factors. *Transplantation* 1991;51(2):343–347.

49. Siraj ES, Abacan C, Chinnappa P, Wojtowicz J, Braun W. Risk factors and outcomes associated with posttransplant diabetes mellitus in kidney transplant recipients. *Transplantation Proc* 2010;42(5):1685–1689.

50. Ollech JE, Kramer MR, Peled N, Ollech A, Amital A, Medalion B, et al. Post-transplant diabetes mellitus in lung transplant recipients: incidence and risk factors. *Eur J Cardio-Thoracic Surg* 2008;33(5):844–848.

51. Ammori JB, Sigakis M, Englesbe MJ, O'Reilly M, Pelletier SJ. Effect of intraoperative hyperglycemia during liver transplantation. *J Surg Res* 2007; 140(2):227–233.

52. Park C, Hsu C, Neelakanta G, Nourmand H, Braunfeld M, Wray C, et al. Severe intraoperative hyperglycemia is independently associated with surgical site infection after liver transplantation. *Transplantation* 2009;87(7):1031–1036.

53. Malmberg K. Prospective randomised study of intensive insulin treatment on long term survival after acute myocardial infarction in patients with diabetes mellitus. DIGAMI (Diabetes Mellitus, Insulin Glucose Infusion in Acute Myocardial Infarction) study group. *BMJ* 1997;314(7093):1512–1515.

54. Furnary AP, Zerr KJ, Grunkemeier GL, Starr A. Continuous intravenous insulin infusion reduces the incidence of deep sternal wound infection in diabetic patients after cardiac surgical procedures. *Ann Thorac Surg* 1999;67(2):352–360; discussion 360–352.

55. Malmberg K, Norhammar A, Wedel H, Ryden L. Glycometabolic state at admission: Important risk marker of mortality in conventionally treated patients with diabetes mellitus and acute myocardial infarction: long-term results from the Diabetes and Insulin-Glucose Infusion in Acute Myocardial Infarction (DIGAMI) study. *Circulation* 1999;99(20):2626–2632.

56. Ishihara M, Kojima S, Sakamoto T, Asada Y, Tei C, Kimura K, et al. Acute hyperglycemia is associated with adverse outcome after acute myocardial infarction in the coronary intervention era. *Am Heart J* 2005;150(4):814–820.

57. Finfer S, Chittock DR, Su SY, Blair D, Foster D, Dhingra V, et al. Intensive versus conventional glucose control in critically ill patients. *N Engl J Med* 2009;360(13):1283–1297.

58. Hermayer KL, Egidi MF, Finch NJ, Baliga P, Lin A, Kettinger L, et al. A randomized controlled trial to evaluate the effect of glycemic control on renal transplantation outcomes. *J Clin Endocrinol Metab* 2012;97(12):4399–4406.

59. Larsen J, Goldner W. Approach to the hospitalized patient with severe insulin resistance. *J Clin Endocrinol Metab* 2011;96(9):2652–2662.

60. Kasiske BL, Zeier MG, Chapman JR, Craig JC, Ekberg H, Garvey CA, et al. KDIGO clinical practice guideline for the care of kidney transplant recipients: a summary. *Kidney Int* 2009;77(4):299–311.

61. Sharif A, Moore R, Baboolal K. Influence of lifestyle modification in renal transplant recipients with postprandial hyperglycemia. *Transplantation* 2008;85(3):353–358.

62. Naylor KL, Li AH, Lam NN, Hodsman AB, Jamal SA, Garg AX. Fracture risk in kidney transplant recipients: a systematic review. *Transplantation* 2013;95(12):1461–1470.

63. Guitard J, Rostaing L, Kamar N. New-onset diabetes and nephropathy after renal transplantation. *Contrib Nephrol* 2011;170:247–255.

64. Hamer RA, Chow CL, Ong AC, McKane WS. Polycystic kidney disease is a risk factor for new-onset diabetes after transplantation. *Transplantation* 2007;83(1):36–40.

65. Eckhard M, Schindler RA, Renner FC, Schief W, Padberg W, Weimer R, et al. New-onset diabetes mellitus after renal transplantation. *Transplant Proc* 2009;41(6):2544–2545.

66. Kamar N, Mariat C, Delahousse M, Dantal J, Al Najjar A, Cassuto E, et al. Diabetes mellitus after kidney transplantation: a French multicentre observational study. *Nephrol Dialysis Transplant* 2007;22(7):1986–1993.

67. Valderhaug TG, Jenssen T, Hartmann A, Midtvedt K, Holdaas H, Reisaeter AV, et al. Fasting plasma glucose and glycosylated hemoglobin in the screening for diabetes mellitus after renal transplantation. *Transplantation* 2009;88(3):429–434.

68. Pageaux GP, Faure S, Bouyabrine H, Bismuth M, Assenat E. Long-term outcomes of liver transplantation: diabetes mellitus. *Liver Transplant* 2009; 15(Suppl 2):S79–82.

69. Ye X, Kuo HT, Sampaio MS, Jiang Y, Reddy P, Bunnapradist S. Risk factors for development of new-onset diabetes mellitus in adult heart transplant recipients. *Transplantation* 2010;89(12):1526–1532.

70. Therasse A, Wallia A, Molitch ME. Management of post-transplant diabetes. *Curr Diab Rep* 2013;13(1):121–129.

71. Gueler I, Mueller S, Helmschrott M, Oeing CU, Erbel C, Frankenstein L, et al. Effects of vildagliptin (Galvus(R)) therapy in patients with type 2 diabetes mellitus after heart transplantation. *Drug Des Devel Ther* 2013;7:297–303.

72. Lane JT, Odegaard DE, Haire CE, Collier DS, Wrenshall LE, Stevens RB. Sitagliptin therapy in kidney transplant recipients with new-onset diabetes after transplantation. *Transplantation* 2011;92(10):e56–57.

73. Werzowa J, Hecking M, Haidinger M, Lechner F, Doller D, Pacini G, et al. Vildagliptin and pioglitazone in patients with impaired glucose tolerance

after kidney transplantation: a randomized, placebo-controlled clinical trial. *Transplantation* 2013;95(3):456–462.

74. KDOQI clinical practice guideline for diabetes and CKD: 2012 update. *Am J Kidney Dis* 2012;60(5):850–886.

Chapter 37

Diabetic Ketoacidosis and Hyperglycemic Hyperosmolar State in Adults

Guillermo E. Umpierrez, MD, CDE
Carlos E. Mendez, MD, FACP

INTRODUCTION

Diabetic ketoacidosis (DKA) and hyperglycemic hyperosmolar state (HHS) are the most serious acute metabolic complications of diabetes. In spite of advances in our understanding of their pathogenesis and more uniform agreement about their diagnosis and treatment, DKA and HHS continue to be important causes of morbidity and mortality among patients with diabetes. Both DKA and HHS are characterized by insulinopenia and severe hyperglycemia. Clinically, they differ only by the degree of dehydration and the severity of metabolic acidosis.[1,2] Successful treatment of DKA and HHS require frequent monitoring of patients, improvement in circulatory volume and tissue perfusion, correction of hypovolemia and hyperglycemia, replacement of electrolyte losses, and careful search and management of the precipitating cause.

EPIDEMIOLOGY

Recent data indicate there are ~144,000 hospital admissions per year for DKA in the U.S.,[3] and the number of cases shows an upward trend, with a 30% increase in the annual number of cases between 1995 and 2009.[3,4] Observational studies have reported that DKA accounts for 4–9% of hospital discharges among patients admitted with a primary diagnosis of diabetes.[5,6] In the EURODIAB study, 8.6% of 3,250 subjects with T1D throughout Europe were admitted with DKA in the previous 12 months.[7] The rate of hospital admissions for HHS is lower than for DKA, accounting for <1% of all diabetes-related admissions.[2,5]

Most patients with DKA have autoimmune type 1 diabetes (T1D); however, patients with type 2 diabetes (T2D) are also at risk of developing DKA during the catabolic stress of acute illness, such as trauma, surgery, or infections.[6,8] In contrast to popular belief, DKA is more common in adults than in children.[11] T2D now accounts for up to one-half of all newly diagnosed diabetes in children ages 10 to 21 years.[8,9] In the U.S., the SEARCH for Diabetes in Youth Study found that 29.4% of participants <20 years of age with T1D presented with DKA as compared with 9.7% of youth with T2D.[10] In community-based studies, >40% of adult patients with DKA are >40 years old and >20% are >55 years old.[5,11,12] HHS occurs most commonly in older patients with T2D,[2,13] but it also occurs in children and young adults.[14–16] As many as 20% of patients with HHS are <30 years of age.[15]

In children and adult subjects with DKA, the overall mortality is <1%, but a mortality rate higher than 5% is reported in the elderly and in patients with con-

DOI: 10.2337/9781580405096.37

comitant life-threatening illnesses.[4,17,18] Death in these conditions rarely is due to the metabolic complications of hyperglycemia or ketoacidosis, but rather it relates to the underlying precipitating illness. Mortality in patients with HHS is higher than in DKA, ranging between 5 and 16% of patients.[1,2,4,19] The prognosis of both conditions is worsened substantially at the extremes of age, particularly in the presence of coma, hypotension, and severe comorbidities.[1,19–22] In adult patients with DKA and HHS, mortality increases substantially with aging, with mortality rates for those >65–75 years reaching 20–40%.[3,21,23] In the older age-groups, the major cause of death relates to the underlying medical illness (e.g., trauma, infection) that precipitated the metabolic decompensation,[23,24] but in the younger patient, mortality is more likely to be due to the metabolic disarray.[8,25,26]

PRECIPITATING CAUSE

DKA is the initial manifestation of diabetes in 20% of adult patients and in 30–40% of children with T1D.[8,10,27] In patients with a known history of diabetes, precipitating factors for DKA include infections, intercurrent illnesses, psychological stress, and poor compliance with therapy.[5,14,28,29] Worldwide, infection is the most common precipitating factor for DKA, occurring in 20–50% of cases. Urinary tract infection and pneumonia account for the majority of infections. Other acute conditions that may precipitate DKA include acute stroke, alcohol abuse, acute pancreatitis, pulmonary embolism, myocardial infarction, and trauma.[6,30] Drugs that affect carbohydrate metabolism such as corticosteroids, sympathomimetic agents, and pentamidine also may precipitate the development of DKA.[6,31,32] Antipsychotic agents also have been associated with increased risk of severe hyperglycemia and DKA.[31] The weight gain observed with the use of antipsychotic drugs, such as clozapine or olanzapine, has been suggested as the potential underlying mechanism leading to impaired glucose metabolism.[33] Newer atypical antipsychotic medications, such as apiriprazole or quetiapine, also have been reported to significantly increase the risk of DKA without a notable increase in weight.[33,34]

The importance of noncompliance and psychological factors in the incidence of DKA has been emphasized in young patients and in inner-city populations. In adult patients with T1D, poor adherence to insulin therapy is reported as the major precipitating cause of DKA in inner-city populations.[11,33–37] A recent study determined clinical, socioeconomic, and psychological factors associated with recurrence of DKA in urban minority patients.[11] Discontinuation of insulin therapy accounted for more than two-thirds of all DKA admissions. Several behavioral, socioeconomic, and psychosocial factors contributed to poor treatment adherence. Among patients with poor compliance with insulin therapy, one-third of patients gave no clear reason for stopping insulin, one-third reported financial troubles, and most of the rest reported being away from supply or did not know how to handle insulin on sick days.[11] Other studies have reported psychological risk factors, including eating disorders, in up to 20% of recurrent episodes of ketoacidosis in young women.[38,39]

HHS is the initial manifestation of diabetes in 7–17% of patients.[2,5] HHS commonly occurs in older adults with T2D who are residents of nursing homes. These patients are at particularly high risk for dehydration because of the age-related impairment of thirst mechanisms and the limited access to fluids.[40] Infection is the major precipitating factor occurring in 30–60% of HHS patients, with urinary tract infections and pneumonia being the most common infections.[2,41] Other common precipitating causes of HHS include acute cerebrovascular events, acute myocardial infarction, surgery, acute pancreatitis, and use of drugs that affect carbohydrate metabolism, such as corticosteroids, sympathomimetic agents, pentamidine, and antipsychotic drugs.[6,31,32]

PATHOGENESIS OF DKA AND HHS

The mechanisms that trigger DKA and HHS are multifactorial and include a combination of reduced secretion and action of insulin and raised levels of counterregulatory hormones (glucagon, catecholamines, cortisol, and growth hormone) (Figure 37.1).[1,42,43] The association of insulin deficiency and increased counterregulatory hormones leads to altered glucose production and disposal and to increased lipolysis and production of ketone bodies.[44,45] Hyperglycemia results from increased hepatic and renal glucose production and impaired glucose utilization in peripheral tissues.[43] Increased gluconeogenesis results from the high availability of noncarbohydrate substrates (alanine, lactate, and glycerol in the liver and glutamine in the kidney)[46] and from the increased activity of gluconeogenic enzymes (phosphoenol pyruvate carboxykinase, fructose-1,6-bisphosphatase, and pyruvate carboxylase).[42,47] From a quantitative standpoint, increased hepatic glu-

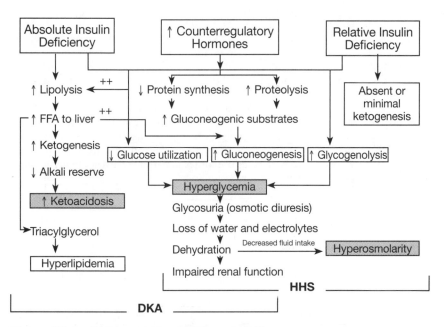

Figure 37.1 — Pathogenesis of DKA and HHS.
++Accelerated pathway. FFA, free fatty acids.

cose production represents the major pathogenic disturbance responsible for hyperglycemia in patients with DKA.[1] In addition, both hyperglycemia and high ketone levels cause osmotic diuresis that leads to hypovolemia and decreased glomerular filtration rate; the latter further aggravates hyperglycemia.[1,43]

Insulinopenia and increased counterregulatory hormones lead to increased lipolysis and increased ketone production in DKA.[42,44,48,49] Insulin deficiency causes the activation of hormone-sensitive lipase in adipose tissue that causes breakdown of triglyceride into glycerol and free fatty acids. Although glycerol becomes an important substrate for gluconeogenesis in the liver, the massive release of free fatty acids serves as a precursor of the ketoacids. In the liver, free fatty acids are oxidized to ketone bodies, a process predominantly stimulated by glucagon. Increased concentration of glucagon lowers the hepatic levels of malonyl coenzyme A, which inhibits carnitine palmitoyl-transferase I (CPT I), the rate-limiting enzyme for transesterification of fatty acyl CoA to fatty acyl carnitine.[50] CPT I is required for movement of free fatty acid into the mitochondria where fatty acid oxidation takes place.[51] Increased production of ketone bodies (acetoacetate, acetone, and β-hydroxybutarate) leads to ketonemia and metabolic acidosis.

HHS is characterized by a relative deficiency of insulin concentration to maintain normoglycemia, but adequate levels to prevent lipolysis and ketogenesis.[43,52] Patients with HHS have been shown to have higher insulin concentration (demonstrated by basal and stimulated C-peptide levels) than those with DKA.[52,53] To date, however, few studies have been performed comparing differences in counterregulatory response in DKA versus HHS.

The excessive levels of circulating nutrients, including glucose and fatty acids, are associated with a proinflammatory and oxidative state.[54] Previous studies have reported significant elevation of interleukin (IL)-6, IL-1B, and IL-8, and tumor necrosis factor (TNF)-α and increased counterregulatory hormones in patients with uncontrolled diabetes and ketoacidosis.[55,56] Of interest, similar high levels of these markers occurred in patients with DKA and HHS, indicating that hyperglycemia, independent of the presence of ketoacidosis, induces changes in proinflammatory cytokines.[55] These elevations of circulating proinflammatory cytokines promptly result in reduced-to-normal levels in response to insulin therapy and normalization of blood glucose concentration.[55,57] The increased cytokine release during DKA and HHS results in capillary perturbation and may explain why hyperglycemia is associated with poor outcomes in patients with acute myocardial infarction, stroke, and cardiac surgery.[54]

DIAGNOSIS OF DKA AND HHS

SYMPTOMS AND SIGNS

The clinical presentation of DKA usually develops rapidly, over a time span of <24 hours. Polyuria, polydipsia, and weight loss may be present for several days before the development of ketoacidosis, while vomiting and abdominal pain are frequently the presenting symptoms. Abdominal pain is reported in 40–75% of cases of DKA.[26,58,59] A prospective study of 189 consecutive patients with DKA reported that abdominal pain was present in 46% of patients with DKA, and its presence related to the severity of metabolic acidosis and not to the severity of hyperglycemia or dehydration.[38] In DKA subjects with abdominal pain, the mean serum bicarbonate (9 ± 1 mmol/l) and blood pH (7.12 ± 0.02) were lower than in patients without pain (15 ± 1 mmol/l and 7.24 ± 0.09, respectively). Delayed gastric emptying and ileus induced by electrolyte disturbance and metabolic acidosis have been implicated as possible causes of abdominal pain in DKA.[39] In the majority of patients, the abdominal pain spontaneously resolves after correction of metabolic disturbance; thus, in the absence of an overt cause for abdominal pain, allowing several hours to treat the underlying acidosis constitutes the best diagnostic tool to elucidate the etiology of abdominal pain in DKA.

Physical examination reveals signs of dehydration, such as dry mucous membranes, tachycardia, and hypotension. Mental status can vary from full alertness to profound lethargy; however, <20% of patients are hospitalized with loss of consciousness.[5,60] Most patients are normothermic or even hypothermic at presentation. Acetone on breath and labored Kussmaul respiration also may be present on admission, particularly in patients with severe metabolic acidosis.[4,26]

The typical patient with HHS is between 55 and 70 years of age and frequently is a nursing home resident with T2D. Most patients who develop HHS do so over days to weeks during which they experience polyuria, dehydration, and progressive decline in the level of consciousness.[5,19] Physical examination reveals signs of volume depletion. Fever due to underlying infection is common, and signs of metabolic acidosis (Kussmaul breathing, acetone breath) usually are absent. Gastrointestinal manifestations (abdominal pain, nausea, vomiting) are not part of HHS.[58] In some patients, focal neurologic signs (hemiparesis, hemianopsia) and seizures (partial motor seizures more common than generalized) may be the dominant clinical features, resulting in a common misdiagnosis of stroke.[61,62] The degree of mental obtundation correlates with increased serum osmolality,[5,15,41] and the majority of patients with impaired mental status or coma have an effective serum osmolality >330 mOsm/kg.

LABORATORY FINDINGS

The syndrome of DKA consists of the triad of hyperglycemia, hyperketonemia, and high anion gap metabolic acidosis. As indicated in Table 37.1, DKA can be classified as mild, moderate, or severe, depending on the extent of metabolic acidosis and level of sensorium.[1,4] The diagnostic criteria for HHS include a plasma glucose concentration >600 mg/dl, an effective serum osmolality >320 mOsm/kg of water, and the absence of significant metabolic acidosis. The effective serum osmolality is calculated with the formula: 2[Na] [mEq/l] + glucose [mg/dl]/18). Although by definition, patients with HHS have a serum pH >7.3, a serum bicarbonate >18 mEq/L, and negative ketone bodies in urine and plasma, mild ketonemia may be present. Approximately 50% of the patients with HHS have an increased anion gap metabolic acidosis as the result of concomitant ketoacidosis or an increase in serum lactate levels.[60]

The assessment of augmented ketonemia, the key diagnostic feature of ketoacidosis, frequently is performed by the nitroprusside reaction. Clinicians, however, should be aware that the nitroprusside reaction provides a semiquantitative estimation of acetoacetate and acetone levels, but it does not recognize the pres-

Table 37.1. Diagnostic Criteria for DKA and HHS[1]

	Mild DKA	Moderate DKA	Severe DKA	HHS
Glucose (mg/dl)	>250	>250	>250	>600
Arterial pH	7.25–7.30	7.00 to <7.24	<7.00	>7.30
Serum bicarbonate (mEq/l)	15–18	10 to <15	<10	>18
Urine ketone	Positive	Positive	Positive	Small
Serum ketone	Positive	Positive	Positive	Small
Effective serum osmolality (mOsm/kg)†	Variable	Variable	Variable	>320
Alteration in sensoria	Alert	Alert/drowsy	Stupor/coma	Stupor/coma

†Effective serum osmolality: 2[measured Na^+ (mEq/l)] + glucose (mg/dl)/18.

ence of β-hydroxybutyrate, which is the main ketoacid in DKA.[63] Therefore, this test can underestimate the level of ketosis. Direct measurement of β-hydroxybutyrate is now available by finger-stick method, which is a more accurate indicator of ketoacidosis and response to medical treatment.[64]

The admission serum sodium is usually low because of the osmotic flux of water from the intracellular to the extracellular space in the presence of hyperglycemia. To assess the severity of sodium and water deficit, serum sodium may be corrected by adding 1.6 mg/dl to the measured serum sodium for each 100 mg/dl of glucose >100 mg/dl.[1] An increase in serum sodium concentration in the presence of hyperglycemia indicates a rather profound degree of water loss.

The admission serum potassium concentration usually is elevated in patients with DKA. The mean serum potassium in patients with DKA and HHS was 5.6 mEq/l and 5.7 mEq/l, respectively.[65] These high levels occur because of a shift of potassium from the intracellular to the extracellular space because of acidemia, insulin deficiency, and hypertonicity. Similarly, the admission serum phosphate level may be normal or elevated because of metabolic acidosis.[43]

Patients with DKA frequently present with leukocytosis in the absence of infection.[66] Because most patients with DKA present with abdominal pain, nausea, or vomiting, the potential diagnosis of acute pancreatitis should be considered.[58,59] Hyperamylasemia has been reported in 21 to 79% of patients with DKA; however, there is little correlation between amylase levels and the presence of symptoms in pancreatic imaging studies.[67,68] Nonspecific serum lipase elevation also has been reported in about one-third of patients with DKA in the absence of clinical and radiological evidence of acute pancreatitis.[69]

TREATMENT

Figure 37.2 shows the recommended algorithm suggested by the most recent position statement from the American Diabetes Association for treatment of DKA

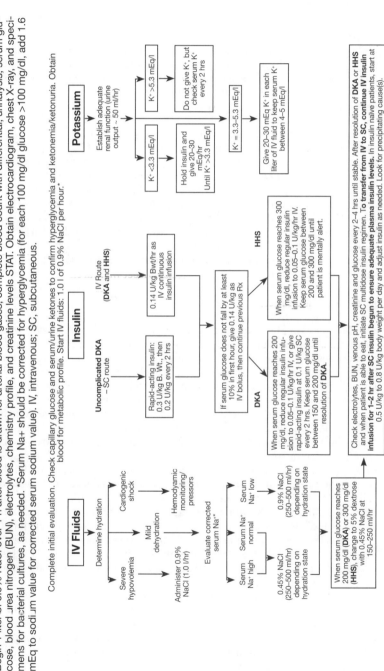

Figure 37.2— Protocol for management of adult patients with DKA or HHS. **DKA diagnostic criteria:** serum glucose >250 mg/dl, arterial pH <7.3, serum bicarbonate <18 mEq/l, and moderate ketonuria or ketonemia. **HHS diagnostic criteria:** serum glucose >600 mg/dl, arterial pH >7.3, serum bicarbonate >15 mEq/l, and minimal ketonuria and ketonemia. Normal laboratory values vary; check local lab normal ranges for all electrolytes. After history and physical exam, obtain capillary glucose and serum or urine ketones (nitroprusside method). Begin 1 liter of 0.9% NaCl over 1 h after blood is drawn for arterial blood gases, complete blood count with differential, urinalysis, serum glucose, blood urea nitrogen (BUN), electrolytes, chemistry profile, and creatinine levels STAT. Obtain electrocardiogram, chest X-ray, and specimens for bacterial cultures, as needed. *Serum Na+ should be corrected for hyperglycemia (for each 100 mg/dl glucose >100 mg/dl, add 1.6 mEq to sodium value for corrected serum sodium value). IV, intravenous; SC, subcutaneous.

and HHS.[1,4] The goals of DKA therapy are *1*) to improve circulatory volume and ultimately tissue perfusion, *2*) to correct hyperglycemia by gradually decreasing serum glucose and plasma osmolality, *3*) to correct electrolyte imbalance and reduce serum and urine ketone bodies to normal, and *4*) to identify and treat precipitating events. Frequent monitoring of vital signs, volume and rate of fluid administration, insulin dosage, and urine output are essential to assess response to medical treatment and to document resolution of hyperglycemia or metabolic acidosis.

In many institutions, patients with DKA are admitted routinely to an intensive care unit (ICU). Several observational and prospective studies, however, have indicated no benefits from treating DKA patients in the ICU compared with step-down units or general medicine wards.[70-72] The mortality rate, length of hospital stay, or time to resolve ketoacidosis are similar between patients treated in ICU and non-ICU settings.[70,72] In addition, ICU admission has been shown to be associated with more testing and significantly higher hospitalization cost in patients with DKA.[70] Thus, the majority of patients with mild to moderate DKA can be safely managed in the emergency department or in step-down units, and only patients with severe DKA, comatose state, or those with a critical illness as precipitating cause (e.g., myocardial infarction, gastrointestinal bleeding, sepsis) should be treated in the ICU.

FLUID THERAPY

Patients with DKA and HHS have severe volume depletion with an estimated water deficit of ~100 ml/kg of body weight.[1] Expansion of extracellular fluid with intravenous (IV) fluids results in significant improvement of hyperglycemia, hypertonicity, and metabolic acidosis led by a decline in counterregulatory hormone levels.[37,56] The severity of dehydration and volume depletion can be estimated by clinical examination and by calculating plasma osmolality.[58,59] An effective plasma osmolality >320 mOsm/kg H_2O is associated with significant fluid deficits.

The initial fluid of choice is isotonic saline (0.9% NaCl) infused at a rate of 500–1,000 ml/hour during the first 2 hours, but in patients with hypovolemic shock, a third or fourth liter of isotonic saline may be needed to restore blood pressure and tissue perfusion. After intravascular volume depletion has been corrected, the rate of normal saline infusion should be reduced or changed to 0.45% saline (250–500 ml/hour) depending on the serum sodium concentration and state of hydration.[4] The choice and rate of subsequent fluid will be based on the patient's sodium concentration and hydration status. The water deficit can be estimated, based on corrected serum sodium concentration, using the following equation: **Water deficit = (0.6)(body weight in kilograms) × (1 – [corrected sodium / 140]).**[1] The goal is to replace half of the estimated water deficit over a period of 24 hours.

During treatment of DKA, hyperglycemia is corrected faster than ketoacidosis. The mean duration of treatment until blood glucose reaches <250 mg/dl and ketoacidosis is corrected is ~6 and 12 hours, respectively.[5,11] Once the plasma glucose is ~250 mg/dl, 5–10% dextrose should be added to the replacement fluids to allow for continued insulin administration until ketoacidosis is resolved, while at the same time avoiding hypoglycemia.[4] An additional important aspect of fluid management is to replace the volume of urinary losses, especially in those subjects with excessive polyuria. Failure to adjust fluid replacement for urinary losses may delay correction of water deficit.[4,26]

INSULIN THERAPY

The cornerstone of DKA management after initial hydration is insulin administration. Insulin increases peripheral glucose utilization and decreases hepatic glucose production, thereby lowering blood glucose concentration. In addition, insulin therapy inhibits the release of free fatty acids from adipose tissue and decreases ketogenesis, both of which lead to the reversal of ketogenesis. In critically ill and mentally obtunded patients, regular insulin given intravenously by continuous infusion is the treatment of choice. Most treatment algorithms have recommended an initial IV bolus of regular insulin at a dose of 0.1 U/kg/hour, followed by continuous infusion of regular insulin at a dose of 0.1 U/kg/hour (5–10 U/hour).[11,74,75] An initial bolus of insulin is not necessary if the hourly insulin infusion rate is 0.14 U/kg body weight.[76] The optimal rate of glucose decrement should be between 50 and 150 mg/hour. Once the serum glucose has declined to ~250 mg/dl an infusion of glucose (D5% 0.45% normal saline) should be started at 150–200 ml/hour, and the insulin infusion rate should be reduced to 0.05 U/kg/hour. Thereafter, the rate of insulin administration may need to be adjusted to maintain glucose levels at ~200 mg/dl and continued until ketoacidosis is resolved.

A patient with uncomplicated DKA can be treated with subcutaneous (SC) rapid-acting insulin analogs. Recent studies have shown that for mild to moderate cases of DKA, the use of SC lispro[70,78] or insulin aspart[79] given every 1 to 2 hours is as effective as the use of regular insulin given intravenously in the ICU. After an initial SC dose of 0.2–0.3 U/kg of lispro or aspart, these analogs can be given in doses of 8–10 units every 2 hours on general medical wards. This is done with the caveat that adequate personnel are available for frequent measuring of blood glucose by finger-stick testing every 2 hours and frequent monitoring of electrolytes and venous pH (every 4–6 hours) with adequate administration of hydrating fluid.

POTASSIUM

Patients with DKA and HHS have total-body potassium deficit of ~3–5 mEq/ kg of body weight.[65] Despite this noted deficit, most patients with DKA have a serum potassium level at or above the upper limits of normal.[80,81] These high levels occur because of a shift of potassium from the intracellular to the extracellular space because of acidemia, insulin deficiency, and hypertonicity. Both insulin therapy and correction of acidosis decrease serum potassium levels by stimulating cellular potassium uptake in peripheral tissues. Therefore, it is important that potassium be monitored carefully during the therapy. IV potassium should be initiated as soon as the serum potassium concentration is <5.0 mEq/l. The treatment goal is to maintain serum potassium levels within the normal range of 4–5 mEq/l.[4] In some hyperglycemic patients admitted with severe potassium deficiency, insulin administration may precipitate profound hypokalemia, which can induce ventricular arrhythmias and respiratory muscle weakness.[82,83] Thus, if the initial serum potassium is <3.3 mEq/l, potassium replacement should begin immediately by an infusion of potassium chloride at a rate of 10–20 mEq/hour, and insulin therapy should be delayed until serum potassium is >3.3 mEq/l.[4,26]

BICARBONATE

Severe metabolic acidosis can lead to impaired myocardial contractility, cerebral vasodilatation and coma, and several gastrointestinal complications,[84,85] but several studies have reported that bicarbonate therapy for DKA offers no advantage in improving clinical outcome or in the rate of recovery of hyperglycemia and ketoacidosis.[86,87] Moreover, several deleterious effects of bicarbonate therapy have been reported, such as increased risk of hypokalemia, decreased tissue oxygen uptake, and cerebral edema.[87–89] Despite that lack of evidence in support of the use of bicarbonate therapy in DKA, clinical guidelines recommend that in patients with severe metabolic acidosis (pH <6.9), 50–100 mmol of sodium bicarbonate should be given as isotonic solution (in 200 ml of water) every 2 hours until pH rises to ~6.9–7.0.[1,4] In patients with arterial pH ≥7.0, no bicarbonate therapy is necessary. There is no indication for bicarbonate treatment in patients with HHS as such patients do not have significant metabolic acidosis. DKA in children usually is not treated with bicarbonate, even when pH is low, as its use has been associated with increased the risk of brain edema.[8,90]

PHOSPHATE

Total body phosphate deficiency is universally present in patients with DKA, but its clinical relevance and benefits of replacement therapy remain uncertain.[91] Severe hypophosphatemia may lead to rhabdomyolysis, hemolytic uremia, muscle weakness, and paralysis,[92] but several studies have failed to show any beneficial effect of phosphate replacement on clinical outcome.[91–93] During insulin therapy and fluid replacement, phosphate reenters the intracellular compartment, leading to mild to moderate reductions in serum phosphate concentrations. Prospective randomized studies have failed to show any beneficial effect of phosphate replacement on the clinical outcome in patients with DKA, and overzealous phosphate therapy can cause severe hypocalcemia. In the presence of severe hypophosphatemia, 20–30 mEq/l of potassium phosphate can be added to replacement fluids.[85]

Patients with DKA and HHS frequently have large magnesium deficits, but there are no data to determine whether replacement of magnesium is beneficial. Replacement of magnesium should be considered in the occasional patient who experiences severe hypomagnesemia and hypocalcemia during therapy.[83] The recommended dose is 25–50 mg/kg per dose for 3–4 doses given every 4–6 hours with a maximum infusion rate of 150 mg/minute and 2 g/hour.

CRITERIA FOR RESOLUTION OF DKA AND HHS

Criteria for resolution of DKA include a blood glucose <200 mg/dl, a serum bicarbonate level ≥18 mEq/l, a pH ≥7.3, and a calculated anion gap ≤14 mEq/l.[4]

The resolution of HHS is indicated when total serum osmolality is <320 mOsm/kg and blood glucose is ≤250 mg/dl with a gradual recovery to mental alertness.

IMMEDIATE FOLLOW-UP CARE AFTER HYPERGLYCEMIC CRISIS

Patients with DKA should be treated with continuous IV insulin until keto-acidosis is resolved. The half-life of regular IV insulin is very short (5–7 minutes); therefore, the IV infusion of insulin must be continued for 2–4 hours after SC insulin is started. A recent study reported that the administration of SC basal insulin early in the course of treatment and several hours before transition prevents rebound hyperglycemia after discontinuation of IV insulin therapy.[94,95]

The best time to transition from SC insulin is once the patient is alert and able to take food by mouth. Patients with DKA who have a previous history of diabetes treated with insulin can be restarted on their previous regimen. Insulin-naïve adult patients with DKA can be started on 0.5–0.7 U/kg/day, in divided doses, to achieve adequate glycemic control.[1,5,31,74] Patients with HHS usually require lower insulin dosage and can be treated at a starting dose between 0.3–0.5 U/kg/day. The American Diabetes Association (ADA) position statement recommends a transition to a multidose regimen of basal and rapid-acting insulin analogs or to split-mixed regimen with neutral protamine Hagedorn (NPH) and regular insulin twice daily.[4] Several observational studies have reported higher rates of hypoglycemic events with the use of NPH and regular insulin during the transition period.[74,96] A recent randomized study compared the safety and efficacy of insulin analogs versus human insulin during the transition from IV to SC insulin in patients with DKA. During the transition to SC insulin, there were no differences in mean daily glucose levels, but 41% of patients treated with NPH and regular insulin had higher rates of hypoglycemia compared with 15% of patients treated with glargine once daily and glulisine before meals.[74] Thus, a basal-bolus regimen with insulin analogs is safer and should be preferred over NPH and regular insulin following the resolution of DKA.

COMPLICATIONS OF THERAPY

The two most common acute complications associated with the treatment of DKA in adult subjects are hypoglycemia and hypokalemia. Hypoglycemia is reported in 10–25% of patients during insulin therapy.[5,24] Hypoglycemic events most commonly occur after several hours of insulin infusion (between 8 and 16 hours) or during the transition phase. The failure to reduce the insulin infusion rate or to use dextrose-containing solutions when glucose levels reach 250 mg/dl are the two most common causes of hypoglycemia during insulin therapy.[5] Because many patients with DKA who develop hypoglycemia during treatment do not experience adrenergic manifestations of sweating, nervousness, fatigue, hunger, and tachycardia, frequent blood glucose monitoring (every 1–2 hours) is mandatory for the early detection of hypoglycemia.

Both insulin therapy and correction of acidosis decrease serum potassium levels by stimulating cellular potassium uptake in peripheral tissues and may lead to hypokalemia.[97] To prevent hypokalemia, initiating replacement with intravenous potassium as soon as the serum potassium concentration is <5.5 mEq/l is recommended. In addition, in patients who present with reduced serum potassium, aggressive IV potassium replacement should begin immediately and insulin therapy should be held until serum potassium is ≥3.3 mEq/l.[98]

Relapse of DKA may occur after sudden interruption of IV insulin therapy or without concomitant use of SC insulin administration or frequent monitoring. To prevent recurrence of ketoacidosis during the transition period to SC insulin, it is important to allow an overlap between discontinuation of IV insulin and the administration of SC insulin. Other complications include hyperchloremic acidosis with an excessive use of NaCl or KCl, resulting in a nonanionic gap metabolic acidosis.[80] This acidosis has no adverse clinical effects and gradually is corrected over the subsequent 24–48 hours by enhanced renal acid excretion. The development of hyperchloremia can be prevented with reduction of the chloride load by judicious use of hydration solutions.[80]

Cerebral edema is a rare complication in adult patients with DKA.[8,96] Symptoms and signs of cerebral edema are variable and include onset of headache, gradual deterioration in level of consciousness, seizures, sphincter incontinence, pupillary changes, papilledema, bradycardia, elevation in blood pressure, and respiratory arrest.[8,9] Cerebral edema typically occurs 4–12 hours after treatment is activated, but it can be present before treatment has begun or may develop any time during treatment for DKA. Although no single factor has been identified that can be used to predict the development of cerebral edema, a number of mechanisms have been proposed, including the role of cerebral ischemia and hypoxia, the generation of various inflammatory mediators, increased cerebral blood flow, disruption of cell membrane ion transport, and rapid shift in extracellular and intracellular fluids resulting in changes in osmolality.[4]

PREVENTION

The majority of DKA and HHS cases occur in patients with known diabetes; therefore, most cases are potentially preventable with proper outpatient treatment programs, patient education, and adherence to self-care.[99,100] The frequency of hospitalizations for DKA has been reduced following diabetes education programs, improved follow-up care, and access to medical advice. Many patients with recurrent DKA are unaware of sick-day management or the consequences of skipping or discontinuing insulin therapy.[101] Quarterly visits to the endocrine clinic will reduce the number of emergency department admissions for DKA. An important feature of patient education is how to deal with illness. This includes *1*) communicating the importance of insulin therapy during illness and emphasizing that insulin should never be discontinued, *2*) early contact with health care providers, *3*) initiation of early management of fevers and infections, and *4*) adequate fluid intake.[1] Patients with diabetes should be instructed on sick-day management, when to contact the health care provider, blood glucose and A1C target, use of supplemental short- or rapid-acting insulin during illness, and, most important, the importance of never discontinuing insulin and of seeking immediate medical attention in the case of severe hyperglycemia. In addition, patients with T1D should be instructed on the use of home ketone monitoring during illness and persistent hyperglycemia, which may allow for early recognition of impending ketoacidosis and the use of intensified insulin therapy, which may prevent hospitalizations.[1,35] A recent study in adolescents reported that an intensive home-based multidisciplinary intervention resulted in a significant decrease in DKA admissions over 2 years.[102] Finally, the alarming rise in insulin discontinuation because of economic reasons as the precipitating cause for DKA in urban patients illustrates the need for health care legislation to ensure reimbursement for medications to treat diabetes. Novel approaches to patient education incorporating a variety of health care beliefs and socioeconomic issues are critical to an effective prevention program.

REFERENCES

1. Kitabchi AE, Umpierrez GE, Murphy MB, Barrett EJ, Kreisberg RA, Malone JI, Wall BM. Management of hyperglycemic crises in patients with diabetes. *Diabetes Care* 2001;24:131–153.

2. Ennis ED, Stahl EJVB, Kreisberg RA. The hyperosmolar hyperglycemic syndrome. *Diabetes Rev* 1994;2:115–126.

3. Centers for Disease Control and Prevention, Department of Health and Human Services. Diabetes data and trends. Crude and age-adjusted hospital discharge rates for diabetic ketoacidosis as first-listed diagnosis per 1,000 diabetic population, United States, 1988–2009. Available at www.cdc.gov/diabetes/statistics/dkafirst/. Accessed January 2013.

4. Kitabchi AE, Umpierrez GE, Miles JM, Fisher JN. Hyperglycemic crises in adult patients with diabetes. *Diabetes Care* 2009;32:1335–1343.

5. Umpierrez GE, Kelly JP, Navarrete JE, Casals MM, Kitabchi AE. Hyperglycemic crises in urban blacks. *Arch Intern Med* 1997;157:669–675.

6. Davis SN, Umpierrez GE. Diabetic ketoacidosis in type 2 diabetes mellitus—pathophysiology and clinical presentation. *Nat Clin Pract Endocrinol Metab* 2007;3:730–731.

7. The EURODIAB IDDM Complications Study Group. Microvascular and acute complications in IDDM patients: the EURODIAB IDDM Complications Study. *Diabetologia* 1994;37:278–285

8. Wolfsdorf J, Craig ME, Daneman D, Dunger D, Edge J, Lee W, Rosenbloom A, Sperling M, Hanas R. Diabetic ketoacidosis in children and adolescents with diabetes. *Pediatr Diabetes* 2009;10(Suppl 12):118–133.

9. Wolfsdorf J, Glaser N, Sperling MA. Diabetic ketoacidosis in infants, children, and adolescents: a consensus statement from the American Diabetes Association. *Diabetes Care* 2006;29:1150–1159.

10. Rewers A, Klingensmith G, Davis C, Petitti DB, Pihoker C, Rodriguez B, Schwartz ID, Imperatore G, Williams D, Dolan LM, Dabelea D. Presence of diabetic ketoacidosis at diagnosis of diabetes mellitus in youth: the Search for Diabetes in Youth study. *Pediatrics* 2008;121:e1258–1266.

11. Randall L, Begovic J, Hudson M, Smiley D, Peng L, Pitre N, Umpierrez D, Umpierrez G. Recurrent diabetic ketoacidosis in inner-city minority patients: behavioral, socioeconomic, and psychosocial factors. *Diabetes Care* 2011;34:1891–1896.

12. Balasubramanyam A, Zern JW, Hyman DJ, Pavlik V. New profiles of diabetic ketoacidosis: type 1 vs type 2 diabetes and the effect of ethnicity. *Arch Intern Med* 1999;159:2317–2322.

13. Cruz-Caudillo JC, Sabatini S. Diabetic hyperosmolar syndrome. *Nephron* 1995;69:201–210.

14. Johnson DD, Palumbo PJ, Chu CP. Diabetic ketoacidosis in a community-based population. *Mayo Clin Proc* 1980;55:83–88.

15. Wachtel TJ, Tetu-Mouradjian LM, Goldman DL, Ellis SE, O'Sullivan PS. Hyperosmolarity and acidosis in diabetes mellitus: a three-year experience in Rhode Island. *J Gen Intern Med* 1991;6:495–502.

16. Fourtner SH, Weinzimer SA, Levitt Katz LE. Hyperglycemic hyperosmolar non-ketotic syndrome in children with type 2 diabetes. *Pediatr Diabetes* 2005;6:129–135.

17. Graves EJ, Gillium BS: Detailed diagnosis and procedures. National Discharge Survey, 1995. National Center for Health Statistics. *Vital Health Stat* 1997;13:1–146

18. Wagner A, Risse A, Brill HL, Wienhausen-Wilke V, Rottmann M, Sondern K, Angelkort B. Therapy of severe diabetic ketoacidosis. Zero-mortality under very-low-dose insulin application. *Diabetes Care* 1999;22:674–677.

19. Fadini GP, de Kreutzenberg SV, Rigato M, Brocco S, Marchesan M, Tiengo A, Avogaro A. Characteristics and outcomes of the hyperglycemic hyperosmolar non-ketotic syndrome in a cohort of 51 consecutive cases at a single center. *Diabet Res Clin Pract* 2011;94:172–179.

20. Kreisberg RA. Diabetic ketoacidosis: an update. *Crit Care Clin* 1987;3:817–834.

21. Basu A, Close CF, Jenkins D, Krentz AJ, Nattrass M, Wright AD. Persisting mortality in diabetic ketoacidosis. *Diabet Med* 1993;10:282–284.

22. Bhowmick SK, Levens KL, Rettig KR. Hyperosmolar hyperglycemic crisis: an acute life-threatening event in children and adolescents with type 2 diabetes mellitus. *Endocr Pract* 2005;11:23–29.

23. Malone ML, Gennis V, Goodwin JS. Characteristics of diabetic ketoacidosis in older versus younger adults. *J Am Geriatr Soc* 1992;40:1100–1104.

24. Fishbein HA, Palumbo PJ. Acute metabolic complications in diabetes. In *Diabetes in America* (NIH publ. no. 95–1468). Bethesda, MD, National Diabetes Data Group, National Institutes of Health, 1995, p. 283–291.

25. White NH. Diabetic ketoacidosis in children. *Endocrinol Metab Clin North Am* 2000;29:657–682.

26. Umpierrez GE, Kitabchi AE. Diabetic ketoacidosis: risk factors and management strategies. *Treat Endocrinol* 2003;2:95–108.

27. Kaufman FR, Halvorson M. The treatment and prevention of diabetic ketoacidosis in children and adolescents with type I diabetes mellitus. *Pediatr Ann* 1999;28:576–582.

28. Ellemann K, Soerensen JN, Pedersen L, Edsberg B, Andersen OO. Epidemiology and treatment of diabetic ketoacidosis in a community population. *Diabetes Care* 1984;7:528–532.

29. Beigelman PM. Severe diabetic ketoacidosis (diabetic "coma"). 482 episodes in 257 patients; experience of three years. *Diabetes* 1971;20:490–500.

30. Delaney MF, Zisman A, Kettyle WM. Diabetic ketoacidosis and hyperglycemic hyperosmolar nonketotic syndrome. *Endocrinol Metab Clin North Am* 2000;29:683–705.

31. McDonnell ME, Umpierrez GE. Insulin therapy for the management of hyperglycemia in hospitalized patients. *Endocrinol Metab Clin North Am* 2012;41:175–201.

32. Jin H, Meyer JM, Jeste DV. Atypical antipsychotics and glucose dysregulation: a systematic review. *Schizophrenia Research* 2004;71:195–212.

33. Allison DB, Mentore JL, Heo M, Chandler LP, Cappelleri JC, Infante MC, Weiden PJ. Antipsychotic-induced weight gain: a comprehensive research synthesis. *Am J Psychiatr* 1999;156:1686–1696.

34. Guenette MD, Hahn M, Cohn TA, Teo C, Remington GJ. Atypical antipsychotics and diabetic ketoacidosis: a review. *Psychopharmacology* 2013;226:1–12.

35. MacGillivray MH, Li PK, Lee JT, Mills BJ, Voorhess ML, Putnam TI, Schaefer PA. Elevated plasma beta-hydroxybutyrate concentrations without ketonuria in healthy insulin-dependent diabetic patients. *J Clin Endocrinol Metab* 1982;54:665–668.

36. Musey VC, Lee JK, Crawford R, Klatka MA, McAdams D, Phillips LS. Diabetes in urban African-Americans. I. Cessation of insulin therapy is the major precipitating cause of diabetic ketoacidosis. *Diabetes Care* 1995;18:483–489.

37. Maldonado MR, Chong ER, Oehl MA, Balasubramanyam A. Economic impact of diabetic ketoacidosis in a multiethnic indigent population: analysis of costs based on the precipitating cause. *Diabetes Care* 2003;26:1265–1269.

38. Polonsky WH, Anderson BJ, Lohrer PA, Aponte JE, Jacobson AM, Cole CF. Insulin omission in women with IDDM. *Diabetes Care* 1994;17:1178–1185.

39. Rewers A. Current concepts and controversies in prevention and treatment of diabetic ketoacidosis in children. *Curr Diabetes Rep* 2012;12:524–532.

40. Phillips PA, Rolls BJ, Ledingham JG, Forsling ML, Morton JJ, Crowe MJ, Wollner L. Reduced thirst after water deprivation in healthy elderly men. *N Engl J Med* 1984;311:753–759.

41. Wachtel TJ. The diabetic hyperosmolar state. *Clin Geriatr Med* 1990;6:797–806.

42. Foster DW, McGarry JD. The metabolic derangements and treatment of diabetic ketoacidosis. *N Engl J Med* 1983;309:159–169.

43. DeFronzo RA, Matzuda M, Barret E. Diabetic ketoacidosis: a combined metabolic-nephrologic approach to therapy. *Diabetes Rev* 1994;2:209–238.

44. Gerich JE, Lorenzi M, Bier DM, Tsalikian E, Schneider V, Karam JH, Forsham PH. Effects of physiologic levels of glucagon and growth hormone on human carbohydrate and lipid metabolism. Studies involving administration of exogenous hormone during suppression of endogenous hormone secretion with somatostatin. *J Clin Invest* 1976;57:875–884.

45. Exton JH. Mechanisms of hormonal regulation of hepatic glucose metabolism. *Diabetes Metab Rev* 1987;3:163–183.

46. Felig P, Sherwin RS, Soman V, Wahren J, Hendler R, Sacca L, Eigler N, Goldberg D, Walesky M. Hormonal interactions in the regulation of blood glucose. *Recent Prog Horm Res* 1979;35:501–532.

47. van de Werve G, Jeanrenaud B. Liver glycogen metabolism: an overview. *Diabetes Metab Rev* 1987;3:47–78.

48. McGarry JD. Lilly Lecture 1978. New perspectives in the regulation of ketogenesis. *Diabetes* 1979;28:517–523.

49. McGarry JD, Foster DW. Regulation of hepatic fatty acid oxidation and ketone body production. *Annu Rev Biochem* 1980;49:395–420.

50. Miles JM, Haymond MW, Nissen SL, Gerich JE. Effects of free fatty acid availability, glucagon excess, and insulin deficiency on ketone body production in postabsorptive man. *J Clin Invest* 1983;71:1554–1561.

51. McGarry JD, Woeltje KF, Kuwajima M, Foster DW. Regulation of ketogenesis and the renaissance of carnitine palmitoyltransferase. *Diabetes Metab Rev* 1989;5:271–284.

52. Gerich JE, Martin MM, Recant L. Clinical and metabolic characteristics of hyperosmolar nonketotic coma. *Diabetes* 1971;20:228–238.

53. Chupin M, Charbonnel B, Chupin F. C-peptide blood levels in keto-acidosis and in hyperosmolar non-ketotic diabetic coma. *Acta Diabetol Lat* 1981;18:123–128.

54. Chaudhuri A, Umpierrez GE. Oxidative stress and inflammation in hyperglycemic crises and resolution with insulin: implications for the acute and chronic complications of hyperglycemia. *J Diabetes Complications* 2012;26:257–258.

55. Stentz FB, Umpierrez GE, Cuervo R, Kitabchi AE. Proinflammatory cytokines, markers of cardiovascular risks, oxidative stress, and lipid peroxidation in patients with hyperglycemic crises. *Diabetes* 2004;53:2079–2086.

56. Hoffman WH, Burek CL, Waller JL, Fisher LE, Khichi M, Mellick LB. Cytokine response to diabetic ketoacidosis and its treatment. *Clin Immunol* 2003;108:175–181.

57. Shen XP, Li J, Zou S, Wu HJ, Zhang Y. The relationship between oxidative stress and the levels of serum circulating adhesion molecules in patients with hyperglycemia crises. *J Diabetes Complications* 2012;26:291–295.

58. Umpierrez G, Freire AX. Abdominal pain in patients with hyperglycemic crises. *J Crit Care* 2002;17:63–67.

59. Pant N, Kadaria D, Murillo LC, Yataco JC, Headley AS, Freire AX. Abdominal pathology in patients with diabetes ketoacidosis. *Am J Med Sci* 2012;344:341–344.

60. Kitabchi AE, Wall BM. Diabetic ketoacidosis. *Med Clin North Am* 1995;79:9–37.

61. Harden CL, Rosenbaum DH, Daras M. Hyperglycemia presenting with occipital seizures. *Epilepsia* 1991;32:215–220.

62. Maccario M. Neurological dysfunction associated with nonketotic hyperglycemia. *Archives of Neurology* 1968;19:525–534.

63. Stephens JM, Sulway MJ, Watkins PJ. Relationship of blood acetoacetate and 3-hydroxybutyrate in diabetes. *Diabetes* 1971;20:485–489.

64. Sheikh-Ali M, Karon BS, Basu A, Kudva YC, Muller LA, Xu J, Schwenk WF, Miles JM. Can serum beta-hydroxybutyrate be used to diagnose diabetic ketoacidosis? *Diabetes Care* 2008;31:643–647.

65. Adrogue HJ, Lederer ED, Suki WN, Eknoyan G. Determinants of plasma potassium levels in diabetic ketoacidosis. *Medicine* 1986;65:163–172.

66. Flood RG, Chiang VW. Rate and prediction of infection in children with diabetic ketoacidosis. *Am J Emerg Med* 2001;19:270–273.

67. Vinicor F, Lehrner LM, Karn RC, Merritt AD. Hyperamylasemia in diabetic ketoacidosis: sources and significance. *Ann Intern Med* 1979;91:200–204.

68. Vantyghem MC, Haye S, Balduyck M, Hober C, Degand PM, Lefebvre J. Changes in serum amylase, lipase and leukocyte elastase during diabetic ketoacidosis and poorly controlled diabetes. *Acta Diabetologica* 1999;36:39–44.

69. Nair S, Yadav D, Pitchumoni CS. Association of diabetic ketoacidosis and acute pancreatitis: observations in 100 consecutive episodes of DKA. *Am J Gastroenterol* 2000;95:2795–2800.

70. Freire AX, Umpierrez GE, Afessa B, Latif KA, Bridges L, Kitabchi AE. Predictors of intensive care unit and hospital length of stay in diabetic ketoacidosis. *J Crit Care* 2002;17:207–211.

71. Moss JM. Diabetic ketoacidosis: effective low-cost treatment in a community hospital. *South Med J* 1987;80:875–881.

72. May ME, Young C, King J. Resource utilization in treatment of diabetic ketoacidosis in adults. *Am J Med Sci* 1993;306:287–294.

73. Umpierrez GE, Isaacs SD, Bazargan N, You X, Thaler LM, Kitabchi AE. Hyperglycemia: an independent marker of in-hospital mortality in patients with undiagnosed diabetes. *J Clin Endocrinol Metab* 2002;87:978–982.

74. Umpierrez GE, Jones S, Smiley D, Mulligan P, Keyler T, Temponi A, Semakula C, Umpierrez D, Peng L, Ceron M, Robalino G. Insulin analogs versus human insulin in the treatment of patients with diabetic ketoacidosis: a randomized controlled trial. *Diabetes Care* 2009;32:1164–1169.

75. Kitabchi AE, Umpierrez GE, Fisher JN, Murphy MB, Stentz FB. Thirty years of personal experience in hyperglycemic crises: diabetic ketoacidosis and hyperglycemic hyperosmolar state. *J Clin Endocrinol Metab* 2008;93: 1541–1552.

76. Kitabchi AE, Murphy MB, Spencer J, Matteri R, Karas J. Is a priming dose of insulin necessary in a low-dose insulin protocol for the treatment of diabetic ketoacidosis? *Diabetes Care* 2008;31:2081–2085.

77. Umpierrez GE, Latif K, Stoever J, Cuervo R, Park L, Freire AX, Kitabchi AE. Efficacy of subcutaneous insulin lispro versus continuous intravenous regular insulin for the treatment of patients with diabetic ketoacidosis. *Am J Med* 2004;117:291–296.

78. Della Manna T, Steinmetz L, Campos PR, Farhat SC, Schvartsman C, Kuperman H, Setian N, Damiani D. Subcutaneous use of a fast-acting insulin analog: an alternative treatment for pediatric patients with diabetic ketoacidosis. *Diabetes Care* 2005;28:1856–1861.

79. Umpierrez GE, Latif KA, Cuervo R, Karabell A, Freire AX, Kitabchi AE. Treatment of diabetic ketoacidosis with subcutaneous insulin aspart. *Diabetes Care* 2004;27(8):1873–1878.

80. Adrogue HJ, Wilson H, Boyd AE, 3rd, Suki WN, Eknoyan G. Plasma acid-base patterns in diabetic ketoacidosis. *N Engl J Med* 1982;307:1603–1610.

81. Arora S, Cheng D, Wyler B, Menchine M. Prevalence of hypokalemia in ED patients with diabetic ketoacidosis. *Am J Emerg Med* 2012;30:481–484.

82. Abramson E, Arky R. Diabetic acidosis with initial hypokalemia. Therapeutic implications. *JAMA* 1966;196:401–403.

83. Matz R. Risk of hypokalemia developing during the therapy of DKA. *J Diabetes Complications* 1995;9:130–131.

84. Mitchell JH, Wildenthal K, Johnson RL Jr. The effects of acid-base disturbances on cardiovascular and pulmonary function. *Kidney Int* 1972;1:375–389.

85. Housley E, Clarke SW, Hedworth-Whitty RB, Bishop JM. Effect of acute and chronic acidaemia and associated hypoxia on the pulmonary circulation of patients with chronic bronchitis. *Cardiovasc Res* 1970;4:482–489.

86. Soler NG, Bennett MA, Dixon K, FitzGerald MG, Malins JM. Potassium balance during treatment of diabetic ketoacidosis with special reference to the use of bicarbonate. *Lancet* 1972;2:665–667.

87. Morris LR, Murphy MB, Kitabchi AE. Bicarbonate therapy in severe diabetic ketoacidosis. *Ann Intern Med* 1986;105:836–840.

88. Lever E, Jaspan JB. Sodium bicarbonate therapy in severe diabetic ketoacidosis. *Am J Med* 1983;75:263–268.

89. Rose KL, Pin CL, Wang R, Fraser DD. Combined insulin and bicarbonate therapy elicits cerebral edema in a juvenile mouse model of diabetic ketoacidosis. *Pediatr Res* 2007;61:301–306.

90. Edge JA, Jakes RW, Roy Y, Hawkins M, Winter D, Ford-Adams ME, Murphy NP, Bergomi A, Widmer B, Dunger DB. The UK case-control study of cerebral oedema complicating diabetic ketoacidosis in children. *Diabetologia* 2006;49:2002–2009.

91. Shen T, Braude S. Changes in serum phosphate during treatment of diabetic ketoacidosis: predictive significance of severity of acidosis on presentation. *Int Med J* 2012;42:1347–1350.

92. Miller DW, Slovis CM. Hypophosphatemia in the emergency department therapeutics. *Am J Emerg Med* 2000;18:457–461.

93. Fisher JN, Kitabchi AE. A randomized study of phosphate therapy in the treatment of diabetic ketoacidosis. *J Clin Endocrinol Metab* 1983;57:177–180.

94. Hsia E, Seggelke S, Gibbs J, Hawkins RM, Cohlmia E, Rasouli N, Wang C, Kam I, Draznin B. Subcutaneous administration of glargine to diabetic patients receiving insulin infusion prevents rebound hyperglycemia. *J Clin Endocrinol Metab* 2012;97:3132–3137.

95. Shankar V, Haque A, Churchwell KB, Russell W. Insulin glargine supplementation during early management phase of diabetic ketoacidosis in children. *Intens Care Med* 2007;33:1173–1178.

96. Rosenbloom AL. Hyperglycemic crises and their complications in children. *J Pediatr Endocrinol Metab* 2007;20:5–18.

97. Sacks HS, Shahshahani M, Kitabchi AE, Fisher JN, Young RT. Similar responsiveness of diabetic ketoacidosis to low-dose insulin by intramuscular injection and albumin-free infusion. *Ann Intern Med* 1979;90:36–42.

98. Kitabchi AE, Umpierrez GE, Murphy MB, Barrett EJ, Kreisberg RA, Malone JI, Wall BM. Hyperglycemic crises in patients with diabetes mellitus. *Diabetes Care* 2003;26(Suppl 1):S109–117.

99. Umpierrez GE, Murphy MB, Kitabchi AE. Diabetic ketoacidosis and hyperglycemic hyperosmolar syndrome. *Diabetes Spectrum* 2002;15:28–36.

100. Laffel LM, Brackett J, Ho J, Anderson BJ. Changing the process of diabetes care improves metabolic outcomes and reduces hospitalizations. *Qual Manag Health Care* 1998;6:53–62.

101. Laffel L. Sick-day management in type 1 diabetes. *Endocrinol Metab Clin North Am* 2000;29:707–723.

102. Ellis D, Naar-King S, Templin T, Frey M, Cunningham P, Sheidow A, Cakan N, Idalski A. Multisystemic therapy for adolescents with poorly controlled type 1 diabetes: reduced diabetic ketoacidosis admissions and related costs over 24 months. *Diabetes Care* 2008;31:1746–1747.

Chapter 38

Diabetic Ketoacidosis in Infants, Children, and Adolescents

Joseph I. Wolfsdorf, MB, BCh

INTRODUCTION

Diabetic ketoacidosis (DKA) is a clinical syndrome resulting from severe insulin deficiency, increased levels of counterregulatory hormones, and proinflammatory cytokines that impair insulin action. The fundamental pathophysiology of this potentially life-threatening complication is the same as in adults (for details, see Chapter 37, Diabetic Ketoacidosis and Hyperglycemic Hyperosmolar State in Adults); however, there are also several important differences between children and adults. The younger the child, the more difficult it is to obtain the classical history of polyuria, polydipsia, and weight loss. Infants and toddlers in DKA are frequently misdiagnosed as having pneumonia, reactive airways disease (asthma), or bronchiolitis, and they receive treatment with glucocorticoids or sympathomimetic agents, which compound and exacerbate the metabolic derangements.

EPIDEMIOLOGY

Because the diagnosis of diabetes often is not suspected, 15–70% of all newly diagnosed infants and children with diabetes present with DKA. Worldwide incidence rates correlate with the regional incidence of type 1 diabetes (T1D). DKA at diagnosis is more common in younger children (<5 years of age) and in children whose families do not have ready access to medical care for social or economic reasons.[1-4] Lower income and lower parental education achievement are associated with higher risk of DKA. Lack of health insurance also is associated with higher rates (and greater severity) of DKA at diagnosis, presumably because uninsured patients delay seeking timely medical care.[4] In the U.S., the overall rates of DKA at diagnosis are ~29.4–34%[5,6] and have not changed appreciably over the past 25 years. Rates of DKA at diabetes onset are higher in the U.S. than in other industrialized countries—for example, Canada, Finland, and Germany—where rates are 18.6%, 19.4%, and 21.1%, respectively.[7-9]

The risk of DKA in children and adolescents with established T1D ranges from 1 to 10 per 100 person-years.[2,10-13] Among 13,005 participants in the Type 1 Diabetes Exchange Registry, 9.9% reported at least one episode of DKA within the preceding 12 months.[14] Risk is increased in children with poor metabolic control or previous episodes of DKA; peripubertal and adolescent girls; children with clinical depression or other psychiatric disorders, including those with eating disorders; children with dysfunctional families or unstable family circumstances (e.g.,

DOI: 10.2337/9781580405096.38

parental abuse); and children with limited access to medical services.[2,13] Whereas delay in diagnosis is the major cause of DKA in previously unrecognized disease, especially in younger children,[7,15,16] omission of insulin or unrecognized failure to deliver insulin (e.g., as a result of pump failure or cannula occlusion) is the leading cause of recurrent DKA, which is most prevalent among adolescents. In one recent study, 6% of patients accounted for 27% of all admissions for DKA. [17] In most cases, insulin omission occurs for psychosocial reasons. An intercurrent infection is seldom the cause when the patient or family is educated properly in diabetes management, is receiving appropriate follow-up care, and has 24-hour telephone access to a diabetes care team.[18–21]

For reasons still incompletely understood, young children with severe DKA, in contrast to adults, are at increased risk of cerebral edema, which is the most common cause of mortality in children with DKA. Clinically significant cerebral edema occurs in ~0.5–1% of all episodes of DKA in children.[22–25] Only a small fraction of deaths in DKA are attributable to other causes, such as sepsis, or other infections, such as mucormycosis, aspiration pneumonia, pulmonary edema, acute respiratory distress syndrome (ARDS), pneumomediastinum, hypo- or hyperkalemia, cardiac arrhythmias, cerebrovascular thrombosis, and rhabdomyolysis.

The reported mortality rates in children with DKA are constant in national population-based studies, varying from ~0.15–0.3%. Once cerebral edema develops, death occurs in 20–25% of cases, and significant morbidity occurs in 10–25% of survivors. In cases in which medical services are less well developed, the risk of dying from DKA is significantly greater, and children may die before receiving treatment. Overall, cerebral edema accounts for ~60–90% of all DKA-related deaths in children.[22,24]

DEFINITION OF DKA

Biochemical criteria for the diagnosis of DKA adopted by the European Society of Pediatric Endocrinology and the Pediatric Endocrine Society include the following:[26]

■ Hyperglycemia (plasma glucose >200 mg/dl)
■ Venous pH <7.3 or bicarbonate <15 mmol/l
■ Ketonemia or ketonuria

A recent comparison of pH and serum bicarbonate concentrations in 300 children with DKA showed that a serum bicarbonate concentration ≤18.5 mmol/l predicts a pH <7.3.[27] Therefore, a serum bicarbonate concentration of <15 mmol/l is a conservative criterion for acidosis.

The severity of DKA is defined by the degree of acidosis: mild, venous pH 7.2–7.3 or bicarbonate <15 mmol/l; moderate, pH 7.1–7.2 or bicarbonate <10 mmol/l; severe, pH <7.1 or bicarbonate <5 mmol/l.[28]

Hyperglycemic hyperosmolar state (HHS), characterized by extreme elevations in serum glucose concentrations and hyperosmolality without significant ketosis, may occur in young patients with type 2 diabetes (T2D). Recent reports suggest an increasing incidence of this disorder in children and adolescents (see Zeitler et al. for a recent review of this topic).[29] Criteria for the diagnosis of HHS include the following:

- Plasma glucose >600 mg/dl
- Serum osmolality >330 mOsm/kg
- No significant ketosis and acidosis (serum bicarbonate >15 mmol/l; urine ketone concentration <15 mg/dl; negative or trace ketonuria)

Features of both HHS and DKA may occur in the same patient, and some patients with HHS, especially those with severe dehydration, experience mild or moderate (lactic) acidosis. Children with T1D who have consumed high carbohydrate–containing beverages to quench their thirst may present with extreme hyperglycemia.[30] Therapy must be appropriately modified to address the unique pathophysiologic and biochemical disturbances of each patient.[28]

PATHOPHYSIOLOGY

The pathophysiology of DKA in children is summarized in Figure 38.1. Absolute insulin deficiency occurs in patients previously undiagnosed with T1D and when established patients deliberately or inadvertently do not take insulin, especially the long-acting component of a basal-bolus regimen.[31] Patients who use an insulin pump can rapidly develop DKA when insulin delivery fails for any reason.[13] Relative insulin deficiency occurs when physiologic stress (e.g., sepsis, trauma, gastrointestinal illness with diarrhea and vomiting) causes an increased concentration of counterregulatory hormones.

Severe insulin deficiency and increased counterregulatory hormone concentrations cause increased glucose production from glycogenolysis and gluconeogenesis while limiting glucose utilization, resulting in hyperglycemia, osmotic diuresis, electrolyte loss, dehydration, decreased glomerular filtration, and hyper-

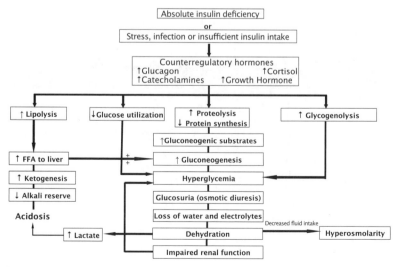

Figure 38.1 — Pathophysiology of Diabetic Ketoacidosis

osmolarity. Lipolysis increases free fatty acid levels and β-oxidation in the liver facilitates gluconeogenesis and generates acetoacetic and β-hydroxybutyric acids (ketones), which overwhelm the body's buffering capacity resulting in metabolic acidosis. Poor tissue perfusion or sepsis may cause lactic acidosis. Progressive dehydration, hyperosmolarity, acidosis, and electrolyte disturbances further stimulate stress hormone secretion, which leads to progressive metabolic decompensation.[32]

CLINICAL MANIFESTATIONS

The clinical manifestations of DKA include polyuria, polydipsia, signs of dehydration, Kussmaul breathing (rapid deep, sighing respirations to eliminate carbon dioxide in response to metabolic acidosis), and progressive obtundation leading to coma. Water and electrolytes are lost from both the intra- and extracellular fluid compartments; usual losses are shown in Table 38.1. Despite dehydration, patients maintain normal blood pressure and children with severe DKA may have mild hypertension.[33] Urine output occurs until extreme volume depletion leads to a critical decrease in renal blood flow and glomerular filtration. The magnitude of specific deficits in an individual patient varies depending on the duration and severity of illness, the extent to which the patient was able to maintain intake of fluid and electrolytes, and the content of food and fluids consumed before coming to medical attention.[32] Consumption of juices or sugar-containing soft drinks with a high carbohydrate content exacerbates hyperglycemia and patients may present with extreme hyperglycemia and hyperosmolality.[30]

Table 38.1 Usual Losses of Fluids and Electrolytes in DKA and Maintenance Requirements in Children

	Average (range) losses per kg	24-hour maintenance requirements
Water	70 ml (30–100)	**≤10 kg:** 100 ml/kg/24 hours **11–20 kg:** 1,000 ml + 50 ml/kg/24 hours for each kg from 11–20 **>20 kg:** 1,500 ml + 20 ml/kg/24 hours for each kg >20
Sodium	6 mmol (5–13)	2–4 mmol†
Potassium	5 mmol (3–6)	2–3 mmol
Chloride	4 mmol (3–9)	2–3 mmol
Phosphate	(0.5–2.5) mmol	1–2 mmol*

Note: Data are from measurements in only a few children and adolescents.[77–79,152,153] In any individual patient, actual losses may be less or greater than the ranges.
†per 100 mL of maintenance fluid.

*Ref. 154

Patients with DKA usually have a fluid volume deficit ranging from ~4 to 10%. The severity of dehydration typically is more severe in patients with mixed DKA and HHS.[29] Children ≤2 years of age often are more dehydrated than older children; however, shock is rare in pediatric DKA. Clinical estimates of the volume deficit are subjective and the magnitude of dehydration cannot be assessed accurately by either clinical or biochemical parameters.[34,35] Additional clinical manifestations of DKA include nausea, vomiting, and abdominal pain that may mimic an acute abdomen; progressive obtundation and loss of consciousness; increased leukocyte count with left shift; and nonspecific elevation of serum amylase. Fever is not a manifestation of DKA and indicates there is an infection.

PRESENTATION: DIFFERENTIAL DIAGNOSIS

Starvation ketosis and alcoholic ketoacidosis are distinguished by clinical history and plasma glucose concentrations ranging from hypoglycemia in the former to mildly increased (but rarely >200 mg/dl) in the latter condition.[36] DKA also must be distinguished from other causes of increased anion gap metabolic acidosis, including lactic acidosis and ingestion of drugs and toxins, such as salicylate, methanol, ethylene glycol, and paraldehyde. These low-molecular-weight organic compounds can produce an osmolar gap in addition to an anion gap acidosis.[37] In infancy, rare inborn errors of metabolism, such as propionic acidemia,[38] the chronic intermittent form of isovaleric acidemia,[39] and defects of ketolysis (succinyl-CoA 3-oxoacid CoA transferase deficiency and mitochondrial acetoacetyl-CoA thiolase deficiency), present with recurrent episodes of severe ketoacidosis. They usually are accompanied by normoglycemia or hypoglycemia, but in older children, hyperglycemia mimicking DKA occurs rarely.[40,41]

MANAGEMENT OF DKA

EMERGENCY ASSESSMENT

The following emergency assessment of DKA should be made:

- Immediately measure blood glucose and, if possible, β-hydroxybutyrate (BOHB) concentrations with bedside meters. Measurement of blood BOHB concentration with a point-of-care meter is useful to confirm ketoacidosis (≥3 mmol/l in children)[42] and to monitor the response to treatment.[43–45]
- Perform a clinical evaluation to identify a possible infection. In recurrent DKA, insulin omission or failure to follow sick-day or pump failure management guidelines accounts for most episodes.
- Weigh the patient (if body surface area is used for fluid therapy calculations, measure height or length to determine surface area) and use this weight for calculations and not the weight from a previous office visit or hospital record.
- Look for acanthosis nigricans suggesting insulin resistance and T2D.
- Clinical assessment of dehydration is inaccurate and generally shows only fair to moderate agreement among examiners. The three most useful signs

for assessing dehydration in young children and predicting at least 5% dehydration and acidosis are as follows:
- Prolonged capillary refill time (normal is ≤1.5–2 seconds)
- Abnormal skin turgor (tenting or inelastic skin)
- Hyperpnea

Other useful signs include dry mucous membranes, sunken eyes, absent tears, weak pulses, and cool extremities; more signs of dehydration tend to be associated with more severe dehydration.

- >10% dehydration is suggested by weak or impalpable peripheral pulses, hypotension, and oliguria.
- Assess level of consciousness (Glasgow coma scale).[46,47]
- Obtain a blood sample for laboratory measurement of serum or plasma glucose, electrolytes (including bicarbonate or total carbon dioxide [TCO_2]), urea nitrogen, creatinine, serum osmolality, venous (arterial only in critically ill patient) pH, PCO_2, hemoglobin and hematocrit or complete blood count (an increased white blood cell count in response to stress is characteristic of DKA and is not indicative of infection[18]), calcium, phosphorus, and magnesium concentrations, blood BOHB concentration,[43–45,48] and A1C.
- Perform a urinalysis for ketones; in severely dehydrated patients, the first void may occur only several hours after presentation.
- If there is evidence of infection (fever), obtain appropriate specimens for culture (blood, urine, throat).
- If laboratory measurement of serum potassium is delayed, perform an electrocardiogram for baseline evaluation of potassium status.[49,50]

SUPPORTIVE MEASURES

The following supportive measures should be taken:

- In the unconscious or severely obtunded patient, secure the airway and empty the stomach by continuous nasogastric suction to prevent pulmonary aspiration.
- A peripheral intravenous (IV) catheter should be placed for blood sampling.
- Use continuous electrocardiographic monitoring to assess T waves for evidence of hyper- or hypokalemia and monitor for arrhythmias.[49,50]
- Give oxygen to patients with air hunger, severe circulatory impairment, or shock.
- Give antibiotics to febrile patients after obtaining appropriate cultures of body fluids.
- Bladder catheterization usually is not necessary, but if the child is unconscious or unable to void on demand (e.g., infants and very ill young children), catheterize the bladder.
- Central venous pressure monitoring rarely may be required to guide fluid management in the critically ill, obtunded, or neurologically compromised patient. Central lines in children with DKA frequently are associated with thrombosis and should be used only when absolutely necessary.

WHERE SHOULD THE CHILD BE MANAGED?

The child should receive care in a unit that has the following resources:

- Experienced nursing staff trained in monitoring and management.
- Access to a laboratory that can provide frequent and timely measurements of biochemical variables.
- A specialist with expertise in the management of DKA should direct management.
- Written guidelines for DKA management in children.
- Children with severe DKA (long duration of symptoms, compromised circulation, or depressed level of consciousness) or those who are at increased risk for cerebral edema (e.g., <5 years of age, low PCO_2, high urea nitrogen concentration) should be treated in a pediatric intensive care unit.[51]

CLINICAL AND BIOCHEMICAL MONITORING

Management of DKA and HHS requires meticulous monitoring of the clinical and biochemical response to treatment so that timely adjustments in treatment can be made when indicated.[32]

Monitoring and documentation on a flow chart should include the following:

- Hourly (or more frequently as indicated) vital signs (heart rate, respiratory rate, blood pressure).
- Hourly (or more frequently as indicated) neurological observations for warning signs and symptoms of cerebral edema (see following signs and symptoms suggestive of cerebral edema).
- Noninvasive end-tidal CO_2 monitoring (capnography) is a valuable and reliable tool to continuously monitor acidosis in pediatric patients with DKA. Continuous end-total CO_2 monitoring supplements data obtained from intermittent blood gas determinations and provides early warning of unexpected changes in acidosis.[52]
- Amount of administered insulin.
- Hourly (or more frequently if indicated) fluid input and output.
- Capillary blood glucose concentration should be measured hourly (but must be cross-checked against laboratory venous plasma glucose measurements because capillary methods may be inaccurate in the presence of poor peripheral circulation and acidosis).
- Laboratory tests: serum electrolytes, glucose, calcium, magnesium, phosphorus, and blood gases should be repeated every 2–4 hours, or more frequently, as clinically indicated, in more severe cases; blood urea nitrogen, creatinine, and hematocrit should be repeated at 6- to 8-hour intervals until they are normal.
- Bedside measurement of blood βOHB concentrations every 2–4 hours, if available
- Urine ketones until cleared.
- If the laboratory cannot provide timely results, a portable biochemical analyzer that measures plasma glucose, serum electrolytes, and blood ketones

on finger-stick blood samples at the bedside is a useful adjunct to laboratory-based determinations.

■ Calculations:
  • Anion gap = Na – (Cl + HCO_3 or TCO_2): normal is 12 ± 2 mmol/l
  • Corrected sodium = measured Na + 0.02 × (plasma glucose mg/dl)
  • Effective osmolality = 2 × (Na) + glucose mmol/l (mg/dl ÷ 18)

MANAGEMENT

The goals of therapy are as follows:

■ Slowly correct dehydration.
■ Correct acidosis and reverse ketosis.
■ Restore blood glucose to near normal.
■ Monitor for complications of DKA and its treatment.
■ Identify and treat any precipitating event.

VOLUME EXPANSION: FLUID AND SALT REPLACEMENT

Fluid replacement alone will reverse many of the clinical and biochemical derangements of DKA.[53] The principles described in the following paragraphs have been accepted and endorsed by a panel of expert physicians representing the Pediatric Endocrine Society, the European Society for Paediatric Endocrinology, and the International Society for Pediatric and Adolescent Diabetes.[51].

Begin fluid replacement before starting insulin therapy. If needed to restore peripheral circulation, volume expansion (resuscitation) should begin immediately with 0.9% saline. The volume and rate of fluid administration depends on circulatory status. The volume administered typically is 10–20 ml/kg over 1–2 hours and may be repeated if necessary. Assume 5–7% dehydration in moderate DKA, and 10% dehydration in severe DKA. Subsequent fluid administration should aim to rehydrate evenly over 48 hours at a rate seldom >1.5–2 times the usual daily maintenance requirement, beginning with 0.9% saline for at least 4–6 hours. Thereafter, deficit replacement should be with a solution that has a tonicity at least ≥0.45% saline with added potassium (see the following section Potassium).[54–58] See Table 38.2 for an example.

Calculation of effective osmolality is a valuable guide to fluid and electrolyte therapy. Urinary losses should not be added routinely to the calculation of replacement fluid. This may be necessary, however, in the profoundly dehydrated patient with mixed DKA and HHS.[29] It is important to calculate the corrected sodium (previous formula) and monitor its changes throughout the course of therapy. As the plasma glucose concentration decreases after administering fluid and insulin, the measured and corrected serum sodium concentration should increase appropriately. The sodium content of the fluid may need to be increased if the measured serum sodium concentration is low and does not rise appropriately as the plasma glucose concentration falls.[55,59] Hyperchloremic metabolic acidosis from large volumes of 0.9% saline is a frequent complication of treatment.[60,61]

Table 38.2 Fluid and Electrolyte Replacement for a Child (30 kg, 1 m²) with Severe DKA Estimated to be 10% Dehydrated

Approximate duration and rate	Fluid composition and volume	Sodium mEq	Potassium mEq	Chloride mEq	Phosphate mmol
Hour 1 (300 ml/hour)	300 ml 0.9% NaCl (normal saline)	46	-	46	-
Hours 2–4 (125 ml/hour) Start regular insulin at 0.1 U/kg/hour	375 ml (normal saline) + 20 mEq K acetate/l + 20 mEq K phosphate/l	58	15	58	5.1
Hours 5–48 (125 ml/hour) Continue regular insulin 0.1 U/kg/hour until pH ≥7.3, anion gap 12±2 or HCO₃ ≥15 mEq/l	5,500 ml (1/2 normal saline + dextrose) +20 mEq K acetate/l + 20 mEq K phosphate/l	424	220	424	75
Total in 48 hours	6,175 ml fluid	528	235	528	80

Normal saline 10 ml/kg is given over 1 hour for initial volume expansion; thereafter, the child is rehydrated over 48 hours at an even rate at two times the maintenance rate of fluid requirement. Potassium phosphate 4.4 mEq potassium and 3 mmol phosphate (1 mEq K and 0.68 mmol phosphate).

INSULIN

Although rehydration alone causes a significant decrease in blood glucose concentration,[53,62] insulin therapy is essential to normalize blood glucose, suppress lipolysis and ketogenesis, and reverse acidosis.[63] Prospective data from randomized trials in pediatric DKA are almost nonexistent;[64] nonetheless, extensive evidence indicates that low-dose IV insulin administration is safe and effective.[65]

IV insulin infusion should commence 1–2 hours after starting fluid replacement therapy (i.e., after the patient has received initial volume expansion).[66] A commonly recommended starting dose is 0.1 U/kg/hour (dilute 50 units regular [soluble] insulin in 50 ml normal saline, 1 unit = 1 ml).[65] An IV priming dose or bolus is unnecessary,[67] may increase the risk of cerebral edema,[66] and should *not* be used at the start of therapy. The dose of insulin usually should remain in the range of 0.05–0.1 U/kg/hour until resolution of DKA (pH >7.30, anion gap normal, bicarbonate >15 mmol/l, BOHB <1 mmol/l), which invariably takes longer than normalization of blood glucose concentrations.[68] If the patient appears to be sensitive to insulin (e.g., some young children, mild DKA, and patients with HHS) or there is difficulty maintaining normal serum potassium concentrations, the dose should be decreased to ≤0.05 U/kg/hour, provided that metabolic acidosis continues to resolve.[28] Recent nonrandomized, observational, and retrospective studies have shown that 0.05 U/kg/hour appears to be as effective as 0.1 U/kg/hour IV insulin infusion in the initial treatment (<6 hours) of DKA in children.[69,70]

The plasma glucose concentration may fall steeply during initial volume expansion;[53] thereafter, and after commencing insulin therapy, the plasma glucose concentration typically decreases at a rate of ~40–90 mg/dl/hour, depending on the timing and amount of glucose administration.[71] Adding dextrose to the IV fluid infusion moderates the rate of decline in glucose concentrations. To prevent an unduly rapid decrease in plasma glucose concentration and reduce the risk of hypoglycemia, 5% glucose should be added to the IV fluid when the plasma glucose is ~250–300 mg/dl, or sooner if the rate of fall is precipitous. It may be necessary to use 10 or even 12.5% dextrose to prevent hypoglycemia while continuing to infuse the amount of insulin necessary to correct metabolic acidosis.

If biochemical parameters of DKA (pH, anion gap, BOHB) do not improve, consider possible causes of impaired response to insulin (e.g., infection) or an error in insulin preparation, and if no obvious cause is found, increase the insulin infusion rate.[28]

When continuous IV administration is not possible and in patients with uncomplicated DKA, hourly or twice hourly subcutaneous (SC) or intramuscular administration of a rapid-acting insulin analog is safe and may be as effective as IV regular insulin infusion,[71–75] but this is not recommended in patients with severe DKA and poor perfusion. A recommended SC regimen consists of an initial SC dose of 0.3 U/kg, followed 1 hour later by SC rapid-acting insulin analog at a dose of 0.1 U/kg/every hour or 0.15–0.2 U/kg every 2 hours. If blood glucose decreases to 250 mg/dl before DKA has resolved, reduce the dose of SC insulin to 0.05 U/kg/hour to keep blood glucose ~200 mg/dl until DKA resolves.

POTASSIUM

Serum potassium levels may be normal, increased, or decreased at the time of presentation. Potassium is driven back into cells by insulin replacement and the correction of acidosis, which may cause an abrupt decrease in potassium concentration and predispose the patient to a cardiac arrhythmia. Potassium replacement therapy is required regardless of the serum potassium concentration. If the patient's serum potassium concentration is low at presentation, start potassium replacement *at the time of* initial volume expansion and *before* starting insulin therapy. If potassium is given with the initial volume expansion, use 20–40 mmol/l. If the patient presents with hyperkalemia, *defer* potassium replacement therapy until urine output is documented. Otherwise, only start replacing potassium *after* initial volume expansion.

If immediate serum potassium measurements are unavailable, an electrocardiograph may help to determine whether the child has hyper- or hypokalemia.[49,50] Flattening of the T wave, widening of the QT interval, and the appearance of U waves indicate hypokalemia. Tall, peaked, symmetrical T waves and shortening of the QT interval are signs of hyperkalemia. Prolonged QTc (the measured QT interval divided by the square root of the R-R interval to correct for heart rate) of unclear significance frequently occurs during DKA and correlates with ketosis in children.[76]

The starting potassium concentration should be 40 mmol/l. Potassium phosphate may be used together with potassium chloride or acetate (e.g., 20 mmol/l potassium chloride and 20 mmol/l potassium phosphate or 20 mmol/l potassium phosphate and 20 mmol/l potassium acetate). Subsequent potassium replacement therapy should be based on serial serum potassium measurements and should continue throughout IV fluid therapy. The maximum recommended rate of IV potassium replacement is usually 0.5 mmol/kg/hour. If hypokalemia persists despite a maximum rate of potassium replacement, reduce the rate of insulin infusion.[28]

PHOSPHATE

Osmotic diuresis results in urinary phosphate loss[77-79] and intracellular phosphate depletion. Insulin promotes phosphate entry into cells,[80-82] and plasma phosphate levels fall after starting treatment. Total body phosphate depletion has been associated with a variety of metabolic disturbances;[83-85] however, prospective studies have not shown clinical benefit from phosphate replacement.[86-91] Nonetheless, severe hypophosphatemia (<1 mg/dl), which may manifest as muscle weakness, should be treated even in the absence of symptoms.[92] Potassium phosphate may be administered safely provided that careful monitoring is performed to avoid hypocalcemia.[93,94]

ACIDOSIS

Insulin stops further ketoacid production and allows ketoacids to be metabolized, which generates bicarbonate. Treatment of hypovolemia improves tissue perfusion and renal function, thereby decreasing lactic acidosis and increasing organic acid excretion. Controlled trials have shown no clinical benefit from bicarbonate administration,[95-98], and bicarbonate therapy may cause paradoxical central nervous system acidosis.[99,100] Rapid correction of acidosis with bicarbonate causes hypokalemia.[99,101,102] There is no evidence that bicarbonate is necessary and its routine administration is not recommended. Rare patients, however, may benefit from *cautious* alkali therapy. These include patients with severe acidemia in whom decreased cardiac contractility and peripheral vasodilatation can further impair tissue perfusion and in patients with life-threatening hyperkalemia.[103] If bicarbonate is considered necessary, cautiously give 1–2 mmol/kg over 60 minutes.

INTRODUCTION OF ORAL FLUIDS AND TRANSITION TO SC INSULIN INJECTIONS

Serial measurements of point-of-care blood BOHB concentrations have been used to monitor biochemical resolution of DKA and to determine when IV insulin infusion should be stopped.[43-45] Blood BOHB concentrations decrease to <1 mmol/l many hours before ketones disappear from the urine. Absence of ketonuria should *not* be used as an endpoint for determining resolution of DKA.

Oral fluids should be introduced after ketoacidosis has resolved (venous pH >7.3, serum bicarbonate ≥15 mEq/l, normal anion gap, BOHB <0.6 mmol/l) and plasma glucose <200 mg/dl. In children receiving large amounts of saline, the anion gap invariably normalizes before the bicarbonate concentration. The most convenient time to change to SC insulin is just before a meal. To prevent rebound hyperglycemia, the first SC injection of rapid-acting insulin should be given at least 15–30 minutes (1 hour if using regular insulin) before stopping the insulin infusion to allow sufficient time for the injected insulin to be absorbed. For patients who will be managed using a multiple dose or basal-bolus insulin regimen, the first dose of basal insulin (glargine or detemir) may be administered on the preceding evening, while the patient is still receiving IV insulin, and the insulin infusion may be stopped the following morning. See Chapter 29 for guidelines on starting SC insulin therapy.

After transitioning to SC insulin, frequent blood glucose monitoring is required to avoid recurrence of hyperglycemia and to prevent hypoglycemia. Supplemental rapid-acting insulin is given at ~3- to 4-hour intervals to correct blood glucose levels that are >200 mg/dl.

COMPLICATIONS OF TREATMENT

The mortality rate from DKA in children is 0.15–0.30% in national population studies[104,105] and cerebral edema accounts for 60–90% of all DKA deaths.[22,24]

CEREBRAL EDEMA

The incidence of cerebral edema in national population studies is ~0.5–1% and the mortality rate is 21–24%.[22,24,25] The etiology of DKA-related cerebral edema continues to be controversial, and its pathogenesis is still incompletely understood.[106] Evidence for disruption of the blood-brain barrier has been found in cases of fatal cerebral edema.[107] In a series of recent studies, the degree of edema formation during DKA in children was found to correlate with the degree of dehydration and hyperventilation at presentation, but not with factors related to initial osmolality or osmotic changes during treatment. There is no convincing evidence of an association between the rate of fluid or sodium administration used to treat DKA and the development of cerebral edema.[108] Although not definitively proven, evidence suggests that the pathophysiology of cerebral edema is not the result of acute changes in serum osmolality, but rather may be a consequence of cerebral ischemia from hypoperfusion and reperfusion leading to vasogenic edema.[106]

Demographic factors that have been associated with an increased risk of cerebral edema include the following:

- Younger age[109]
- New-onset diabetes[105,109]
- Longer duration of symptoms[23]

These risk associations simply may reflect the greater likelihood of severe DKA.

Epidemiological studies have identified several potential risk factors at diagnosis or during treatment of DKA. These include the following:

- Greater hypocapnia at presentation after adjusting for degree of acidosis[22,110,111]
- Increased serum urea nitrogen at presentation[22,111]
- More severe acidosis at presentation [66,112]
- Bicarbonate treatment for correction of acidosis[22,113]
- An attenuated rise in measured serum sodium concentrations during therapy[22,55,114]
- Greater volumes of fluid given in the first 4 hours[66]
- Administration of insulin in the first hour of fluid treatment[66]

Clinically significant cerebral edema usually develops 4–12 hours after treatment has started but can occur even before treatment has begun.[22,25,115–118] Rarely, it may develop as late as 24–48 hours after the start of treatment.[22,109,119] Symptoms and signs are variable. Following is a method of clinical diagnosis based on a bedside evaluation of neurological state.[120]

Diagnostic Criteria

- Abnormal motor or verbal response to pain
- Decorticate or decerebrate posture
- Cranial nerve palsy (especially III, IV, and VI)
- Abnormal neurogenic respiratory pattern (e.g., grunting, tachypnea, Cheyne–Stokes respiration, apneusis)

Major Criteria

- Altered mentation or fluctuating level of consciousness
- Sustained heart rate deceleration (decrease >20 beats/minute) not attributable to improved intravascular volume or sleep state
- Age-inappropriate incontinence

Minor Criteria

- Vomiting
- Headache
- Lethargy or not easily aroused
- Diastolic blood pressure >90 mmHg
- Age <5 years

One diagnostic criterion, two major criteria, or one major and two minor criteria have a sensitivity of 92% and a false positive rate of only 4%. Signs present before starting treatment are not considered in the diagnosis of cerebral edema. A chart with the reference ranges for blood pressure and heart rate, which vary depending on height, weight, and gender, should be readily available at the bedside.

Treatment of Cerebral Edema

- Initiate treatment as soon as the condition is suspected.
- Reduce the rate of fluid administration by one-third.

■ Give mannitol 0.5–1 g/kg IV over 10–15 minutes and repeat if there is no initial response in 30 minutes.[121–123]

■ Hypertonic saline (3%), suggested dose 2.5–5 ml/kg over 10–15 minutes, may be an alternative to mannitol, especially if there is no initial response to mannitol.[124,125] Mannitol or hypertonic saline should be available at the bedside.

■ Elevate the head of the bed to 30°.

■ Intubation may be necessary for the patient with impending respiratory failure.

■ *After* treatment for cerebral edema has been started, cranial imaging may be considered as with any critically ill patient with encephalopathy or acute focal neurologic deficit. The primary concern is whether the patient has a lesion requiring emergency neurosurgery (e.g., intracranial hemorrhage) or a lesion that may necessitate anticoagulation (e.g., cerebrovascular thrombosis).[126–134]

Other Causes of Morbidity and Mortality

Following are other causes of morbidity and mortality in the patient with DKA:

■ Hypoglycemia

■ Hypokalemia

■ Hyperchloremic metabolic acidosis

■ Prothrombotic tendency and peripheral venous thrombosis,[135,136] especially with central venous catheters

■ Sepsis

■ Rhino-orbital-cerebral, auricular, or pulmonary mucormycosis

■ Aspiration pneumonia

■ Pulmonary edema

■ ARDS

■ Pneumothorax, pneumomediastinum, and SC emphysema

■ Rhabdomyolysis

■ Acute renal failure

■ Acute pancreatitis

PREVENTION OF DKA

PRIMARY PREVENTION IN UNDIAGNOSED PATIENTS

Programs to Raise Awareness

Progression of metabolic deterioration to DKA generally is related to a long duration of ignored or misdiagnosed hyperglycemia-related symptoms. In the Parma area of Italy, Vanelli et al. implemented a highly successful DKA prevention program in children ages 6–14 years.[137,138] A poster showing the classic symptoms of diabetes (and highlighting the special significance of nocturnal enuresis in a previously dry child) was displayed in schools. Pediatricians working in the area were given equipment to measure glucosuria and blood glucose levels, as well as cards listing guidelines for the early diagnosis of diabetes to be given to patients. A toll-free number provided free access to health care providers experienced in diabetes diagnosis. This intervention resulted in a decrease in the cumulative frequency of DKA in new-onset diabetes from 78% during the 4-year period before initiation to 12.5% during the subsequent 8 years after the information about diabetes was introduced to teachers, students, parents, and pediatricians. The campaign to prevent DKA was still effective 8 years after it was promoted and confirmed that enuresis is the most important symptom for the early diagnosis of T1D. To maintain its effectiveness, the campaign should be renewed periodically (possibly every 5 years).[139]

SCREENING IN HIGH-RISK INDIVIDUALS

When children at increased risk of developing T1D (e.g., family history of T1D, positive pancreatic autoantibodies, or expression of diabetes-associated human leukocyte antigen genotypes) are screened regularly and followed prospectively, many are asymptomatic and have a normal A1C concentration at the time of diagnosis.[140] DKA is infrequent, the onset of diabetes is less severe, A1C is lower at diagnosis, fewer patients are hospitalized, and patients have a milder clinical course in the first year after diagnosis.[140–143] In one study, however, no substantial benefit with respect to A1C and insulin dose was observed during the first 5 years after diagnosis.[143]

SECONDARY PREVENTION IN ESTABLISHED PATIENTS

Prevention of Recurrent DKA

Insulin omission is the cause of recurrent DKA in most cases and management of an episode of DKA should not be considered complete until its cause has been identified and an attempt has been made to address it. A psychiatric social worker or clinical psychologist should be consulted to identify possible psychosocial reasons that may be contributing to DKA. Some reasons for insulin omission include an attempt to lose weight in an adolescent with an eating disorder; a means of escaping an intolerable or abusive home situation; financial constraints leading to a deliberate decrease in insulin dosing to reduce the need to buy insulin as often; and clinical depression causing inability of the patient to manage diabetes unassisted. An infection that is not associated with vomiting and diarrhea is seldom the cause when the patient or family is educated properly in diabetes management, is receiving appropriate follow-up care, and has 24-hour telephone access to a diabetes team for assistance when ketosis develops.[144]

Insulin omission can be prevented by education, psychosocial evaluation, and treatment combined with adult supervision of insulin administration.[145] When a responsible adult administers insulin, there may be as much as a tenfold reduction in frequency of recurrent DKA,[145] and a more recent study has shown that intensive behavioral intervention reduces admissions for DKA and related costs in high-risk youth with poorly controlled diabetes.[146]

The most common cause of DKA in patients who use insulin pumps is failure to take extra insulin with a pen or syringe when hyperglycemia and hyperketonemia or ketonuria occur. Home measurement of blood BOHB concentrations, when compared with urine ketone testing, decreases diabetes-related hospital visits by the early identification and treatment of ketosis.[147] Blood BOHB measurements may be especially valuable to prevent DKA in patients who use a pump because interrupted insulin delivery rapidly leads to ketosis,[148,149] and serum BOHB concentrations may be increased to levels consistent with DKA when urine is still ketone negative or shows only trace or small ketonuria.[150]

Parents and patients should learn how to recognize and treat impending DKA with additional rapid- or short-acting insulin and oral fluids, and patients should have access to a 24-hour telephone helpline for emergency advice and treatment.[19]

SICK-DAY MANAGEMENT

Illness and stress can trigger counterregulation and subsequent metabolic deterioration. Sick-day management requires increased monitoring of blood glucose levels and measurement of blood or urine ketones. Urine testing for ketones had been the standard approach to sick-day management until the advent of self-monitoring of blood BOHB levels.[150,151]

Because the majority of patients presenting with DKA have established diabetes, outpatient education directed at sick-day management and the early identification and treatment of impending DKA are important elements of a comprehensive diabetes education program. Teaching and reinforcing sick-day rules—especially, the vital importance of frequent self-monitoring of blood glucose and ketone levels—and timely administration of supplemental rapid-acting insulin, as well as oral salt and water, reduce episodes of DKA in patients with established T1D.

REFERENCES

1. Pinkey JH, Bingley PJ, Sawtell PA, Dunger DB, Gale EA. Presentation and progress of childhood diabetes mellitus: a prospective population-based study. The Bart's-Oxford Study Group. *Diabetologia* 1994;37:70–74.

2. Rewers A, Chase HP, Mackenzie T, et al. Predictors of acute complications in children with type 1 diabetes. *JAMA* 2002;287:2511–2518.

3. Komulainen J, Kulmala P, Savola K, et al. Clinical, autoimmune, and genetic characteristics of very young children with type 1 diabetes. Childhood Diabetes in Finland (DiMe) Study Group. *Diabetes Care* 1999;22:1950–1955.

4. Maniatis AK, Goehrig SH, Gao D, Rewers A, Walravens P, Klingensmith GJ. Increased incidence and severity of diabetic ketoacidosis among uninsured children with newly diagnosed type 1 diabetes mellitus. *Pediatr Diabetes* 2005;6:79–83.

5. Rewers A, Klingensmith G, Davis C, et al. Presence of diabetic ketoacidosis at diagnosis of diabetes mellitus in youth: the Search for Diabetes in Youth Study. *Pediatrics* 2008;121:e1258–1266.

6. Klingensmith GJ, Tamborlane WV, Wood J, et al. Diabetic ketoacidosis at diabetes onset: still an all too common threat in youth. *J Pediatr* 2013;162:330–334 e1.

7. Bui H, To T, Stein R, Fung K, Daneman D. Is diabetic ketoacidosis at disease onset a result of missed diagnosis? *J Pediatr* 2010;156:472–477.

8. Hekkala A, Knip M, Veijola R. Ketoacidosis at diagnosis of type 1 diabetes in children in northern Finland: temporal changes over 20 years. *Diabetes Care* 2007;30:861–866.

9. Neu A, Hofer SE, Karges B, Oeverink R, Rosenbauer J, Holl RW. Ketoacidosis at diabetes onset is still frequent in children and adolescents: a multicenter analysis of 14,664 patients from 106 institutions. *Diabetes Care* 2009;32:1647–1648.

10. Rosilio M, Cotton JB, Wieliczko MC, et al. Factors associated with glycemic control. A cross-sectional nationwide study in 2,579 French children with type 1 diabetes. The French Pediatric Diabetes Group [see comments]. *Diabetes Care* 1998;21:1146–1153.

11. Smith CP, Firth D, Bennett S, Howard C, Chisholm P. Ketoacidosis occurring in newly diagnosed and established diabetic children. *Acta Paediatr* 1998;87:537–541.

12. Morris AD, Boyle DI, McMahon AD, Greene SA, MacDonald TM, Newton RW. Adherence to insulin treatment, glycaemic control, and ketoacidosis in insulin-dependent diabetes mellitus. The DARTS/MEMO Collaboration. Diabetes Audit and Research in Tayside Scotland. Medicines Monitoring Unit. *Lancet* 1997;350:1505–1510.

13. Hanas R, Lindgren F, Lindblad B. A 2-yr national population study of pediatric ketoacidosis in Sweden: predisposing conditions and insulin pump use. *Pediatr Diabetes* 2009;10:33–37.

14. Cengiz E, Xing D, Wong JC, et al. Severe hypoglycemia and diabetic ketoacidosis among youth with type 1 diabetes in the T1D Exchange clinic registry. *Pediatr Diabetes* 2013;14:447–454.

15. Quinn M, Fleischman A, Rosner B, Nigrin DJ, Wolfsdorf JI. Characteristics at diagnosis of type 1 diabetes in children younger than 6 years. *J Pediatr* 2006;148:366–371.

16. Pawlowicz M, Birkholz D, Niedzwiecki M, Balcerska A. Difficulties or mistakes in diagnosing type 1 diabetes in children?—demographic factors influencing delayed diagnosis. *Pediatr Diabetes* 2009;10:542–549.

17. White PC, Dickson BA. Low morbidity and mortality in children with diabetic ketoacidosis treated with isotonic fluids. *J Pediatr* 2013;163:761–766.

18. Flood RG, Chiang VW. Rate and prediction of infection in children with diabetic ketoacidosis. *Am J Emerg Med* 2001;19:270–273.

19. Hoffman WH, O'Neill P, Khoury C, Bernstein SS. Service and education for the insulin-dependent child. *Diabetes Care* 1978;1:285–288.

20. Drozda DJ, Dawson VA, Long DJ, Freson LS, Sperling MA. Assessment of the effect of a comprehensive diabetes management program on hospital admission rates of children with diabetes mellitus. *Diabetes Educ* 1990;16:389–393.

21. Grey M, Boland EA, Davidson M, Li J, Tamborlane WV. Coping skills training for youth with diabetes mellitus has long-lasting effects on metabolic control and quality of life. *J Pediatr* 2000;137:107–113.

22. Glaser N, Barnett P, McCaslin I, et al. Risk factors for cerebral edema in children with diabetic ketoacidosis. The Pediatric Emergency Medicine Collaborative Research Committee of the American Academy of Pediatrics. *N Engl J Med* 2001;344:264–269.

23. Bello FA, Sotos JF. Cerebral oedema in diabetic ketoacidosis in children [letter]. *Lancet* 1990;336:64.

24. Edge JA, Hawkins MM, Winter DL, Dunger DB. The risk and outcome of cerebral oedema developing during diabetic ketoacidosis. *Arch Dis Child* 2001;85:16–22.

25. Lawrence SE, Cummings EA, Gaboury I, Daneman D. Population-based study of incidence and risk factors for cerebral edema in pediatric diabetic ketoacidosis. *J Pediatr* 2005;146:688–692.

26. Dunger DB, Sperling MA, Acerini CL, et al. European Society for Paediatric Endocrinology/Lawson Wilkins Pediatric Endocrine Society consensus statement on diabetic ketoacidosis in children and adolescents. *Pediatrics* 2004;113:e133–140.

27. Nadler OA, Finkelstein MJ, Reid SR. How well does serum bicarbonate concentration predict the venous pH in children being evaluated for diabetic ketoacidosis? *Pediatr Emerg Care* 2011;27:907–910.

28. Wolfsdorf J, Craig ME, Daneman D, et al. Diabetic ketoacidosis in children and adolescents with diabetes. *Pediatr Diabetes* 2009;10(Suppl 12):118–133.

29. Zeitler P, Haqq A, Rosenbloom A, Glaser N. Hyperglycemic hyperosmolar syndrome in children: pathophysiological considerations and suggested guidelines for treatment. *J Pediatr* 2011;158:9–14, e1–2.

30. McDonnell CM, Pedreira CC, Vadamalayan B, Cameron FJ, Werther GA. Diabetic ketoacidosis, hyperosmolarity and hypernatremia: are high-carbohydrate drinks worsening initial presentation? *Pediatr Diabetes* 2005;6:90–94.

31. Karges B, Kapellen T, Neu A, et al. Long-acting insulin analogs and the risk of diabetic ketoacidosis in children and adolescents with type 1 diabetes:

a prospective study of 10,682 patients from 271 institutions. *Diabetes Care* 2010;33:1031–1033.

32. Wolfsdorf J, Glaser N, Sperling MA. Diabetic ketoacidosis in infants, children, and adolescents: A consensus statement from the American Diabetes Association. *Diabetes Care* 2006;29:1150–1159.

33. Deeter KH, Roberts JS, Bradford H, et al. Hypertension despite dehydration during severe pediatric diabetic ketoacidosis. *Pediatr Diabetes* 2011;12:295–301.

34. Koves IH, Neutze J, Donath S, et al. The accuracy of clinical assessment of dehydration during diabetic ketoacidosis in childhood. *Diabetes Care* 2004;27:2485–2487.

35. Sottosanti M, Morrison GC, Singh RN, et al. Dehydration in children with diabetic ketoacidosis: a prospective study. *Arch Dis Child* 2012;97:96–100.

36. Umpierrez GE, DiGirolamo M, Tuvlin JA, Isaacs SD, Bhoola SM, Kokko JP. Differences in metabolic and hormonal milieu in diabetic- and alcohol-induced ketoacidosis. *J Crit Care* 2000;15:52–59.

37. DeFronzo RA, Matsuda M, Barrett EJ. Diabetic ketoacidosis: a combined metabolic-nephrologic approach to therapy. *Diabetes Reviews* 1994;2:209–238.

38. Dweikat IM, Naser EN, Abu Libdeh AI, et al. Propionic acidemia mimicking diabetic ketoacidosis. *Brain Dev* 2011;33:428–431.

39. Erdem E, Cayonu N, Uysalol E, Yildirmak ZY. Chronic intermittent form of isovaleric acidemia mimicking diabetic ketoacidosis. *J Pediatr Endocrinol Metab* 2010;23:503–505.

40. Saudubray JM, Specola N, Middleton B, et al. Hyperketotic states due to inherited defects of ketolysis. *Enzyme* 1987;38:80–90.

41. Fukao T, Scriver CR, Kondo N. The clinical phenotype and outcome of mitochondrial acetoacetyl-CoA thiolase deficiency (beta-ketothiolase or T2 deficiency) in 26 enzymatically proved and mutation-defined patients. *Mol Genet Metab* 2001;72:109–114.

42. Sheikh-Ali M, Karon BS, Basu A, et al. Can serum beta-hydroxybutyrate be used to diagnose diabetic ketoacidosis? *Diabetes Care* 2008;31:643–647.

43. Ham MR, Okada P, White PC. Bedside ketone determination in diabetic children with hyperglycemia and ketosis in the acute care setting. *Pediatr Diabetes* 2004;5:39–43.

44. Noyes KJ, Crofton P, Bath LE, et al. Hydroxybutyrate near-patient testing to evaluate a new end-point for intravenous insulin therapy in the treatment of diabetic ketoacidosis in children. *Pediatr Diabetes* 2007;8:150–156.

45. Rewers A, McFann K, Chase HP. Bedside monitoring of blood beta-hydroxybutyrate levels in the management of diabetic ketoacidosis in children. *Diabetes Technol Ther* 2006;8:671–676.

46. Teasdale G, Jennett B. Assessment of coma and impaired consciousness. A practical scale. *Lancet* 1974;2:81–84.

47. Reilly PL, Simpson DA, Sprod R, Thomas L. Assessing the conscious level in infants and young children: a paediatric version of the Glasgow Coma Scale. *Childs Nerv Syst* 1988;4:30–33.

48. Wiggam MI, O'Kane MJ, Harper R, et al. Treatment of diabetic ketoacidosis using normalization of blood 3- hydroxybutyrate concentration as the endpoint of emergency management. A randomized controlled study. *Diabetes Care* 1997;20:1347–1352.

49. Malone JI, Brodsky SJ. The value of electrocardiogram monitoring in diabetic ketoacidosis. *Diabetes Care* 1980;3:543–547.

50. Soler NG, Bennett MA, Fitzgerald MG, Malins JM. Electrocardiogram as a guide to potassium replacement in diabetic ketoacidosis. *Diabetes* 1974;23:610–615.

51. Dunger DB, Sperling MA, Acerini CL, et al. ESPE/LWPES consensus statement on diabetic ketoacidosis in children and adolescents. *Arch Dis Child* 2004;89:188–194.

52. Agus MS, Alexander JL, Mantell PA. Continuous non-invasive end-tidal CO_2 monitoring in pediatric inpatients with diabetic ketoacidosis. *Pediatr Diabetes* 2006;7:196–200.

53. Waldhausl W, Kleinberger G, Korn A, Dudczak R, Bratusch-Marrain P, Nowotny P. Severe hyperglycemia: effects of rehydration on endocrine derangements and blood glucose concentration. *Diabetes* 1979;28:577–584.

54. Adrogue HJ, Barrero J, Eknoyan G. Salutary effects of modest fluid replacement in the treatment of adults with diabetic ketoacidosis. Use in patients without extreme volume deficit. *JAMA* 1989;262:2108–2113.

55. Harris GD, Fiordalisi I, Harris WL, Mosovich LL, Finberg L. Minimizing the risk of brain herniation during treatment of diabetic ketoacidemia: a retrospective and prospective study. *J Pediatr* 1990;117:22–31.

56. Harris GD, Fiordalisi I. Physiologic management of diabetic ketoacidemia. A 5-year prospective pediatric experience in 231 episodes. *Arch Pediatr Adolesc Med* 1994;148:1046–1052.

57. Rother KI, Schwenk WF, 2nd. Effect of rehydration fluid with 75 mmol/L of sodium on serum sodium concentration and serum osmolality in young patients with diabetic ketoacidosis. *Mayo Clin Proc* 1994;69:1149–1153.

58. Felner EI, White PC. Improving management of diabetic ketoacidosis in children. *Pediatrics* 2001;108:735–740.

59. Duck SC, Wyatt DT. Factors associated with brain herniation in the treatment of diabetic ketoacidosis. *J Pediatr* 1988;113:10–14.

60. Adrogue HJ, Eknoyan G, Suki WK. Diabetic ketoacidosis: role of the kidney in the acid-base homeostasis re-evaluated. *Kidney Int* 1984;25:591–598.

61. Oh MS, Carroll HJ, Uribarri J. Mechanism of normochloremic and hyperchloremic acidosis in diabetic ketoacidosis. *Nephron* 1990;54:1–6.

62. Owen OE, Licht JH, Sapir DG. Renal function and effects of partial rehydration during diabetic ketoacidosis. *Diabetes* 1981;30:510–518.

63. Luzi L, Barrett EJ, Groop LC, Ferrannini E, DeFronzo RA. Metabolic effects of low-dose insulin therapy on glucose metabolism in diabetic ketoacidosis. *Diabetes* 1988;37:1470–1477.

64. Burghen GA, Etteldorf JN, Fisher JN, Kitabchi AQ. Comparison of high-dose and low-dose insulin by continuous intravenous infusion in the treatment of diabetic ketoacidosis in children. *Diabetes Care* 1980;3:15–20.

65. Kitabchi AE, Umpierrez GE, Fisher JN, Murphy MB, Stentz FB. Thirty years of personal experience in hyperglycemic crises: diabetic ketoacidosis and hyperglycemic hyperosmolar state. *J Clin Endocrinol Metab* 2008;93:1541–1552.

66. Edge JA, Jakes RW, Roy Y, et al. The UK case-control study of cerebral oedema complicating diabetic ketoacidosis in children. *Diabetologia* 2006;49:2002–2009.

67. Lindsay R, Bolte RG. The use of an insulin bolus in low-dose insulin infusion for pediatric diabetic ketoacidosis. *Pediatr Emerg Care* 1989;5:77–79.

68. Soler NG, FitzGerald MG, Wright AD, Malins JM. Comparative study of different insulin regimens in management of diabetic ketoacidosis. *Lancet* 1975;2:1221–1224.

69. Puttha R, Cooke D, Subbarayan A, et al. Low dose (0.05 units/kg/h) is comparable with standard dose (0.1 units/kg/h) intravenous insulin infusion for the initial treatment of diabetic ketoacidosis in children with type 1 diabetes: an observational study. *Pediatr Diabetes* 2010;11:12–17.

70. Al Hanshi S, Shann F. Insulin infused at 0.05 versus 0.1 units/kg/hr in children admitted to intensive care with diabetic ketoacidosis. *Pediatr Crit Care Med* 2011;12:137–140.

71. Fisher JN, Shahshahani MN, Kitabchi AE. Diabetic ketoacidosis: low-dose insulin therapy by various routes. *N Engl J Med* 1977;297:238–241.

72. Sacks HS, Shahshahani M, Kitabchi AE, Fisher JN, Young RT. Similar responsiveness of diabetic ketoacidosis to low-dose insulin by intramuscular injection and albumin-free infusion. *Ann Intern Med* 1979;90:36–42.

73. Umpierrez GE, Latif K, Stoever J, et al. Efficacy of subcutaneous insulin lispro versus continuous intravenous regular insulin for the treatment of patients with diabetic ketoacidosis. *Am J Med* 2004;117:291–296.

74. Umpierrez GE, Cuervo R, Karabell A, Latif K, Freire AX, Kitabchi AE. Treatment of diabetic ketoacidosis with subcutaneous insulin aspart. *Diabetes Care* 2004;27:1873–1878.

75. Della Manna T, Steinmetz L, Campos PR, et al. Subcutaneous use of a fast-acting insulin analog: an alternative treatment for pediatric patients with diabetic ketoacidosis. *Diabetes Care* 2005;28:1856–1861.

76. Kuppermann N, Park J, Glatter K, Marcin JP, Glaser NS. Prolonged QT interval corrected for heart rate during diabetic ketoacidosis in children. *Arch Pediatr Adolesc Med* 2008;162:544–549.

77. Atchley D, Loeb R, Richards D, Jr., Benedict E, Driscoll M. On diabetic ketoacidosis: a detailed study of electrolyte balances following the withdrawal and reestablishment of insulin therapy. *J Clin Invest* 1933;12:297–326.

78. Butler A, Talbot N, Burnett C, Stanbury J, MacLachlan E. Metabolic studies in diabetic coma. *Trans Assoc Am Physicians* 1947;60:102–109.

79. Nabarro J, Spencer A, Stowers J. Metabolic studies in severe diabetic ketosis. *Q J Med* 1952;82:225–248.

80. Guest G. Organic phosphates of the blood and mineral metabolism in diabetic acidosis. *Am J Dis Child* 1942;64.

81. Guest G, Rapoport S. Electrolytes of blood plasma and cells in diabetic acidosis and during recovery. *Proc Am Diabetes Assoc* 1947;7:95–115.

82. Riley MS, Schade DS, Eaton RP. Effects of insulin infusion on plasma phosphate in diabetic patients. *Metabolism* 1979;28:191–194.

83. Alberti KG, Emerson PM, Darley JH, Hockaday TD. 2,3-Diphosphoglycerate and tissue oxygenation in uncontrolled diabetes mellitus. *Lancet* 1972;2:391–395.

84. Knochel JP. The pathophysiology and clinical characteristics of severe hypophosphatemia. *Arch Intern Med* 1977;137:203–220.

85. O'Connor LR, Wheeler WS, Bethune JE. Effect of hypophosphatemia on myocardial performance in man. *N Engl J Med* 1977;297:901–903.

86. Gibby OM, Veale KE, Hayes TM, Jones JG, Wardrop CA. Oxygen availability from the blood and the effect of phosphate replacement on erythrocyte 2,3-diphosphoglycerate and haemoglobin-oxygen affinity in diabetic ketoacidosis. *Diabetologia* 1978;15:381–385.

87. Keller U, Berger W. Prevention of hypophosphatemia by phosphate infusion during treatment of diabetic ketoacidosis and hyperosmolar coma. *Diabetes* 1980;29:87–95.

88. Wilson HK, Keuer SP, Lea AS, Boyd AE 3rd, Eknoyan G. Phosphate therapy in diabetic ketoacidosis. *Arch Intern Med* 1982;142:517–520.

89. Becker DJ, Brown DR, Steranka BH, Drash AL. Phosphate replacement during treatment of diabetic ketosis. Effects on calcium and phosphorus homeostasis. *Am J Dis Child* 1983;137:241–246.

90. Fisher JN, Kitabchi AE. A randomized study of phosphate therapy in the treatment of diabetic ketoacidosis. *J Clin Endocrinol Metab* 1983;57:177–180.

91. Clerbaux T, Reynaert M, Willems E, Frans A. Effect of phosphate on oxygen-hemoglobin affinity, diphosphoglycerate and blood gases during recovery from diabetic ketoacidosis. *Intens Care Med* 1989;15:495–498.

92. Bohannon NJ. Large phosphate shifts with treatment for hyperglycemia. *Arch Intern Med* 1989;149:1423–1425.

93. Zipf WB, Bacon GE, Spencer ML, Kelch RP, Hopwood NJ, Hawker CD. Hypocalcemia, hypomagnesemia, and transient hypoparathyroidism during therapy with potassium phosphate in diabetic ketoacidosis. *Diabetes Care* 1979;2:265–268.

94. Winter RJ, Harris CJ, Phillips LS, Green OC. Diabetic ketoacidosis. Induction of hypocalcemia and hypomagnesemia by phosphate therapy. *Am J Med* 1979;67:897–900.

95. Hale PJ, Crase J, Nattrass M. Metabolic effects of bicarbonate in the treatment of diabetic ketoacidosis. *BMJ* 1984;289:1035–1038.

96. Morris LR, Murphy MB, Kitabchi AE. Bicarbonate therapy in severe diabetic ketoacidosis. *Ann Intern Med* 1986;105:836–840.

97. Okuda Y, Adrogue HJ, Field JB, Nohara H, Yamashita K. Counterproductive effects of sodium bicarbonate in diabetic ketoacidosis. *J Clin Endocrinol Metab* 1996;81:314–320.

98. Green SM, Rothrock SG, Ho JD, et al. Failure of adjunctive bicarbonate to improve outcome in severe pediatric diabetic ketoacidosis. *Ann Emerg Med* 1998;31:41–48.

99. Assal JP, Aoki TT, Manzano FM, Kozak GP. Metabolic effects of sodium bicarbonate in management of diabetic ketoacidosis. *Diabetes* 1974;23:405–411.

100. Ohman JL, Jr., Marliss EB, Aoki TT, Munichoodappa CS, Khanna VV, Kozak GP. The cerebrospinal fluid in diabetic ketoacidosis. *N Engl J Med* 1971;284:283–290.

101. Soler NG, Bennett MA, Dixon K, FitzGerald MG, Malins JM. Potassium balance during treatment of diabetic ketoacidosis with special reference to the use of bicarbonate. *Lancet* 1972;2:665–667.

102. Lever E, Jaspan JB. Sodium bicarbonate therapy in severe diabetic ketoacidosis. *Am J Med* 1983;75:263–268.

103. Narins RG, Cohen JJ. Bicarbonate therapy for organic acidosis: the case for its continued use. *Ann Intern Med* 1987;106:615–618.

104. Curtis JR, To T, Muirhead S, Cummings E, Daneman D. Recent trends in hospitalization for diabetic ketoacidosis in Ontario children. *Diabetes Care* 2002;25:1591–1596.

105. Edge JA, Ford-Adams ME, Dunger DB. Causes of death in children with insulin dependent diabetes 1990–96. *Arch Dis Child* 1999;81:318–323.

106. Glaser N. Cerebral injury and cerebral edema in children with diabetic keto-acidosis: could cerebral ischemia and reperfusion injury be involved? *Pediatr Diabetes* 2009;10:534-541.

107. Hoffman WH, Stamatovic SM, Andjelkovic AV. Inflammatory mediators and blood brain barrier disruption in fatal brain edema of diabetic ketoacidosis. *Brain Res* 2009;1254:138-148.

108. Brown TB. Cerebral oedema in childhood diabetic ketoacidosis: is treatment a factor? *Emerg Med J* 2004;21:141-144.

109. Rosenbloom AL. Intracerebral crises during treatment of diabetic ketoacidosis. *Diabetes Care* 1990;13:22-33.

110. Mahoney CP, Vlcek BW, DelAguila M. Risk factors for developing brain herniation during diabetic ketoacidosis. *Pediatr Neurol* 1999;21:721-727.

111. Glaser NS, Marcin JP, Wootton-Gorges SL, et al. Correlation of clinical and biochemical findings with diabetic ketoacidosis-related cerebral edema in children using magnetic resonance diffusion-weighted imaging. *J Pediatr* 2008;153:541-546.

112. Durr JA, Hoffman WH, Sklar AH, el Gammal T, Steinhart CM. Correlates of brain edema in uncontrolled IDDM. *Diabetes* 1992;41:627-632.

113. Bureau MA, Begin R, Berthiaume Y, Shapcott D, Khoury K, Gagnon N. Cerebral hypoxia from bicarbonate infusion in diabetic acidosis. *J Pediatr* 1980;96:968-973.

114. Hale PM, Rezvani I, Braunstein AW, Lipman TH, Martinez N, Garibaldi L. Factors predicting cerebral edema in young children with diabetic ketoacidosis and new onset type I diabetes. *Acta Paediatr* 1997;86:626-631.

115. Deeb L. Development of fatal cerebral edema during outpatient therapy for diabetic ketoacidosis. *Pract Diab* 1989;6:212-213.

116. Glasgow AM. Devastating cerebral edema in diabetic ketoacidosis before therapy [letter]. *Diabetes Care* 1991;14:77-78.

117. Couch RM, Acott PD, Wong GW. Early onset fatal cerebral edema in diabetic ketoacidosis. *Diabetes Care* 1991;14:78-79.

118. Fiordalisi I, Harris GD, Gilliland MG. Prehospital cardiac arrest in diabetic ketoacidemia: why brain swelling may lead to death before treatment. *J Diabetes Complications* 2002;16:214-219.

119. Edge JA. Cerebral oedema during treatment of diabetic ketoacidosis: are we any nearer finding a cause? *Diabetes Metab Res Rev* 2000;16:316-324.

120. Muir AB, Quisling RG, Yang MC, Rosenbloom AL. Cerebral edema in childhood diabetic ketoacidosis: natural history, radiographic findings, and early identification. *Diabetes Care* 2004;27:1541-1546.

121. Franklin B, Liu J, Ginsberg-Fellner F. Cerebral edema and ophthalmoplegia reversed by mannitol in a new case of insulin-dependent diabetes mellitus. *Pediatrics* 1982;69:87–90.

122. Shabbir N, Oberfield SE, Corrales R, Kairam R, Levine LS. Recovery from symptomatic brain swelling in diabetic ketoacidosis. *Clin Pediatr (Phila)* 1992;31:570–573.

123. Roberts MD, Slover RH, Chase HP. Diabetic ketoacidosis with intracerebral complications. *Pediatr Diabetes* 2001;2:109–114.

124. Curtis JR, Bohn D, Daneman D. Use of hypertonic saline in the treatment of cerebral edema in diabetic ketoacidosis (DKA). *Pediatr Diabetes* 2001;2:191–194.

125. Kamat P, Vats A, Gross M, Checchia PA. Use of hypertonic saline for the treatment of altered mental status associated with diabetic ketoacidosis. *Pediatr Crit Care Med* 2003;4:239–242.

126. Kanter RK, Oliphant M, Zimmerman JJ, Stuart MJ. Arterial thrombosis causing cerebral edema in association with diabetic ketoacidosis. *Crit Care Med* 1987;15:175–176.

127. Roe TF, Crawford TO, Huff KR, Costin G, Kaufman FR, Nelson MD Jr. Brain infarction in children with diabetic ketoacidosis. *J Diabetes Complications* 1996;10:100–108.

128. Keane S, Gallagher A, Ackroyd S, McShane MA, Edge JA. Cerebral venous thrombosis during diabetic ketoacidosis. *Arch Dis Child* 2002;86:204–205.

129. Rosenbloom AL. Fatal cerebral infarctions in diabetic ketoacidosis in a child with previously unknown heterozygosity for factor V Leiden deficiency. *J Pediatr* 2004;145:561–562.

130. Lee HS, Hwang JS. Cerebral infarction associated with transient visual loss in child with diabetic ketoacidosis. *Diabet Med* 2011;28:516–518.

131. Lin JJ, Lin KL, Wang HS, Wong AM, Hsia SH. Occult infarct with acute hemorrhagic stroke in juvenile diabetic ketoacidosis. *Brain Dev* 2008;30:91–93.

132. Foster JR, Morrison G, Fraser DD. Diabetic ketoacidosis-associated stroke in children and youth. *Stroke Res Treat* 2011;2011:219706.

133. Mahmud FH, Ramsay DA, Levin SD, Singh RN, Kotylak T, Fraser DD. Coma with diffuse white matter hemorrhages in juvenile diabetic ketoacidosis. *Pediatrics* 2007;120:e1540–1546.

134. Zerah M, Patterson R, Hansen I, Briones M, Dion J, Renfroe B. Resolution of severe sinus vein thrombosis with super selective thrombolysis in a pre-adolescent with diabetic ketoacidosis and a prothrombin gene mutation. *J Pediatr Endocrinol Metab* 2007;20:725–731.

135. Gutierrez JA, Bagatell R, Samson MP, Theodorou AA, Berg RA. Femoral central venous catheter-associated deep venous thrombosis in children with diabetic ketoacidosis. *Crit Care Med* 2003;31:80–83.

136. Worly JM, Fortenberry JD, Hansen I, Chambliss CR, Stockwell J. Deep venous thrombosis in children with diabetic ketoacidosis and femoral central venous catheters. *Pediatrics* 2004;113:e57–e60.

137. Vanelli M, Chiari G, Ghizzoni L, Costi G, Giacalone T, Chiarelli F. Effectiveness of a prevention program for diabetic ketoacidosis in children. An 8-year study in schools and private practices. *Diabetes Care* 1999;22:7–9.

138. Vanelli M, Scarabello C, Fainardi V. Available tools for primary ketoacidosis prevention at diabetes diagnosis in children and adolescents. "The Parma campaign." *Acta Biomed* 2008;79:73–78.

139. Vanelli M, Chiari G, Lacava S, Iovane B. Campaign for diabetic ketoacidosis prevention still effective 8 years later. *Diabetes Care* 2007;30:e12.

140. Triolo TM, Chase HP, Barker JM. Diabetic subjects diagnosed through the Diabetes Prevention Trial-Type 1 (DPT-1) are often asymptomatic with normal A1C at diabetes onset. *Diabetes Care* 2009;32:769–773.

141. Barker JM, Goehrig SH, Barriga K, et al. Clinical characteristics of children diagnosed with type 1 diabetes through intensive screening and follow-up. *Diabetes Care* 2004;27:1399–1404.

142. Elding Larsson H, Vehik K, Bell R, et al. Reduced prevalence of diabetic ketoacidosis at diagnosis of type 1 diabetes in young children participating in longitudinal follow-up. *Diabetes Care* 2011;34:2347–2352.

143. Winkler C, Schober E, Ziegler AG, Holl RW. Markedly reduced rate of diabetic ketoacidosis at onset of type 1 diabetes in relatives screened for islet autoantibodies. *Pediatr Diabetes* 2012;13:308–313.

144. Farrell K, Holmes-Walker DJ. Mobile phone support is associated with reduced ketoacidosis in young adults. *Diabet Med* 2011;28:1001–1004.

145. Golden MP, Herrold AJ, Orr DP. An approach to prevention of recurrent diabetic ketoacidosis in the pediatric population. *J Pediatr* 1985;107:195–200.

146. Ellis D, Naar-King S, Templin T, et al. Multisystemic therapy for adolescents with poorly controlled type 1 diabetes: reduced diabetic ketoacidosis admissions and related costs over 24 months. *Diabetes Care* 2008;31:1746–1747.

147. Laffel LM, Wentzell K, Loughlin C, Tovar A, Moltz K, Brink S. Sick day management using blood 3-hydroxybutyrate (3-OHB) compared with urine ketone monitoring reduces hospital visits in young people with T1DM: a randomized clinical trial. *Diabet Med* 2006;23:278–284.

148. Attia N, Jones TW, Holcombe J, Tamborlane WV. Comparison of human regular and lispro insulins after interruption of continuous subcutaneous

insulin infusion and in the treatment of acutely decompensated IDDM. *Diabetes Care* 1998;21:817–821.

149. Guerci B, Meyer L, Salle A, et al. Comparison of metabolic deterioration between insulin analog and regular insulin after a 5-hour interruption of a continuous subcutaneous insulin infusion in type 1 diabetic patients. *J Clin Endocrinol Metab* 1999;84:2673–2678.

150. Laffel L. Sick-day management in type 1 diabetes. *Endocrinol Metab Clin North Am* 2000;29:707–723.

151. Bismuth E, Laffel L. Can we prevent diabetic ketoacidosis in children? *Pediatr Diabetes* 2007;8(Suppl 6):24–33.

152. Danowski T, Peters J, Rathbun J, Quashnock J, Greenman L. Studies in diabetic acidosis and coma, with particular emphasis on the retention of administered potassium. *J Clin Invest* 1949;28:1–9.

153. Darrow D, Pratt E. Retention of water and electrolyte during recovery in a patient with diabetic acidosis. *J Pediatr* 1952;41:688–696.

154. Taketomo C, Hodding J, Kraus D. *Pediatric Dosage Handbook.* 12th ed. Lexi-Comp; 2005.

Chapter 39

Glycemic Control and Chronic Diabetes Complications

Samuel Dagogo-Jack, MD

INTRODUCTION

The chronic complications of diabetes include microvascular and macrovascular disorders. The microvascular complications include diabetic retinopathy, nephropathy, and neuropathy. Diabetic retinopathy is a leading cause of blindness in adults in the industrial world, nephropathy may progress to end-stage renal disease, and neuropathy is a major risk factor for foot ulceration and amputation. Owing to the long period (several years) between onset and diagnosis, up to 25% of type 2 diabetes (T2D) patients already have developed one or more microvascular complications by the time of diagnosis (Table 39.1).[1] Although the microvascular complications typically develop on a background of chronic exposure to hyperglycemia, atypical and early presenting forms can occur,[2] and microvascular lesions have been reported even at the prediabetic stage.[3-5] According to the Centers for Disease Control and Prevention, in 2005–2008, 4.2 million (28.5%) people with diabetes age ≥40 years had diabetic retinopathy, and of these, 655,000 (4.4% of those with diabetes) had vision-threatening advanced diabetic retinopathy.[6] About 60–70% of people with diabetes have mild to severe forms of neuropathy, and diabetes accounts for >60% of nontraumatic lower limb amputations.[6] Furthermore, 44% of new cases of end-stage kidney disease in 2008 were diabetes related, which is consistent with the historical ~50% contribution of diabetes to the end-stage kidney disease burden. The macrovascular complications include cardiovascular disease (CVD), stroke, and peripheral vascular disease (PVD). The risks for stroke and CVD are increased two- to fourfold in adults with diabetes compared with adults without diabetes.[6] Unlike the microvascular complications, where hyperglycemia is the major etiologic factor, the etiology of macrovascular complications is multifactorial, with important contributions from hypertension, dyslipidemia, dysfibrinolysis, atheroinflammation, and other traditional and nontraditional CVD risk factors.[7] The economic costs of diabetes in 2012 in the U.S. amounted to $245 billion.[8] These high costs were driven principally by chronic diabetes complications.[9] There is a direct relationship between the degree of poor diabetic control and the development of microvascular complications and the prohibitive rise in health care costs. Other complications of diabetes, such as periodontal disease, local and systemic infections, depression, musculoskeletal disorders, and pregnancy-related morbidities will not be considered further in this chapter. Although the link between several of the aforementioned complications and poor glycemic control is undoubted,[6] a

DOI: 10.2337/9781580405096.39

fuller treatment of these nonclassical complications is beyond the scope of this chapter.

DIABETES COMPLICATIONS IN PEOPLE DIAGNOSED WITH PREDIABETES

Emerging data indicate that the "long-term" complications of diabetes can manifest during the prediabetes stage.[3-5] In the Diabetes Prevention Program (DPP), 7.9% of people with prediabetes, and 12.6% with newly diagnosed T2D, had retinopathy.[3] During National Health and Nutrition Examination Survey (NHANES) III, fundus photography with a nonmydriatic camera revealed that the prevalence of diabetic retinopathy was 46% higher in African Americans and 84% higher in Mexican Americans than in non-Hispanic whites.[9] A recent analysis of the NHANES 2005–2008 data indicated a retinopathy prevalence of 6.3% for white people and 13.1% for black people, and a higher risk for retinopathy among black people with A1C levels of 5.5–5.9%.[10] Increased risks for microalbuminuria,[4] neuropathy,[5] and macrovascular complications[11-13] have been documented in subjects with prediabetes. Some 25–62% of patients with idiopathic peripheral neuropathy have prediabetes; 11–25% of subjects with prediabetes show evidence of peripheral neuropathy (with 13–21% manifesting neuropathic pain).[5] Glycemia is believed to underlie the pathogenesis of prediabetic microvascular complications, and there appears to be a toxicity gradient beginning during prediabetes.[5]

Table 39.1 Screening for Diabetes Complications in Adults

Complication	Screening method	Frequency	Goals
CVD PVD CVA	Blood pressure measurement	Every routine visit	<130/80 mmHg
Dyslipidemia	LDL, HDL, and triglyceride measurement	Annually; every 2 years in patients with values at goal who are not receiving treatment and who have no CVD	Patients without overt CVD: LDL <100 mg/dl Patients with overt CVD: consider LDL <70 mg/dl; HDL >40 mg/dl in men, >50 mg/dl in women; triglycerides <150 mg/dl
Nephropathy	Urine microalbumin	Annually*	Normal albumin <30 mg/24 hours or albumin-creatinine ratio <30 mg/g in a random urine specimen
	Serum creatinine for estimation of GFR	Annually	Normal GFR >90 ml/minute/1.73 m²

(continued)

Table 39.1 Screening for Diabetes Complications in Adults (*continued*)

Complication	Screening method	Frequency	Goals
Retinopathy	Dilated and comprehensive eye examination	T1D: 3–5 years after onset; T2D, shortly after diagnosis; repeat annually, more often if retinopathy is progressing or during pregnancy	Prevention of irreversible damage and vision loss
Neuropathy	Examination for DPN	At diagnosis and annually	Early detection
	Assessment for autonomic neuropathy	T1D: 5 years after diagnosis T2D: at diagnosis	Early detection
	Inspection of insensate feet	Every visit	Intact skin
	Comprehensive foot examination	Annually	Normal examination

Note: CVD = cardiovascular disease; DPN = distal symmetrical polyneuropathy; GFR = glomerular filtration rate; HDL = high-density lipoprotein; LDL = low-density lipoprotein.

*In patients with T1D who have had diabetes for ≥5 years and in all patients with T2D starting at diagnosis and during pregnancy.

Source: American Diabetes Association.[121]

Although CVD,[11–13] endothelial dysfunction,[14] and PVD[15] can occur in prediabetes, their etiologies tend to be multifactorial and the specific role of glycemia is less clear. A cross-section of U.S. adults (age ≥40 years) examined in the NHANES 2001–2004, whose mean fasting plasma glucose (FPG) was 112 mg/dl, showed a prevalence of PVD (ankle brachial blood pressure index <0.9) of 8.5%; obesity increased the odds of PVD (3.10 [1.84–5.22]).[15] Endothelium, the largest end organ in the body by surface area, is the target of numerous noxious stimuli, including shear stress from blood pressure, inflammatory and oxidative stress, glycemia, and lipidemia. Endothelial dysfunction precedes fatty streaking, the well-known initiator of atherosclerosis, and is therefore an early macrovascular disease risk marker.[16–18] Compared with lean normoglycemic subjects, age-matched obese individuals with prediabetes (FPG 106 mg/dl) have been reported to show evidence of endothelial dysfunction (as indicated by impaired flow-mediated dilatation).[14] The occurrence of diabetes complications in patients with prediabetes argues for increased surveillance and further research to unravel the pathophysiological mechanisms and direct appropriate interventions.[19,20]

PATHOPHYSIOLOGICAL MECHANISMS OF DIABETES COMPLICATIONS

Although not fully understood, key components in the pathogenesis of chronic diabetes complications include genetic predisposition and intracellular hyperglycemia leading to alterations in the polyol, hexosamine, and protein kinase C pathways.[21-23] Advanced glycated end products and their interactions with their receptors also serve as mediators of target organ damage,[24] glomerular hyperfiltration,[25] aberrant growth factor expression,[26] hypoxia,[27] inflammation, and oxidative stress, as well as alterations in endothelial, pericyte, and mesangial structure or function.[28-30] Familial clustering has been reported for diabetic nephropathy and severe retinopathy.[31,32] With regard to nephropathy, genetic susceptibility (or protection) may explain the fact that only 30–40% of patients with diabetes develop this complication. The specific genes and the mechanisms whereby those genes confer susceptibility to (or protection from) kidney disease are under investigation.[33-35] Promising insights are emerging that link variants within the coding region *APOL1*, a gene that protects against trypanosomiasis (African sleeping sickness), with increased risk for kidney disease in African Americans.[35]

The selective nature of the tissues that develop chronic diabetes complications (retina, glomerulus, peripheral neurons) is remarkable, given that all perfused tissues of the body are exposed to hyperglycemia in people with diabetes. Brownlee has suggested that the cells that escape hyperglycemic damage are those that are able to limit their exposure to glucose influx from plasma, whereas cells susceptible to diabetic complications (such as retinal endothelial cells, glomerular mesangial cells, and Schwann cells of peripheral neurons) lack an efficient mechanism for limiting intracellular glucose influx during exposure to hyperglycemia.[23,36,37] Because cytosolic glucose concentration in such cells mirrors ambient plasma glucose levels, those cell types may be described as "poikiloglycemic" (analogous to poikilothermic organisms that take on ambient temperature because of their inability to regulate body temperature). Exposure to sustained intracellular hyperglycemia is linked to tissue damage via four toxic pathways: *1)* increased flux through the aldose reductase (polyol) pathway, *2)* formation of advanced glycosylation end products, *3)* protein kinase C (PKC) activation, and *4)* increased hexosamine pathway activity (see Figure 39.1).[23] Aldose reductase is a cytosolic enzyme that normally catalyzes the conversion of toxic aldehydes to inactive alcohols.[38] Aldose reductase also reduces cytoplasmic glucose to sorbitol, which is further oxidized to fructose by sorbitol dehydrogenase. With rising intracellular hyperglycemia, these chemical reactions consume nicotinamide adenine dinucleotide phosphate (NADPH), which depletes reduced glutathione, an intracellular antioxidant.[39] The decrease in reduced glutathione exposes the cell to oxidative damage.[23] The toxic pathway can be limited by lowering ambient glycemia (which decreases intracellular hyperglycemia) and by inhibition of aldose reductase. The latter has been reported to prevent neuropathy in dogs with diabetes.[40]

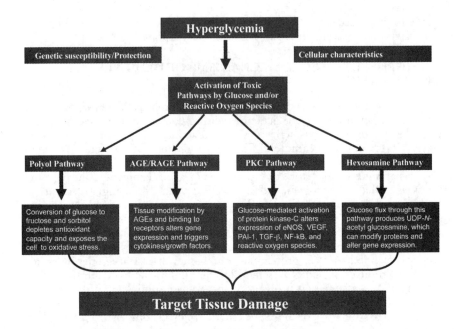

Figure 39.1—Multiple pathways have been described that link high blood glucose levels to the microvascular and neuropathic complications of diabetes (see text). Primary genetic susceptibility to or protection from complications probably exists. The specific tissues damaged by hyperglycemia also have a unique susceptibility in that they lack mechanisms for limiting influx of glucose. Once inside the cell, glucose can drive four toxic mechanisms that mediate downstream activation of inflammatory cytokines, growth factors, reactive oxygen species, and other processes that lead to fibrosis, vascular permeability, angiogenesis, and tissue damage.

Note: AGE = advanced glycosylation end products; RAGE = receptor for AGE; PKC = protein kinase C; eNOS = endothelial nitric oxide synthase; VEGF = vascular endothelial growth factor; PAI-1-plasminogen activator inhibitor-1; TGF-β = transforming growth factor–β; NF-kB = nuclear factor-κB.

Source: Adapted from Dagogo-Jack S. Complications of diabetes mellitus, in Section 9, Metabolism. In *ACP Medicine.* Nabel EG, Ed. Philadelphia, Decker Intellectual Properties, 2012, chap. 3.

Advanced glycated end products (AGEs) are formed from dicarbonyl precursors, whose levels increase in proportion to intracellular glucose levels. AGEs modify intracellular proteins and nuclear DNA and can diffuse out of the cell to modify extracellular matrix and circulating proteins.[23,41–43] The AGE-modified proteins and macromolecules bind to receptors for AGEs (RAGEs), which triggers inflammatory reactions, which induces generation of reactive oxygen species at various sites (endothelial cells, mesangial cells, and macrophages). The AGE–RAGE interaction also leads to alteration of gene expression of various cytokines and growth factors, with dire consequences for basement membrane and vascular integrity.[23,24,41–43] Skin levels of AGEs correlate with A1C and predict the occurrence of diabetic retinopathy, nephropathy, and neuropathy.[44] Similarly, levels of glycated collagen and carboxymethyl-lysine predicted 10-year progression of retinopathy and nephropathy during the Epidemiology of Diabetes Interventions and Complications (EDIC) study.[45] Chemical inhibition of the formation of AGEs can prevent diabetic retinopathy in experimental animals.[46]

Intracellular hyperglycemia upregulates diacylglycerol levels, resulting in the activation of protein kinase-C.[23,47] The PKC activation alters the expression of several downstream genes that regulate vascular function (e.g., nitric oxide synthase, endothelin-1, vascular endothelial growth factor), collagen synthesis and fibrosis (transforming growth factor-β), inflammation (nuclear factor–κB, fibrinolysis, plasminogen activator inhibitor-1), and generation of reactive oxygen species.[23,47–50] The net result is increased vascular permeability, vascular endothelial growth factor expression, and aberrant angiogenesis, neovascularization, and fibrosis (see Figure 39.1).[47–50] The toxic consequences of the PKC pathway can be mitigated by decreasing ambient hyperglycemia or by inhibiting PKC, which has been shown to prevent microvascular complications in mice with diabetes.[51]

Under normal conditions, most of the glucose that enters the cell is processed through the Krebs cycle, with a small fraction (~3%) passing through the nutrient-sensing hexosamine (glucosamine) pathway.[52] Intracellular glucose enters the hexosamine pathway after the second phosphorylation step (glucose → glucose-6-phosphate → fructose-6-phosphate). The fructose-6-phosphate is converted to glucosamine-6-phosphate, and ultimately to uridine diphosphate (UDP) N-acetyl glucosamine. The UDP-N-acetyl glucosamine can induce tissue damage through modification of intracellular proteins and alteration of gene expression. In "poikiloglycemic" cell types, chronic intracellular hyperglycemia increases glucose flux through the hexosamine pathway, thereby increasing the risk for tissue damage.[53–55] Notably, each of the four major toxic pathways linking hyperglycemia to tissue damage can be triggered by reactive oxygen species, independent of glycemia.[23,56,57]

Increased understanding of the mechanisms and mediators of microvascular complications has opened up novel targets for drug development. Pharmacological interventions targeting one or more of the known toxic pathways potentially could prevent diabetes complications or complement the effects of glycemic control, the latter currently being the only proven approach of preventing microvascular complications. Inhibitors of PKC, aldose reductase, and AGE formation have been shown to have salutary effects in preclinical models, although human data are limited.[46,51,58,59]

GLYCEMIC CONTROL AND CHRONIC DIABETES COMPLICATIONS

The preceding section underscores the central role of hyperglycemia in the pathogenesis of microvascular complications ("glucose hypothesis"). The corollary to the "glucose hypothesis" (i.e., control of hyperglycemia should prevent the development of microvascular complications) has been demonstrated in several landmark studies.[60–62] The Diabetes Control and Complications Trial (DCCT) randomized 1,441 patients with type 1 diabetes (T1D) to receive conventional treatment (i.e., no more than two insulin injections a day) or intensive treatment (three or four insulin injections a day or continuous subcutaneous insulin infusion by pump).[60] During the study, the A1C values stabilized at 8.9% in the conventional-treatment group, as compared with 7.1% in the intensive-treatment group. Over a mean follow-up period of 6.5 years, intensive treatment resulted in risk reductions of 27–76% for the occurrence or progression of retinopathy, 35% for the development of microalbuminuria, 56% for albuminuria, and 60% for the development of clinical neuropathy.[60] The relationship between decreasing A1C levels and declining risk of microvascular complications was curvilinear, without evidence of a lower threshold for benefit. There was a threefold increase in the risk of severe hypoglycemia, however, as A1C decreased from ~9% to ~7% in the intensive-treatment group.[60,63]

The EDIC study is a long-term observational follow-up study of the original DCCT cohort. Upon completion of the DCCT 1,349 out of the original 1,441 participants (93.6%) enrolled in EDIC. Within 2 years of EDIC, the A1C levels in the original intensive-treatment group and the conventional-treatment group converged around a mean value of 8%. Despite this convergence in ambient post-DCCT glycemia, patients in the early intensive control group have showed a sustained 43–84% reduction in the risks for all complications of diabetes.[64] The Kumamoto study adopted a design similar to that of the DCCT, albeit in patients with T2D, and achieved similar results.[61]

Following a 3-month dietary run-in period, the U.K. Prospective Diabetes Study (UKPDS) randomized patients with newly diagnosed T2D to conventional treatment consisting of dietary modification ($n = 1,138$) or intensive treatment ($n = 2,729$), using sulfonylurea drugs ($n = 1,573$), insulin ($n = 1,156$), or metformin ($n = 342$).[62,65] The goal of intensive treatment was an FPG level of <108 mg/dl. Most of the patients in the conventional-treatment group ultimately required medications to keep their FPG <270 mg/dl, but treatment was not intensified and time spent on diet therapy alone constituted nearly 60% of the total treatment time. Also, the intensive-treatment group required the use of multiple drug combinations to maintain the treatment goal. After 10 years of follow-up, intensive treatment was associated with a 25% reduction in the risk of serious microvascular complications (i.e., vitreous hemorrhage, need for laser treatment, and renal failure), compared with conventional treatment.[62,65] The median A1C levels were 7% in the intensive therapy group and 7.9% in the conventional therapy group. Severe hypoglycemia occurred in ~2% of patients on intensive treatment, which was much lower than the rates seen with intensive treatment in patients with T1D in the DCCT. In 2008, the UKPDS investigators reported 10-year follow-up data. As was observed post-DCCT, the 0.9% difference in A1C between treatment groups during UKPDS disappeared after 1 year of additional follow-up. Despite the glycemic convergence, the 10-year poststudy follow-up data showed persistence of the benefits of intensive glucose control on microvascular endpoints (24% risk reduction, $P = 0.01$).[66] In contrast, the benefits of previously improved blood pressure control were not sustained when between-group differences in blood pressure were lost during the 10-year poststudy period.[67] These results support the concept of "metabolic memory" or "legacy effect"[68,69] and emphasize the importance of early intervention.

In the Action in Diabetes and Vascular Disease (ADVANCE) study,[70] 11,140 patients with T2D were assigned randomly to a standard glucose control or an intensive glucose control arm. The intensive glucose control arm consisted of treatment with a sulfonylurea (modified-release gliclazide) plus other drugs as required to achieve A1C values of ≤6.5%. After a median follow-up period of 5 years, the mean A1C level was 6.5% in the intensive control group compared with 7.3% in the standard control group. Intensive control resulted in a 21% relative reduction in the development of new or worsening nephropathy, but there was no significant difference in the incidence of new or worsening retinopathy between the intensive- and the standard-treatment groups, perhaps because of the low overall event rates.[70] In the Veterans Affairs Diabetes Trial (VADT), 1,791 military veterans with T2D (mean duration since diagnosis of diabetes 11.5 years) were assigned randomly to receive either intensive or standard glucose control.[71,72] After a median follow-up of 5.6 years, the median A1C levels were 8.4% in the standard-therapy group and 6.9% in the intensive-therapy group. Although the primary outcome was the development of major cardiovascular events, microvascular complications were prespecified secondary endpoints. Compared with standard therapy, intensive treatment was associated with a decreased incidence of microalbuminuria and macroalbuminuria, a trend toward a reduction in the risk of diabetic retinopathy, and no significant difference in the incidence of neuropathy.[71,72] The VADT data showed variable benefits of decreasing the A1C level from 8.4% to 6.9% on microvascular end points, perhaps owing to the shorter follow-up period and the unique study population compared with the DCCT and UKPDS participants.

The Action to Control Cardiovascular Risk in Diabetes (ACCORD) study had a substudy (ACCORD-Eye), whose goal was to determine the effects of intensive glycemic control, combination therapy for dyslipidemia, and intensive blood pressure control on the progression of diabetic retinopathy.[73] The latter was defined as the occurrence of a three or more step increase on the Early Treatment Diabetic Retinopathy Study Severity Scale (based on seven-field stereoscopic fundus photographs) or the development of diabetic retinopathy requiring photocoagulation or vitrectomy. Of the 10,251 participants with T2D enrolled in the main ACCORD study, a subgroup of 2,856 participants was evaluated for retinopathy outcomes at 4 years. Compared with standard therapy (A1C target 7–7.9%), intensive glycemic control (A1C target <6.0%) resulted in a significant 23% reduction in the rate of progression of diabetic retinopathy. Interestingly, use of fenofibrate for intensive dyslipidemia therapy was associated with a significant 40% reduction in retinopathy risk compared with placebo-treated subjects.[73] Retinopathy outcomes, however, did not differ significantly between the intensive and standard blood pressure treatment arms.[73] The finding of decreased retinopathy risk in the fenofibrate-treated group supports a growing body of observations indicating that fibrates might have a protective effect against microvascular complications.[74–76] In the Fenofibrate and Event Lowering in Diabetes study, patients with diabetes treated with fenofibrate experienced reductions in the risks of developing microalbuminuria, proliferative retinopathy, and minor amputations.[75,76]

The mechanisms whereby fibrates decrease microvascular risk are not fully understood, but they might involve lipid and nonlipid pathways.[77]

In an expanded report on microvascular outcomes from the ACCORD group,[78] there was no significant effect of intensive glycemic control on the pre-specified composite end points of advanced microvascular complications, including end-stage renal failure requiring dialysis or renal transplantation, increased serum creatinine >3.3 mg/dl (>291.7 µmol/l), retinal photocoagulation, or vitrectomy after a median follow-up of 3.7 years.[78] Intensive therapy, however, delayed the onset of albuminuria and peripheral neuropathy, and decreased the risk of cataract extraction.[78] The differences in the scope and magnitude of the effects of glycemic control on microvascular complications between the ACCORD study and the UKPDS[64,66] might be due to the older age, more advanced diabetes, and shorter duration of intensive glycemic therapy among participants in the ACCORD study.

Clearly, the microvascular and neuropathic complications of diabetes can be prevented by optimization of glycemic control (A1C ≤7%). In the DCCT, the risk of retinopathy was decreased by ~44% for each proportional 10% decrease in A1C (e.g., a decrease in A1C from 10% to 9%).[60,79] Microalbuminuria and neuropathy showed glycemic risk patterns similar to those of retinopathy. In the UKPDS, the risk of microvascular complications decreased by ~37% for every absolute decrease of 1% in A1C.[30,62,80] The Kumamoto investigators calculated that the glycemic thresholds to prevent the onset or progression of diabetic microvascular complications were as follows: A1C <6.5%, FBG <110 mg/dl, and 2-hour postprandial blood glucose concentration <180 mg/dl.[61] Neither the UKPDS nor the DCCT analyses, however, indicated any glycemic threshold in the diabetic range of A1C below which there was no further risk reduction for microvascular complications.[79,80]

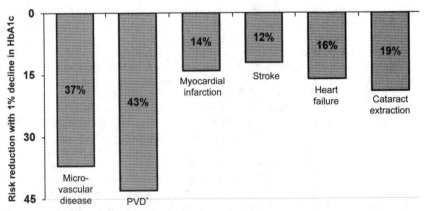

Figure 39.2—Effect of a 1% absolute reduction of A1C on microvascular and macrovascular complications and cataract extraction in patients with T2D in the United Kingdom Prospective Diabetes Study.[74]

Note: PVD = peripheral vascular disease/lower extremity amputation.

These findings argue strongly in favor of early glycemic control as a powerful means of preventing microvascular complications. Moreover, the long-term follow-up data from the EDIC study and the UKPDS showed that the benefits of previous intensive treatment (or the adverse effects of previous conventional treatment) persist well beyond the period of active intervention, despite convergence of between-group A1C values.[64,66,68] Thus, early sustained glycemic control confers an enduring legacy of protection from microangiopathic complications. Conversely, previous sustained exposure to poor glycemic control continues to exert a legacy of adverse effects even after some improvement in metabolic control has occurred.

CLINICAL MANIFESTATIONS

RETINOPATHY

The lesions of diabetic retinopathy evolve as background or nonproliferative retinopathy, preproliferative retinopathy, and proliferative retinopathy. Over several years, diabetic retinopathy develops in most patients with T2D with suboptimal glycemic control.[81,82] In T1D, where the date of onset of clinical disease is easier to determine, ~50% of patients have evidence of background retinopathy after 7 years, and nearly all patients have some form of retinopathy after 20 years.[22,81,82] In the DPP, 7.9% of subjects with impaired glucose tolerance were found to have lesions consistent with diabetic retinopathy.[3] Transient worsening of diabetic retinopathy has been noted during intensification of glycemic control.[83] The mechanisms underlying such exacerbation are not fully understood. During the first year of initiation of the DCCT, early worsening of retinopathy was observed in 13.1% of 711 patients assigned to intensive treatment and in 7.6% of 728 patients assigned to conventional treatment (odds ratio, 2.06; $P < 0.001$). No case of early worsening was associated with serious visual loss (high-risk proliferative retinopathy developed in two patients and clinically significant macular edema occurred in three, all of whom responded well to treatment).[83] By the 18-month visit, recovery had occurred in the majority of patients who had experienced early worsening of retinopathy. The significant predictors of early worsening were a higher A1C level at screening and reduction of this level during the initial 6 months after randomization.[83] The DCCT findings are consistent with previous reports of paradoxical worsening of retinopathy following rapid glycemic improvement in patients with long-standing poor glycemic control and preexisting retinopathy.[84,85] There is no evidence that more gradual reduction of glycemia might be associated with less risk of early worsening.[83] Close ophthalmologic monitoring, however, is prudent in patients with preexisting retinopathy and poor glycemic control who are undergoing glycemic optimization. Preemptive photocoagulation may be considered in patients with vision-threatening retinopathy before initiation of intensive treatment.[83]

Epidemiological assessment of the association between glycemic exposure (A1C) before and during the DCCT with the risk of retinopathy showed that the initial A1C level and the duration of diabetes were major predictors of the risk of retinopathy progression.[79] In both the intensive- and standard-treatment groups, the mean A1C during the trial was the dominant predictor of retinopathy progression: A 10% relative decrease in A1C (e.g., 8% vs. 7.2%) was associated with a 43% retinopathy risk reduction in the intensive group and a 45% risk reduction in the conventional group.[79] Patients with shorter duration of diabetes experienced greater benefits of intensive therapy.[79] Thus, optimization of glycemic control should be instituted as early as possible to maximize the benefits of prevention of retinopathy and other microvascular complications.

NEPHROPATHY

Diabetic nephropathy, which affects ~40% of patients with T1D and ~20% of patients with T2D, accounts for 50% of patients with end-stage kidney disease requiring dialysis treatment.[86–89] Albuminuria (30–299 mg/24 hours; historically, called microalbuminuria) is a marker of incipient nephropathy; progression to higher-grade albuminuria (>300 mg/24 hours; historically, called macroalbuminuria) and decline in glomerular filtration rate (GFR) occurs over several years.[89] Decreases in microalbuminuria are ready demonstrable following improved glycemic control,[60–62] but data demonstrating that glycemic control slows the decline in GFR are scant. Fewer than 1% of UKPDS participants developed renal failure during the study, because the study enrolled only subjects with newly diagnosed diabetes. Nonetheless, the UKPDS showed benefits of improved glycemic control on significant renal end points: A 0.9% reduction in median A1C was associated with decreased albuminuria, a 67% risk reduction in the proportion of patients who had a twofold increase in plasma creatinine, and 74% risk reduction in those who had a doubling of their plasma urea levels.[62]

In the DCCT/EDIC study, the rate of disease progression, as defined by a serum creatinine concentration >2 mg/dl, was decreased by intensive glycemic control.[90] A subsequent report on the combined DCCT/EDIC cohort followed up for a median period of 22 years showed that intensive glycemic control during DCCT was associated with a 50% risk reduction (95% confidence interval [CI], 18–69; P = 0.006) in the incidence of impaired GFR (<60 ml/minute/1.73 m^2 of body surface area at two consecutive study visits).[91] End-stage kidney disease developed in 8 participants in the intensive-therapy group versus 16 patients in the conventional-therapy group.

On the basis of the DCCT data, intensive glycemic control in 29 patients with T1D treated for 6.5 years prevented one case of impaired GFR over a total follow-up period of 20 years.[91] Interestingly, intensive glycemic control was associated with a modest early decline in GFR during the DCCT years (possibly due to amelioration of hyperfiltration). After 10 years (the EDIC phase), intensive glucose control was associated with a slower decline in the GFR and higher mean estimated GFR compared with conventional therapy. The effect of improved glycemic control on the GFR remained significant after adjustments for blood pressure, BMI, and the use of antihypertensive agents (including inhibitors of the renin–angiotensin–aldosterone system) and was fully attenuated after adjustment for A1C.[91] Together, the results from the landmark clinical trials demonstrate that achieving A1C levels of ~7% early in the course of diabetes is specifically associated with decreased risk of diabetic nephropathy.[60-62,90,91] Furthermore, even in the setting of preexisting nephropathy, improved glycemic control can slow the rate of progression of kidney disease.[62,90]

NEUROPATHY

The occurrence of diabetic neuropathy is duration dependent, although early presenting forms are recognized.[2] The most common form of diabetic neuropathy (i.e., peripheral, symmetrical, sensorimotor polyneuropathy) affects up to 50% of patients.[92–94] The hallmark symptoms include paresthesias, numbness, tingling, and burning sensation in a glove and stocking distribution. Some patients with diabetic neuropathy present with severe pain[92]; hyperglycemia is known to decrease pain threshold, thereby exacerbating the severity of neuropathic symptoms.[95,96] Diabetes accounts for >60% of cases of nontraumatic lower extremity amputations in the U.S. and loss of protective sensation from peripheral neuropathy is the major risk factor for amputation. Other contributory factors include PVD, foot deformities, trauma, and deep tissue infections. Most of these risk factors are affected by the state of glycemic control. Suboptimal glycemic control is associated with increased risks of infections, impaired wound healing, and development of microangiopathy and PVD.

Involvement of the autonomic nervous system is common in diabetic neuropathy.[93,97] Autonomic neuropathy involving the heart is a risk factor for abnormal cardiac reflexes, resting tachycardia, and sudden death.[97] In the DCCT/EDIC study, intensive therapy with insulin in subjects with T1D was associated with a 53% reduction in the incidence of cardiovascular autonomic neuropathy and the benefit persisted during prolonged follow-up.[98,99]

Hypoglycemia-associated autonomic failure (HAAF) is a reversible form of hypoglycemia unawareness and defective glucose counterregulation that is induced by recurrent episodes of hypoglycemia in insulin-treated patients.[100–102] As a consequence of the loss of the autonomic warning symptoms of hypoglycemia (and impaired glucose counterregulation), patients with HAAF are prone to recurrent episodes of severe life-threating hypoglycemia. The scrupulous avoidance of iatrogenic hypoglycemia can restore recognition of hypoglycemic symptoms and may improve counterregulatory function within several weeks.[101,102] This approach might entail a deliberate policy of allowing the A1C level to increase modestly in patients with HAAF who are undergoing intensive glycemic control.[103,104]

GLYCEMIC CONTROL AND MACROVASCULAR COMPLICATIONS

Data from several observational studies[105–113] and the UKPDS[74] have shown that glycemic burden is a risk factor for cardiovascular events and death. Other observational studies, however, have not found the same relationship.[114,115] If a causal relationship between glycemic burden and CVD risk exists, then interventions to decrease glucose levels should decrease CVD risk. The latter effect has been demonstrated in the DCCT/EDIC.[116] During ~20 years of extended follow-up of the patients with T1D enrolled in the DCCT/EDIC study, it was observed that the participants who had received prior intensive therapy (mean A1C during DCCT ~7%) experienced a 42% reduction in first macrovascular events and a 57% reduction in nonfatal myocardial infarction (MI), stroke, and cardiovascular death compared with the conventional group (mean A1C during DCCT ~9%)[30,116] (see Figure 39.3). In the UKPDS, intensive treatment with insulin or a sulfonylurea showed a trend toward decreasing MI (risk reduction 16%, $P = 0.052$) during the active phase of the study[62] that reached statistical significance during a 10-year follow-up period.[66] Intensive treatment with sulfonylurea or insulin resulted in

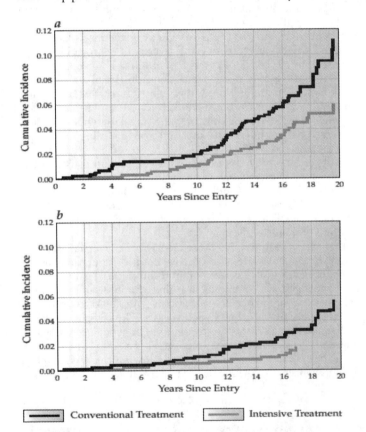

Figure 39.3—(a) Cumulative incidence of the first cardiovascular event that included clinical findings or the need for revascularization and (b) cumulative incidence of the first occurrence of nonfatal MI, stroke, or death from cardiovascular disease in patients with T1D enrolled in the DCCT/EDIC.[60]

Source: Reproduced with permission from Dagogo-Jack S. Complications of diabetes mellitus, in Section 9, Metabolism. In *ACP Medicine.* Nabel EG, Ed. Philadelphia, Decker Intellectual Properties, 2012, chap. 3.

reductions in the risks for MI (15%, $P = 0.01$) and all-cause mortality (13%, $P = 0.007$).[66] Also, the metformin-treated subgroup continued to show reductions in the risks for MI (33%, $P = 0.005$) and death from any cause (27%, $P = 0.002$) 10 years poststudy.[66]

In contrast, three recent studies failed to show significant reduction in CVD events (and one of them showed increased mortality) following intensive glycemic control to A1C targets of <6–6.5% in patients with T2D.[70–72,117] In the ACCORD study,[117] 10,251 patients with longstanding T2D (mean age, 62.2 years) were assigned randomly to receive intensive therapy (A1C target of <6.0%) or standard therapy (A1C target of 7 to 7.9%). The study population was 62% male, and 35% had had prior cardiovascular events. After a mean follow-up of 3.5 years, the intensive glucose control arm of the ACCORD study was abruptly discontinued due to higher mortality compared with standard therapy (257 deaths versus 203 deaths, hazard ratio [HR], 1.22; 95% CI, 1.01–1.46; $P = 0.04$). The mean A1C level attained during the study was 6.4% in the intensive-therapy group and 7.5% in the standard-therapy group. In the intensive-therapy group, 352 patients reached the prespecified primary outcome of composite nonfatal cardiovascular events, as compared with 371 in the standard-therapy group (HR 0.90; 95% CI, 0.78–1.04; $P = 0.16$). Severe hypoglycemia and weight gain of >10 kg occurred more frequently in the intensive-therapy group than in the standard-therapy group. To date, the ACCORD investigators have not been able to determine the reasons for the excess mortality in the intensive-therapy group; contribution from the adverse effects of hypoglycemia in high-risk patients is widely suspected but difficult to prove, retrospectively.[118,119]

In the ADVANCE study,[70] intensive control (mean A1C 6.5%) decreased the incidence of combined major macrovascular and microvascular events (18.1%, vs. 20.0%; HR 0.90 [0.82–0.98], $P = 0.01$), as compared with standard control (mean A1C 7.3%). When assessed separately, however, intensive treatment did not significantly decrease major macrovascular events (HR 0.88 [0.74–1.04], $P = 0.12$) or mortality (HR 0.93 [0.83–1.06], $P = 0.28$).[70] Similar to the findings of the ACCORD and ADVANCE studies, the VADT investigators reported that intensive glucose control to a median A1C level of 6.9% (versus standard therapy; median A1C 8.4%) for a mean duration of 5.6 years did not significantly decrease the incidence of major macrovascular end points.[71,72] There was no increased mortality from intensive glycemic control in VADT (HR of death from any cause, 1.07 [0.81–1.42], $P = 0.62$), similar to the findings in ADVANCE.

Together, the data from the ACCORD, VADT, and ADVANCE studies indicate that aggressive attempts aimed at normalizing or near-normalizing A1C levels do not significantly decrease CVD events in people with T2D. This is in contrast to the findings of the DCCT/EDIC[110] and the UKPDS[66] long-term follow-up studies that showed significant reductions in fatal and nonfatal cardiovascular events one decade or more following prior intensive glycemic control. Table 39.2 summarizes the major differences among the DCCT/EDIC, UKPDS, ACCORD, VADT, and ADVANCE studies. In general, the patients enrolled in DCCT were younger, had minimal CVD risk factors and no prior CVD events, had had diabetes for a shorter duration, and were followed up over a much longer period before CVD events were assessed. In contrast, the ACCORD, VADT, and ADVANCE studies enrolled older patients with T2D, one-third of whom had had prior CVD events and more than half of whom harbored two or more CVD risk factors. Furthermore, insulin was the only antidiabetic agent used in DCCT, whereas multiple oral agents (often in combination with insulin) were prescribed in the other studies. Importantly, the concurrent use of medications that modify CVD risk (e.g., statins, angiotensin-converting-enzyme [ACE] inhibitors, angiotensin-receptor blockers [ARBs], aspirin) was more frequent among participants in the VADT and ACCORD studies compared with those in the DCCT or UKPDS.

OPTIMAL GLYCEMIC TARGETS

Current evidence from the DCCT/EDIC and the UKDPS supports an A1C goal of ≤7%, to prevent microvascular complications in patients with T1D or

Table 39.2 Comparison of Major Trials of Intensive Glucose Control and CVD Outcomes

	DCCT/EDIC	UKPDS	ACCORD	ADVANCE	VADT
Participant characteristics					
Number (Type)	1,394 (T1D)	3,277 (T2D)	10,251 (T2D)	11,140 (T2D)	1,791 (T2D)
Mean age (years)	27.7	53	62	66	60
Caucasian (%)	96	76.1	64.6	ND*	62
Duration of diabetes (years)	2.6	Newly diagnosed	10	8	11.5
History of CVD (%)	Excluded subjects with CVD or major risk factors	Excluded subjects with CVD or major risk factors	35	32	40
Insulin treated (%) (IC vs. SC)	100 vs. 100	38 vs. 16**	77 vs. 55	40 vs. 24	89 vs. 74
Final A1C (%) (IC vs. SC)	7.1 vs. 8.9	7.0 vs. 7.9	6.4 vs. 7.5	6.3 vs. 7.0	6.9 vs. 8.5
Weight change IC – SC (kg)	4.6 (at 5 yr)	2.9	3.1	0.9	5.4
Severe hypoglycemia (subjects >1 episode) (%) IC arm	62***	1–1.8	16.2	2.7	21.2
SC arm	19***	0.7	5.1	1.5	9.9

T2D.[120-122] The specific treatment target should be individualized, however, based on the characteristics and risk profile of patients.[120] The risk of hypoglycemia always must be balanced against the benefits of an intensified glucose control regimen. The glycemic target (A1C ≤7%) that significantly decreased the risk of microvascular complications was associated with decreased risk of macrovascular events in patients with T1D.[116] Maintenance of A1C levels of ~7% was not associated with significant CVD risk reduction among patients with T2D during the active intervention phase of the UKPDS.[62] CVD risk reduction was observed during follow-up evaluation at 10 years poststudy among UKPDS participants with prior intensive control (median A1C ~7%) compared with patients in the conventional policy arm (median A1C 7.9%).[66] More aggressive glycemic targets (A1C 6–6.5%) have not been shown to decrease CVD risk and are not recommended for

	DCCT/EDIC	UKPDS	ACCORD	ADVANCE	VADT
CVD outcomes					
Events reduction with IC (%)	42% (first CVD event + re-vascularization)	SU/Insulin: 15% for MI Metformin: 33% for MI	NS	NS	NS
Risk reduction for death with IC (%)	57% (nonfatal MI, stroke, or CV death)	SU/Insulin: 13% Metformin: 27%	Increased deaths†	NS	NS

Note: ACCORD = Action to Control Cardiovascular Risk in Diabetes; ADVANCE = Action in Diabetes and Vascular Disease; CVD = cardiovascular disease; DCCT = Diabetes Control and Complications Trial; EDIC = Epidemiology of Diabetes Interventions and Complications Study; IC = intensive glycemic control; NS = not significant; SC = standard glycemic control; SU = sulfonylurea; T1D = type 1 diabetes; T2D = type 2 diabetes; VADT = Veterans Affairs Diabetes Trial; UKPDS = U.K. Prospective Diabetes Study.

*ND = no data; subjects were enrolled from Australia, Europe, Asia, and North America.

**Approximate figures; UKPDS medications schedule was complex, with much crossover. At least 50% of patients in the sulfonylurea arm required add-on insulin therapy.

***Episodes per 100 patient-years during DCCT.

†In ACCORD, intensive treatment was associated with increased death (hazard ratio 1.22 [95% CI 1.01–1.46]).

Sources: Adapted from Dagogo-Jack S. Complications of diabetes mellitus, in Section 9, Metabolism. In *ACP Medicine*. Nabel EG, Ed. Philadelphia, Decker Intellectual Properties., 2012, chap. 3. Data were compiled from Holman RR, Paul SK, Bethel MA, Matthews DR, Neil HA: 10-year follow-up of intensive glucose control in type 2 diabetes. *N Eng J Med* 2008;359:1577–1589; The ADVANCE Collaborative Group. Intensive blood glucose control and vascular outcomes in patients with type 2 diabetes. *N Eng J Med* 2008;358:2560–2672; Duckworth W, Abraira C, Moritz T, et al. VADT Investigators. Glucose control and vascular complications in veterans with type 2 diabetes. *N Eng J Med* 2009;360:129–139; Moss OE, Klein R, Klein BE, Meuer SM. The association of glycemia and cause-specific mortality in a diabetic population. *Arch Intern Med* 1994;154:2473–2479; Andersson DK, Svärdsudd K. Long-term glycemic control relates to mortality in type II diabetes. *Diabetes Care* 1995;18:1534–1543; Uusitupa MI, Niskanen LK, Siitonen O, Voutilainen E, Pyörälä K. Ten-year cardiovascular mortality in relation to risk factors and abnormalities in lipoprotein composition in type 2 (non-insulin-dependent) diabetic and non-diabetic subjects. *Diabetologia* 1993;36:1175–1184.

the prevention of macrovascular complications in diabetes.[70–72,117] Given the multi-factorial etiology of macrovascular disease in diabetes, a comprehensive policy targeting glycemia, lipids, blood pressure, and other known risk factors, is the best approach to the prevention of macrovascular disease in patients with diabetes.[123]

CONCLUSION

In conclusion, secular trends show downward patterns in the occurrence of diabetes-related complications and mortality.[124–128] The improvements have been particularly striking with regard to microvascular complications, including retinopathy, nephropathy, and amputation. For instance, during the 12 years between 1996 and 2008, hospitalization for nontraumatic lower extremity amputations among U.S. adults with diabetes age ≥40 years decreased by 65%.[129] It is highly unlikely that these secular trends occurred by chance, given the progressive, predictive, and pernicious relationship between uncontrolled diabetes and adverse long-term complications. Increased awareness of the benefits of controlling glycemia (and other risk factors), triggered by the results of the DCCT, UKPDS, and other outcome studies, likely had a kindling effect in producing these salutary secular trends in diabetes complications.[130] Despite these hopeful trends, the magnitude of the recent improvements in diabetes complications, such as amputation, has been less pronounced in older persons (≥75 years) and African Americans.[129] Moreover, the increasing burden of T2D in children and adolescents presents unique challenges regarding optimal glycemic control that will require an expansion of the evidence base.[131,132] Therefore, clinicians are urged to maintain surveillance for diabetes complications (Table 39.1) and institute prompt intervention to optimize glycemic control and consolidate the downward secular trends in the burden of chronic diabetes complications across all demographic groups.[123–129,133]

REFERENCES

1. U.K. Prospective Diabetes Study Group: UK Prospective Diabetes Study VIII: study design, progress and performance. *Diabetologia* 1991;34:877–890.

2. Said G, Goulon-Goeau C, Slama G, Tchobroutsky G. Severe early-onset polyneuropathy in insulin-dependent diabetes mellitus: a clinical and pathological study. *N Engl J Med* 1992;326:1257–1263.

3. Diabetes Prevention Program Research Group. The prevalence of retinopathy in impaired glucose tolerance and recent-onset diabetes in the Diabetes Prevention Program. *Diabet Med* 2007;24:137–144.

4. Haffner SM, Gonzales C, Valdez RA, Mykkänen L, Hazuda HP, Mitchell BD, Monterrosa A, Stern MP. Is microalbuminuria part of the prediabetic state? The Mexico City Diabetes Study. *Diabetologia* 1993;36:1002–1006.

5. Papanas N, Vinik AI, Ziegler D. Neuropathy in prediabetes: does the clock start ticking early? *Nat Rev Endocrinol* 2011;7:682–690.

6. Centers for Disease Control and Prevention. 2011 National Diabetes Fact Sheet. Available at www.cdc.gov/diabetes/pubs/factsheet11.htm. Accessed 29 September 2013.

7. Ridker PM, Danielson E, Fonseca FA, Genest J, Gotto AM Jr, Kastelein JJ, Koenig W, Libby P, Lorenzatti AJ, MacFadyen JG, Nordestgaard BG, Shepherd J, Willerson JT, Glynn RJ; JUPITER Study Group. Rosuvastatin to prevent vascular events in men and women with elevated C-reactive protein. *N Engl J Med* 2008;359:2195–2207.

8. American Diabetes Association. Economic costs of diabetes in the U.S. in 2012. *Diabetes Care* 2013;36:1033–1046.

9. Harris MI, Klein R, Cowie CC, et al. Is the risk of diabetic retinopathy greater in non-Hispanic blacks and Mexican Americans than in non-Hispanic whites with type 2 diabetes? A U.S. population study. *Diabetes Care* 1998;21:1230–1235.

10. Tsugawa Y, Mukamal KJ, Davis RB, Taylor WC, Wee CC. Should the hemoglobin A1c diagnostic cutoff differ between blacks and whites? A cross-sectional study. *Ann Intern Med* 2012;157:153–159.

11. Eschwege E, Richard JL, Thibult N, Ducimetiere P, Warnet JM, Claude JR, Rosselin GE. Coronary heart disease mortality in relation with diabetes, blood glucose and plasma insulin levels. The Paris Prospective Study, ten years later. *Horm Metab Res* 1985;(Suppl 15):41–46.

12. Khaw KT, Wareham N, Bingham S, Luben R, Welch A, Day N. Association of hemoglobin A1c with cardiovascular disease and mortality in adults: the European prospective investigation into cancer in Norfolk. *Ann Intern Med* 2004;141:413–420.

13. DeFronzo RA, Abdul-Ghani M. Assessment and treatment of cardiovascular risk in prediabetes: impaired glucose tolerance and impaired fasting glucose. *Am J Cardiol* 2011;108(Suppl):3B–24B.

14. Gupta AK, Ravussin E, Johannsen DL, Stull AJ, Cefalu WT, Johnson WD. Endothelial dysfunction: an early cardiovascular risk marker in asymptomatic obese individuals with prediabetes. *Br J Med Med Res* 2012;2:413–423.

15. Ylitalo KR, Sowers M, Heeringa S. Peripheral vascular disease and peripheral neuropathy in individuals with cardiometabolic clustering and obesity: National Health and Nutrition Examination Survey 2001–2004. *Diabetes Care* 2011;34:1642–1647.

16. Vita JA, Keaney JF. Endothelial function: a barometer for cardiovascular risk? *Circulation* 2002;106:640–642.

17. Deanfield JE, Halcox JP, Rabelink TJ. Endothelial function and dysfunction: testing and clinical relevance. *Circulation* 2007;115:1285–1295.

18. Corrado E, Rizzo M, Coppola G, Muratori I, Carella M, Novo S. Endothelial dysfunction and carotid lesions are strong predictors of clinical events in patients with early stages of atherosclerosis: a 24-month follow-up study. *Coron Artery Dis* 2008;19:139–144.

19. Rad Pour O, Dagogo-Jack S. Prediabetes as a therapeutic target. *Clin Chem* 2011;57:215–220.

20. Dagogo-Jack S. Primary prevention of cardiovascular disease in pre-diabetes: the glass is half-full and half-empty (Editorial). *Diabetes Care* 2005; 28:971–972.

21. Greene DA, Lattimer SA, Sima AAF. Sorbitol, phosphoinosotides, and sodium-potassium-ATPase in the pathogenesis of diabetic complications. *N Engl J Med* 1987;316:599–606.

22. Nathan DM. Long-term complications of diabetes mellitus. *N Engl J Med* 1993;328:1676–1685.

23. Brownlee M. Banting Lecture 2004. The pathobiology of diabetic complications: a unifying mechanism. *Diabetes* 2005;54:1615–1625.

24. Vlassara H. Receptor-mediated interaction of advanced glycosylation end products with cellular components within diabetic tissues. *Diabetes* 1992;41(Suppl 2):52–56.

25. Hostetter TH. Diabetic nephropathy, metabolic versus hemodynamic considerations. *Diabetes Care* 1992;15:1205–1215.

26. Sharp PS. Growth factors in the pathogenesis of diabetic retinopathy. *Diabetes Rev* 1995;3:164–176.

27. Arden GB, Sivaprasad S. Hypoxia and oxidative stress in the causation of diabetic retinopathy. *Curr Diabetes Rev* 2011;7:291–304.

28. Al-Kateb H, Mirea L, Xie X, et al. Multiple variants in vascular endothelial growth factor (VEGFA) are risk factors for time to severe retinopathy in type 1 diabetes: the DCCT/EDIC genetics study. *Diabetes* 2007;56:2161–2168.

29. Dagogo-Jack S, Santiago JV. Pathophysiology of type 2 diabetes and modes of action of therapeutic interventions. *Arch Intern Med* 1997;157:1802–1817.

30. Dagogo-Jack S. Complications of diabetes mellitus, in Section 9, Metabolism. In *ACP Medicine*. Nabel EG, Ed. Philadelphia, Decker Intellectual Properties, 2012, chap. 3.

31. Quinn M, Angelico MC, Warram JH, et al. Familial factors determine the development of diabetic nephropathy in patients with IDDM. *Diabetologia* 1996;39:940–945.

32. Diabetes Control and Complications Trial Research Group. Clustering of long-term complications in families with diabetes in the Diabetes Control and Complications Trial. *Diabetes* 1997;46:1829–1839.

33. Boright AP, Paterson AD, Mirea L, Bull SB, Mowjoodi A, Scherer SW, Zinman B; DCCT/EDIC Research Group. Genetic variation at the ACE gene is associated with persistent microalbuminuria and severe nephropathy in type 1 diabetes: the DCCT/EDIC Genetics Study. *Diabetes* 2005;54:1238–1244.

34. Freedman BI, Divers J, Palmer ND. Population ancestry and genetic risk for diabetes and kidney, cardiovascular, and bone disease: modifiable environmental factors may produce the cures. *Am J Kidney Dis* 2013 [Epub ahead of print July 26, 2013].

35. Genovese G, Friedman DJ, Pollak MR. APOL1 variants and kidney disease in people of recent African ancestry. *Nat Rev Nephrol* 2013;9:240–244.

36. Kaiser N, Sasson S, Feener EP, Boukobza-Vardi N, Higashi S, Moller DE, Davidheiser S, Przybylski RJ, King GL. Differential regulation of glucose transport and transporters by glucose in vascular endothelial and smooth muscle cells. *Diabetes* 1993;42:80–89.

37. Heilig CW, Concepcion LA, Riser BL, Freytag SO, Zhu M, Cortes P. Overexpression of glucose transporters in rat mesangial cells cultured in a normal glucose milieu mimics the diabetic phenotype. *J Clin Invest* 1995;96:1802–1814.

38. Gabbay KH, Merola LO, Field RA. Sorbitol pathway: presence in nerve and cord with substrate accumulation in diabetes. *Science* 1966;151:209–210.

39. Lee AY, Chung SS. Contributions of polyol pathway to oxidative stress in diabetic cataract. *FASEB* 1999;J13:23–30.

40. Engerman RL, Kern TS, Larson ME. Nerve conduction and aldose reductase inhibition during 5 years of diabetes or galactosaemia in dogs. *Diabetologia* 1994;37:141–144.

41. Giardino I, Edelstein D, Brownlee M. Nonenzymatic glycosylation in vitro and in bovine endothelial cells alters basic fibroblast growth factor activity: a model for intracellular glycosylation in diabetes. *J Clin Invest* 1994;94:110–117.

42. McLellan AC, Thornalley PJ, Benn J, Sonksen PH. Glyoxalase system in clinical diabetes mellitus and correlation with diabetic complications. *Clin Sci* 1994;87:21–29.

43. Charonis AS, Reger LA, Dege JE, Kouzi-Koliakos K, Furcht LT, Wohlhueter RM, Tsilibary EC. Laminin alterations after in vitro nonenzymatic glycosylation. *Diabetes* 1990;39:807–814.

44. Monnier VM, Bautista O, Kenny D, et al. Skin collagen glycation, glycoxidation, and crosslinking are lower in subjects with long-term intensive versus conventional therapy of type 1 diabetes. Relevance of glycated collagen products versus HbA1c as markers of diabetic complications. *Diabetes* 1999;48:870–880.

45. Genuth S, Sun W, Cleary P, et al. Glycation and carboxymethyllysine levels in skin collagen predict the risk of future 10-year progression of diabetic retinopathy and nephropathy in the Diabetes Control and Complications Trial and Epidemiology of Diabetes Interventions and Complications participants with type 1 diabetes. *Diabetes* 2005;54:3103–3111.

46. Hammes HP, Martin S, Federlin K, Geisen K, Brownlee M. Aminoguanidine treatment inhibits the development of experimental diabetic retinopathy. *Proc Natl Acad Sci* 1991;88:11555–11558.

47. Koya D, King GL. Protein kinase C activation and the development of diabetic complications. *Diabetes* 1988;47:859–866.

48. DeRubertis FR, Craven PA. Activation of protein kinase C in glomerular cells in diabetes: mechanisms and potential links to the pathogenesis of diabetic glomerulopathy. *Diabetes* 1994;43:1–8.

49. Studer RK, Craven PA, Derubertis FR. Role for protein kinase C in the mediation of increased fibronectin accumulation by mesangial cells grown in high-glucose medium. *Diabetes* 1993;42:118–126.

50. Koya D, Jirousek MR, Lin YW, Ishii H, Kuboki K, King GL. Characterization of protein kinase C beta isoform activation on the gene expression of transforming growth factor-beta, extracellular matrix components, and prostanoids in the glomeruli of diabetic rats. *J Clin Invest* 1997;100:115–126.

51. Ishii H, Jirousek MR, Koya D, Takagi C, Xia P, Clermont A, Bursell SE, Kern TS, Ballas LM, Heath WF, Stramm LE, Feener EP, King GL. Amelioration of vascular dysfunctions in diabetic rats by an oral PKC beta inhibitor. *Science* 1996;272:728–731.

52. Rossetti L. Perspective. Hexosamines and nutrient sensing. *Endocrinology* 2000;141:1922–1925.

53. Kolm-Litty V, Sauer U, Nerlich A, Lehmann R, Schleicher ED. High glucose-induced transforming growth factor beta1 production is mediated by the hexosamine pathway in porcine glomerular mesangial cells. *J Clin Invest* 1998;101:160–169.

54. Sayeski PP, Kudlow JE. Glucose metabolism to glucosamine is necessary for glucose stimulation of transforming growth factor-alpha gene transcription. *J Biol Chem* 1996;271:15237–15243.

55. Wells L, Hart G. O-GlcNAc turns twenty: functional implications for post-translational modification of nuclear and cytosolic protein with a sugar. *FEBS Lett* 2003;546:154–158.

56. Brownlee M. Biochemistry and molecular cell biology of diabetic complications. *Nature* 2001;414:813–820.

57. Giugliano D, Ceriello A, Paolisso G. Oxidative stress and diabetic vascular complications. *Diabetes Care* 1996;19:257–267.

58. Cohen SY, Dubois L, Tadayoni R, Fajnkuchen F, Nghiem-Buffet S, Delahaye-Mazza C, Guiberteau B, Quentel G. Results of one-year's treatment with ranibizumab for exudative age-related macular degeneration in a clinical setting. *Am J Ophthalmol* 2009;148:409–413.

59. Danis RP, Sheetz MJ. Ruboxistaurin: PKC-beta inhibition for complications of diabetes. *Expert Opin Pharmacother* 2009;10:2913–2925.

60. Diabetes Control and Complications Trial Research Group. The effect of intensive treatment of diabetes on the development and progression of long-term complications in insulin-dependent diabetes mellitus. *N Engl J Med* 1993;329:977–986.

61. Ohkubo Y, Kishikawa H, Araki E, Miyata T, Isami S, Motoyoshi S, Kojima Y, Furuyoshi N, Shichiri M. Intensive insulin therapy prevents the progression of diabetic microvascular complications in Japanese patients with non-insulin-dependent diabetes mellitus: a randomized prospective 6-year study. *Diabetes Res Clin Pract* 1995;28:103–117.

62. U.K. Prospective Diabetes Study Group. Intensive blood-glucose control with sulfophonylurea or insulin compared with conventional treatment and risk of complications in patients with type 2 diabetes (UKPDS 33). *Lancet* 1998;352:837–853.

63. Diabetes Control and Complications Trial Research Group. Adverse events and their association with treatment regimens in the Diabetes Control and Complications Trial. *Diabetes Care* 1995;18:1415–1427.

64. Diabetes Control and Complications Trial/Epidemiology of Diabetes Interventions and Complications Research Group. Effect of intensive therapy on the microvascular complications of type 1 diabetes mellitus. *JAMA* 2002;287:2563–2569.

65. U.K. Prospective Diabetes Study (UKPDS) Group. Effect of intensive blood-glucose control with metformin on complications in overweight patients with type 2 diabetes (UKPDS 34). *Lancet* 1998;352:854–865.

66. Holman RR, Paul SK, Bethel MA, Matthews DR, Neil HA. 10-year follow-up of intensive glucose control in type 2 diabetes. *N Engl J Med* 2008;359:1577–1589.

67. Holman RR, Paul SK, Bethel MA, Neil HA, Matthews DR. Long-term follow-up after tight control of blood pressure in type 2 diabetes. *N Engl J Med* 2008;359:1565–1576.

68. White NH, Sun W, Cleary PA, Danis RP, Davis MD, Hainsworth DP, Hubbard LD, Lachin JM, Nathan DM. Prolonged effect of intensive therapy on the risk of retinopathy complications in patients with type 1 diabetes mellitus: 10 years after the Diabetes Control and Complications Trial. *Arch Ophthalmol* 2008;26:1707–1715.

69. Murray P, Chune GW, Raghavan VA. Legacy effects from DCCT and UKPDS: what they mean and implications for future diabetes trials. *Curr Atheroscler Rep* 2010;12:432–439.

70. The ADVANCE Collaborative Group. Intensive blood glucose control and vascular outcomes in patients with type 2 diabetes. *N Eng J Med* 2008;358:2560–2572.

71. Duckworth W, Abraira C, Moritz T, et al. VADT Investigators. Glucose control and vascular complications in veterans with type 2 diabetes. *N Eng J Med* 2009;360:129–139.

72. Moritz T, Duckworth W, Abraira C. Veterans Affairs Diabetes Trial—corrections. *N Engl J Med* 2009;361:1024–1025.

73. The ACCORD Study Group and ACCORD Eye Study Group. Effects of medical therapies on retinopathy progression in type 2 diabetes. *N Engl J Med* 2010;363:233–244.

74. Davis TM, Yeap BB, Davis WA, Bruce DG. Lipid-lowering therapy and peripheral sensory neuropathy in type 2 diabetes: the Fremantle Diabetes Study. *Diabetologia* 2008;51:562–566.

75. Keech AC, Mitchell P, Summanen PA, et al.; FIELD study investigators. Effect of fenofibrate on the need for laser treatment for diabetic retinopathy (FIELD study): a randomised controlled trial. *Lancet* 2007;370:1687–1697.

76. Rajamani K, Colman PG, Li LP, Best JD, Voysey M, D'Emden MC, Laakso M, Baker JR, Keech AC; FIELD study investigators. Effect of fenofibrate on amputation events in people with type 2 diabetes mellitus (FIELD study): a prespecified analysis of a randomised controlled trial. *Lancet* 2009;373:1780–1788.

77. Simó R, Roy S, Behar-Cohen F, Keech A, Mitchell P, Wong TY. Fenofibrate: a new treatment for diabetic retinopathy. Molecular mechanisms and future perspectives. *Curr Med Chem* 2013;20:3258–3266.

78. Ismail-Beigi F, Craven T, Banerji MA, Basile J, Calles J, Cohen RM, Cuddihy R, Cushman WC, Genuth S, Grimm RH Jr, Hamilton BP, Hoogwerf B, Karl D, Katz L, Krikorian A, O'Connor P, Pop-Busui R, Schubart U, Simmons D, Taylor H, Thomas A, Weiss D, Hramiak I; ACCORD trial group. Effect of intensive treatment of hyperglycaemia on microvascular outcomes in type 2 diabetes: an analysis of the ACCORD randomised trial. *Lancet* 2010;376:419–430.

79. The Diabetes Control and Complications Trial Research Group. The relationship of glycemic exposure (HbA1c) to the risk of development and progression of retinopathy in the Diabetes Control and Complications Trial. *Diabetes* 1995;44:968–983.

80. Stratton IM, Adler AI, Neil HA, et al. Association of glycaemia with macrovascular and microvascular complications of type 2 diabetes (UKPDS 35): prospective observational study. *Br Med J* 2000;321:405–412.

81. Fong DS, Aiello L, Gardner TW, et al. Diabetic retinopathy. *Diabetes Care* 26(Suppl 1),S99–S102.

82. Williams R, Airey M, Baxter H, et al. Epidemiology of diabetic retinopathy and macular edema: a systematic review. *Eye* 2004;18:963–983.

83. The Diabetes Control and Complications Trial Research Group. Early worsening of diabetic retinopathy in the Diabetes Control and Complications Trial. *Arch Ophthalmol* 1988;116:874–886.

84. Lauritzen T, Frost-Larsen K, Larsen HW, Deckert T; Steno Study Group. Effect of one year of near-normal blood glucose levels on retinopathy in insulin-dependent diabetics. *Lancet* 1983;1200–1204.

85. Dandona P, Bolger JP, Boag F, Fonesca V, Abrams JD. Rapid development and progression of proliferative retinopathy after strict diabetic control. *BMJ (Clin Res Ed)* 1985;290895–290896.

86. Andersen AR, Christiansen JS, Andersen JK, et al. Diabetic nephropathy in type 1 (insulin-dependent) diabetes: an epidemiological study. *Diabetologia* 1983;25:496–501.

87. Adler AI, Stevens RJ, Manley SE, et al. Development and progression of nephropathy in type 2 diabetes: the United Kingdom Prospective Diabetes Study (UKPDS 64). *Kidney Int* 2003;63:225–232.

88. Mogensen CE, Cooper ME. Diabetic renal disease: from recent studies to improved clinical practice. *Diabet Med* 2004;21:4–17.

89. Rossing P, Rossing K, Gaede P, Pedersen O, Parving HH. Monitoring kidney function in type 2 diabetic patients with incipient and overt diabetic nephropathy. *Diabetes Care* 2006;29:1024–1030.

90. DCCT/EDIC Research Group. Sustained effects of intensive treatment of type 1 diabetes mellitus on the development and progression of diabetic nephropathy. *JAMA* 2003;290:2159–2167.

91. DCCT/EDIC Research Group. Intensive diabetes therapy and glomerular filtration rate in type 1 diabetes. *N Engl J Med* 2011;365:2366–2376.

92. Argoff CE, Cole BE, Fishbain DA. Diabetic peripheral neuropathic pain: clinical and quality-of-life issues. *Mayo Clin Proc* 81(Suppl 4):S3–S11.

93. Vinik AI. Diabetic neuropathy: pathogenesis and therapy. *Am J Med* 1999;107(Suppl 2B):17S–26S.

94. Eaton S, Tesfaye S. Clinical manifestations and measurement of somatic neuropathy. *Diabetes Rev* 1999;7:312–325.

95. Lee JH, McCarty R. Glycemic control of pain threshold in diabetic and control rats. *Physiol Behav* 1990;47:225–230.

96. Morley GK, Mooradian AD, Levine AS, Morley JE. Mechanism of pain in diabetic peripheral neuropathy: effect of glucose on pain perception in humans. *Am J Med* 1984;77:79–82.

97. Maser RE, Mitchell BD, Vinik AI, et al. The association between cardiovascular autonomic neuropathy and mortality in individuals with diabetes: a meta-analysis. *Diabetes Care* 2003;26:1895–1901.

98. Diabetes Control and Complications Trial Research Group. The effect of intensive diabetes therapy on measures of autonomic nervous system function in the Diabetes Control and Complications Trial (DCCT). *Diabetologia* 1998;41:416–423.

99. Pop-Busui R, Low PA, Waberski BH, et al. Effects of prior intensive insulin therapy on cardiac autonomic nervous system function in type 1 diabetes mellitus: the Diabetes Control and Complications Trial/Epidemiology of Diabetes Interventions and Complications study (DCCT/EDIC). *Circulation* 2009;119:2886–2893.

100. Dagogo-Jack SE, Craft S, Cryer PE. Hypoglycemia-associated autonomic failure in insulin-dependent diabetes mellitus. *J Clin Invest* 1993;91:819–828.

101. Fanelli CG, Epifano L, Rambotti AM, et al. Meticulous prevention of hypoglycemia normalizes the glycemic thresholds and magnitude of most of the neuroendocrine responses to, symptoms of, and cognitive function during hypoglycemia in intensively treated patients with short-term IDDM. *Diabetes* 1993;42:1683–1689.

102. Dagogo-Jack S, Rattarasarn C, Cryer PE. Reversal of hypoglycemia unawareness, but not defective glucose counterregulation, in IDDM. *Diabetes* 1994;43:1426–1434.

103. Dagogo-Jack S. Hypoglycemia in type 1 diabetes mellitus. Pathophysiology and prevention. *Treat Endocrinol* 2004;3:91–103.

104. Seaquist ER, Anderson J, Childs B, Cryer P, Dagogo-Jack S, Fish L, Heller SR, Rodriguez H, Rosenzweig J, Vigersky R. Hypoglycemia and diabetes: a report of a workgroup of the American Diabetes Association and the Endocrine Society. *Diabetes Care* 2013;36:1384–1395.

105. Moss SE, Klein R, Klein BE, et al. The association of glycemia and cause-specific mortality in a diabetic population. *Arch Intern Med* 1994;154:2473–2479.

106. Kuusisto J, Mykkänen L, Pyörälä K, et al. NIDDM and its metabolic control predict coronary heart disease in elderly subjects. *Diabetes* 1994;43:960–967.

107. Andersson DK, Svärdsudd K. Long-term glycemic control relates to mortality in type II diabetes. *Diabetes Care* 1995;18:1534–1543.

108. Khaw KT, Wareham N, Bingham S, Luben R, Welch A, Day N. Association of hemoglobin A1c with cardiovascular disease and mortality in adults: the European prospective investigation into cancer in Norfolk. *Ann Intern Med* 2004;141:413–420.

109. Knuiman MW, Welborn TA, McCann VJ, Stanton KG, Constable IJ. Prevalence of diabetic complications in relation to risk factors. *Diabetes* 1986;35:1332–1339.

110. Moss SE, Klein R, Klein BE, Meuer SM. The association of glycemia and cause-specific mortality in a diabetic population. *Arch Intern Med* 1994;154:2473–2479.

111. Andersson DK, Svärdsudd K. Long-term glycemic control relates to mortality in type II diabetes. *Diabetes Care* 1995;18:1534–1543.

112. Uusitupa MI, Niskanen LK, Siitonen O, Voutilainen E, Pyörälä K. Ten-year cardiovascular mortality in relation to risk factors and abnormalities in lipoprotein composition in type 2 (non-insulin-dependent) diabetic and non-diabetic subjects. *Diabetologia* 1993;36:1175–1184.

113. von Gunten E, Braun J, Bopp M, Keller U, Faeh D. J-shaped association between plasma glucose concentration and cardiovascular disease mortality over a follow-up of 32 years. *Prev Med* 2013 [Epub Aug 28, 2013].

114. Borch-Johnsen K, Kreiner S. Proteinuria: value as predictor of cardiovascular mortality in insulin dependent diabetes mellitus. *BMJ (Clin Res Ed)* 1987;294:1651–1654.

115. Nelson RG, Sievers ML, Knowler WC, Swinburn BA, Pettitt DJ, Saad MF, Liebow IM, Howard BV, Bennett PH. Low incidence of fatal coronary heart disease in Pima Indians despite high prevalence of non-insulin-dependent diabetes. *Circulation* 1990;81:987–995.

116. Nathan DM, Cleary PA, Backlund JY, et al. Intensive diabetes treatment and cardiovascular disease in patients with type 1 diabetes. Diabetes Control and Complications Trial/Epidemiology of Diabetes Interventions and Complications (DCCT/EDIC) Study Research Group. *N Engl J Med* 2005;353:2643–2653.

117. The Action to Control Cardiovascular Risk in Diabetes Study Group. Effects of intensive glucose lowering in type 2 diabetes. *N Eng J Med* 2008;358:2545–2559.

118. Bonds DE, Miller ME, Bergenstal RM, Buse JB, Byington RP, Cutler JA, Dudl RJ, Ismail-Beigi F, Kimel AR, Hoogwerf B, Horowitz KR, Savage PJ, Seaquist ER, Simmons DL, Sivitz WI, Speril-Hillen JM, Sweeney ME. The association between symptomatic, severe hypoglycaemia and mortality in type 2 diabetes: retrospective epidemiological analysis of the ACCORD study. *BMJ* 2010 Jan 8;340:b4909. doi: 10.1136/bmj.b4909.

119. Miller ME, Bonds DE, Gerstein HC, Seaquist ER, Bergenstal RM, Calles-Escandon J, Childress RD, Craven TE, Cuddihy RM, Dailey G, Feinglos MN, Ismail-Beigi F, Largay JF, O'Connor PJ, Paul T, Savage PJ, Schubart UK, Sood A, Genuth S. The effects of baseline characteristics, glycaemia treatment approach, and glycated haemoglobin concentration on the risk of severe hypoglycaemia: post hoc epidemiological analysis of the ACCORD study. *BMJ* 2010 Jan 8;340:b5444. doi: 10.1136/bmj.b5444.

120. Inzucchi SE, Bergenstal RM, Buse JB, Diamant M, Ferrannini E, Nauck M, Peters AL, Tsapas A, Wender R, Matthews DR; American Diabetes Association (ADA); European Association for the Study of Diabetes (EASD). Man-

agement of hyperglycemia in type 2 diabetes: a patient-centered approach: position statement of the American Diabetes Association (ADA) and the European Association for the Study of Diabetes (EASD). *Diabetes Care* 2012;35:1364–1379.

121. American Diabetes Association. Clinical practice recommendations–2013. *Diabetes Care* 2013;36:S1–S110.

122. American Association of Clinical Endocrinologists. AACE comprehensive diabetes management algorithm 2013. *Endocr Pract* 2013;19(2):327–336.

123. Gaede P, Lund-Andersen H, Parving HH, Pedersen O. Effect of a multifactorial intervention on mortality in type 2 diabetes. *N Engl J Med* 2008;358:580–591.

124. Hovind P, Tarnow L, Rossing K, Rossing P, Eising S, Larsen N, Binder C, Parving H-H. Decreasing incidence of severe diabetic microangiopathy in type 1 diabetes. *Diabetes Care* 2003;26:1258–1264.

125. Nordwall M, Bojestig M, Arnqvist HJ, Ludvigsson J. Declining incidence of severe retinopathy and persisting decrease of nephropathy in an unselected population of type 1 diabetes: the Linkoping Diabetes Complications Study. *Diabetologia* 2004;46:1266–1272.

126. Bojestig M, Arnqvist HJ, Hermansson G, Karlberg BE, Ludvigsson J. Declining incidence of nephropathy in insulin-dependent diabetes mellitus. *N Engl J Med* 1994;330:15–18.

127. Pambianco G, Costacou T, Ellis D, Becker DJ, Klein R, Orchard TJ. The 30-year natural history of type 1 diabetes complications: the Pittsburgh Epidemiology of Diabetes Complications Study experience. *Diabetes* 2006;55:1463–1469.

128. Miller RG, Secrest AM, Sharma RK, Songer TJ, Orchard TJ. Improvements in the life expectancy of type 1 diabetes: the Pittsburgh Epidemiology of Diabetes Complications study cohort. *Diabetes* 2012;61:2987–2992.

129. Li Y, Burrows NR, Gregg EW, Albright A, Geiss LS. Declining rates of hospitalization for nontraumatic lower-extremity amputation in the diabetic population aged 40 years or older: U.S., 1988–2008. *Diabetes Care* 2012;35:273–277.

130. Nathan DM, Zinman B, Cleary PA, et al. DCCT/EDIC Research Group. Modern-day clinical course of type 1 diabetes mellitus after 30 years' duration: the Diabetes Control and Complications Trial/Epidemiology of Diabetes Interventions and Complications and Pittsburgh Epidemiology of Diabetes Complications experience (1983–2005). *Arch Intern Med* 2009;169:1307–1316.

131. Chen LH, Zhu WF, Liang L, Yang XZ, Wang CL, Zhu YR, Fu JF. Relationship between glycated haemoglobin and subclinical atherosclerosis in obese children and adolescents. *Arch Dis Child* 2014;99:39–45.

132. TODAY Study Group, Zeitler P, Hirst K, Pyle L, Linder B, Copeland K, Arslanian S, Cuttler L, Nathan DM, Tollefsen S, Wilfley D, Kaufman F. A clinical trial to maintain glycemic control in youth with type 2 diabetes. *N Engl J Med* 2012;366:2247–2256.

133. Dagogo-Jack S. Preventing diabetes-related morbidity and mortality in the primary care setting. *J Natl Med Assoc* 2002;94:549–560.

ACKNOWLEDGMENTS

Dr. Dagogo-Jack is supported in part by grants from the National Institutes of Health (R01 DK067269, DK62203, and U01-DK098246).

Chapter 40

Hypoglycemia in Diabetes

Anthony L. McCall, MD, PhD, FACP

INTRODUCTION

Hypoglycemia is the most common acute side effect of diabetes treatment. It is due to the use of insulin and sulfonylurea receptor (SUR) binding insulin secretagogues alone or in combination with other agents.[1,2] It is the most important barrier to safely attaining optimum glycemic control. Hypoglycemia is implicated as a major risk factor that may cause and can be linked to severe morbidity and mortality. Repeated moderate hypoglycemia may have both favorable and unfavorable adaptations. Adaptations include greater tolerance of low blood glucose as well as reduced recognition and defenses against them. Moreover, hypoglycemia is something patients and health care providers fear. It is nearly universal in type 1 diabetes (T1D), although it is less frequent in type 2 diabetes (T2D), often estimated to be about one-third as common). Nonetheless, because of the far greater number of patients affected, it is a much more common problem overall in T2D. Hypoglycemia often has been underestimated in its importance in T2D.[3] Recent studies, including Action to Control Cardiovascular Risk in Diabetes (ACCORD),[4] Action in Diabetes and Vascular Disease (ADVANCE),[5] and Veterans Affairs Diabetes Trial (VADT),[6] have indicated that hypoglycemia causes and likely also serves as a powerful risk marker for adverse outcomes and may increase the risk of ischemic events and arrhythmias and cause neurological damage, which can cause increased mortality and morbidity.

FEAR OF HYPOGLYCEMIA

The fear of hypoglycemia, especially in patients who live alone and in the parents of young children, is often quite intense.[7] Fear of hypoglycemia and hypoglycemia symptoms may be barriers to optimal self-care.[8] Recent, frequent, or severe hypoglycemia (SH) episodes tend to exacerbate this fear, while useful strategies to reduce the frequency of hypoglycemia, such as insulin pump adjustments or continuous glucose monitoring, may alleviate such fear. There is clearly concern about the adverse consequences of hypoglycemia. These concerns primarily include damage to the brain and increased cardiovascular risk. Fear of hypoglycemia sometimes leads to deliberate undertreatment with insulin therapy. Paradoxically, poor glycemic control does not reliably protect against hypoglycemia,[9] and there may be an increased danger of SH in those who have poor glycemic control. This belief is suggested by analysis of the relative risk of SH in those with T2D with good control versus those with poor control in the ACCORD and ADVANCE trials.[9,10]

 DOI: 10.2337/9781580405096.40

GLYCEMIC STANDARDS

The standards of care suggested for glycemic control by the American Diabetes Association (ADA)[11] have been modified as a result of such studies as ACCORD, ADVANCE, and VADT, which failed to show reliable protection against cardiovascular risk and found an increased risk in the ACCORD trial. The standards thus are individualized to a much greater degree,[12,13] and recognize adjustment based on risk factors for hypoglycemia. Table 40.1, adapted from the annual ADA standards of care, indicates the 2014 glycemic targets. The ADA and European Association for the Study of Diabetes (EASD) have suggested management advice to take a patient-centered approach[12] for those with T2D, and these suggestions have been updated in light of these considerations to individualize goals and strategies for glycemia control. The individualization is based on normal life expectancy[14] and a number of other factors, most of which are summarized in Table 40.1.

HYPOGLYCEMIA FREQUENCY

The frequency of hypoglycemia is about threefold greater in T1D than in T2D. Nonetheless, it would be mistaken to trivialize the importance of hypoglycemia in T2D because the absolute number of events is greater in T2D, and these events may lead to significant morbidity and mortality. The severity and frequency of hypoglycemia correlates with the degree to which endogenous insulin production is lost in both types of diabetes. Figure 40.1 illustrates the frequency of SH reported in a number of classic studies in both T1D and T2D.[15–27]

Within the experience of individuals with T1D, hypoglycemia that is mild or moderate symptomatically is a regular and expected part of life,[28] on average hap-

---

Table 40.1 Summary of General Glycemic Recommendation for Many Nonpregnant Adults with Diabetes

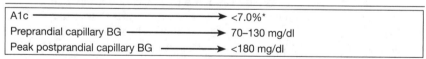

A1c	<7.0%*
Preprandial capillary BG	70–130 mg/dl
Peak postprandial capillary BG	<180 mg/dl

Individualization:
*Individualize goals based on:
- duration of diabetes
- age/life expectancy
- comorbid conditions
- known CVD or advanced microvascular complications
- hypoglycemia unawareness
- individual patient considerations

ALSO
- More or less stringent glycemic goals may be appropriate for individual patients.
- Postprandial glucose may be targeted if A1C goals are not met despite reaching preprandial glucose goals.

Source: Adapted from American Diabetes Association. Standards of medical care. *Diabetes Care* 2014;37(Suppl 1):S26.

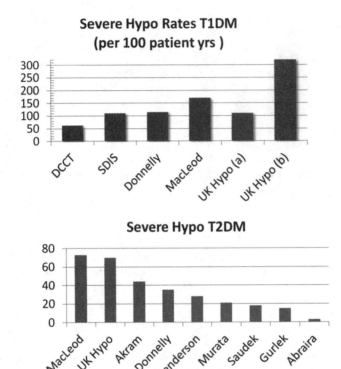

Figure 40.1—Rates of severe hypoglycemia in T1D (top) and T2D (bottom). Studies shown are of glycemic control and diabetes complications before the ACCORD, ADVANCE, and VADT studies.[4-6] Severe hypoglycemia is less common with tight glycemic control in T2D when compared with T1D. Note that the scales of frequency are not the same for T1D and T2D. Studies of T1D, such as the Diabetes Control and Complications Trial (DCCT),[15,16] show lower severe hypoglycemia rates than other T1D studies in part because of studying early-onset T1D and screening out subjects who had a history of severe hypoglycemia. Nonetheless, DCCT rates were >60 per 100 patient-years and had a threefold increased risk relative to those with less intensive glucose control. By contrast, studies of T2D found a risk of severe hypoglycemia with tight glycemic control that was substantially lower. Nonetheless, some studies found an overlap in frequency, indicating that some patients with T2D have a risk comparable to that seen with intensive control in T1D. There is a suggestion that the duration of insulin therapy may be a risk factor for hypoglycemia in both T1D and T2D.

pening twice a week, adding up to thousands of episodes over many years. Averages do not capture the marked variability within one person or that of certain people for whom symptomatic hypoglycemia is a recurring burden that adversely affects their quality of life on a daily basis.[1] Although many come to accept it and view it as a minor nuisance, others feel constant dread and fear of the inability to reliably predict and successfully manage prevention and proper treatment of hypoglycemia. Such fears may inhibit willingness to engage in exercise and can lead to deliberate and inappropriate reduction of insulin doses. Similarly, those who live alone may make themselves hyperglycemic deliberately to avoid hypoglycemia. Often there are considerable concerns about overnight hypoglycemia during sleep, a known vulnerability.[29–32]

Individuals with T1D experience severe hypoglycemia, defined as requiring assistance from another person, 1–1.7 times per year on average. Thirty to 40% of people with T1D experience severe hypoglycemia in a year.[28] This finding is compared with the DCCT in which there were 0.6 episodes per year; in the DCCT, however, those individuals who had a history of severe hypoglycemia were excluded. The averages fail to capture that some people experience multiple 911 calls or emergency room visits or admissions. The psychological and monetary costs are large and may dominate the experience of caring for diabetes for some patients and their families.

HYPOGLYCEMIA: DEFINITIONS AND CLASSIFICATION

A joint workgroup from the ADA and the Endocrine Society[33] recently updated information on definitions of hypoglycemia, and many of the short- and long-term implications of and outcomes from hypoglycemia. They appropriately argued that because hypoglycemia risks injury and death, the definition of hypoglycemia should be linked to this risk. No one threshold value, however, adequately captures this risk, given adaptations of the body to recent lows and to poor control that lead to a range of values that might create symptoms. An alert value of ≤70 mg/dl (3.9 mmol/l) is recommended that draws attention to possible harm from hypoglycemia. Although in the past it has been suggested that a threshold approximating when neuroglycopenic symptoms and thus brain fuel starvation begin (~54 mg/dl or 3.0 mmol/l) should be used, such a threshold likely would allow too little buffer to permit reliable self-treatment.

In the workgroup paper,[33] five important aspects of hypoglycemia classification are given. The first is for *severe hypoglycemia*, defined as an event requiring assistance of another person to administer treatment (e.g., carbohydrate, glucagon). A confirming blood glucose test need not be required, but characteristic symptoms such as neurological symptom recovery are considered adequate evidence for the role of hypoglycemia (two of the three classic Whipple's diagnostic triad). The second is *documented symptomatic hypoglycemia* in which typical symptoms are associated with a measured plasma glucose of ≤70 mg/dl (3.9 mmol/l). The third is *asymptomatic hypoglycemia*, which means a documented value of ≤70 mg/dl without the usual symptoms. The meaning and import of such asymptomatic low glucose values are several. Most worrisome, it may augur the onset of hypoglycemia unawareness and its associated weakened hormonal defenses. Because of this, such episodes require thorough assessment. More benign explanations also may occur. Some well-controlled patients without reduced awareness or impairment of counterregulation may have few or no symptoms until they are in the low 60 mg/dl range. Patients with T2D not on insulin secretagogue or insulin therapy and those without diabetes occasionally may be observed to have blood glucose in the 60 mg/dl range or even lower without symptoms or serious concern.

Self-monitored blood glucose (SMBG) measurements at home are notoriously imprecise especially in the low range, complicating interpretation of "lows" without symptoms. Moreover, blood glucose values sometimes are referred to as levels, but in reality, as revealed by frequent sampling using continuous glucose monitoring or in some studies, they should be more properly thought of conceptually as "vectors," as they seldom stay around the same levels over time. A fourth classification is *probable symptomatic hypoglycemia* during which typical symptoms develop and are relieved with treatment but are never documented to meet the alert threshold of 70 mg/dl.

Many patients favor treatment of hypoglycemia symptoms over documentation of their blood glucose values. Thus, review of their downloaded glucose meters or insulin pumps may fail to reflect the frequency and severity of their hypoglycemia episodes. Providers need to ask about the frequency, the severity, the symptoms (autonomic vs. neuroglycopenic), and the blood glucose concentrations at which symptoms usually tend to occur. Treating hypoglycemia first and immediately documenting the level is a reasonable tactic for patients, but failure to document may miss a chance to determine how low the values are and to amend how much treatment is given for very low values. Often values significantly <50 mg/dl indicate the need for more aggressive treatment and to document that glucose values have risen to safe levels. A final, fifth classification delineated by the work group is termed *pseudohypoglycemia*, which is an episode with typical hypoglycemia symptoms but measured plasma glucose values that are >70 mg/dl, although they usually approach that level. The experience of hypoglycemia despite documented values that are not truly low under usual circumstances (as in those without diabetes) is common, particularly in poorly controlled diabetes. Patients usually describe experience of typical, sometimes quite intense, autonomic symptoms and seem to respond to treatment but have documented values significantly >70 mg/dl. Some of these events may be nonspecific, whereas others often represent a rapid fall from usually very high usual blood glucose to high normal or slightly elevated values.

ADAPTATIONS TO ALTERED GLYCEMIA

Poor Versus Tight Glycemic Control

The phenomenon referred to as pseudohypoglycemia points out that adaptations of multiple types appear to occur in those with diabetes. In addition to the intolerance to "normal" blood glucose in those with very poor control, it is clear contrariwise that those with very tightly controlled diabetes may tolerate frankly low blood glucose with few or only subtle symptoms, and that those symptoms are often neuroglycopenic in origin.[29,30] The initial observations of greater tolerance of low blood glucose in tight glycemic control versus those in poor glucose control led to further observations. It was largely antecedent hypoglycemia per se rather than simply tight control that was the usual cause of the greater tolerance.[34,35] This finding led to the original concept of the hypoglycemia-associated autonomic failure (HAAF) syndrome, including hypoglycemic unawareness, altered thresholds for symptoms and for counterregulatory hormone release, as well as delayed and often deficient hormone responses.[30,31] An analogy to explain this concept to patients is that "the horn and the brakes" do not work at the same time. HAAF syndrome has several causes (e.g., prior hypoglycemia, sleep, with exercise early and late) that affect many counterinsulin hormone defenses and is reversible, at least in part.

One early aspect of counterregulation failure in T1D that occurs is glucagon failure in response to hypoglycemia.[36] This may occur despite glucagon increases due to stress, poor glycemic control, and inappropriate glucagon excess with meals. Originally identified by Gerich,[36] it appears in humans to be irreversible and is a key component of the increased risk of severe hypoglycemia in insulin-deficient diabetes.

A reversal of symptom order (i.e., neuroglycopenic then later autonomic symptoms) or simply a loss of autonomic (also called neurogenic) symptoms occurs in hypoglycemia-unaware patients (part of the HAAF syndrome).[30,31] For example, some patients will sweat when markedly hypoglycemic only after an hour or more of mental slowing. Table 40.2 shows the two major types of hypoglycemia symptoms; the autonomic symptoms usually permit early warning and allow self-treatment, whereas with neuroglycopenic symptoms, patients often are not able to self-treat. Training patients and families to recognize changing symptoms may be helpful.[37,38] Blood glucose awareness training shows promise as treatment for patients with problematic hypoglycemia and is available online.

Table 40.2 Common Symptoms of Hypoglycemia

Autonomic	Neuroglycopenic
Cold sweats	Confusion of slow mentation
Parasthesias	Blurred vision or diplopia
Fine tremor	General fatigue or weakness
Hunger	Faint or dizzy feeling
Palpitations	Mood disturbance
Anxiety	Feeling of warmth

Note: The common symptoms of hypoglycemia are divided into autonomic (associated with hypoglycemia awareness) and neuroglycopenic (likely related to fuel deprivation of the brain) symptoms. When neuroglycopenic symptoms predominate, there is greater concern for the ability to self-treat and often blood glucose is more severely decreased (<50 mg/dl). In addition, the usual oral treatment with carbohydrate of 15 grams may be insufficient to reverse hypoglycemia fully.

Sources: McCall, AL. Insulin therapy and hypoglycemia. *Endocrinol Metab Clin North Am* 2012;41(1):57–87; Cryer PE. *Hypoglycemia in Diabetes: Pathophysiology, Prevalence, and Prevention.* Alexandria, VA, American Diabetes Association, 2009.

The HAAF syndrome originally was thought to be primarily due to antecedent hypoglycemia. HAAF components included altered thresholds for counterregulatory hormone responses and absent or diminished hormone defenses, including—for all counterregulatory hormones but perhaps most notably for the early responders—glucagon and epinephrine.[31] Ordinarily, epinephrine does not play a critical or major glucoregulatory role, but when glucagon responses are lost in response to hypoglycemia, as appears to be the case in T1D and likely also in late T2D of long duration, glucagon responses are not just reversibly lost as a result of the HAAF syndrome. Glucagon responses to hypoglycemia appear to be lost in a stimulus-specific irreversible manner when there is more severe insulin deficiency. By contrast, in the HAAF syndrome, which affects all of the counterregulatory hormones, epinephrine, cortisol, growth hormone, and others are (at least to some degree) reversibly lost in response to conditions that impair counterregulation. These include prior hypoglycemia, often in clusters or overnight, as well as sleep-related and exercise-related HAAF with similar or overlapping physiology that may lead to a vicious cycle and dangerous risk of severe hypoglycemic damage.

CONSEQUENCES OF SEVERE HYPOGLYCEMIA

There are several major concerns about the risks of bodily damage resulting from hypoglycemia. One vulnerable organ is the brain, which is markedly dependent on glucose as fuel for normal functioning. Brain dysfunction or damage of several types may be observed and some neurological manifestations are listed in Table 40.3.[1]

Severe hypoglycemia may injure the brain permanently. Another critical issue is that among the severe manifestations of hypoglycemia is sudden death, which may not be linked directly to neurological effects of hypoglycemia. Although the brain is at risk from hypoglycemia, other organs, particularly the heart, also may be affected, perhaps to a greater degree in T2D.[39]

Cardiovascular consequences of hypoglycemia include possible alterations in cardiac ventricular repolarization that could underlie sudden death.[40] Hypoglycemia creates a prothrombotic state[41] and may predispose to acute cardiac ischemia, as suggested in the dual assessment of continuous glucose monitoring and Holter monitors in the study of Desouza et al.;[42] ischemia may occur either in the coronary or cerebral circulation. Ischemic events may be more common in patients with T2D or in those with long-standing T1D because of underlying

Table 40.3 Neurological Manifestations of Acute Hypoglycemia

Decortication	Locked-in syndrome
Decerebration	Amnesia
Transient hemiplegia	Stroke
Choreoathetosis	Cortical atrophy
Ataxia	Peripheral neuropathy
Generalized or focal convulsions	Focal neurological signs (e.g., pons, visual pathways)

Reprinted with permission from the publisher.[1]

atherosclerosis. Surprisingly few reports of such events occur in the literature, although they occasionally are noted in practice,[33,39,43,44] with an acute hypoglycemic event appearing to trigger a myocardial infarction or a thrombotic stroke. One of the most feared consequences of hypoglycemia is the dead-in-bed syndrome.[45] The potentially atherogenic effect of hypoglycemia and abnormalities in the QT interval,[46] which may predispose to arrhythmias, after severe hypoglycemia, are both clear concerns raised by several investigators, with the latter perhaps being important in light of the 22% increased mortality observed in the ACCORD trial.[4]

Although recurring hypoglycemia clearly leads to the vicious cycle of the HAAF syndrome and even to the risk of sudden death, there are reasons to believe that hypoglycemia may have some favorable adaptations as well. In both the ACCORD[9,47] and ADVANCE[10] studies, the risks associated with severe hypoglycemia were substantial and varied. Noteworthy, however, was an apparent tendency of subjects with severe hypoglycemia to have less severe consequences if they had been in better overall control. Conversely, when study participants had poor glycemic control, the outcomes of a severe hypoglycemia reaction appear to be relatively worse. One may speculate that either through central nervous system adaptation or perhaps effects on the heart that might be analogous to ischemic preconditioning, a history of better glycemic control augured a less severe outcome of severe hypoglycemia. It is not clear to what degree such protection would be offered in a first-event situation; it could be that repeated low blood glucose values may provide protection in those with better glycemic control. The risks and the benefits of some hypoglycemia (tolerance that may help vs. risk) need further delineation. Risk factors for hypoglycemia and HAAF are shown in Table 40.4.

Table 40.4 Risk Factors for Hypoglycemia in Diabetes

Relative or absolute insulin excess:

1. Insulin or insulin secretagogue doses are excessive, ill-timed, or of the wrong type.
2. Exogenous glucose delivery is decreased (e.g., after missed meals and during the overnight fast).
3. Endogenous glucose production is decreased (e.g., after alcohol ingestion).
4. Glucose utilization is increased (e.g., during and shortly after exercise).
5. Sensitivity to insulin is increased (e.g., after weight loss or improved glycemic control and in the middle of the night).
6. Insulin clearance is decreased (e.g., with renal failure).

Hypoglycemia-associated autonomic failure (defective glucose counterregulation and hypoglycemia unawareness):

1. Absolute endogenous insulin deficiency
2. A history of severe hypoglycemia, hypoglycemia unawareness, or both as well as recent antecedent hypoglycemia, prior exercise, and sleep
3. Aggressive glycemic therapy per se (lower A1C levels, lower glycemic goals, or both)

Source: From Cryer.[31]

RISK FACTORS FOR HYPOGLYCEMIA

The need to identify underlying causes (behavioral, hormonal, counterregulatory, and other medical reasons) is an important aspect of hypoglycemia evaluation and management. Inadvertent overtreatment with insulin is the primary cause, but other factors should be identified that are critical to address as well (Table 40.4). Behavioral issues include infrequent testing of self-monitored glucose, skipping meals or eating much less than usual without appropriate insulin adjustment, use of sliding-scale insulin, imbalance between meal and basal insulin, and mistiming insulin (such as taking meal insulin before or after going out to eat in a restaurant) all represent several commonly encountered behavioral issues.[37] Other hormonal factors or risks for hypoglycemia are important to address. For example, concomitant untreated hypothyroidism, adrenal insufficiency, or pituitary disease are common hormonal issues. Worsening of kidney dysfunction, worsening heart failure, or liver disease are a few of the many other medical issues that may have an impact on the risk of hypoglycemia. Normal counterregulation defenses, often lost in insulin-deficient diabetes, are outlined in Table 40.5 below. Counterregulatory defects may come in a variety of ways as delineated throughout this chapter.

Table 40.5 Altered Defenses Against Hypoglycemia in Diabetes

Defense	Comment
Reduction and cessation of endogenous insulin secretion	Loss of β-cells removes this defense and may help impair glucagon responses
*Loss of glucagon pulses	Early response; appears stimulus-specific and irreversible[†]
*Reduced epinephrine	Early response; critical when glucagon has been lost
Cortisol	Important late response**; increases gluconeogenesis
Growth hormone	Late response
Hepatic autoregulation	Late response
Brain areas	VMH‡, hindbrain (regulate insulin counterregulation and appetite)

Note:

*Hypothesized to be important in HAAF.

†Recent information in animal models suggests that reversibility may actually be possible.[1]

**Cortisol responses to hypoglycemia have been found in some studies to potentially be a factor in genesis of HAAF.

‡Several of the counterregulatory responses appear to be organized within the ventromedial hypothalamus (VMH) by a variety of signaling pathways including local activity of AMPK (adenosine monophosphate kinase), which is a fuel sensor enzyme, while other brain areas such as the hindbrain are important by causing hunger.

PHYSIOLOGY OF GLYCEMIC CONTROL, PATHOPHYSIOLOGY IN DIABETES, AND PRESENTATION: NORMAL DEFENSES AGAINST HYPOGLYCEMIA

ROLE OF ENDOGENOUS INSULIN

As extensively delineated by several researchers over many years,[29,31] there is a hierarchy of responses to acute lowering of glucose both within the physiological euglycemic range and into the hypoglycemic range. Hypoglycemia hormonal defenses are quite redundant, and they begin to adjust within the nonhypoglycemic range—both of these aspects are quite important. There are both early (primarily altered insulin, glucagon, and epinephrine secretion) and later defenses (see Table 40.5). In the hierarchy of defenses against hypoglycemia, the reduction in endogenous pancreatic release of insulin into the portal vein, of which about half or more is extracted by the liver, is the earliest response as blood glucose falls into the low normal range before frank hypoglycemia. It appears that the inhibitory effect of insulin (perhaps other β-cell products as well) is able to normally suppress glucagon secretion. When endogenous insulin secretion is reduced, it helps to ensure that glucagon will increase its secretion during hypoglycemia through a combination of direct and indirect mechanisms.

ROLE OF GLUCAGON

Ordinarily, pancreatic glucagon is in balance with insulin and a primary control mechanism for glucoregulation in the fasting and postprandial state. Glucagon largely works by regulating glucose release from the liver through fostering glycogen breakdown and thus increasing hepatic glucose output. It is an early key responder in hypoglycemia defenses along with epinephrine. Either of these two hormones alone seems adequate to maintain early counterregulation defenses against severe hypoglycemia.[31] When both are lost, however, hormone defenses against hypoglycemia are too little and too late to prevent rapid descent into severe hypoglycemia. Moreover, symptoms of hypoglycemia tied to the release of catecholamines from the adrenal gland and sympathetic nerve activity are markedly reduced, a condition referred to as hypoglycemia unawareness. This may limit adequate self-treatment of hypoglycemia and is an important component of and risk factor for HAAF, a syndrome that creates risk for severe hypoglycemia. Table 50.4 shows several risk factors for hypoglycemia and HAAF.

THE IMPORTANCE OF EPINEPHRINE

In the normal state of physiological defenses against hypoglycemia, epinephrine and glucagon are arguably the most important early response mechanisms of hypoglycemic counterregulation. Either hormone alone is usually sufficient to reduce the rate of descent of glucose after insulin overdose and to help the glucose to increase after hypoglycemia. Because it is common for glucagon responses to be weakened or absent within a few years after the onset of insulin lack in T1D, epinephrine assumes a particularly important role.

CLINICAL MANIFESTATIONS

Behavioral abnormalities often are associated with hypoglycemia risk.[37] There is a surprising stubbornness to change insulin strategies in people who exhibit a common phenotype associated with HAAF, which is extreme variability. There can be confusion about what is the appropriate focus of treatment, that is, whether to be more concerned with high or low blood glucose. This extreme variability,[48] sometimes called the 40/400 club, indicates a high and imminent risk of severe hypoglycemia. Thus, the focus routinely should be reducing the risk of lows. Overcorrection of both highs and lows can contribute to this variability, and there can be a marked behavioral resistance to reducing excessive insulin doses. One has the impression that this resistance is almost as if there is a difficulty with complex reasoning temporarily in those with erratic control. Because therapeutic hyperinsulinemia is routinely present, the most important adjustment is typically to make moderate and often repeated adjustments downward in the insulin (occasionally the insulin secretagogue) dose deemed most likely to be the root cause of the hypoglycemia. On the other hand, one also occasionally notes people who make very large changes in the dose of insulin, such as omitting it altogether or taking a markedly lower than needed dose. Typically, reductions of 10–20%, which are necessary to repeat with the reemergence of hypoglycemia, are a safe way to reduce the risk of further hypoglycemia. More severe hypoglycemia may require more aggressive dose reductions.

SLEEP AND HYPOGLYCEMIA

It has been estimated that about one-half of hypoglycemia episodes occur during sleep. Hypoglycemia during sleep is common and leads to one version of the HAAF syndrome with typically a reduction in epinephrine protection against a descent into hypoglycemia.[32] Values overnight into the 60 mg/dl range may occur without obvious symptoms, but with a twice-weekly occurrence can cause defective hypoglycemia awareness and defective counterregulation.[1] There is an important diurnal rhythm in insulin sensitivity that occurs with sleep. In the middle of the night, insulin sensitivity in enhanced. Bedtime snacks traditionally have been used; however, because they do not last long enough (typically 1–2 hours), they offer only partial protection against overnight lows.

Recognition of hypoglycemia frequently is reduced already in T1D and late T2D and nocturnal hypoglycemia is less readily recognized. By the early hours of the morning, there is sometimes decreased insulin sensitivity (the so-called early morning or dawn phenomenon), which in part is mediated by delayed effects of growth hormone secretion. For those seeking safe overnight control, it may be important to set their clocks and wake up sometime at night to ensure that nocturnal hypoglycemia is not occurring. Attempts to tightly control overnight glycemia may result in poorly symptomatic hypoglycemia with delayed recognition and treatment.

Insulin injection therapy with basal insulin can be problematic because of such nocturnal hypoglycemia. It is one reason why insulin pump treatment may be preferred. Basal insulin doses with pumps can be reduced overnight and increased if necessary to deal with dawn phenomenon. An increase in basal insulin rates 1–2 hours before awakening may be helpful. Experience suggests that the dawn phenomenon is not uniform in daily appearance and thus some caution is needed in attempts to aggressively control fasting glycemia when caused by the dawn phenomenon. Similarly, aggressive correction dosing in response to the dawn phenomenon also can result in late morning hypoglycemia because of the effects of waning insulin resistance by late morning. Recent information suggests nocturnal hypoglycemia also may disrupt restful sleep and lead to daytime sleepiness.

EXERCISE

Physical activity may increase glucose transport and utilization acutely and chronically.[1,29,31] People with diabetes should be taught that increased activity may cause hypoglycemia during or shortly after the activity and that there is an important delayed effect. The response to intense physical activity, contrariwise, actually may increase hyperglycemia, as moderate activity also may do if poor glycemic control is established. As many people are recommended to stay active as a part of managing their diabetes mellitus, avoidance of hypoglycemia becomes a major problem.

Several approaches are used to minimize hypoglycemia risk with exercise. In those injecting insulin, meal insulin doses taken several hours before exercising often are reduced by one-half for moderate activity (such as a 30-minute walk) to one-quarter or less for vigorous activity, such as running or bicycling.[49] Both the intensity and the duration of activity influence the need for adjustments. The meal after exercising also usually will require some reduction in dose. A recent study in young men with T1D found that a 45-minute run on a treadmill 1 hour after breakfast required a reduction to one-quarter the usual dose at breakfast and to one-half the usual dose for the noon meal to avoid hypoglycemia during and shortly after exercise.[49] Nonetheless, overnight hypoglycemia still occurred in a substantial minority, suggesting that either a reduction of supper insulin or snacking at bedtime, or potentially, a reduction of basal insulin doses may be required. There is little firm guidance on the best approaches to avoid late-exercise hypoglycemia and good comparative studies are not yet available. One potentially promising approach may be the "artificial pancreas," which can reduce the risk of overnight lows.

With insulin pumps, a major additional benefit is the ability to reduce basal rates using the temporary basal rate function. During and for a period of time after vigorous exercise, reductions of 40–90% are not uncommon. It is important to have hypoglycemia treatment close at hand. Many athletes with diabetes will titrate glucose-containing sports drinks to keep their frequently measured blood glucose values within a desirable range. Hypoglycemia avoidance with insulin pumps can be superior to injections in individuals, but this tool is not clearly superior in all people, perhaps because of the need for adequate monitoring and proper dose adjustment, which is not always superior in insulin pump users. Similarly, it is not always the case that the use of continuous glucose monitoring reduces hypoglycemia risk. Perhaps this emphasizes that the technology is promising but has some intrinsic flaws, for example, reliability of glucose estimation. Again, for certain patients, the use of continuous glucose monitoring is clearly helpful in the avoidance of hypoglycemia, although it is not a universal panacea.

Snacks taken before exercise may provide protection against hypoglycemia episodes during exercise or for a short time afterward. Some people prefer not to use fast-acting carbohydrate but instead use a mixed snack with protein, fat, and a carbohydrate. It is important to make the distinction between eating to prevent hypoglycemia (mixed snack) and treatment of hypoglycemia. Mixed snacks are less rapidly effective in raising low blood glucose and should not be preferred to pure dextrose or other rapidly effective treatment when hypoglycemia is occurring. It remains remarkable how frequently people erroneously believe that peanut butter, for example, is an appropriate treatment for acute hypoglycemia.

ALCOHOL AND HYPOGLYCEMIA RISK

Alcohol excess, especially in the fasting state, is a major risk factor for severe hypoglycemia.[29,31] By contrast, moderate alcohol consumption usually taken with food need not be restricted and seems likely to have moderate cardiovascular risk benefits in people with and without diabetes, although it may be contraindicated in the presence of liver disease or for other reasons, such as hypertriglyceridemia. Many alcoholic beverages have carbohydrates in them so there may be a biphasic effect on glycemic control (hyper- then hypoglycemia). Binge drinking without food intake is dangerous because alcohol metabolism reduces the flow of carbon into gluconeogenic pathways.

INPATIENT HYPOGLYCEMIA

It is beyond the scope of this review to comment extensively on inpatient hypoglycemia, but a few comments are worth noting. It is clear that as in the outpatient setting, hospital hypoglycemia may be deadly and is all too common.[50,51] Studies of inpatient glycemic control clearly are limited by the inability to avoid hypoglycemia with intensive treatment, and this is an area for future improvement as protocols and algorithms are developed. Inappropriate dosing or timing of insulin in relationship to nutrition is probably the most common cause for inpatient hypoglycemia. Tube feeding, whether continuous (often unintentionally discontinuous) or episodically scheduled, creates hypoglycemic risk. Holding insulin doses when inpatients are well controlled often leads later to excessive correction doses and high hypoglycemia risk. Administration of meal (or more generally nutritional) insulin when there is no meal or tube feeds are skipped, stopped, or not given without compensatory dextrose infusion are among the avoidable hypoglycemia risk situations. Using basal insulin as an insulin infusion to treat meals is a common avoidable cause of hypoglycemia, as many protocols do not permit meal boluses when patients on insulin infusions are eating meals. This creates marked therapeutic hyperinsulinemia often followed by postabsorptive hypoglycemia.

BRAIN VULNERABILITY TO HYPOGLYCEMIA

Repeated severe hypoglycemia over time may impair cognitive function or damage the brain.[52-54] Patients with T1D and a history of severe hypoglycemia have a slight but significant decline in intelligence scores in comparison with matched controls.[55,56] Magnetic resonance imaging (MRI) in small studies[57] of people with T1D with no history of severe hypoglycemia when compared with patients with T1D with a history of five or more episodes of severe hypoglycemia have found cortical atrophy in nearly half of those who had a history of severe hypoglycemia. Computed tomography and MRI have been used to show that the basal ganglia, cerebral cortex, substantia nigra, and hippocampus are vulnerable brain areas after profound, but sublethal, hypoglycemia.[1,18] Hypoglycemia with seizures predicts cognitive dysfunction in diabetic children, and early onset (<5 years old) of diabetes also portends cognitive problems.[55,56,58] One clinical concern raised by such findings is that repeated hypoglycemia may interfere with the complex task of managing insulin therapy in T1D. This interference may result in a vicious cycle during which subtle neurocognitive dysfunction increases the risk of subsequent hypoglycemia.[59]

DEMENTIA, DIABETES, AND HYPOGLYCEMIA

A number of studies have observed a relationship between dementing illness and diabetes.[54,60–63] Both hyperglycemia and hypoglycemia potentially are implicated in the increased risk of dementing illness most commonly observed in elderly patients.[64,65] Vascular dementia certainly explains some of the relationship and would be expected to be associated primarily with hyperglycemia. Hypoglycemia also has some plausibility as a risk and a number of studies specifically have found hypoglycemia to be an important risk factor for dementia.[66] It is clear that severe brain injury occasionally does occur with severe hypoglycemia. One difficulty in interpreting the association of dementia and hypoglycemia is that in those who are demented, the ability to adhere to regimens with insulin and insulin secretagogues like sulfonylureas already is impaired. In the DCCT cohort, hyperglycemia and complications of neuropathy related to hyperglycemia had a much greater link to cognitive loss than did a tight control in which no clear association was manifest.[67]

It has been argued that tight control of diabetes is seldom warranted in the elderly,[68] but this may represent an oversimplification.[66] Moderate control with individualized recommendations for glycemia is the current standard of care, and overtreatment with insulin and lack of adequate treatment in older patients both create a potential for the risk of cognitive change. A focus on matching therapy to meals is probably one of the most important interventions, and keeping therapy regimens supervised by others (such as family members) and as clear and uncomplicated as possible are important aspects of therapy in the older person with diabetes.

MANAGEMENT AND TREATMENT

Skillful use and adjustment of insulin therapy based on home monitoring of blood glucose is the key to management of hypoglycemia risk. Patient education is critical to this task and working with skilled clinicians including certified diabetes educators is invaluable. The discussion below reviews several aspects of clinical insulin adjustment and suggestions to improve the therapy to reduce hypoglycemia risk.

NEUTRAL PROTAMINE HAGEDORN–BASED REGIMENS

Neutral protamine Hagedorn (NPH) and regular insulin often are prescribed partly based on their lower cost. They often are given together as a predinner and prebreakfast strategy (referred to a split-mix insulin). A nonpeaking basal insulin strategy based on the Treat-to-Target trial in T2D with either insulin glargine or insulin detemir increasingly is used because of the potential reduction of nocturnal hypoglycemia.[69,70] When NPH insulin is used, it should be given preferably at bedtime[71] (although not with meal insulin) to reduce hypoglycemia risk from middle-of-the-night peaks of insulin action. Also, rapid analog insulin may create less risk of late-postmeal hypoglycemia then does regular insulin, especially with low-fat meals.[1]

FIXED-RATIO INSULIN

Fixed-ratio insulin preparations, such as 70/30 insulin (NPH/regular), are popular because of their potential convenience and presumed greater dosing accuracy. They are, however, inflexible when used with different size meals. Their higher risk of hypoglycemia (about threefold) when compared with basal insulin alone mitigates their possible benefits. Both NPH and regular insulin have the potential to increase risk of hypoglycemia. Regular insulin should be timed 30 to 40 minutes before eating—this often is not done, making dosing less effective and more risky because of the inappropriate timing of its peak action and duration.[1] Regular insulin lasts longer than most low-fat meals, and thus it risks late-postmeal hypoglycemia. Its extended action for up to 8 hours also may require snacking between meals to avoid hypoglycemia, especially when one is physically active. NPH insulin often is given at dinnertime for people with T2D, especially obese people who require higher doses that peak later than those who use lower doses and are less overweight. Dinnertime NPH insulin used with lean T2D patients and those with insulin deficiency from T1D or pancreatic diabetes is notoriously problematic because of increased nocturnal hypoglycemia. Nocturnal hypoglycemia is expected when the peak action of NPH insulin in glucose lowering occurs within 8 hours of administration, sometimes earlier. If dinnertime is 6:00 P.M., then peak insulin action occurs often after midnight, when patients are asleep and less able to recognize and effectively treat hypoglycemia. For T1D, basal-bolus regimens with analog insulin are considered the standard of care. NPH insulin and fixed-ratio preparations are seldom if ever a good choice in T1D, primarily because they present too high a risk of hypoglycemia.

PREVENTING NOCTURNAL HYPOGLYCEMIA ON NPH AND NPH-LIKE INSULIN REGIMENS

One remedy for nocturnal hypoglycemia from dinnertime NPH is to move the NPH (but not the short-acting meal insulin) to near bedtime. If the patient is on fixed-ratio insulin preparation (e.g., 70/30 or 75/25), this means individual dosing of intermediate-acting and short- or rapid-acting insulins (e.g., regular or lispro). NPH-like effects of analog insulin mixes should be similarly avoided, in the case of nocturnal hypoglycemia, because of neutral protamine aspart or lispro. For patients who reliably eat on time and similar amounts, the use of fixed-ratio insulins may be helpful; however, often one sees an increase in hypoglycemia risk. To determine the correct starting dose, the total dose of 70/30 is multiplied by 0.7 to determine NPH amount and by 0.3 to determine the regular insulin dose. The need to separate evening NPH and regular insulin applies particularly to patients with T1D not on basal-bolus therapy and to leaner patients with T2D. Table 40.6 suggests ways to decrease hypoglycemia risk.

TIMING MISMATCH WITH FIXED-RATIO INSULINS

Similarly, fixed-ratio insulin preparations (e.g., 50/50 NPH and regular or analog combinations) may increase hypoglycemia risk with tighter control as inflexible dosing often does not match the meal content. A high-carbohydrate low-fat meal may have a mismatch in postprandial glycemia or nocturnal hypoglycemia if the ratio is wrong for the meal composition. The remedy is individual dosing and optimal timing of the insulin. It has been suggested that preprandial combinations of short-acting and intermediate-acting insulin at each meal will provide adequate basal insulin and bolus insulin, but in the author's experience this is too complex a strategy for most patients or providers to adequately assess patterns of glycemia to manage dose adjustments.[72]

Fixed-ratio insulin (NPH and regular as well as analog mixes) has convenience in avoiding mixing of insulin and separately drawing them up. Nonetheless, fixed-ratio insulin in several studies,[1] although more effective in glucose and A1C low-

---

Table 40.6—Reducing Hypoglycemia Risk with Insulin Therapy

- Change sliding-scale insulin to carb counting or pattern management[72]
- Stop fixed-ratio insulin and go to individual doses or basal plus bolus therapy
- Move NPH insulin to bedtime, but leave short-acting insulin at mealtime
- Use correction doses, but avoid insulin stacking; wait 4–6 hours after last dose
- No correction dose at bedtime; expect double drop in blood glucose, if it must be done
- Prioritize avoiding hypoglycemia before adjusting for hyperglycemia
- Avoid big changes in basal insulin and keep it usually <50% with basal-bolus Rx
- Ensure hypoglycemia recovers to >100 mg/dl; check blood glucose 15 minutes after treatment
- Give snacks or reduce insulin to reduce lows with exercise
- Balance meal and basal insulin; too much of either increases hypoglycemia risk postmeal or overnight
- Change lag time for safety when low or if uncertain how much you will eat
- Switch from NPH or fixed-ratio insulin to basal plus bolus (1, 2, or 3)
- Switch from regular to analog insulin with low-fat meals
- Base meal insulin on carbs and fat and your experience—adjust to postmeal target[73]
- Decrease total daily doses by 10–20% when going from simple to complex regimens
- Use insulin pumps in appropriately trained and motivated people

ering overall, leads to more hypoglycemia and weight gain. It seems likely that it is the NPH-like effect that is often responsible for middle-of-the-night peaks. There are also problems with patients who use such fixed-ratio insulin if they miss or delay meals because of the meal insulin.

ERRATIC SCHEDULES AND INTERMEDIATE INSULIN

Patients with erratic schedules, such as variable mealtimes or activities, changing work shifts, and so forth, often struggle to avoid hypoglycemia on NPH-based (or neutral protamine aspart/lispro) insulin regimens, paying the price with frequent hypoglycemia or poor glycemic control to avoid hypoglycemia. Switching to a basal-bolus regimen may remedy this kind of problem with hypoglycemia. The use of insulin glargine and insulin detemir thus may help patients reduce the frequency of hypoglycemia, especially at night, and may be a superior basal insulin strategy, in part due to greater reproducibility. Some trade-offs occur, however, because neither glargine nor detemir can be mixed with other insulins. Long-acting insulin analogs are not without peak effects in all, and the peak of effect seems higher the larger the dose that is given. Higher cost also may be a barrier. The efficacy in treat-to-target trials is equal to that of NPH, but consistently the risk of hypoglycemia, largely overnight, is reduced in frequency.[69,70]

REVERSING THE HAAF SYNDROME

Hormonal, HAAF-related, nutritional, and other medical issues increase hypoglycemia risk (see Table 40.7 for a brief summary). The initially described cause of HAAF was prior recent hypoglycemia, often observed in clusters. The primary role of practitioners is to encourage and show people with HAAF how to reverse the syndrome. Avoidance of hypoglycemia is the primary goal. Decreasing

Table 40.7 Factors Influencing Hypoglycemia Risk

HAAF related	Nutrition related
Prior hypoglycemia	Gastroparesis
Exercise (early and late)	Alcohol intake
Sleep	Fasting or skipped meals
Hypoglycemia unawareness	Low-carb fad diets
Autonomic neuropathy	Malnutrition
Hormonal factors	**Medical and lifestyle issues**
Excessive insulin	Extremes of age (young and old)
Adrenal insufficiency	Renal and hepatic insufficiency
Hypopituitarism	Sliding-scale insulin therapy
Hypothyroidism	Poor balance or timing of insulin
Pregnancy/breast feeding	Erratic schedules
Glucocorticoid excess?	

insulin doses is the only certain way to achieve this. Because patients cannot reliably tell when they are becoming hypoglycemic, it is critical for them to test through SMBG frequently enough (sometimes with use of diagnostic continuous glucose monitoring to help) to avoid all hypoglycemia. The goal is to not get <100 mg/dl if possible continuously for days to weeks. In several studies improved hypoglycemic recognition can occur, although full restoration of hormone counterregulation may not occur.[31] Because of the failure of counterregulation, it is important to recognize that people must treat themselves with a greater amount of glucose to reverse hypoglycemia. In practice, this often takes two to three times as much glucose as usual. A period of 24–48 hours of instability persists in which the risk of severe hypoglycemia remains and beyond that an improved stability in glycemia often occurs.[48] Thus, an initial goal of strict hypoglycemia avoidance for about 3 days (including especially overnight and after exercise) is critical. If this can be maintained for 2–3 weeks, symptomatic recognition of hypoglycemia appears to be improved enough to enter into a safer period. Patterns of glycemia often change within days of strict hypoglycemia avoidance with both fewer highs as well as lows. The following mnemonic is given to advise patients on the general approach to HAAF reversal:

- Test SMBG more than three times daily (4–7 times daily including overnight needed)
- Treatment needs up to three times usual to reverse hypoglycemia (usual is 15 grams and may increase temporarily up to 30–45 grams to reach >100 mg/dl)
- Initial goal: avoid all hypoglycemia for 3 days; new glycemic patterns emerge
- Next goal: avoid hypoglycemia for 3 weeks; associated with some recovery of awareness or counterregulation responses if no diabetic autonomic neuropathy exists

BASAL INSULIN STRATEGIES TO PREVENT HYPOGLYCEMIA OR REDUCE ITS RISK

The standard of care to a large degree with T1D is basal insulin plus rapid analog meal insulin. The basal-bolus strategy is with the use of analog insulin, which is somewhat easier to use and seems to cause fewer hypoglycemia reactions in between meals and overnight than NPH and regular insulin. For those with T2D, basal analogs often are used in primary care practice. They are especially useful with erratic eating schedules or with hypoglycemia when on NPH and regular or other short-acting insulin. A switch to analog basal insulin may reduce hypoglycemia frequency and severity. Basal insulin normally includes a little less than half of the total daily insulin dose in adults and a lower proportion in adolescents whose insulin resistance seems to show up markedly with meals. The precise ratio cannot be mandated as it must be individualized depending on how much carbohydrate people eat and how much exercise someone gets. A characteristic glycemic pattern (glucose staircase and cliff) often is observed in those overtreated with basal insulin alone or when basal insulin far exceeds the meal insulin dose and is illustrated in Figure 40.2. A similar staircase and cliff effect (Figure 40.3) can be observed in insulin pump users when they inadvertently use basal insulin to aid in the treatment of

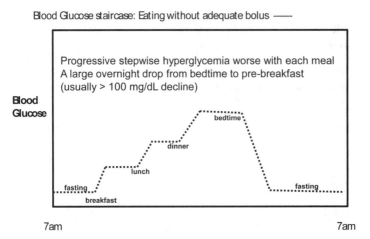

Blood Glucose staircase: Eating without adequate bolus -----

Progressive stepwise hyperglycemia worse with each meal
A large overnight drop from bedtime to pre-breakfast
(usually > 100 mg/dL decline)

Blood
Glucose

bedtime

dinner

lunch

fasting

breakfast

fasting

7am   7am

Figure 40.2—A glycemic pattern is observed in those on either basal insulin therapy only or basal-bolus therapy with an imbalance between basal (too much) and meal insulin (too little). Meal insulin will be needed or increased, but to safely do so, it is necessary to reduce the basal insulin as meal control improves, especially with dinner insulin. A reciprocal decrease in basal insulin and an increase in meal insulin usually will help to avoid overnight hypoglycemia when correcting this pattern. Patients may note that they cannot take much meal insulin as it tends to precipitate hypoglycemia because of high basal insulin. No increase in overall insulin is required with a gradual stepwise redistribution transferred from basal to meal insulin, which usually improves overall hyperglycemia while reducing the risk of overnight hypoglycemia.

meal control. Again, one often sees an overuse overall of basal insulin but sometimes it is restricted to a single large meal, such as supper. Basal insulin doses rise at around mealtime. This is a high-risk situation for hypoglycemia, particularly when meals or snacks are delayed. It is also common to observe that people who do this may note the need to have frequent snacks between meals or "graze" during the day. Lower insulin doses overnight are recognized as important, but it may not be clear unless there has been a formal validation of basal rates recently.

Inadvertent overreliance on basal insulin risks delayed hypoglycemia typically overnight; this commonly is seen when basal insulin far exceeds 50% of the total daily dosage with basal-bolus therapy in T1D. Basal-bolus therapy now usually means once- or twice-daily dosing of insulin glargine or insulin detemir while rapid-acting analog insulin is used for meal coverage. We anticipate that this same issue potentially will be applicable to the use of long-acting analog insulins, such as insulin degludec in the future. Although bolus insulin in theory could be regular or any of the three rapid analogs (lispro, aspart, or glu-

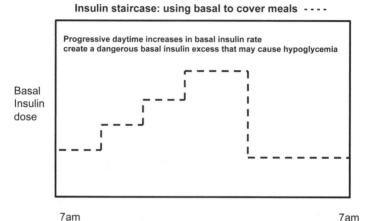

Figure 40.3—Insulin staircase and cliff effect in insulin pump users: This pattern suggests the use of basal insulin to treat meals. This commonly is observed in those needing extended bolus configurations with insulin pump (simple extended bolus or combination boluses). Most patients have not validated their basal rates. The marked drop in basal rate overnight may help indicate the daytime overdose of basal insulin as well. To improve this situation, one should start reducing the high daytime basal rates so that adequate mealtime boluses can be given safely. Thus, the total daily dose may not be incorrect, but a high risk of hypoglycemia is associated with an imbalance between meal and basal insulin.

lisine), in practice, it is most common to use the rapid analogs because of a reduced risk of hypoglycemia between meals. This strategy is effective and flexible but requires proper timing and dosing of rapid analog insulin at each mealtime, usually. In outpatient practice, long-acting basal insulin doses usually are adjusted gradually, from every few days to once weekly to minimize overinsulinization as doses are adjusted upward to control fasting glycemia. Meal insulin doses are intended to be adjusted based primarily on the amount and glycemic impact of the food to be consumed. Suppertime meal insulin and basal insulin may both influence the fasting glycemic control, which may be confusing as to which to adjust.

To avoid hypoglycemia with basal insulin overtreatment, individuals must snack frequently or "graze" during the day and eat a large meal and snack at bedtime (Figure 40.4). Even so, basal insulin overdose usually shows up in the early morning with a timing somewhat similar to that observed in the Treat-to-Target study. If a meal is skipped such as lunch then a long period without food in the middle of the day is also likely to risk hypoglycemia.

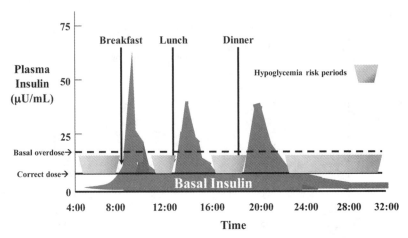

Figure 40.4—Depicted is a pattern of basal insulin overdose against a background of normal peripheral plasma insulin levels. The shaded spaces between normal insulin dosage needs indicate times of vulnerability to hypoglycemia. These depend (darker shading = greater risk) on the duration of time during which food consumption is stopped, with the longest at-risk period being overnight and early morning.

Source: Adapted from Polonsky KS, et al. Non-insulin-dependent diabetes mellitus—a genetically programmed failure of the beta cell to compensate for insulin resistance. *N Engl J Med* 1996;334(12):777–783.

PROBLEMS WITH SLIDING SCALES

Adjusting insulin therapy based on SMBG can be done in several ways. Part of the adjustment involves the art of diabetes medicine. Many patients primarily base their insulin adjustments (including sometimes their long-acting basal doses, a significant error) primarily on the current blood glucose concentrations. This approach is similar to the use of sliding-scale insulin therapy often used in the hospital setting.[75,76] As with hospitalized patients, it usually is a poor choice, often causing poor and erratic control with unpredictable hypoglycemia. Although this approach is nowhere near as effective as carbohydrate counting as the primary basis for meal administration of insulin, so-called correction dosing with refinement of the dose or the timing (adjustment of lag time) is legitimate and useful for short-acting insulin adjustment, especially at meals. Table 40.8 lists some of the problems with sliding-scale insulin.

Sliding-scale insulin works poorly in matching insulin needs and timing. It removes context from the interpretation of SMBG testing (e.g., rebound hyperglycemia), although supplemental correction doses of insulin may be important, particularly on sick days. As a primary strategy, however, it leads to erratic control, with alternating hyperglycemia and hypoglycemia.

Table 40.8—Problems with Sliding-Scale Insulin

- Never use with long-acting insulin
- Cannot change past hyperglycemia
- Doses insulin based on a single glucose value
- Ignores patterns of therapy response to insulin
- Leads to unstable and variable response
- Ignores or minimizes what the meal effects will be
- Requires hyperglycemia to start insulin especially when given without use of basal insulin

BOLUS INSULIN STRATEGIES

Matching bolus insulin to meals represents an ongoing challenge for many patients with diabetes, particularly those who are markedly insulin deficient. Important variables often not attended to include those factors mentioned in Table 40.9. It is clear from older studies that the timing of insulin can be as important as the dose of insulin. Rapid-acting analogs may have their timing manipulated to reduce hypoglycemia risk (postmeal dosing or negative lag time) or to enhance glycemic control without increasing dose for premeal hyperglycemia (e.g., administer bolus 30–45 minutes before eating instead of the more typical 10–20 minutes).

MANIPULATION OF THE LAG TIME TO AVOID HYPOGLYCEMIA

Altering the lag time, the time between insulin injection and meal ingestion, can help achieve good postprandial glycemic control and avoid hypoglycemia. Those who are hypoglycemic are understandably concerned about injection of

Table 40.9 Summary of Approaches to Reduce Hypoglycemia Risk

- Reducing hypoglycemia risk in insulin-deficient diabetes
- Mimic normal β-cell basal and meal responses (basal-bolus or insulin pump therapy)
- Balance basal and meal insulin in all patients
- Adequate treatment of hypoglycemia should always be available, in easy reach
- Family and friends should be taught to use glucagon
- Set individual glycemic goals for SMBG and A1C with a focus on lowest blood glucose[77]
- Modify glycemic goals with HAAF or any of its components and in those with risk factors for severe hypoglycemia or severe consequences (e.g., coronary disease)
- Recognize overtreatment early, especially nocturnal hypoglycemia
- Alter insulin therapy for those not doing well on current therapy (reduce doses for hypoglycemia)
- If current insulin tactics do not work well, refer to a diabetes educator or diabetes specialist
- Ensure medical identification is always on hand

rapid-acting analog insulins. Often insulin is omitted (instead of slightly reduced) from fear of hypoglycemia. This can be counterproductive as the omission or marked reduction of a meal insulin dose may risk hypoglycemia because of rebound hyperglycemia and, often, subsequent overcorrection. An alternative approach for bolus dosing in the face of hypoglycemia is to reduce the lag time (for regular insulin) or make it a negative (i.e., take a rapid analog, lispro, glulisine, or aspart) shortly after the meal to minimize hypoglycemia. This action avoids the excessive hyperglycemia that undertreatment of the meal insulin would permit. On the other hand, one can help avoid delayed hypoglycemia from excessive insulin bolus (prandial) doses by simply allowing increased time for the insulin to work instead of a taking a large increase in insulin to catch up. In practice, the lag time for regular insulin may be from 1 hour before to 30 minutes after meals (the latter usually in patients with gastroparesis), with that for the rapid analogs being from a half hour before to a half hour after meals.

INCONSISTENCY OF BOLUS TIMING

It is important to ask about the specifics of the timing and consistency of the interval between insulin administration and meals. Many patients do not reliably time their insulin therapy consistently before meals. For regular insulin, it is often taken 5 to 10 minutes before meals, with later hyperglycemia. Rapid analog insulin often is taken right at mealtime or afterward, whereas a lag time of about 20 minutes appears better. This timing also may differ when patients eat out. If the dose is increased to prevent postprandial hyperglycemia, the result sometimes is late-postprandial hypoglycemia, as there is a mismatch between the timing of insulin and food absorption. For example, in patients who eat a high-fat meal, however, the usual lag time for regular insulin may be shortened because a high-fat meal slows carbohydrate absorption and better matches insulin to meal absorption–related hyperglycemia. High-fat meals create insulin resistance and delay hyperglycemia.[78]

RAPID-ACTING INSULIN ANALOGS

Use of rapid analogs for a high-fat meal may both come on too soon and wear off too soon. Increasing the dose to prevent late postprandial hyperglycemia may give too concentrated an effect with early postprandial hypoglycemia. To rectify such a problem, some practitioners will combine regular with rapid analog insulin in a 1:1 proportion with a high-carbohydrate, high-fat meal (typically dinner) that partly mimics combination boluses with insulin pumps. People who use insulin pumps have the option with higher-fat meals of using an extended bolus (either simple or compound) to accomplish a similar objective of more physiologic matching of bolus insulin to meal composition.

CARBOHYDRATE COUNTING

The total carbohydrate content of a meal is an important guide to the amount of insulin needed as a bolus to cover the meal. Less sophisticated patients can be introduced to this concept, but they may not be able to count grams of carbohydrate formally at each meal with sufficient precision. An alternate strategy is to ask patients to assess their meal-related insulin's effects 2 or 4 hours postprandially (analog or regular, respectively) and observe patterns of glycemic response.[72,73] When hypoglycemia occurs with meals containing lower carbohydrate, the patient can reduce standard bolus doses subsequently to prevent postprandial hypoglycemia. Insulin-to-carbohydrate ratios can be estimated in most patients based on standard ranges (1:10–1:20, i.e., 1 unit of bolus insulin for every 10–20 grams of total carbohydrate in the meal) for insulin-sensitive patients and a lower ratio for those who are more insulin resistant. Use of a 450 rule (450/total daily dose of insulin) can help estimate the insulin-to-carbohydrate ratio, and other proprietary calculators are available for smartphones.

Strategies for carbohydrate counting are used often with insulin-pump therapy and with basal-bolus therapy in both T1D and T2D. Teaching "carb counting" requires motivation and attention to detail. Several visits with a registered dietician or certified diabetes educator skilled in dealing with bolus insulin adjustments for diabetes usually are required. Many patients with T1D require about 1 unit of short-acting insulin for every 10–15 grams of carbohydrate. The individual range, however, is wide. Although relative consistency is observed in individuals, insulin-to-carbohydrate ratios also can change according to circumstances. For example, they may be markedly increased after exercise or may be reduced as a result of the dawn phenomenon. Some patients carry books on carbohydrates with them and, increasingly, patients use a variety of smartphone applications for use with diabetes to aid in carbohydrate counting and to estimate accurate carbohydrate content in meals. Carb counting is not entirely accurate even if done with consistency and skill. This partly is due to greater glycemic effects of different carbohydrates as well as to the effects of fats on timing and the dose needs for insulin at meals.

CORRECTION DOSES OF INSULIN

In general, the use of an 1800 (older rule and more conservative) or 1700 rule to calculate insulin sensitivity and thus correction doses of insulin, often is done based on the total daily dose (TDD) of insulin.[1] The author prefers the 1800 rule, which means dividing the TDD of all insulins into 1800 to estimate the drop in glucose from the premeal time to the 2-hour postmeal glucose level of 1 unit extra insulin to correct hyperglycemia premeal. With patients who have frequent hypoglycemia and unawareness, it often is best to be conservative because they are more likely to have a TDD that is in excess of their needs. It is sometimes quite remarkable that a patient with repeated hypoglycemia may be required on several occasions to reduce their dose of insulin to find out the actual need. Correction dosing at bedtime is strongly discouraged on a routine basis. Repeated use of a correction dose before a meal typically indicates the need to adjust the prior meals' insulin dosing to be more accurate, a procedure known as pattern therapy or pattern management.

CORRECTION DOSING AND RISK OF HYPOGLYCEMIA

There is an important relationship between glycemic variability and hypoglycemia risk. This can be observed for the outpatient and the inpatient setting. Both glycemic variability and antecedent hyperglycemia may increase the risk of hypoglycemia, the latter largely through attempts to lower marked hyperglycemia. A few other aspects of correction dosing may help minimize hypoglycemia risk and are important. The elements of a correction dose include judgments about when to correct. For example, how high do you have to be before extra short-acting insulin is given? Typically, correction doses are considered when there is a 50–100 mg/dl rise about target glycemia. When correction doses routinely are given at any meal, one has to recognize that this means that there is a failure to anticipate the meal dose needed at the prior meal.

When should you use correction doses? Usually, it is best done at mealtimes. It is important to largely avoid at bedtime and be judicious and somewhat selective in postmeal dosing on a routine basis. Postmeal dosing is okay sometimes, but it is important to remember that postmeal dosing may lead to later lows because of insulin stacking (peaks overlapping). People who use insulin pumps have an advantage now that all pumps remember the insulin on board for them, although that only works when you are using the bolus calculator and not a manual bolus.

Correction doses at bedtime are fraught with risk of lows during sleep because the peak effect is less likely to be safe as insulin sensitivity often is enhanced, and during deep sleep, there is delayed recognition of hypoglycemia and defenses against lows may be compromised. If a bedtime correction really is needed because of a very high value, our practice and that of many diabetes physicians is to assume that glucose will drop up to twice as much as usual when given at bedtime (increased ISF [insulin sensitivity factor] twofold). Another consideration in avoiding hypoglycemia due to overcorrection is how aggressive your target of correction is. Many people try to get their blood glucose down to 80–100 but because correction doses are intrinsically imprecise, it is important to be careful not to shoot for too aggressive a target. A final consideration is that it is also important to recognize in someone with high glycemic variability that may be a result of a marked low, that it is helpful to be conservative in correction doses for later highs. This can help correct a "cycling" with episodic highs and lows related to overcorrection of both.

Gastroparesis is a difficult complication in diabetes. It is a challenge to achieve stable glycemic control and avoid hypoglycemia. It is important to remember that absorption of liquids is much less affected than absorption of solids. Administration of regular insulin either with no lag time or after meals may be required to avoid early postprandial hypoglycemia. Unfortunately, hyperglycemia itself tends to worsen gastroparesis.

A trial of metoclopramide or erythromycin may be warranted in some patients with erratic control and problematic hypoglycemia to see whether it can improve and stabilize glycemic control. The long-term use of these medications, however, is problematic because of modest efficacy, central nervous system side effects with metoclopramide (such as tardive dyskinesia), and the P-glycoprotein 3A4 drug interaction effects with erythromycin. For patients who use rapid analog injections or an insulin pump, manipulation of the lag time can be helpful in dealing with gastroparesis. In addition, pumps allow extended boluses, either simple or combination (which is an immediate bolus often of 50% of the total followed by a slower bolus of the rest equivalent to an infusion for 1 to several hours) or a square-wave or rectangular bolus, which may be helpful in achieving control with reduced risk of hypoglycemia.

For patients with gastroparesis the use of high-fat, high-fiber meals may exacerbate symptoms. Ultimately, for appropriate trained patients with severe hypoglycemia or extreme variability with marked highs and lows, insulin-pump therapy (with or without continuous glucose monitoring) will be the best solution, with sufficient power and flexibility to achieve more stable glycemic control. In appropriately motivated patients who are willing to monitor frequently and learn carbohydrate counting and pattern management, it will be the best solution for avoidance of severe hypoglycemia.

COMBINATION THERAPY

When combining insulin with tablets, it may be important to recognize that certain combinations result in different hypoglycemia patterns. Certain sulfonylureas such as glyburide and chlorpropamide seem to have a high propensity to cause hypoglycemia especially in the daytime but sometimes also overnight. Metformin seems to have less propensity to do so in combination, but certainly may require downward insulin dosage adjustment to avoid hypoglycemia. Thiazolidinediones (TZDs) and sodium-glucose cotransporter inhibitors often cause hypoglycemia if doses of insulin (or sulfonylureas) are not reduced. Because this may take a month or more with TZDs to become clinically manifest, some patients find the hypoglycemia unexpected. Combining insulin therapy with glucagon-like peptide-1 agonists and pramlintide usually leads to the need to reduce basal and meal insulin doses.

CONCLUSION

Hypoglycemia remains the critical obstacle to safe and excellent control of diabetes with insulin and sulfonylurea secretagogues. The largely acquired physiologic defects that create much of the risk of overtreatment, namely, the hypoglycemia unawareness and defective insulin counterregulation components of HAAF syndrome, appear to be partially reversible except for deficient glucagon responses. The solution is strictly avoiding even moderate hypoglycemia, especially at night, as a useful strategy to avoid severe hypoglycemia with little warning and thus no chance of self-treating. Identifying patients at risk is crucial because their glucose and A1C goals should be individualized to reduce their risk,[13] and their monitoring frequency should be conducted to lead to the recognition of poorly symptomatic hypoglycemia. Full treatment of hypoglycemia, especially in those with few symptoms, is crucial for patient safety. Physiologic mimicry with basal-bolus injection therapy or insulin pumps is essential for those with marked insulin deficiency.

Avoiding peaks of insulin when not needed and adapting the use of self-monitoring information to aid therapy adjustment can help in the key task of avoiding nocturnal hypoglycemia.[79] Nonetheless, basal insulin overtreatment with analogs can and does occur, and often is not recognized promptly. Its masking by undertreatment at meals can be deduced from patterns of glucose, thus helping to guide the patient to safer therapy. Although frequent adjustments and correction of dosing are important, when looking at the big picture, pattern management can enhance safety and exploit the benefit of modern insulins and administration to reduce glycemic variability and accurately provide safe and effective therapy by copying the body's own physiology of insulin delivery.

REFERENCES

1. McCall AL. Insulin therapy and hypoglycemia. *Endocrinol Metab Clin North Am* 2012;41(1):57–87.

2. Wright AD, Cull CA, Macleod KM, Holman RR. Hypoglycemia in type 2 diabetic patients randomized to and maintained on monotherapy with diet, sulfonylurea, metformin, or insulin for 6 years from diagnosis: UKPDS 73. *J Diabetes Complications* 2006;20:395–401.

3. Bloomgarden Z, Einhorn D. Hypoglycemia in type 2 diabetes: current controversies and changing practices. *Front Endocrinol (Lausanne)* 2012;3:1–5.

4. Action to Control Cardiovascular Risk in Diabetes Study Group. Effects of intensive glucose lowering in type 2 diabetes. *N Engl J Med* 2008;358:2545–2559.

5. ADVANCE collaborative group. Intensive blood glucose control and vascular outcomes in patients with type 2 diabetes. *New Engl J Med* 2008;358(24):2560–2572.

6. Duckworth W, Abraira C, Moritz T, Reda D, Emanuele N, Reaven PD, Zieve FJ, Marks J, Davis SN, Hayward R, Warren SR, Goldman S, McCarren M, Vitek ME, Henderson WG, Huang GD. Glucose control and vascular complications in veterans with type 2 diabetes. *New Engl J Med* 2009;360(2):129–139.

7. Gonder-Frederick L, Nyer M, Shepard JA, Vajda K, Clarke W. Assessing fear of hypoglycemia in children with type 1 diabetes and their parents. *Diabetes Manag* 2011;1(6):627–639.

8. Wild D, von Maltzahn R, Brohan E, Christensen T, Clauson P, Gonder-Frederick L. A critical review of the literature on fear of hypoglycemia in diabetes: implications for diabetes management and patient education. *Patient Educ Couns* 2007;68(1):10–15.

9. Bonds DE, Miller ME, Bergenstal RM, Buse JB, Byington RP, Cutler JA, Dudl RJ, Ismail-Beigi F, Kimel AR, Hoogwerf B, Horowitz KR, Savage PJ, Seaquist ER, Simmons DL, Sivitz WI, Speril-Hillen JM, Sweeney ME. The association between symptomatic, severe hypoglycaemia and mortality in type 2 diabetes: retrospective epidemiological analysis of the ACCORD study. *BMJ* 2010;340:1–9.

10. Zoungas S, Patel A, Chalmers J, de Galan BE, Li Q, Billot L, Woodward M, Ninomiya T, Neal B, MacMahon S, Grobbee DE, Kengne AP, Marre M, Heller S. Severe hypoglycemia and risks of vascular events and death. *N Engl J Med* 2010;363(15):1410–1418.

11. American Diabetes Association. Standards of medical care. *Diabetes Care* 2013;36(Suppl 1):S21.

12. Inzucchi SE, Bergenstal RM, Buse JB, Diamant M, Ferrannini E, Nauck M, Peters AL, Tsapas A, Wender R, Matthews DR. Management of hyperglycemia in type 2 diabetes: a patient-centered approach: position statement of the American Diabetes Association (ADA) and the European Association for the Study of Diabetes (EASD). *Diabetes Care* 2012;35(6):1364–1379.

13. Ismail-Beigi F, Moghissi E, Tiktin M, Hirsch IB, Inzucchi SE, Genuth S. Individualizing glycemic targets in type 2 diabetes mellitus: implications of recent clinical trials. *Ann Intern Med* 2011;154(8):554–559.

14. Lutgers HL, Gerrits EG, Sluiter WJ, et al. Life expectancy in a large cohort of type 2 diabetes patients treated in primary care (ZODIAC-10). *PLoS One* 2009;4:e6817

15. Diabetes Control and Complications Trial Research Group. The effect of intensive treatment of diabetes on the development and progression of long-term complications in insulin-dependent diabetes mellitus. *N Engl J Med* 1993;329:977–986.

16. Diabetes Control and Complications Trial Research Group. Hypoglycemia in the Diabetes Control and Complications Trial. *Diabetes* 1997;46:271–286.

17. Reichard P, Pihl M. Mortality and treatment side-effects during longterm intensified conventional insulin treatment in the Stockholm Diabetes Intervention Study. *Diabetes* 1994;43:313–317.

18. MacLeod KM, Hepburn DA, Frier BM. Frequency and morbidity of severe hypoglycaemia in insulin-treated diabetic patients. *Diabet Med* 1993;10:238–245.

19. U.K. Hypoglycaemia Study Group. Risk of hypoglycaemia in types 1 and 2 diabetes: effects of treatment modalities and their duration. *Diabetologia* 2007;50:1140–1147.

20. Akram K, Pedersen-Bjergaard U, Carstensen B, Borch-Johnsen K, Thorsteinsson B. Frequency and risk factors of severe hypoglycaemia in insulin-treated type 2 diabetes: a cross-sectional survey. *Diabet Med* 2006;23:750–756.

21. Donnelly LA, Morris AD, Frier BM, Ellis JD, Donnan PT, Durrant R, Band MM, Reekie G, Leese GP. Frequency and predictors of hypoglycaemia in type 1 and insulin-treated type 2 diabetes: a population-based study. *Diabet Med* 2005;22:749–755.

22. Henderson JN, Allen KV, Deary IJ, Frier BM. Hypoglycaemia in insulin-treated type 2 diabetes: frequency, symptoms and impaired awareness. *Diabet Med* 2003;20:1016–1021.

23. Murata GH, Duckworth WC, Shah JH, et al. Hypoglycemia in stable, insulin treated veterans with type 2 diabetes: a prospective study of 1662 episodes. *J Diabetes Complications* 2005;19(1):10–17.

24. Ohkubo Y, Kishikawa H, Araki E, Miyata T, Isami S, Motoyoshi S, Kojima Y, Furuyoshi N, Shichiri M. Intensive insulin therapy prevents the progression of diabetic microvascular complications in Japanese patients with non-insulin-dependent diabetes mellitus: a randomized prospective 6-year study. *Diabetes Res Clin Pract* 1995;28:103–117.

25. Saudek CD, Duckworth WC, Giobbie-Hurder A, Henderson WG, Henry RR, Kelley DE, Edelman SV, Zieve FJ, Adler RA, Anderson JW, Anderson RJ, Hamilton BP, Donner TW, Kirkman MS, Morgan NA. Implantable insulin pump vs multiple-dose insulin for non-insulin-dependent diabetes mellitus: a randomized clinical trial. Department of Veterans Affairs Implantable Insulin Pump Study Group. *JAMA* 1996;276:1322–1327.

26. Gurlek A, Erbas T, Gedik O. Frequency of severe hypoglycaemia in type 1 and type 2 diabetes during conventional insulin therapy. *Exp Clin Endocrinol Diabetes* 1999;107:220–224.

27. Abraira C, Colwell JA, Nuttall FQ, Sawin CT, Nagel NJ, Comstock JP, Emanuele NV, Levin SR, Henderson W, Lee HS. Veterans Affairs Cooperative Study on glycemic control and complications in type II diabetes (VA CSDM). Results of the feasibility trial. Veterans Affairs Cooperative Study in Type II Diabetes. *Diabetes Care* 1995;18:1113–1123.

28. Frier BM. How hypoglycaemia can affect the life of a person with diabetes. *Diabetes Metab Res Rev* 2007;24:87–92.

29. Amiel SA. Hypoglycemia in patients with type 1 diabetes. In *Therapy for Diabetes Mellitus and Related Disorders*, 5th ed. Lebovitz HE, Ed. Alexandria, VA, American Diabetes Association, 2009, p. 369–384.

30. Cryer PE. *Hypoglycemia: Pathophysiology, Diagnosis and Treatment.* New York: Oxford University Press, 1997.

31. Cryer PE. *Hypoglycemia in Diabetes: Pathophysiology, Prevalence, and Prevention.* 2nd ed. Alexandria, VA, American Diabetes Association, 2012.

32. Jones TW, Porter P, Sherwin RS, Davis EA, O'Leary P, Frazer F, et al. Decreased epinephrine responses to hypoglycemia during sleep. *N Engl J Med* 1998;338:1657–1662.

33. Seaquist ER, Anderson J, Childs B, Cryer P, Dagogo-Jack S, Fish L, Heller SR, Rodriguez H, Rosenzweig J, Vigersky R. Hypoglycemia and diabetes: a report of a workgroup of the American Diabetes Association and the Endocrine Society. *Diabetes Care* 2013;36(5):1384–1395.

34. Dagogo-Jack SE, Craft S, Cryer PE. Hypoglycemia-associated autonomic failure in insulin-dependent diabetes mellitus. Recent antecedent hypoglycemia reduces autonomic responses to, symptoms of, and defense against subsequent hypoglycemia. *J Clin Invest* 1993;91(3):819–828.

35. Heller SR, Cryer PE. Reduced neuroendocrine and symptomatic responses to subsequent hypoglycemia after 1 episode of hypoglycemia in nondiabetic humans. *Diabetes* 1991;40:223–226.

36. Gerich JE, Langlois M, Noacco C, Karam JH, Forsham PH. Lack of glucagon response to hypoglycemia in diabetes: evidence for an intrinsic pancreatic alpha cell defect. *Science* 1973;182(4108):171–173.

37. Cox DJ, Gonder-Frederick LA, Kovatchev BP, et al. Biopsychobehavioral model of severe hypoglycemia. II. Understanding the risk of severe hypoglycemia. *Diabetes Care* 1999;22(12):2018–2025.

38. Cox D, Ritterband L, Magee J, et al. Blood glucose awareness training delivered over the Internet. *Diabetes Care* 2008;31(8):1527–1528.

39. Frier BM, Schernthaner G, Heller SR. Hypoglycemia and cardiovascular risks. *Diabetes Care* 2011;34(Suppl 1):S132–137.

40. Marques JL, George E, Peacey SR, et al. Altered ventricular repolarization during hypoglycaemia in patients with diabetes. *Diabet Med* 1997;14(8):648–654.

41. Trovati M, Anfossi G, Cavalot F, et al. Studies on mechanisms involved in hypoglycemia-induced platelet activation. *Diabetes* 1986;35(7):818–825.

42. Desouza C, Salazar H, Cheong B, et al. Association of hypoglycemia and cardiac ischemia: a study based on continuous monitoring. *Diabetes Care* 2003;26:1485–1489.

43. Duh E, Feinglos M. Hypoglycemia-induced angina pectoris in a patient with diabetes mellitus. *Ann Intern Med* 1996;44(7):751–755.

44. Kamijo Y, Soma K, Aoyama N, et al. Myocardial infarction with acute insulin poisoning—a case report. *Angiology* 2000;51(8):689–693.

45. Sovik O, Thordarson H. Dead-in-bed syndrome in young diabetic patients. *Diabetes Care* 1999;22(Suppl 2):B40–42.

46. Robinson RT, Harris ND, Ireland RH, et al. Mechanisms of abnormal cardiac repolarization during insulin-induced hypoglycemia. *Diabetes* 2003;52(6):1469–1474.

47. Riddle MC. Counterpoint: intensive glucose control and mortality in ACCORD—still looking for clues. *Diabetes Care* 2010;33(12):2722–2724.

48. Breton MD. Bio-behavioral control, glucose variability, and hypoglycemia-associated autonomic failure in type 1 diabetes (T1DM). *Conf Proc IEEE Eng Med Biol Soc* 2006;1:315–318.

49. Campbell MD, Walker M, Trenell MI, Jakovljevic DG, Stevenson EJ, Bracken RM, Bain SC, West DJ. Large pre- and postexercise rapid-acting insulin reductions preserves glycemia and prevents early- but not late-onset hypoglycemia in patients with type 1 diabetes. *Diabetes Care* 2013;36(8):2217–2224.

50. McDonnell ME, Umpierrez GE. Insulin therapy for the management of hyperglycemia in hospitalized patients. *Endocrinol Metab Clin North Am* 2012;41(1):175–201.

51. Umpierrez GE, Smiley D, Zisman A, et al. Randomized study of basal-bolus insulin therapy in the inpatient management of patients with type 2 diabetes (RABBIT 2 Trial). *Diabetes Care* 2007;30(9):2181–2186.

52. Fujioka M, Okuchi K, Hiramatsu KI, et al. Specific changes in human brain after hypoglycemic injury. *Stroke* 1997;28(3):584–587.

53. Languren G, Montiel T, Julio-Amilpas A, Massieu L. Neuronal damage and cognitive impairment associated with hypoglycemia: an integrated view. *Neurochemistry International* 2013;63(4):331–343.

54. Lin CH, Sheu WH. Hypoglycaemic episodes and risk of dementia in diabetes mellitus: 7-year follow-up study. *J Intern Med* 2013;273(1):102–110.

55. Rovet JF, Ehrlich RM, Czuchta D. Intellectual characteristics of diabetic children at diagnosis and one year later. *J Pediatr Psychol* 1990;15:775–788.

56. Rovet JF, Ehrlich RM. The effect of hypoglycemic seizures on cognitive function in children with diabetes: a 7-year prospective study. *J Pediatr* 1999;134(4):503–506.

57. Perros P, Deary IJ, Sellar RJ, et al. Brain abnormalities demonstrated by magnetic resonance imaging in adult IDDM patients with and without a history of recurrent severe hypoglycemia. *Diabetes Care* 1997;20(6):1013–1018.

58. Kaufman FR, Epport K, Engilman R, et al. Neurocognitive functioning in children diagnosed with diabetes before age 10 years. *J Diabetes Complications* 1999;13(1):31–38.

59. Gold AE, MacLeod KM, Deary IJ, et al. Hypoglycemia-induced cognitive dysfunction in diabetes mellitus: effect of hypoglycemia unawareness. *Physiol Behav* 1995;58(3):501–511.

60. Strachan MW, Deary IJ, Ewing FM, et al. Recovery of cognitive function and mood after severe hypoglycemia in adults with insulin-treated diabetes. *Diabetes Care* 2000;23(3):305–312.

61. Strachan MW, Reynolds RM, Marioni, RE, Price JF. Cognitive function, dementia and type 2 diabetes mellitus in the elderly. *Nat Rev Endocrinol* 2011;7(2):108–114.

62. Wessels AM, Lane KA, Gao S, et al. Diabetes and cognitive decline in elderly African Americans: a 15-year follow-up study. *Alzheimers Dement* 2011;7(4):418–424.

63. Yaffe K, Falvey CM, Hamilton N, Harris TB, Simonsick EM, Strotmeyer ES, Shorr RI, Metti A, Schwartz AV; for the Health ABC Study. Association between hypoglycemia and dementia in a biracial cohort of older adults with diabetes mellitus. *JAMA Intern Med* 2013;173(14):1300–1306.

64. Daviglus ML, Plassman BL, Pirzada A, et al. Risk factors and preventive interventions for Alzheimer disease: state of the science. *Arch Neurol* 2011;68(9):1185–1190.

65. Deary IJ, Crawford JR, Hepburn DA, et al. Severe hypoglycemia and intelligence in adult patients with insulin-treated diabetes. *Diabetes* 1993;42(2):341–334.

66. Biessels GJ. Diabetes: hypoglycemia and dementia in type 2 diabetes: chick or egg? *Nat Rev Endocrinol* 2009;5(10):532–534.

67. Diabetes Control and Complications Trial/Epidemiology of Diabetes Interventions and Complications Study Research Group; Jacobson AM, Musen G, Ryan CM, Silvers N, Cleary P, Waberski B, Burwood A, Weinger K, Bayless M, Dahms W, Harth J. Long-term effect of diabetes and its treatment on cognitive function. *N Engl J Med* 2007;356:1842–1852.

68. Montori VM, Fernández-Balsells M. Glycemic control in type 2 diabetes: time for an evidence-based about-face? *Ann Intern Med* 2009;150:803–808.

69. Riddle MC, Rosenstock J, Gerich J. The Treat-to-Target trial: randomized addition of glargine or human NPH insulin to oral therapy of type 2 diabetic patients. *Diabetes Care* 2003;26(11):3080–3086.

70. Hermansen K, Davies M, Derezinski T, et al. A 26-week, randomized, parallel, treat-to-target trial comparing insulin detemir with NPH insulin as add-on therapy to oral glucose-lowering drugs in insulin-naive people with type 2 diabetes. *Diabetes Care* 2006;29(6):1269–1274.

71. Yki-Jarvinen H, Ryysy L, Nikkila K, Tulokas T, Vanamo R, Heikkila M. Comparison of bedtime insulin regimens in patients with type 2 diabetes mellitus. A randomized, controlled trial. *Ann Intern Med* 1999;130:389–396.

72. Guthrie DW, Guthrie RA. Approach to management. *Diabetes Educ* 2000;16(5):401–406.

73. Bergenstal RM, Johnson M, Powers MA, et al. Adjust to target in type 2 diabetes. *Diabetes Care* 2008;31(7):1305–1310.

74. Polonsky KS, et al. Non-insulin-dependent diabetes mellitus: a genetically programmed failure of the beta cell to compensate for insulin resistance. *N Engl J Med* 1996;334(12):777–783.

75. Gearhart JG, Ducan JL 3rd, Replogle JH, et al. Efficacy of sliding-scale insulin therapy: a comparison with prospective regimens. *Fam Pract Res J* 1994;14(4):313–322.

76. Sawin CT. Action without benefit. The sliding scale of insulin use. *Arch Intern Med* 1997;157(5):489.

77. Lipska KJ, Warton EM, Huang ES, et al. HbA1c and risk of severe hypoglycemia in type 2 diabetes: the Diabetes and Aging Study. *Diabetes Care* 2013;36(11):3535–3542.

78. Wolpert HA, Atakov-Castillo A, Smith SA, Steil GM. Dietary fat acutely increases glucose concentrations and insulin requirements in patients with type 1 diabetes: implications for carbohydrate-based bolus dose calculation and intensive diabetes management. *Diabetes Care* 2013;36(4):810–816.

79. Holman RR, Farmer AJ, Davies MJ, Levy JC, Darbyshire JL, Keenan JF, Paul SK; for the 4-T Study Group. Three-year efficacy of complex insulin regimens in type 2 diabetes. *N Engl J Med* 2009;361(18):1736–1747.

Chapter 41

Ocular Complications

PAOLO S. SILVA, MD
JERRY D. CAVALLERANO, OD, PHD
LLOYD M. AIELLO, MD
LLOYD PAUL AIELLO, MD, PHD

Diabetes will affect >592 million people worldwide by the year 2035. Diabetic retinopathy (DR) is the most prevalent of the diabetes complications, affecting nearly half of all people with diabetes at any point in time. Almost all people with diabetes eventually will develop some degree of DR. Today, DR remains one of the leading causes of new-onset blindness, severe visual loss, and moderate visual loss in people of working age in almost all industrial countries worldwide.

DR and diabetic macular edema (DME) affect individuals with both type 1 diabetes (T1D) and type 2 diabetes (T2D). Patients with T1D, because of the earlier onset and longer duration of DM, experience more frequent and severe ocular complications. After 5 years of DM, 23% of patients with T1D have DR. After 10 and 15 years, this prevalence increases to almost 60 and 80%, respectively. Proliferative diabetic retinopathy (PDR), the most sight-threatening stage of the disease, is present in 25 and 56% of patients with T1D after 15 and 20 years, respectively, and often remains asymptomatic until it has progressed substantially beyond the optimal stage for initiating treatment (Figure 41.1).

In T2D, DR was present in 20% of cases at diagnosis, increasing to 60–85% after 15 years, as assessed by the Wisconsin Epidemiologic Study of Diabetic Retinopathy (WESDR). PDR was present in 3–4% of patients within 4 years and 5–20% of T2D after 15 years and >50% after ≥20 years. Thus, patients with T2D are more likely to have DR at diagnosis and are more likely to develop DR sooner after diagnosis than patients with T1D (Figure 41.2).

Globally, it is estimated that >93 million people have DR, 17 million have PDR, 21 million have DME, and 28 million have vision-threatening DR. In the U.S. during 2005–2008, among people with diabetes ≥40 years, the estimated prevalence of DR was 28.5% and vision-threatening retinopathy was 4.4%. During that same time period, the prevalence of nonrefractive visual impairment increased by 21%, with the risk for nonrefractive visual impairment being more than three times greater in people with diabetes compared with those without diabetes (1.4 vs. 5.3%, P <0.001). Fortunately, multiple landmark clinical trials have demonstrated that interventions can have a significant benefit in preventing visual loss and preserving vision in people with diabetes. The Diabetes Control and Complications Trial (DCCT) and the United Kingdom Prospective Diabetes Study (UKPDS) demonstrated that adherence to intensive blood glucose control regimens can reduce the rates of onset and progression of DR. The Diabetic Retinopathy Study (DRS) and the Early Treatment Diabetic Retinopathy Study (ETDRS) showed that laser photocoagulation greatly reduced severe visual loss from diabetic retinal disease, particularly when laser surgery was initiated

DOI: 10.2337/9781580405096.41

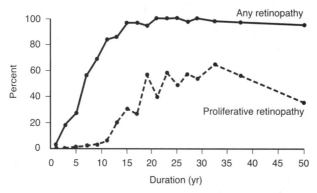

Figure 41.1—Frequency of retinopathy or proliferative retinopathy by duration of diabetes (years) in 996 insulin-taking persons in whom diabetes was diagnosed when <30 years of age and who participated in the Wisconsin Epidemiologic Study of Diabetic Retinopathy (WESDR), 1980–1982. *Source:* Klein R, Klein BEK, Moss SE, et al. The Wisconsin Epidemiologic Study of Diabetic Retinopathy. II. Prevalence and risk of diabetic retinopathy when age at diagnosis is less than 30 years. *Arch Ophthalmol* 1984:102:520–526.

promptly. Timely laser photocoagulation may reduce the risk of severe visual loss (best vision of 5/200 or worse) from high-risk PDR to <4% and can reduce the risk of moderate visual loss (a doubling of the visual angle, e.g., 20/20 reduced to 20/40) from DME by ≥50%. Vitrectomy surgery can restore useful vision by removing vitreous hemorrhage (VH) or by relieving retinal traction threatening the macula. Intravitreal injection of anti–vascular endothelial growth factor (VEGF) medications when performed according to protocols, such as done in the Diabetic Retinopathy Clinical Research Network (DRCR.net), has become standard care for patients with center-involved DME with reduced vision, further reducing the risk of moderate vision loss from DME.

Despite these advances, the early detection and treatment of DR are critical. Because only 40–60% of the people with diabetes in the U.S. population receive adequate ophthalmic care, emphasis must be placed on early detection of retinal disorders, with appropriate referral for management and treatment. In addition, careful control of blood glucose levels and concurrent systemic conditions, such as hypertension, renal disease, and dyslipidemia, is critical.

DIABETIC RETINOPATHY

PATHOPHYSIOLOGY

Elevated blood glucose levels result in structural, physiological, and biochemical changes that alter cellular metabolism, retinal blood flow, and retinal capillary

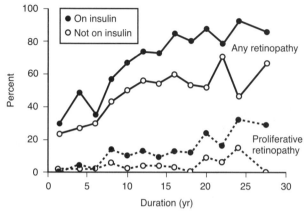

Figure 41.2—The frequency of retinopathy or proliferative retinopathy by duration of diabetes (years) in 673 people taking insulin and 697 people not taking insulin in whom diabetes was diagnosed when >29 years and who participated in the Wisconsin Epidemiologic Study of Diabetic Retinopathy (WESDR), 1980–1982. *Source:* Klein R, Klein BEK, Moss SE, et al. The Wisconsin Epidemiologic Study of Diabetic Retinopathy. III. Prevalence and risk of diabetic retinopathy when age at diagnosis is 30 or more years. *Arch Ophthalmol* 1984:102:527–532.

competency. Classic pathophysiologic processes characterize DR and include biochemical changes affecting cellular metabolism, decreased retinal blood flow, impaired vascular autoregulation, loss of retinal pericytes, outpouchings of the capillary walls to form microaneurysms, closure of retinal capillaries and arterioles resulting in retinal ischemia, increased vascular permeability of retinal capillaries sometimes leading to retinal edema, proliferation of new vessels (with or without VH), development of fibrous tissue, and contraction of vitreous and fibrous proliferation with subsequent retinal traction and detachment.

Clinically, these processes are manifested as either PDR, nonproliferative diabetic retinopathy (NPDR), or DME (Table 41.1). These and other processes of DR may affect the macula, significantly altering function and reading vision. Loss of vision from diabetes usually results from VH, PDR leading to fibrous tissue formation, and subsequent traction retinal detachment, or DME.

CLINICAL CARE

Current management strategies for DR are guided by results of large, well-designed clinical trials. These landmark studies currently guide the standard of diabetes eye care to optimally preserve vision and reduce the threat of visual loss (Table 41.2).

The DRS (1971–1975) definitively established the beneficial effects of scatter (panretinal) laser photocoagulation for PDR. The ETDRS (1979–1990) demonstrated the benefit of focal laser treatment for DME and provided insight into the

Table 41.1—Clinical Manifestations of Retinopathy

Diabetic macular edema (DME) may occur at any level of diabetic retinopathy, although it is more common with more advanced retinopathy.

Nonproliferative diabetic retinopathy (NPDR)

Mild—one or both of the following:
   –Few scattered retinal microaneurysms and hemorrhages
   –Hard exudate

Moderate—one or more of the following:
   –More extensive retinal hemorrhages and/or microaneurysms
   –Mild intraretinal microvascular abnormalities (IRMA)
   –Early venous beading

Severe to very severe—one or more of the following:
   –Severe hemorrhages or microaneurysms in all four quadrants (Figure 41.3)
   –More extensive IRMA in at least one quadrant (Figure 41.5)
   –Venous beading in at least two quadrants (Figure 41.4)

Proliferative diabetic retinopathy (PDR)

Early—one or more of the following:
   –Minimal new vessels on disk (NVD) less than one-quarter disk area without preretinal or
   vitreous hemorrhage
   –New vessels elsewhere on retina (NVE) without preretinal or vitreous hemorrhage

High risk—one or more of the following:
   –NVD one-quarter or more disk area with or without preretinal or vitreous hemorrhage
   (Figure 41.6)
   –NVD less than one-quarter disk area in extent accompanied by fresh hemorrhage
   –NVE one-half or more disk area with preretinal or vitreous hemorrhage

Table 41.2—Management Recommendations

Diabetic retinopathy and macular edema severity	Follow-up (months)	Retinal imaging*	Fluorescein angiography	Panretinal laser	Focal laser	Intravitreal anti-VEGF
Normal or minimal NPDR	12	No	No	No	No	No
Mild to moderate NPDR	6–12	Occasionally	No	No	No	No
Mild to moderate NPDR with DME	4–6	Often	No	No	No	No

Diabetic retinopathy and macular edema severity	Follow-up (months)	Retinal imaging*	Fluorescein angiography	Panretinal laser	Focal laser	Intravitreal anti-VEGF
Mild to moderate NPDR with CSME						
Center not involved	3–4	Yes	Occasionally	No	Consider	No
Center involved	1 (3–4)†	Yes	Consider	No	Occasionally	Yes
Severe to very severe NPDR	3–4	Yes	No	Consider	No	No
Severe to very severe NPDR with DME	3–4	Yes	No	Consider	No	No
Severe to very severe NPDR with CSME						
Center not involved	3–4	Yes	Occasionally	Consider	Consider	No
Center involved	1 (3–4)†	Yes	Consider	Consider	Occasionally	Yes
Non-high-risk PDR	2–3	Yes	No	Consider	No	No
Non-high-risk PDR with DME	2–3	Yes	No	Consider	No	No
Non-high-risk PDR with CSME						
Center not involved	2–3	Yes	Occasionally	Consider	Consider	No
Center involved	1 (2–3)†	Yes	Consider	Consider	Occasionally	Yes
High-risk PDR	1–3	Yes	No	Yes	No	No
High-risk PDR with DME	1–3	Yes	No	Yes	No	No
High-risk PDR with CSME						
Center not involved	1–3	Yes	Occasionally	Yes	Consider	No
Center involved	1 (1–3)†	Yes	Consider	Yes	Occasionally	Yes
High-risk PDR not amenable to photocoagulation	1–6	Yes	Yes, if CSME	In connection with vitrectomy		Consider in adjunct to vitrectomy

Note: NPDR = nonproliferative diabetic retinopathy; DME = diabetic macular edema; CSME = clinically significant macular edema; PDR = proliferative diabetic retinopathy; VEGF = vascular endothelial growth factor.

*Retinal imaging: color fundus photography, optical coherence tomography, and other validated methods of imaging.

†One month if following anti VEGF treatment.

Source: Adapted from American Academy of Ophthalmology preferred practice patterns for diabetic retinopathy.

most appropriate timing for retinal laser surgery for DR and DME. The study also demonstrated that the use of 650 mg/day aspirin is unlikely to have any effect on the progression of DR or the risk of VH in the presence of DR. The Diabetic Retinopathy Vitrectomy Study (1977–1987) established early guidelines on the timing of surgical intervention after visual loss from VH. The DCCT (1983–1993) demonstrated that intensive control of blood glucose levels in patients with T1D, resulting in at least a 1% drop in glycosylated hemoglobin levels, reduces the risk of onset of any DR, the progression of retinopathy, and the need for laser surgery. The UKPDS (1977–1999) found similar results of intensive blood glucose control for patients with T2D. Additionally, the UKPDS found that more intensive control of blood pressure, with either a β-blocking agent or an angiotensin-converting enzyme inhibitor, reduced the risk of progression of retinopathy. DRCR.net and pharmaceutical studies have established the clear benefit of a defined regimen of intravitreal anti-VEGF injections for center-involved DME, reducing the risk for moderate visual loss to <5% with nearly 50% of patients experiencing recovery of two or more lines of vision.

DIAGNOSIS: CLINICAL LEVELS OF DR AND DME

DR can be classified broadly into NPDR and PDR. On the basis of the presence and degree of retinal lesions, NPDR is classified clinically as mild, moderate, severe, or very severe. PDR is marked by proliferation of new vessels on the optic disc (NVD), new vessels elsewhere on the retina (NVE), preretinal hemorrhage (PRH), VH, or fibrous tissue proliferation (FP). DME can be present with any level of DR, but it is more frequent with increasing DR severity. Accurate diagnosis of the severity of DR is essential because the risk of progression to PDR and high-risk PDR is correlated closely with specific NPDR level. Proper diagnosis of DR severity establishes the risk of progression to sight-threatening retinopathy and appropriate clinical management both in terms of follow-up schedule and therapeutic options.

NONPROLIFERATIVE DIABETIC RETINOPATHY

Mild NPDR, characterized by microaneurysms with or without occasional blot hemorrhages, is virtually ubiquitous after 15–17 years of DM. Microaneurysms may resolve slowly with time or show little or no change. Dot hemorrhages and microaneurysms can be considered together clinically as one type of lesion. They frequently are indistinguishable from one another by ophthalmoscopic examination without fluorescein angiography, and identifying them separately does not add any benefit in terms of predicting progression risk. The invasive fluorescein angiography testing is not warranted at this stage of DR unless macular edema threatening central vision is present. The microaneurysms represent outpouchings of blood vessel walls, possibly secondary to weakness of the capillary wall from loss of pericytes or from increased intraluminal pressure or because of endothelial proliferation.

Rare flecks of hard exudates, representing small white or yellowish white deposits generally with sharp borders, may be present in the intermediate layers of the retina. Hard exudates are lipid deposits leaked from microaneurysms or compromised capillary beds and may be present at any stage of NPDR and PDR.

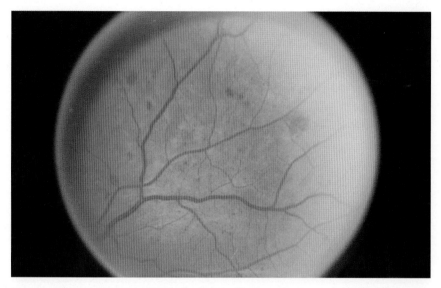

Figure 41.3—This severity and extent of hemorrhages or microaneurysms in all four quadrants constitutes severe nonproliferative diabetic retinopathy. Standard photograph 2A.

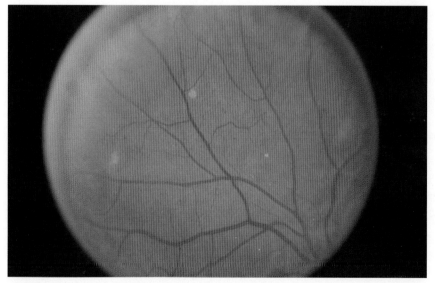

Figure 41.4—This extent of intraretinal microvascular abnormalities in one or more quadrants constitutes severe nonproliferative diabetic retinopathy. Standard photograph 8A.

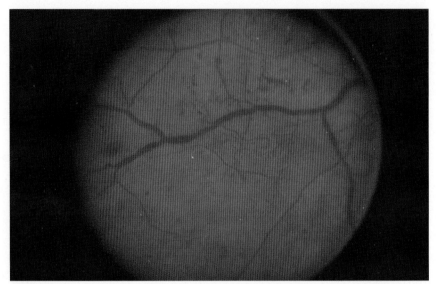

Figure 41.5—Venous beading in two or more quadrants constitutes severe nonproliferative diabetic retinopathy. Standard photograph 6B.

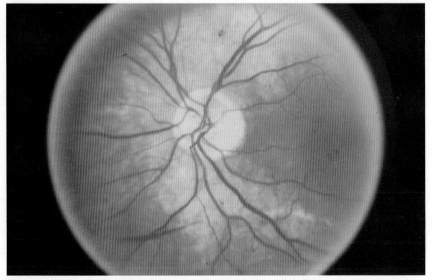

Figure 41.6—This extent of new vessels on the disk (one-quarter or more disk area) with or without preretinal or vitreous hemorrhage constitutes high-risk diabetic retinopathy. Standard photograph 10A.

Patients with mild NPDR can safely be followed every 9–12 months unless macular edema is present (Table 41.1).

Moderate NPDR is characterized by more severe retinal lesions. These lesions represent not only changes in vascular and perivascular tissue, but also changes within the retina associated with the effects of relative retinal hypoxia and circulatory changes. More abundant retinal hemorrhages and microaneurysms are present (Figure 41.3). Early venous caliber abnormalities also may be present, reflected clinically as tortuous vasculature with varying lumen size. Venous caliber abnormalities may be caused by either sluggish blood flow, blood vessel wall weakening, or hypoxia.

Another vascular change observed in moderate NPDR is intraretinal microvascular abnormalities (IRMA). IRMA is a type of intraretinal neovascularization. Cotton-wool spots may be present at this stage and represent microinfarct-induced stasis of axoplasmic flow in the nerve fiber layer of the retina. Cotton-wool spots tend to disappear as NPDR becomes more severe.

Patients with moderate NPDR have more significant retinal disease. These patients are at greater risk for progression to vision-threatening DR and should be monitored every 4–6 months.

Severe or very severe NPDR is characterized by an abundance of nonproliferative lesions that include venous beading (Figure 41.5), IRMA (Figure 41.4), or extensive hemorrhages and microaneurysms (Figure 41.3). The risk for progression to PDR is high because of the widespread retinal ischemia, but frank new vessel growth on the retina is not present. Consultation with an ophthalmologist experienced in the management of diabetic eye disease for possible early laser surgery is urgent, particularly if exacerbating conditions exist (e.g., hypertension, renal disease, pregnancy) or if the patient seems to be nonadherent or untimely with follow-up examination. Rates of progression to high-risk PDR approach 45–50% in 2 years and 75% in 5 years if untreated. Patients with T2D may be candidates for scatter laser photocoagulation at this time (i.e., before developing high-risk PDR).

PROLIFERATIVE DIABETIC RETINOPATHY

PDR represents a severe form of retinopathy. It is characterized by the growth of new vessels on or within 1 disk diameter of the optic disk (NVD), the growth of NVE on the retina, VH or PRH, or preretinal FP. These vessels grow over the retinal surface and on the posterior surface of the vitreous. They are fragile and rupture easily, causing PRH and VH. The vessels can rupture spontaneously, even while a person is asleep, or with vigorous exercise, straining, coughing, or sneezing.

High-risk PDR puts a person at significant risk of visual loss (Table 41.1). The DRS revealed a 25–40% risk of severe visual loss (<20/400, worse than legal blindness) over a 2-year period if high-risk PDR is present. Scatter laser treatment can reduce this risk by ~60%. High-risk PDR is characterized by any one of the following lesions:

- NVD greater than standard photo 10A of the modified Airlie House classification of DR (i.e., NVD that covers more than one-fourth to one-third of the disk area) (Figure 41.6)

- NVD less than standard photo 10A if PRH or VH is present
- NVE greater than or equal to one-half of the disk area if PRH or VH is present

Patients with high-risk PDR are candidates for immediate scatter laser photocoagulation. These patients should be referred immediately for laser treatment by an ophthalmologist skilled in the treatment of DR. These patients generally should not wait more than a few days for laser surgery.

The ETDRS demonstrated that scatter laser treatment applied when a person approaches or reaches high-risk PDR can reduce the 5-year risk of severe visual loss to <4%. In full scatter treatment, 1,200–2,400 lesions are applied to the posterior pole. One or more sessions normally are required to complete the treatment. Typically, the treating ophthalmologist applies the 500 μm laser burns 500 μm apart. Major retinal vessels, the optic nerve and the central macula are avoided.

The response to full scatter photocoagulation varies depending on the retinal and medical status of the patient. There may be 1) regression of active neovascularization, 2) persistent neovascularization without further progression, 3) continued growth of the neovascularization, or 4) recurrent VH. Careful follow-up evaluation by the treating ophthalmologist with additional scatter or local laser photocoagulation or vitrectomy may be indicated, especially if continued new vessel growth or recurrent VH occurs.

FP may lead to traction, which may cause a retinal detachment. If a view of the posterior pole is obscured by VH, ultrasound examination may be necessary. Non-resolving VH and traction retinal detachments, particularly those threatening detachment of the macula, may be indications for vitrectomy surgery.

Following the natural history of DR, PDR usually progresses through an active phase, followed by remission. In the remission phase, fibrous tissue usually forms along abnormal vessels but also may form between the retina and posterior vitreous surface. A goal of panretinal laser photocoagulation is to shorten the active phase of DR, leading to remission before major VH or FP compromises vision. Patients who undergo panretinal laser photocoagulation for PDR may experience a reactivation of DR in the future and may require further laser treatments or vitrectomy.

Laser photocoagulation is not without potential side effects and complications. The DRS documented occasional minor decreases in visual acuity levels and peripheral visual fields, particularly in eyes treated with the xenon-arc photocoagulator, a system no longer in use. Today, panretinal laser photocoagulation is performed with newer, more efficient laser systems that may minimize adverse effects, but as with any surgical procedure, the risks need to be weighed against the potential benefits of laser surgery.

Poor diabetes control, hypertension, kidney disease, high cholesterol, and anemia are documented risk factors for the progression of DR. Many factors affect the progression of DR in patients with T1D, including duration of DM, DR status, pregnancy, the use of diuretics, and glycosylated hemoglobin levels. In patients with T2D, the age of the patient, severity of DR, glycosylated hemoglobin levels, diuretic usage, lower intraocular pressure, smoking, and lower diastolic blood pressure may be risk factors.

DIABETIC MACULAR EDEMA

DME can be present at any stage of DR and is a leading cause of moderate visual loss from DM. Proper evaluation requires stereoscopic examination of the macula with slit-lamp biomicroscope, fundus photography, or optical coherence tomography. DME is a collection of fluid or thickening in the macula. Hard exudates within the macula area, nonperfusion of the retina inside the temporal vessel arcades, or any combination of these lesions may be present. Patients with or suspected of having DME should be referred to an ophthalmologist for evaluation for clinically significant DME (CSME) because, at this stage, laser photocoagulation frequently is indicated. CSME is macular edema that involves or threatens the center of the macula and is characterized by any of the following retinal lesions:

- Retinal thickening at or within 500 µm from the center of the macula
- Hard exudates at or within 500 µm from the center of the macula if accompanied by thickening of the adjacent retina
- A zone(s) of thickening greater than or equal to one disk area in size, if any portion of that is within one disk diameter from the center of the macula

Patients with CSME should be referred to an ophthalmologist experienced in the care of diabetic eye disease. The urgency for treatment of DME is not as acute as for high-risk PDR, but consultation and referral preferably should occur within 1 month.

The term CSME was introduced in the ETDRS to signify an increased risk for moderate visual loss. Data from the ETDRS evaluating eyes with DME have shown that the presence or absence of thickening involving the center of the macula (center-involved DME) was the primary important factor in determining short- and long-term visual acuity outcomes. Eyes with center-involved DME had nearly a 10-fold greater risk for developing moderate visual loss compared with eyes without center involvement. Thus, current DME evaluation is more focused on the presence or absence of edema at the center of the macula.

Patients with non–center-involved CSME are candidates for focal laser photocoagulation. The goal of this laser treatment is to maintain acuity at approximately the same level as before treatment by preventing or limiting further leakage in the retina and allowing the leakage already present to resorb. Fluorescein angiography often is used to determine whether treatable lesions are present and to guide the application of focal or grid laser surgery. Focal treatment is applied to focal leaks contributing to DME. Grid treatment is applied to areas of diffuse leakage or areas of nonperfusion in the macula area. The ETDRS demonstrated that in eyes with CSME, the risk of moderate visual loss was 50–60% less for eyes treated with focal laser compared with eyes assigned to deferral of treatment, being reduced from 32 to 15% after 3 years of follow-up. Focal photocoagulation reduced the risk of moderate visual loss, increased the chance of visual improvement, decreased retinal thickening, and was not associated with any major adverse effects.

The standard care for patients with center-involved DME with visual impairment is intravitreal injections of anti-VEGF agents. This therapeutic approach both reduces the risk of moderate visual loss to <5% and improves visual acuity by two lines or more in nearly 50% of patients at 1 year. An average of eight to nine intravitreal injections are needed in the first year of treatment. This number is reduced to two to three and one or two injections in the second and third years of follow-up, respectively.

Given the number of patients who may develop DME and the number of injections administered as part of the treatment regimens for DME, health care providers caring for people with diabetes should be aware of the potential ocular and systemic adverse effects that may occur following these injections. These ocular adverse events include endophthalmitis, ocular inflammation, retinal detachment, VH, and traumatic cataract. These severe complications are estimated to occur in <1 in 1,000 injections. Systemic VEGF levels play a role in promoting collateral vessel formation following ischemic events. This role is particularly important in people with diabetes who are at increased risk of having cardiovascular and peripheral vascular ischemic events. An increased risk of ischemic and thromboembolic events has been observed in as many as 5% of patients receiving systemic VEGF inhibition for cancer chemotherapy. These patients, however, received intravenous anti-VEGF doses that are several hundredfold greater than those typically given intravitreally in the eye. Multicenter ophthalmic clinical trials have not found a clear association with ischemic and thromboembolic events when anti-VEGF medications are administered intravitreally, but this risk is potentially a concern and part of the treatment decision process.

NONRETINAL OCULAR COMPLICATIONS

The ocular manifestations of diabetes that receive the most attention are those related to DR and macular edema because these changes are usually responsible for the most devastating visual threat from diabetes. Diabetic eye disease, however, represents an end-organ response to a systemic medical condition. Consequently, all structures of the eye are susceptible to the deleterious effects of diabetes. Following are some of the ocular problems in addition to DR that are associated with diabetes:

- Mononeuropathies of cranial nerves III, IV, or VI
- Higher incidence of glaucoma
- Earlier and more rapidly progressing cataracts
- Susceptibility to corneal abrasions and recurrent corneal erosions
- Early presbyopia
- Blurred or fluctuating vision

LENTICULAR OPACITIES

Cataracts may occur at a younger age and progress more rapidly in the presence of diabetes. Compared with similarly aged individuals without diabetes, cataracts are 60% more common in people with diabetes. This increased risk of cataract development occurs in populations with both T1D and T2D.

Reversible lenticular opacities related to DM can occur in different layers of the lens and most frequently are related to poor glycemic control. The so-called true diabetic cataracts usually are bilateral and are characterized by dense bands of white subcapsular spots that look like snowflakes or fine needle-shaped opacities. Because diabetic cataracts are related to prolonged periods of severe hyperglycemia and untreated diabetes, they seldom are seen in the U.S. and other industrial countries.

Management of cataracts in patients with diabetes involves the same treatment strategies as management of age-related cataracts. For visual impairment not requiring surgery, optimum refraction for maximum visual acuity is recommended. Glare-control lenses and the use of sunglasses may relieve cataract-induced visual symptoms. Fortunately, cataract extraction with intraocular lens implantation is 90–95% successful in restoring useful vision, but the surgery has potential complications unique to diabetes. Intraocular lens implants provide the most natural postsurgical refractive correction. Careful patient education and consultation with the cataract surgeon is indicated.

The level of DR and DME severity needs to be evaluated carefully before planned cataract surgery because of the potential risk of worsening during the postoperative period. Diabetes is associated with an increased incidence of postoperative neovascularization on the iris (NVI) and neovascular glaucoma (NVG) after cataract extractions, regardless of the degree of retinopathy before surgery. If active PDR is present before cataract surgery, the risk of subsequently developing NVI, NVG, and VH is greater. Scatter laser photocoagulation is indicated for patients with high-risk PDR. With cataracts developing in the presence of severe NPDR or PDR without high-risk PDR, early laser treatment may be indicated. Laser treatment may be required a few days after surgery if active PDR is present. Preoperative evaluation may require optical coherence tomography to evaluate the vitreoretinal interface to assess subtle vitreoretinal traction. Presurgical evaluation may influence the decision to perform cataract surgery in conjunction with vitrectomy or intravitreal injection intraocular steroids or anti-VEGF agents to optimize postsurgical visual outcomes.

GLAUCOMA

Open-angle glaucoma is 1.2–2.7 times more common in the diabetic than in the nondiabetic population. The prevalence of glaucoma increases with age and duration of diabetes, but medical therapy for open-angle glaucoma is generally effective. Argon laser trabeculoplasty may normalize intraocular pressures in some patients if medical therapy proves ineffective. Treatment of open-angle glaucoma for the diabetes patient is essentially the same as for the nondiabetic patient.

NVG is a severe problem and sometimes occurs in eyes with severe DR or retinal detachments or occasionally after cataract surgery. NVG results from a proliferation of new vessels on the surface of the iris. These vessels usually are first observed at the pupillary border. As these new vessels progress, a fine network of vessels and fibrous tissue grows over the iris tissue and into the filtration angle of the eye. This fibrovascular growth results in peripheral anterior synechiae and closure of the filtration angle, resulting in NVG. In some cases, intraocular pressure may be elevated before angle involvement because of protein and cellular leakage from the proliferative vessels. Occasionally, iris neovascularization may be present in the filtration angle while not observed at the pupillary border.

NVG may be difficult to manage and generally requires aggressive treatment. Treatment modalities for NVI and NVG include scatter laser photocoagulation, intraocular anti-VEGF agents, topical antiglaucoma drugs, topical steroids, topical atropine, systemic antiglaucoma drugs, laser and glaucoma surgery, or a combination of these therapies. Early recognition and prompt retinal photocoagulation with or without pretreatment with an intravitreal anti-VEGF agent may help ameliorate this otherwise devastating condition.

EXAMINATION CRITERIA AND FREQUENCY

Current American Diabetes Association (ADA) recommendations for pediatric patients with T1D include the following: *1*) an initial dilated and comprehensive eye examination for the child at the start of puberty or at >10 years old, whichever is earlier, once the youth has had diabetes for 3–5 years; and *2*) after the initial examination, annual routine follow-up generally is recommended. Less frequent examinations may be acceptable on the advice of an eye care professional. ADA recommendations for adults include the following: *1*) for those with T1D, an initial dilated and comprehensive eye examination by an ophthalmologist or optometrist within 5 years after the onset of diabetes; *2*) for patients with T2D, an initial dilated and comprehensive eye examination by an ophthalmologist or optometrist shortly after the diagnosis of diabetes; and *3*) women with preexisting diabetes who are planning pregnancy or who have become pregnant should have a comprehensive eye examination and be counseled on the risk of development or progression of DR. Eye examination should occur in the first trimester with close follow-up throughout pregnancy and for 1 year postpartum.

If evidence of retinopathy is lacking for one or more eye exams, then exams every 2 years may be considered. If DR is present, subsequent examinations for patients with T1D and T2D should be repeated annually by an ophthalmologist or optometrist. If retinopathy is progressing or sight-threatening, then examinations will be required more frequently.

The 2014 ADA Standards of Medical Care (S45) state "high-quality fundus photographs can detect most clinically significant diabetic retinopathy. Interpretation of the images should be performed by a trained eye care provider, and while retinal photography may serve as a screening tool for retinopathy, it is not a substitute for a comprehensive eye exam, which should be performed at least initially and at intervals thereafter as recommended by an eye care professional."

Pregnancy, nephropathy, hypertension, hypercholesterolemia, anemia, and other medical conditions may dictate more frequent examination. The presence of DME or DR more advanced than mild NPDR indicates a need for more frequent examination. Table 41.3 outlines the examination schedule and guidelines for the care of patients with diabetes.

Table 41.3—Eye Examination Schedule

Age of diabetes onset (years)	Recommended time for first examination	Routine minimum follow-up*
0–29	3–5 years after onset†	Yearly
≥30 and older	At time of diagnosis	Yearly
During pregnancy	During first trimester	At discretion of the ophthalmologist but often each trimester and 6–8 weeks postpartum

Note:
*Abnormal findings dictate more frequent follow-up examinations.
†Once age ≥10 years, <3–5 years if in immediate postpubescent stage.

Source: Adapted from the American Diabetes Association clinical recommendations.

VISUAL AND PSYCHOSOCIAL REHABILITATION

All patients with diabetes should be advised that proven methods are in place to preserve vision. These methods include regular comprehensive eye and retinal examination; intensive control of blood glucose (as evaluated by glycosylated hemoglobin A1C levels); control of comorbidities such as hypertension, kidney disease, or dyslipidemia; and appropriate and timely laser surgery or other interventions when indicated for DME or DR. As a routine part of the health history, all patients with diabetes should be asked whether they have any visual symptoms (Table 41.1), such as any reduction in vision (either at a distance or near), fluctuation of vision, floating spots in field of view, flashing lights in field of view, any metamorphopsia or apparent warping of straight lines, eye redness or pain, or diplopia (double vision).

There are numerous etiologies for reduced vision—some benign and others requiring immediate treatment. In general, patients who report floating spots in their view, flashing lights, or the sensation of a curtain or veil crossing their vision should be referred for immediate ophthalmological attention because they may be experiencing symptoms of a VH, retinal detachment, or retinal hole. Patients with metamorphopsia or distorted vision may have significant macular edema or traction in the macular area and should be referred for prompt ophthalmological evaluation, preferably within 1 week.

Fluctuating vision is frequently the result of poor blood glucose control. Elevated blood glucose levels may lead to a myopic shift, enabling presbyopic individuals to read without their glasses, while their distance vision becomes blurred. For some people who never have worn glasses, distance vision may become blurred, and for those with hyperopia, glasses may no longer be needed for clear distance vision. Blurred vision may be the presenting symptom for a wide range of ocular conditions, such as macular edema and cataracts. In general, if the vision clears with a pinhole, the condition is most likely refractive and referral is less urgent.

Patients complaining of pain in or above the eye should be evaluated for possible neovascular or angle-closure glaucoma, especially if there is a loss of corneal reflex, irregularity in shape and response of the pupil, or acute redness of the eye. Also, a painful or red eye may reflect a corneal abrasion or corneal erosion. In most cases, patients with anterior-segment complaints should be examined promptly with a slit-lamp biomicroscope to rule out any form of glaucoma, foreign body, corneal abrasion, or iritis. Tonometry to measure intraocular pressure also is advisable. An emergency referral to an ophthalmologist may be critical in these cases.

Patients with new-onset double vision require neuro-ophthalmic and often neurological evaluation. Any patient who shows neovascularization of the optic nerve head or elsewhere in the retina or hard exudates or microaneurysms in the macula area should be referred promptly for complete ophthalmological evaluation. If proliferative retinopathy is present, immediate referral is warranted (Table 41.2).

For those patients who experience significant vision loss, referral for visual rehabilitation (low vision) is beneficial to help maximize visual function. A variety of handheld, stand, spectacle-borne, and electronic magnifiers are useful to assist distance and near vision. Nonoptical aids, such as large-print books, audio books, specially designed computer software, closed-circuit television, and other electronic aids allow a person to perform tasks otherwise prevented by reduced vision. Counseling and support groups may be beneficial for both patients and their families.

Although the DCCT and UKPDS demonstrated that intensive control of glycemic levels can delay the onset and slow the progression of DR, there is still no proven method to prevent DR. Consequently, current therapeutic strategies focus on addressing avenues to delay the onset and slow the progression of eye disease and ensure proper management of proliferative retinopathy and DME when these conditions are present. All patients should be informed of the potential ocular complications of diabetes and should be advised to have a regular comprehensive eye examination with pupil dilation and appropriate referral for management and treatment as indicated to preserve vision.

Patients with significant retinal disease or those who have lost vision from DR should be encouraged to continue with regular eye care. Vitrectomy surgery can restore useful vision for some individuals who have lost sight from VHs or FP with traction retinal detachment. Proper refraction, visual rehabilitation (low-vision evaluation), optical aids, and other techniques and devices are available to enable a person to use even severely limited vision. Referral to visual rehabilitation specialists may be appropriate. Support groups for the visually impaired and organizations providing vocational rehabilitation exist in most areas. All practitioners should be familiar with appropriate referral sources for their patients with visual impairment.

Unlike many other eye conditions, DR is not solely an eye problem but an end-organ response to a chronic systemic condition also affecting other organs (e.g., the heart and kidney). Multiple psychological and social issues also may be present. Health care providers should be aware of these issues and assist in their appropriate management. Close communication among all members of a patient's health care team is of paramount importance in dealing with the physical and psychological stresses of visual loss from diabetes.

CONCLUSION

Diabetes remains the leading cause of new-onset blindness in industrial countries. In its earliest stages, DR is asymptomatic. Visual acuity may be excellent and, on evaluation and diagnosis, a patient may deny the presence or significance of retinopathy. At this stage, the physician should initiate a careful program of education and follow-up. Early institution of routine lifelong follow-up; intensive systemic control of blood glucose, hypertension, and dyslipidemia; and timely therapeutic intervention when required are the hallmarks of appropriate diabetic eye care— and can prevent the majority of vision loss from diabetes.

BIBLIOGRAPHY

Aiello LM. Perspectives on diabetic retinopathy. *Am J Ophthalmol* 2003;136(1):122–135.

Aiello LM, Cavallerano J, Aiello LP. Diagnosis, management and treatment of nonproliferative diabetic retinopathy and macular edema. In *The Principles and Practices of Ophthalmology: The Harvard System*. Philadelphia, Saunders, 2000, p. 1900–1914.

Aiello LP, Cahill MT, Wong JS. Systemic considerations in the management of diabetic retinopathy. *Am J Ophthalmol* 2001;132:760–776.

Aiello LP, Gardner TW, King GL, Blankenship G, Cavallerano JD, Ferris FL III, Klein R. Diabetic retinopathy (technical review). *Diabetes Care* 1998;21:143–156.

American Diabetes Association. Retinopathy in diabetes (Position Statement). *Diabetes Care* 2004;27(Suppl 1):S84–S87.

Centers for Disease Control and Prevention. The prevention and treatment of complications of diabetes mellitus: a guide for primary care practitioners. *Prevention Guidelines* 1991;01:01. Available at http://wonder.cdc.gov/wonder/prevguid/p0000063/p0000063.asp. Accessed 28 March 2014.

Early Treatment Diabetic Retinopathy Study Research Group. Fundus photographic risk factors for progression of diabetic retinopathy: ETDRS report no. 12. *Ophthalmology* 1991;98:823–833.

Early Treatment Diabetic Retinopathy Study Research Group. Early photocoagulation for diabetic retinopathy: ETDRS report no. 9. *Ophthalmology* 1991;98:766–785.

Early Treatment Diabetic Retinopathy Study Research Group. Effects of aspirin treatment on diabetic retinopathy: ETDRS report no. 8. *Ophthalmology* 1991;98:757–765.

Early Treatment Diabetic Retinopathy Study Research Group. Photocoagulation for diabetic macular edema: ETDRS report no. 1. *Arch Ophthalmol* 1985;103:1796–1806.

Elman MJ, Aiello LP, Beck RW, Bressler NM, Bressler SB, Edwards AR, Ferris FL III, Friedman SM, Glassman AR, Miller KM, Scott IU, Stockdale CR, Sun JK. Randomized trial evaluating ranibizumab plus prompt or deferred laser or triamcinolone plus prompt laser for diabetic macular edema. *Ophthalmology* 2010;117:1064–1077.

Elman MJ, Bressler NM, Qin H, Beck RW, Ferris FL III, Friedman SM, Glassman AR, Scott IU, Stockdale CR, Sun JK. Expanded 2-year follow-up of ranibizumab plus prompt or deferred laser or triamcinolone plus prompt laser for diabetic macular edema. *Ophthalmology* 2011;118:609–614.

Elman MJ, Qin H, Aiello LP, Beck RW, Bressler NM, Ferris FL III, Glassman AR, Maturi RK, Melia M. Intravitreal ranibizumab for diabetic macular edema with prompt versus deferred laser treatment: three-year randomized trial results. *Ophthalmology* 2012;119:2312–2318.

Ferris FL III. Early photocoagulation in patients with either type I or type II diabetes. *Trans Am Ophthalmol Soc* 1996;94:505–537.

International Diabetes Federation. *IDF Diabetes Atlas.* 6th ed. Brussels, International Diabetes Federation, 2013.

Javitt JC, Aiello LP, Bassi LJ, Canner JK. Detecting and treating diabetic retinopathy: financial and visual savings associated with improved implementation of current guidelines. *Ophthalmology* 1990;98:1565–1574.

Klein R, Klein BEK, Moss SE, Davis MD, DeMets DL. The Wisconsin Epidemiologic Study of Diabetic Retinopathy. II. Prevalence and risk of diabetic retinopathy when age at diagnosis is less than 30 years. *Arch Ophthalmol* 1984;102:520–526.

Klein R, Klein BEK, Moss SE, Davis MD, DeMets DL. The Wisconsin Epidemiologic Study of Diabetic Retinopathy. III. Prevalence and risk of diabetic retinopathy when age at diagnosis is 30 or more years. *Arch Ophthalmol* 1984;102:527–532.

Ko F, Vitale S, Chou CF, Cotch MF, Saaddine J, Friedman DS. Prevalence of nonrefractive visual impairment in US adults and associated risk factors, 1999–2002 and 2005–2008. *JAMA* 2012;308:2361–2368.

U.K. Prospective Diabetes Study (UKPDS) Group. Intensive blood-glucose control with sulphonylureas or insulin compared with conventional treatment and risk of complications in patients with type 2 diabetes (UKPDS 33). *Lancet* 1998;352:837–853.

Yau JW, Rogers SL, Kawasaki R, Lamoureux EL, Kowalski JW, Bek T, Chen SJ, Dekker JM, Fletcher A, Grauslund J, Haffner S, Hamman RF, Ikram MK, Kayama T, Klein BE, Klein R, Krishnaiah S, Mayurasakorn K, O'Hare JP, Orchard TJ, Porta M, Rema M, Roy MS, Sharma T, Shaw J, Taylor H, Tielsch JM, Varma R, Wang JJ, Wang N, West S, Xu L, Yasuda M, Zhang X, Mitchell P, Wong TY. Global prevalence and major risk factors of diabetic retinopathy. *Diabetes Care* 2012;35:556–564.

Zhang X, Saaddine JB, Chou CF, Cotch MF, Cheng YJ, Geiss LS, Gregg EW, Albright AL, Klein BE, Klein R. Prevalence of diabetic retinopathy in the United States, 2005–2008. *JAMA* 2010;304:649–656.

Chapter 42

Management of Diabetic Retinopathy

Maxwell S. Stem, MD
Thomas W. Gardner, MD, MS
Grant M. Comer, MD, MS

INTRODUCTION

Diabetic retinopathy (DR) is a leading cause of vision loss in the Western world, and recent predictions suggest the number of people with DR will triple by 2050[1] in parallel with the rise in type 2 diabetes (T2D). The diagnosis and treatment of this complication requires tools not found in the offices of primary care physicians, but the combination of improved diabetes care and treatments for vision-threatening retinopathy have made DR the most treatable of the major diabetes complications.

Management strategies for DR have evolved tremendously since the ophthalmic manifestations of diabetes were first described by the Austrian ophthalmologist Eduard Jaeger in 1855. Systemic control of risk factors for retinopathy (e.g., hyperglycemia and hypertension) is currently the primary method for preventing the onset and slowing the progression of DR. Two eye-specific treatments for DR, laser photocoagulation and intraocular injections, have been successful at preventing blindness, but they are limited to advanced stages of DR when vision is already endangered or compromised. For example, panretinal photocoagulation (PRP) has been the mainstay of therapy for proliferative diabetic retinopathy (PDR) for five decades, but its main benefit lies in preserving existing vision rather than restoring lost vision. Diabetic macular edema (DME), another advanced form of DR, often is treated with focal argon laser photocoagulation to prevent further visual loss from retinal swelling. Recently, the introduction of intravitreal injections of antivascular endothelial growth factor (anti-VEGF) antibodies has advanced the therapy for DME by providing a specific pharmacotherapy and may be used for PDR treatment in the future. These agents work by inactivating the molecule largely responsible for disrupting the blood–retinal barrier and promoting diabetes-related neovascularization. Unlike intraocular corticosteroid injections, which also have been used to treat DME, anti-VEGF agents are not associated with the side effects of glaucoma and cataract.

Despite the success of PRP, focal laser, anti-VEGF antibodies, and intraocular steroids in preserving vision in people with advanced DR, a need remains for new therapies to treat early stages of DR and to prevent or ameliorate the progression of the disease. Current treatment of early DR emphasizes controlling systemic risk factors for retinopathy, such as hyperglycemia, hyperlipidemia, and hypertension. Efforts are under way, however, to develop local treatments for early stage DR that can be delivered noninvasively. Such therapies potentially could obviate

DOI: 10.2337/9781580405096.42

much of the need for the expensive and invasive treatments for advanced DR by preserving vision in people living with diabetes.

PROLIFERATIVE DIABETIC RETINOPATHY

Retinal neovascularization is the hallmark of PDR. As retinopathy progresses, the retinal tissue presumably becomes hypoxic and liberates angiogenic growth factors, such as VEGF, to restore retinal perfusion. Unfortunately, the newly formed blood vessels lack fully developed blood–retinal barrier properties and are prone to bleeding, fibrosis, and retinal membrane formation that can lead to blinding consequences, such as vitreous hemorrhage, tractional retinal detachment, and neovascular glaucoma.

PRP has been used to treat patients with PDR for more than five decades. During PRP, ophthalmologists create laser burns in the peripheral retina (Figure 42.1) to reduce the metabolic demand of the retina, which in turn reduces the stimulus for retinal neovascularization.

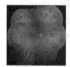

Figure 42.1—Fundus photograph of the right eye of a patient with regressed PDR who has undergone PRP. The dark spots in the retinal periphery correspond to areas of laser treatment.

PRP became the standard treatment for PDR after the Diabetic Retinopathy Study showed that PRP-treated eyes with advanced PDR had a 50% reduction in the risk of severe visual loss at 6 years relative to fellow nontreated eyes.[2] To determine the optimal time to administer PRP, the Early Treatment for Diabetic Retinopathy Study (ETDRS) randomized 3,711 patients with nonproliferative diabetic retinopathy (NPDR) and early PDR (without high-risk characteristics) to either prompt PRP or defer PRP until high-risk characteristics developed.[3] The investigators found that after 5 years of follow-up, severe vision loss was rare in both the early and deferred treatment groups (2.6% vs. 3.7%, respectively).[4] Because PRP can be associated with undesirable visual side effects, such as macular edema,[5] reduced peripheral vision,[4,6,7] prolonged dark adaptation,[8–10] and deficits in color vision,[11] it typically is reserved for patients with high-risk PDR. People with early PDR or severe to very severe NPDR, however, also may warrant PRP if they have neovascularization of the iris (rubeosis), a high degree of retinal ischemia and capillary nonperfusion, or retinal neovascularization.

Importantly, the level of glycemic control before, during, and after PRP can influence the success of treatment. In a study of 76 patients with T2D, the odds of having a satisfactory response to PRP was 72% greater in individuals with A1C values <8% relative to those with A1C values ≥8%.[12] This point shows the importance of maintaining optimal metabolic control throughout the course of diabetes.

Two primary complications of PDR include vitreous hemorrhage and tractional retinal detachment. In eyes with PDR, separation of the vitreous from the retina causes the fragile new blood vessels to bleed into the vitreous gel. Although blood located between the posterior face of the vitreous and the retina can be absorbed over weeks to months, blood in the vitreous may turn white over time and never resolve. In addition to causing preretinal bleeding, contraction of the vitreous in the setting of fibrovascular proliferation during PDR can lead to tractional retinal detachments. A detachment that involves the fovea or displaces the macula severely impairs visual acuity. In such cases, PRP alone is an insufficient treatment modality, so vitrectomy is required to relieve the tractional retinal detachment. Vitrectomy also can be used to remove nonclearing vitreous hemorrhage. During pars plana vitrectomy, surgeons enter the vitreous cavity through 20- to 25-gauge scleral incisions in the pars plana of the ciliary body. The vitreous gel is cut and aspirated, thus removing the blood and eliminating tractional forces on the retina.

The question of when to perform a vitrectomy in eyes with vitreous hemorrhage from advanced DR was partly answered by the Diabetic Retinopathy Vitrectomy Study, in which 616 eyes of patients with diabetes and new vitreous hemorrhage were assigned to either early vitrectomy (within 6 months of hemorrhage onset) or deferred vitrectomy for at least 1 year.[13] The percentage of eyes with 20/40 or better vision was consistently higher in the early vitrectomy group compared with the delayed group over the 4-year follow-up period (25% vs. 15%, respectively). Early vitrectomy appeared to be more beneficial in patients with type 1 diabetes (T1D) and severe PDR compared with those with T2D and less severe retinopathy. Improved instruments have enabled earlier, more rapid, and more successful vitrectomy over the past 10 years.

The current standard of care for nonclearing vitreous hemorrhage or tractional retinal detachment is a surgical vitrectomy. Some pharmaceutical agents, however, have shown promise in achieving enzymatic vitreolysis in cases of vitreous hemorrhage, thus obviating the need for anesthesia and the risks inherent to vitreoretinal surgery. For example, ocriplasmin recently received approval by the U.S. Food and Drug Administration (FDA) for treatment of idiopathic vitreomacular traction and related disorders, although its effectiveness in people with DR has not been evaluated. Alternatively, hyaluronidase injections have been evaluated in clearing vitreous hemorrhages in several randomized studies involving patients with diabetes[14] but have not gained regulatory approval.

Although PRP and vitrectomy have been instrumental in improving the visual prognosis for people with PDR, intravitreal anti-VEGF agents such as ranibizumab and bevacizumab have the potential to revolutionize the treatment of ocular neovascularization in diabetes. Bevacizumab is a full-length monoclonal antibody that binds to and inactivates all forms of the VEGF protein, and ranibizumab is a truncated (Fc) antibody that also recognizes all the VEGF isoforms.

Most prospective trials and case series that have examined the efficacy of intravitreal anti-VEGF agents for PDR have used the drugs as adjuncts to PRP or vitrectomy. For example, a randomized, prospective study evaluating the effects of PRP versus PRP and a single 0.5 mg ranibizumab injection found that treatment with combined PRP-ranibizumab reduced vascular leakage and protected against a decrease in visual acuity compared with the PRP-only group.[15] In a similarly designed trial comparing a single 1.25 mg bevacizumab injection and PRP to PRP alone, the combined-treatment group had a higher percentage of eyes with complete regression of neovascularization at 6 weeks (88% vs. 25%).[16] At 16 weeks follow-up, however, there was no difference in the proportion of eyes with complete regression between the groups because neovascularization frequently recurred once the bevacizumab presumably was cleared from the eye. Previtrectomy treatment with bevacizumab appears to reduce the rate of early postoperative recurrent vitreous hemorrhage[17] and may be associated with fewer intraoperative complications and better final visual acuity[18] compared with vitrectomy alone.

The Diabetic Retinopathy Clinical Research Network currently is evaluating the relative merits of ranibizumab versus PRP in people with PDR. The results of this and other similar studies could change the way that PDR is managed in the anti-VEGF era, but questions such as treatment frequency, duration, and long-term effects on retinal function need to be answered before anti-VEGF therapy becomes part of the standard management of PDR.

DIABETIC MACULAR EDEMA

DME is the principal cause of moderate vision loss (equivalent to difficulty with reading or driving) in patients with diabetes[19] and affects roughly 3% of adults with diabetes in the United States.[20] DME was defined in early clinical trials as the presence of retinal thickening or hard exudates within 1.5 mm of the center of the macula (Figure 42.2).[21]

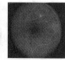

Figure 42.2—The left panel is a fundus photograph of the right eye of a patient with DME. The ring of lipid exudates is characteristic of focal DME emanating from central microaneurysms. The right panel is a late-phase fluorescein angiogram demonstrating the leaky microaneurysms as focal bright areas along a superior retinal vessel.

The ETDRS[21] demonstrated that focal laser treatment preserves visual acuity in eyes with clinically significant DME. Eyes that received prompt laser treatment were half as likely to lose three or more lines of vision after 3 years compared with eyes assigned to delayed treatment (12% vs. 24%, respectively). Thus, it appears that in the natural history of DME, if left untreated, roughly one-quarter of eyes will lose significant vision within 3 years.

Currently, intravitreal injections of pharmaceutical agents often are used as the primary treatment, or in addition to focal laser treatment, for DME. Intravitreal triamcinolone sometimes is used in patients with DME refractory to treatment with laser or in patients in whom laser is contraindicated. Intravitreal triamcinolone can be a viable option in patients with DME refractory to laser photocoagulation,[22] but its transient effect, need for repeated injections, and side effects of cataract and glaucoma preclude it from being a first-line treatment for patients with DME.

Unlike intraocular steroid injections, anti-VEGF agents are not associated with accelerated cataract formation or the development of glaucoma. Anti-VEGF agents such as ranibizumab and bevacizumab commonly are used in the treatment of DME, either alone or in combination with laser photocoagulation. The question of how to best combine focal laser with anti-VEGF injections to optimize visual acuity in patients with DME is a difficult one, but the results of a recent meta-analysis[23] may provide some potential answers. The authors of the meta-analysis evaluated four randomized clinic trials[24–27] comparing different permutations of ranibizumab and laser to laser alone. They concluded that ranibizumab, used alone or in combination with focal laser treatment, more effectively improves visual acuity and reduces central macular thickness after 1 and 2 years of follow-up compared with focal laser photocoagulation alone. In phase III studies in which focal laser was available to each study arm, monthly ranibizumab injections were superior to sham injections in improving visual acuity during DME.[28] Although other trials have similarly shown bevacizumab[29] to be efficacious in the treatment of DME, ranibizumab remains the only FDA-approved therapy for this condition. The major disadvantages of bevacizumab and ranibizumab are the need for monthly injections for a year or more, and the high cost of ranibizumab (~$2,000 per injection). Several outbreaks of infectious endophthalmitis after use of bevacizumab prepared in compounding pharmacies have curtailed the availability of this less expensive agent.

Despite the relative success of anti-VEGF agents in treating DME, a substantial proportion of patients (~50%)[25,27,28] will not experience a significant increase in visual acuity with ranibizumab. Thus, continued research is needed into the mechanisms underlying the pathogenesis of DME so that other targeted therapies can be developed for patients who do not respond to current treatments. Furthermore, questions such as how best to combine focal laser therapy with intravitreal VEGF injections will need to be addressed in future large clinical trials.

NONPROLIFERATIVE DIABETIC RETINOPATHY

NPDR refers to the presence of microaneurysms, hemorrhages, cotton wool spots, or DME, without neovascularization. No eye-specific treatments are yet available for patients with NPDR who do not have DME. As mentioned, however, PRP can be considered for people with severe to very severe NPDR who have a high likelihood of progressing to high-risk PDR. Currently, the treatment for patients with mild to moderate DR is directed solely at controlling systemic risk factors, such as hyperglycemia[30] and hypertension.[31] Dyslipidemia is a more controversial risk factor for DR, with some studies showing a reduced risk of DR development and progression with treatment[32,33] and others showing no difference despite treatment.[34]

Hypertension is clearly a risk factor for DR progression, but there is no consensus as to which antihypertensive agents may be able to delay DR progression independently of their effects on blood pressure. Angiotensin-converting enzyme (ACE) inhibitors or angiotensin-receptor blockers (ARB) showed promise in reducing DR development or progression in patients with T1D in one study[35] but not others[36,37] after adjusting for blood pressure and glycemic control. Thus, currently, there are no recommendations regarding specific antihypertensive therapy in patients with diabetes with regard to slowing the development or progression of DR.

Therapy aimed at reducing lipid levels in diabetes is vitally important to preventing cardiovascular disease, but the effects of lipid reduction on DR are less well established. One small study that randomized 50 patients with diabetes to simvastatin or placebo found that the placebo group had more patients with decreased visual acuity after 6 months.[32] Fenofibrate, which lowers triglyceride levels by promoting the activity of lipoprotein lipase, was shown in the Action to Control Cardiovascular Risk in Diabetes (ACCORD) Eye Study to reduce the progression of DR ~40% compared to placebo.[33] Nevertheless, fenofibrate is seldom prescribed for retinopathy, perhaps because it lacks a commercial sponsor.

Without question, primary and secondary prevention of DR starts with controlling systemic risk factors for retinopathy, such as hyperglycemia and hypertension. Eye-specific treatments for early NPDR are lacking, but patients with diabetes and mild retinopathy should receive annual eye examinations to monitor for signs of progressive retinopathy, even in the absence of symptoms. The recommended frequency of eye examinations for patients with T1D and T2D is outlined in Table 42.1.[38,39] Notably, women with pregestational diabetes who become pregnant appear to be at increased risk for DR progression relative to their nonpregnant peers. The mechanisms underlying this acceleration of retinal damage during pregnancy remain unclear but could be related to alterations in retinal blood flow. Risk factors for progression of DR during pregnancy are similar to those affecting nonpregnant patients and include hypertension and poor glycemic control.[40]

EMERGING THERAPIES FOR THE TREATMENT OF EARLY STAGE DR

Diabetes clearly has deleterious effects on the retinal vasculature, and accumulating evidence suggests that diabetes also damages the neural component of the retina.[41-44] Patients with diabetes and no or minimal clinical signs of DR may exhibit reduced neuroretinal thickness,[43] impaired color vision,[45] decreased contrast sensitivity,[46] abnormal dark adaptation,[47] and reduced visual field sensitivity[42] (Figure 42.3). Importantly, a large proportion of these patients display abnormalities by electrophysiological testing, and the dysfunctional retinal areas identified during these examinations are more likely to develop microaneurysms or

Table 42.1 Suggested Schedule for Dilated Fundus Exams in Patients with T1D or T2D

Diabetes type	Recommended time of first examination	Recommended follow-up
T1D	Age >10 years: Within 5 years of diabetes onset Age ≤10 years: 5 years from time of diagnosis or at age 10, whichever occurs later	No DR: Annually[38] or biennially[39] DR: At least yearly (or more frequently depending on severity of DR)
T2D	At time of diagnosis or very shortly thereafter	No DR: Annually[38] or biennially[39] DR: At least yearly (or more frequently depending on severity of DR)
Pregnancy (T1D or T2D)	Prior to conception and early in the first trimester	No DR to moderate NPDR: every 3–12 months Severe NPDR or worse: every 1–3 months

Note: Screening examinations should be performed by an eye care professional. DR = diabetic retinopathy; NPDR = nonproliferative diabetic retinopathy. Reprinted with permission from American Academy of Ophthalmology.[38]

hemorrhages.[48] Furthermore, the vasodilatory response to flickering light is reduced in early diabetes,[49] which suggests that the disease impairs neurovascular coupling in the retina. Taken together, these findings suggest that neuroretinal damage during diabetes may precede and perhaps even contribute to the development of the vascular lesions associated with DR.

Currently, the European Consortium of the Early Treatment of Diabetic Retinopathy is attempting to determine whether the neuroprotective agents brimonidine or somatostatin (administered topically) can slow or eliminate the neurodegenerative changes observed in early DR.[50] The primary endpoint being used in this study is the implicit time of the multifocal electroretinogram. Neuroprotective therapies, if shown to be successful at arresting neurodegeneration and

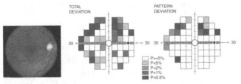

Figure 42.3—Fundus photograph and frequency-doubling technology perimetry visual field results from the right eye of a 28-year-old patient with T1D, visual acuity of 20/20, and minimal DR. The visual field results indicate moderate neuroretinal dysfunction that is not readily apparent on ophthalmoscopy.

visual dysfunction, have the potential to change the treatment of DR from a surgical to a neurobiological approach. Such treatments could obviate the need for more destructive treatments, such as laser photocoagulation, if fewer people develop the advanced stages of DR.

CONCLUSION

DR is a devastating complication of diabetes that progresses through relatively asymptomatic stages to severe levels that threaten vision. Current eye-specific treatments for DR are limited to the advanced stages of the condition. All patients with diabetes, however, should strive to achieve excellent control of blood glucose and blood pressure to minimize the development of complications. In most cases, patients with diabetes should be screened by an eye care professional yearly to assess for signs of vision-threatening retinopathy.

The recommended management strategies for PDR and DME continue to include laser photocoagulation, but anti-VEGF agents often are indicated for patients with diffuse DME or DME that lies in proximity to the central macula. Anti-VEGF injections are being explored as an alternative or adjunct to PRP for patients with PDR. Vitrectomy is used to manage the complications of PDR, such as vitreous hemorrhage and tractional retinal detachment.

Clearly, treatments for DR have progressed since the disease was first characterized in the mid-1800s. Nevertheless, eye-specific therapies are needed that can be delivered noninvasively to patients with early stage DR. Such treatments may involve neuroprotective strategies that, if proven effective, may greatly reduce the incidence of vision-threatening retinopathy among patients with diabetes.

REFERENCES

1. Saaddine JB, Honeycutt AA, Narayan KM, Zhang X, Klein R, Boyle JP. Projection of diabetic retinopathy and other major eye diseases among people with diabetes mellitus: United States, 2005-2050. *Arch Ophthalmol* 2008;126(12):1740–1747.

2. The Diabetic Retinopathy Study Research Group. Photocoagulation treatment of proliferative diabetic retinopathy. Clinical application of Diabetic Retinopathy Study (DRS) findings, DRS report number 8. *Ophthalmology* 1981;88(7):583–600.

3. Early Treatment Diabetic Retinopathy Study design and baseline patient characteristics. ETDRS report number 7. *Ophthalmology* 1991; 98(5Suppl):741–756.

4. Early Treatment Diabetic Retinopathy Study Research Group. Early photocoagulation for diabetic retinopathy. ETDRS report number 9. *Ophthalmology* 1991;98(5Suppl):766–785.

5. Soman M, Ganekal S, Nair U, Nair K. Effect of panretinal photocoagulation on macular morphology and thickness in eyes with proliferative diabetic retinopathy without clinically significant macular edema. *Clin Ophthalmol* 2012;6:2013–2017.

6. Doft BH, Blankenship GW. Single versus multiple treatment sessions of argon laser panretinal photocoagulation for proliferative diabetic retinopathy. *Ophthalmology* 1982;89(7):772–779.

7. Pahor D. Visual field loss after argon laser panretinal photocoagulation in diabetic retinopathy: full- versus mild-scatter coagulation. *Int Ophthalmol* 1998;22(5):313–319.

8. Seiberth V, Alexandridis E, Feng W. Function of the diabetic retina after panretinal argon laser coagulation. *Graefes Arch Clin Exp Ophthalmol* 1987;225(6):385–390.

9. Russell PW, Sekuler R, Fetkenhour C. Visual function after pan-retinal photocoagulation: a survey. *Diabetes Care* 1985;8(1):57–63.

10. Pender PM, Benson WE, Compton H, Cox GB. The effects of panretinal photocoagulation on dark adaptation in diabetics with proliferative retinopathy. *Ophthalmology* 1981;88(7):635–638.

11. Birch-Cox J. Defective colour vision in diabetic retinopathy before and after laser photocoagulation. *Mod Probl Ophthalmol* 1978;19:326–329.

12. Kotoula MG, Koukoulis GN, Zintzaras E, Karabatsas CH, Chatzoulis DZ. Metabolic control of diabetes is associated with an improved response of diabetic retinopathy to panretinal photocoagulation. *Diabetes Care* 2005;28(10):2454–2457.

13. Early vitrectomy for severe vitreous hemorrhage in diabetic retinopathy. Four-year results of a randomized trial: Diabetic Retinopathy Vitrectomy Study report 5. *Arch Ophthalmol* 1990;108(7):958–964.

14. Kuppermann BD, Thomas EL, de Smet MD, Grillone LR. Pooled efficacy results from two multinational randomized controlled clinical trials of a single intravitreous injection of highly purified ovine hyaluronidase (Vitrase) for the management of vitreous hemorrhage. *Am J Ophthalmol* 2005;140(4):573–584.

15. Filho JA, Messias A, Almeida FP, et al. Panretinal photocoagulation (PRP) versus PRP plus intravitreal ranibizumab for high-risk proliferative diabetic retinopathy. *Acta Ophthalmol* 2011;89(7):e567–572.

16. Mirshahi A, Roohipoor R, Lashay A, Mohammadi SF, Abdoallahi A, Faghihi H. Bevacizumab-augmented retinal laser photocoagulation in proliferative diabetic retinopathy: a randomized double-masked clinical trial. *Eur J Ophthalmol* 2008;18(2):263–269.

17. Smith JM, Steel DH. Anti-vascular endothelial growth factor for prevention of postoperative vitreous cavity haemorrhage after vitrectomy for proliferative diabetic retinopathy. *Cochrane Database Syst Rev* 2011(5):CD008214.

18. Zhao LQ, Zhu H, Zhao PQ, Hu YQ. A systematic review and meta-analysis of clinical outcomes of vitrectomy with or without intravitreal bevacizumab pretreatment for severe diabetic retinopathy. *Br J Ophthalmol* 2011; 95(9):1216–1222.

19. Ding J, Wong TY. Current epidemiology of diabetic retinopathy and diabetic macular edema. *Curr Diab Rep* 2012;12(4):346–354.

20. Zhang X, Saaddine JB, Chou CF, et al. Prevalence of diabetic retinopathy in the United States, 2005-2008. *JAMA* 2010;304(6):649–656.

21. Early Treatment Diabetic Retinopathy Study Research Group. Photocoagulation for diabetic macular edema. Early Treatment Diabetic Retinopathy Study report number 1. *Arch Ophthalmol* 1985;103(12):1796–1806.

22. Gillies MC, Sutter FK, Simpson JM, Larsson J, Ali H, Zhu M. Intravitreal triamcinolone for refractory diabetic macular edema: two-year results of a double-masked, placebo-controlled, randomized clinical trial. *Ophthalmology* 2006;113(9):1533–1538.

23. Wang H, Sun X, Liu K, Xu X. Intravitreal ranibizumab (lucentis) for the treatment of diabetic macular edema: a systematic review and meta-analysis of randomized clinical control trials. *Curr Eye Res* 2012;37(8):661–670.

24. Massin P, Bandello F, Garweg JG, et al. Safety and efficacy of ranibizumab in diabetic macular edema (RESOLVE Study): a 12-month, randomized, controlled, double-masked, multicenter phase II study. *Diabetes Care* 2010;33(11):2399–2405.

25. Mitchell P, Bandello F, Schmidt-Erfurth U, et al. The RESTORE Study: ranibizumab monotherapy or combined with laser versus laser monotherapy for diabetic macular edema. *Ophthalmology* 2011;118(4):615–625.

26. Elman MJ, Aiello LP, Beck RW, et al. Randomized trial evaluating ranibizumab plus prompt or deferred laser or triamcinolone plus prompt laser for diabetic macular edema. *Ophthalmology* 2010;117(6):1064–1077, e1035.

27. Nguyen QD, Shah SM, Khwaja AA, et al. Two-year outcomes of the Ranibizumab for Edema of the Macula in Diabetes (READ-2) study. *Ophthalmology* 2010;117(11):2146–2151.

28. Nguyen QD, Brown DM, Marcus DM, et al. Ranibizumab for diabetic macular edema: Results from 2 phase III randomized trials: RISE and RIDE. *Ophthalmology* 2012;119(4):789–801.

29. Rajendram R, Fraser-Bell S, Kaines A, et al. A 2-year prospective randomized controlled trial of intravitreal bevacizumab or laser therapy (BOLT) in the management of diabetic macular edema: 24-month data: report 3. *Arch Ophthalmol* 2012;130(8):972–979.

30. The Diabetes Control and Complications Trial Research Group. The effect of intensive treatment of diabetes on the development and progression of long-term complications in insulin-dependent diabetes mellitus. *N Engl J Med* 1993;329(14):977–986.

31. U.K. Prospective Diabetes Study Group. Tight blood pressure control and risk of macrovascular and microvascular complications in type 2 diabetes: UKPDS 38. *BMJ* 1998;317(7160):703–713.

32. Sen K, Misra A, Kumar A, Pandey RM. Simvastatin retards progression of retinopathy in diabetic patients with hypercholesterolemia. *Diabetes Res Clin Pract* 2002;56(1):1–11.

33. Chew EY, Ambrosius WT, Davis MD, et al. Effects of medical therapies on retinopathy progression in type 2 diabetes. *N Engl J Med* 2010;363(3):233–244.

34. Colhoun HM, Betteridge DJ, Durrington PN, et al. Primary prevention of cardiovascular disease with atorvastatin in type 2 diabetes in the Collaborative Atorvastatin Diabetes Study (CARDS): multicentre randomised placebo-controlled trial. *Lancet* 2004;364(9435):685–696.

35. Mauer M, Zinman B, Gardiner R, et al. Renal and retinal effects of enalapril and losartan in type 1 diabetes. *N Engl J Med* 2009;361(1):40–51.

36. Chaturvedi N, Sjolie AK, Stephenson JM, et al. Effect of lisinopril on progression of retinopathy in normotensive people with type 1 diabetes. The EUCLID Study Group. EURODIAB Controlled Trial of Lisinopril in Insulin-Dependent Diabetes Mellitus. *Lancet* 1998;351(9095):28–31.

37. Chaturvedi N, Porta M, Klein R, et al. Effect of candesartan on prevention (DIRECT-Prevent 1) and progression (DIRECT-Protect 1) of retinopathy in type 1 diabetes: randomised, placebo-controlled trials. *Lancet* 2008;372(9647):1394–1402.

38. American Academy of Ophthalmology Retina Panel. *Preferred Practice Pattern Guidelines. Diabetic Retinopathy*. San Francisco, American Academy of Ophthalmology, 2008. Available at: www.aao.org/ppp.

39. American Diabetes Association. Standards of medical care in diabetes—2014. *Diabetes Care* 2014;37(Suppl 1):S14–S80.

40. Sheth BP. Does pregnancy accelerate the rate of progression of diabetic retinopathy? An update. *Curr Diab Rep* 2008;8(4):270–273.

41. Barber AJ, Lieth E, Khin SA, Antonetti DA, Buchanan AG, Gardner TW. Neural apoptosis in the retina during experimental and human diabetes. Early onset and effect of insulin. *J Clin Invest* 1998;102(4):783–791.

42. Parravano M, Oddone F, Mineo D, et al. The role of Humphrey Matrix testing in the early diagnosis of retinopathy in type 1 diabetes. *Br J Ophthalmol* 2008;92(12):1656–1660.

43. van Dijk HW, Verbraak FD, Kok PH, et al. Decreased retinal ganglion cell layer thickness in patients with type 1 diabetes. *Invest Ophth Vis Sci* 2010;51(7):3660–3665.

44. Jackson GR, Scott IU, Quillen DA, Walter LE, Gardner TW. Inner retinal visual dysfunction is a sensitive marker of non-proliferative diabetic retinopathy. *Br J Ophthalmol* 2012;96(5):699–703

45. Hardy KJ, Lipton J, Scase MO, Foster DH, Scarpello JH. Detection of colour vision abnormalities in uncomplicated type 1 diabetic patients with angiographically normal retinas. *Br J Ophthalmol* 1992;76(8):461–464.

46. Di Leo MA, Caputo S, Falsini B, et al. Nonselective loss of contrast sensitivity in visual system testing in early type I diabetes. *Diabetes Care* 1992;15(5):620–625.

47. Henson DB, North RV. Dark adaptation in diabetes mellitus. *Br J Ophthalmol* 1979;63(8):539–541.

48. Harrison WW, Bearse MA Jr, Ng JS, et al. Multifocal electroretinograms predict onset of diabetic retinopathy in adult patients with diabetes. *Invest Ophthalmol Vis Sci* 2011;52(2):772–777.

49. Garhofer G, Zawinka C, Resch H, Kothy P, Schmetterer L, Dorner GT. Reduced response of retinal vessel diameters to flicker stimulation in patients with diabetes. *Br J Ophthalmol* 2004;88(7):887–891.

50. Cunha-Vaz J. Neurodegeneration as an early event in the pathogenesis of diabetic retinopathy: a multicentric, prospective, phase II-III, randomised controlled trial to assess the efficacy of neuroprotective drugs administered topically to prevent or arrest diabetic retinopathy. EUROCONDOR–EU FP7 Project. *Acta Ophthalmol* 2012;90(Suppl 249):0. doi: 10.1111/1755-3768.2012.2825.x

Chapter 43

Chronic Kidney Disease Complicating Diabetes

MARY C. MALLAPPALLIL, MD
ELI A. FRIEDMAN, MD, MACP, FRCP

INTRODUCTION

Continuously, over the past half-century, the increasing global pandemic of kidney failure attributed to diabetes mellitus has provoked anxiety and continual reassessment of treatment strategies in the belief that micro- and macrovascular complications of diabetes are preventable. Drug regimens for metabolic and blood pressure (BP) regulation have been revised and sometimes reversed due to inferences from prospective, controlled, properly populated trials. Illustrating this trend is the current "less stringent" target for glycosylated hemoglobin (A1C) of <8% in selected individual patients, especially with advanced age or "a history of hypoglycemia or other adverse effects of treatment,"[1] because of an observed greater rate of cardiovascular complications noted when striving to reduce attained A1C to the prior target of ≤6.5%. Our concept of the natural history of kidney disease in diabetes has repeatedly been modified,[2] in large part due to a rising median age of those who develop end-stage renal disease (ESRD) to 64 years,[3] underscoring the reality that the majority of diabetic ESRD patients now fall within the geriatric age-group. An encouraging finding, first reported in 2005, and continuing through 2010, is a declining incidence rate of irreversible advanced kidney failure in individuals known to have diabetes. Although not yet evidence based, there is a belief that this "good news" is the product of properly utilized renoprotective management throughout the course of chronic kidney disease (CKD) in those with diabetes,[4] as advocated in this chapter.

CHRONIC KIDNEY DISEASE AND ITS STAGES AS APPLIED TO DIABETES

CKD's definition and staging were introduced by the National Kidney Foundation (NKF) to signify the presence of kidney damage noted by urinary abnormalities or decreased kidney function with a low glomerular filtration rate (GFR), either of which has to be present for at least 3 months irrespective of cause.[5] Kidney injury is signaled by markers of pathology, such as proteinuria, or morphologic evidence of disease evidenced by findings on radiographic or sonographic imaging or a history of kidney transplantation. CKD staging was proposed in the NKF Outcomes Quality Initiative (KDOQI) in 2002 (stages 1–5), modified by the Kidney Disease Improving Global Outcomes (KDIGO) in 2004 and fur-

 DOI: 10.2337/9781580405096.43

ther updated to include the cause of disease when known, six categories of residual GFR, and three categories of proteinuria.[5,6]

Currently, an estimated GFR (eGFR) may be calculated based on the Modification of Diet in Renal Disease (MDRD) equation, and most laboratories now commonly report eGFR along with the serum creatinine level to recognize the presence of CKD, which otherwise might be overlooked.[7] Over the past few years, due to an increasing awareness of CKD prevalence, concerns regarding its diagnoses and significance have increased. The CKD-Epidemiology Collaboration Equation (CKD-EPI), based on the same four components (age, gender, serum creatinine, and race) as the MDRD equation, reclassified 24% of patients to less severe CKD classifications.[8] Ohsawa et al. found that using the estimated CKD-EPI equation to reclassify 24,000 Japanese patients with early CKD stages 1 to 3B enabled a better prediction of mortality than did the use of the eGFR (MDRD) equation.[9] Despite this report, current staging of CKD continues to be based most commonly on eGFR (MDRD).

The premise underlying complex CKD staging is the hope that inclusion of cause, development, and extent of lost renal function will stimulate patient awareness and preparation for impending irreversible renal failure, while prompting testing of strategies that might delay CKD progression, thereby improving outcomes.[10] For example, in CKD resulting from diabetes, staging would include GFR categories and quantification of proteinuria that reflect both current kidney function and extent of pathologic damage, respectively. Stages included are based on GFR: G1 (normal GFR >90 ml/minute), G2 (mildly decreased GFR at 60–89 ml/minute), G3A (mild to moderately decreased GFR, 45–59 ml/minute), G3B (moderately to severely decreased, 30–44 ml/minute), G4 (GFR of 15–29 ml/minute), and G5 (kidney failure with GFR <15 ml/minute). The addition of G5D would signify current reliance on supportive dialysis therapies. Besides this classification of GFR, substages quantifying albuminuria also have been added: A1 is normal to mildly increased albuminuria (<30 mg albumin/g creatinine), A2 moderately increased (30–300 mg albumin/g creatinine), and A3 severely increased (>300 mg albumin/g creatinine). The term "microalbuminuria," which, in the past, was defined as a 24-hour urinary albumin excretion rate of 20–200 µg/minute (30–300 mg/24 hour), has been dropped because of the evident confusion it caused (see Table 43.1).

The reasoning underlying staging of CKD is that its progression will benefit recognition of the risk of complications that might be prevented by altering prescribed medications or other management components. Timing of patient preparation for consideration of renal replacement therapy is contingent on correct evaluation of present renal function along with an estimated rate of its subsequent decline. Critics of reliance on CKD staging argue that it cannot be applied to predict prognosis nor does it accurately determine present severity of CKD.

EPIDEMIOLOGY

In 2011, at the United Nations (UN) summit on chronic diseases, the World Health Organization (WHO) added CKD to its list of major chronic diseases that are a primary threat to public health. The other conditions on the list that account for a majority of worldwide deaths include diabetes, cardiovascular disease (CVD),

Table 43.1 Chronic Kidney Disease Stages in Diabetes Based on Estimated Glomerular Filtration Rate and Proteinuria

Stages	eGFR (based on serum creatinine concentration)
G1	>90 ml/minute
G2	60–89 ml/minute
G3A	45–59 ml/minute
G3B	30–44 ml/minute
G4	15–29 ml/minute
G5	<15 ml/minute
G5D	<15 ml/minute on dialysis

Albuminuria	Quantification of albuminuria.
A1	<30 mg albumin/g creatinine
A2	30–300 mg albumin/g creatinine
A3	>300 mg albumin/g creatinine

Source: Modified from Kidney Disease: Improving Global Outcomes (KDIGO). Summary of recommendation statements. *Kidney Int* 2013;3(Suppl 5):1–150.
Note: eGFR = estimated glomerular filtration rate.
ADA 2013 guidelines suggest referral to a nephrologist early when the diagnosis of diabetic nephropathy is in doubt, at any stage when there is difficulty managing the complication of CKD, or later in CKD4 for preparation for renal replacement therapy.

chronic lung disease, and cancer. According to the WHO, "Renal, oral and eye diseases pose a major health burden for many countries and…these diseases share common risk factors and can benefit from common responses to non-communicable diseases."[11] This was the first time the importance of kidney disease was acknowledged in UN or WHO plans to address the growing burden of noncommunicable diseases (NCD).[11]

The U.S. Renal Data System (USRDS) reports the prevalence of diabetic nephropathy in the general U.S. adult population based on the National Health and Nutrition Examination Survey (NHANES). The NHANES reports on eGFR or albuminuria using either the CKD-EPI equation for an eGFR <60 ml/minute/1.73 m^2 or a urine albumin-creatinine ratio (ACR) of ≥30 mg/gram. When defined by eGFR, the prevalence of CKD in 2005–2010 was 6.3%, compared with 9.3 and 8.5% for diabetes and CVD, respectively. If kidney disease is defined, however, by ACR, the prevalence of CKD rises to 9.2%. The USRDS 2012 Annual Data Report (ADR), which looked at 2010 data, stated that 13.1% had CKD, defined by an eGFR <60 ml/minute/1.73 m^2 or an ACR of 30 mg/gram or higher.[3] The most recent Centers for Disease Control and Prevention report based on NHANES data states that 26 million Americans have CKD.[12]

Data sets from NHANES report that among the prevalent CKD population, 40.1% had diabetes in the 2005–2010 period, which is a slight decrease from 43.1% reported over the 1988–1994 period.[3] Since 2000, the rate of new CKD5D cases caused by diabetes has been stable, reaching 152 per million in the general population in 2010. In comparison, the rate of CKD5D due to hypertension is 7.7% higher than it was in 2000, at 99 per million individuals, and the rate of CKD5D due to glomerulonephritis has fallen 27%, to 22.7 per million individuals. Among non-Hispanic whites between 30 and 39 years old, the incident rate has fallen just 1% since 2000, and in 2010, was 35.4 per million individuals. For African Americans of the same age, the rate has increased 69% since 2000, to reach 133.8. Rates among Asians, although low, has doubled among those 30–39 years old since 2000, reaching 32.6 per million individuals in 2010. In the U.S., CKD expenditure was $41 billion from Medicare, which accounted for 17% of total Medicare expenditure and CKD with diabetes accounted for 27% of Medicare expenditure or ~$81.4 billion.[3]

CURRENT THINKING IN PATHOPHYSIOLOGY OF DIABETIC NEPHROPATHY

In the kidney, hyperfiltration is noted with an increase in eGFR when the eGFR exceeds normal, and this occurs early in the course of both type 1 diabetes (T1D) and type 2 diabetes (T2D).[13,14] The connection between glycemic control and hyperfiltration was shown in a study of Pima Indians using iothalamate clearance. Hyperfiltration was noted to be increasingly greater with the presence of impaired glucose tolerance, newly diagnosed T2D, and in patients who had diabetes for 5 years and those with diabetes and overt proteinuria.[15] There was subsequent progression at 4 years in hyperfiltration in the groups. The group with overt proteinuria also was noted to have a decrease in GFR by ~35%, signaling the start of decline of renal function. The hypothesis for progressive loss of kidney function includes glomerular hypertension, which increases GFR and glomerular hypertrophy, which subsequently places shear stress on the glomerulus leading to nephropathy with glomerulosclerosis or ischemic injury from hyaline narrowing of the vessels that supply the glomeruli.[15] It now is reported that this sequential progression may not occur and that nephropathy may be present even without significant proteinuria. Several mechanisms seem to be involved in the development of diabetic nephropathy, and there is an interaction between these risk factors that can worsen progression of the disease.

Renin angiotensin blockade has a role in reducing the effect of glomerular hyperfiltration and glomerular hypertension. In addition, angiotensin II has profibrotic effects that can lead to sclerosis, which can decrease with the use of angiotensin-converting-enzyme (ACE) inhibitors or angiotensin-receptor blockers (ARBs).[16,17]

Hyperglycemia and advanced glycosylated end products (AGEs) may induce mesangial expansion and injury by increasing glycation of matrix proteins and mesangial cell apoptosis.[18] In the setting of hyperglycemia, other mechanisms that have been postulated include increased prorenin activity that binds to mitogen-activated protein kinase (MAPK). The significance for the role of prorenin has been suggested in the streptozotocin diabetic mouse model, in which blockage of the prorenin receptor decreased MAPK activation and prevented the development of diabetic nephropathy despite high angiotensin II activity.[19] Other suggested pathophysiologic roles for diabetic nephropathy include proinflammatory cytokines like vascular endothelial growth factor, protein kinase C, and transforming growth factor β.

The role of nephrin also may be impaired in diabetic nephropathy.[20] Nephrin is a transmembrane protein expressed by podocytes, with deficiencies noted in some congenital diseases that result in severe congenital nephrotic syndrome of the Finnish type. In vitro studies on human-cultured podocytes demonstrated that glycated albumin and angiotensin II reduced nephrin expression. Glycated albumin inhibited nephrin synthesis through the engagement of a receptor for AGEs, whereas angiotensin II acted on cytoskeleton redistribution, inducing the shedding of nephrin. This study suggested that the alteration in nephrin expression may be an early event in proteinuric patients with diabetes and suggests that glycated albumin and angiotensin II contribute to nephrin downregulation.[21]

OTHER RISK FACTORS IN PATHOPHYSIOLOGY

Genetic risk is an important factor in both the presence and severity of diabetic nephropathy, and those with diabetes who have a first-degree relative with diabetic nephropathy have a higher likelihood of developing diabetic nephropathy themselves, which has been noted in both subjects with T1D and T2D.[22,23]

In T2D, the ACE gene DD polymorphism may increase the risk of developing diabetic nephropathy, more severe proteinuria, a greater likelihood of progressive renal failure, and greater mortality on dialysis.[24,25] No such association has been defined in T1D. An additional genetic factor that contributes to risk is race. Being African American in comparison with non-Hispanic white increases the risk of developing diabetic nephropathy three- to sixfold.[26,27]

In diabetes, renal autoregulation is impaired, resulting in the transmission of the elevated systemic BP to the glomerulus.[28] Progression of kidney disease in the setting of hypertension and T2D in African American patients was implied in a study of 194 African American patients with T2D who developed hypertension after their diagnosis of diabetes. These patients (17 of 20 [85%]), were likely to have evidence of nephropathy as compared with subjects whose hypertension was diagnosed before or simultaneously diagnosed with their diabetes (7 of 13 [54%]).[29] Additionally obesity and smoking have been shown to contribute to proteinuria.[30,31]

CURRENT DEBATE AS TO WHETHER CKD STAGES MAY REVERT

Previous assumptions that persistent proteinuria leads to increasing quantities of albuminuria and subsequent decrease in GFR in T1D have been challenged after studies documented its reversion to normal proteinuria—even lacking specific treatment with an ACE inhibitor.[32] Further confirmation of the unpredictable course of microalbuminuria derives from analysis of the Diabetes Control and Complications Trial (DCCT) Epidemiology of Diabetes Intervention and Complication study.[33] Surprisingly, it is now clear that severe loss of GFR may occur without any increase in the amount of proteinuria, as previously had been detailed as a component of the course of progressive diabetic nephropathy.[34] Because renal lesions in T2D are more heterogeneous than in T1D and timed protocol biopsies are not performed during progression of kidney disease in T2D, correlation of renal histopathology with the extent of proteinuria is less predictable. Lowering proteinuria in T2D, however, may be predictive of renal outcomes and until more accurate markers of renal functional deterioration in diabetic nephropathy are validated, the urinary ACR remains the defining standard for assigning severity.[35]

That effective drug therapy might retard progression of renal disease in diabetes was a major finding in the 1993 Captopril Collaborative Study. It demonstrated an 11% decline in GFR per year in patients with T1D who were treated with an ACE inhibitor as compared with 17% per year in those untreated with an ACE inhibitor.[36] Similar benefit was noted in patients with T2D in whom the rate of decline of GFR without renin-angiotensin-system (RAS) blockade was ~6 ml/minute versus 4 ml/minute per year with ACE inhibitor treatment.[37,38] A long-term benefit of an ACE inhibitor was inferred from a study in which 6 out of 40 patients with T1D maintained on the ACE inhibitor captopril for 7.7 years had clinical remission to non–nephrotic-range proteinuria <1 gram/day and with a stable plasma creatinine. In addition, Hovind et al. reported a graded effect in BP control among patients with T1D who were treated with captopril in which the cohort attaining a lower mean arterial pressure of 113 mmHg had remission and regression rates of 17 and 7% compared with those who had a mean arterial pressure of 93 mmHg with regression rates of 58 and 42%, respectively.[39]

REFERRAL TO A NEPHROLOGIST AND THE RELATION BETWEEN FAMILY PHYSICIAN, ENDOCRINOLOGIST, NEPHROLOGIST, AND GERIATRICIAN

Initial referral of a patient with diabetes to a nephrologist is advisable when urinary protein excretion exceeds 1 gram/day, because other causes of proteinuria need to be identified and the potential benefit of a percutaneous kidney biopsy must be weighed. For example, in a patient with diabetes and proteinuria with kidney disease, a percutaneous kidney biopsy may lead to a diagnosis other than diabetic nephropathy in a significant percentage. As noted by Christenson et al., of 347 patients with T2D and albuminuria without diabetic retinopathy, kidney biopsies revealed normal glomerular structure or nondiabetic kidney diseases in 30%.[40]

The question of when a kidney biopsy is appropriate to gain a specific diagnosis depends on atypical findings not frequently seen in diabetic nephropathy, including but not limited to the absence of retinopathy, presence of gross hematuria, or pyuria.

In CKD patients, factors that contributed to late referrals were combinations of patient and health system characteristics, including being older, belonging to a racial minority group, being less educated, being uninsured, or suffering from multiple comorbidities, and importantly, the lack of communication between primary care physicians and nephrologists. A major inference of the large Dialysis Outcomes and Practice Patterns Study (DOPPS) was that both primary care physicians and nephrologists need to engage in collaborative efforts to ensure patient education and enhance physician awareness to improve kidney patient care.[41]

Patients with CKD and diabetes are most effectively followed by a team, including physicians of various specialties, for effective care. Appropriate early referral decreases overall health care costs and mortality.[42] KDOQI 2006 guidelines proposed early referral to a nephrologist. At initial diagnosis, care must be taken to ensure that the patient does not have a rapidly progressive condition with accelerated GFR loss. Once a patient with diabetes is noted to have stable CKD, the frequency of follow-up visits to a nephrologist is based on the stage of CKD. Those in CKD stage 2 (GFR 60–90 ml/minute) are unlikely to have other coexisting conditions, such as secondary hyperparathyroidism or anemia and can be followed annually to monitor progression of disease. Protective therapy (renoprotection) is most effective if started early before eGFR declines to <60 ml/minute/1.73m^2. Those with CKD stage 3A (eGFR of 45–60 ml/minute) can be seen every 6–12 months, while those in stage 3B (eGFR 30–45 ml/minute), who are more likely to progress, need to be seen at a minimum of every 6 months. In CKD stage 4, with a GFR of 15–30 ml/minute, several decisions have to be made, including timing for vascular access placement if maintenance hemodialysis (HD) is planned, which needs a minimum of 3–6 months to mature. Optimally, a vascular access should be placed in time to be ready for initiation of dialysis (see Table 43.2).

Table 43.2 Stage-Specific Problems and Management

Stages	Problems to be addressed
G1–G2	Determine diagnosis based on findings and if needed refer to nephrologist for kidney biopsy. With a normal eGFR and abnormal findings on urinalysis or incidental findings on imaging, further evaluation may be needed. In hypertensive patients, angiotensin blockade is most effective starting early.
G2	Address the possible need for further work-up or monitoring to determine whether decreased renal function is acute and will resolve or is likely to progress to CKD. Etiology and need for renal biopsy are considered. At this stage, comorbidities of anemia and secondary hyperparathyroidism are absent.
G3A	Determine initiation of anemia treatment, including supplemental iron and erythropoiesis-stimulating agents (ESA) to minimize blood transfusion and unnecessary antigen exposure from avoidable blood transfusions, which could compromise a successful future kidney transplant.
G3B	Weigh value of sodium bicarbonate and diuretics if acidosis and hypertension or volume overload may be present.
G4	Preparation for renal replacement therapy options, including family discussion. Vein mapping and access placement if hemodialysis selected. Social workers' assessment of home suitability for home hemodialysis. Peritoneal dialysis arrangements, including preparing home and caregiver selection. Once eGFR has decreased <20 ml/minute, referral to a transplant center for listing for deceased donor transplantation. Potential live donor assessment is also appropriate in this phase.
G5	May be seen every 1–2 months; decide when to start renal replacement therapy based on patient status and wishes.

Note: CKD = chronic kidney disease; eGFR = estimated glomerular filtration rate. Stages may be accelerated by episodic acute kidney injury (AKI) induced by infection, periods of poor diabetes control, or hospitalization. Reassessment of renal function is needed after all adverse events.

Other decisions include exploring the important option of preemptive kidney transplantation from a living donor. As shown by Wolfe in a landmark study, every patient with advanced CKD and diabetes who does not have absolute contraindication for kidney transplantation should be evaluated, as it is the optimal renal replacement therapy, improving the quality and length of life in people with diabetes with CKD; recipients of a kidney transplant had better long-term survival than those on the deceased donor kidney waiting list, and people with diabetes and younger patients gained the greatest survival benefits.[43] Major lifestyle changes require that patient, family, nephrologist, primary care physician or geriatrician, and endocrinologist work collaboratively. Once renal function in a diabetic CKD patient declines to a GFR of 20 ml/minute, many transplant centers will list the patient for a deceased donor kidney transplant. For patients with a potential live kidney donor, the evaluation is deferred to the time that dialysis would be initiated. Dialysis generally is initiated when GFR declines <15 ml/minute unless the patient becomes symptomatic sooner.[44]

Importantly, CKD stage deterioration may be accelerated with intermittent episodes of acute kidney injury (AKI), which often is seen after bouts of infection, periods of poor diabetes control, or hospitalization, and assessment of kidney function needs to be done after such events. KDIGO 2013 guidelines suggest that all patients with CKD be considered at risk of AKI because of observational data that suggest a strong association between preexisting CKD and AKI.[3]

Late referral to a nephrologist, before CKD5D, continues to be a concern. Despite the introduction of "new" medical evidence forms by Medicare in 2005 that asked about pre-ESRD care, little progress has been made to improve this deficiency. As an example, 43% of new ESRD patients in 2010 had not seen a nephrologist before beginning dialysis therapy. Further to the point, of those initiating HD, 88% were begun on HD via a catheter, compared with 54% of those who had received ≥1 year of nephrology care. Among those with ≥1 year of pre-ESRD nephrologist care, 26% began therapy with an arterio-venous fistula (AVF) (the preferred access for HD patients), a rate eight times higher than that among nonreferred patients.[3]

WHEN SHOULD THERAPY FOR AZOTEMIA IN DIABETES BE INITIATED?

In general, there is no absolute GFR value at which dialysis therapies need to be started. It is a joint decision by nephrologist and patient, based on subjective and objective clinical evidence and prevalent Medicare guidelines. Patients with diabetes in CKD5 usually are started on dialysis when the eGFR declines to 15 ml/minute or higher if symptomatic. For example, uremic pericarditis would be an indication to start dialysis even at higher eGFR. Urgent indications to start dialysis therapies in CKD include uremic encephalopathy, bleeding diathesis, and medically resistant disturbances like uncontrolled hypertension, hyperkalemia, fluid overload, and acidosis. Dialysis should be started before the patient becomes malnourished and starts to lose weight, which is a sign of uremia.

Comparisons of eGFR at the initiation of ESRD therapy indicate that patients are now starting treatment earlier than in the past. In 2010, 29% initiated treatment with an eGFR of 10–15 ml/minute/1.73 m², compared with 17.7% in 2000.

In 2010, 16% began with an eGFR of ≥15 ml/minute/1.73 m², in contrast to 7.4% in 2000.[21]

Kidney transplantation is the preferred option of renal replacement therapy in eligible diabetic nephropathy patients with ESRD as it yields much higher survival than either HD or peritoneal dialysis (PD). Advances in kidney transplantation have improved both kidney and patient survival. Moving from an era when corticosteroids, azathioprine, and the calcineurin inhibitors were among the few immunosuppressive choices available, new options such as monoclonal antibodies, antilymphocyte antibodies, rapamycin, and mycophenolate are approved for general use. Preemptive transplantation, in which patients who are in CKD5 but not yet on dialysis may directly receive a kidney transplant instead of first proceeding with dialysis, has been shown to reduce mortality.[45] Although the debate as to whether this reduction in mortality is due to the use of live versus deceased kidney donors continues, the reality is that few patients will get a preemptive deceased donor kidney transplantation, because of long wait times that exceed 8 years in some regions such as New York City. Other advances that improved transplant outcome include laparoscopic kidney retrieval from a live donor, which decreases morbidity for the donor with fewer hospital days, fewer lost workdays, and a smaller surgical scar. Making kidney donation attractive by decreasing morbidity is important, as the greatest concern about transplantation today is the meager supply of donor organs facing a continuously increasing demand.

Efforts to increase the number of living donors include kidney-paired donation programs in which living donors who are incompatible with their intended recipients, either because of ABO incompatibility or because of sensitization, may donate to another recipient, whose organs then may be given to the primary recipients, thus expanding available donors.[46]

There is now an active national paired kidney exchange pilot program that intends to increase the mathematical probability of getting a kidney transplant. In addition, another method to increase the donor pool is to encourage nondirected live kidney donation by altruistic donors. In the 2005 Scientific Registry of Transplant Recipients Report, there were 88 nondirected donations out of a total of 2,343 living unrelated donors.[47]

The timing of referrals to the various ESRD therapies varies considerably and requires a strong effort to improve coordination from all involved physicians. Preemptive transplantation can occur as early as an eGFR of 20 ml/minute, as can listing for a deceased donor organ. In the case of HD and PD, the readiness of access placement ideally has to predate the initiation of therapy. In turn, the date to initiate therapy is a complex decision made jointly by the nephrologist and the patient. It now is considered ideal to have vein mapping done before AVF placement, which determines the size and location of placement of the access, thereby improving success rates in establishing a working access. Native AVFs are preferred over other forms of chronic HD access because of fewer problems with infection and clotting; however, not all patients are candidates for an AVF placement. In patients with poor anatomy, unsuitable body habitus, or comorbid conditions, where an AVF is less likely to mature and be functional, benefit may be derived from an arterio-venous graft (AVG), a connection between veins using synthetic material, which is less desirable than an AVF but better than a dialysis catheter. Hemodialysis catheters may provide inadequate dialysis clearance because of lower blood flows and pose a higher risk of infection. The Fistula First Initiative, designed to increase the number of AVFs, may have caused more attempts at AVF placement but also may have resulted in suboptimal AVF, inducing longer duration of dialysis catheter use.[48] One essential technique to increase the number of successful AVF creations is the preoperative evaluation of forearm veins by imaging, usually ultrasonography, for ideal access placement. Routine preoperative sonographic evaluation of upper-extremity arteries and veins compared with historic controls resulted in doubling the rate (64 vs. 34%) of resulting functional AVF, and the subgroups that benefited most were women and patients with diabetes.[49]

Timing of PD catheter placement is advocated at ~2 weeks before the start of therapy, but challenges include a requirement for 6–8 weeks of patient training and education. It is an option chosen by dedicated patients who have a significant amount of family support. Plantinga et al. found that in 949 patients from 77 clinics, the mean social support scores in this population were significantly higher in PD than HD patients.[50] After adjustment, highest versus lowest overall support predicted greater 1-year satisfaction and quality-of-life scores in all patients. PD is cheaper, and the choice between the two dialysis modalities often is made on the basis of socioeconomic factors rather than any medical advantage. The initial survival advantage seen in PD is lost after the first year, which coincides with the loss of the residual renal function. In a large study of 35,265 patients from the Canadian Organ Replacement Register comparing mortality between HD and PD, the overall survival for the entire study period favored PD in the first 18 months and HD after 36 months. Among women >65 years with diabetes, PD had a 27% higher mortality rate.[51] Overall, substantive differences in long-term outcome with PD compared with in-center HD have not been documented. PD may offer a slight advantage in younger patients without diabetes in the early phase of renal replacement therapy. PD has not been found to be advantageous for elderly patients with diabetes, an increasingly large cohort of the U.S. dialysis population.[52]

In the U.S., an additional cause for the underuse of PD may be a lack of confidence in the nephrology trainee who has had only minimal experience using this dialysis modality.[53] PD, nevertheless, is selected more commonly than is home HD.

COMPREHENSIVE MANAGEMENT OF DECLINING RENAL FUNCTION IN PATIENTS WITH DIABETES

As CKD afflicting diabetic patients progresses, two emerging clinical facets become obvious: First, the care of patients' preexisting conditions changes, including fewer options in medications for glycemic control of diabetes, while goals for glycemic and BP control are moving targets as CKD progresses; and, second, complications of uremia have to be managed medically until renal replacement therapy is initiated.

AVOIDING IATROGENIC INJURY

With decreasing eGFR, treatment options for diabetes management become fewer. Additionally, caution must be exercised to avoid exposing the patient to toxins that might induce iatrogenic injury. As ESRD nears, it is essential to minimize use of all nonsteroidal anti-inflammatory drugs (NSAIDs), aminoglycosides, intravenous contrast, and large doses of phosphate (even as enemas or bowel-cleansing preparations). NSAIDS commonly are started by patients without medical supervision for the very aches and pains that may have resulted from CKD-associated hyperparathyroidism and that could accelerate loss of eGFR in patients taking a combination of NSAIDS, diuretics, and ACE inhibitors and ARBs.

AKI noted after large phosphorus loads has been implicated in phosphate nephropathy.[54] The phosphorus content in these agents commonly used, such as sodium phosphate, are severalfold the normal daily intake of phosphorus, which is ~1 gram/day, and may overwhelm the kidney's excretory capacity in CKD. Other risk factors for increased drug toxicity include advanced age, dehydration, and concurrent use of ACE inhibitors or ARBs. Kidney biopsy in phosphate nephropathy typically shows tubular and interstitial deposition of calcium phosphate. No effective treatment for acute phosphate deposition has as yet been devised.

Abruptly deteriorating renal function may be due to interstitial nephritis related to other medications, including cimetidine, methicillin sodium chloride, allopurinol, phenylhydantoin, NSAIDs, and furosemide. The ACE inhibitors may reversibly worsen azotemia or precipitate hyperkalemia and incapacitating nonproductive cough in up to 20% of individuals with diabetes. ARBs regulate hypertensive BP, reduce proteinuria, and slow the course of nephropathy, but they also may trigger renal functional deterioration and, less often, nonproductive cough. Dosage reductions according to residual GFR of cyclophosphamide, cimetidine, clofibrate, digoxin, and many antibiotics (particularly aminoglycosides) are required for azotemic patients with worsening GFR.

Debate over radio contrast agent–induced nephropathy (CI-AKI) has increased because of the lack of an effective management plan. Despite the multiple possible therapies tried, the question of optimal protection against radio-contrast media nephropathy remains open. Prior data has been limited by the lack of a definition of acute renal failure in addition to the other challenges, as demonstrated by a recent Australian meta-analysis of 1,489 CI-AKI studies, which found only 13 of these studies to meet the criteria for inclusion in a study seeking an end point of AKI, death, or resort to dialysis. Interestingly, the investigators concluded that of 13 randomized studies on contrast medium–induced nephropathy, there was a similar incidence of AKI, dialysis, and death between the contrast medium group and the control group.[55]

Currently, the optimal strategy appears to be avoiding use of radio contrast agents, whenever possible. Conflicting data exist about previously accepted preventive measures, such as administration of *N*-acetylcysteine previously given twice a day, on the day before and the day of the contrast exposure. Data on the effect of hydration also have conflicting results, with the best type of fluid course still under debate. The available choices are isotonic saline or isotonic fluid with bicarbonate; amount of time and volume used for hydration are also subject to discussion. The optimal strategy for preventing CI-AKI is not established. Accepted practice at present is to keep the patient in optimal fluid balance and avoid volume overload, while minimizing the amount of low or iso-osmolar contrast medium and use of *N*-acetylcysteine. Some nephrologists would hold off on agents like ACE inhibitors and ARBs in addition to any potential nephrotoxins when there is planned contrast use in CKD patients.

Nephrogenic systemic fibrosis (NSF) is an irreversible complication seen in advanced CKD patients who have been given gadolinium-containing contrast agents (GCCA), most often in a magnetic resonance imaging (MRI) study. The incidence of NSF was 4.3 cases per 1,000 patient-years, with each radiologic study using gadolinium having a 2.4% risk for NSF.[56] The risk of NSF after gadolinium exposure varies by eGFR, with most reported cases found in chronic dialysis patients. The risk in individuals with an estimated GFR of 15–59 ml/minute/1.73 m² remains unclear, although cases have been reported in these stages as well as with AKI. Skin disease in NSF typically presents as symmetrical, bilateral fibrotic indurated papules, plaques, or subcutaneous nodules, afflicting the limbs and abdomen. Diagnosis is made clinically and confirmed by skin biopsy. Convinced of the association of NSF and gadolinium in advanced CKD in most cases, the U.S. Food and Drug Administration (FDA) has recommended that in patients with an estimated GFR <30 ml/minute/1.73 m², or receiving dialysis, or with AKI, GCCA should be given only if clearly necessary.[57] Gadolinium should be avoided in patients with a diagnosis or clinical suspicion of NSF. If an MRI is indicated in advanced CKD, dialysis should be arranged immediately after the MRI, which results in significant removal of the contrast agent.[58] For dialysis patients, this usually means having a dialysis session right after the gadolinium exposure.

Lee et al. noted a fourfold increase in urinary tract infection in critically ill diabetic patients when compared with nondiabetic patients after bladder catheterizations. The authors proposed that unless the benefit clearly outweighs this risk, bladder catheterization should be avoided.[59]

TARGET GOALS IN THERAPY OF PATIENTS WITH DIABETES AND CKD

Data for slowing progression of CKD in diabetes began with the DCCT trial in the U.S. and the U.K. Prospective Diabetes Study (UKPDS) in the United Kingdom. In T2D, a linear relationship has been identified between the degree of hyperglycemia and development and progression of kidney damage.[9,60]

With advancing CKD and declining renal function, insulin clearance does not change significantly because of compensatory peritubular insulin uptake, and this compensation persists until the eGFR is <20 ml/minute resulting in a longer half-life of insulin and a decline in insulin requirement.[61,62]

A1C

A1C is the most accurate long-term glycemic control assessment tool in non-CKD patients; however, it is less reliable in patients with CKD. False elevations may be noted because of testing methods that are used to measure the glycated hemoglobin. A1C is affected by renal failure because of interference from the carbamylated hemoglobin that forms in the presence of elevated serum urea (noted with urea levels >84 mg/dl). A false reduction in A1C may be seen with reduced red blood cell life span and accelerated erythropoiesis because of the administration of erythropoietin-stimulating agents (ESAs) for anemia. Both of the latter situations are common in CKD patients, prompting the exploration of glycated albumin in CKD patients.[63,64]

Once CKD is present in diabetes, the target for glycemic control still is not defined sharply. Slinin et al. found that in people with diabetes, intensive glycemic control and lipid interventions did not improve clinical outcomes in patients with T2D; outcomes included death from cardiovascular causes, incident kidney failure, and nonfatal cardiovascular events.[65] Currently the KDOQI 2012 guidelines suggest a target A1C of 7% to prevent or delay progression of the microvascular complications of diabetes such as diabetic kidney disease. In addition, the Dialysis Outcomes and Practice Patterns Study (DOPPS) concluded that A1C levels strongly predicted mortality in HD patients with T1D or T2D. Mortality increased as the A1C moved farther from 7–7.9%, either lower or higher, confirming that the current target for people with diabetes with varying stages of CKD probably needs to be in this range (see Table 43.3).[66]

Problems that arise include managing CVD, hypertension, and bone mineral disease, including hyperparathyroidism, hypo-vitamin D levels, hypocalcemia,

Table 43.3 New Goals in Treatment of Diabetic Kidney Disease

Targets	Goals and outcomes
Blood Pressure	If a target blood pressure <140/90 mmHg is selected, therapy must be individualized considering age and risk of adverse events. First line: drugs are generally an ACE inhibitor or ARB but not the combination. A diuretic, calcium channel blocker, or β-blocker can be added.
Hemoglobin A1C	KDOQI 2012: A1C of 7% prevents or delays onset of microvascular disease, including diabetic nephropathy. DOPPS: Mortality lowers as A1C increases from 7 to 7.9% in dialysis patients with T1D and T2D. ADA 2013: A1C should be performed twice a year in those meeting goals, quarterly with medication changes or in those not meeting goals. First antihyperglycemic drug in early CKD is metformin.
Proteinuria	ADA suggests no longer using the confusing term "microalbuminuria." Progression of CKD does not necessarily follow increasing amounts of proteinuria, and advanced CKD can occur with minimal proteinuria. ADA 2013 recommends the use of ACE inhibitors or ARBs in nonpregnant patients with proteinuria >30 mg/day.
Hyperlipidemia	An LDL goal is similar to non-CKD patients. KDOQI clinical practice guidelines for managing dyslipidemias in early CKD advise striving for an LDL cholesterol level <100 mg. No consensus guides drug therapy to lower serum triglycerides. Patients with CKD may increase the risk of muscle toxicity when treated with statins.
Hemoglobin	Federal reimbursement requires a hemoglobin between 10 and 11.5 grams/dl but not >12 grams/dl in patients receiving ESAs. During ESA use, the benefits of avoiding transfusions should be weighed against a risk of strokes and hypertensive complications and the need for caution if malignancy risk present.

Note: ACE = angiotensin-converting-enzyme; ADA = American Diabetes Association; ARB = angiotensin-receptor blockers; CKD = chronic kidney disease; DOPPS = Dialysis Outcomes and Practice Patterns Study; ESA = erythropoiesis-stimulating agents; KDOQI = National Kidney Foundation Outcomes Quality Initiative; LDL = low-density lipoprotein.

hyperphosphatemia, dyslipidemia, protein restriction, hyperurecemia, metabolic acidosis, anemia, and hyperkalemia.

CKD AND CVD

Patients with CKD have a higher risk of CVD, because traditional risk factors overlap both conditions such as hypertension, diabetes, hypercholesterolemia, and metabolic syndrome. CKD by itself is also an independent risk factor for CVD and with moderate CKD the chances of death from CVD are greater than progression to renal replacement therapy. There is a suggestion, on the basis of observational data, that CKD should be considered a "coronary equivalent," meaning that these patients should be aggressively treated. In addition, exposure to the large load of calcium used as a phosphate binder, hyperphosphatemia, elevated serum calcium phosphate product, and parathyroid hormone have been indicted as increasing cardiac mortality in chronic HD patients.[67]

According to the USRDS 2010 ADR, mortality in the CKD population of almost 550,000 patients under treatment with renal replacement therapy in 2008 included 50% who died from CVD; it was especially noted that even those with less advanced stages of CKD were at greater risk of death from coronary artery disease (CAD) than of reaching the final stages of renal failure that eventually would require renal replacement therapy.[68] In these patients, ~50–60% of all cardiovascular deaths are due to acute myocardial infarction, sudden death, or ischemic heart disease.[69] The interplay between CKD and CAD is complex and can be explained only partly by the fact that patients with CKD share many of the so-called traditional risk factors also linked to CAD, such as long-standing diabetes, hypertension, low levels of high-density lipoprotein cholesterol, and hypertriglyceridemia.[70] Additionally, a proinflammatory state and high oxidative stress levels usually are seen in patients with advanced CKD, which may contribute to accelerated atherosclerosis, plaque instability, acute coronary syndromes, and myocardial fibrosis.[71] Despite this reality, there is concern that patients with CVD and CKD are undertreated for their CKD, as many CVD studies exclude patients with CKD. Current KDIGO guidelines suggest that patients with CKD be given the same level of care for CVD as those without CKD (see Table 43.3).[3]

BLOOD PRESSURE CONTROL

The Joint National Committee 7 in 2003 suggested that some patients may benefit from lowering BP <130/80 mmHg, acknowledging that the data for such a recommendation was sparse.[72] Current KDIGO guidelines have a more conservative approach based on the few available prospective randomized controlled trials, such as the Action to Control Cardiovascular Risk in Diabetes (ACCORD) study,[73] in patients with diabetes who have CKD and who do not have increased albuminuria. The ACCORD trial assessed 4,733 diabetic patients in two groups with target systolic BP of <120 mmHg compared with <140 mmHg and found no difference in primary end point of death or cardiovascular events, but it did note a reduction in the risk of stroke that was a secondary endpoint at the expense of adverse events like elevation in serum creatinine and hyperkalemia. Current KDIGO and American Diabetes Association (ADA) recommendations for patients with diabetes without increased albuminuria call for a target BP of ≤140/90 mmHg and lower in those in whom the benefit would be greater than the harm that might be induced in very old persons at high risk for strokes, nonadherent younger individuals, and those with persistent hypertension who are not being treated with an overall plan employing several antihypertensive medications.

In patients with diabetes who have high urine albumin excretion, the Steno-2 study was a randomized controlled trial in 160 patients with T2D and persistent microalbuminuria over a period of 13 years, listing all-cause mortality as the primary endpoint. The two arms included intensive BP control or conventional BP control. Intensive control achieved a BP of ≤130/80 mmHg with either ACE inhibitors or ARBs compared with the conventional group, which achieved a BP of ≤135/85 mmHg. The intensive group had a reduced risk of CVD; nephropathy, with fewer patients progressing to CKD5D (one patient compared with six patients); retinopathy; and autonomic neuropathy. Additionally, the intensive group had other interventions, including intensive glucose control, lipid-lowering therapy, aspirin, and lifestyle modification advice (see Table 43.3).[74]

METABOLIC BONE DISEASE

The KDOQI 2003 guidelines[75] and the KDIGO 2009 guidelines[76] for bone disease in CKD not yet on dialysis do not agree as to what an optimal target level of intact parathyroid hormone (iPTH) should be. According to the KDOQI practice guidelines, the target plasma levels of iPTH vary based on the stage of CKD, with a suggested goal of 35–70 pg/ml in CKD3, 70–110 pg/ml in CKD4, and 150–300 pg/ml in CKD5. This iPTH is based on a second-generation assay that is no longer available, which is one of the reasons why the KDIGO guidelines avoid using absolute iPTH levels. In addition, based on concern over CVD, compared with KDIGO 2009 guidelines, KDOQI poses more stringent phosphorus (between 2.7 and 4.6 mg/dl), normal calcium levels, and a calcium phosphorus product of <55 mg^2/dl^2. The KDIGO guidelines do not list any absolute PTH values, but instead they require demonstration of a persistently elevated PTH that is rising for treatment. KDIGO suggests that serum calcium and phosphate be kept in the normal range. Clinically, in CKD3A–5A, baseline measurement of PTH, serum calcium, phosphorus, and alkaline phosphatase are suggested by the KDIGO 2009 guidelines.

In the clinical setting, once hyperphosphatemia occurs in CKD patients, dietary phosphate restriction should be initiated and if not successful (as dietary restriction of phosphate includes protein restriction as well), phosphate binders are added in the form of calcium acetate or carbonate, sevelamer, or lanthanum. Correction of phosphate and calcium levels can be achieved in this single step if a calcium-containing agent is used. With limited observational data, patients in CKD3A–5 phosphorus levels should be maintained in the normal range. Vitamin D levels in the form of cacidiol vitamin D2 should be monitored and supplemented, as needed, in the form of ergocalciferol. PTH levels are treated based on trends of hyperparathyroidism as noted earlier. Cinacalcet has not been approved as yet for use in CKD patients not yet on dialysis.

DYSLIPIDEMIA

Dyslipidemia is common in people with diabetes and CKD. Cardiovascular events are a frequent cause of morbidity and mortality in this population. Lowering low-density lipoprotein cholesterol (LDL-C) with statin-based therapies reduces risk of major atherosclerotic events, but not all-cause mortality, in patients with CKD including those with diabetes.[77]

Data on the benefits of statins in CKD are conflicting. A recent meta-analysis by Nikolic et al. explored the impact of short- and long-term statin therapy on lipid profiles in 3,594 CKD patients not on dialysis and noted that statin therapy significantly reduced total cholesterol, triglycerides, and LDL-C.[78]

Commonly accepted recommendations include the use of statins or statins with ezetimibe in CKD patients with diabetes, including those with a kidney transplant. Because the lipid profiles are different and the cause of death in patients on dialysis frequently is not attributed to atherosclerotic complications, the use of statins is not routinely initiated in dialysis patients.

DIETARY PROTEIN RESTRICTION

Although dietary protein restriction has been shown to be beneficial in slowing CKD progression, the amount of employed protein restriction has varied. Severe protein restriction reported in two studies to ~0.6 grams/kg/day, which was 30–40% lower than the control group in patients with T1D with nephropathy, induced a 75% reduction in the rate of loss of GFR at 18–36 months.[79] This severe level of protein restriction, however, is difficult to maintain and might lead to nutritional deficiencies. Emphasis on the source of protein is now thought to be relevant to the degree of restriction advised. A high total protein intake of nondairy animal protein may accelerate renal decline in CKD. The most recent KDIGO guidelines suggest lowering protein intake to 0.8 grams/kg/day in adults with or without diabetes, eGFR <30 ml/minute, and avoiding a high protein diet >1.3 grams/kg/day in CKD patients who are at risk for disease progression.[80] Current ADA guidelines suggest reducing protein intake to 0.8–1 grams/kg body weight/day in individuals with diabetes in the early stages of CKD. It further suggests protein restriction to 0.8 grams/kg body weight/day in later stages of CKD to preserve renal function.[81]

HYPERURICEMIA AND TREATMENT

Kuo et al. noted a greater annual decline in eGFR in those with higher uric acid levels in 63,785 patients over a 12-year period compared with those with normal uric acid levels.[82] With limited studies to support the use of agents to lower serum uric acid to prevent progression of CKD, the KDIGO 2013 guidelines have neither supported nor refuted their use.[3] On the basis of these data, we recommend that symptomatic elevation of uric acid be treated and recurrences prevented. In addition, uric acid levels >10 mg/dl should be treated with allopurinol after obtaining informed consent from the patient noting risks and potential benefits of the medication.

ACIDOSIS

Even though the efficacy of treatment of acidosis with oral bicarbonate has been known since the 1930s, it was only in 2009 that data on its benefits in a randomized controlled study, in 134 patients with CKD4 and serum bicarbonate levels between 16 and 20 mmol/l with oral sodium bicarbonate over a 2-year period, became available. The treated group had higher serum bicarbonate levels without an increase in BP. CKD progression was significantly slower in the treated group compared with controls, while fewer treated patients reached ESRD.[83] Additional trials will help define the extent of bicarbonate use.

HYPERKALEMIA

In the presence of aldosterone and distal tubular flow, serum potassium can be maintained in the normal range even with advanced CKD.[84] In people with diabetes, hyperkalemia can arise from aldosterone reduction either in the form of drugs that inhibit the angiotensin system or with hyporeninemic hypoaldosteronism. Dehydration with a decrease in urine flow to the distal tubule is another mechanism for hyperkalemia. Hyperkalemia also can occur in the setting of decreased cellular uptake because of the effect of medications that inhibit the sodium potassium pump such as nonselective β-blockers. Treatment in most situations would include the use of a diuretic to increase distal tubular sodium. Diuretics also would decrease plasma volume and stimulate renin and aldosterone leading to potassium excretion. Patients with CKD should consult with a dietitian, in most cases, to be on a low-potassium diet (<2 grams/day; see Table 43.4).

EFFECTIVE DRUGS FOR TREATMENT OF DIABETES

Metformin is the tier one–validated core therapy for T2D according to the consensus statement of the ADA and the European Association for the Study of Diabetes (ADA/EASD). It follows that metformin is the most commonly prescribed oral agent for diabetes.[85] Metformin is not protein bound and is eliminated by the kidney both via glomerular filtration and by tubular secretion. With advancing CKD, metformin accumulates and the risk of lactic acidosis increases. The exact eGFR cutoff at which metformin should be avoided is still under debate. Although the manufacturer's package insert suggests a serum creatinine <1.5 mg/dl in men and <1.4 mg/dl in women, and in Canada, an eGFR >60 ml/minute, the most recent KDIGO guideline includes those with an eGFR >45 ml/minute and reviews its use in those with an eGFR between 30–44 ml/minute.[3]

The first-generation sulfonylureas are eliminated to a large extent by the kidney and should be avoided in those with CKD to prevent hypoglycemia. Second-generation sulfonylurea agents, including glyburide, should be avoided because of active metabolites that are excreted by the kidney and that may accumulate in patients with CKD. Glimepiride mainly is metabolized by the liver with some renal excretion of active metabolites and may be used with caution starting at low doses. Glipizide is the preferred drug since it undergoes metabolism within the liver.[86] Glyburide should be avoided in patients with advanced CKD in or greater

Table 43.4 Checklist of Medications in Diabetic Nephropathy

Medication	Recommendation
Metformin	KDIGO suggests metformin use in patients with eGFR >45 ml/minute as first-line medication.
ACE inhibitor or ARB	First-line therapy for diabetic nephropathy. Either ACE inhibitor or ARB but not in combination due to increased risk of cardiovascular disease, hyperkalemia, and death.
Sodium bicarbonate	KDIGO 2013 guidelines suggest maintaining serum bicarbonate in the normal range of 23–29 meq/l with oral sodium bicarbonate. There is less sodium retention with sodium bicarbonate than with sodium chloride.
Allopurinol	For therapy in gout and prevention of joint pain, in addition if serum uric acid is >10 grams/dl, although its use is still controversial.
Phosphate binders	Usually needed once the eGFR <40 ml/minute when serum phosphorus is noted to rise.
Vitamin D supplementation	Check vitamin D levels and replace orally as needed, when eGFR decreases <40 ml/minute, 1,25-vitamin D levels decrease.
Vitamin D analogs	Monitor parathyroid hormone levels and treat trends toward secondary hyperparathyroidism to prevent renal osteodystrophy.
Statins	Treat hypercholesterolemia and monitor for muscle toxicity.
Vaccinations	KDIGO 2012 guidelines suggest an annual influenza vaccine unless contraindicated. Polyvalent pneumococcal vaccine every 5 years unless contraindicated. CKD4–5 immunized against hepatitis B and the response confirmed by immunologic testing.

Note: ACE = angiotensin converting enzyme; ARB = angiotensin-receptor blockers; CKD = chronic kidney disease; eGFR = estimated glomerular filtration rate; KDIGO = Kidney Disease Improving Global Outcomes.

than stage 3B. Meglitinides such as repaglinide require no dose adjustment. Nateglinide may be started at a low dose before meals. With the FDA's intervention to decrease use of rosiglitazone[87] and a black-box warning for pioglitazone in heart failure, both of these drugs are best not given in CKD with volume overload issues in a population that has a high risk of CVD. In addition, an FDA alert informed the public that the agency has approved updated drug labels for pioglitazone-containing medicines, including a safety alert that use of pioglitazone for >1 year may be associated with an increased risk of bladder cancer.[88]

Amylin analogs such as pramlintide need no dose adjustment for eGFR between 20–50 ml/minute. Among the incretin-based insulin secretagogues, glucagon-like peptide-1 (GLP-1) analogs, including exenatide and liraglutide, are not recommended once the serum creatinine concentration is >2 mg/dl or the eGFR is <30 ml/minute, while caution should be applied with initiating or increasing dosage in patients with an eGFR between 30 and 50 ml/minute, primarily because of reduced renal drug clearance.[89] Sitagliptin, one of several dipeptidyl peptidase-4 (DPP-4) inhibitors, is excreted in the urine and thus reduced doses are recommended in patients with CKD stages 3–5 to 50 mg/day and with an eGFR of <30–25 mg/day.[90] Linagliptin is metabolized by the liver and does not require dose adjustment for CKD.[91]

It is important when using insulin to individualize dosage for patients whose dose is based on eGFR. Usually, no dose adjustment is needed with an eGFR >50 ml/minute. In those with an eGFR between 10 and 50 ml/minute, the insulin dose can be decreased by 25% while in patients with an eGFR <10 ml/minute, the insulin dose should be lowered by 50%. Blood glucose levels must be monitored closely as there is a substantive risk of hypoglycemia.[92]

CHOOSING ANGIOTENSIN SYSTEM BLOCKERS IN PATIENTS WITH T1D AND T2D WITH CKD

T1D and Angiotensin System Blockade

That blocking angiotensin with captopril was protective of kidney function in T1D was the main finding in a remarkable 1994 report by Viberti et al.[93] Treatment with captopril versus placebo, for 2 years, in a cohort of 92 normotensive subjects with T1D with albuminuria noted that the captopril-treated group had slower progression to overt diabetic nephropathy. Renoprotection was evident even in those with a serum creatinine <2.5 mg/dl who were treated with captopril for 4 years, gaining BP control equivalent to that of other antihypertensive agents. Benefits were noted even in those patients with an initial creatinine >1.5 mg/dl in whom the rate of increase of serum creatinine was 1.4 mg/dl/year in the noncaptopril group compared with 0.6 mg/dl in the captopril group. There were no demonstrable benefits over the 4-year period in individuals who began the study with a lower baseline serum creatinine, as the rate of progression was too slow in this group.[94]

Although some authors, based on small short-term studies,[95] argue that it is the degree of BP reduction rather than the agent administered that yields a beneficial effect of ACE inhibition on diabetic nephropathy in normotensive patients with T1D, we interpret overall reports as sustaining use of an ACE inhibitor or ARB as first-line treatment to slow progression of diabetic nephropathy for all patients with T1D and albuminuria, with or without hypertension.

The benefits of maximal blockade of the renin angiotensin system has been addressed in small studies over a short term. Jacobsen et al. administered two agents to block the renin-angiotensin system compared with giving just the maximal dose of an ACE inhibitor in diabetic nephropathy. The authors treated small cohorts of patients with T1D nephropathy for 8 weeks with either an ACE inhibitor or placebo versus an ACE inhibitor plus ARB, concluding that dual blockade had greater benefits, including lower albuminuria, lower systolic and diastolic BPs, and unchanged eGFR and serum potassium.[96]

T2D and Angiotensin System Blockade

In T2D, two large trials have noted the benefits of ARBs. The first was the Irbesartan Diabetic Nephropathy Trial (IDNT)[97] conducted in ~1,700 patients with T2D with diabetic nephropathy and a mean serum creatinine of 1.7 mg/dl. Subjects were randomized to one of three groups receiving an ARB-irbesartan, a calcium channel blocker (amlodipine), or placebo. Of note, no direct comparison between an ACE inhibitor and ARB was made. At 2.6 years, the ARB group had a significantly lower risk of reaching end points of death or progression to CKD as noted by a doubling of serum creatinine, reaching ESRD, or death from any cause. These outcomes were independent of BP reduction between the groups. CKD progression was noted to be slowest in the group with systolic BP <134 mmHg.

The RENAAL trial[98] looked at 1,513 patients with T2D and a mean serum creatinine of 1.9 mg/dl who were randomized to receive either the ARB-losartan or placebo. The trial noted that at a mean follow-up of 3.4 years, there was a significant reduction in CKD progression in those treated with losartan. Again no direct comparison between an ARB and ACE inhibitor was made.

A direct comparison between an ACE inhibitor and ARB was made in the trial that compared enalapril to telmisartan in 250 patients with T2D and nephropathy over 5 years, finding no difference in benefit for either cohort in terms of CKD progression by decline in GFR; enalapril had a 15 ml/minute decline in GFR compared with 17.5 ml/minute in the telmisartan group.[99]

Combination of ACE Inhibition Plus ACE Receptor Blockage in Diabetes

The ONTARGET trial combined an ARB (telmisartan) and an ACE inhibitor (ramipril) compared with using telmisartan alone in ~15,000 patients with T2D for a median period of 56 months to study primary outcomes of death or cardiac morbidity. The trial found no difference between the groups except for adverse events. The ramipril group had more cough and angioedema and the combination group had more hypotension and renal dysfunction. The authors concluded that telmisartan was equivalent to ramipril in patients with vascular disease or high-risk diabetes, and the combination of the two drugs was associated with more adverse events without any increase in benefit.[100]

NEED FOR TARGET HEMOGLOBIN DURING ADMINISTRATION OF RECOMBINANT ERYTHROPOIETIN

Anemia as defined by a hemoglobin (Hb) level <13 grams/dl in men and <12 grams/dl in women is a common coexisting condition seen with CKD. As GFR decreases in progressive CKD, hemoglobin levels also decrease. Many symptoms of uremia in the past have been attributed to anemia with resolution once the anemia is corrected. Anemia seen in CKD is hypoproliferative, normochromic, and normocytic, with similar characteristics to and undistinguishable from anemia noted in other chronic diseases. Despite the low erythropoietic nature of CKD, erythropoietin levels are not measured and not recommended because they frequently are not helpful, although reticulocyte counts are considered to be more helpful to determine proliferative activity.[101,102] Serum ferritin levels are helpful in determining iron stores; however, because serum ferritin is also an acute phase reactant, unless the levels are low, it needs to be interpreted with caution. In general, if the ferritin level is <30 ng/ml indicative of severe iron deficiency—normal to high levels do not necessarily indicate adequate stores and should be used along with transferrin saturation values. For example, intravenous iron replacement can be considered when the ferritin is <500 ng/ml and transferrin saturation is <30%.

FREQUENCY OF TESTING FOR ANEMIA

There is a paucity of data to define the progression of anemia and ideal hemoglobin levels in CKD prior to initiation of dialysis. The following suggestions are from the KDIGO 2012 guidelines for anemia management in CKD[107] and are based on observations that hemoglobin levels decline following loss of GFR. There is the need to monitor for the presence of anemia to determine whether iron administration and an ESA administration are needed. In the absence of anemia and before CKD stage 3, hemoglobin can be measured only as needed. By CKD stages 4–5, in the absence of anemia, monitoring for anemia should be done two to four times a year. Once patients require ESA therapy, however, measurement of hemoglobin should be performed at least monthly. In patients with CKD3–5, before dialysis but after ensuring that other causes of anemia have been excluded, hemoglobin can be checked monthly when on ESA therapy.[83] Physicians need to carefully weigh the risk of CVD and hypertension, which may be side effects of the therapy, against the benefit of avoiding blood transfusions, which could prevent future kidney transplantation because of unnecessary antigen exposure. In addition ESA should be used cautiously if at all in patients with malignancy.

In CKD5D, hemoglobin measurements, even in those who are not anemic, are done once a month and more frequently on ESA therapy as mandated by federal guidelines. In addition, any change to the clinical needs of the patient, such as from bleeding or surgery, warrants further monitoring.

Treatment with an ESA

Before initiation of ESA therapy in CKD, all other correctable causes of anemia need to be addressed because the anemia attributed to CKD is often a diagnosis made by exclusion. Risks associated with ESA therapy include cerebrovascular accidents and concerns of malignancy in those at high risk for these two conditions. In those with a hemoglobin level >10 grams/dl, ESA is not recommended; in those with a hemoglobin <10 grams/dl, decisions should be made on an individual basis, to avoid blood transfusion if left untreated as well as the risk of the therapy. The goal of therapy is a moving target, and currently, patients with CKD who are not yet on dialysis are started on ESA when the hemoglobin is consistently <10 grams/dl with symptoms of anemia, fatigue, or inability to function. In general, ESA is not used to maintain a hemoglobin >11.5 grams/dl (see Table 43.4).[103]

Once iron stores are corrected, ESA can be administered, with the generally accepted goal being a hemoglobin between 10 and 12 grams/dl with the medication being held once hemoglobin exceeds 11.5 grams/dl.

CHANGING PARADIGMS IN CARING FOR KIDNEY FAILURE IN DIABETES

The 2012 USRDS ADR noted a mild increase in the prevalence of CKD (based on estimated GFR <60 ml/minute) to 6.7% in 2005–2010 compared with 4.9% in 1988–1994. If CKD is defined by either a decrease in eGFR to <60 ml/minute or an ACR of >30 mg/gram, then the CKD prevalence rose from 12.3 to 14%

between those respective periods. First- and second-year mortality decreased by 14 and 16.5% in the ESRD CKD5D population between 2003 and 2009 compared with the period between 1993 and 2003. The mortality, however, in the first few months of therapy continues to stay high, at ~10-fold, when compared with age-matched controls not on dialysis. In addition to late referrals and access-related infections, other causes of mortality are also high. From 2000 onward, there has been a 19% decline in mortality of prevalent ESRD CKD5D patients. Despite these relative improvements, only 51% of dialysis and 82% of preemptive transplant patients were alive after 3 years of therapy.

The cost of CKD treatments is high and consumes a significant portion of funds spent by Medicare for diabetes. Among Medicare beneficiaries alone, the costs in 2007 for CKD reached 4% or $7.5 billion, which was a 10% increase from the previous year. In 2007, Medicare costs for patients with diabetes reached $80.5 billion; the subset of patients with diabetes and CKD accounted for 39% of these costs.[104]

Data on patient care at the start of ESRD therapy show that the percentage of patients receiving an ESA before initiation continues to decline, reaching just 20% in 2010 compared with one-third in the early part of the decade. This may reflect concern over potential adverse events when hemoglobin levels are targeted to a level >12 grams/dl. The mean hemoglobin at initiation of ESRD treatment is now 9.73 grams/dl. These changes place different demands on care after the initiation of dialysis and may alter the likelihood of a patient receiving a blood transfusion. The balance between cardiovascular risk in the setting of a hemoglobin >12 grams/dl and the risk of transfusion with lower hemoglobin levels needs to be addressed by patients and their physicians, particularly in the case of patients contemplating a kidney transplant, for whom sensitization from blood transfusions is to be avoided, if at all possible.

The number of patients with diabetic kidney disease is expected to increase in the near future and the number of specialty caregivers, including nephrologists, is expected to decrease. Patient demand therefore would require primary caregivers to take over many of the services provided by the nephrologist and to be comfortable managing CKD in its early stages to effectively arrest progression early on in the disease process. Shortages in the field were predicted as early as 2004 with reports of a sluggish increase in the number of nephrologists being trained and a concurrent rise in the number of patients with CKD.

Because of rising cost, the federal government has attempted to limit expenditures by changing guidelines and reimbursements in CKD anemia management. With an emphasis on the growing economic burden in caring for ESRD patients, it is urgent that we seek new approaches to treat the expanding population. At present, besides slowing CKD progression, there are no practical therapeutic options.

Prevention of diabetes would be an ideal intervention to prevent diabetic nephropathy; the public health benefits from pursuing a healthy lifestyle are promising. The Diabetes Prevention Program research group compared 3,234 patients without diabetes who had elevated fasting and postload plasma glucose concentrations in three groups: placebo, metformin 850 mg twice a day, or lifestyle changes with a goal of 7% weight loss and at least 150 minutes/week of physical activity along with encouragement to follow the food pyramid guide and the National Cholesterol Education Program Step 1 diet. The study participants had an average follow-up of 2.8 years. The lifestyle changes group had the lowest incidence of diabetes compared with the other groups, which were reported as cases of diabetes per 100 patient-years: 11 in the placebo group, 7.8 in the metformin group, and 4.8 in the lifestyle modification group.[105]

Treatment of diabetic nephropathy with methyl bardoxolone, thiazolidinediones, direct renin inhibitors, and endothelin antagonists has not been successful.[106] Newer therapies under investigation include protein kinase C inhibitors and inhibitors of AGEs, transforming growth factor-β inhibitors, sulodexie, and connective tissue inhibitors.[107]

Table 43.5 Preventing Iatrogenic Complication in Diabetic Nephropathy

Complication	Prevention measure
NSAIDS COX 2 inhibitors	Avoid or discontinue especially before additional nephrotoxicity (such as intravenous contrast) planned or in dehydration.
Intravenous radio-contrast agents	Avoid contrast agents intravenously to prevent contrast-induced nephropathy, if possible. If required, hydrate patient with isotonic intravenous fluid at 0.5 ml/kg/hour for 12–24 hours before the radiographic procedure. In addition, *N*-acetylcysteine 600 mg orally twice a day should be given on the day before and the day of the radiographic procedure. The benefit of seeking protection by administering isotonic intravenous bicarbonate is controversial but can be given as 3 ml/kg 1 hour before the contrast exposure.
Aminoglycosides	The affinity of the drug class for renal proximal tubule proteins results in damage. To minimize tubular injury, minimize the number of doses of the drug and monitor serum drug levels. Affinity of the drug also predicts toxicity, with neomycin having a greater toxicity than gentamycin and tobramycin, which has greater toxicity than amikacin; the least nephrotoxic is streptomycin.
Urinary tract infections	Avoid bladder catheterization and an indwelling catheter, if possible.
Gadolinium-induced nephrotoxicity	Avoid gadolinium when eGFR is <30 ml/minute or with AKI to prevent nephrogenic systemic fibrosis. If needed, remove gadolinium with back-to-back dialysis sessions. The American Society of Radiology suggests avoiding gadolinium even if eGFR ranges between 30 and 44 ml/minute.
Hyperphosphatemic nephropathy	Bowel-cleansing preparations with phosphorus should be avoided in CKD and AKI as injury from undiagnosed hyperphosphatemia may result.
Arteriovenous hemodialysis fistula (AVF)	If eGFR is <30 ml/minute, vasculature in the nondominant arm should be protected for an AVF. Avoid blood pressure monitoring and phlebotomy in that arm. Vein mapping and hemodialysis access placement performed when eGFR is <20 ml/minute.

Note: AKI = acute kidney injury; CKD = chronic kidney disease; eGFR = estimated glomerular filtration rate; NSAID = nonsteroidal anti-inflammatory drugs.

The question of using the bowel as a substitute kidney is being revisited,[108] this time with the use of probiotics in patients on dialysis to assist in nitrogen waste removal. Microbes in the colon produce compounds, normally excreted by the kidneys, which are potential uremic toxins, examples of which include *p*-cresol and indoxyl sulfate. Aronov et al. compared plasma from HD patients with and without colons to identify and further characterize colon-derived uremic solutes and found the colonic origin of *p*-cresol sulfate and indoxyl sulfate.[109] Compared with patients with colons, >30 individual substances in patients without colons were either absent or present in lower concentration. Almost all of these chemicals were more prominent in plasma from dialysis patients than normal subjects, suggesting that they represented uremic solutes. These results suggest that colonic microbes may produce an important component of "toxic" uremic solutes, many of which remain unidentified.

Removal of uremic toxins induced by oral administration of specific probiotic bacteria is a promising approach to the management of symptomatic CKD and ESRD, which ultimately may replace the need for dialysis therapy as well as kidney transplantation.[110]

CONCLUSION

A relatively small subset of patients with CKD and diabetes will progress to CKD5 needing renal replacement therapy, whereas the majority of patients with earlier stages of CKD will die of cardiovascular complications before progressing to ESRD. Proven therapies to slow down progression of CKD still remain: seeking to optimize BP with ACE inhibitors and striving to restore euglycemia. The predicted shortage of nephrologists will require more non-nephrologists to treat these patients striving to arrest the progression of the disease. Referrals to nephrologists should be considered in the setting of a possible alternate diagnosis, or later to manage complications of CKD as it progresses (see Table 43.5). Among the options of renal replacement therapy, the optimal choice for diabetic nephropathy continues to be kidney transplantation.

REFERENCES

1. American Diabetes Association. Executive summary: standards of medical care in diabetes—2013. *Diabetes Care* 2013;36;(Suppl 1):S4–5.

2. Mogensen CE. Twelve shifting paradigms in diabetic renal disease and hypertension. *Diabetes Res Clin Pract* 2008;82(Suppl 1):S2–9.

3. U.S. Renal Data System. *USRDS 2012 Annual Data Report: Atlas of Chronic Kidney Disease and End-Stage Renal Disease in the United States*, Bethesda, MD, National Institutes of Health, National Institute of Diabetes and Digestive and Kidney Diseases, 2012, Table A7, p. 362.

4. Friedman EA. Continuously evolving management concepts for diabetic CKD and ESRD. *Semin Dial* 2010;23:134–139.

5. National Kidney Foundation. K/DOQI clinical practice guidelines for CKD: evaluation, classification and stratification. *Am J Kidney Dis* 2002;(S1):39:1–266.

6. Kidney Disease: Improving Global Outcomes (KDIGO). Summary of recommendation statements. *Kidney Int* 2013;3(S5)1–150.

7. Levey AS, Bosch JP, Lewis JB. A more accurate method to estimate glomerular filtration rate from serum creatinine. *Ann Intern Med* 1999;130(6): 461–470.

8. Matsushita K. Mahmoodi BK, Woodward M, Emberson JR, Jafar TH, Jee SH, Polkinghorne KR, Shankar A, Smith DH, Tonelli M, Warnock DG, Wen CP, Coresh J, Gansevoort RT, Hemmelgarn BR, Levey AS; for the Chronic Kidney Disease Prognosis Consortium. Comparison of risk prediction using CKD EPI equation and the MDRD Study equation for estimated GFR. *JAMA* 2012;307(18):1941–1951.

9. Ohsawa M, Tanno K, Itai K, Turin TC, Okamura T, Ogawa A, Ogasawara K, Fujioka T, Onoda T, Yoshida Y, Omama SI, Ishibashi Y, Nakamura M, Makita S, Tanaka F, Kuribayashi T, Koyama T, Sakata K, Okayama A. Comparison of predictability of future cardiovascular events between chronic kidney disease (CKD) stage based on CKD epidemiology collaboration equation and that based on modification of diet in renal disease equation in the Japanese general population. *Circ J* 2013;77(5):1315–1325.

10. Levey AS, Stevens LA, Coresh J. Conceptual model of CKD: applications and implications. *Am J Kidney Dis* 2009;53(Suppl 3):S4–16.

11. Horspool, S. Kidney disease acknowledged as NCD at UN meeting. Available at www.theisn.org. Posted 28 September 2011. Accessed 7 March 2014.

12. Centers for Disease Control and Prevention. An estimated 26 million adults in the United States have chronic kidney disease. Available at www.cdc.gov/Features/dsChronicKidneyDisease. Accessed 7 March 2014.

13. Vora JP, Dolben J, Dean JD, Thomas D, Williams JD, Owens DR, Peters JR. Renal hemodynamics in newly presenting non-insulin dependent diabetes mellitus. *Kidney Int* 1992;41(4):829–835.

14. Nelson RG, Bennett PH, Beck GJ, Tan M, Knowler WC, Mitch WE, Hirschman GH, Myers BD. Development and progression of renal disease in Pima Indians with non-insulin-dependent diabetes mellitus. *N Engl J Med* 1996;335(22):1636–1642.

15. Fliser D, Wagner KK, Loos A, Tsikas D, Haller H. Chronic angiotensin II receptor blockade reduces (intra)renal vascular resistance in patients with type 2 diabetes. *J Am Soc Nephrol* 2005;16(4):1135–1140.

16. Hilgers KF, Veelken R. Type 2 diabetic nephropathy: never too early to treat? *J Am Soc Nephrol* 2005;16:574–575.

17. Nagai Y, Yao L, Kobori H, et al. Temporary angiotensin II blockade at the prediabetic stage attenuates the development of renal injury in type 2 diabetic rats. *J Am Soc Nephrol* 2005;16:703–711.

18. Harris RD, Steffes MW, Bilous RW, et al. Global glomerular sclerosis and glomerular arteriolar hyalinosis in insulin dependent diabetes. *Kidney Int* 1991;40:107–114.

19. Ichihara A, Suzuki F, Nakagawa T, Kaneshiro Y, Takemitsu T, Sakoda M, Nabi AH, Nishiyama A, Sugaya T, Hayashi M, Inagami T. Prorenin receptor blockade inhibits development of glomerulosclerosis in diabetic angiotensin II type 1a receptor-deficient mice. *J Am Soc Nephrol* 2006;17(7):1950–1961.

20. Doublier S, Salvidio G, Lupia E, Ruotsalainen V, Verzola D, Deferrari G, Camussi G. Nephrin expression is reduced in human diabetic nephropathy: evidence for a distinct role for glycated albumin and angiotensin II. *Diabetes* 2003;52(4):1023–1030.

21. Doublier S, Salvidio G, Lupia E, Ruotsalainen V, Verzola D, Deferrari G, Camussi G. Nephrin expression is reduced in human diabetic nephropathy—evidence for a distinct role for glycated albumin and angiotensin II. *Diabetes* 2003;52:1023–1030.

22. Trevisan R, Viberti G. Genetic factors in the development of diabetic nephropathy. *J Lab Clin Med* 1995;126:342–349.

23. Satko SG, Langefeld CD, Daeihagh P, et al. Nephropathy in siblings of African Americans with overt type 2 diabetic nephropathy. *Am J Kidney Dis* 2002;40:489–494.

24. Jeffers BW, Estacio RO, Raynolds MV, Schrier RW. Angiotensin-converting enzyme gene polymorphism in non-insulin dependent diabetes mellitus and its relationship with diabetic nephropathy. *Kidney Int* 1997;52:473–477.

25. Kuramoto N, Iizuka T, Ito H, et al. Effect of ACE gene on diabetic nephropathy in NIDDM patients with insulin resistance. *Am J Kidney Dis* 1999;33:276–281.

26. Brancati FL, Whittle JC, Whelton PK, Seidler AJ, Klag MJ. The excess incidence of diabetic end-stage renal disease among blacks. A population-based study of potential explanatory factors. *JAMA* 1992;268(21):3079–3084.

27. Smith SR, Svetkey LP, Dennis VW. Racial differences in the incidence and progression of renal diseases. *Kidney Int* 1991;40(5):815–822.

28. Hayashi K, Epstein M, Loutzenhiser R, Forster H. Impaired myogenic responsiveness of the afferent arteriole in streptozotocin-induced diabetic rats: role of eicosanoid derangements. *J Am Soc Nephrol* 1992;2(11):1578–1586.

29. Chaiken RL, Palmisano J, Norton ME, Banerji MA, Bard M, Sachimechi I, Behzadi H, Lebovitz HE. Interaction of hypertension and diabetes on renal function in black NIDDM subjects. *Kidney Int* 1995;47(6):1697–1702.

30. Ejerblad E, Fored CM, Lindblad P, Fryzek J, McLaughlin JK, Nyrén O. Obesity and risk for chronic renal failure. *J Am Soc Nephrol* 2006;17(6):1695–1702.

31. Chase HP, Garg SK, Marshall G, Berg CL, Harris S, Jackson WE, Hamman RE. Cigarette smoking increases the risk of albuminuria among subjects with type I diabetes. *JAMA* 1991;265(5):614–617.

32. Perkins BA, Ficociello LH, Silva KH, Finkelstein DM, Warram JH, Krolewski AS. Regression of microalbuminuria in type I DM. *N Engl J Med* 2003;(348):2285–2293.

33. de Boer IH, Rue TC, Cleary PA, Lachin JM, Molitch ME, Steffes MW, Sun W, Zinman B, Brunzell JD; Diabetes Control and Complications Trial/Epidemiology of Diabetes Interventions and Complications Study Research Group, White NH, Danis RP, Davis MD, Hainsworth D, Hubbard LD, Nathan DM. Long term renal outcomes in type I DM and microalbuminuria: an analysis of the Diabetes Control and Complications Trial/Epidemiology of Diabetes Interventions and Complications cohort. *Arch Intern Med* 2011;171(5):412–420.

34. Perkins BA, Ficociello LH, Roshan B, Warram JH, Krolewski AS. Patients with type I DM and new onset microabluminuria and the developement of advanced CKD may not have progression to proteinuria. *Kidney Int* 77(1):57–64.

35. Eijkelkamp WB, Zhang Z, Remuzzi G, Parving HH, Cooper ME, Keane WF, Shahinfar S, Gleim GW, Weir MR, Brenner BM, de Zeeuw D. Albuminuria is a target for renoprotective therapy independent from blood pressure in patients with type 2 DM nephropathy: post hoc analysis of the RENAAL trial. *J Am Soc Nephrol* 2007;18(5):1540–1546.

36. Lewis EJ, Hunsicker LG, Bain RP, Rohde RD and the Collaborative Study Group. The effect of ACE inhibition on diabetic nephropathy. *N Engl J Med* 1993;329(20):1456–1462.

37. Brenner BM, Cooper ME, de Zeeuw D, Keane WF, Mitch WE, Parving HH, Remuzzi G, Snapinn SM, Zhang Z, Shahinfar S; RENAAL Study Investigators. Effect of losartan on renal and cardiovascular outcomes in patients with type 2 diabetes and nephropathy. *N Engl J Med* 2001;345(12):861–869.

38. Wilmer WA, Hebert LA, Lewis EJ, Rohde RD, Whittier F, Cattran D, Levey AS, Lewis JB, Spitalewitz S, Blumenthal S, Bain RP. Remission of nephrotic syndrome in type 1 diabetes: long-term follow-up of patients in the Captopril Study. *Am J Kidney Dis* 1999;34(2):308–314.

39. Hovind P, Rossing P, Tarnow L, Smidt UM, Parving HH. Remission and regression in the nephropathy of type 1 diabetes when blood pressure is controlled aggressively. *Kidney Int* 2001;60(1):277–283.

40. Christensen PK, Larsen S, Horn T, Olsen S, Parving HH. Causes of albuminuria in patients with type 2 diabetes without diabetic retinopathy. *Kidney Int* 2000;58(4):1719–1731.

41. Bradbury BD, Fissell RB, Albert JM, Anthony MS, Critchlow CW, Pisoni RL, Port FK, Gillespie BW. Predictors of early mortality among incident US hemodialysis patients in the Dialysis Outcomes and Practice Patterns Study (DOPPS). *Clin J Am Soc Nephrol* 2007;2(1):89–99.

42. Astor BC, Eustace JA, Powe NR, Klag MJ, Sadler JH, Fink NE, Coresh J. Timing of nephrologist referral and arteriovenous access use: the CHOICE Study. *Am J Kidney Dis* 2001;38(3):494–501.

43. Wolfe RA, Ashby VB, Milford EL, Ojo AO, Ettenger RE, Agodoa LY, Held PJ, Port FK. Comparison of mortality in all patients on dialysis, patients on dialysis awaiting transplantation, and recipients of a first cadaveric transplant. *N Engl J Med* 1999;341(23):1725–1730.

44. Nelson RG, Tuttle KR. The new KDOQI 2006 clinical practice guidelines and clinical practice recommendations for diabetes and CKD. *Blood Purif* 2007;25(1):112–114.

45. Meier-Kriesche HU, Port FK, Ojo AO, Rudich SM, Hanson JA, Cibrik DM, Leichtman AB, Kaplan B. Effect of waiting time on renal transplant outcome. *Kidney Int* 2000;58(3):1311–1317.

46. Delmonico FL. Exchanging kidneys—advances in living-donor transplantation. *N Engl J Med* 2004;350(18):1812–1814.

47. Marks WH, Wagner D, Pearson TC, Orlowski JP, Nelson PW, McGowan JJ, Guidinger MK, Burdick J. Organ donation and utilization, 1995-2004: entering the collaborative era. *Am J Transplant* 2006;6(5 Pt 2):1101–1110.

48. Patel ST, Hughes J, Mills JL Sr. Failure of arteriovenous fistula maturation: an unintended consequence of exceeding dialysis outcome quality initiative guidelines for hemodialysis access. *J Vasc Surg* 2003;38(3):439–445.

49. Allon M, Lockhart ME, Lilly RZ, Gallichio MH, Young CJ, Barker J, Deierhoi MH, Robbin ML. Effect of preoperative sonographic mapping on vascular access outcomes in hemodialysis patients. *Kidney Int* 2001;60(5):2013–2020.

50. Plantinga LC, Fink NE, Harrington-Levey R, Finkelstein FO, Hebah N, Powe NR, Jaar BG. Association of social support with outcomes in incident dialysis patients. *Clin J Am Soc Nephrol* 2010;5(8):1480–1488.

51. Yeates K, Zhu N, Vonesh E, Trpeski L, Blake P, Fenton S. Hemodialysis and peritoneal dialysis are associated with similar outcomes for end-stage renal disease treatment in Canada. *Nephrol Dial Transplant* 2012;27(9):3568–3575.

52. Mallappallil M, Patel A, Friedman EA. Peritoneal dialysis should not be the first choice for renal replacement therapy in the elderly. *Semin Dial* 2012;25(6):671–674.

53. Berns JS. A survey-based evaluation of self-perceived competency after nephrology fellowship training. *Clin J Am Soc Nephrol* 2010;5(3):490–496.

54. Markowitz GS, Stokes MB, Radhakrishnan J, D'Agati VD. Acute phosphate nephropathy following oral sodium phosphate bowel purgative: an under-recognized cause of chronic renal failure. *J Am Soc Nephrol* 2005;16(11):3389–3396.

55. McDonald JS, McDonald RJ, Comin J, Williamson EE, Katzberg RW, Murad MH, Kallmes DF. Frequency of acute kidney injury following intravenous contrast medium administration: a systematic review and meta-analysis. *Radiology* 2013 Apr;267(1):119–128.

56. Deo A, Fogel M, Cowper SE. Nephrogenic systemic fibrosis: a population study examining the relationship of disease development to gadolinium exposure. *Clin J Am Soc Nephrol* 2007;2(2):264–267.

57. United States Federal Drug Administration. Posting Date 5/18/2011. Available at www.fda.gov/cder/drug/infoSheets/HCP/gcca_200705.htm. Accessed 7 March 2014.

58. Okada S, Katagiri K, Kumazaki T, Yokoyama H. Safety of gadolinium contrast agent in hemodialysis patients. *Acta Radiol* 2001;42(3):339–341.

59. Lee JH, Kim SW, Yoon BI, Ha US, Sohn DW, Cho YH. Factors that affect nosocomial catheter-associated urinary tract infection in intensive care units: 2-year experience at a single center. *Korean J Urol* 2013;54(1):59–65.

60. U.K. Prospective Diabetes Study (UKPDS) Group. Intensive blood-glucose control with sulphonylureas or insulin compared with conventional treatment and risk of complications in patients with type 2 diabetes. *Lancet* 1998 Sep 12;352(9131):837–853.

61. Rabkin R, Simon NM, Steiner S, Colwell JA. Effects of renal disease on renal uptake and excretion of insulin in man. *N Engl J Med* 1970;282:182–187.

62. Shrishrimal K, Hart P, Michota F. Managing diabetes in hemodialysis patients: observations and recommendations. *Cleve Clin J Med* 2009;76(11):649–655.

63. Freedman BI, Shihabi ZK, Andries L, Cardona CY, Peacock TP, Byers JR, Russell GB, Stratta RJ, Bleyer AJ. Relationship between assays of glycemia in diabetic subjects with advanced chronic kidney disease. *Am J Nephrol* 2010;31(5):375–379.

64. Freedman BI, Shenoy RN, Planer JA, Clay KD, Shihabi ZK, Burkart JM, Cardona CY, Andries L, Peacock TP, Sabio H, Byers JR, Russell GB, Bleyer AJ. Comparison of glycated albumin and hemoglobin A1c concentrations in diabetic subjects on peritoneal and hemodialysis. *Perit Dial Int* 2010;30(1):72–79.

65. Slinin Y, Ishani A, Rector T, Fitzgerald P, MacDonald R, Tacklind J, Rutks I, Wilt TJ. Management of hyperglycemia, dyslipidemia, and albuminuria in

patients with diabetes and CKD: a systematic review for a KDOQI clinical practice guideline. *Am J Kidney Dis* 2012;60(5):747–769.

66. Ramirez SP, McCullough KP, Thumma JR, Nelson RG, Morgenstern H, Gillespie BW, Inaba M, Jacobson SH, Vanholder R, Pisoni RL, Port FK, Robinson BM. Hemoglobin A(1c) levels and mortality in the diabetic hemodialysis population: findings from the Dialysis Outcomes and Practice Patterns Study (DOPPS). *Diabetes Care* 2012;35(12):2527–2532.

67. Ganesh SK, Stack AG, Levin NW, Hulbert-Shearon T, Port FK. Association of elevated serum PO(4), Ca x PO(4) product, and parathyroid hormone with cardiac mortality risk in chronic hemodialysis patients. *J Am Soc Nephrol* 2001;12(10):2131–2138.

68. Sarnak MJ, Levey AS, Schoolwerth AC, Coresh J, Culleton B, Hamm LL, McCullough PA, Kasiske BL, Kelepouris E, Klag MJ, Parfrey P, Pfeffer M, Raij L, Spinosa DJ, Wilson PW; American Heart Association Councils on Kidney in Cardiovascular Disease, High Blood Pressure Research, Clinical Cardiology, and Epidemiology and Prevention. Kidney disease as a risk factor for development of cardiovascular disease: a statement from the American Heart Association Councils on Kidney in Cardiovascular Disease, High Blood Pressure Research, Clinical Cardiology, and Epidemiology and Prevention. *Circulation* 2003;108(17):2154–2169.

69. Herzog CA, Mangrum JM, Passman R. Sudden cardiac death and dialysis patients. *Seminars in Dialysis* 2008;21(4):300–307.

70. McCullough PA, Nowak RM, Foreback C, Tokarski G, Tomlanovich MC, Khoury N, Weaver WD, Sandberg KR, McCord J. Emergency evaluation of chest pain in patients with advanced kidney disease. *Arch Intern Med* 2002;162(21):2464–2468.

71. Yerkey MW, Kernis SJ, Franklin BA, Sandberg KR, McCullough PA. Renal dysfunction and acceleration of coronary disease. *Heart* 2004;90(8):961–966.

72. Chobanian AV, Bakris GL, Black HR, Cushman WC, Green LA, Izzo JL Jr, Jones DW, Materson BJ, Oparil S, Wright JT Jr, Roccella EJ; National Heart, Lung, and Blood Institute Joint National Committee on Prevention, Detection, Evaluation, and Treatment of High Blood Pressure; National High Blood Pressure Education Program Coordinating Committee. The seventh report of the Joint National Committee on Prevention, Detection, Evaluation, and Treatment of High Blood Pressure: the JNC 7 report. *JAMA* 2003;289(19):2560–2572.

73. ACCORD Study Group, Cushman WC, Evans GW, Byington RP, Goff DC Jr, Grimm RH Jr, Cutler JA, Simons-Morton DG, Basile JN, Corson MA, Probstfield JL, Katz L, Peterson KA, Friedewald WT, Buse JB, Bigger JT, Gerstein HC, Ismail-Beigi F. Effects of intensive blood-pressure control in type 2 diabetes mellitus. *N Engl J Med* 2010;362(17):1575–1585.

74. Gaede P, Lund-Andersen H, Parving HH, Pedersen O. Effect of a multifactorial intervention on mortality in type 2 diabetes. *N Engl J Med* 2008;358(6):580–591.

75. National Kidney Foundation. K/DOQI clinical practice guidelines for bone metabolism and disease in chronic kidney disease. *Am J Kidney Dis* 2003;42(4Suppl 3):S1–S206.

76. Kidney Disease: Improving Global Outcomes (KDIGO). Clinical practice guidelines for the diagnosis, evaluation, prevention, and treatment of chronic kidney disease-mineral and bone disorder (CKD-MBD). *Kidney Int* 2009;76(Suppl 13):S1–S140.

77. Slinin Y, Ishani A, Rector T, Fitzgerald P, MacDonald R, Tacklind J, Rutks I, Wilt TJ. Management of hyperglycemia, dyslipidemia, and albuminuria in patients with diabetes and CKD: a systematic review for a KDOQI clinical practice guideline. *Am J Kidney Dis* 2012;60(5):747–769.

78. Nikolic D, Nikfar S, Salari P, Rizzo M, Ray KK, Pencina MJ, Mikhailidis DP, Toth PP, Nicholls SJ, Rysz J, Abdollahi M, Banach M; Lipid and Blood Pressure Meta-Analysis Collaboration Group. Effects of statins on lipid profile in chronic kidney disease patients: a meta-analysis of randomized controlled trials. *Curr Med Res Opin* 2013;29(5):435–451.

79. Walker JD, Bending JJ, Dodds RA, Mattock MB, Murrells TJ, Keen H, Viberti GC. Restriction of dietary protein and progression of renal failure in diabetic nephropathy. *Lancet* 1989;2(8677):1411–1415.

80. Kidney Disease: Improving Global Outcomes (KDIGO). Clinical practice guidelines for the evaluation and management of chronic kidney disease. *Kidney Int* 2013;3(Suppl 1)1–150.

81. American Diabetes Association. Standards of medical care in diabetes—2013. *Diabetes Care* 2013;36(Suppl 1)S11–S66.

82. Kuo CF, Luo SF, See LC, Ko YS, Chen YM, Hwang JS, Chou IJ, Chang HC, Chen HW, Yu KH. Hyperuricaemia and accelerated reduction in renal function. *Scand J Rheumatol* 2011;40(2):116–121.

83. De Brito-Ashurst I, Varagunam M, Raftery MJ. Bicarbonate supplementation slows progression of CKD and improves nutritional status. *J Am Soc Nephrol* 2009;20:2075–2084.

84. Allon MSO. Hyperkalemia in end-stage renal disease: mechanisms and management. *J Am Soc Nephrol* 1995;6(4):1134–1142.

85. Inzucchi SE, Bergenstal RM, Buse JB, Diamant M, Ferrannini E, Nauck M, Peters AL, Tsapas A, Wender R, Matthews DR; American Diabetes Association (ADA); European Association for the Study of Diabetes (EASD). Management of hyperglycemia in type 2 diabetes: a patient-centered approach. Position statement of the American Diabetes Association (ADA) and the European Association for the Study of Diabetes (EASD). *Diabetes Care* 2012;35:1364–1379.

86. Snyder RW, Berns JS. Use of insulin and oral hypoglycemic medications in patients with diabetes mellitus and advanced kidney disease. *Semin Dial* 2004;17(5):365–370.

87. U.S. Food and Drug Administration significantly restricted the use of rosiglitazone to patients with type 2 diabetes due to the response to data that suggest an elevated risk of CVD in those treated with rosiglitazone, 2010. Available at www.fda.gov/ForConsumers/ConsumerUpdates/ucm049063. htm. Accessed 18 May 2011.

88. U.S. Food and Drug Administration. Update on pioglitazone, 2011. Available at www.fda.gov/ForConsumers/ConsumerUpdates/ucm266555.htm. Accessed 7 March 2014.

89. Lubowsky ND, Siegel R, Pittas AG. Management of glycemia in patients with diabetes mellitus and CKD. *Am J Kidney Dis* 2007;50:865–879.

90. Bergman AJ, Cote J, Yi B, et al. Effect of renal insufficiency on the pharmacokinetics of sitagliptin, a dipeptidyl peptidase-4 inhibitor. *Diabetes Care* 2007;30:1862–1864.

91. Graefe-Mody U, Friedrich C, Port A. Linagliptin a novel DPP4 inhibitor: no need for dose adjustment in patients with renal impairment. Poster No. 822-P, European Association for the Study of Diabetes Annual Meeting, 20–24 September 2010, Stockholm, Sweden.

92. Charpentier G, Riveline JP, Varroud-Vial M. Management of drugs affecting blood glucose in diabetic patients with renal failure. *Diabetes Metab* 2000;26(Suppl 4):73–85.

93. Viberti G, Mogensen CE, Groop LC, Pauls JF; European Microalbuminuria Captopril Study Group. Effect of captopril on progression to clinical proteinuria in patients with insulin-dependent diabetes mellitus and microalbuminuria. *JAMA* 1994;271(4):275–279.

94. Lewis EJ, Hunsicker LG, Bain RP, Rohde RD; Collaborative Study Group. The effect of angiotensin-converting-enzyme inhibition on diabetic nephropathy. *N Engl J Med* 1993;329(20):1456–1462.

95. Parving HH, Hommel E, Jensen BR, Hansen HP. The purpose of this study was to assess whether long-term (8 years) inhibition of angiotensin-converting enzyme (ACE) protects kidney function in normotensive type 1 diabetic patients with diabetic nephropathy. *Kidney Int* 2001;60(1):228–284.

96. Jacobsen P, Andersen S, Rossing K, Jensen BR, Parving HH. Dual blockade of the renin-angiotensin system versus maximal recommended dose of ACE inhibition in diabetic nephropathy. *Kidney Int* 2003;63(5):1874–1880.

97. Lewis EJ, Hunsicker LG, Clarke WR, Berl T, Pohl MA, Lewis JB, Ritz E, Atkins RC, Rohde R, Raz I; Collaborative Study Group. Renoprotective effect of the angiotensin-receptor antagonist irbesartan in patients with nephropathy due to type 2 diabetes. *N Engl J Med* 2001;345(12):851–860.

98. Brenner BM, Cooper ME, de Zeeuw D, Keane WF, Mitch WE, Parving HH, Remuzzi G, Snapinn SM, Zhang Z, Shahinfar S; RENAAL Study Investigators. Effects of losartan on renal and cardiovascular outcomes in patients with type 2 diabetes and nephropathy. *N Engl J Med* 2001;345(12):861–869.

99. Barnett AH, Bain SC, Bouter P, Karlberg B, Madsbad S, Jervell J, Mustonen J; Diabetics Exposed to Telmisartan and Enalapril Study Group. *N Engl J Med* 2004;351(19):1952–1961.

100. ONTARGET Investigators, Yusuf S, Teo KK, Pogue J, Dyal L, Copland I, Schumacher H, Dagenais G, Sleight P, Anderson C. Telmisartan, ramipril, or both in patients at high risk for vascular events. *N Engl J Med* 2008;358(15):1547–1559.

101. Fehr T, Ammann P, Garzoni D, Korte W, Fierz W, Rickli H, Wüthrich RP. Interpretation of erythropoietin levels in patients with various degrees of renal insufficiency and anemia. *Kidney Int* 2004;66(3):1206–1211.

102. Ross RP, McCrea JB, Besarab A. Erythropoietin response to blood loss in hemodialysis patients is blunted but preserved. *ASAIO J* 1994;40(3):M880–8885.

103. Kidney Disease: Improving Global Outcomes (KDIGO) Anemia Work Group. KDIGO clinical practice guideline for anemia in chronic kidney disease. *Kidney Inter* 2012;(Suppl 2):279–335.

104. U.S. Renal Data System. Bethesda, MD, *USRDS 2010 Annual Data Report: Atlas of Chronic Kidney Disease and End-Stage Renal Disease in the United States.* National Institutes of Health, National Institute of Diabetes and Digestive and Kidney Disease, 2010.

105. Knowler WC, Barrett-Connor E, Fowler SE, Hamman RF, Lachin JM, Walker EA, Nathan DM; Diabetes Prevention Program Research Group. Reduction in the incidence of type 2 diabetes with lifestyle intervention or metformin. *N Engl J Med* 2002;346(6):393–403.

106. Thomas MC. Emerging drugs for managing kidney disease in patients with diabetes. *Expert Opin Emerg Drugs* 2013;18(1):55–70.

107. Reeves WB, Rawal BB, Abdel-Rahman EM, Awad AS. Therapeutic modalities in diabetic nephropathy: future approaches. *Open J Nephrol* 2012;2(2):5–18.

108. Friedman EA, Mallappallil M. *Present and Future Therapies for End-Stage Renal Disease.* Hackensack, NJ, World Scientific Publishing, 2010.

109. Aronov PA, Luo FJ-G, Plummer NS, Quan Z, Holmes S, Hostetter TH, Meyer TW. Colonic contribution to uremic solutes. *J Am Soc Nephrol* 2011;22:1769–1776.

110. Ranganathan N, Vyas U. Probiotics, prebiotics and synbiotics: Gut and beyond. *Gasteroenterol Res Prac* 2012;2012:872716doi;10.1155/1012/872716.

Chapter 44

Peripheral Neuropathy in Diabetes

Rodica Pop-Busui, MD, PhD
James W. Albers, MD, PhD
Eva L. Feldman, MD, PhD

INTRODUCTION

D iabetic peripheral neuropathy (DPN) is a common complication of diabetes with multiple manifestations, diverse pathogenetic mechanisms, and a complex natural history. The late complications of neuropathy such as foot problems, including ulceration[1] and nontraumatic amputations,[2] represent the most common causes of hospitalization among patients with diabetes in most western countries. Unsurprisingly, DPN often has an adverse effect on quality of life.[3–5] Given the epidemic explosion of diabetes worldwide (www.who.org), the high prevalence of this complication, and its clinical and socioeconomic consequences, effective therapeutic and preventive measures are paramount.

This chapter includes a classification system for DPNs as a basis for better understanding the disorder and for discussing the current state of knowledge with respect to the natural history, pathogenesis, clinical manifestations, morbidity, diagnostic evaluations, and available treatment. It outlines knowledge gaps that need to be targeted for more sensitive assessments and development of effective therapies to prevent or reverse DPN and its consequences.

DEFINITION OF DPN

DPN complicates both type 1 diabetes (T1D) and type 2 diabetes (T2D) and is characterized by the presence of symptoms or signs of peripheral nerve dysfunction, after the exclusion of other causes.[6,7] A large number of people with DPN may be asymptomatic. The 2009 Toronto Consensus Panel on Diabetic Neuropathies updated the definitions and diagnostic criteria fto include possible, probable, confirmed, and subclinical categories, as well as typical DPN and atypical DPN.[7,8]

The typical DPN is a distal (length-dependent) symmetrical sensorimotor polyneuropathy (DSP) attributable to chronic hyperglycemia, associated metabolic derangements, cardiovascular risk covariates, and microvessel alterations.[8] Data from cohort and population-based epidemiologic studies show that this is the most common variety of DPN. Any variation from this description, such as acute onset, asymmetry, proximal involvement, or motor prominence, suggests an "atypical" neuropathy.[7] The possible, probable, confirmed, and subclinical forms of DSP are discussed in more detail in the following sections. Exclusion of nondiabetic causes in the diagnosis of DPN is important, as up to 10% of peripheral neuropathies in patients with diabetes have a nondiabetic etiology.[6,9]

DOI: 10.2337/9781580405096.44

CLASSIFICATION OF DPN

Because DPN may have quite heterogeneous patterns of symptoms, neurologic signs, temporal course, risk covariates, pathologic alterations, and underlying mechanisms, multiple classifications have been proposed over time. DPNs can be classified in terms of their anatomical distribution (e.g., proximal or distal, symmetric or asymmetric, focal or multifocal), temporal onset (e.g., acute, subacute, or chronic), clinical course (e.g., progressive or monophasic), characteristic features (e.g., painful or nonpainful, sensory, motor, or autonomic), or pathophysiology. Classification into "typical" or "atypical" forms is based on their prevalence.[8] Chronic DSP is the most frequent (typical) form, which accounts for ~75% of diabetic neuropathies.[7,8] Atypical DPNs usually are superimposed on a DSP and may develop at any time during the course of a patient's diabetes. These atypical subtypes most often have subacute onset with a monophasic or fluctuating course over time, and some tend to preferentially involve small sensory nerve fibers or motor nerve fibers.[8] A variety of diabetic mononeuropathies are included among the atypical DPNs; these forms may have an acute, subacute, or chronic onset, and their features depend on the individual nerve involved. Atypical DPN has not been as well characterized and studied as has typical DPN, but some have suggested that it may not be necessarily associated with chronic hyperglycemia.[8] Table 44.1 provides a summary of most common forms of DPN and classifications. Note, however, that most all forms of neuropathy listed also occur in patients without diabetes.

Whereas DSP is the most common form of DPN,[8] the focal and multifocal neuropathies account for no more than 10% of all the neuropathies. They tend to occur in older patients, and in general, their clinical course includes either partial or complete recovery of the deficits and the concomitant pain. A rapid onset of symptoms and signs and the focal nature of the deficits are suggestive of a vascular etiology. Exclusion of nondiabetic causes is important for all forms, but particularly in the atypical, rapid-onset neuropathies. Conversely, any patient without diabetes presenting with one of these forms of neuropathy should be screened for diabetes.

To enhance clarity and avoid redundancy, this chapter describes these various forms of DPN following the outline shown in Table 44.2.

TYPICAL FORMS OF DPN

DISTAL SYMMETRIC POLYNEUROPATHY

The distal symmetric polyneuropathy (DSP) is the most common form of all diabetic neuropathies and essentially almost all information regarding the epidemiology, natural history, pathogenesis, diagnostic, and therapeutic approaches apply to DSP. The hallmark of the DSP is a progressive loss of sensory nerve fibers. The most distal portions of longest nerves are affected first, creating the typical "stocking" pattern.[6,7] Over time, the deficits proceed proximally, eventually resulting in a "stocking-glove" pattern that promotes the presence of symptoms and sensory loss (Figure 44.1). Although there are no major structural differences

---

Table 44.1 — Common DPN Classifications

Thomas et al. Classification[187]
1. Distal symmetric sensorimotor polyneuropathy
2. Focal and multifocal neuropathies
   - Cranial neuropathies
   - Limb mononeuropathies (median, ulnar, radial, femoral, peroneal, lateral femoral, cutaneous)
   - Trunk mononeuropathy
   - Mononeuropathy multiplex
   - Asymmetric lower limb motor neuropathy (amyotrophy)
3. Mixed forms

American Diabetes Association (ADA) Adapted Classification of Diabetic Neuropathy[6,7]
1. Generalized symmetric polyneuropathies
   - Acute sensory
   - Chronic sensorimotor
   - Autonomic
2. Focal and multifocal neuropathies
   - Cranial
   - Truncal
   - Focal limb
   - Proximal motor (amyotrophy)
   - Coexisting chronic inflammatory demyelinating polyneuropathy (CIDP)

Toronto Expert Panel on Diabetic Neuropathy[8]
1. Typical DPN
2. Atypical DPN

---

in nerve pathology between T1D and T2D, clinical differences do exist, with symptomatic autonomic syndromes usually occurring in longstanding T1D patients.[10]

EPIDEMIOLOGY OF DSP

The epidemiology and natural history of DSP, and of diabetic neuropathies in general, remain poorly defined mainly because of variable diagnostic criteria and patient population studies.

Incidence and Prevalence

DSP is the most common complication of both T1D and T2D, with an estimated lifetime prevalence exceeding 50%.[6,7] Approximately 20% of newly diagnosed T2D patients show evidence of DSP at the time diabetes is diagnosed.[11] When a DSP is identified in a patient who has abnormal glucose metabolism that is insufficient to establish a diagnosis of diabetes, the neuropathy is sometimes classified as "impaired glucose tolerance" or "prediabetic" neuropathy.[11] Persistent

Table 44.2—Chapter Outline

Typical DPN: Distal Symmetric Polyneuropathy (DSP)
Epidemiology of DSP
Incidence and Prevalence
Natural History
Risk Factors
Clinical Diagnosis of DSP
History
Symptoms and Signs
Limitations
Diagnostic Tests
Electrophysiology
Quantitative Sensory Testing (QST)
Skin Biopsy and Intraepidermal Nerve Fiber Density (IENFD)
Corneal Confocal Microscopy
Nerve Axon Reflex/Flare Response
Sudomotor Function
Late Complications of DSP
Pathogenesis
Treatment
Charcot Neuroarthropathy

Atypical Forms of DPN
Diabetic Radiculoplexus Neuropathy
Acute Small Fiber Neuropathy
Chronic Inflammatory Demyelinating Polyneuropathy
Diabetic Focal Mononeuropathies

neuropathic pain develops in as many as 20% of diabetic patients.[12,13] In the U.S., DSP is the primary cause of diabetic foot problems and ulcerations, which are the leading causes of diabetes-related hospital admissions and nontraumatic amputations.[6,7,9]

Although there are no major structural differences in nerve pathology between T1D and T2D, some differences in epidemiology and clinical presentation do exist. As demonstrated by the Diabetes Control and Complications Trial (DCCT), the prevalence of DSP is quite low in patients with early T1D, ~5% at baseline.[14,15] Among DCCT participants who were considered to be non-neuropathic at baseline, however, the prevalence of an abnormal neurologic exam was almost 20% in those on conventional treatment and almost 10% in those on intensive treatment after ~5 years of follow-up.[14,15] The prevalence of DSP increased during the observational follow-up of the DCCT cohort, Epidemiology of Diabetes Interventions and Complications (EDIC). At EDIC years 13–14, after a mean T1D duration of 26 years, reported prevalence rates were 25 and 35% for DSP in the former intensive and conventional control treatment groups, respectively.[16] The EURODIAB IDDM Complications Study found that the prevalence of DSP, across randomly

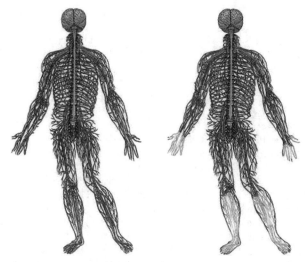

Figure 44.1—Progressive axonal loss in DPN. Adapted from Edwards JL, et al., *Pharmacol Ther* 2008;120:1—34. Used with permission.

selected patients with T1D from 16 European countries, was 28%, with no significant geographic differences.[17]

At the diagnosis of T2D, DSP is present in at least ≥10%[1] of patients with T2D,[18] and up to 50% of older T2D patients will have signs or symptoms of DSP during their life,[19] although estimates vary from 10 to 90%, depending on the diagnostic criteria used.[6,7,9] In a cohort of >1,500 individuals with screen-detected T2D participating in the ADDITION-Denmark Study, the prevalence of DSP was ~30% after 6 years of follow-up.[20] One prospective study of outpatients that included patients with both T1D and T2D reported an increase in the prevalence of DSP from 10 (at the time of diagnosis) to 50% after 25 years of diabetes.[21] The Rochester Diabetic Study reported prevalence rates of 59% in patients with T2D and 66% of patients with T1D,[22,23] and a large cross-sectional study that included T1D and T2D patients in the U.K. reported prevalence rates for DSP of 29%.[18] The Bypass Angioplasty Revascularization Intervention 2 Diabetes (BARI 2D), a large study that enrolled >2,300 participants with T2D with a mean diabetes duration of ~10 years and confirmed coronary artery disease, found that the prevalence of DSP was ~50%.[24,25] In the NHANES study,[26] the prevalence of painful DSP was found to be 27%. In this survey, however, an appreciable proportion of those without diabetes also had painful symptoms. Thus, the difference between these estimates could be a better indication of the prevalence of painful neuropathy attributable to diabetes. In other studies, estimates of painful symptoms have ranged from 3 to >20%.[1,6,9,27] Last, although in the past it was in general assumed that children and youth with diabetes are somewhat protected against developing DSP, one study reported higher vibration thresholds in children and adolescents with T1D compared with those who did not have diabetes.[28] More recent evidence from the SEARCH for Diabetes in Youth study reported that signs of DSP are found in youth with T1D at similar rates observed in adults with T1D.[29]

Incidence estimates of DSP for T1D have been obtained in several large studies, although the most comprehensive data emerged from the DCCT. Among DCCT participants who were considered to be nonneuropathic at baseline, 20% of those on conventional treatment and almost 10% of those on intensive treatment developed an abnormal neurologic examination after ~5 years of follow-up.[14] The incidence was higher for developing an abnormal nerve conduction study: >30% in those on conventional treatment and almost 20% in those on intensive treatment.[14,30] In the observational EDIC follow-up of the DCCT cohort, among participants free of DSP at DCCT closeout, 29 and 34%, respectively, of the former intensive- and conventional-treatment groups had confirmed DSP at EDIC year 13–14.[16,30] In the Wisconsin Epidemiologic Study of Diabetic Retinopathy,[31] depending on characteristics of the T1D patients who were studied, tactile sensation was decreased in 19–25%, and temperature sensitivity was decreased in 11–19% after 10 years of follow-up. In the Pittsburgh Epidemiology of Diabetes Complications Study, in which patients with T1D were followed over a period of 5.3 years, the cumulative incidence of DSP was 29%.[32] For T2D, among BARI 2D participants who were free of DSP at baseline, the cumulative incidence of DSP over 4 years of follow-up was 69%.[25]

As observed from these data, the prevalence of DSP varies widely, mainly because of differences in diagnostic criteria and the type of testing used. For instance, marked differences in the presence of hypoesthesia have been observed with the use of various quantitative sensory tests (QSTs), reporting DSP prevalence rates anywhere from 8 to 34%, according to the specific sensory test.[33] Studies using combined assessments of neuropathy also have shown marked differences in the prevalence of DSP. In one such study, the EURODIAB IDDM Complications Study,[17] the prevalence ranged from <20% at certain sites to >50% at other sites. Ethnicity also may affect DSP prevalence. In a large cohort of 15,692 patients with diabetes receiving community-based care in northwest England, signs of DSP were less prevalent in South Asians compared with Europeans or African Caribbean, but symptoms were greater in South Asians.[34] Even within the American Indian population of the Strong Heart Study,[35] there was marked variation, with rates varying from 22% in Arizona to only 8% in Oklahoma.[35] The importance of methodology was particularly evident in one study of patients with T1D in which the incidence of DSP without a confirmatory examination was ~5/100 person-years, whereas the incidence was <1/100 person-years with a confirmatory examination.[36] Thus, studies of the natural history and epidemiology of diabetic neuropathy should be examined with attention to the specific assessments and criteria for neuropathy that were used. Other factors to be considered include characteristics of the study population, the type of diabetes, and study design.

Natural History

The natural history of DSP is still not fully clear. It is, however, likely that the pathologic processes of DSP begin even before the onset of overt diabetes as some abnormalities are described relatively early in the course of both T1D and T2D.[18] In addition, both clinical evidence of DSP and neuropathic changes in small nerve fibers were reported in individuals with impaired glucose tolerance.[37–40] Among individuals newly diagnosed with T2D, there were decreases in vibration and thermal sensitivities after 2 years of follow-up.[41] This is not surprising, because it is common for T2D to go undiagnosed for years before diagnosis. In a different study of patients with T2D that utilized the 10-gram monofilament test as the outcome measure, no progression was observed for several years following diagnosis.[35] In another T1D study, thermal thresholds increased more than vibration thresholds among those followed for 5 years after diagnosis.[42]

DSP usually persists once it occurs. This is especially evident from such measures as QST and nerve conduction studies (NCSs). Pain from neuropathy, however, can remit. In one study,[43] a slight improvement in electrophysiologic and cardiovascular autonomic testing with pain remission was evident. Those whose pain remitted tended to develop their pain after a sudden metabolic change or weight loss, when the duration of diabetes was short. In a clinical trial of Japanese patients with T2D, the group receiving more intensive insulin therapy had an increase in the median nerve conduction velocity, although no improvement was observed in vibration thresholds.[44] In contrast, those receiving less intensive insulin therapy (fewer injections) had a decrease in these measures. Some evidence indicates that the rate of deterioration in vibration and thermal thresholds increases after impaired sensation is first evident.[45,46]

Risk Factors

There is no longer a controversy as to whether higher glucose levels and the duration of exposure to hyperglycemia contribute to the development of DSP. This conclusion is based largely on the findings obtained in patients with T1D participating in the DCCT.[14,47] Several observational studies have shown associations between the occurrence of DSP and glucose levels.[17,31] The evidence is not as strong for T2D as for T1D, however. In terms of T2D, the Kumamoto trial that enrolled Japanese patients with T2D reported better DSP outcome with intensive insulin treatment.[44] In the UKDPS trial, however, that tested the effects of an intensive glucose lowering, targeting A1C levels <7% versus conventional treatment in a large cohort of newly diagnosed T2D patients, results were not as definitive, showing only a trend for the conventional treatment group to have a greater occurrence of vibration insensitivity.[48] The Action to Control Cardiovascular Risk in Diabetes (ACCORD) trial reported that an intensive glucose-lowering strategy, targeting an A1C <6%, delayed the progression of DSP in patients with T2D at high risk of cardiovascular disease events.[49] Although some T2D studies have demonstrated a rather modest slowing of progression with intensive glycemic control, reversal of neuronal loss was not reported.[49,50]

Despite the clear evidence that DSP is associated with the degree of glycemia, there is still much more to be learned about the nature of that relationship. For instance, it has been postulated that higher glucose levels early in the course of the disease, even if for a limited period, could have a marked impact on the risk of DSP, so-called metabolic memory. These observations are mainly a result from the follow-up data obtained during EDIC study of former DCCT patients.[16,30] DSP continued to be more prevalent in the conventional treatment group 8 years later when first reassessed during EDIC, even though the difference in A1C between the groups had narrowed and, over time, no longer was different.[51] Because the neurologic assessments at EDIC year 8 were less comprehensive than they were in the DCCT, complete neurological assessments comparable to the DCCT assessments were performed at EDIC year 13/14.[16,52] Although there was a significant difference in the unadjusted incidence of DSP, after adjustment for differences in NCS results at the end of the DCCT, a "metabolic memory" effect on the primary DSP endpoint was no longer evident. A persistent treatment group effect was observed for several NCS measures, however, and longitudinal analyses showed a significant association between mean A1C and measures of incident and prevalent neuropathy.[16,52]

Glucose variability also has been assessed as a risk factor for DSP, but in studies that have examined the possible impact of such variability so far, the findings have been inconsistent.[53,54] Alternatively, some studies have shown associations of DSP with blood pressure and lipid indexes in both T1D and T2D, although these could have been possible surrogates of vascular disease. The EURODIAB IDDM trial found that hypertension and hyperlipidemia accelerated the effects of hyperglycemia on the risk of DSP in people with T1D.[55] Similarly, data from the U.K. Prospective Diabetes Study (UKPDS) suggest that hypertension, obesity, and smoking contribute to the development of DSP in T2D.[48,56–58] Other studies found that elevated triglycerides were independently associated with development of DSP.[59,60]

Constitutional factors also can influence the risk of DSP. Height has been shown to be a risk factor,[27,35,61,62] with an increasing effect for more distal assessments.[62] The basis for this is not known, but height is a surrogate for nerve length; hence, longer nerves could be more susceptible to metabolic factors. In addition, age always should be considered, as neurologic function is known to decline with age in populations both with and without diabetes.[63] Moreover, associations of DSP with other risk factors can vary with age.[32] Findings involving associations of DSP with alcohol consumption[35,61,62] and cigarette smoking,[35,61,62,64] however, have been inconsistent. Last, studies describing associations between DSP and genetic factors in patients with both T1D and T2D are emerging.[65,66]

Diagnosis of DSP

The diagnosis and staging of DSP are important for day-to-day clinical practice, as well as for assessing etiology and natural history, and for the design and conduct of clinical trials to test new treatments. The Peripheral Nerve Society issued a Consensus Statement on measures to assess efficacy in controlled trials of new therapies for neuropathy,[67] and the more recent Toronto Consensus on diabetic neuropathies reviewed the definitions, diagnostic criteria, and estimation of severity of DPN[8] and outlined principles of management. DSP remains a clinical diagnosis and equipment requiring an electrical power source usually is not needed in the assessment of peripheral nerve function.[6,19] Simple observation of the feet and legs with shoes and socks removed can identify signs of a neuropathic foot: small muscle wasting, clawing of toes, prominent metatarsal heads, dry skin and calluses, and occasionally bony deformity secondary to a Charcot neuroarthropathy. The clinical features of DSP are paralleling the "stocking-glove" pattern of the nerve fiber damage and sensory loss[6,7] that promotes the presence of symptoms and signs (Figure 44.1).

CLINICAL DIAGNOSIS OF DSP

History

The history may reveal the presence of risk factors strongly associated with DSP, including duration of diabetes, older age (e.g., >70 years), tall stature, and poorly controlled hyperglycemia.[14,15,48] History of dyslipidemia with elevated triglycerides and hypertension also may be present.[55] In addition, a history of recent falls should be elicited, which may reflect gait and balance disorders. In recording symptoms, the location, precipitating factors, and character are important as well as specific enquiry about nocturnal exacerbation. A brief enquiry about the patient's emotional affect particularly relating to the presence of anxiety or depressive symptomatology also is indicated.[9]

Symptoms and Signs. The symptoms associated with a diabetic DSP vary according to the class of sensory fibers involved (Table 44.3). Symptoms induced by the involvement of small nerve fibers include pain and dysesthesias (unpleasant abnormal sensations of burning, prickling, and stabbing). The intensity varies from minor discomfort to disabling pain that is worse at night and disturbs sleep (Table 44.3). Pain is often the reason patients with DSP seek medical care. Numbness symptoms (a perception that the feet feel "numb or asleep") usually are experienced in the same "stocking" pattern but may extend to the fingers and hands in more severe cases, resulting in the so-called stocking-glove neuropathy. The stocking distribution sensory "asleep or numb" sensory sensation usually is not particularly painful. These symptoms reflect large nerve fiber involvement and develop in the setting of distally impaired vibration, joint position, and touch-pressure sensations and abnormal (unequivocally diminished or absent) ankle reflexes.[68] The presence of the described DSP symptoms also have been linked to sleep disturbances and to additional adverse physical and psychological impairment, including balance loss, falls, and depression in association with a perception of poor quality of life.[4,5]

Table 44.3—Symptoms of DSP

Predominantly Small Fiber
- Pain
  - Sticking
  - Lancinating
  - Prickling
  - Burning
  - Aching
  - Boring
  - Excessively sensitive
- Dysesthesias (burning, tingling)
- Numbness

Predominantly Large Fiber
- Numbness
- Unsteady gait
- Balance loss

Some patients with a diabetic DSP may be asymptomatic, with the neurological deficits discovered by chance during a routine clinical examination,[68] while others who are initially aware of neuropathic symptoms become asymptomatic late in the course of the disease. A consequence of severe sensory loss resulting from diabetic DSP is painless injury and an increased risk of foot ulcerations, sometimes leading to amputation.[68] Objects lodged in the shoe, including a wrinkled stocking, frequently cause injury; unrecognized increased pressure during walking and weight bearing produces a blister that erodes through the skin. When the DSP is severe, distal weakness with foot drop may develop over time, as well as variable amounts of autonomic dysfunction.[8,69]

A clinical diagnosis of diabetic DSP is based on symptoms and signs of neuropathy in a patient with diabetes in whom other causes of neuropathy have been excluded.[8] The 2009 Toronto Consensus Panel on Diabetic Neuropathies updated the definitions and diagnostic criteria for DSP to represent several different categories of diagnostic "certainty," including possible, probable, confirmed, and subclinical.[8] *Possible DSP* was defined to require sensory symptoms appropriate for a length-dependent neuropathy *or* signs (including symmetrical decrease in distal sensation or unequivocally abnormal ankle reflexes). *Probable DSP* was defined to require at least two abnormalities among sensory symptoms, sensory signs, or ankle reflexes (again, representing appropriate symptoms and signs for a length-dependent neuropathy). *Confirmed DSP* required symptoms *or* signs (sensory or ankle reflexes) *and* an abnormal NCS, whereas *subclinical DSP* was defined as an abnormal NCS, with neither signs nor symptoms of DSP. An abnormal NCS requires evidence of abnormalities based on appropriate reference values and not limited to a single nerve (e.g., evidence consistent with a diffuse process).

Diagnosing a DSP that preferentially involves small nerve fibers can be challenging[11] and cannot be assessed by NCSs. The 2009 Toronto Consensus Panel–proposed definition of small fiber neuropathy (SFN)[7,70] included the following categories: *possible* (length-dependent symptoms or signs of small fiber damage), *probable* (length-dependent symptoms, clinical signs, and normal sural NCS), and *definite* (fulfilling definition of *probable and* an altered intraepidermal nerve fiber density [IENFD] density at the ankle or abnormal quantitative thermal threshold [foot]).[7,70] Markers of DSP that focus on small nerve fibers include nerve biopsy (invasive, highly specialized, and no longer utilized except in special situations), QST (for temperature discrimination and pain, covered previously), skin biopsy (for evaluation of IENFD), corneal confocal microscopy (CCM; potential surrogate for SFN), and nerve axon reflex or flare response (requires further validation).[7]

Several simple instruments can be used in clinical practice or for clinical trial assessment. The Michigan Neuropathy Screening Instrument (MNSI) developed by Feldman et al.[71] is a two-step instrument, which includes a 15-item yes-no symptom questionnaire followed by a clinical examination.[10,71] The clinical examination part has a high sensitivity and specificity for identifying DSP.[71,72] The MNSI, and especially the clinical examination, has been used most extensively, including in major large clinical trials such as the DCCT/EDIC,[51,72] ACCORD, and BARI 2D.[25,73] The Toronto Clinical Neuropathy Score[74] and the Utah Neuropathy Scale[75] are two other similar instruments that were validated against morphological criteria or nerve conduction velocities and nerve conduction amplitude. Likewise, the simplified Neuropathy Disability Score requires a simple clinical examination that sums abnormalities of reflexes and sensory assessments and has been used in clinical practice and in epidemiological studies.[10,19,76] The McGill Pain Questionnaire, which consists of descriptive symptoms from which the patients select those that best describe their experience, was found to be a sensitive measure for diabetic neuropathy pain.[10] Finally, because neuropathic symptoms are a source of severe emotional distress, an assessment of the patient's psychological status and quality of life also are emerging as part of the assessment of DPN; specific instruments have been developed and validated for use in diabetic neuropathy, such as NeuroQol[77] and the Norfolk Quality of Life Instrument.[78]

Overall, accurate recording of symptoms (see previous section and Table 44.3) as described by the patient and a careful clinical examination are essential for diagnosis in both clinical practice and clinical trials.

Limitations of the Clinical Diagnosis. Although most physicians probably assume that the clinical diagnosis of DSP is straightforward, this assumption recently was challenged by the results of a study in which 12 physicians (diabetologists and neurologists) who were all experienced in the assessment of diabetic neuropathy were required to evaluate 24 diabetic subjects on two occasions.[79] The physicians were masked to the identity and characteristics of the patients, who wore gowns and had their faces covered and their voices distorted, and the results of the two evaluations were used to determine diagnostic proficiency (based on accuracy and intra- or inter-evaluator variability). The study results were surprising and showed that evaluators showed poor proficiency, overestimating DSP compared to gold-standard 75% group diagnosis and summated electrophysiological scores. In a second study of the same physicians, in which specific instructions were provided to base clinical diagnoses only on unequivocally abnormal symptoms and signs, while taking age (~50% of the diabetic subjects were >70 years old), sex, and physical variables into account, proficiency improved greatly and abnormal clinical signs were not overreported.[80,81]

Last, the diagnosis of DSP requires exclusion of other causes, because no distinguishing features are unique to DSP. Therefore, all other possible causes of the observed neuropathy (e.g., hypothyroidism, cyanocobalamin deficiency, uremia, chronic alcoholism) must be ruled out by careful history and then must be confirmed by physical examination and laboratory tests. Some of these conditions occur more frequently in people with diabetes and, therefore, may coexist.

DIAGNOSTIC TESTS

Nerve Conduction Studies

NCS have for years been considered the gold-standard diagnostic tests for DPN, as they include objective measures, do not rely on a patient's response, and presumably have high reliability. An abnormal NCS is considered one of the first quantitative indicators of diabetic DSP,[7] an impression that is reinforced by the regular finding of motor conduction velocity slowing near the lower limit of normal among asymptomatic, neurologically intact diabetic patients or among individuals without known diabetes, leading to the diagnosis of diabetes.[11] The 2009 Toronto Consensus Panel reviewed the use of NCSs in the evaluation of diabetic DSP.[8] The panel concluded that composite sum scores based off normal deviations involving several nerves (from percentiles) employing NCS attributes known to be sensitive to DPS (e.g., fibular and tibial conduction velocity, sural amplitude) performed "best" in diagnosing DSP, recognizing that a single gold standard is lacking. Unfortunately, this recommended approach is not available to most physicians. The panel also considered more easily applied criteria, including use of at least one abnormal NCS attribute (e.g., amplitude or conduction velocity) in two separate lower-extremity nerves based on 1st and 99th percentile reference values), a criterion that also performed well.[8] Further requiring that the sural nerve be included among the nerves studied[82] produced similar favorable results. The panel further emphasized that to produce reliable results, NCSs must be done rigorously, with careful attention to measuring and maintaining appropriate limb temperature, electrode placement, "just supramaximal" stimulation levels, and accurate measurement of distances, and establishing evidence of "abnormality" using reference values corrected for appropriate variables.[7,8] Just as clinical proficiency performed below expectations, however, an extension of the clinical study of diabetic DSP[79] to include an evaluation of NCS proficiency showed similar, somewhat disappointing results, challenging the assumption that carefully performed NCS results are reliable indicators of abnormality. The study showed that individual electromyographers showed high intraobserver agreement without significant differences on repeat testing. Statistically significant interobserver differences, however, were observed for most NCS attributes,[80] a finding that was reduced but not eliminated by the use of uniform NCS technique, standard references, and broader categorization of abnormality. The small but statistically significant interexaminer differences were unlikely to be clinically meaningful in terms of use in medical practice involving the evaluation of diabetic DSP. The finding raised concern, however, for use in therapeutic trials and supported the conclusion of previous investigators[83] who concluded that the same clinical electrophysiologists should perform serial NCSs for a given subject to obtain the most ideal results.

Quantitative Sensory Testing. QST assesses the patient's ability to detect sensory stimuli including light touch, vibration, and temperature discrimination. Most QST results are a function of the patient's concentration and cooperation, however, and therefore involve a certain degree of subjectivity. An abnormal finding may not necessarily indicate DSP, as the abnormality may lie anywhere in the afferent neural pathway. QSTs vary in complexity. Simpler instruments such as monofilaments and tuning forks can be used in day-to-day clinical practice. More sophisticated instruments, usually requiring more expensive equipment and an external power source, commonly are used for more detailed assessment and for follow-up assessments in clinical trials.[10] The more commonly used techniques are briefly described in the following sections.

Semmes-Weinstein Monofilaments. These monofilaments test light-touch pressure, a function of large myelinated fibers, and include sets of nylon filaments of variable diameter that buckle at a predefined force when applied to the testing site, usually the halluces and plantar surfaces of the metatarsal-phalangeal joints area. They are used widely in clinical practice and are particularly helpful in identifying individuals who are at risk of neuropathic foot ulceration. The inability to perceive pressure of 10 grams (5.07-g) monofilaments has been shown in prospective studies to be indicative of risk for neuropathic ulceration.[84]

Vibration Perception. A number of devices have been designed specifically to assess the vibration perception threshold, indicative of large myelinated fiber function.[10] In clinical practice, it usually is evaluated using a simple, 128 Hz tuning fork applied at the big toe bilaterally, using a forced choice algorithm. Alternatively, a variety of more sophisticated instruments (e.g., Vibratron II, Neurothesiometer, computer-assisted sensory examinations [CASE IV]) may be used for clinical research that follow specific algorithms developed to facilitate sensory threshold determination. The vibration perception threshold increases with age in individuals without diabetes and also tends to be higher in the lower extremities. More recently, a simple pocket-size disposable device, the Vibratrip, has been developed to test vibration sensation in the clinical setting and may be useful for the prediction of patients at risk for foot ulceration.[85]

Thermal and Cooling Thresholds. Warm and cold sensations are transmitted by small myelinated and unmyelinated fibers and can be assessed using a number of devices. Usually these are CASEs (CASE IV, Medoc), using a forced-choice algorithm.[8] Because these tests tend to be expensive, they are used mostly for clinical research and for detailed clinical assessment.[8,19]

Skin Biopsy and Intraepidermal Nerve Fiber Density. Immunohistochemical quantification of IENFD using punch skin biopsies has been used increasingly to quantify SFNs in diabetes.[86] The distal leg skin biopsy, with quantification of the linear density of IENFD using generally agreed-on counting rules, is a reliable technique for SFN.[87-89] Intra- and interobserver variability for the assessment of IENFD demonstrates good agreement.[89,90] IENFD declines with age and does not appear to be influenced by weight or height,[91] and therefore, the analysis of IENFD always should refer to normative values matched for age.[89] No study assessing the sensitivity and specificity of IENFD in DSN is available. Several studies in SFN, however, have included patients with DSP. In 58 patients with pure SFN, a cutoff IENFD of ≤8.8/mm at the ankle was associated with a sensitivity of 77.2% and a specificity of 79.6%.[7,92] In a study of 210 patients with SFN, which included 65 diabetic patients, the receiver operating characteristic (ROC) curve analysis had the highest specificity and sensitivity.[7,70,93] A reduced IENFD was shown to be associated with the risk of developing neuropathic pain, although it does not correlate with its intensity,[88-90] and correlates inversely with thermal thresholds.[70]

The use of IENFD is not yet recommended as a routine in the clinical practice, but it has emerged as an objective small fiber measure for clinical trials evaluating new therapeutic interventions for DSP.[7,11,70,89,94-96]

Corneal Confocal Microscopy. CCM is a novel reiterative in vivo noninvasive clinical examination technique that is capable of imaging corneal nerve fibers.[97] Corneal nerve fiber damage correlates with IENFD loss and severity of neuropathy in patients with diabetes and is more marked in patients with painful diabetic neuropathy.[79,98] CCM has been shown to improve 6 months after restoration of euglycemia following pancreas transplantation in patients with T1D.[99] As with IENFD, this technique is not recommended for use in routine clinical care and requires further validation studies for larger implementation in clinical studies.

Nerve Axon Reflex and Flare Response. Nerve axon reflex and flare response is a technique based on the stimulation of the nociceptive C fibers, resulting in both orthodromic conduction to the spinal cord and antidromic conduction to other axon branches (i.e., the axon reflex). This stimulates the release of peptides, such as substance P and calcitonin gene–related peptide, resulting in vasodilation and increased permeability.[70] Studies have shown that this neurovascular response mediated by the nerve axon reflex is reduced in patients with diabetic neuropathy, correlates with other nerve function measurements, and has reasonable sensitivity and specificity in identifying patients with diabetic neuropathy. Similarly with CCM, the use of this technique as a potential surrogate for SFN requires further validation.

Assessment of Sudomotor Function. Assessment of sudomotor function may be done with a variety of more or less complex techniques and equipment. Quantitative sudomotor axon reflex testing (QSART) evaluates sudomotor function by assessing the local sweat response to iontophoresis of acetylcholine, evaluating the postganglionic axon function. The complexity of the technique and requirements for highly specialized infrastructure and personnel limits the use of QSART in both clinical practice and research.[100] Alternatively, the Neuropad test is a simple visual indicator test, which uses a color change to define the integrity of skin sympathetic cholinergic innervation. Neuropad responses have been shown to correlate with some measure of DPN, but this test has relatively low sensitivity and specificity.[100] Other devices also can provide a quantitative assessment of sudomotor function using direct current stimulation and reverse iontophoresis. These devices measure the ability of sweat glands to release chloride ions in response to electrochemical activation by recording local skin conductance.[101]

LATE COMPLICATIONS OF DSP

Diabetic Foot Ulcers

Several longitudinal studies have confirmed that DSP is a major contributory factor in the pathogenesis of foot ulceration in diabetes.[2,19,76,84] Therefore, screening of all patients with diabetes at least annually is recommended for the identification of the neuropathic foot at risk of ulceration.[84] The American Diabetes Association (ADA) recommends that an annual comprehensive foot examination should be performed in all patients with diabetes to identify risk factors predictive of ulcers or amputations.[102] The foot examination should include inspection, assessment of foot pulses, and testing for loss of protective sensation with the use of 10-gram monofilaments plus one other test that might include 128 Hz tuning fork, pin-prick, or ankle reflexes.[102] The identification of the high-risk foot is different from the early diagnosis of neuropathy. Once the foot examination reveals the presence of risk factors for foot ulceration, comprehensive quantitative testing for DPN is not required to make this diagnosis. Any patient found to have neuropathy of sufficient severity to put them at risk of foot ulceration requires education and preventive foot care and podiatric care.[84]

Charcot Neuroarthropathy

Charcot neuroarthropathy is much less common than foot ulceration but is a clinically important and potentially devastating disorder that commonly leads to ulceration.[103] In the 21st century, diabetes is the most common cause of this condition in countries in the Western hemisphere.[104] It is more frequent than commonly perceived, with a prevalence of 0.8—7.5% of all patients with diabetes also having neuropathy, and in up 35% of cases, it may become bilateral.[103] A high degree of awareness and suspicion may enable early diagnosis and effective intervention. Permissive factors for the development of Charcot neuroarthropathy include history of poor glucose control, DPN, sympathetic denervation in the foot, and an intact peripheral circulation.[103,104] Mild unperceived or repetitive traumas are often the precipitating event.[10] It is believed that following repetitive minor trauma, osteoblastic activity is stimulated with remodeling of bones.[10,105] A neurovascular theory involving an increase in bone blood flow, perhaps associated with increased arteriovenous shunting because of a reduction in tone of vasoconstrictor innervations, with subsequent bone resorption ultimately leading to fracture and deformities, was also invoked.[105] More recent data indicate that bone remodeling is increased in subjects with Charcot neuroarthropathy. Levels of urinary cross-linked N-telopeptides and pyridinoline cross-linked carboxy-terminal telopeptide of type I collagen consistent with increased bone resorption and alkaline phosphatase (a marker of osteoblast activity) have been shown to be increased in patients with acute Charcot neuroarthopathy.[106,107]

Any patient with known DPN who has a unilateral, unexplained swollen, warm foot should be considered to have acute Charcot neuroarthropathy until proven otherwise.[107] Asymptomatic fractures are discovered in 22% of patients with diabetes and with neuropathy.

The location of the radiological bony changes can give good clues as to the underlying diagnosis. For example, neuropathic osteoarthropathy is primarily an articular disease and is most common at the Lisfranc (tarsometatarsal) joint, which can lead to lateral and superior subluxation of the metatarsal heads and the development of a rocker-bottom foot deformity (Figure 44.2).[107] Involvement of Chopart (transverse tarsal) joints is also common and initial pathology often affects the medial column of the foot. Finally, neuropathic arthropathy tends to involve several joints in a region, whereas infection tends to remain localized or spread contiguously. Secondary ulceration and infection of the Charcot foot is common, however, and can create considerable difficulties in distinguishing osteomyelitis from neuroarthopathy.[107]

PATHOGENESIS

As with the epidemiology and diagnosis, most of the available information regarding the pathogenesis of DPN refers to DSP. The development and progression of DSP occur within the heterogeneous environment of the peripheral nerve and involves a complex interplay between the nerve and surrounding cells and

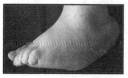

Figure 44.2—Charcot foot image. Obtained from the personal collection of Dr. Crystal Holmes, DPM.

tissue.[108] The disease pathogenesis, however, continues to be incompletely understood, which is one of the reasons for the paucity of therapeutic options.

Hyperglycemia plays a key role in the activation of various biochemical pathways related to the metabolic or redox state of the cell, which, in concert with impaired nerve perfusion, contribute to the development and progression of diabetic neuropathies. The importance of hyperglycemia in the pathogenesis of neuropathy has received strong support from landmark studies, such as the DCCT.[14,15,109] In the DCCT, the benefits of 6.5 years of intensive control were maintained for at least 13–14 years after the end of the study.[16,110]

Hyperglycemia-induced increased oxidative and nitrosative stress, with a subsequent increase in free radical production, is a major mechanism of DSP in animal models and in human disease.[111–115] The increased generation of free radicals and the compromised endogenous antioxidant defenses in diabetes were shown to lead to injurious oxidation of proteins and lipids, a process that was involved in promoting cellular apoptosis and the activation of other important pathways, including activation of polyADP ribosylation or activation of genes involved in neuronal damage, in dorsal root ganglia neurons.[111,116,117] In addition to hyperglycemia, decreased nerve blood flow,[118–121] dyslipidemia,[122,123] and lack of insulin signaling[113] also contribute to the activation of several pathogenic pathways with an impact on the peripheral and autonomic neuronal function in diabetes. Other important mechanisms involve formation of advanced glycation end products (AGEs) and downregulation of the soluble receptor for AGE (sRAGE), activation of polyol aldose reductase signaling, activation of the protein kinase C pathways, impaired Na^+/K^+-ATPase activity, and mitochondrial dysfunction.[111,116,117,124–128] C-peptide–related signaling pathways also have been shown to be associated with beneficial outcomes on measures of DSP in animal models.[128] C-peptide provides an insulin-like signaling function that modulates early metabolic perturbations of neural Na^+/K^+-ATPase and nitric oxide, with subsequent preventive effects on early nerve dysfunction, that is relevant to DSP. Further corrective consequences resulting from this signaling cascade may have beneficial effects on gene regulation of early gene responses, neurotrophic factors, their receptors, and the insulin receptor itself.[129–132] Recent evidence suggests that low-grade inflammation also may play an important role in the pathogenesis of diabetic neuropathies, mediated by NF-κB activation and downstream effects,[133,134] inducing deficits in peripheral and autonomic nerve fibers.[133,135] An ample overview of recent findings linking the role of inflammatory cytokines and adipocytokines on neural and autonomic imbalance in diabetes and prediabetes was covered by Vinik.[125]

Others have described an important role played by mitochondria in the development of experimental DSP. For instance, altered mitochondrial bioenergetics[127] or impaired mitochondrial function in adult sensory neurons or dorsal root ganglia have been described by several groups of investigators[127,136,137] and appeared to be modulated by the heat shock protein (Hsp) 70.[137] Recent experimental evidence obtained in rodent models of T1D and T2D also implicates endoplasmic reticulum (ER) stress as a novel mechanism in the onset and progression of DPN.[108] ER homeostasis may be disrupted by a variety of stressors, including hyperglycemia, altered redox status, increases in unsaturated fatty acids or cholesterol, nutrient deprivation, and perturbation of calcium balance. These may lead to the accumulation of unfolded or misfolded proteins within the luminal space of the ER and activation of the unfolded protein response (UPR), a well-orchestrated signaling cascade responsible for relieving stress and restoring normal ER function.[108] During times of extreme or chronic stress, the capacity of the UPR is overwhelmed, and the resulting failure to alleviate ER stress triggers apoptotic processes via several pathways, including association with tumor necrosis factor receptor–associated factor 2 (TRAF2) and apoptosis signal-regulating kinase 1 (ASK1), with subsequent c-jun-N-terminal-kinase (JNK) activation;[138] activation of the ER calcium channel inositol 1,4,5–triphosphate (IP3) triggering release of calcium stores into the cytosol, mitochondrial membrane depolarization, and cytochrome c release;[139] or via cleavage of pro-caspase-12 within the ER and caspase signaling initiation.[140] In animal models of diabetes, treatment with chemical chaperones or ER stress inhibitors was shown to alleviate ER stress and improve peripheral nerve function,[108] although these outcomes could have been the result of an improvement in ER stress in pancreatic β-cells and improvement in the metabolic profile.[141,142]

Emerging data in human studies also have reported that peripheral nerve dysfunction may occur before the development of diabetic-range hyperglycemia in individuals with features of the metabolic syndrome or in patients with impaired glucose tolerance.[39,96] These changes appear to correlate with an increase in adipose tissue–derived inflammatory markers.[143,144] It is generally accepted that in human diabetes, the development of DPNs is a function of complex interactions among the degree of glycemic control, disease duration, age-related neuronal attrition, and other risk factors, including systolic and diastolic blood pressure, lipid variables, and weight.[55,60,145,146] These promote progressive peripheral and autonomic neural dysfunction in a fashion that begins distally and progresses proximally. A detailed review of each of these mechanisms and pathways and their complex interactions, however, is beyond the scope of this chapter.

TREATMENT

Treatment for DSP includes therapies that might alter (slow) the progressive loss of nerve function and otherwise are known as pathogenetic or disease-modifying agents and therapies for symptomatic relief.[13] Some medications have efficacy in both these areas. This section primarily covers the management of painful symptomatic DSP. Although there are no specific therapies for painless neuropathy, all these patients warrant foot care education and regular podiatric care as part of DSP treatment to prevent ulcers and late complications.[84]

Disease-Modifying Therapies

Glycemic Control. Of all the therapies for DSP, tight and stable glycemic control is to date the only approach that was shown to prevent and/or delay DSP development in T1D and may possibly have an effect in in preventing progression of neuropathy and provide symptomatic relief in some patients with T2D.[14–16,25,31,32,44,48,49,50] Some evidence suggests that rapid changes in blood glucose may induce neuropathic pain; therefore, glycemic stability may be important in pain relief or pain prevention.[27]

Multiple Risk Factor Intervention. An intensive multifactorial cardiovascular risk intervention targeting glucose, blood pressure, lipids, smoking, and other lifestyle factors in a European cohort of patients with T2D had no effect on the development or progression of DSP, although it reduced the progression or the development of autonomic neuropathy.[147]

Lifestyle Interventions. Lifestyle changes including healthy diet and exercise were shown to significantly reduce the prevalence of diabetes and complications, including DSP.[148] Large, randomized controlled trials also have established that the type of exercise is important. Specifically, a combination of aerobic and resistance exercise not only improves physical fitness, glycemic control, and insulin sensitivity in people with diabetes,[149] but also could affect complications risk. For instance, in a clinical trial that enrolled patients with DSP associated with impaired glucose tolerance, a prediabetic state, lifestyle interventions including diet and exercise have been shown to improve both neuropathic symptoms and IENFD and also may beneficially affect complications risk.[96] A more recent pilot study that enrolled patients with diabetes and with DSP, also described improvements in IENFD measures with a supervised moderately intense aerobic and resistance training.[150]

α-Lipoic Acid. Experimental evidence suggests that free radical–mediated oxidative stress is implicated in the pathogenesis of DSP and that treatment with the antioxidant α-lipoic acid (ALA) might help prevent these abnormalities, slow the development of DSP, and improve painful symptoms.[151,152] This agent therefore is regarded as a pathogenetic therapy that also helps symptoms. An earlier meta-analysis of the use of intravenous ALA supported some efficacy in painful DSP,[153] an effect that was confirmed in a more recent long-term study of oral ALA that reported a clinically meaningful improvement of symptoms.[151] No difference was identified between ALA and placebo, however, in the primary DSP composite endpoint (a composite of the Neuropathy Impairment Score [NIS]-Lower Limb and seven neurophysiologic tests) or in secondary endpoints that included NCS or QST.[151] Most recently, a smaller randomized double-blind clinical trial comparing a triple antioxidant combination that included ALA versus placebo in patients with T1D had no effect on any objective measures of DPN, including NCSs and IENFD.[154]

C-Peptide. The potential mechanisms of C-peptide in preventing DSP have been discussed. Several small-scale clinical trials reported beneficial effects on measures of DSP and cardiac autonomic neuropathy (CAN) in men.[155,156] A larger phase 3 clinical trial evaluating the effects of C-peptide in patients with T1D and mild-to-moderate DPN is currently ongoing (ClinicalTrials.gov Identifier:NCT01681290).

Other Agents. Additional pathogenic therapies include aldose-reductase inhibitors, various other antioxidants including vitamins E and C, recombinant nerve growth factors, acetyl-carnitine, and actovegin. At present, randomized, controlled studies generally have shown a lack of efficacy on objective measures of DSP.[157,158] Similarly, a recent small randomized trial comparing the effectiveness of a combination of L-methylfolate, methylcobalamin, and pyridoxal-5'-phosphate versus placebo in patients with T2D also failed to show a benefit on objective measures of DSP, although some participants reported some improvement in neuropathic symptoms.[159]

Symptomatic Therapies

A major challenge to effective therapies for the relief of symptoms in DSP involves the lack of strong clinical evidence regarding which treatments are likely to work for which patients, given the wide range of available medications. Specific symptomatic therapies, however, generally are recommended, as they are thought to improve the patient's quality of life.

Pain is usually the symptom that triggers medical care attention for most patients. Because neuropathic pain affects many areas of the patient's life, a multidisciplinary approach is essential in managing the condition. In many cases, the clinical assessment will indicate the need for psychological or physical therapy in addition to standard pharmacologic treatments. Similarly, support and information on practical measures, such as using a bed cradle to lift the bedclothes off hyperaesthetic skin, often prove invaluable. Although the achievement of stable glycemic control and a full patient assessment are crucial first steps in the management of neuropathy, most patients with painful symptoms, often with sleep disturbance, will require pharmacologic therapy.

Table 44.4—Main Agents for Treating Neuropathic Pain

Anticonvulsants

Pregabalin[150–152]
- Is FDA approved for treatment of DPN pain.
- Binds to and modulates voltage-gated calcium channels.
- Is a more potent regulator of calcium channels than gabapentin (it is this mode of action that may modulate neuropathic pain).
- Has been found to significantly decrease mean pain score in people with painful DPN compared with placebo.
- Main adverse effects include dizziness, somnolence, weight gain, peripheral edema, blurred vision, and constipation.
- It is a controlled (scheduled) drug in the U.S., and, unlike its predecessor gabapentin, there is a possibility it could be habit-forming.
- The maximum approved dose for DPN pain is 300 mg/day in divided doses; stepwise titration is recommended.

Gabapentin[150,151]
- Has been found to improve pain in people with DPN in several studies.
- Although not FDA approved for the treatment of pain associated with DPN, it is one of the most widely used agents in clinical practice.
- Adverse effects that may require discontinuation of therapy include dizziness, ataxia, somnolence or confusion (especially in older people), headache, nausea, diarrhea, weight gain.
- Dose titration usually starts with 300 mg three times/day, but doses as high as 3,600 mg/day may be required in some patients because of tachyphylaxis.

Serotonin and norepinephrine reuptake inhibitors (SNRIs)

Duloxetine[150,153]
- It is the second FDA-approved agent for use in painful DPN.
- It is a selective dual SNRI and is relatively balanced in its affinity for reuptake inhibition.

(continued)

Table 44.4—Main Agents for Treating Neuropathic Pain *(continued)*

- The spectrum of side effects is superior to the tricyclic agents but less favorable compared with pregabalin.
- Patients frequently experience nausea with initiation of therapy; a slow titration of the drug usually can avoid this common adverse effect.
- Most common adverse effects, besides nausea, are sedation and generalized sleepiness.
- Duloxetine does not usually require dose titration, with most patients requiring 60 mg daily, occasionally 60 mg twice daily.
- May be combined with pregabalin or gabapentin, which usually require lower doses for all.

Venlafaxine[150]
- Venlafaxine has been found to be probably effective in lessening the pain of DPN and is recommended to be considered for treatment.[150]
- Dose should be progressively titrated, selecting the minimum effective dose to mitigate side effects.
- Most common adverse effects include nausea, sedation, dizziness, and generalized sleepiness.

Tricyclic antidepressants (TCAs)[150]
- Act by blocking neuronal reuptake of norepinephrine and serotonin, thereby potentiating the inhibitory effect of these neurotransmitters in nociceptive pathways.
- Amitriptyline, imipramine, and desipramine have all been found, in small RCTs, to relieve pain better than placebo in patients with DPN.[150]
- Additional support for the efficacy of TCAs was provided by a meta-analysis of 21 clinical trials.
- Adverse effects are common and sometime troublesome with TCAs and may lead to treatment withdrawal.
- In clinical trials of TCAs, ~20% of participants withdrew because of intolerable adverse effects, such as severe sedation, confusion, and anticholinergic adverse effects. Suicidal ideation also was described.
- Side effects are particularly problematic in older patients, in whom it is advisable to start at low dosages nightly.
- The most commonly used TCAs may be ranked in order from most to least associated with anticholinergic effects as follows: amitriptyline, imipramine, nortriptyline, and desipramine.

Opioid analgesics[85,150]
- They are considered second-line approaches.
- Suppress pain by activating μ-receptors, which are present on the pre- and postsynaptic membranes of primary afferent nerve fibers, second-order neurons in the dorsal horn of the spinal cord, and neurons in pain-relevant supraspinal centers.
- May be considered either in combination with existing therapies or for use alone.
- Are used commonly for DPN pain, but have significant adverse effects with long-term use.
- Dependence may occur.
- Oxycodone has been found to be superior to placebo in the treatment of DPN pain.
- Tramadol (a weak opioid that acts through low-affinity binding to micro-opioid receptors and weak inhibition of norepinephrine and serotonin reuptake) also has been found to be effective in treatment of pain in DPN. It is often good treatment for breakthrough or refractory pain.

Topical capsaicin cream
- May be used in combination with other therapies or alone for pain that is refractory.
- Stimulates the release and subsequent depletion of substance P from sensory nerve fibers.
- A few small studies have demonstrated the effectiveness of capsaicin cream in control of pain and improvement in daily activities.[85]

- Poor adherence is common because of the need for frequent applications, an initial exacerbation of symptoms, and frequent burning and redness at the application site.

Transcutaneous electrical nerve stimulation (TENS) or acupuncture
- May be added on to existing therapy or used alone in refractory cases.
- Uncontrolled studies of TENS and of acupuncture have been reported to decrease pain in patients with DPN.
- A report of the Therapeutics and Technology Assessment Subcommittee of the American Academy of Neurology, based on a review of the literature up to April 2009, concluded that TENS may have some effectiveness for reducing pain caused by diabetic peripheral neuropathy, but there is no evidence for confirmed efficacy in well-designed randomized trials.[13]

Anticonvulsants. Pregabalin is one of the two drugs currently approved for relief of DSP pain in the U.S. Pregabalin (highest level of evidence) and gabapentin have proven efficacy in large, randomized controlled trials for the relief of neuropathic pain,[160] but neither of these affords complete relief. In addition, pregabalin is known to have an antianxiolytic effect, which also may be helpful.[161,162] Their adverse effects seem to be less pronounced than those associated with tricyclic agents.[161,162] There is little evidence to support the use of any other anticonvulsant agents in the therapy of neuropathic pain.[160]

Serotonin and Norepinephrine Reuptake Inhibitors. The serotonin and norepinephrine reuptake inhibitor (SNRI) duloxetine is the other drug approved by the U.S. Food and Drug Administration for pain associated with DSP. It has both analgesic and antidepressive effects that can be useful in the treatment of neuropathic pain.[163] Duloxetine usually does not require dose titration, with most patients requiring once-daily dosing. As with pregabalin, when used as monotherapy in most cases, it may not provide complete pain relief. The side-effect profile is superior to that of the tricyclic agents. Venlafaxine has been found to be probably effective in lessening the pain associated with DSP and is recommended to be considered for treatment.[160] Pregabalin-duloxetin combination therapy recently has been assessed in a double-blind, parallel-group study in patients with painful DSP who are not responding to standard doses of duloxetine or pregabalin alone.[164] Although not significantly superior to high-dose monotherapy, combination therapy was considered to be effective for DSP pain and was well tolerated.[164]

Tricyclic Antidepressants. Tricyclic drugs such as amitriptyline and imipramine remain useful agents for painful neuropathy. Their efficacy, confirmed only in small randomized placebo controlled trials,[160] is related to plasma drug level, and the onset of symptomatic relief is faster than the antidepressant effect. Although with proven efficacy, these agents have troublesome, sedating, and anticholinergic side effects, which are also dose related and often restrict their use. Side effects are particularly problematic in older patients in whom it is advisable to start at low dosages nightly.[10,13]

Other Treatment Approaches. Second-line approaches include the use of opiates such as the synthetic opioid tramadol, or for more severe discomfort, controlled-release oxycodone.[13,160] Alternatively, topical and physical treatments may offer several theoretical advantages, including minimal systemic side effects and lack of drug interactions; however, few have been evaluated in well-designed randomized controlled trials. Agents that have been used include capsaicin, lidocaine patches, and isosorbide dinitrate spray.[13] Similarly, a number of nonpharmacological agents have been proposed, including acupuncture and various electrical stimulation therapies, but none has confirmed efficacy in well-designed randomized trials.[13]

A major problem in the area of the treatment of neuropathic pain in diabetes is a relative lack of head-to-head studies that also include quality-of-life outcomes. Most cited studies have compared active agents against placebo, and there is a need for more comparisons of two potentially active agents. As previously mentioned, the recently reported study comparing high doses of pregabalin and duloxetine as monotherapies or in combination for 8 weeks in patients with painful DSP found no significant differences between combination and high-dose monotherapy regarding average pain change or response rate.[164] Given the range of partially effective treatment options, a tailored and stepwise pharmacologic strategy, often combining several agents, with careful attention to relative symptom improvement, medication adherence, and medication side effects, may be necessary to achieve pain reduction and improve quality of life.[165]

ATYPICAL FORMS OF DPN

Atypical subtypes of DPN generally have distinguishing features such as subacute onset with a monophasic or fluctuating course over time, with various combinations of preferential involvement of small sensory nerves or motor nerves,[8] prominent pain, or asymmetry. The diabetic mononeuropathies are included among the atypical DPNs.

DIABETIC RADICULOPLEXUS NEUROPATHY

Diabetic radiculoplexus neuropathy (DRPN), also called proximal motor neuropathy, most often presents with a lumbosacral distribution (where it is also known as diabetic amyotrophy). Less frequently, a DRPN presents in acervical or thoracic distribution. DRPN is thought to affect ~1% of patients with diabetes and includes those who are typically middle age or older, are more likely to have T2D, and may be otherwise asymptomatic.[69,166] DRPN is not related to the duration or severity of diabetes, initiation of diabetes treatment, level of glycemic control, or presence or absence of an underlying DSP or other consequences of diabetes.[11,22,69] DRPN typically presents over days with severe proximal pain that, in the case of a lumbosacral DRPN, involves the low back, hip, and anterior thigh. The onset may be unilateral or bilateral, but when it is bilateral, it presents asymmetrically, involving one side predominantly.[11,69,167] The pain at times is severe and difficult to manage, sometimes requiring opioids that have limited effectiveness. Following the onset of pain, progressive weakness appears shortly thereafter in a similar distribution involving the proximal leg. The pain and weakness spread in a progressive or stepwise manner over weeks to months, involving nearby and contralateral segments. As an approximation, ~50% of patients with a unilateral

DRPN develop contralateral symptoms within ~6 months, and occasional patients go on to develop an asymmetric quadriparesis.[168] This asymmetric painful condition almost always shows an initial proximal predilection, but distal limb segments eventually become involved to some extent in most patients.[11] Weak muscles, such as those in the thigh, develop profound atrophy, and bilateral weakness may result in wheelchair dependence. Weight loss is common, in association with anorexia resulting from severe pain and loss of muscle mass in the involved muscles. Among patients with DRPN, about half experience prominent dysautonomia with combinations of orthostatic intolerance and change in sexual, bladder, and bowel function.[11,69] Unlike DSP, DRPN has a monophasic course, with improvement beginning within 9–12 months of onset and with a prolonged recovery over years that is often incomplete recovery.[11,69]

DRPN is thought to reflect a multifocal ischemic injury due to an immune-mediated microvasculitis involving motor, sensory, and autonomic fibers in the plexus, nerve root, and individual nerves.[169,170] This impression is supported by the frequent appearance of stepwise deterioration, with clinical and electromyography (EMG) evidence of multifocal distribution. This presumed pathogenesis has resulted in use of immunotherapy treatments and anecdotal reports that intravenous (IV) immunoglobulin (Ig)[171] or IV methylprednisolone[166] reduces pain and weakness. Nevertheless, efficacy is unproven and no controlled studies convincingly support the use of immunotherapy treatment.[172,173]

A painless form of DRPN also has been described. This condition resembles "diabetic amyotrophy" in all ways aside from absence of the characteristic pain and greater clinical symmetry.[174] It is unclear whether this painless radiculoplexus neuropathy is a variant of DRPN or a chronic inflammatory demyelinating polyneuropathy (CIDP).[174] Painful forms of radiculoplexus neuropathy (e.g., idiopathic brachial plexus neuropathy) that are indistinguishable from DRPN also occur in the absence of diabetes,[166] but they alternatively may be the presenting condition leading to a diagnosis of diabetes.[172]

ACUTE SMALL FIBER NEUROPATHY

Several atypical neuropathies associated with diabetes are characterized by subacute onset (days) and prominent involvement of small fibers. These so-called SFNs present with painful sensations in the legs. They progress over days to weeks to constant burning dysesthesias and allodynia (excessive sensitivity to touch)[12,69] involving the legs in a stocking distribution with occasional spread to proximal sites including the trunk or more diffusely.[11] Autonomic features may be prominent. Despite the prominent pain, sensory loss may be mild or absent, there is no weakness, and reflexes are preserved unless there is an underlying DSP.[12] The clinical course is a brief monophasic crescendo[11] followed by improvement and resolving within 3–18 months.[12,175] Because these SFNs preferentially involve small nerve fibers, they are not readily assessed by NCSs[175] but require other measures, such as assessment of thermal thresholds, R-R variation, sweat production, orthostatic blood pressure, or skin biopsy to assess IENFD.[176] Furthermore, although acute SFNs often present in a length-dependent distribution, their monophasic course makes it very unlikely that they are part of the DSP spectrum.[11,69] The only known treatment involves control of pain and symptomatic attention to dysautonomia, when severe.[32] Two closely related subtypes of diabetic SFN differ mostly in associated factors (e.g., weight loss or initiation of intensive glycemic control) and in the degree of autonomic involvement.[11,12,69]

SFN with weight loss is a painful SFN associated with profound weight loss (e.g., >25%) and sometimes is referred to as diabetic cachexia. The weight loss usually precedes the onset of severe burning pain and allodynia but sometimes develops at the onset of pain or even as the pain subsides.[11,69] Patients with T2D are afflicted most often, and most, but not all, cases are unrelated to initiation or change in treatment or degree of glycemic control.[177] The mechanism associating weight loss and a severe diabetic SFN is unknown. The prognosis is good with full recovery and pain resolving in the setting of adequate glycemic control and weight gain.[11]

Treatment-induced SFN (at times described as "insulin neuritis") is another painful SFN with sudden onset. This SFN, however, is linked temporally to the onset of intensive treatment, developing within 2–4 weeks (occasionally up to 6 weeks) after rapid and sustained glycemic control with insulin, oral hypoglycemic agents, or diet.[176,178] It is experienced by patients with either T1D or T2D.[176] Aside from the timing of onset relative to rapid glycemic control, no abnormal laboratory values or other evaluations suggest other causes. Weight loss is not a major feature of this SFN, although some patients report a past history of withholding insulin for weight loss (diabetic anorexia).[176] As mentioned previously, occasional patients experience profound weight loss after initiating intensive treatment but before the onset of pain,[177] blurring the distinction between treatment-induced and weight-loss SFN. Dysautonomia frequently is a prominent feature of treatment-induced SFN. A recent study of 16 subjects with treatment-induced SFN showed that all had autonomic symptoms and signs, including orthostatic hypotension and parasympathetic dysfunction in two-thirds of the patients.[176] This SFN generally is self-limited with continued glycemic control,[178] but some patients (especially those with T2D) experience residual pain and dysautonomia.[176] The causal role of treatment in developing this SFN is supported by reports of recurrence in some individuals after lapse of diabetic control followed by once again rapidly initiated intensive treatment.[11] The unlikely risk of developing treatment-induced SFN, however, is not a valid reason to discourage attaining A1C levels approaching normal.[165] The mechanism by which rapid normalization of hyperglycemia causes a SFN is unknown. Studies do not support the hypothesis that it is explained by episodes of hypoglycemia.[179] Possible explanations based on sural nerve biopsies showing arteriolar attenuation and epineural arteriovenous shunting with proliferating "new vessels" are similar to those found in the retina and suggest a possible "steal" effect that results in an ischemic endoneurium.[178] The observation that diabetic retinopathy as evaluated by ophthalmoscopy examinations deteriorates in parallel with treatment-induced diabetic SFN supports a common pathophysiology.[176]

CHRONIC INFLAMMATORY DEMYELINATING POLYNEUROPATHY

CIDP is an immune-mediated neuropathy frequently diagnosed by neuromuscular specialists. The purported association between CIDP and diabetes initially was based on observational studies and is controversial,[11] and whether the association between CIDP and diabetes represents the chance occurrence of two common disorders or the unmasking of mild diabetes among some patients with CIDP who are treated with corticosteroids is unclear. One study of 1,827 patients concluded that patients with diabetes were 11-fold more likely to fulfill EMG and clinical criteria for CIDP compared with those without diabetes (*P* <0.001).[180,181] More recent studies, including one involving review of 1,581 medical records involving patients from Olmsted County, Minnesota, a community where cases of CIDP are unlikely to have been misdiagnosed, failed to confirm an increased risk of CIDP in diabetic populations.[182] Nevertheless, the coexistence of diabetes, substantial weakness, slow motor nerve conduction, and an elevated cerebrospinal fluid protein makes the distinction between a severe diabetic DSP and CIDP difficult. Assuming, for discussion, that the relationship between diabetes and CIDP represents a chance association, the coexistence of diabetes and a severe DPN with weakness nonetheless poses a therapeutic challenge. As a general rule, marked weakness and pronounced slowing of motor conduction velocity with abnormal temporal dispersion or partial conduction block rarely occurs as part of a DSP. Such findings should prompt additional testing for conditions associated with CIPD (e.g., investigation for an underlying monoclonal gammopathy). A trial of therapeutic plasma exchange, corticosteroids, or IVIg that results in dramatically improved strength confirms the presence of an immune-mediated CIDP in a patient with diabetes.

DIABETIC FOCAL MONONEUROPATHIES

Diabetes is associated with a number of focal mononeuropathies involving cranial, thoracic, or extremity nerves. An oculomotor palsy (CN III) is the most common cranial neuropathy, presenting suddenly of unilateral headache, orbital pain, ptosis, and diplopia owing to impaired eye movements (with the involved eye turned down and out) but a normally responsive pupil (partial third nerve palsy with pupillary sparing).[11,69] Exclusion of other causes such as neoplasms, aneurysms, and brain stem infarcts is nonetheless important. The relationship to diabetes and other cranial mononeuropathies in diabetes, including trochlear and facial nerves, is less clear.[11]

A common complication of diabetes is the sudden onset of a unilateral truncal (thoracic) radiculopathy. Technically a radiculopathy, not a mononeuropathy, this condition presents with sensory loss and neuropathic pain in a dermatome band-like distribution circling the chest or abdomen. At times, the pain suggests an intraabdominal process or is indistinguishable from herpes zoster (absent the rash) or a structural (spinal) process.[11] The needle EMG examination may help to secure the diagnosis of a thoracic radiculopathy, especially if there is a motor involvement with bulging of abdominal muscles.[183]

Many peripheral nerves are susceptible to compression or cumulative trauma, including the median, ulnar, radial, lateral femoral cutaneous, fibular, and plantar nerves. These nerves commonly are injured in patients with diabetes ("sick" nerves are prone to injury).[11] The exact explanation for the seemingly increased predisposition to injury in diabetes is undoubtedly multifactorial, involving metabolic factors, ischemia, and impaired nerve repair. Obesity also is a factor in some situations, as BMI is an independent risk factor for carpal tunnel syndrome (CTS). The frequency of "entrapment" mononeuropathies undoubtedly is increased in diabetes, although this may involve to some extent how electrodiagnostic findings are interpreted. An NCS showing evidence of a "median mononeuropathy at the wrist" is not equivalent to a diagnosis of CTS, which is a clinical diagnosis requiring appropriate clinical symptoms. Standard NCS criteria for median mononeuropathy are based on reference values from normal subjects, not asymptomatic, neurological patients with diabetes. When patients with mild diabetic DSP are evaluated randomly, more than one-fifth show "positive results" for a median mononeuropathy, despite having no symptoms of CTS.[184] The reason for this high frequency of false-positive results involving the median nerve at the wrist is not fully understood, but it indicates that patients with diabetes require special consideration when diagnosing entrapment, specifically involving the median nerve but probably other nerves as well. A patient with diabetes presenting with a mononeuropathy should be investigated for entrapment.[11,185] In fact, patients with diabetes and CTS are thought to have the same beneficial outcome after carpal tunnel release surgery as patients without diabetes,[186] but vague symptoms suggesting a possible entrapment neuropathy and equivocal NCS abnormalities supporting the diagnosis are likely insufficient. Treatment decisions involving a diagnosis of entrapment mononeuropathy in a patient with diabetes should be based on robust agreement between clinical and NCS/EMG findings, and not automatic reliance on equivocal NCS abnormalities.

CONCLUSION

DPNs are prevalent and have a diverse clinical spectrum of symptoms and signs. By far the most common form is the distal symmetrical sensorimotor polyneuropathy, and pain is the usual symptom that triggers medical attention. Given its high morbidity and mortality risk, an earlier diagnosis is recommended. In most cases, accurate recording of symptoms, as described by the patient, a careful clinical examination, use of simple instruments (e.g., the MNSI), and foot inspection are sufficient for daily clinical practice. More sophisticated diagnostic tests or procedures, including referral to neurologists or electrophysiology, rarely are needed and are reserved for atypical and rapidly progressing cases. Treatment of diabetic neuropathies is challenging, often requiring a team approach. Glucose control (especially for patients with T1D), effective treatment of pain, and measures to prevent foot ulcerations continue to remain the mainstream of treatment.

REFERENCES

1. Partanen J, Niskanen L, Lehtinen J, Mervaala E, Siitonen O, Uusitupa M. Natural history of peripheral neuropathy in patients with non-insulin-dependent diabetes mellitus. *N Engl J Med* 1995;333:89–94.

2. Boulton AJ, Vileikyte L, Ragnarson-Tennvall G, Apelqvist J. The global burden of diabetic foot disease. *Lancet* 2005;366:1719–1724.

3. Vileikyte L. Diabetic foot ulcers: a quality of life issue. *Diabetes Metab Res Rev* 2001;17:246–249.

4. Vileikyte L, Leventhal H, Gonzalez JS, Peyrot M, Rubin RR, Ulbrecht JS, Garrow A, Waterman C, Cavanagh PR, Boulton AJ. Diabetic peripheral neuropathy and depressive symptoms: the association revisited. *Diabetes Care* 2005;28:2378–2383.

5. Vileikyte L, Rubin RR, Leventhal H. Psychological aspects of diabetic neuropathic foot complications: an overview. *Diabetes Metab Res Rev* 2004;20(Suppl 1):S13–18.

6. Boulton AJ, Vinik AI, Arezzo JC, Bril V, Feldman EL, Freeman R, Malik RA, Maser RE, Sosenko JM, Ziegler D. Diabetic neuropathies: a statement by the American Diabetes Association. *Diabetes Care* 2005;28:956–962.

7. Tesfaye S, Boulton AJ, Dyck PJ, Freeman R, Horowitz M, Kempler P, Lauria G, Malik RA, Spallone V, Vinik A, Bernardi L, Valensi P. Diabetic neuropathies: update on definitions, diagnostic criteria, estimation of severity, and treatments. *Diabetes Care* 2010;33:2285–2293.

8. Dyck PJ, Albers JW, Andersen H, Arezzo JC, Biessels GJ, Bril V, Feldman EL, Litchy WJ, O'Brien PC, Russell JW. Diabetic polyneuropathies: update on research definition, diagnostic criteria and estimation of severity. *Diabetes Metab Res Rev* 2011;27:620–628.

9. Boulton AJ, Valensi P, Tesfaye S. The diabetic neuropathies: reports from the Diabetic Neuropathy Expert Panel Meeting on Neuropathy, Toronto, October 2009: Introduction. *Diabetes Metab Res Rev* 2011;27:617–619.

10. Boulton A, Malik R. Diabetes mellitus: neuropathy. In *Endocrinology: Adult and Pediatric.* Jameson JL, De Groot LJ, Eds. Philadelphia, Saunders Elsevier, 2010, p. 984–998.

11. Smith AG, Singleton JR. Diabetic neuropathy. *Continuum* 2012;18:60–84.

12. Tesfaye S, Kempler P. Painful diabetic neuropathy. *Diabetologia* 2005;48:805–807.

13. Tesfaye S, Vileikyte L, Rayman G, Sindrup S, Perkins B, Baconja M, Vinik A, Boulton A. Painful diabetic peripheral neuropathy: consensus recommendations on diagnosis, assessment and management. *Diabetes Metab Res Rev* 2011;27:629–638.

14. Diabetes Control and Complications Trial (DCCT) Research Group. The effect of intensive treatment of diabetes on the development and progression of long-term complications in insulin-dependent diabetes mellitus. *N Engl J Med* 1993;329:977–986.

15. Diabetes Control and Complications Trial (DCCT) Research Group. Effect of intensive diabetes treatment on nerve conduction in the Diabetes Control and Complications Trial. *Ann Neurol* 1995;38:869–880.

16. Albers JW, Herman WH, Pop-Busui R, Feldman EL, Martin CL, Cleary PA, Waberski BH, Lachin JM. Effect of prior intensive insulin treatment during the Diabetes Control and Complications Trial (DCCT) on peripheral neuropathy in type 1 diabetes during the Epidemiology of Diabetes Interventions and Complications (EDIC) Study. *Diabetes Care* 2010;33:1090–1096.

17. Tesfaye S, Stevens LK, Stephenson JM, Fuller JH, Plater M, Ionescu-Tirgoviste C, Nuber A, Pozza G, Ward JD. Prevalence of diabetic peripheral neuropathy and its relation to glycaemic control and potential risk factors: the EURODIAB IDDM Complications Study. *Diabetologia* 1996;39:1377–1384.

18. Young MJ, Boulton AJ, MacLeod AF, Williams DR, Sonksen PH. A multicentre study of the prevalence of diabetic peripheral neuropathy in the United Kingdom hospital clinic population. *Diabetologia* 1993;36:150–154.

19. Boulton AJ, Malik RA, Arezzo JC, Sosenko JM. Diabetic somatic neuropathies. *Diabetes Care* 2004;27:1458–1486.

20. Charles M, Ejskjaer N, Witte DR, Borch-Johnsen K, Lauritzen T, Sandbaek A. Prevalence of neuropathy and peripheral arterial disease and the impact of treatment in people with screen-detected type 2 diabetes: the ADDITION-Denmark study. *Diabetes Care* 2011;34:2244–2249.

21. Pirart J. Diabetes mellitus and its degenerative complications: a prospective study of 4,400 patients observed between 1947 and 1973. *Diabetes Metab* 1977;3:97–107.

22. Dyck PJ, Kratz KM, Karnes JL, Litchy WJ, Klein R, Pach JM, Wilson DM, O'Brien PC, Melton LJ 3rd, Service FJ. The prevalence by staged severity of various types of diabetic neuropathy, retinopathy, and nephropathy in a population-based cohort: the Rochester Diabetic Neuropathy Study. *Neurology* 1993;43:817–824.

23. Dyck PJ, Kratz KM, Lehman KA, Karnes JL, Melton LJ, O'Brien PC, Litchy WJ, Windebank AJ, Smith BE, Low PA, Service FJ, Rizza RA, Zimmerman BR. The Rochester Diabetic Neuropathy Study: design, criteria for types of neuropathy, selection bias, and reproducibility of neuropathic tests. *Neurology* 1991;41:799–807.

24. Pop-Busui R, Low PA, Waberski BH, Martin CL, Albers JW, Feldman EL, Sommer C, Cleary PA, Lachin JM, Herman WH. Effects of prior intensive insulin therapy on cardiac autonomic nervous system function in type 1 diabetes mellitus: the Diabetes Control and Complications Trial/Epidemiology of Diabetes Interventions and Complications study (DCCT/EDIC). *Circulation* 2009;119:2886–2893.

25. Pop-Busui R, Lu J, Brooks MM, Albert S, Althouse AD, Escobedo J, Green J, Palumbo P, Perkins BA, Whitehouse F, Jones TL. Impact of glycemic control strategies on the progression of diabetic peripheral neuropathy in the Bypass Angioplasty Revascularization Investigation 2 Diabetes (BARI 2D) cohort. *Diabetes Care* 2013;36:3208–3215.

26. Harris M, Eastman R, Cowie C. Symptoms of sensory neuropathy in adults with NIDDM in the U.S. population. *Diabetes Care* 1993;16:1446–1452

27. Sorensen L, Molyneaux L, Yue DK. Insensate versus painful diabetic neuropathy: the effects of height, gender, ethnicity and glycaemic control. *Diabetes Res Clin Pract* 2002;57:45–51.

28. Sosenko JM, Boulton AJ, Kubrusly DB, Weintraub JK, Skyler JS. The vibratory perception threshold in young diabetic patients: associations with glycemia and puberty. *Diabetes Care* 1985;8:605–607.

29. Jaiswal M, Lauer A, Martin CL, Bell RA, Divers J, Dabelea D, Pettitt DJ, Saydah S, Pihoker C, Standiford DA, Rodriguez BL, Pop-Busui R, Feldman EL. Peripheral neuropathy in adolescents and young adults with type 1 and type 2 diabetes from the SEARCH for Diabetes in Youth follow-up cohort: a pilot study. *Diabetes Care* 2013;36:3903–3908.

30. Martin CL, Albers JW, Pop-Busui R. Neuropathy and related findings in the Diabetes Control and Complications Trial/Epidemiology of Diabetes Interventions and Complications study. *Diabetes Care* 2014;37:31–38.

31. Klein R, Klein BE, Moss SE. Relation of glycemic control to diabetic microvascular complications in diabetes mellitus. *Ann Intern Med* 1996;124:90–96.

32. Maser RE, Steenkiste AR, Dorman JS, Nielsen VK, Bass EB, Manjoo Q, Drash AL, Becker DJ, Kuller LH, Greene DA, et al. Epidemiological correlates of diabetic neuropathy. Report from Pittsburgh Epidemiology of Diabetes Complications Study. *Diabetes* 1989;38:1456–1461.

33. Cheng WY, Jiang YD, Chuang LM, Huang CN, Heng LT, Wu HP, Tai TY, Lin BJ. Quantitative sensory testing and risk factors of diabetic sensory neuropathy. *J Neurol* 1999;246:394–398.

34. Abbott CA, Malik RA, van Ross ER, Kulkarni J, Boulton AJ. Prevalence and characteristics of painful diabetic neuropathy in a large community-based diabetic population in the U.K. *Diabetes Care* 2011;34:2220–2224.

35. Sosenko JM, Sparling YH, Hu D, Welty T, Howard BV, Lee E, Robbins DC. Use of the Semmes-Weinstein monofilament in the Strong Heart Study. Risk factors for clinical neuropathy. *Diabetes Care* 1999;22:1715–1721.

36. Sands ML, Shetterly SM, Franklin GM, Hamman RF. Incidence of distal symmetric (sensory) neuropathy in NIDDM. The San Luis Valley Diabetes Study. *Diabetes Care* 1997;20:322–329.

37. Grandinetti A, Chow DC, Sletten DM, Oyama JK, Theriault AG, Schatz IJ, Low PA. Impaired glucose tolerance is associated with postganglionic sudomotor impairment. *Clin Auton Res* 2007;17:231–233.

38. Singleton JR, Smith AG, Bromberg MB. Painful sensory polyneuropathy associated with impaired glucose tolerance. *Muscle Nerve* 2001;24:1225–1228.

39. Singleton JR, Smith AG, Russell J, Feldman EL. Polyneuropathy with impaired glucose tolerance: implications for diagnosis and therapy. *Curr Treat Options Neurol* 2005;7:33–42.

40. Ziegler D, Rathmann W, Dickhaus T, Meisinger C, Mielck A, Group KS. Prevalence of polyneuropathy in pre-diabetes and diabetes is associated with abdominal obesity and macroangiopathy: the MONICA/KORA Augsburg Surveys S2 and S3. *Diabetes Care* 2008;31:464–469.

41. Sosenko JM, Kato M, Soto R, Goldberg RB. Sensory function at diagnosis and in early stages of NIDDM in patients detected through screening. *Diabetes Care* 1992;15:847–852.

42. Ziegler D, Mayer P, Muhlen H, Gries FA. The natural history of somatosensory and autonomic nerve dysfunction in relation to glycaemic control during the first 5 years after diagnosis of type 1 (insulin-dependent) diabetes mellitus. *Diabetologia* 1991;34:822–829.

43. Young RJ, Ewing DJ, Clarke BF. Chronic and remitting painful diabetic polyneuropathy. Correlations with clinical features and subsequent changes in neurophysiology. *Diabetes Care* 1988;11:34–40.

44. Ohkubo Y, Kishikawa H, Araki E, Miyata T, Isami S, Motoyoshi S, Kojima Y, Furuyoshi N, Shichiri M. Intensive insulin therapy prevents the progression of diabetic microvascular complications in Japanese patients with non-insulin-dependent diabetes mellitus: a randomized prospective 6–year study *Diabetes Res Clin Pract* 1995;28:103–117.

45. Laudadio C, Sima AA. Progression rates of diabetic neuropathy in placebo patients in an 18–month clinical trial. Ponalrestat Study Group. *J Diabetes Complications* 1998;12:121–127.

46. Sosenko JM, Kato M, Soto R, Bild DE. A prospective study of sensory function in patients with type 2 diabetes. *Diabet Med* 1993;10:110–114.

47. Diabetes Control and Complications Trial (DCCT) Research Group. Factors in development of diabetic neuropathy. Baseline analysis of neuropathy in feasibility phase of Diabetes Control and Complications Trial (DCCT). *Diabetes* 1988;37:476–481.

48. UK Prospective Diabetes Study (UKPDS) Group. Intensive blood-glucose control with sulphonylureas or insulin compared with conventional treatment and risk of complications in patients with type 2 diabetes (UKPDS 33). *Lancet* 1998;352:837–853.

49. Ismail-Beigi F, Craven T, Banerji MA, Basile J, Calles J, Cohen RM, Cuddihy R, Cushman WC, Genuth S, Grimm RH Jr, Hamilton BP, Hoogwerf B, Karl D, Katz L, Krikorian A, O'Connor P, Pop-Busui R, Schubart U, Simmons D, Taylor H, Thomas A, Weiss D, Hramiak I. Effect of intensive treatment of hyperglycaemia on microvascular outcomes in type 2 diabetes: an analysis of the ACCORD randomised trial. *Lancet* 2010;376:419–430.

50. Callaghan BC, Little AA, Feldman EL, Hughes RA. Enhanced glucose control for preventing and treating diabetic neuropathy. *Cochrane Database Syst Rev* 2012;6:CD007543.

51. Martin CL, Albers J, Herman WH, Cleary P, Waberski B, Greene DA, Stevens MJ, Feldman EL. Neuropathy among the Diabetes Control and Complications Trial cohort 8 years after trial completion. *Diabetes Care* 2006;29:340–344.

52. Pop-Busui R, Herman WH, Feldman EL, Low PA, Martin CL, Cleary PA, Waberski BH, Lachin JM, Albers JW. DCCT and EDIC studies in type 1 diabetes: lessons for diabetic neuropathy regarding metabolic memory and natural history. *Curr Diab Rep* 2010;10:276–282.

53. Bragd J, Adamson U, Backlund LB, Lins PE, Moberg E, Oskarsson P. Can glycaemic variability, as calculated from blood glucose self-monitoring, predict the development of complications in type 1 diabetes over a decade? *Diabetes Metab* 2008;34:612–616.

54. Siegelaar SE, Kilpatrick ES, Rigby AS, Atkin SL, Hoekstra JB, Devries JH. Glucose variability does not contribute to the development of peripheral and autonomic neuropathy in type 1 diabetes: data from the DCCT. *Diabetologia* 2009;52:2229–2232.

55. Tesfaye S, Chaturvedi N, Eaton SE, Ward JD, Manes C, Ionescu-Tirgoviste C, Witte DR, Fuller JH. Vascular risk factors and diabetic neuropathy. *N Engl J Med* 2005;352:341–350.

56. U.K. Prospective Diabetes Study Group. Efficacy of atenolol and captopril in reducing risk of macrovascular and microvascular complications in type 2 diabetes: UKPDS 39. [See comments.] *BMJ* 1998;317:713–720.

57. The Long-Term Intervention with Pravastatin in Ischaemic Disease (LIPID) Study Group. Prevention of cardiovascular events and death with pravastatin in patients with coronary heart disease and a broad range of initial cholesterol levels. [See comments.] *N Engl J Med* 1998;339:1349–1357.

58. U.K. Prospective Diabetes Study (UKPDS) Group. Effect of intensive blood-glucose control with metformin on complications in overweight patients with type 2 diabetes (UKPDS 34). *Lancet* 1998;352:854–865.

59. Rajamani K, Colman PG, Li LP, Best JD, Voysey M, D'Emden MC, Laakso M, Baker JR, Keech AC. Effect of fenofibrate on amputation events in people with type 2 diabetes mellitus (FIELD study): a prespecified analysis of a randomised controlled trial. *Lancet* 2009;373:1780–1788.

60. Wiggin TD, Sullivan KA, Pop-Busui R, Amato A, Sima AA, Feldman EL. Elevated triglycerides correlate with progression of diabetic neuropathy. *Diabetes* 2009;58:1634–1640.

61. Adler AI, Boyko EJ, Ahroni JH, Stensel V, Forsberg RC, Smith DG. Risk factors for diabetic peripheral sensory neuropathy. Results of the Seattle Prospective Diabetic Foot Study. *Diabetes Care* 1997;20:1162–1167.

62. Sosenko JM, Gadia MT, Fournier AM, O'Connell MT, Aguiar MC, Skyler JS. Body stature as a risk factor for diabetic sensory neuropathy. *Am J Med* 1986;80:1031–1034.

63. Wiles PG, Pearce SM, Rice PJ, Mitchell JM. Vibration perception threshold: influence of age, height, sex, and smoking, and calculation of accurate centile values. *Diabet Med* 1991;8:157–161.

64. Mitchell BD, Hawthorne VM, Vinik AI. Cigarette smoking and neuropathy in diabetic patients. *Diabetes Care* 1990;13:434–437.

65. Gragnoli C. PSMD9 is linked to type 2 diabetes neuropathy. *J Diabetes Complications* 2011;25:329–331.

66. Strokov IA, Bursa TR, Drepa OI, Zotova EV, Nosikov VV, Ametov AS. Predisposing genetic factors for diabetic polyneuropathy in patients with type 1 diabetes: a population-based case-control study. *Acta Diabetologica* 2003;40(Suppl 2):S375–S379.

67. Diabetic polyneuropathy in controlled clinical trials: consensus report of the Peripheral Nerve Society. *Ann Neurol* 1995;38:478–482.

68. Boulton AJ, Kirsner RS, Vileikyte L. Clinical practice. Neuropathic diabetic foot ulcers. *N Engl J Med* 2004;351:48–55.

69. Sinnreich M, Taylor BV, Dyck PJ. Diabetic neuropathies. Classification, clinical features, and pathophysiological basis. *Neurologist* 2005;11:63–79.

70. Malik R, Veves A, Tesfaye S, Smith G, Cameron N, Zochodne D, Lauria G. Small fiber neuropathy: role in the diagnosis of diabetic sensorimotor polyneuropathy. *Diabetes Metab Res Rev* 2011;27:678–684.

71. Feldman EL, Stevens MJ, Thomas PK, Brown MB, Canal N, Greene DA. A practical two-step quantitative clinical and electrophysiological assessment for the diagnosis and staging of diabetic neuropathy. *Diabetes Care* 1994;17:1281–1289.

72. Herman WH, Pop-Busui R, Braffett BH, Martin CL, Cleary PA, Albers JW, Feldman EL. Use of the Michigan Neuropathy Screening Instrument as a measure of distal symmetrical peripheral neuropathy in type 1 diabetes: results from the Diabetes Control and Complications Trial/Epidemiology of Diabetes Interventions and Complications. *Diabet Med* 2012;29:937–944.

73. Pop-Busui R, Lu J, Lopes N, Jones TL. Prevalence of diabetic peripheral neuropathy and relation to glycemic control therapies at baseline in the BARI 2D cohort. *J Peripher Nerv Syst* 2009;14:1–13.

74. Perkins BA, Olaleye D, Zinman B, Bril V. Simple screening tests for peripheral neuropathy in the diabetes clinic. *Diabetes Care* 2001;24:250–256.

75. Singleton JR, Bixby B, Russell JW, Feldman EL, Peltier A, Goldstein J, Howard J, Smith AG. The Utah Early Neuropathy Scale: a sensitive clinical scale for early sensory predominant neuropathy. *J Peripher Nerv Syst* 2008;13:218–227.

76. Abbott CA, Carrington AL, Ashe H, Bath S, Every LC, Griffiths J, Hann AW, Hussein A, Jackson N, Johnson KE, Ryder CH, Torkington R, Van Ross ER, Whalley AM, Widdows P, Williamson S, Boulton AJ. The North-West Diabetes Foot Care Study: incidence of, and risk factors for, new diabetic foot ulceration in a community-based patient cohort. *Diabet Med* 2002;19:377–384.

77. Vileikyte L, Peyrot M, Bundy C, Rubin RR, Leventhal H, Mora P, Shaw JE, Baker P, Boulton AJ. The development and validation of a neuropathy- and foot ulcer-specific quality of life instrument. *Diabetes Care* 2003;26:2549–2555.

78. Vinik EJ, Hayes RP, Oglesby A, Bastyr E, Barlow P, Ford-Molvik SL, Vinik AI. The development and validation of the Norfolk QOL-DN, a new measure of patients' perception of the effects of diabetes and diabetic neuropathy. *Diabetes Technol Ther* 2005;7:497–508.

79. Dyck PJ, Overland CJ, Low PA, Litchy WJ, Davies JL, O'Brien PC, Albers JW, Andersen H, Bolton CF, England JD, Klein CJ, Llewelyn JG, Mauermann ML, Russell JW, Singer W, Smith AG, Tesfaye S, Vella A. Signs and symptoms versus nerve conduction studies to diagnose diabetic sensorimotor polyneuropathy: Cl vs. NPhys trial. *Muscle Nerve* 2010;42:157–164.

80. Dyck PJ, Albers JW, Wolfe J, Bolton CF, Walsh N, Klein CJ, Zafft AJ, Russell JW, Thomas K, Davies JL, Carter RE, Melton LJ, Litchy WJ. A trial of proficiency of nerve conduction: greater standardization still needed. *Muscle Nerve* 2013;48:369–374.

81. Dyck PJ, Overland CJ, Low PA, Litchy WJ, Davies JL, Carter RE, Melton LJ, Andersen H, Albers JW, Bolton CF, England JD, Klein CJ, Llewelyn G, Mauermann ML, Russell JW, Selvarajah D, Singer W, Smith AG, Tesfaye S, Vella A. "Unequivocally abnormal" vs. "usual" signs and symptoms for proficient diagnosis of diabetic polyneuropathy: Cl vs N Phys Trial. *Arch Neurol* 2012;69:1609–1614.

82. American Association of Neuromuscular & Electrodiagnostic Medicine (AANEM). Proper performance and interpretation of electrodiagnostic studies. *Muscle Nerve* 2006;33:436–439.

83. Chaudhry V, Cornblath DR, Mellits ED, Avila O, Freimer ML, Glass JD, Reim J, Ronnett GV, Quaskey SA, Kuncl RW. Inter- and intra-examiner reliability of nerve conduction measurements in normal subjects. *Ann Neurol* 1991;30:841–843.

84. Boulton AJ, Armstrong DG, Albert SF, Frykberg RG, Hellman R, Kirkman MS; Lavery LA, Lemaster JW, Mills JL Sr, Mueller MJ, Sheehan P, Wukich DK, American Diabetes Association, American Association of Clinical Endocrinologists. Comprehensive foot examination and risk assessment. a report of the task force of the foot care interest group of the American Diabetes Association, with endorsement by the American Association of Clinical Endocrinologists. *Diabetes Care* 2008;31:1679–1685.

85. Bowling FL, Abbott CA, Harris WE, Atanasov S, Malik RA, Boulton AJ. A pocket-sized disposable device for testing the integrity of sensation in the outpatient setting. *Diabet Med* 2012;29:1550–1552.

86. Quattrini C, Harris ND, Malik RA, Tesfaye S. Impaired skin microvascular reactivity in painful diabetic neuropathy. *Diabetes Care* 2007;30:655–659.

87. Lauria G, Cazzato D, Porretta-Serapiglia C, Casanova-Molla J, Taiana M, Penza P, Lombardi R, Faber CG, Merkies IS. Morphometry of dermal nerve fibers in human skin. *Neurology* 2011;77:242–249.

88. Lauria G, Devigili G. Skin biopsy as a diagnostic tool in peripheral neuropathy. *Nat Clin Pract Neurol* 2007;3:546–557.

89. Lauria G, Hsieh ST, Johansson O, Kennedy WR, Leger JM, Mellgren SI, Nolano M, Merkies IS, Polydefkis M, Smith AG, Sommer C, Valls-Sole J. European Federation of Neurological Societies/Peripheral Nerve Society guideline on the use of skin biopsy in the diagnosis of small fiber neuropathy. Report of a joint task force of the European Federation of Neurological Societies and the Peripheral Nerve Society. *Eur J Neurol* 2010;17:903–912, e944–909.

90. Smith AG, Howard JR, Kroll R, Ramachandran P, Hauer P, Singleton JR, McArthur J. The reliability of skin biopsy with measurement of intraepidermal nerve fiber density. *J Neurol Sci* 2005;228:65–69.

91. Bakkers M, Merkies IS, Lauria G, Devigili G, Penza P, Lombardi R, Hermans MC, van Nes SI, De Baets M, Faber CG. Intraepidermal nerve fiber density and its application in sarcoidosis. *Neurology* 2009;73:1142–1148.

92. Vlckova-Moravcova E, Bednarik J, Dusek L, Toyka KV, Sommer C. Diagnostic validity of epidermal nerve fiber densities in painful sensory neuropathies. *Muscle Nerve* 2008;37:50–60.

93. Nebuchennykh M, Loseth S, Lindal S, Mellgren SI. The value of skin biopsy with recording of intraepidermal nerve fiber density and quantitative sensory testing in the assessment of small fiber involvement in patients with different causes of polyneuropathy. *J Neurol* 2009;256:1067–1075.

94. Polydefkis M, Hauer P, Griffin JW, McArthur JC. Skin biopsy as a tool to assess distal small fiber innervation in diabetic neuropathy. *Diabetes Technol Ther* 2001;3:23–28.

95. Polydefkis M, Hauer P, Sheth S, Sirdofsky M, Griffin JW, McArthur JC. The time course of epidermal nerve fibre regeneration: Studies in normal controls and in people with diabetes, with and without neuropathy. *Brain* 2004;127:1606–1615.

96. Smith AG, Russell J, Feldman EL, Goldstein J, Peltier A, Smith S, Hamwi J, Pollari D, Bixby B, Howard J, Singleton JR. Lifestyle intervention for prediabetic neuropathy. *Diabetes Care* 2006;29:1294–1299.

97. Malik RA, Kallinikos P, Abbott CA, van Schie CH, Morgan P, Efron N, Boulton AJ. Corneal confocal microscopy: a non-invasive surrogate of nerve fibre damage and repair in diabetic patients. *Diabetologia* 2003;46:683–688.

98. Quattrini C, Tavakoli M, Jeziorska M, Kallinikos P, Tesfaye S, Finnigan J, Marshall A, Boulton AJ, Efron N, Malik RA. Surrogate markers of small fiber damage in human diabetic neuropathy. *Diabetes* 2007;56:2148–2154.

99. Mehra S, Tavakoli M, Kallinikos PA, Efron N, Boulton AJ, Augustine T, Malik RA. Corneal confocal microscopy detects early nerve regeneration after pancreas transplantation in patients with type 1 diabetes. *Diabetes Care* 2007;30:2608–2612.

100. Kempler P, Amarenco G, Freeman R, Frontoni S, Horowitz M, Stevens M, Low P, Pop-Busui R, Tahrani A, Tesfaye S, Varkonyi T, Ziegler D, Valensi P. Gastrointestinal autonomic neuropathy, erectile-, bladder- and sudomotor dysfunction in patients with diabetes mellitus: clinical impact, assessment, diagnosis, and management. *Diabetes Metab Res Rev* 2011;27:665–677.

101. Mayaudon H, Miloche PO, Bauduceau B. A new simple method for assessing sudomotor function: relevance in type 2 diabetes. *Diabetes Metab* 2010;36:450–454.

102. American Diabetes Association. Standards of medical care in diabetes—2013. *Diabetes Care* 2013;36(Suppl 1):S11–S66.

103. Armstrong DG, Todd WF, Lavery LA, Harkless LB, Bushman TR. The natural history of acute Charcot's arthropathy in a diabetic foot specialty clinic. *Diabet Med* 1997;14:357–363.

104. Jeffcoate WJ. Charcot neuro-osteoarthropathy. *Diabetes Metab Res Rev* 2008;24(Suppl 1):S62–S65.

105. Rajbhandari SM, Jenkins RC, Davies C, Tesfaye S. Charcot neuroarthropathy in diabetes mellitus. *Diabetologia* 2002;45:1085–1096.

106. Gough A, Abraha H, Li F, Purewal TS, Foster AV, Watkins PJ, Moniz C, Edmonds ME. Measurement of markers of osteoclast and osteoblast activity in patients with acute and chronic diabetic Charcot neuroarthropathy. *Diabet Med* 1997;14:527–531.

107. Rogers LC, Frykberg RG, Armstrong DG, Boulton AJ, Edmonds M, Van GH, Hartemann A, Game F, Jeffcoate W, Jirkovska A, Jude E, Morbach S, Morrison WB, Pinzur M, Pitocco D, Sanders L, Wukich DK, Uccioli L. The Charcot foot in diabetes. *J Am Podiatr Med Assoc* 2011;101:437–446.

108. O'Brien PD, Hinder LM, Sakowski SA, Feldman EL. ER stress in diabetic peripheral neuropathy: a new therapeutic target. *Antioxid Redox Signal* 2014. PMID: 24382087, published online.

109. Diabetes Control and Complications Trial (DCCT) Research Group. The effect of intensive diabetes therapy on measures of autonomic nervous system function in the Diabetes Control and Complications Trial (DCCT). *Diabetologia* 1998;41:416–423.

110. Pop-Busui R, Evans G, Gerstein HC, Fonseca V, Hoogwerf B, Fleg J, Corson MA, Grimm RH Jr, Prineas RJ. Cardiac autonomic dysfunction predicts cardiovascular mortality in the Action to Control Cardiovascular Risk in Diabetes (ACCORD) trial. *Diabetes* 2009;58(Suppl 1):A58.

111. Edwards JL, Vincent AM, Cheng HT, Feldman EL. Diabetic neuropathy: mechanisms to management. *Pharmacol Ther* 2008;120:1–34.

112. Vincent AM, Brownlee M, Russell JW. Oxidative stress and programmed cell death in diabetic neuropathy. *Ann N Y Acad Sci* 2002;959:368–383.

113. Vincent AM, Callaghan BC, Smith AL, Feldman EL. Diabetic neuropathy: cellular mechanisms as therapeutic targets. *Nat Rev Neurol* 2011;7:573–583.

114. Vincent AM, McLean LL, Backus C, Feldman EL. Short-term hyperglycemia produces oxidative damage and apoptosis in neurons. *FASEB J* 2005; 19:638–640.

115. Vincent AM, Russell JW, Low P, Feldman EL. Oxidative stress in the pathogenesis of diabetic neuropathy. *Endocr Rev* 2004;25:612–628.

116. Pacher P, Liaudet L, Soriano FG, Mabley JG, Szabo E, Szabo C. The role of poly(ADP-ribose) polymerase activation in the development of myocardial and endothelial dysfunction in diabetes. *Diabetes* 2002;51:514–521.

117. Pop-Busui R. What do we know and we do not know about cardiovascular autonomic neuropathy in diabetes. *J Cardiovasc Transl Res* 2012;5:463–478.

118. Cameron NE, Cotter MA, Jack AM, Basso MD, Hohman TC. Protein kinase C effects on nerve function, perfusion, Na(+), K(+)-ATPase activity and glutathione content in diabetic rats. *Diabetologia* 1999;42:1120–1130.

119. Cameron NE, Cotter MA, Low PA. Nerve blood flow in early experimental diabetes in rats: relation to conduction deficits. *Am J Physiol* 1991;261:E1–E8.

120. Low PA, Nickander KK, Tritschler HJ. The roles of oxidative stress and antioxidant treatment in experimental diabetic neuropathy. *Diabetes* 1997;46(Suppl 2):S38–S42.

121. Stevens MJ, Van Huysen C, Beyer L, Thomas T, Yorek M. Amelioration of nerve blood flow deficits by myo-inositol in streptozotocin-diabetic rats. *Diabetes* 1996;45(Suppl 1):A775.

122. Hinder LM, Vincent AM, Hayes JM, McLean LL, Feldman EL. Apolipoprotein E knockout as the basis for mouse models of dyslipidemia-induced neuropathy. *Exp Neurol* 2013;239:102–110.

123. Vincent AM, Hayes JM, McLean LL, Vivekanandan-Giri A, Pennathur S, Feldman EL. Dyslipidemia-induced neuropathy in mice: the role of oxLDL/LOX-1. *Diabetes* 2009;58:2376–2385.

124. Vinik AI, Maser RE, Mitchell BD, Freeman R. Diabetic autonomic neuropathy. *Diabetes Care* 2003;26:1553–1579.

125. Vinik AI, Maser RE, Ziegler D. Autonomic imbalance: prophet of doom or scope for hope? *Diabet Med* 2011;28:643–651.

126. Witzke KA, Vinik AI, Grant LM, Grant WP, Parson HK, Pittenger GL, Burcus N. Loss of RAGE defense: a cause of Charcot neuroarthropathy? *Diabetes Care* 2011;34:1617–1621.

127. Fernyhough P, Roy Chowdhury SK, Schmidt RE. Mitochondrial stress and the pathogenesis of diabetic neuropathy. *Expert Rev Endocrinol Metab* 2010;5:39–49.

128. Sima A, Kamiya H. C-peptide and diabetic neuropathy. *Science Med* 2004;10:308–319.

129. Kamiya H, Zhang W, Sima AA. C-peptide prevents nociceptive sensory neuropathy in type 1 diabetes. *Ann Neurol* 2004;56:827–835.

130. Kamiya H, Zhang W, Sima AA. Degeneration of the Golgi and neuronal loss in dorsal root ganglia in diabetic BioBreeding/Worcester rats. *Diabetologia* 2006;49:2763–2774.

131. Sima A. Physiological and pathophysiological significance of C-peptide action. *Exp Diab Res* 2004;5:1–96.

132. Kamiya H, Zhang W, Sima AA. The beneficial effects of C-peptide on diabetic polyneuropathy. *Rev Diabet Stud* 2009;6:187–202.

133. Cameron NE, Cotter MA. Pro-inflammatory mechanisms in diabetic neuropathy: focus on the nuclear factor kappa B pathway. *Curr Drug Targets* 2008;9:60–67.

134. Wang Y, Schmeichel AM, Iida H, Schmelzer JD, Low PA. Enhanced inflammatory response via activation of NF-kappaB in acute experimental diabetic neuropathy subjected to ischemia-reperfusion injury. *J Neurol Sci* 2006;247:47–52.

135. Kellogg AP, Wiggin T, Larkin D, Hayes J, Stevens M, Pop-Busui R. Protective effects of cyclooxygenase-2 gene inactivation against peripheral nerve dysfunction and intraepidermal nerve fibers loss in experimental diabetes. *Diabetes* 2007;56:2997–3005.

136. Chowdhury SK, Zherebitskaya E, Smith DR, Akude E, Chattopadhyay S, Jolivalt CG, Calcutt NA, Fernyhough P. Mitochondrial respiratory chain dysfunction in dorsal root ganglia of streptozotocin-induced diabetic rats and its correction by insulin treatment. *Diabetes* 2010;59:1082–1091.

137. Ma J, Farmer KL, Pan P, Urban MJ, Zhao H, Blagg BS, Dobrowsky RT. Heat shock protein 70 is necessary to improve mitochondrial bioenergetics and reverse diabetic sensory neuropathy following KU-32 therapy. *J Pharmacol Exp Ther* 2014;348:281–292.

138. Urano F, Wang X, Bertolotti A, Zhang Y, Chung P, Harding HP, Ron D. Coupling of stress in the ER to activation of JNK protein kinases by transmembrane protein kinase IRE1. *Science* 2000;287:664–666.

139. Timmins JM, Ozcan L, Seimon TA, Li G, Malagelada C, Backs J, Backs T, Bassel-Duby R, Olson EN, Anderson ME, Tabas I. Calcium/calmodulin-dependent protein kinase II links ER stress with Fas and mitochondrial apoptosis pathways. *J Clin Invest* 2009;119:2925–2941.

140. Nakagawa T, Zhu H, Morishima N, Li E, Xu J, Yankner BA, Yuan J. Caspase-12 mediates endoplasmic-reticulum-specific apoptosis and cytotoxicity by amyloid-beta. *Nature* 2000;403:98–103.

141. Ozawa K, Miyazaki M, Matsuhisa M, Takano K, Nakatani Y, Hatazaki M, Tamatani T, Yamagata K, Miyagawa J, Kitao Y, Hori O, Yamasaki Y, Ogawa S. The endoplasmic reticulum chaperone improves insulin resistance in type 2 diabetes. *Diabetes* 2005;54:657–663.

142. Ozcan U, Yilmaz E, Ozcan L, Furuhashi M, Vaillancourt E, Smith RO, Gorgun CZ, Hotamisligil GS. Chemical chaperones reduce ER stress and restore glucose homeostasis in a mouse model of type 2 diabetes. *Science* 2006;313:1137–1140.

143. Chang CJ, Yang YC, Lu FH, Lin TS, Chen JJ, Yeh TL, Wu CH, Wu JS. Altered cardiac autonomic function may precede insulin resistance in metabolic syndrome. *Am J Med* 2010;123:432–438.

144. Lieb DC, Parson HK, Mamikunian G, Vinik AI. Cardiac autonomic imbalance in newly diagnosed and established diabetes is associated with markers of adipose tissue inflammation. *Exp Diabetes Res* 2012;2012:878760.

145. Stella P, Ellis D, Maser RE, Orchard TJ. Cardiovascular autonomic neuropathy (expiration and inspiration ratio) in type 1 diabetes. Incidence and predictors. *J Diabetes Complications* 2000;14:1–6.

146. Witte DR, Tesfaye S, Chaturvedi N, Eaton SE, Kempler P, Fuller JH. Risk factors for cardiac autonomic neuropathy in type 1 diabetes mellitus. *Diabetologia* 2005;48:164–171.

147. Gaede P, Vedel P, Larsen N, Jensen GV, Parving HH, Pedersen O. Multifactorial intervention and cardiovascular disease in patients with type 2 diabetes. *N Engl J Med* 2003;348:383–393.

148. Balducci S, Iacobellis G, Parisi L, Di Biase N, Calandriello E, Leonetti F, Fallucca F. Exercise training can modify the natural history of diabetic peripheral neuropathy. *J Diabetes Complications* 2006;20:216–223.

149. Davidson LE, Hudson R, Kilpatrick K, Kuk JL, McMillan K, Janiszewski PM, Lee S, Lam M, Ross R. Effects of exercise modality on insulin resistance and functional limitation in older adults: a randomized controlled trial. *Arch Intern Med* 2009;169:122–131.

150. Kluding PM, Pasnoor M, Singh R, Jernigan S, Farmer K, Rucker J, Sharma NK, Wright DE. The effect of exercise on neuropathic symptoms, nerve function, and cutaneous innervation in people with diabetic peripheral neuropathy. *J Diabetes Complications* 2012;26:424–429.

151. Ziegler D, Low PA, Litchy WJ, Boulton AJ, Vinik AI, Freeman R, Samigullin R, Tritschler H, Munzel U, Maus J, Schutte K, Dyck PJ. Efficacy and safety of antioxidant treatment with alpha-lipoic acid over 4 years in diabetic polyneuropathy: the NATHAN 1 trial. *Diabetes Care* 2011;34:2054–2060.

152. Ziegler D, Nowak H, Kempler P, Vargha P, Low PA. Treatment of symptomatic diabetic polyneuropathy with the antioxidant alpha-lipoic acid: a meta-analysis. *Diabet Med* 2004;21:114–121.

153. Ziegler D. Thioctic acid for patients with symptomatic diabetic polyneuropathy: a critical review. *Treat Endocrinol* 2004;3:173–189.

154. Pop-Busui R, Stevens MJ, Raffel DM, White EA, Mehta M, Plunkett CD, Brown MB, Feldman EL. Effects of triple antioxidant therapy on measures of cardiovascular autonomic neuropathy and on myocardial blood flow in type 1 diabetes: a randomised controlled trial. *Diabetologia* 2013;56:1835–1844.

155. Ekberg K, Brismar T, Johansson BL, Jonsson B, Lindstrom P, Wahren J. Amelioration of sensory nerve dysfunction by C-peptide in patients with type 1 diabetes. *Diabetes* 2003;52:536–541.

156. Ekberg K, Brismar T, Johansson BL, Lindstrom P, Juntti-Berggren L, Norrby A, Berne C, Arnqvist HJ, Bolinder J, Wahren J. C-peptide replacement therapy and sensory nerve function in type 1 diabetic neuropathy. *Diabetes Care* 2007;30:71–76.

157. Boulton AJ, Kempler P, Ametov A, Ziegler D. Whither pathogenetic treatments for diabetic polyneuropathy? *Diabetes Metab Res Rev* 2013;29:327–333.

158. Ziegler D, Luft D. Clinical trials for drugs against diabetic neuropathy: can we combine scientific needs with clinical practicalities? *Int Rev Neurobiol* 2002;50:431–463.

159. Fonseca VA, Lavery LA, Thethi TK, Daoud Y, DeSouza C, Ovalle F, Denham DS, Bottiglieri T, Sheehan P, Rosenstock J. Metanx in type 2 diabetes with peripheral neuropathy: a randomized trial. *Am J Med* 2013;126:141–149.

160. Bril V, England JD, Franklin GM, Backonja M, Cohen JA, Del Toro DR, Feldman EL, Iverson DJ, Perkins B, Russell JW, Zochodne DW. Evidence-based guideline: treatment of painful diabetic neuropathy—report of the American Association of Neuromuscular and Electrodiagnostic Medicine, the American Academy of Neurology, and the American Academy of Physical Medicine & Rehabilitation. *Muscle Nerve* 2011;43:910–917.

161. Backonja M, Glanzman RL. Gabapentin dosing for neuropathic pain: evidence from randomized, placebo-controlled clinical trials. *Clin Ther* 2003;25:81–104.

162. Freeman R, Durso-Decruz E, Emir B. Efficacy, safety, and tolerability of pregabalin treatment for painful diabetic peripheral neuropathy: findings

from seven randomized, controlled trials across a range of doses. *Diabetes Care* 2008;31:1448–1454.

163. Kajdasz DK, Iyengar S, Desaiah D, Backonja MM, Farrar JT, Fishbain DA, Jensen TS, Rowbotham MC, Sang CN, Ziegler D, McQuay HJ. Duloxetine for the management of diabetic peripheral neuropathic pain: evidence-based findings from post hoc analysis of three multicenter, randomized, double-blind, placebo-controlled, parallel-group studies. *Clin Ther* 2007;29(Suppl):2536–2546.

164. Tesfaye S, Wilhelm S, Lledo A, Schacht A, Tolle T, Bouhassira D, Cruccu G, Skljarevski V, Freynhagen R. Duloxetine and pregabalin: high-dose mono-therapy or their combination? The "COMBO-DN study"—a multinational, randomized, double-blind, parallel-group study in patients with diabetic peripheral neuropathic pain. *Pain* 2013;154:2616–2625.

165. American Diabetes Association. Professional practice committee for the 2014 clinical practice recommendations. *Diabetes Care* 2014;37(Suppl 1): S154–S155.

166. Dyck PJ, Windebank AJ. Diabetic and nondiabetic lumbosacral radiculo-plexus neuropathies: new insights into pathophysiology and treatment. *Muscle Nerve* 2002;25:477–491.

167. Barohn RJ, Sahenk Z, Warmolts JR, Mendell JR. The Bruns-Garland syndrome (diabetic amyotrophy). Revisited 100 years later. *Arch Neurol* 1991;48:1130–1135.

168. Taylor BV, Dunne JW. Diabetic amyotrophy progressing to severe quadriparesis. *Muscle Nerve* 2004;30:505–509.

169. Massie R, Mauermann ML, Staff NP, Amrami KK, Mandrekar JN, Dyck PJ, Klein CJ. Diabetic cervical radiculoplexus neuropathy: a distinct syndrome expanding the spectrum of diabetic radiculoplexus neuropathies. *Brain* 2012;135:3074–3088.

170. Younger DS. Diabetic lumbosacral radiculoplexus neuropathy: a postmortem studied patient and review of the literature. *J Neurol* 2011;258:1364–1367.

171. Wada Y, Yanagihara C, Nishimura Y, Oka N. A case of diabetic amyotrophy with severe atrophy and weakness of shoulder girdle muscles showing good response to intravenous immune globulin. *Diabetes Res Clin Pract* 2007;75:107–110.

172. Chan YC, Lo YL, Chan ES. Immunotherapy for diabetic amyotrophy. *Cochrane Database Syst Rev* 2012;6:CD006521.

173. Donofrio PD, Berger A, Brannagan TH 3rd, Bromberg MB, Howard JF, Latov N, Quick A, Tandan R. Consensus statement: the use of intravenous immunoglobulin in the treatment of neuromuscular conditions. Report of the AANEM ad hoc committee. *Muscle Nerve* 2009;40:890–900.

174. Garces-Sanchez M, Laughlin RS, Dyck PJ, Engelstad JK, Norell JE. Painless diabetic motor neuropathy: a variant of diabetic lumbosacral radiculoplexus neuropathy? *Ann Neurol* 2011;69:1043–1054.

175. Gemignani F. Acute painful diabetic neuropathy induced by strict glycemic control ("insulin neuritis"): the old enigma is still unsolved. *Biomed Pharmacother* 2009;63:249–250.

176. Gibbons CH, Freeman R. Treatment-induced diabetic neuropathy: a reversible painful autonomic neuropathy. *Ann Neurol* 2010;67:534–541.

177. Grewal J, Bril V, Lewis GF, Perkins BA. Objective evidence for the reversibility of nerve injury in diabetic neuropathic cachexia. *Diabetes Care* 2006;29:473–474.

178. Tesfaye S, Malik R, Harris N, Jakubowski JJ, Mody C, Rennie IG, Ward JD. Arterio-venous shunting and proliferating new vessels in acute painful neuropathy of rapid glycaemic control (insulin neuritis). *Diabetologia* 1996; 39:329–335.

179. Dabby R, Sadeh M, Lampl Y, Gilad R, Watemberg N. Acute painful neuropathy induced by rapid correction of serum glucose levels in diabetic patients. *Biomed Pharmacother* 2009;63:707–709.

180. Sharma KR, Cross J, Ayyar DR, Martinez-Arizala A, Bradley WG. Diabetic demyelinating polyneuropathy responsive to intravenous immunoglobulin therapy. *Arch Neurol* 2002;59:751–757.

181. Sharma KR, Cross J, Farronay O, Ayyar DR, Shebert RT, Bradley WG. Demyelinating neuropathy in diabetes mellitus. *Arch Neurol* 2002;59:758–765.

182. Laughlin RS, Dyck PJ, Melton LJ 3rd, Leibson C, Ransom J. Incidence and prevalence of CIDP and the association of diabetes mellitus. *Neurology* 2009;73:39–45.

183. Chaudhuri KR, Wren DR, Werring D, Watkins PJ. Unilateral abdominal muscle herniation with pain: a distinctive variant of diabetic radiculopathy. *Diabet Med* 1997;14:803–807.

184. Albers JW, Brown MB, Sima AA, Greene DA. Frequency of median mononeuropathy in patients with mild diabetic neuropathy in the early diabetes intervention trial (EDIT). Tolrestat Study Group For EDIT (Early Diabetes Intervention Trial). *Muscle Nerve* 1996;19:140–146.

185. Bansal V, Kalita J, Misra UK. Diabetic neuropathy. *Postgrad Med J* 2006; 82:95–100.

186. Thomsen N, Cederlund R, Rosen I. Clinical outcomes of surgical release among diabetic patients with carpal tunnel syndrome. prospective follow up with matched controls. *J Hand Surg* 2006;34:1177–1187.

187. Thomas PK. Classification, differential diagnosis, and staging of diabetic peripheral neuropathy. *Diabetes* 1997;46(Suppl 2):S54–S57.

Chapter 45

Autonomic Neuropathy in Diabetes

Rodica Pop-Busui, MD, PhD
Martin Stevens, MD

INTRODUCTION

This chapter summarizes the various forms of diabetic autonomic neuropathy, provides a brief overview of its pathogenesis and natural history, and discusses the main clinical manifestations and diagnosis procedures for both research and clinical care. It also provides an update on most recent treatment recommendations. The chapter serves as a reference for the current state of knowledge in that it melds information from a wide range of different sources.

DIABETIC AUTONOMIC NEUROPATHY

Diabetic autonomic neuropathy can involve a number of different systems including the cardiovascular, gastrointestinal, urogenital, and sudomotor (Table 45.1). This can result in an array of abnormalities from milder forms, such as subclinical impaired heart rate variability (HRV), to more severe clinically apparent forms, such as resting tachycardia, increased propensity for arrhythmias, postural hypotension, altered bowel motility, decreased bladder contractility, erectile dysfunction (ED), lower urinary tract symptoms, and sweating disorders.

Although the entire constellation of symptoms and forms of autonomic neuropathy occurs less frequently than other complications, once manifested, it is extremely debilitating and difficult to treat.

EPIDEMIOLOGY AND NATURAL HISTORY

Considering the broad spectrum of autonomic neuropathies and the number of methods by which the presence and degree of severity of each form can be assessed, studies of the natural history and epidemiology of diabetic autonomic

Table 45.1 Forms of Autonomic Neuropathies in Diabetes

Cardiovascular
Gastrointestinal
Genitourinary
Sudomotor
Other

DOI: 10.2337/9781580405096.45

neuropathy should be examined with attention to the specific assessments and criteria that were used. Other factors also should be considered, such as characteristics of the study population, the type of diabetes, and study design.

Some diagnostic tests such as questionnaires or indices of HRV can be performed in large numbers of individuals, on repeat occasions, and with relatively little difficulty. Relying on instruments that collect information on symptoms alone may result in bias, however, as there is a degree of subjectivity in many of these instruments, and there are also many instances in which patients may be completely asymptomatic yet have changes in some diagnostic tests.

INCIDENCE AND PREVALENCE

The incidence and prevalence of cardiovascular autonomic neuropathy (CAN) has varied substantially among studies. Such data are highly dependent on the diagnostic criteria, type of tests, definitions of normal, and patient characteristics.[1] The prevalence of CAN, diagnosed using standard cardiovascular reflex tests, was as low as 2.5% in patients with newly diagnosed type 1 diabetes (T1D) enrolled in the primary prevention cohort of the Diabetes Control and Complications Trial (DCCT).[2,3] After ~5 years of follow-up <10% of DCCT participants who had normal autonomic function at baseline, were found to have CAN.[2,4] These findings contrast with a longitudinal study of new-onset T1D patients in whom HRV was abnormal in 27% at diagnosis and in 56% after 10 years of follow-up.[5] Overall the prevalence of CAN is thought to be ~20%.[1]

CAN does increase substantially with the duration of diabetes regardless of diabetes type.[1,6,7] Evaluations done after 13–14 years of follow-up of the DCCT participants enrolled in the observational Epidemiology of Diabetes Interventions and Complications (EDIC) study, found CAN prevalence rates as high as 35% in the prior conventionally treated DCCT cohort.[7] In the EURODIAB IDDM Complications Study, autonomic dysfunction was present in one-third of T1D subjects at follow-up.[3,8] Prevalence rates of ≥60% were reported in cohorts of patients with long-standing type 2 diabetes (T2D),[1,3,9,10] and in patients with long-standing T1D who were potential candidates for a pancreas transplantation.[11] CAN was found to develop in 35% of subjects with T2D over 7 years in a prospective cohort study in Korea.[12] The impact of gender on CAN is unclear. For example, one report suggested that CAN prevalence was similar in 3,250 men and women with T1D in a multicenter, cross-sectional study.[8] In contrast, in the Action to Control Cardiovascular Risk in Diabetes (ACCORD) trial of >8,000 patients with T2D, CAN was more prevalent in women.[13]

Estimates of prevalence for other manifestations of diabetic autonomic neuropathy, such as gastrointestinal manifestations, bladder dysfunction, and ED, have been reported to be ≥25% in populations with long-standing T1D or T2D.[14] Gastroparesis, defined as a delayed gastric emptying in the absence of an obstructive etiology, is arguably the most important gastrointestinal manifestation. Older reports described prevalence rates as high as 50% in patients with long-standing T1D or T2D.[15] Many studies, however, have included small samples of selected populations, without adequate controls for other comorbidities or medication. More recent studies have described lower rates and lack of agreement between objective measures of gastroparesis and reported symptoms.[16] For instance, in a large cohort of >1,000 patients with T1D attending specialized diabetes clinics in Denmark, the prevalence of symptoms associated with gastroparesis was ~ 9%.[17]

ED prevalence among diabetic men varies broadly, from 35 to 90%, depending on the population studied and the instruments used for diagnosis. In T1D, probably the best data were obtained from UroEDIC, an ancillary study to DCCT/EDIC to study urologic complications in men and women with T1D. Among 713 men with T1D participating in the DCCT/EDIC, ED was present in 34%, orgasmic dysfunction in 20%, and decreased libido in 55% at year 10 of EDIC follow-up and after a mean duration of diabetes for the cohort of 22 years.[18] In the EURODIAB IDDM Complications Study, between 16 and 18% of patients had difficulties with intercourse, obtaining an erection, or sustaining an erection.[16] Estimates of the prevalence of bladder dysfunction are also ≥25% in patients with either T1D or T2D.[16] Among women with T1D participating in the DCCT/EDIC, 38% of women reported any incontinence and 17% reported weekly or greater incontinence.[19]

NATURAL HISTORY

The natural history of autonomic neuropathy is not well understood. Although clinical manifestations of overt autonomic neuropathy usually are not present at the time of diagnosis of diabetes, abnormalities in HRV or cardiovascular reflex testing can be present early in its course.[3] For instance, in the Framingham Heart Study, changes in measures of CAN with a possible shift in the sympathetic–parasympathetic balance favoring sympathetic tone were described in individuals who had glucose values in a prediabetes range.[3,20] Similarly, abnormalities in HRV also were observed in another large cohort of individuals with impaired glucose tolerance.[21]

Several studies also have described that children with diabetes consistently have been found to have higher average heart rates than those without diabetes.[22,23] The basis for the increased heart rate is unknown, but it possibly is related to autonomic dysfunction. Resting tachycardia, however, in children or adults, may occur as a consequence of other conditions, such as anemia, thyroid dysfunction, an underlying cardiovascular disease (CVD), obesity, and poor fitness. Therefore, these conditions should be excluded before a diagnosis of CAN is considered.[3] A fixed heart rate that is unresponsive to moderate exercise, stress, hypoglycemia, or sleep suggests almost complete cardiac denervation.[3]

Although data suggest that subtle autonomic dysfunction is an explanation for the elevated heart rate in diabetes, direct effects of hyperglycemia on heart rate and myocardial dysfunction also could be factors.

RISK FACTORS

The association between CAN and glycemia has been examined in several studies. The DCCT demonstrated that intensive insulin therapy for T1D reduced the incidence of CAN by 53% compared with conventional therapy.[2,4] During EDIC, CAN progressed substantially in both former treatment groups, but the prevalence and incidence of CAN in EDIC remained significantly lower in the former intensive group than in the former conventional group, despite convergent levels of glycemic control.[7] This suggests that "metabolic memory" could be a determinant for CAN. Treatment group differences in the mean A1C level during

DCCT and EDIC explained virtually all of the beneficial effects of intensive versus conventional therapy on the risk of incident CAN. This supports the view that intensive treatment of T1D should be initiated as early as is safely possible.[3]

In T2D, the impact of glycemic control on CAN is less conclusive. The Veterans Affairs Cooperative Study demonstrated no difference in the prevalence of autonomic neuropathy in T2D patients after 2 years of tight glycemic control compared to those without tight control.[24] Similar results were reported by the Veterans Affairs Diabetes Trial (VADT),[25] although some might question whether the CAN outcome measures were sufficiently sensitive.[3] In a trial of Japanese patients with T2D,[26] no significant differences were found in the prevalence of postural hypotension or abnormal heart rate variation between the intensively treated group and the conventional group.

Associations between CAN and glucose levels have been observed in several other studies.[8,27,28] Data pertaining to a role of glucose variability in the pathophysiology of CAN are limited. In one study, however, CAN was not associated with glucose variability.[29]

In studies of other risk factors, CAN has been observed to be associated with hypertension, lipid indexes, smoking, and adiposity indexes.[8,28] Several cross-sectional studies in adults without diabetes have provided evidence that markers of autonomic function are associated inversely with obesity, insulin resistance, and fasting glucose,[30–33] all components of the metabolic syndrome. In the Finnish Diabetes Prevention Study, measures of CAN were associated with higher triglycerides and higher waist circumference, both features of metabolic syndrome.[3,34]

In the Steno-2 study, an intensive multifactorial cardiovascular risk intervention targeting glucose, blood pressure (BP), lipids, smoking, and other lifestyle factors reduced the progression or the development of CAN among T2D patients with microalbuminuria.[35] A beneficial effect of the intensive glycemic intervention alone on CAN was not clearly evident.[3]

Data from the Diabetes Prevention Program showed that lifestyle interventions consisting of diet and exercise may be beneficial for preventing CAN, as indexes of CAN improved more in the lifestyle modification arm than either the metformin or placebo arm.[3] Other studies have reported that improved heart rate variation was associated with strictly supervised endurance training[36] and that weight loss in obese patients was accompanied by improvement in cardiovascular autonomic function.[37] A recent study demonstrated an association between CAN and lower financial income.[38]

PATHOGENESIS

The various pathways involved in the pathogenesis of neuropathy are amply discussed in Chapter 44. It generally is accepted that the development of diabetic neuropathies is a function of complex interactions between the degree of glycemic control, disease duration, age-related neuronal attrition, and other risk factors, including systolic and diastolic BP, lipid variables, and weight.[20–42] These factors promote progressive autonomic neural dysfunction in a fashion that begins distally and progresses proximally.[3] For instance, several studies have reported that early in the progression of CAN complicating T1D, there is a compensatory increase in the cardiac sympathetic tone in response to subclinical peripheral denervation.[43,44] Later, sympathetic denervation follows beginning at the apex of the ventricles and progressing toward the base.[3] A detailed review of these mechanisms and their complex interactions, however, is beyond the scope of this chapter.

CLINICAL FEATURES AND IMPLICATIONS

In its early stages, autonomic neuropathy can be completely asymptomatic, which could delay implementation of an appropriate therapeutic algorithm. The advanced disease may be indicated by orthostasis, fixed tachycardia, or severe diarrhea and potentially an impaired response to hypoglycemia. CAN is the most studied and clinically important form of diabetic autonomic neuropathy because of its independent association with mortality risk and overall CVD morbidity.[45]

Cardiovascular Autonomic Neuropathy

Impaired Heart Rate Variability. Impaired HRV is considered to be the earliest sign of CAN and may be completely unassociated with symptoms.[1,3,36]

Resting Tachycardia and Exercise Intolerance. In more advanced cases, patients may present with resting tachycardia and exercise intolerance because of a reduced response in heart rate and BP, as well as blunted increases in cardiac output in response to exercise (Table 45.2).[1,3,36] Resting tachycardia may occur in several other conditions, such as anemia, thyroid dysfunction, underlying cardiovascular

Table 45.2 Symptoms of Diabetic Autonomic Neuropathies

Cardiovascular autonomic neuropathy	Gastrointestinal	Urogenital
Impaired rate variability	Gastroparesis ■ Nausea	Bladder dysfunction ■ Frequency
Exercise intolerance	■ Bloating ■ Loss of appetite	■ Urgency ■ Nocturia
Resting tachycardia	■ Early satiety ■ Postprandial vomiting	■ Hesitancy ■ Weak stream
Abnormal blood pressure regulation ■ Nondipping ■ Reverse dipping	■ Dribbling Esophageal dysfunction ■ Heartburn ■ Dysphagia for solids	■ Urinary incontinence ■ Urinary retention
Orthostatic hypotension (all with standing) ■ Lightheadedness ■ Weakness ■ Faintness ■ Dizziness ■ Visual impairment ■ Syncope	Diabetic diarrhea ■ Profuse and watery diarrhea ■ Fecal incontinence Constipation	Male sexual dysfunction ■ Erectile dysfunction ■ Decreased libido ■ Abnormal ejaculation Female sexual dysfunction ■ Decreased sexual desire ■ Increased pain during intercourse ■ Decreased sexual arousal ■ Inadequate lubrication

disease (including heart failure), obesity, and poor fitness. These conditions should be excluded before a diagnosis of CAN is considered.[3] Resting tachycardia with a fixed heart rate >100 beats/minute (bpm) that is unresponsive to moderate exercise, stress, or sleep indicates more advanced disease.[3,36]

Silent Ischemia. In a meta-analysis involving 12 cross-sectional studies, CAN was found to be associated with silent ischemia in diabetes (prevalence rate risk of 1.96, 95% confidence interval [CI] of 1.53–2.51).[46] In the Detection of Ischemia in Asymptomatic Diabetics (DIAD) study of 1,123 patients with T2D, CAN was a strong predictor of silent ischemia and subsequent cardiovascular events.[47] A slow heart rate recovery after exercise, which is proposed to indirectly reflect CAN, also was shown to be associated with silent myocardial ischemia.[48] The association between CAN and silent ischemia has important implications, as reduced appreciation for ischemic pain impairs timely recognition of myocardial ischemia or infarction, thereby delaying appropriate therapy.[3]

Myocardial Dysfunction. The presence of CAN also was linked to development of diabetic cardiomyopathy. Diastolic dysfunction, characterized by impairment in left ventricle (LV) relaxation and passive filling, was reported as the earliest manifestation of diabetic cardiomyopathy.[49,50] Early in the natural history of CAN, isolated diastolic dysfunction may contribute to impaired exercise tolerance.[51] Studies in patients with T1D reported that LV dysfunction may precede or occur in the absence of coronary artery disease or hypertension, often seen in the setting of a normal ejection fraction.[43,52] This was confirmed recently in a large cohort (~900) of patients with T1D participants in the DCCT/EDIC. In this cohort, the presence of CAN, confirmed by comprehensive cardiovascular reflex testing, was associated with increased LV mass and with concentric remodeling as assessed by cardiac magnetic resonance imaging independent of age, sex, and other factors.[53] Sacre et al. reported that in patients with T2D, measures of both systolic and diastolic function were associated with measures of CAN.[54] In a subgroup analysis of ~300 patients with T2D enrolled in the prospective AdreView Myocardial Imaging for Risk Evaluation in Heart Failure (ADMIRE-HF), the presence of CAN at baseline, as assessed by I-123 metaiodobenzylguanidine imaging, was associated with a significantly greater 2-year rate of heart failure progression, compared with patients with no CAN enrolled in the same trial.[3,55] Recent studies also have described that patients with T1D may present with increased LV torsion, an early measure of LV dysfunction, which is associated with the presence of CAN.[56,57] The contribution of this abnormality to adverse clinical outcomes remains to be established.

Abnormal Blood Pressure Regulation. In normal situations, at night, a predominance of vagal tone and a decreased sympathetic tone are associated with a reduction in nocturnal BP.[58] In diabetic CAN, this pattern is altered, resulting in nocturnal sympathetic predominance during sleep and subsequent nocturnal hypertension, also known as nondipping and reverse dipping.[3,59]

Orthostatic Hypotension. Orthostatic hypotension (a fall in systolic or diastolic BP in response to a postural change from supine to standing) occurs in diabetes largely as a consequence of efferent sympathetic vasomotor denervation, causing reduced vasoconstriction of the splanchnic and other peripheral vascular beds. It occurs late in the progression of CAN and is a poor prognostic indicator. Symptoms associated with orthostatic hypotension are shown in Table 45.2.[1,3,36] Intractable lower-limb edema also can be a troublesome complication of peripheral sympathetic denervation, which can result in ulceration.

CAN and Chronic Kidney Disease. The sympathetic activation associated with CAN also may play a central role in the pathogenesis of chronic kidney disease (CKD), due to changes in glomerular hemodynamics and in the circadian rhythms of BP and albuminuria.[3,60-63] A higher resting heart rate was reported to be associated with overt nephropathy development in patients with T1D. In the Atherosclerosis Risk in Communities (ARIC) Study, which included >1,500 adults with diabetes followed for 16 years, higher resting heart rate and lower HRV indexes were associated with the highest risk of developing end-stage renal disease.[3,63,64]

Mortality Risk. One of the most serious consequences of CAN is its relationship with mortality risk.[3] A meta-analysis of 15 studies that included 2,900 subjects with diabetes reported a pooled relative risk of mortality of 3.45 (95% CI 2.66–4.47) in patients with CAN.[65]

In a prospective cohort study of T1D patients participating in the EURODIAB IDDM Complications Study, CAN was the strongest predictor for mortality during a 7-year follow-up.[66] A higher predictive value of increased number of CAN abnormalities was described in patients with both T1D and T2D.[67,68] Given that CAN is associated with multiple factors including duration of diabetes, severity of hyperglycemia, the presence of coronary artery disease, and other diabetes chronic complications, the exact contribution of CAN to the increased mortality risk has been difficult to quantify in most studies because of relatively small sample size that prevented adjustments for multiple covariates.[3] Recently, however, in a large and carefully characterized cohort of >8,000 participants with T2D enrolled in the ACCORD trial, it was confirmed that the presence of CAN strongly predicts all-cause (hazard ratio [HR] = 2.14, 95% CI 1.37–3.37) and CVD mortality (HR = 2.62, 95% CI 1.4–4.91) independently of baseline CVD, diabetes duration, multiple traditional CVD risk factors, and medications (Table 45.3).[3,13]

A proposed sequence in the progression of CAN and its clinical consequences is shown in Figure 45.1.

Gastrointestinal Autonomic Neuropathy

The effect of autonomic neuropathy on the gastrointestinal system can have several manifestations.

Esophageal Dysfunction. Esophageal dysfunction results, at least in part, from vagal dysfunction. Associated symptoms include heartburn and dysphagia for solids (Table 45.2).

Gastroparesis. Gastroparesis, due to delayed gastric emptying, has been observed in up to 50% of patients with long-standing diabetes. The range of symptoms is broad (Table 45.2) but nonspecific.[16] Advanced cases dominated by severe nausea and postprandial vomiting can complicate diabetes control and reduce the quality of life.[16]

Diabetic Diarrhea. Diabetic diarrhea is typically intermittent and occurs in up to 20% of diabetic patients, particularly those with other forms of autonomic dysfunction. Profuse and watery diarrhea, typically occurring at night, also has been described, especially in patients with T1D. It may alternate with constipation and is extremely difficult to treat. History should rule out diarrhea secondary to ingestion of lactose, nonabsorbable hexitols, or medication.

Table 45.3 Hazard Ratios and 95% Confidence Intervals for All-Cause and CVD Mortality in ACCORD Participants with CAN Versus Participants Without CAN

Measure	All-cause mortality*			CVD mortality*		
	Hazard Ratio (CAN+/CAN-)	95% CI	P-value	Hazard Ratio (CAN+/CAN-)	95% CI	P-value
CAN1	1.55	1.09, 2.21	0.016	1.94	1.20, 3.12	0.007
CAN2	2.14	1.37, 3.37	0.0009	2.62	1.40, 4.91	0.003
CAN3	2.07	1.14, 3.76	0.02	2.95	1.33, 6.53	0.008

Note: CAN1 = the lowest quartile of standard deviation of normally conducted R-R intervals (SDNN) + highest quartile of QTI; CAN2 = CAN1 + highest quartile of heart rate; CAN3 = CAN2 + DPN.

*Adjusted for treatment allocation, CVD history, baseline age, gender, ethnicity, diabetes duration, A1C, BMI, systolic and diastolic blood pressure, low-density lipoprotein cholesterol, triglycerides, albumin-to-creatinine ratio, and use of thiazolidinedione, insulin, β-blockers, angiotensin-converting enzyme inhibitors and angiotensin-receptor blockers, statins, alcohol, and cigarettes.

Source: Pop-Busui R. What do we know and we do not know about cardiovascular autonomic neuropathy in diabetes. *J Cardiovasc Transl Res* 2012;5:463–478; Pop-Busui R, Evans GW, Gerstein HC, Fonseca V, Fleg JL, Hoogwerf BJ, Genuth S, Grimm RH, Corson MA, Prineas R. Effects of cardiac autonomic dysfunction on mortality risk in the Action to Control Cardiovascular Risk in Diabetes (ACCORD) trial. *Diabetes Care* 2010;33:1578–1584.

Other Manifestations. People with diabetes also may experience fecal incontinence due to poor sphincter tone or severe constipation.

Urogenital Autonomic Neuropathy

Bladder Dysfunction. Bladder dysfunction occurs in up to 50% of people with diabetes.[16] Symptoms are diverse and include frequency, urgency, nocturia, hesitancy, a weak stream, dribbling and urinary incontinence, and urinary retention (Table 45.2).

Erectile Dysfunction. ED is present in 30 to 75% of men with diabetes.[16] It has a multifactorial etiology that includes autonomic neuropathy, other vascular risk factors such as hypertension, hyperlipidemia, obesity, endothelial dysfunction, smoking, CVD, concomitant medication, and psychogenic factors.

Female Sexual Dysfunction. Female sexual dysfunction may occur in diabetic women and present as decreased sexual desire, increased pain during intercourse, and decreased sexual arousal; inadequate lubrication also may occur (Table 45.2).

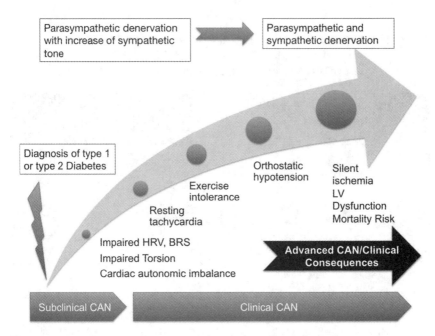

Figure 45.1—Proposed sequence for progression of cardiovascular autonomic neuropathy and its clinical consequences.

Source: Adapted with permission from Kuehl M, Stevens MJ. Cardiovascular autonomic neuropathies as complications of diabetes mellitus. *Nat Rev Endocrinol* 2012;8:405–416.

Note: CAN = cardiovascular autonomic neuropathy; HRV = heart rate variability; BRS = baroreflex sensitivity.

Other Manifestations of Autonomic Neuropathy

Autonomic neuropathy can lead to sudomotor dysfunction with such manifestations as anhidrosis, heat intolerance, dry skin, and hyperhidrosis.[69] An unawareness of hypoglycemia also possibly could be related to autonomic neuropathy.

DIAGNOSIS

CARDIOVASCULAR AUTONOMIC NEUROPATHY

Several diagnostic approaches with varying degrees of complexity are available to diagnose CAN in clinical practice or research, including the assessment of cardiovascular reflexes, HRV, 24-hour BP profiles, orthostatic hypotension, baroreflex sensitivity (BRS), cardiac sympathetic imaging, microneurography or occlusion plethysmography, and head-up tilt-table testing (HUTT).[3] Although some societies have developed guidelines for screening for CAN, the benefits of sophisticated testing beyond risk stratification are not clear.[45]

ASSESSMENT OF SYMPTOMS

Symptoms associated with CAN include exercise intolerance, orthostatic intolerance, and syncope (Table 45.2).[10] The correlation between symptom scores and deficits generally is weak in mild CAN, as these symptoms usually occur late in the disease process. Low et al., using a validated self-report measure of autonomic symptoms in a population-based study, found that autonomic symptoms were present more commonly in T1D than in T2D.[3,10]

Cardiovascular Autonomic Reflex Tests

On the basis of the strongest evidence available to date, the recent Toronto Consensus Panel on Diabetic Neuropathy concluded that the cardiovascular autonomic reflex tests (CARTs) are sensitive, specific, reproducible, safe, and standardized.[1,3,36,69,70] Their use was recommended as the gold standard for clinical autonomic testing.[1,3]

These tests, first described in the 1970s,[71,72] assess the cardiovascular autonomic function using provocative physiological maneuvers and include *1*) changes in R-R interval with deep breathing, a measure of sinus arrhythmia during quiet respiration reflecting primarily parasympathetic function;[69] *2*) the R-R response to standing, inducing reflex tachycardia followed by bradycardia, which is jointly vagal and baroreflex-mediated; *3*) the Valsalva ratio, which evaluates cardiovagal function in response to a standardized increase in intrathoracic pressure (the Valsalva maneuver); *4*) orthostatic hypotension; and *5*) the BP response to a Valsalva maneuver and sustained isometric muscular strain, which is now used in clinical research only.[1,3] Although no test is clearly superior,[1] the deep breathing test is the most widely used test because of its high reproducibility, ~80% specificity,[73] and ease of use.[1,69,73] The Valsalva maneuver requires greater patient cooperation. Because of the associated increase in intrathoracic, intraocular, and intracranial pressure, it theoretically could result in intraocular hemorrhage or lens dislocation; thus, it cannot be performed universally.[1] Test abnormalities should be defined using age-based and technique-specific normative data.[1,3] A detailed description of CART's standardization, analysis, and staging is provided in Spallone et al.[1]

Heart Rate Variability

A decrease in HRV is the earliest clinical indicator of CAN. In normal individuals, beat-to-beat variability with respiration, increasing with inspiration and decreasing with expiration, is due to the direct influence of sympathetic and parasympathetic stimuli. HRV can be evaluated in the time and frequency domain, derived from electrocardiogram (ECG) recordings, ideally under paced breathing. Longer ECG recordings (e.g., 24-hour) initially were used exclusively, but shorter recordings also were shown to provide reliable information on cardiovascular autonomic function.[3,74,75]

Time domain measures of the normal R-R intervals, basically reflecting parasympathetic activity, include the difference between the longest and shortest R-R interval, standard deviation of 5-minute average of normal R-R intervals

(SDANN), and root-mean square of the difference of successive R-R intervals (rMSSD).[74] The accuracy of these measures is affected by various arrhythmias, and the analysis requires normal sinus rhythm and atrioventricular-nodal function.[3]

The frequency domain measures are obtained by spectral analysis of R-R intervals and other respiratory and cardiovascular signals.[75] It traditionally is accepted that the parasympathetic system affects the high-frequency components (0.15–0.4 Hz), sympathetic activity essentially influences a rather narrow band around 0.1 Hz, and the very low-frequency components (<0.04 Hz) essentially are related to fluctuations in vasomotor tone associated with thermoregulation or activity.[75] A variety of mathematical methods used to analyze HRV and the commercially available software programs for assessment of HRV are covered broadly in Bernardi et al.[75] It generally is recommended that HRV testing be used for research and in conjunction with the cardiovascular autonomic reflex testing.[3,75]

Baroreflex Sensitivity

The BRS technique evaluates the capability to reflexively increase vagal activity and decrease sympathetic activity in response to a sudden increase in BP. Currently, this technique is used exclusively in research protocols. An increase in BP reduces the firing of sympathetic vascular and cardiac efferents and increases the firing of vagal cardiac efferents, resulting in a rapid reduction in heart rate and BP. The reduction in BP is due to both a reduction in cardiac output caused by bradycardia and to a slower direct vasodilation secondary to sympathetic withdrawal.[75] The cardiac-vagal arm of the BRS can be assessed with drugs or by physical maneuvers; alternatively, the spontaneous BP variations can be used. In all cases, the response in heart rate to the changes in BP is quantified. These methods have been described in detail.[3,75]

BRS can detect subclinical CAN[76] and may be abnormal before other tests of CAN.[77] The BRS was a significant independent risk predictor of cardiac mortality in large cohorts of patients with heart failure, a recent myocardial infarction, or diabetes.[3,78–80]

Imaging Techniques for CAN

Quantitative scintigraphic assessment of sympathetic innervation of the human heart is possible with positron emission tomography (PET) and either [123I]*meta*-iodobenzylguanidine (MIBG) [11C]-*meta*-hydroxy-ephedrine [11C] HED, 6-[18F] dopamine, and [11C]-epinephrine.[36,81]

Deficits of LV [123I]MIBG and [11C]HED retention have been identified in subjects with T1D and T2D[82–84] and in subject with[82–84] and without[43] abnormal cardiovascular reflex testing. The delivery of tracers is influenced critically by myocardial perfusion, so the myocardial retention of tracers should be performed with a quantitative analysis of myocardial blood flow.[3,75]

Regional myocardial [123I]-MIBG "uptake" is semiquantitative and not a clean index of neuronal uptake. It is further complicated by an increased BMI and diastolic BP, which have been reported to reduce myocardial MIBG uptake.[75] Metabolically stable [11C]HED undergoes highly specific uptake into sympathetic nerve varicosities via norepinephrine transporters, and quantitative [11C]HED retention may be assessed in 480 independent LV regions.[81] The striking consistency of the evolution of the pattern of denervation in T1D supports the reliability of [^{11}C]HED to monitor changes in cardiac sympathetic nerve populations and to evaluate early anatomical regional deficits of sympathetic denervation.[3,43,81,82] Although a valuable research tool, due to their high costs and the need for highly specialized infrastructure and personnel, the use of these techniques is not yet recommended for standard clinical care.[3]

Muscle Sympathetic Nerve Activity

The muscle sympathetic nerve activity (MSNA) technique is based on recording electrical activity emitted by skeletal muscle (peroneal, tibial, radial) at rest or in response to various physiological perturbations, via microelectrodes inserted into a fascicle of a distal sympathetic nerve to the skin or muscle (microneurography), and identification of sympathetic bursts.[85] Recently available fully automated sympathetic neurogram techniques provide a more rapid and objective method that is affected minimally by signal quality and that preserves beat-by-beat sympathetic neurograms.[3,85] Because of its invasiveness and the time-consuming nature of the procedure, MSNA is not indicated for routine autonomic assessment but rather remains an important research tool.[3,75]

Head-Up Tilt-Table Testing

Head-up tilt-table testing (HUTT) with and without pharmacological provocation is another tool used to investigate CAN or a predisposition to neurally mediated (vasovagal) syncope. HUTT records a wide range of changes in the autonomic input to the heart and in the R-R intervals induced by the rapid postural changes during the test. This test requires specialized personnel and is not readily available in general practice.[3]

GASTROINTESTINAL AUTONOMIC NEUROPATHY (GASTROPARESIS)

Symptoms

The Diabetes Bowel Symptom Questionnaire (DBSQ) has been validated in a diabetic population to quantify gastrointestinal symptoms; however, the predictive value is poor.[75] Quality-of-life measures have not focused specifically on the gastrointestinal tract.[75] Therefore, objective measurements of gastric emptying are recommended for the diagnosis of gastroparesis.

Gastric Emptying Studies

The evaluation of solid emptying is probably more sensitive than that of low-nutrient liquid or semisolid meals.[16] Gastric emptying can be affected by many factors, including medications, smoking, and blood glucose concentrations, and standardization of testing is important as described in Kempler et al.[16] Utility of testing is limited by poor correlation with symptoms and intraindividual variability of test results. A barium meal or upper-endoscopy studies always are recommended to rule out mucosal lesions or obstruction.

Scintigraphy still is regarded as the gold standard technique for the measurement of gastric emptying. It also helps to assess the intragastric distribution of a meal, which frequently is abnormal in diabetic patients. Standardization of the technique between centers is important, and recent consensus guidelines recommend a low-fat egg white meal labeled with 99mTc sulfur colloid and consumed with jam and toast as a sandwich, along with a glass of water.[86] The limitations of scintigraphy are exposure to a modest dose of radiation, the relative expense, and the need for specialist centers.

Breath tests using nonradioactive ^{13}C-acetate or octanoic acid as a label are safe and inexpensive. The results correlate well with scintigraphy results.[16,86] Ultrasonography is a noninvasive diagnostic method. Two- and three-dimensional ultrasound have been validated for measuring emptying of liquids and semisolids.[16,86] MRI has been used to measure gastric emptying and motility with excellent reproductivity, but its use is limited to research purposes.[16] Surface electrogastrography to detect abnormal gastric electric activity currently is recommended as research tool.[16] Manometry is used to assess motor function of the stomach, small intestine, and colon; manometry and scintigraphy results correlate relatively well.[16,86] Manometry should be considered as a research technique to investigate gastric and intestinal motility. Tests of anorectal motor and sensory functions are well developed for clinical use.

ERECTILE DYSFUNCTION

Clinical Evaluation

A comprehensive interview is a key diagnostic procedure for assessing ED and includes information on sexual and medical history, drug use for associated comorbidities (tranquillizers, antidepressants, antihypertensives), and psychological and organic factors. It is helpful to confirm the nature of the erectile problem and to distinguish it from other forms of sexual difficulty, such as penile curvature or premature ejaculation. An interview with the partner is advisable and will confirm the problem but also may reveal other causes of the difficulties (e.g., vaginal dryness).[16] The use of validated questionnaires, such as the International Index of Erectile Function and the Sexual Encounter Profile, is the most appropriate method to characterize frequency and severity of ED symptoms.[16]

Laboratory

Routine laboratory tests should include A1C, fasting blood glucose, and lipid profile. Measurements for bioavailable testosterone are recommended (if not available, total or free testosterone instead) to rule out primary or hypogonadotropic hypogonadism, especially in patients who do not respond to phosphodiesterase type 5 (PDE-5) inhibitors.

ED tests may be useful in patients who do not respond to PDE-5 inhibitors and include evaluations of nocturnal penile tumescence, penile Doppler ultrasound, bulbocavernosus reflex, dorsal sensory nerve conduction of the penis, amplitude and latency of penile sympathetic skin response, pudendal nerve somatosensory evoked potentials, assessment of prostaglandin E1 (PGE1) effect on erection, psychological evaluation, and urodynamic studies.[16]

BLADDER DYSFUNCTION

Clinical Evaluation

Lower urinary tract symptoms (LUTS) severity can be assessed by comprehensive interview to include specific questions about urinary symptoms, ideally using a validated questionnaire for incontinence and LUTS. The American Urological Association Symptom Index is a standardized seven-item questionnaire that quantifies the presence and frequency of the following LUTS: nocturia, frequency, urgency, weak urinary stream, intermittency, straining, and the sensation of incomplete emptying.[87] Scores on the index range from 0 to 35, with widely accepted cut points of 0–7, 8–19, and 20–35 are designated as none or mild, moderate, and severe LUTS, respectively.

Assessments of perineal sensation, sphincter tone, and the bulbocavernosus reflex may identify peripheral neuropathy consistent with diabetes. Complete urogynaecologic examination is needed to exclude pelvic organ prolapse or other pelvic disorders.[16]

Laboratory

Because diabetic patients are at increased risk of bacterial cystitis, microscopic urinalysis and culture are essential in assessing patients complaining of LUTS. Alterations in polymorphonuclear leukocyte function in the high-glucose state may contribute to an increased risk of urinary tract infection.[16]

Urodynamic Testing

Detailed assessment of bladder function with urodynamic studies is indicated if initial management is unsuccessful, or there is doubt about the diagnosis. This may include cystometry, uroflow, simultaneous pressure and flow studies, sphincter electromyography, urethral pressure profilometry with evaluation of leak-point pressures, measurement of peak urinary flow rate, and postvoid residual (PVR) volume.[16] Urodynamic findings associated with autonomic dysfunction include impaired bladder sensation, increased cystometric capacity, decreased detrusor contractility, and increased PVR volume.[16]

SUDOMOTOR DYSFUNCTION

Several methods have been developed to assess sudomotor function with variable degree of complexity and accuracy, including the quantitative sudomotor axon reflex test (which evaluates postganglionic sudomotor function by acetylcholine iontophoresis), thermoregulatory sweat testing, sympathetic skin response, quantitative direct and indirect axon reflex testing. Limitations of all these techniques include fair test sensitivity, high costs for specialized equipment and personnel time, and the lack of good normative data.[16] The Sudoscan+ (Impeto Medical SAS), a noninvasive device that uses reverse iontophoresis and chronoamperometry to test for sudomotor dysfunction, recently became available and may emerge as an easier-to-implement technique.

Microvascular Function Assessment

The skin offers an accessible organ to assess microvascular blood flow (MBF) and endothelial function, which correlate with systemic measurements of endothelial function and myocardial microcirculation.[16] Several methods are available to assess skin MBF. Laser Doppler (LD) determines blood flow under basal conditions or following physical (e.g., heating) or pharmacological (e.g., acetylcholine or sodium nitroprusside) stimulation. This differentiates endothelial-dependent and independent responses.[16,88] Furthermore, LD measures nerve axon reflex-related vasodilation following acetylcholine iontophoresis, which is the result of C-fiber stimulation. LD techniques include LD flowmetry, LD perfusion imaging, and laser speckle contrast imaging.[16]

TREATMENT

Tight and stable glycemic control implemented as early as possible in the course of disease, as well as aggressive management of other cardiovascular risk factors remain the mainstay of therapy, as other effective disease-modifying therapies are not available.[45] A timely referral to specialists should be sought as soon as possible, once the signs of established disease are identified.[45]

DISEASE-MODIFYING THERAPIES

Glycemic Control

Intensive control of hyperglycemia early in the course of T1D has been shown to prevent or reverse CAN or to delay its progression as demonstrated by the DCCT.[4] EDIC has shown persistent beneficial effects of past glucose control on microvascular complications, including neuropathic complications, despite the loss of glycemic separation.[89] CAN was reevaluated recently in >1,200 well-characterized EDIC participants during the 13th and 14th year of EDIC follow-up. During EDIC, CAN progressed substantially in both former treatment groups; however, the prevalence and incidence of CAN in EDIC remained significantly lower in the former intensive group than in the former conventional group, despite similar levels of glycemic control.[7] Treatment group differences in the mean A1C level during DCCT and EDIC explained virtually all of the beneficial effects of intensive versus conventional therapy on the risk of incident CAN. These results support the finding that intensive treatment of T1D should be initiated as early as is safely possible.[3,7,45]

In T2D, the effects of glycemic control are less conclusive. The Veterans Affairs Cooperative Study demonstrated no difference in the prevalence of autonomic neuropathy in T2D patients after 2 years of tight glycemic control compared with those without tight control.[24] Similar results were reported by the VADT.[3,25]

Multiple Risk Factor Intervention

As mentioned previously, an intensive multifactorial cardiovascular risk intervention targeting glucose, BP, lipids, smoking, and other lifestyle factors, reduced the progression or the development of CAN among patients with T2D.[35] Data regarding the impact of lifestyle interventions in preventing progression of CAN were reported by the Diabetes Prevention Program, where indexes of CAN improved most in the lifestyle modification arm.[90,91] Others reported improvement in cardiovascular autonomic function in obese patients after weight loss,[37] or after strictly supervised endurance training combined with dietary changes.[36] A few small, mostly open, interventional studies in diabetes showed a beneficial effect of aerobic training on cardiovascular autonomic indexes, with some indication that mild physical exercise may be effective only in patients with less severe CAN.[1,3]

Other Therapies Targeting Pathogenetic Pathways

Evidence is limited on the effects of agents targeting pathogenetic pathways shown to contribute to CAN development. Phase II randomized controlled trials have shown favorable effects on HRV indexes using the antioxidant α-lipoic acid, vitamin E, and C-peptide.[1,3] However, a recent trial using PET and [^{11}C]HED evaluating the efficacy of a combination of antioxidant approaches including allopurinol, α-lipoic acid, and nicotinamide in 44 subjects with T1D did not show any benefit.[92] Further studies are needed to confirm these findings as well as to unveil new and effective potential pathogenetic treatments.

A number of drugs may adversely affect the autonomic tone by reducing HRV with a consequent potential proarrhythmic effect.[1,3] On the other hand, an increase in HRV has been described, with some controversy, in patients who have diabetes with angiotensin-converting enzyme inhibitors, angiotensin II type 1 receptor blockers, cardioselective β-blockers without intrinsic sympathomimetic activity (e.g., metoprolol, nebivolol, bisoprolol), digoxin, and verapamil.[1,6,36] Some have proposed the use of cardioselective β-blockers to treat resting tachycardia associated with CAN, but to date, there is no clear evidence on their efficacy in diabetic CAN.[3]

SYMPTOMATIC TREATMENT

Orthostatic Hypotension

The therapeutic goal is to minimize postural symptoms rather than to restore normotension. In severe cases, treatment is challenging and, in most cases, requires the use of both nonpharmacological and pharmacological measures (described in brief in Table 45.4).[3]

Gastroparesis

The approach to gastroparesis usually requires a combination of dietary changes and drug therapy (Table 45.4), but the rate of success declines with recurrent and advanced disease.[16] Nonpharmacological approaches, such as gastric pacing and surgery, may be needed for refractory cases although randomized trials demonstrating efficacy are lacking (Table 45.4).

Diabetic Diarrhea

Broad-spectrum antibiotics commonly are used to treat diabetic diarrhea. Other agents such as cholestyramine and somatostatin analogs may be used in severe cases (Table 45.4).

Table 45.4 Symptomatic Treatment of Autonomic Neuropathy

1. Orthostatic Hypotension
  A. Lifestyle and supportive measures[3]
  - Avoid sudden changes in body posture to the head-up position.
  - Avoid medications that aggravate hypotension (i.e., tricyclic antidepressants, phenothiazines, diuretics).
  - Eat small, frequent meals.
  - Avoid activities that involve straining.
  - Elevate the head of the bed 18 inches at night.
  - Use a compressive garment over the legs and abdomen.
  - Use an inflatable abdominal band.
  - Use a low portable chair, as needed for symptoms.
  - Avoid physical countermaneuvers, such as leg crossing, squatting, and muscle pumping.
  - Increase fluid and salt intake if not contraindicated.

  B. Pharmacologic therapy[3]
  Midodrine
  - A peripheral-selective direct α-1-adrenoreceptor agonist.
  - Activates α-1 receptors on arterioles and veins, thereby increasing total peripheral resistance; several double-blind, placebo-controlled studies have documented its efficacy in the treatment of orthostatic hypotension.[3]
  - The only Food and Drug Administration (FDA)-approved agent approved for the treatment of orthostatic hypotension.
  - Doses of 2.5–10 mg three to four times a day usually are recommended.[3]
  - First dose to be taken before arising.
  - Avoid taking several hours before planned recumbent position.
  - Does not cross the blood-brain barrier.
  - Main adverse effects include piloerection, pruritus, paresthesias, supine hypertension, urinary retention.

  Fludrocortisone
  - A synthetic mineralocorticoid, with a long duration of action, which induces plasma expansion.
  - Also may enhance the sensitivity of blood vessels to circulating catecholamines.
  - The effects are not immediate; occur over a 1- to 2-week period.[3]
  - Treatment usually begins with 0.05 mg at bedtime, and may be titrated gradually to a maximum of 0.2 mg/day; higher doses are associated with higher risk for side effects.
  - Main adverse advents include supine hypertension, hypokalemia, hypomagnesemia, congestive heart failure, and peripheral edema.
  - Caution must be used in patients with congestive heart failure to avoid fluid overload.

  Erythropoietin
  - May improve standing blood pressure in patients with orthostatic hypotension.
  - Possible mechanisms of action include increase in red cell mass and central blood volume; correction of the normochromic normocytic anemia that frequently accompanies diabetic autonomic neuropathy; alterations in blood viscosity; and a direct or indirect neurohumoral effect on the vascular wall and vascular tone regulation, which are mediated by the interaction between hemoglobin and the vasodilator nitric oxide.

(continued)

Table 45.4 Symptomatic Treatment of Autonomic Neuropathy *(continued)*

■ Can be administered in patients with diabetes with orthostatic hypotension and hemoglobin levels <11 g/dl subcutaneously or intravenously at doses between 25 and 75 U/kg three times a week until the hemoglobin reaches target of 12 grams/dl followed by lower maintenance doses.
■ Risk of serious cardiovascular events should be considered.

Somatostatin analogs
■ May attenuate the postprandial blood pressure fall and reduce orthostatic hypotension in patients with autonomic failure.
■ Mechanisms of action include a local effect on splanchnic vasculature, by inhibiting the release of vasoactive gastrointestinal peptides; enhanced cardiac output; and an increase in forearm and splanchnic vascular resistance.
■ Usually 25–200 μg/day octreotide are given subcutaneously in divided doses every 8 hours.
■ Long-acting depot preparation may be used, 20–30 mg intramuscularly once monthly.
■ Adverse events include severe hypertension.

Caffeine citrate
■ A methylxanthine with well-established pressor effect, primarily due to blockade of vasodilating adenosine receptors.
■ May improve orthostatic hypotension and attenuate postprandial hypotension.
■ Recommended dose 100–250 mg orally three times daily; dose expressed as anhydrous-caffeine.
■ May be taken as tablets or caffeinated beverage.
■ Tachyphylaxis occurs with continuing use of caffeine.

2. Gastroparesis
A. Dietary changes
■ Eat multiple small meals.
■ Decrease dietary fat and fiber.
B. Drug therapy (prokinetic agents)
Metoclopramide (Reglan)
■ Has antiemetic properties, stimulates acetylcholine release in the myenteric plexus, and is a dopamine antagonist.[93]
■ Open, single-blind, and double-blind trials have shown mild benefit.[93]
■ Possible adverse effects include extrapyramidal symptoms, such as acute dystonic reactions (drug-induced parkinsonism, akathisia, tardive dyskinesia), galactorrhea, amenorrhea, gynecomastia, and hyperprolactinemia.
■ Recent evidence from the European Medicine Agency[94] confirmed that risks of extrapyramidal symptoms are high and outweigh benefits. Therefore, in the European Union, metoclopramide use is restricted to a maximum of 5 days and is no longer indicated for the long-term treatment of gastroparesis. It should be reserved to most severe cases, that are unresponsive to other therapies and side effects would be closely monitored. The FDA decision is pending.
Domperidone (not FDA approved in the U.S.)
■ Is a peripheral dopamine receptor antagonist.[95]
■ Has been shown to stimulate gastric motility and to possess antiemetic properties. It acts as a prokinetic agent, increasing the number and the intensity of gastric contractions, and improves symptoms in patients with diabetic gastroparesis.[95]
■ Stimulates both liquid- and solid-phase gastric emptying.
■ Its major benefit results from its antiemetic properties and, to a lesser extent, its motor stimulatory actions.

(continued)

Table 45.4 Symptomatic Treatment of Autonomic Neuropathy *(continued)*

- A systematic review of all studies using oral domperidone for the treatment of diabetic gastroparesis demonstrated improvement in gastric emptying and the efficacy of domperidone in treating gastroparesis.[96]
- Its role has become controversial, due to safety concerns, and it has never been approved for marketing by the FDA in the U.S.

Erythromycin
- Is effective in accelerating gastric emptying.[97]
- Is believed to act by stimulating motilin receptors in the gut.[98]
- May be used orally or intravenously.[97,99]

Onabotulinumtoxin A (formerly known as botulinum toxin type A)
- Reserved for severe diabetic gastroparesis refractory to dietary changes and the use of high-dose prokinetic agents.[100,101]
- Few case-reports describe significant symptomatic improvement after intrapyloric injection, performed during upper GI endoscopy.[101]

C. Other nonpharmacological methods

Gastric pacing (stimulation)
- Short-term studies of gastric pacing in humans have demonstrated that it is possible to entrain gastric slow waves and normalize myoelectrical activity with pacing.[102,103]
- Uses high-frequency, low-amplitude signals that do not alter gastric myoelectrical or muscular activity.[102,103]
- Improvements in nausea and vomiting with gastric stimulation in people with gastroparesis have been reported.[102,103]

Surgery
- Persistent vomiting may require a surgical approach.
- Placement of a feeding jejunostomy to bypass an atonic stomach has been advocated, based on clinical practice.[104]
- Radical surgery, consisting of resection of a large portion of the stomach, with performance of a Roux-en-Y loop was successful in a small series of patients.[104]

3. Diabetic Diarrhea
A. Drug therapy

Broad-spectrum antibiotics
- Metronidazole 500 mg every 6 hours for 3 weeks; or 750 mg every 8 hours for 3 weeks.[14,105]
- Ampicillin or tetracycline 250 mg every 6 to 8 hours for 14 days.[14,105]
- Amoxicillin/clavulanate 875 mg twice daily for 14 days (dose refers to the amoxicillin component).[106]
- Cholestyramine.
- Chelates bile salts.
- Used if the hydrogen breath test is normal, or if patients failing an empiric trial of broad-spectrum antibiotics.[14]

Octreotide
- Accelerates gastric emptying, inhibits small bowel transit, reducing ileocolonic bolus transfers, inhibiting postprandial colonic tonic response, and increasing colonic phasic pressure activity in healthy volunteers.
- Was effective, in a case report of a single patient, for diabetic diarrhea.[107]
- May be used if other methods have not helped.[14]

(continued)

Table 45.4 Symptomatic Treatment of Autonomic Neuropathy *(continued)*

4. Erectile Dysfunction
A. Drug therapy
Phosphodiesterase-5 (PDE-5) inhibitors
- Preferred therapy for erectile dysfunction.[16]
- Several agents have been approved (e.g., sildenafil, tadalafil, vardenafil).
- Efficacy demonstrated in randomized placebo-controlled clinical trials,[16,108,109] and in general it is well tolerated.[16]
- Headaches and flushing are most frequent adverse event reported; other adverse events reported in a descending order of frequency may include upper-respiratory tract complaints, flulike syndromes, dyspepsia, myalgias, abnormal vision, and back pain.[16]

B. Nonpharmacological approaches
Intracavernosal injections
- Success rate is high, with nearly 90% of patients achieving erection.[110,111]
- Other therapies
- Vacuum devices
- Rigid penile implants
- Inflatable prostheses for the treatment of erectile dysfunction
- All with mild to modest benefits

5. Bladder Dysfunction
- Bethanechol, a parasympathomimetic agent, may be helpful.
- Bladder training, such as scheduled voiding, may be used particularly for urge incontinence.
- The Crede maneuver may be helpful.

Erectile Dysfunction

A mainstream of treatment involves the use of PDE-5 inhibitors (Table 45.4).[16] Nonpharmacological approaches also can be used alone or in combination with the PDE-5 inhibitors (Table 45.4).

Bladder Dysfunction

Pharmacological and nonpharmacological approaches are shown in Table 45.4.

CONCLUSION

Autonomic neuropathies are a common complication of diabetes with a broad spectrum of clinical manifestations and high morbidity. Recent evidence unveiled important information on the natural history of this complication; however, the pathogenetic mechanisms are still not well understood and the therapeutic options continue to lag behind. Glycemic control remains the only effective disease-modifying treatment strategy, especially for patients with T1D earlier in the course of disease. Lifestyle interventions may be beneficial in some patients with new-onset

T2D or prediabetes. Symptomatic relief may be the only strategy available for the majority of more advanced forms of autonomic neuropathy.

REFERENCES

1. Spallone V, Ziegler D, Freeman R, Bernardi L, Frontoni S, Pop-Busui R, Stevens M, Kempler P, Hilsted J, Tesfaye S, Low P, Valensi P. Cardiovascular autonomic neuropathy in diabetes: clinical impact, assessment, diagnosis, and management. *Diabetes Metab Res Rev* 2011;27:639–653.

2. Diabetes Control and Complications Trial Research Group. The effect of intensive treatment of diabetes on the development and progression of long-term complications in insulin-dependent diabetes mellitus. *N Engl J Med* 1993;329:977–986.

3. Pop-Busui R. What do we know and we do not know about cardiovascular autonomic neuropathy in diabetes. *J Cardiovasc Transl Res* 2012;5:463–478.

4. Diabetes Control and Complications Trial Research Group. The effect of intensive diabetes therapy on measures of autonomic nervous system function in the Diabetes Control and Complications Trial (DCCT). *Diabetologia* 1998;41:416–423.

5. Ziegler D, Gries FA, Spuler M, Lessmann F. The epidemiology of diabetic neuropathy. Diabetic Cardiovascular Autonomic Neuropathy Multicenter Study Group. *J Diabetes Complications* 1992;6:49–57.

6. Pop-Busui R. Cardiac autonomic neuropathy in diabetes: a clinical perspective. *Diabetes Care* 2010;33:434–441.

7. Pop-Busui R, Low PA, Waberski BH, Martin CL, Albers JW, Feldman EL, Sommer C, Cleary PA, Lachin JM, Herman WH. Effects of prior intensive insulin therapy on cardiac autonomic nervous system function in type 1 diabetes mellitus: the Diabetes Control and Complications Trial/Epidemiology of Diabetes Interventions and Complications study (DCCT/EDIC). *Circulation* 2009;119:2886–2893.

8. Kempler P, Tesfaye S, Chaturvedi N, Stevens LK, Webb DJ, Eaton S, Kerenyi Z, Tamas G, Ward JD, Fuller JH. Autonomic neuropathy is associated with increased cardiovascular risk factors: the EURODIAB IDDM Complications Study. *Diabet Med* 2002;19:900–909.

9. Low PA. Diabetic autonomic neuropathy. *Semin Neurol* 1996;16:143–151.

10. Low PA, Benrud-Larson LM, Sletten DM, Opfer-Gehrking TL, Weigand SD, O'Brien PC, Suarez GA, Dyck PJ. Autonomic symptoms and diabetic neuropathy: a population-based study. *Diabetes Care* 2004;27:2942–2947.

11. Kennedy WR, Navarro X, Goetz FC, Sutherland DE, Najarian JS. Effects of pancreatic transplantation on diabetic neuropathy. *N Engl J Med* 1990; 322:1031–1037.

12. Ko SH, Park SA, Cho JH, Song KH, Yoon KH, Cha BY, Son HY, Yoo KD, Moon KW, Park YM, Ahn YB. Progression of cardiovascular autonomic dysfunction in patients with type 2 diabetes: a 7-year follow-up study. *Diabetes Care* 2008;31:1832–1836.

13. Pop-Busui R, Evans GW, Gerstein HC, Fonseca V, Fleg JL, Hoogwerf BJ, Genuth S, Grimm RH, Corson MA, Prineas R. Effects of cardiac autonomic dysfunction on mortality risk in the Action to Control Cardiovascular Risk in Diabetes (ACCORD) trial. *Diabetes Care* 2010;33:1578–1584.

14. Vinik AI, Maser RE, Mitchell BD, Freeman R. Diabetic autonomic neuropathy. *Diabetes Care* 2003;26:1553–1579.

15. Horowitz M, Maddox AF, Wishart JM, Harding PE, Chatterton BE, Shearman DJ. Relationships between oesophageal transit and solid and liquid gastric emptying in diabetes mellitus. *Eur J Nucl Med* 1991;18:229–234.

16. Kempler P, Amarenco G, Freeman R, Frontoni S, Horowitz M, Stevens M, Low P, Pop-Busui R, Tahrani A, Tesfaye S, Varkonyi T, Ziegler D, Valensi P. Gastrointestinal autonomic neuropathy, erectile-, bladder- and sudomotor dysfunction in patients with diabetes mellitus: clinical impact, assessment, diagnosis, and management. *Diabetes Metab Res Rev* 2011;27:665–677.

17. Kofod-Andersen K, Tarnow L. Prevalence of gastroparesis-related symptoms in an unselected cohort of patients with type 1 diabetes. *J Diabetes Complications* 2012;26:89–93.

18. Penson DF, Wessells H, Cleary P, Rutledge BN. Sexual dysfunction and symptom impact in men with long-standing type 1 diabetes in the DCCT/EDIC cohort. *J Sex Med* 2009;6:1969–1978.

19. Sarma AV, Kanaya A, Nyberg LM, Kusek JW, Vittinghoff E, Rutledge B, Cleary PA, Gatcomb P, Brown JS. Risk factors for urinary incontinence among women with type 1 diabetes: findings from the epidemiology of diabetes interventions and complications study. *Urology* 2009;73:1203–1209.

20. Singh JP, Larson MG, O'Donnell CJ, Wilson PF, Tsuji H, Lloyd-Jones DM, Levy D. Association of hyperglycemia with reduced heart rate variability (The Framingham Heart Study). *Am J Cardiol* 2000;86:309–312.

21. Wu JS, Yang YC, Lin TS, Huang YH, Chen JJ, Lu FH, Wu CH, Chang CJ. Epidemiological evidence of altered cardiac autonomic function in subjects with impaired glucose tolerance but not isolated impaired fasting glucose. *J Clin Endocrinol Metab* 2007;92:3885–3889.

22. Barkai L, Madacsy L, Kassay L. Investigation of subclinical signs of autonomic neuropathy in the early stage of childhood diabetes. *Hormone Res* 1990;34:54–59.

23. Sosenko JM, Boulton A, Kubrusly DB, Weintraub JK, Pasin RA, Schneiderman N, Skyler JS. Autonomic function and heart rate in young diabetic patients. *J Pediatr Endocrinol* 1985;1:207–210.

24. Azad N, Emanuele NV, Abraira C, Henderson WG, Colwell J, Levin SR, Nuttall FQ, Comstock JP, Sawin CT, Silbert C, Rubino FA. The effects of intensive glycemic control on neuropathy in the VA cooperative study on type II diabetes mellitus (VA CSDM). *J Diabetes Complications* 1999;13:307–313.

25. Duckworth W, Abraira C, Moritz T, Reda D, Emanuele N, Reaven PD, Zieve FJ, Marks J, Davis SN, Hayward R, Warren SR, Goldman S, McCarren M, Vitek ME, Henderson WG, Huang GD. Glucose control and vascular complications in veterans with type 2 diabetes. *N Engl J Med* 2009;360:129–139.

26. Ohkubo Y, Kishikawa H, Araki E, Miyata T, Isami S, Motoyoshi S, Kojima Y, Furuyoshi N, Shichiri M. Intensive insulin therapy prevents the progression of diabetic microvascular complications in Japanese patients with non-insulin- dependent diabetes mellitus: a randomized prospective 6-year study [see comments]. *Diabetes Res Clin Pract* 1995;28:103–117.

27. Solders G, Thalme B, Aguirre-Aquino M, Brandt L, Berg U, Persson A. Nerve conduction and autonomic nerve function in diabetic children. A 10-year follow-up study. *Acta Paediatrica* 1997;86:361–366.

28. Voulgari C, Psallas M, Kokkinos A, Argiana V, Katsilambros N, Tentolouris N. The association between cardiac autonomic neuropathy with metabolic and other factors in subjects with type 1 and type 2 diabetes. *J Diabetes Complications* 2011;25:159–167.

29. Bragd J, Adamson U, Backlund LB, Lins PE, Moberg E, Oskarsson P. Can glycaemic variability, as calculated from blood glucose self-monitoring, predict the development of complications in type 1 diabetes over a decade? *Diabetes Metab* 2008;34:612–616.

30. Singh K, Communal C, Sawyer DB, Colucci WS. Adrenergic regulation of myocardial apoptosis. *Cardiovasc Res* 2000;45:713–719.

31. Panzer C, Lauer MS, Brieke A, Blackstone E, Hoogwerf B. Association of fasting plasma glucose with heart rate recovery in healthy adults: a population-based study. *Diabetes* 2002;51:803–807.

32. Ziegler D, Zentai C, Perz S, Rathmann W, Haastert B, Meisinger C, Lowel H. Selective contribution of diabetes and other cardiovascular risk factors to cardiac autonomic dysfunction in the general population. *Exp Clin Endocrinol Diabetes* 2006;114:153–159.

33. Vinik AI, Maser RE, Ziegler D. Autonomic imbalance: prophet of doom or scope for hope? *Diabet Med* 2011;28:643–651.

34. Laitinen T, Lindstrom J, Eriksson J, Ilanne-Parikka P, Aunola S, Keinanen-Kiukaanniemi S, Tuomilehto J, Uusitupa M. Cardiovascular autonomic dysfunction is associated with central obesity in persons with impaired glucose tolerance. *Diabet Med* 2011;28:699–704.

35. Gaede P, Vedel P, Larsen N, Jensen GV, Parving HH, Pedersen O. Multifactorial intervention and cardiovascular disease in patients with type 2 diabetes. *N Engl J Med* 2003;348:383–393.

36. Vinik AI, Ziegler D. Diabetic cardiovascular autonomic neuropathy. *Circulation* 2007;115:387–397.

37. Maser RE, Lenhard MJ. An overview of the effect of weight loss on cardiovascular autonomic function. *Curr Diabetes Rev* 2007;3:204–211.

38. Secrest AM, Costacou T, Gutelius B, Miller RG, Songer TJ, Orchard TJ. Associations between socioeconomic status and major complications in type 1 diabetes: the Pittsburgh Epidemiology of Diabetes Complication (EDC) Study. *Ann Epidemiol* 2011;21:374–381.

39. Tesfaye S, Chaturvedi N, Eaton SE, Ward JD, Manes C, Ionescu-Tirgoviste C, Witte DR, Fuller JH. Vascular risk factors and diabetic neuropathy. *N Engl J Med* 2005;352:341–350.

40. Wiggin TD, Sullivan KA, Pop-Busui R, Amato A, Sima AA, Feldman EL. Elevated triglycerides correlate with progression of diabetic neuropathy. *Diabetes* 2009;58:1634–1640.

41. Stella P, Ellis D, Maser RE, Orchard TJ. Cardiovascular autonomic neuropathy (expiration and inspiration ratio) in type 1 diabetes. Incidence and predictors. *J Diabetes Complications* 2000;14:1–6.

42. Witte DR, Tesfaye S, Chaturvedi N, Eaton SE, Kempler P, Fuller JH. Risk factors for cardiac autonomic neuropathy in type 1 diabetes mellitus. *Diabetologia* 2005;48:164–171.

43. Pop-Busui R, Kirkwood I, Schmid H, Marinescu V, Schroeder J, Larkin D, Yamada E, Raffel DM, Stevens MJ. Sympathetic dysfunction in type 1 diabetes: association with impaired myocardial blood flow reserve and diastolic dysfunction. *J Am Coll Cardiol* 2004;44:2368–2374.

44. Taskiran M, Rasmussen V, Rasmussen B, Fritz-Hansen T, Larsson HB, Jensen GB, Hilsted J. Left ventricular dysfunction in normotensive type 1 diabetic patients: the impact of autonomic neuropathy. *Diabet Med* 2004;21:524–530.

45. American Diabetes Association. Professional practice committee for the 2014 clinical practice recommendations. *Diabetes Care* 2014;37(Suppl 1):S154–S155.

46. Vinik AI, Freeman R, Erbas T. Diabetic autonomic neuropathy. *Semin Neurol* 2003;23:365–372.

47. Young LH, Wackers FJ, Chyun DA, Davey JA, Barrett EJ, Taillefer R, Heller GV, Iskandrian AE, Wittlin SD, Filipchuk N, Ratner RE, Inzucchi SE. Cardiac outcomes after screening for asymptomatic coronary artery disease in patients with type 2 diabetes: the DIAD study: a randomized controlled trial. *JAMA* 2009;301:1547–1555.

48. Hage FG, Iskandrian AE. Cardiovascular imaging in diabetes mellitus. *J Nucl Cardiol* 2011;18:959–965.

49. Fang ZY, Prins JB, Marwick TH. Diabetic cardiomyopathy: evidence, mechanisms, and therapeutic implications. *Endocr Rev* 2004;25:543–567.

50. Fang ZY, Yuda S, Anderson V, Short L, Case C, Marwick TH. Echocardiographic detection of early diabetic myocardial disease. *J Am Coll Cardiol* 2003;41:611–617.

51. Vanninen E, Mustonen J, Vainio P, Lansimies E, Uusitupa M. Left ventricular function and dimensions in newly diagnosed non-insulin-dependent diabetes mellitus. *Am J Cardiol* 1992;70:371–378.

52. Fang ZY, Najos-Valencia O, Leano R, Marwick TH. Patients with early diabetic heart disease demonstrate a normal myocardial response to dobutamine. *J Am Coll Cardiol* 2003;42:446–453.

53. Pop-Busui R, Cleary PA, Braffett BH, Martin CL, Herman WH, Low PA, Lima JA, Bluemke DA. Association between cardiovascular autonomic neuropathy and left ventricular dysfunction: DCCT/EDIC study (Diabetes Control and Complications Trial/Epidemiology of Diabetes Interventions and Complications). *J Am Coll Cardiol* 2013;61:447–454.

54. Sacre JW, Franjic B, Jellis CL, Jenkins C, Coombes JS, Marwick TH. Association of cardiac autonomic neuropathy with subclinical myocardial dysfunction in type 2 diabetes. *JACC Cardiovasc Imaging* 2010;3:1207–1215.

55. Gerson MC, Caldwell JH, Ananthasubramaniam K, Clements IP, Henzlova MJ, Amanullah A, Jacobson AF. Influence of diabetes mellitus on prognostic utility of imaging of myocardial sympathetic innervation in heart failure patients. *Circ Cardiovasc Imaging* 2011;4:87–93.

56. Shivu GN, Abozguia K, Phan TT, Ahmed I, Weaver R, Narendran P, Stevens M, Frenneaux M. Increased left ventricular torsion in uncomplicated type 1 diabetic patients: the role of coronary microvascular function. *Diabetes Care* 2009;32:1710–1712.

57. Piya MK, Shivu GN, Tahrani A, Dubb K, Abozguia K, Phan TT, Narendran P, Pop-Busui R, Frenneaux M, Stevens MJ. Abnormal left ventricular torsion and cardiac autonomic dysfunction in subjects with type 1 diabetes mellitus. *Metabolism* 2011;60:1115–1121.

58. Furlan R, Guzzetti S, Crivellaro W, Dassi S, Tinelli M, Baselli G, Cerutti S, Lombardi F, Pagani M, Malliani A. Continuous 24-hour assessment of the neural regulation of systemic arterial pressure and RR variabilities in ambulant subjects. *Circulation* 1990;81:537–547.

59. Spallone V, Bernardi L, Ricordi L, Solda P, Maiello MR, Calciati A, Gambardella S, Fratino P, Menzinger G. Relationship between the circadian rhythms of blood pressure and sympathovagal balance in diabetic autonomic neuropathy. *Diabetes* 1993;42:1745–1752.

60. Axelrod S, Lishner M, Oz O, Bernheim J, Ravid M. Spectral analysis of fluctuations in heart rate: an objective evaluation of autonomic nervous control in chronic renal failure. *Nephron* 1987;45:202–206.

61. Converse RL Jr, Jacobsen TN, Toto RD, Jost CM, Cosentino F, Fouad-Tarazi F, Victor RG. Sympathetic overactivity in patients with chronic renal failure. *N Engl J Med* 1992;327:1912–1918.

62. Siddiqi L, Joles JA, Grassi G, Blankestijn PJ. Is kidney ischemia the central mechanism in parallel activation of the renin and sympathetic system? *J Hypertens* 2009;27:1341–1349.

63. Pop-Busui R, Roberts L, Pennathur S, Kretzler M, Brosius FC, Feldman EL. The management of diabetic neuropathy in CKD. *Am J Kidney Dis* 2010;55:365–385.

64. Brotman DJ, Bash LD, Qayyum R, Crews D, Whitsel EA, Astor BC, Coresh J. Heart rate variability predicts ESRD and CKD-related hospitalization. *J Am Soc Nephrol* 2010;21:1560–1570.

65. Maser RE, Mitchell BD, Vinik AI, Freeman R. The association between cardiovascular autonomic neuropathy and mortality in individuals with diabetes: a meta-analysis. *Diabetes Care* 2003;26:1895–1901.

66. Soedamah-Muthu SS, Chaturvedi N, Witte DR, Stevens LK, Porta M, Fuller JH. Relationship between risk factors and mortality in type 1 diabetic patients in Europe: the EURODIAB Prospective Complications Study (PCS). *Diabetes Care* 2008;31:1360–1366.

67. Lykke JA, Tarnow L, Parving HH, Hilsted J. A combined abnormality in heart rate variation and QT corrected interval is a strong predictor of cardiovascular death in type 1 diabetes. *Scand J Clin Lab Invest* 2008:1–6.

68. Ziegler D, Zentai CP, Perz S, Rathmann W, Haastert B, Doring A, Meisinger C. Prediction of mortality using measures of cardiac autonomic dysfunction in the diabetic and nondiabetic population: the MONICA/KORA Augsburg Cohort Study. *Diabetes Care* 2008;31:556–561.

69. Low PA, Denq JC, Opfer-Gehrking TL, Dyck PJ, O'Brien PC, Slezak JM. Effect of age and gender on sudomotor and cardiovagal function and blood pressure response to tilt in normal subjects. *Muscle Nerve* 1997;20:1561–1568.

70. Assessment: clinical autonomic testing report of the Therapeutics and Technology Assessment Subcommittee of the American Academy of Neurology. *Neurology* 1996;46:873–880.

71. Ewing DJ, Clarke BF. Diagnosis and management of diabetic autonomic neuropathy. *Br Med J (Clin Res Ed)* 1982;285:916–918.

72. Ewing DJ, Campbell IW, Clarke BF. Assessment of cardiovascular effects in diabetic autonomic neuropathy and prognostic implications. *Ann Intern Med* 1980;92:308–311.

73. England JD, Gronseth GS, Franklin G, Carter GT, Kinsella LJ, Cohen JA, Asbury AK, Szigeti K, Lupski JR, Latov N, Lewis RA, Low PA, Fisher MA, Herrmann DN, Howard JF Jr, Lauria G, Miller RG, Polydefkis M, Sumner AJ. Practice parameter: evaluation of distal symmetric polyneuropathy: role of autonomic testing, nerve biopsy, and skin biopsy (an evidence-based review). Report of the American Academy of Neurology, American Association of Neuromuscular and Electrodiagnostic Medicine, and American Academy of Physical Medicine and Rehabilitation. *Neurology* 2009;72:177–184.

74. Task Force of the European Society of Cardiology and the North American Society of Pacing and Electrophysiology. Heart rate variability: standards of measurement, physiological interpretation and clinical use. *Circulation* 1996;93:1043–1065.

75. Bernardi L, Spallone V, Stevens M, Hilsted J, Frontoni S, Pop-Busui R, Ziegler D, Kempler P, Freeman R, Low P, Tesfaye S, Valensi P. Investigation methods for cardiac autonomic function in human research studies. *Diabetes Metab Res Rev* 2011;27:639–653.

76. Kuehl M, Stevens MJ. Cardiovascular autonomic neuropathies as complications of diabetes mellitus. *Nat Rev Endocrinol* 2012;8:405–416.

77. Frattola A, Parati G, Gamba P, Paleari F, Mauri G, Di Rienzo M, Castiglioni P, Mancia G. Time and frequency domain estimates of spontaneous baroreflex sensitivity provide early detection of autonomic dysfunction in diabetes mellitus. *Diabetologia* 1997;40:1470–1475.

78. Gerritsen J, Dekker JM, TenVoorde BJ, Kostense PJ, Heine RJ, Bouter LM, Heethaar RM, Stehouwer CD. Impaired autonomic function is associated with increased mortality, especially in subjects with diabetes, hypertension, or a history of cardiovascular disease: the Hoorn Study. *Diabetes Care* 2001;24:1793–1798.

79. La Rovere MT, Bigger JT, Jr., Marcus FI, Mortara A, Schwartz PJ. Baroreflex sensitivity and heart-rate variability in prediction of total cardiac mortality after myocardial infarction. ATRAMI (Autonomic Tone and Reflexes After Myocardial Infarction) Investigators. *Lancet* 1998;351:478–484.

80. La Rovere MT, Pinna GD, Maestri R, Robbi E, Caporotondi A, Guazzotti G, Sleight P, Febo O. Prognostic implications of baroreflex sensitivity in heart failure patients in the beta-blocking era. *J Am Coll Cardiol* 2009;53:193–199.

81. Raffel DM, Wieland DM. Assessment of cardiac sympathetic nerve integrity with positron emission tomography. *Nucl Med Biol* 2001;28:541–559.

82. Stevens MJ, Dayanikli F, Raffel DM, Allman KC, Sandford T, Feldman EL, Wieland DM, Corbett J, Schwaiger M. Scintigraphic assessment of regionalized defects in myocardial sympathetic innervation and blood flow regulation in diabetic patients with autonomic neuropathy. *J Am Coll Cardiol* 1998;31:1575–1584.

83. Stevens MJ, Raffel DM, Allman KC, Schwaiger M, Wieland DM. Regression and progression of cardiac sympathetic dysinnervation complicating diabetes: an assessment by C-11 hydroxyephedrine and positron emission tomography. *Metabolism* 1999;48:92–101.

84. Schnell O, Muhr D, Weiss M, Dresel S, Haslbeck M, Standl E. Reduced myocardial 123I-metaiodobenzylguanidine uptake in newly diagnosed IDDM patients. *Diabetes* 1996;45:801–805.

85. Hamner JW, Taylor JA. Automated quantification of sympathetic beat-by-beat activity, independent of signal quality. *J Appl Physiol* 2001;91:1199–1206.

86. Parkman HP, Hasler WL, Fisher RS. American Gastroenterological Association technical review on the diagnosis and treatment of gastroparesis. *Gastroenterology* 2004;127:1592–1622.

87. Van Den Eeden SK, Sarma AV, Rutledge BN, Cleary PA, Kusek JW, Nyberg LM, McVary KT, Wessells H. Effect of intensive glycemic control and diabetes complications on lower urinary tract symptoms in men with type 1 diabetes: Diabetes Control and Complications Trial/Epidemiology of Diabetes Interventions and Complications (DCCT/EDIC) study. *Diabetes Care* 2009;32:664–670.

88. Chao CY, Cheing GL. Microvascular dysfunction in diabetic foot disease and ulceration. *Diabetes Metab Res Rev* 2009;25:604–614.

89. DCCT/EDIC Writing Group. Sustained effect of intensive treatment of type 1 diabetes mellitus on development and progression of diabetic nephropathy: the Epidemiology of Diabetes Interventions and Complications (EDIC) study. *JAMA* 2003;290:2159–2167.

90. Carnethon MR, Jacobs DR Jr, Sidney S, Liu K. Influence of autonomic nervous system dysfunction on the development of type 2 diabetes: the CARDIA study. *Diabetes Care* 2003;26:3035–3041.

91. Carnethon MR, Jacobs DR Jr, Sidney S, Sternfeld B, Gidding SS, Shoushtari C, Liu K. A longitudinal study of physical activity and heart rate recovery: CARDIA, 1987–1993. *Med Sci Sports Exerc* 2005;37:606–612.

92. Pop-Busui R, Stevens MJ, Raffel DM, White EA, Mehta M, Plunkett CD, Brown MB, Feldman EL. Effects of triple antioxidant therapy on measures of cardiovascular autonomic neuropathy and on myocardial blood flow in type 1 diabetes: a randomised controlled trial. *Diabetologia* 2013;56:1835–1844.

93. Patterson D, Abell T, Rothstein R, Koch K, Barnett J. A double-blind multicenter comparison of domperidone and metoclopramide in the treatment of diabetic patients with symptoms of gastroparesis. *Am J Gastroenterol* 1999;94:1230 1234.

94. European Medicine Agency. Available at www.ema.europa.eu/docs/en_GB/document_library/Press_release/2013/07/WC500146614.pdf.

95. Horowitz M, Harding PE, Chatterton BE, Collins PJ, Shearman DJ. Acute and chronic effects of domperidone on gastric emptying in diabetic autonomic neuropathy. *Dig Dis Sci* 1985;30:1–9.

96. Ahmad N, Keith-Ferris J, Gooden E, Abell T. Making a case for domperidone in the treatment of gastrointestinal motility disorders. *Curr Opin Pharmacol* 2006;6:571–576.

97. DiBaise JK, Quigley EM. Efficacy of prolonged administration of intravenous erythromycin in an ambulatory setting as treatment of severe gastroparesis: one center's experience. *J Clin Gastroenterol* 1999;28:131–134.

98. Peeters T, Matthijs G, Depoortere I, Cachet T, Hoogmartens J, Vantrappen G. Erythromycin is a motilin receptor agonist. *Am J Physiol* 1989;257:G470–474.

99. Richards RD, Davenport K, McCallum RW. The treatment of idiopathic and diabetic gastroparesis with acute intravenous and chronic oral erythromycin. *Am J Gastroenterol* 1993;88:203–207.

100. Lacy BE, Crowell MD, Schettler-Duncan A, Mathis C, Pasricha PJ. The treatment of diabetic gastroparesis with botulinum toxin injection of the pylorus. *Diabetes Care* 2004;27:2341–2347.

101. Lacy BE, Zayat EN, Crowell MD, Schuster MM. Botulinum toxin for the treatment of gastroparesis: a preliminary report. *Am J Gastroenterol* 2002;97:1548–1552.

102. Forster J, Sarosiek I, Delcore R, Lin Z, Raju GS, McCallum RW. Gastric pacing is a new surgical treatment for gastroparesis. *Am J Surg* 2001;182:676–681.

103. McCallum RW, Chen JD, Lin Z, Schirmer BD, Williams RD, Ross RA. Gastric pacing improves emptying and symptoms in patients with gastroparesis. *Gastroenterology* 1998;114:456–461.

104. Ejskjaer NT, Bradley JL, Buxton-Thomas MS, Edmonds ME, Howard ER, Purewal T, Thomas PK, Watkins PJ. Novel surgical treatment and gastric pathology in diabetic gastroparesis. *Diabet Med* 1999;16:488–495.

105. Vinik A, Erbas T, Pfeifer M, Feldman E, Stevens M, Russell J. Diabetic autonomic neuropathy. In *The Diabetes Mellitus Manual.* Inzucchi S, Porte D Jr, Sherwin R, Baron A, Eds. New York, McGraw-Hill, 2005, p. 347–365.

106. Verne GN, Sninsky CA. Diabetes and the gastrointestinal tract. *Gastroenterol Clin North Am* 1998;27:861–874, vi–vii.

107. Tsai ST, Vinik AI, Brunner JF. Diabetic diarrhea and somatostatin. *Ann Intern Med* 1986;104:894.

108. Goldstein I, Kim E, Steers WD, Pryor JL, Wilde DW, Natanegara F, Wong DG, Ahuja S. Efficacy and safety of tadalafil in men with erectile dysfunction with a high prevalence of comorbid conditions: results from MOMENTUS:

Multiple Observations in Men with Erectile Dysfunction in National Tadalafil Study in the US. *J Sex Med* 2007;4:166–175.

109. Rendell MS, Rajfer J, Wicker PA, Smith MD. Sildenafil for treatment of erectile dysfunction in men with diabetes: a randomized controlled trial. Sildenafil Diabetes Study Group. *JAMA* 1999;281:421–426.

110. Spollett GR. Assessment and management of erectile dysfunction in men with diabetes. *Diabetes Educ* 1999;25:65–73; quiz 75.

111. Virag R, Frydman D, Legman M, Virag H. Intracavernous injection of papaverine as a diagnostic and therapeutic method in erectile failure. *Angiology* 1984;35:79–87.

Chapter 46

The Diabetic Foot

ANDREW J.M. BOULTON, MD, DSc (HON), FACP, FRCP

The importance of diabetic foot disease increasingly has been recognized over the past three decades as this represents one of the most common causes of hospital admission among people with diabetes in Western countries, is responsible for much morbidity and even mortality, and is a major economic drain on the health care system. Diabetic foot ulceration (DFU) ultimately affects up to 25% of those living with diabetes.[1] Patients with DFU have been reported to have morbidity and mortality rates equivalent to many aggressive forms of cancer.[2] It recently was reported that patients who have lost a limb following a foot ulcer who are on dialysis have worse outcomes than almost every form of cancer except for malignant disease of the lung and pancreas. Amputation is a well-recognized complication of DFU in many cases, especially because of the presence of ischemia and infection: Up to 85% of all lower limb amputations in diabetes are preceded by foot ulcers, and diabetes remains the most common cause of nontraumatic amputation in Western countries. Diabetes also is now the most common cause of Charcot neuroarthropathy (CN) in Western countries, another condition that generally should be preventable.[3]

The American Diabetes Association (ADA) and the U.S. Department of Health and Human Services have developed national standards for the prevention and care of diabetic foot problems.[4,5] Despite this, foot ulcers appear to be increasingly more prevalent and represent a frequent and highly expensive complication of diabetes. According to one estimate, nearly $9 billion was spent on DFU treatment in 2001.[6] A more recent study from the U.K. suggests that the cost of care with people for the year after their first ulcer episode is 5.4 times higher than the cost of care of people without a foot ulcer history.[7] In view of the extreme cost of diabetic foot complications, it therefore may seem surprising that of all the National Institutes of Health (NIH)-funded projects in diabetes between 2002 and 2011, only 0.15% were specific to diabetic foot problems. This is despite a 78% increase in publications listed in PubMed on the diabetic foot over the past 30 years.[2]

Foot problems occur in all types of diabetes and in Western countries, and foot ulcers are more common in men and in patients >60 years of age. A large population-based study of >10,000 patients in the northwest of England reported that 5% had past or present foot ulceration and almost 67% had one or more risk factors for foot problems: The annual incidence of foot ulceration in these patients with diabetes was 2.2%.[8] Foot ulceration may be the presenting feature of type 2 diabetes, and any patient with a foot ulcer of undetermined cause should be screened for diabetes.[9]

       DOI: 10.2337/9781580405096.46

This chapter discusses the causal pathways and presentation of foot lesions, followed by the potential for prevention of foot problems. The management of foot ulcers is discussed in brief followed by a short section on CN. The term "diabetic foot" will be used in this chapter to refer to a variety of pathological conditions that might affect the feet of people with diabetes.

CAUSATION OF DIABETIC FOOT ULCERATION

Foot ulceration usually occurs as a result of trauma (often unperceived) in the presence of neuropathy or peripheral vascular disease (PVD). Contrary to popular belief, there is no evidence that infection directly causes foot ulcers: Infection usually occurs after a skin break has occurred. A number of prospective studies have confirmed that the most common variety of diabetic neuropathy, chronic sensorimotor neuropathy, is a major risk factor for ulceration. Those patients with moderate to severe sensorimotor neuropathy have a 5% annual risk of developing their first foot ulcer, seven times higher than those without neuropathy. Peripheral sympathetic autonomic neuropathy typically also is present in those patients with sensorimotor neuropathy and leads to dry skin that cracks and fissures easily and, in the absence of significant PVD, results in increased blood flow to the foot as the result of "autosympathectomy." Thus the warm, insensate foot is very much the "at-risk foot." Altered proprioception and small muscle wasting in the feet in the presence of limited joint mobility leads to altered loading under the foot during standing and walking: Dry skin results in a build-up of callus, and the presence of callus under weight-bearing areas can be a major contributory factor in the genesis of ulceration. It must be remembered, however, that neuropathy alone does not cause ulceration. It is the combination of neuropathy and other factors, such as high pressure or unperceived injury, that leads to skin breakdown and ulceration. The most common contributory factors in the genesis of foot ulceration were shown to be neuropathy, deformity, and trauma.[10] PVD is more common in patients with diabetes and is another major factor in the etiology of ulceration. These, together with other risk factors for foot ulceration, are listed in Table 46.1.

IDENTIFICATION OF THE HIGH-RISK FOOT

As it is well recognized that the majority of foot ulcers should be preventable, the first step in prevention is identification of the at-risk population. Careful inspection and examination of the foot is a pivotal part of the annual medical review that all patients with diabetes should undergo.[9] Because up to 50% of neuropathic patients may have no symptoms whatsoever, a history alone never can be used to identify high-risk patients. Those groups at greatest risk of ulceration are listed in Table 46.1, but on inspection and examination, key points to confirm are as follows:

- Evidence of neuropathies
- Evidence of ischemia
- Foot deformity (e.g., claw toes, hammer toe, Charcot changes)
- Callus at pressure areas

Table 46.1 Factors Increasing Risk of Diabetic Foot Ulceration

- **Peripheral neuropathy**
  - **—Somatic**
  - **—Autonomic**
- **Peripheral vascular disease**
- **Past history of foot ulcers and/or amputation**
- **Other long-term complications**
  - **—End-stage renal disease**
  - —Visual loss
- **Plantar callus**
- **Foot deformity**
- Edema
- Ethnic background
- Poor social background

Note: More common contributory factors shown in boldface.

An ADA task force addressed the question as to what should be included in the annual review for the Comprehensive Diabetic Foot Exam (CDFE).[4] It was agreed that no expensive equipment is required to identify the high-risk foot; indeed, a simple clinical exam is all that is essential. A summary of the key features of the CDFE is provided in Table 46.2. The task force agreed that for neuropathy, insensitivity to the 10-gram monofilaments for sites in each foot is essential plus one other test to confirm any abnormal findings (Table 46.2).

PREVENTION OF FOOT ULCERATION

There is no evidence that patients who have healthy feet and none of the risk factors or findings in Tables 46.1 and 46.2 require specific foot care education. Indeed, it may be counterproductive and it is not economically viable. Those patients with healthy feet should be given general advice on foot hygiene, nail care, and footwear purchase that all of us should follow. Their risk status should be reviewed annually.[9]

Those patients with any risk factors in Table 46.1 or findings from Table 46.2 require more frequent review, podiatry, and education on preventive foot care. The approach to patients with different levels of risk is covered in the ADA task force report.[4]

The question of preventive education is a difficult one because no randomized study actually has shown that such education results in a reduction of subsequent foot ulcers. Several studies, however, have shown that comprehensive foot care education for high-risk patients, together with other factors such as regular podiatry and careful follow-up, might lead to a reduction in ulceration and amputation.[4,11,12]

Table 46.2 Key Components of the Diabetic Foot Exam

Inspection

■ Evidence of past or present ulcers?
■ Foot shape?
  —Prominent metatarsal heads/claw toes
  —Hallux valgus
  —Muscle wasting
  —Charcot deformity
■ Dermatological
  —Callus
  —Erythema
  —Sweating

Neurological

■ 10g monofilament at 4 sites on each foot + 1 of the following:
  —Vibration using 128Hz tuning fork
  —Pinprick sensation
  —Ankle reflexes
  —Vibration perception threshold

Vascular

■ Foot pulses
■ Ankle brachial index, if indicated
■ Doppler wave forms

The prevention of recurrent DFU is also challenging. Again there is some evidence that a multidisciplinary approach may be beneficial,[11] but more recently it has been suggested that education together with self–foot temperature monitoring might help reduce recurrent neuropathic ulcers.[13] In this study, patients checked their foot skin temperatures on a regular basis, and if a significant difference in temperatures was found, the patients were advised to rest and contact their podiatrist. Whereas the ulcer recurrence rate was only 8.5% in those who were in the active treatment group, the standard of care groups reported 30% reulceration rates.[13] Thus the neuropathic foot heats up (due to inflammation) before it breaks down, and this observation may be used to prevent recurrent ulceration.

DIABETIC FOOT ULCERATION

Despite all efforts at prevention, patients still will develop ulcers, and a system of classification is important both for clinical practice and clinical research. One of the most commonly used methods in the U.S. is that known as the University of Texas (UT) classification scheme.[14] This system grades a wound according to depth and each grade has four stages depending on the presence or absence of infection or ischemia (Table 46.3).

Table 46.3 University of Texas (UT) Diabetic Wound Classification System

Stage	Grade			
	0	1	2	3
A	Preulcerative or healed postulcerative lesion	Superficial wound, not involving tendon, capsule, or bone	Wound penetrating to tendon or capsule	Wound penetrating to bone or joint
B	Plus infection	Plus infection	Plus infection	Plus infection
C	Plus ischemia	Plus ischemia	Plus ischemia	Plus ischemia
D	Plus infection and ischemia	Plus infection and ischemia	Plus infection and ischemia	Plus infection and ischemia

GRADE 0

A UT grade 0 foot, whether or not there is ischemia, is at very high risk of ulceration, and preulcerative signs include hemorrhage into a callused area. Patients in this grade require regular podiatry, callus debridement, and appropriate orthoses and shoe gear.

GRADE 1

UT grade 1 ulcers are superficial, but there is full-thickness skin loss. The majority of ulcers in this class are neuropathic either with or without infection (UT 1a and UT 1b). Again, debridement of any callus is essential in the management of such lesions (Figure 46.1 provides one example). Although clinically superficial, radiographs are indicated in grade 1 and all other grades of foot ulcers to exclude unsuspected osteomyelitis. Key management points of grade 1 ulcers include aggressive debridement of callus and dead tissue around the wound margin, and if there is any suspicion of infection (UT 1b or 1d), then tissue from the wound base should be taken for culture. The management of pressure relief and infection are dealt with in detail in the following paragraphs, but all wounds of course require a dressing, remembering that a dressing alone will not heal the wound if there is any loss of sensation because patients continue to weight-bear in the absence of pain. Sadly, there are no randomized controlled trials to confirm the efficacy of any particular dressing: Dressings should be chosen according to the amount of exudation of the wound and cost considerations.

GRADE 2

Grade 2 ulcers are deeper lesions that may penetrate subcutaneous tissue reaching the tendon or capsule, but there is no penetration to bone. Infection is more likely to be present in these wounds (UT 2b or 2d). If situated on weight-bearing areas together with calluses, then neuropathy is almost certainly a con-

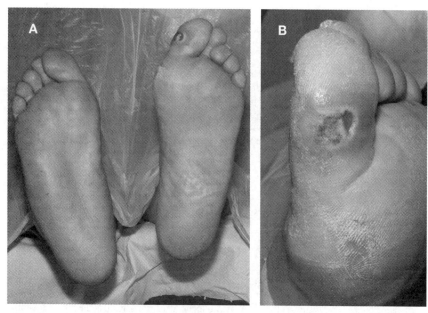

Figure 46.1. *A*: A typical neuropathic foot ulcer on the plantar surface of the left hallux of a patient with diabetic neuropathy. There is a typical build-up of callus in the periulcer area, but this is not clinically infective. *B*: Close-up of neuropathic foot ulcer after debridement. This is clearly noninfective and will heal with appropriate offloading.

tributory factor to the genesis of such ulcers. In contrast, heel ulcers tend to be predominantly neuroischemic: Management principles for grade 2 ulcers are not dissimilar to those for grade 1.

GRADE 3

Grade 3 ulcers are deep ulcers that reach down to bone or joints. The ability to probe to bone using a metal probe strongly suggests the presence of osteomyelitis, although the inability to probe to bone is more reliable in excluding osteomyelitis. Management aspects of grade 3 ulcers are considered in detail under the section on Infection.

OFFLOADING

The failure to offload neuropathic foot ulcers is a major contributory factor in the nonhealing of such lesions: This is permissible because the patient has lost the ability to feel pain, and it has been shown that continued weight-bearing on active ulcers results in persistent chronic inflammation.[15] First used in leprosy, the total contact cast (TCC) has become the gold standard for offloading plantar ulcers occurring on weight-bearing areas.[16] The efficacy of this form of therapy has been confirmed in several randomized controlled trials.[3,16] Although removable cast walkers have been shown to offload equally well to the TCC, their efficacy in clinical practice was demonstrated to be inferior to the TCC. A subsequent study confirmed the reason for this: When instructed to wear the removable cast walker for every footstep taken, it was demonstrated that only 28% of all footsteps were taken with the device on.[18] This was rectified by rendering the removable cast walker nonremovable (by wrapping in cohesive bandage or scotch cast): When this is clearly worn for all footsteps, the removable cast walker had equal efficacy to the TCC.[18]

INFECTION

Infections in the diabetic foot are common and potentially serious, especially in the presence of PVD. If left untreated, infections may spread, leading to rapid deterioration, tissue necrosis, and gangrene, thereby increasing the risk of amputation. Despite the importance of infection, however, there are few well-designed randomized controlled trials to guide us in management and treatment. The Infectious Disease Society of America (IDSA) recently published a clinical practice guideline for the diagnosis and treatment of diabetic foot infection that gives comprehensive coverage to the topic and useful guidance on the classification and antimicrobial therapy for such infections.[20] Foot infections are graded into mild, moderate, or severe depending on clinical signs, as it is well recognized that all wounds are colonized, but the finding of bacteria on its own does not indicate infection. Hence, the clinical classification remains valid. Whereas most diabetic foot infections are polymicrobial, gram-positive cocci, especially staphylococci, remain the most common causative organism. Those wounds without clinical evidence of infection do not require antibiotic treatment. The IDSA guidelines are a source of valuable advice on diagnosis and treatment of foot infections. As stated, there is no clinical trial evidence to guide infection management, but useful antibiotics on an outpatient basis include amoxicillin-clavulanate (Augmentin), clindamycin (which has good bone penetration), and the cephalosporins. Whereas mild infections can be treated safely with oral antibiotics, most severe and many moderate infections may require intravenous treatment.

Osteomyelitis is all too common in infected diabetic foot ulcers especially when longstanding and deep. Whereas traditionally osteomyelitis always has required surgical treatment, evidence is increasing that antibiotic therapy alone might be helpful in osteomyelitis that usually is confined to a digit, for example. A recent randomized controlled trial of antibiotics versus surgery did not find surgery to be superior over antibiotic treatment.[21] Uncertainty remains about the duration of antimicrobial treatment in the management of osteomyelitis.

OTHER THERAPIES

The use of negative pressure wound therapy (NPWT) in both postsurgical and complex diabetic foot wounds has been supported in two randomized trials.[22,23] The strength of these studies has been questioned, however, as they were necessarily nonblinded. NPWT does seem to be a useful therapy in the management of complex wounds that have failed to respond to standard treatments.

The use of hyperbaric oxygen (HBO) in diabetic foot wounds remains highly controversial and has conflicting evidence to support its use. There is no indication whatsoever for the use of HBO in any neuropathic foot ulcers or noninfected ischemic ulcers. A number of other biological therapies and topical treatments, including bioengineered skin substitutes, are used widely, although the clinical trials supporting their use have been criticized as being of questionable quality.[24]

PERIPHERAL VASCULAR DISEASE AND GANGRENE

Neuroischemic ulcers are becoming more common and now are seen more often than purely neuropathic ulcers (see Chapter 48 for a detailed discussion on this and gangrene). The role of the ankle-brachial index (ABI) in screening for vascular disease in the CDFE is controversial (Table 46.2).[4] Vascular calcification is common in patients with diabetes, especially those with neuropathy, and this may result in a false elevation of the ABI, which may give a false sense of security or a false negative. The combination of PVD and infection often results in amputation, so an aggressive approach to the management of infection in those with known vascular disease is essential.

INPATIENT DIABETIC FOOT PROBLEMS

Any patient with diabetes admitted to the hospital is at risk for foot problems, and appropriate care of the feet with special mattresses, protection of the heels, and other pressure areas is vital. Even in the 21st century, it is sadly true that iatrogenic heel ulcers most commonly are caused by inappropriate foot care in hospital. Special guidelines on the inpatient management of diabetic foot disorders recently were published in the ADA's journal *Diabetes Care*.[25]

CHARCOT NEUROARTHROPATHY

Named after the French physician Jean-Martin Charcot, CN is a noninfective arthropathy in well-perfused insensate feet. It is a progressive condition characterized by joint dislocation, pathological fractures, and debilitating deformities that may result in progressive bone destruction as well as soft tissue abnormalities (Fig. 46.2).[9] Although the exact mechanisms resulting in the development of CN remain elusive, progress has been made in our understanding of the etiopathogenesis of this disorder in the past decade. Although characterized by increased local bone resorption, the exact cellular mechanisms contributing to this condition remain unsolved. Recently, a receptor activator of the nuclear factor κB ligand (RANK-L) has been identified as an essential mediator of osteoclast formation and activation.[26] It now is hypothesized that the RANK-L/osteoprotegerin (OPG) pathway may play an important role in the development of acute CN. There are as yet no

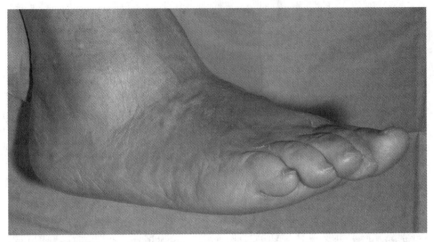

Figure 46.2—Charcot neuroarthropathy in right cuneiform metatarsal area of a patient with diabetic neuropathy. Note the distended dorsal foot veins, a sign of autonomic neuropathy with increased arteriovenous shunting together with dry skin, and a loss of normal architecture of dorsum of foot. There is some swelling distal of the lateral malleolus.

proven medical therapies for the acute phase of CN, although recent evidence that the RANK-L/RANK/OPG signaling pathway is modulated in patients with CN highlights this pathway as a potential target for future therapies.[27]

To date, treatment of CN mainly is based on expert opinion rather than randomized trials, and the rarity of this condition makes the conduct of such trials challenging. Thus, any patient with known neuropathy presenting with a warm, swollen, and occasionally painful foot must be considered to have acute CN until proven otherwise. The recommended treatment at this stage is offloading of the affected foot by use of an appropriate cast that preferably should be nonremovable.[28] The management of advanced CN with bone deformity requiring reconstructive surgery is beyond the scope of this chapter, and the reader is referred to a recent review.[29]

REFERENCES

1. Singh N, Armstrong DG, Lipsky BA. Preventing foot ulcers in patients with diabetes. *JAMA* 2005;293:217–228.

2. Armstrong DG, Kanda VA, Lavery LA, Marston W, Mills JL Sr, Boulton AJM. Mind the gap: disparity between research funding and costs of care for diabetic foot ulcers. *Diabetes Care* 2013;36:1815–1817.

3. Boulton AJM. The diabetic foot: from art to science. The 18th Camillo Golgi lecture. *Diabetologia* 2004;47:1343–1353.

4. Boulton AJM, Armstrong DG, Albert SF, Frykberg RG, Hellman R, Kirkman MS, Lavery LA, LeMaster JW, Mills JL (Sr), Mueller MJ, Sheehan P, Wukich DK; American Diabetes Association; American Association of Clinical Endocrinologists. Comprehensive foot examination and risk assessment: a report of the Task Force of the Foot Care Interest Group of the American Diabetes Association, with endorsement by the American Association of Clinical Endocrinologists. *Diabetes Care* 2008;31:1679–1684.

5. U.S. Department of Health and Human Services. HealthyPeople.gov: 2020 topics and objectives, 2012. Available at www.healthypeople.gov/2020/topicsobjectives2020/objectiveslist.aspx?topicid=8. Accessed 8 December 2012.

6. Sen CK, Gordillo GM, Roy S, Kirsner R, Lambert L, Hunt TK, Gottrup F, Gurtner GC, Longaker MT. Human skin wounds: a major and snowballing threat to public health and the economy. *Wound Repair Regen* 2009;17:763–771.

7. Tan T, Shaw EJ, Siddiqui F, Kandaswamy P, Barry PW, Baker M; Guideline Development Group. Inpatient management of diabetic foot problems: summary of NICE guidance. *BMJ* 2011;342:d1280.

8. Abbott CA, Abbott CA, Carrington AL, Ashe H, Bath S, Every LC, Griffiths J, Hann AW, Hussein A, Jackson N, Johnson KE, Ryder CH, Torkington R, Van Ross ER, Whalley AM, Widdows P, Williamson S, Boulton AJ; North-West Diabetes Foot Care Study. The North-West Diabetes Foot Care Study: incidence of, and risk factors for, new diabetic foot ulceration in a community-based patient cohort. *Diabet Med* 2002;19:377–384.

9. Boulton AJM. The diabetic foot. *Medicine* 2010;38:644–648.

10. Reiber GE, Vileikyte L, Boyko EJ, de Aguila M, Smith DG, Lavery LA, Boulton AJ. Causal pathways for incident lower-extremity ulcers in patients with diabetes from two settings. *Diabetes Care* 1999;22:157–162.

11. Dargis V, Pantelejeva O, Jonushaite A, Vileikyte L, Boulton AJM. Benefits of a multi-disciplinary approach in the management of recurrent diabetic foot ulcers in Lithuania. *Diabetes Care* 1999;22:1428–1431.

12. Krishnan S, Nash F, Baker N, Fowler D, Rayman G. Reduction in diabetic amputations over 11 years in a defined UK population: benefits of multidisciplinary team work and continuous prospective audit. *Diabetes Care* 2008;31:99–101.

13. Lavery LA, Higgins KR, Lanctot DR, Constantinides GP, Zamorano RG, Athanasiou KA, Armstrong DG, Agrawal CM. Preventing diabetic foot ulcer recurrence in high-risk patients: use of temperature monitoring as a self-assessment tool. *Diabetes Care* 2007;30:14–20.

14. Oyibo S, Jude EB, Tarawneh I, Van Schie CH, Boulton AJM, Harkless LB. A comparison of two diabetic foot ulcer classification systems. *Diabetes Care* 2001;24:84–88.

15. Piaggesi A, Viacava P, Rizzo L, Naccarato G, Baccetti F, Romanelli M, Zampa V, Del Prato S. Semi-quantitative analysis of the histopathological features of the neuropathic foot ulcer: effects of pressure relief. *Diabetes Care* 2003;26:3123–3128.

16. Boulton AJM, Kirsner RS, Vileikyte L. Neuropathic diabetic foot ulcers. *N Engl J Med* 2004;351:48–55.

17. Armstrong DG, Nguyen HC, Lavery LA, van Schie CH, Boulton AJM, Harkless LB. Off-loading the diabetic foot wound: a randomized clinical trial. *Diabetes Care* 2001;24:1019–1022.

18. Armstrong DG, Lavery LA, Kimbriel HR, Nixon BP, Boulton AJM. Activity patterns of patients with diabetic foot ulceration: Patients with active ulceration may not adhere to a standard pressure off-loading regimen. *Diabetes Care* 2003;26:2595–2597.

19. Katz I, Harlan A, Miranda-Palma B, Prieto-Sanchez L, Armstrong DG, Bowker JH, Mizel MS, Boulton AJM. A randomized trial of two irremovable off-loading devices in the management of plantar neuropathic diabetic foot ulcers. *Diabetes Care* 2005;28:555–559.

20. Lipsky BA, Berendt AR, Cornia PB, Pile JC, Peters EJ, Armstrong DG, Deery HG, Embil JM, Joseph WS, Karchmer AW, Pinzur MS, Senneville E. 2012 Infectious Disease Society of America clinical practice guidelines for the diagnosis and treatment of diabetic foot infections. *Clin Infect Dis* 2012;54:132–173.

21. Lázaro-Martinez J, Aragón-Sánchez J, Garcia-Morales E. Antibiotics versus conservative therapy for treating diabetic foot osteomyelitis: a randomized comparative trial. *Diabetes Care* 2013, Epub October 15.

22. Armstrong DG, Lavery LA; Diabetic Foot Study Consortium. Negative pressure wound therapy after partial diabetic foot amputation: a multicentre, randomized controlled trial. *Lancet* 2005;366:1704–1710.

23. Blume PA, Walters J, Payne W, Ayala J, Lantis J. Comparison of negative pressure wound therapy utilising vacuum-assisted closure to advance moist wound therapy in the treatment of diabetic foot ulcers. A multicentre randomized controlled trial. *Diabetes Care* 2008;31:631–636.

24. Blozik E, Scherer M. Skin replacement therapies for diabetic foot ulcers: systematic review and meta-analysis. *Diabetes Care* 2008;31:693–694.

25. Wukich DK, Armstrong DG, Attinger CE, Boulton AJ, Burns PR, Frykberg RG, Hellman R, Kim PJ, Lipsky BA, Pile JC, Pinzur MS, Siminerio L. Inpatient management of diabetic foot disorders: a clinical guide. *Diabetes Care* 2013;36:2862–2871.

26. Molines L, Darmon P, Raccah D. Charcot's foot: newest findings on its pathophysiology, diagnosis and treatment. *Diabetes Metab* 2010;36:251–255.

27. Ndip A, Williams A, Jude EB, Serracino-Inglott F, Richardson S, Smyth JV, Boulton AJM, Alexander MY. The RANK-L/RANK/OPG signalling pathway mediates medial arterial calcification in diabetic Charcot neuroarthropathy. *Diabetes* 2011;60:2187–2196.

28. Mascarenhas JV, Jude EB. Pathogenesis and medical management of diabetic Charcot neuroarthropathy. *Med Clin N Amer* 2013;97;857–872.

29. Shen W, Wukich DK. Orthopaedic surgery and the diabetic Charcot foot. *Med Clin N Amer* 2013;97:873–882.

Chapter 47

Macrovascular Complications and Coronary Artery Disease: Primary and Secondary Prevention in Patients with Diabetes

Tina K. Thethi, MD, MPH, FACE
Vivian Fonseca, MD

INTRODUCTION

Diabetes is associated with an increased risk of cardiovascular disease (CVD) including nonfatal and fatal myocardial infarction (MI), heart failure (HF), and cerebrovascular disease (stroke). Whether it is type 1 diabetes (T1D) or type 2 diabetes (T2D), there is substantial evidence to support that increasing hyperglycemia, uncontrolled blood pressure (BP), and hyperlipidemia lead to an increase in CVD risk. The death rate due to CVD in patients with diabetes is two to four times higher than in those without diabetes. Approximately 68% of the deaths in patients age >65 years with diabetes are attributed to CVD.[1] Results from the Steno type 2 randomized study[2] showed that nearly 4 years of intensified multifactorial intervention in patients with T2D and microalbuminuria slowed progression to nephropathy and other microvascular complications, such as retinopathy and autonomic neuropathy. Spanning the past two decades, several large studies have evaluated the potential impact of lowering glucose on cardiovascular (CV) outcomes in both T1D and T2D.[3,4] Trials such as Action to Control Cardiovascular Disease in Diabetes (ACCORD), Action in Diabetes and Vascular Disease: Preterax and Modified Release Controlled Evaluation (ADVANCE), and Veterans Affairs Diabetes Trial (VADT) trials[5-8] specifically addressed the impact of various approaches to intensive glycemic control on CVD outcomes. Several other trials have focused on the impact of different strategies for glycemic control on CVD. Numerous studies have shown the efficacy of controlling individual risk factors such as hypertension and hyperlipidemia in preventing or decreasing CVD in those with diabetes. Several meta-analyses have been conducted that have given further insight into the statistical significance of the results from these trials regarding the number of patients included and the length of these studies,[9,10] all factors that affect the results. The heterogeneity of the results from these trials places an emphasis on the complexity of diabetes and thus has stirred controversy around the effect of intensive glucose control on CVD risk. The purpose of this chapter is to briefly review some of the trials on primary and secondary prevention of macrovascular complications in diabetes.

RELATIONSHIP BETWEEN GLUCOSE AND CARDIOVASCULAR DISEASE IN DIABETES

In spite of the advances in the prevention and treatment of CVD, the outcomes for those patients with diabetes remain suboptimal. Hyperglycemia contin-

DOI: 10.2337/9781580405096.47

ues to remain a risk factor and thus an appropriate therapeutic target.[11] A meta-analysis of 37 prospective studies that included 447,064 people worldwide reported that the age-adjusted risk of fatal coronary heart disease (CHD) was 3.69 (95% confidence interval [CI] 2.64–5.15) in women with T2D and 2.16 (95% CI 1.77–2.64) in men with T2D.[12] The European Prospective Investigation into Cancer in Norfolk (EPIC–NORFOLK) study highlighted the risk of CVD and mortality associated with A1C levels of 5 to 5.4% and from 5.5 to 6.9% as compared with those with A1C <5%. An increase in A1C of 1% was associated with a relative risk of death of 1.24 (95% CI, 1.14–1.34; P <0.001) in men and 1.28 (95% CI 1.063–1.32; P <0.001) in women. Although intensive glycemic control trials have demonstrated a reduction in risk for microvascular complications in patients with T2D, the impact on CVD, stroke, and vascular disease remains uncertain. Yet, studies focusing on intensive glycemic control to reduce A1C levels have had incongruent results.[13,14]

Perhaps it is the U.K. Prospective Diabetes Study (UKPDS) data that lend support to the most extensive analysis of glycemic control and CVD risk. Patients were followed for 10 years comparing outcomes in the intensive glucose-lowering therapy (with either insulin or sulfonylurea) with a diet-based conventional approach. At the end of the study,[4] 3,867 participants with newly diagnosed T2D had a significant decline (P = 0.029) in diabetes-related microvascular endpoints, but a nonsignificant decrease in the incidence of MI. Results from the 753 obese patients who were allocated to intensive glycemic control with metformin demonstrated a significant reduction in MI and all-cause mortality.[15] Secondary analysis of the UKPDS data demonstrated that while there was microvascular risk reduction and a trend toward reduction in MI in the intensive control group, this was offset by a nonsignificant increase in stroke risk. The absolute risk events per 1,000 patient-years were 5.8 for the intensive arm versus 5.0 for the conventional arm (P = 0.52; 95% CI 0.81–1.51). There was no statistically significant effect on macrovascular complications.[4] Long-term follow-up of 3,277 patients demonstrated, however, that although there was no difference in A1C between the intensive and control arm within the first year after the trial ended, the intensive glycemic arm had significant reductions in observed MI and all-cause mortality in all treatment groups (either sulfonylurea, insulin, or metformin) as well as sustained benefit in previously demonstrated microvascular risk reduction.[14,16]

The Diabetes Control and Complications Trial (DCCT) was a landmark study designed to assess the impact of intensive glycemic control on microvascular risk in T1D. The patients in the DCCT were relatively younger (mean age = 26.8 ± 8 years in the conventional arm and 27.7 ± 7 years in the intensive arm of the primary prevention group) with a shorter duration of the disease (mean duration of diabetes ranging from 2.6 to 8.9 years). The younger age-group of the patients made the detection of treatment-related differences in rates of macrovascular events unlikely, although it was not the intention of the trial to evaluate the impact of glycemic outcome on CVD. In the intensive therapy arm, there was decreased incidence of hypercholesterolemia (which was defined as low-density lipoprotein [LDL] cholesterol >160 mg/dl) by 34% (P = 0.02; 95% CI 7–54) in the combined primary and secondary prevention cohorts. After combining all the major CV and peripheral vascular events, however, results showed that intensive therapy resulted in a nonsignificant decrease in the risk of macrovascular disease by 41% (to 0.5

event per 100 patient-years vs. 0.8 event; 95% CI –10 to 68%).[3] The findings from both the UKPDS and DCCT provided support for the premise that intensive glycemic control may perhaps decrease the CV risk in patients with diabetes. The Epidemiology of Diabetes Interventions and Complications (EDIC) study was the 17-year follow-up to the DCCT. Results of the EDIC study showed that intensive treatment reduced the risk of any CVD event by 42% (*P* = 0.02; 95% CI 9–63). The risk for nonfatal MI, stroke, or death from CVD was reduced by 57% (*P* = 0.02; 95% CI 12–79).[16] Thus, some evidence exists for the long-term reduction of CV risk with intensive glycemic control in both T1D and T2D. Longitudinal follow-up of the EDIC cohort[17] for 18 years suggests that the beneficial risk reductions due to intensive therapy as compared with conventional therapy are persistent but decreasing with time. The declining risk reductions are evident for microvascular complications. The risk reduction for further progression of retinopathy has decreased from 70 to 53 to 46% at EDIC year 4, year 10, and year 18, respectively. For confirmed clinical neuropathy, the risk reduction decreased from 64% at DCCT closeout to 30% at EDIC year 14. The risk reduction for albuminuria with intensive therapy decreased from nearly 60% at EDIC year 8 to nearly 40% at EDIC year 18.

In spite of these findings, investigators and clinicians remained cautiously skeptical of the potential impact of glycemic control on future CV outcomes, specifically in T2D. One of the key questions was: Does intensive glycemic control in very-high-risk patients who have experienced complications already and have longer duration of diabetes offer any further benefit in terms of reducing CV risk? Thus, long-term randomized controlled clinical trials to assess the impact of more aggressive glucose control on CVD outcomes in such high-risk populations were conducted in an attempt to give further insight into this conundrum. As a result of these trials, many new questions have been raised regarding the risks and benefits of intensive glucose control on CVD outcomes. An understanding of the distinctive study methods, patient populations, and approach to care in these trials is essential to allow clinicians to comprehend the benefit and potential risk of intensive glucose lowering in patients at risk for CVD. Following is a brief description of some of these trials.

In the VADT, Duckworth et al.[6] assessed CV outcomes in 1,791 veterans with long-standing T2D. The mean age of the subjects was 60.4 years, median A1C was 9.4% at enrollment, with the mean duration of diabetes being 11.5 years. Subjects were randomized to either standard or intensive glucose-lowering therapy. The primary outcome of the study was the occurrence of major CV events, such as MI, stroke, congestive HF, inoperable coronary artery disease (CAD), ischemia leading to lower-extremity amputation, and death from CV causes. After median treatment duration of 5.6 years, subjects in the intensive therapy group had an A1C of 6.4% and those in the standard therapy group had an A1C of 8.4%. There was no significant difference seen between the two groups in the primary outcome and all-cause mortality (29.5 vs. 33.5%; hazard ratio [HR] 0.88; *P* = 0.14; 95% CI 0.74–1.05). Episodes of severe hypoglycemia were significantly more frequent in the intensive therapy group as compared with the standard therapy group (21.2 vs. 9.9%; *P* <0.001).[6] Severe hypoglycemia was associated with increased CV death in both arms and increased CV death in the 180 days following severe hypoglycemia (HR 3.72; *P* = 0.01).[6] There was a decline in the glomerular filtration rate (GFR) to 76 ml/minute by year 6. Worsening of the albuminuria was greater in the standard treatment arm ($P = 0.01$) in addition to progression to macroalbuminuria ($P = 0.04$).[6] Patients in VADT had a history of long-standing diabetes, and therefore, whether intensive glycemic control in such a case translates into any meaningful CV benefit remains unclear. Although intensive glycemic control may yet be beneficial in early diabetes, offering protection against CV events in future years, to expect no further progression of these complications at all with intensive control may yet be unrealistic.[18]

The ACCORD study[7] randomized 10,251 patients with either history of a CVD event (ages 40–79 years) or significant CVD risk (ages 55–79 years) who were at high risk for CVD events. Patients were randomized to either intensive therapy (target A1C <6%) or standard therapy (target A1C 7–7.9%) with the intention of determining whether aggressive glycemic control could significantly reduce the risk of CVD events. Other CVD risk factors including lipids and BP were treated intensively and similarly between groups. A subgroup of the participants in ACCORD also were enrolled in the ACCORD Lipid trial and the ACCORD Blood Pressure trial after undergoing randomization in a 2 × 2 factorial design. Results of these trials are discussed in the sections discussing the relationship of lipids and BP with CVD in diabetes, respectively. Overall, participants in ACCORD had T2D ~10 years before study onset. After a mean follow-up of 3.5 years, patients in the intensive glycemic arm achieved a significantly greater reduction in median A1C: 6.4% as compared with 7.5% in the standard glycemic arm. Given the finding of increased all-cause mortality in the intensively treated patients, the glycemia intervention was terminated in February 2008 after a mean follow-up of 3.5 years instead of the 5.5 years as originally planned. The standard approach to glucose lowering then was applied instead of the intensive approach, which resulted in the A1C increasing from <6 to 7–7.9%. During the 3.5 years of average follow-up, 1.42% of the patients died each year in the intensive am compared with 1.14% a year in the standard intervention arm (HR 1.22; 95% CI 1.01–1.46; $P = 0.04$) and the CV mortality was higher (HR 1.35; 95% CI 1.04–1.76; $P = 0.02$). The underlying cause of the increased mortality in the intensive arm was unclear at the time the intensive intervention was stopped. Interestingly, however, in the first 3.5 years, despite an increased mortality rate in the ACCORD trial, the rates of nonfatal MI were significantly lower in the intensively treated group (HR 0.76; 95% CI 0.62–0.92; $P = 0.004$). Between the two groups, there was no significant difference in the rate of either nonfatal stroke or congestive HF. There was a nonsignificant trend toward a reduction in the primary outcome of the trial (composite of nonfatal MI, nonfatal stroke, or death from CV causes) with the intensive glycemic control (HR 0.90; 95% CI 0.78–1.04; $P = 0.16$).[8]

One of the key questions from the ACCORD study results is whether the results can be applied to the broader population or specific subgroups of patients with T2D. There is a suggestion of a significant benefit of intensive glycemic control on CVD events in those patients who had a lower A1C at entry or absence of history of CVD events, but there was no suggestion of a differential effect on mortality. Both before and after adjustment for other covariates, a higher average A1C was a stronger predictor of mortality than either the final A1C or the decrease in A1C seen in the first year.[19] Higher average A1C was associated with higher risk for death. Each percentage point increase in mean A1C was associated with an ~20% increase in all-cause mortality. With intensive glycemic control, there was a linear increase in the risk for death from A1C levels of 6 to 9%. The original ACCORD conclusion that mortality risk was greater with the intensive strategy than with the standard strategy seemed to occur only when the average A1C was >7%.

HYPOGLYCEMIA MAY WORSEN CARDIOVASCULAR RISK

In the ACCORD trial, one or more hypoglycemic episodes that required assistance were associated with an increased risk of death. In the intensive glycemic control arm, the unadjusted annual mortality was 2.8% in those who had one or more episodes of hypoglycemia requiring any assistance as compared with 1.2% for those with no such episodes (adjusted HR 1.41; 95% CI 1.03–1.93). Similarly, in the standard glycemic control arm, the annual mortality was 3.7% in those with hypoglycemic episodes requiring assistance versus 1% among those without such episodes (adjusted HR 2.30; 95% CI 1.46–3.65). The risk of death, however, was significantly lower in intensively treated patients who had severe hypoglycemia requiring medical assistance (HR 0.55; 95% CI 0.31–0.99) as compared with the standard-treatment group. These paradoxical findings might suggest that with close monitoring, the adverse effects of intensive treatment might be mitigated, resulting in clinical benefits.[20] The underlying mechanism leading to increased mortality in patients with severe hypoglycemia has yet to be clarified. A plausible explanation is that cardiac ischemia or fatal arrhythmia during recognized or unrecognized episodes of hypoglycemia may be responsible for this, particularly in the setting of cardiac autonomic neuropathy.[21] Patients with T2D who experience symptomatic, severe hypoglycemia, however, are at increased risk of death, regardless of the intensity of glycemic control. The reasons for higher mortality in the intensively treated glycemic arm during the pretransition period are still unclear. In the post-transition period (from intensive to the standard approach), the rates of hypoglycemia were similar in both the intensive and standard glycemic control groups. Thus, the increased risk of death among patients in the intensive glycemic control group cannot be attributed to the increased rate of severe hypoglycemia in the intensive-control group participants. Hypoglycemia can impair hormonal and autonomic responses to subsequent hypoglycemia. Adler et al.[21] tested their hypothesis that prior exposure to hypoglycemia leads to impaired CV autonomic function. Twenty healthy subjects (age 28 ± 2 years) underwent two 3-day inpatient visits 1–3 months apart. A 2-hour hyperinsulinemic (hypoglycemic) or euglycemic clamp was performed on day 2 of the inpatient visit. Sympathetic, parasympathetic, and baroreflex testing was done on days 1 and 3. Their results showed that antecedent hypoglycemia led to reduced baroreflex sensitivity ($P = 0.03$), decreased muscle sympathetic nerve activity response to transient nitroprusside-induced hypotension ($P < 0.01$), and reduced plasma norepinephrine response to lower body negative pressure ($P < 0.001$).

Another important question that arises is whether the increased mortality in patients who experience hypoglycemia is seen in clinical practice as well. A retrospective cohort study by Zhao et al.[22] aimed to study the impact of hypoglycemia on vascular events in clinical practice among patients in the Veterans Integrated

Service Network 16. There were an equal number (n = 761) of patients in the hypoglycemia and the propensity score–matched control group with a median follow-up of 3.93 years and preindex A1C of 10.96 ± 2.61% with a similar 1-year change in A1C (hypoglycemia group –0.51 vs. control group –0.32%; P = 0.72). There was a significantly higher risk of CV events in the hypoglycemia group (HR 2.0; 95% CI 1.63–2.44) and microvascular complications (HR 1.76; 95% CI 1.46–2.11). However, no statistically significant increase was seen in mortality. Moreover, patients who had at least two episodes of hypoglycemia were at higher risk of vascular events than those with one episode. Thus, monitoring and prevention of hypoglycemia in all patients remains an important medical management issue in patients with T2D.

Another trial assessing impact of intensive versus standard glycemic control in patients with T2D was the ADVANCE trial.[5] In contrast to ACCORD, patients (n = 11,140) in ADVANCE were moderately older (required to be at least 55 years) with either known vascular disease or at least one other vascular risk factor. Patients also had a relatively shorter duration of diabetes (i.e., 8 years; 2 years shorter than ACCORD subjects). The baseline A1C was lower in ADVANCE, and there was virtually no use of insulin as part of patients' treatment regimen. After a median follow-up of 5 years, the A1C was significantly lower at 6.5% in the intensive glycemic control group compared with 7.3% in the standard glycemic control group. The rate of reduction of A1C was substantially slower in ADVANCE at 0.6% at 12 months versus 0.6% at 6 months in ACCORD.

Severe hypoglycemia was more common in the intensive-control arm, but the rates were considerably lower compared with ACCORD (2.7 vs. 1.5%; HR 1.86; 95% CI 1.42– 24.0, P < 0.001). The combined incidence of major macrovascular and microvascular events was significantly lower in the intensive glycemic control arm (HR 0.90; 95% CI 0.82–0.98; P = 0.01). This mainly was due to a 21% relative reduction in nephropathy.[8] The development of macroalbuminuria was clearly reduced with intensive glycemic control compared with standard glycemic control (2.9 vs. 4.1%; HR 0.70; CI 0.57–0.85; P <0.001). By contrast, the CV component of the endpoint, which was a composite of MI, stroke, and CV death, was not reduced significantly by intensive glycemic control (HR 0.94; 95% CI 0.84–1.06; P = 0.32).[14] An important observation is that there was no evidence that intensive glycemic control led to an increase in CV or all-cause mortality.[8] These results have importance in our understanding and application of intensive glycemic control measures to the appropriate group of patients for CV benefits.

OTHER STUDIES EVALUATING CARDIOVASCULAR DISEASE IN DIABETES

Postprandial hyperglycemia has been associated with CVD independent of the fasting blood glucose or the A1C. The Hyperglycemia and Its Effect After Acute Myocardial Infarction on Cardiovascular Outcomes in Patients with Type 2 Diabetes Mellitus (HEART2D) trial[23] compared the effects of prandial (the PRAN-DIAL arm; three premeal doses of insulin lispro targeting 2-hour postprandial glucose <7.5 mmol/l) or the basal strategy (the BASAL arm; neutral protamine Hagedorn twice daily or insulin glargine once daily targeting fasting/premeal blood glucose to <6.7 mmol/l). The trial was stopped due to lack of efficacy, as the risk of first combined adjudicated primary CV events in the PRANDIAL arm was similar to the BASAL arm (HR 0.98; 95% CI 0.8–1.21). Kilpatrick et al.[24] evaluated the DCCT data to further investigate the question whether glycemic variability plays a role in increasing the risk of microvascular complications in addition to the mean blood glucose. Their analyses showed that within-day and between-day variability in blood glucose levels around a patient's mean value has no effect on the development or progression of retinopathy (P = 0.18 and P = 0.72, respectively) or nephropathy (P = 0.32 and P = 0.57, respectively). Neither preprandial (P = 0.18) nor postprandial (P = 0.31) glucose levels contributed to retinopathy.

Meanwhile, the Bypass Angioplasty Revascularization Investigation 2 Diabetes (BARI 2D) trial[25] was designed to test the effect of prompt revascularization with intensive medical therapy or intensive medical therapy alone (either insulin-sensitization or insulin provision) in patients with CAD and diabetes. The primary endpoints were the rate of death and a composite of death, MI, or stroke. At 5 years, there was no difference in the rate of survival between the revascularization and the medical therapy groups (88.3 vs. 87.8%, respectively; P = 0.97) or between the insulin-sensitization and the insulin-provision groups (88.2 vs. 87.9%, respectively; P = 0.29).

The Prospective Pioglitazone Clinical Trial in Macrovascular Events (PROactive) study[18,26] was not designed as a glucose-lowering trial as such, but it is discussed here due to its implication in the important meta-analyses examining whether CV events are reduced with intensive glucose control. This outcome study randomized 5,238 patients with T2D with preexisting CVD. The PROactive trial was designed to explore whether the addition of pioglitazone or placebo to a patient's normal glucose-lowering medications could reduce CV events. The primary endpoint reduced by 10% with pioglitazone treatment, but it was not statistically significant (HR 0.90; 95% CI 0.8–1.02; P = 0.095). Controversially, the study was presented as having a positive outcome because the main secondary endpoint, which was a composite of all-cause mortality, nonfatal MI, and stroke, was significantly reduced by 16% with pioglitazone treatment (HR 0.84; 95% CI 0.72–0.98, P = 0.027).[8]

Additionally, post hoc analysis (PROactive 08) provided valuable information regarding HF risk. The patients who were included in the study had established macrovascular disease, which put them at high risk for HF. This certainly may be plausible reason for any therapeutic advantage to be possibly lost by associated HF mortality. According to Erdmann et al.,[27] there were more patients who took pioglitazone (5.7%) than placebo (4.1%) who had a serious HF event during the study (P = 0.007). The mortality due to HF, however, was similar in both the groups (25 of 2,605 [0.96%] for pioglitazone vs. 22 of 2,633 [0.84%] for placebo; P = 0.639). Additionally, fewer patients taking pioglitazone with a serious HF event went on to have an event in the primary (47.7% with pioglitazone vs. 57.4% with placebo; P = 0.0593) or main secondary endpoint (34.9% with pioglitazone vs. 47.2% with placebo; P = 0.025). Thus, although the incidence of serious HF was increased with pioglitazone versus placebo in the patients in the PROactive trial, subsequent mortality or morbidity was not increased in patients with serious HF.[26]

The Outcome Reduction with an Initial Glargine Intervention (ORIGIN) trial[28] was designed to test whether provision of sufficient basal insulin to normalize the fasting plasma glucose (target of ≤95 mg/dl) would reduce CV events because an elevated fasting plasma glucose is an independent risk factor for adverse CV outcomes.[29-35] The trial enrolled 12,537 people from 40 countries with CV risk factors plus impaired fasting glucose, impaired glucose tolerance, or T2D. Subjects were randomized to receive either insulin glargine or standard care and to receive n-3 fatty acids or placebo per the 2 × 2 factorial design. There were two coprimary composite CV outcomes. The first was death from CV causes, nonfatal MI, or nonfatal stroke; the second was a composite of any of these events, a revascularization procedure (cardiac, carotid, or peripheral), or hospitalization for HF. The mean age was 36.5 years and the median follow-up was 6.2 years. In the insulin glargine group, more than half (59.3%) of the subjects had a prior CV event and 35.5% had a prior MI. The incidence of both coprimary outcomes did not differ significantly between treatment groups with HRs of 1.02 (95% CI 0.94–1.11; *P* = 0.63) and 1.04 (95% CI 0.97–1.11; *P* = 0.27) for the first and second coprimary outcomes, respectively. Additionally, there was no significant difference in mortality (HR 0.98; 95% CI 0.90–1.08; *P* = 0.70) or microvascular events (HR 0.97; 95% CI 0.90–1.05; *P* = 0.43). Lack of diabetes and lower baseline A1C were independently associated with a 5-year mean A1C <6.5%.[36] Maintaining mean A1C <6.5% was more likely with glargine (OR 2.98; 95% CI 2.67–3.32; *P* <0.001) than standard care after adjusting for other independent predictors. Subjects who had diabetes at baseline had relatively shorter duration (mean = 5.5 years) of the disease. Thus, results from this study cannot be extrapolated to an older population with longer duration of diabetes.

Although the effects of pharmacologic agents on glycemic control in patients with diabetes and the effects on CVD have been studied extensively, the Look AHEAD (Action for Health in Diabetes) trial[37] investigated the long-term impact of an intensive lifestyle intervention on CVD in overweight and obese adults with T2D. Some 5,145 patients were assigned randomly to participate either in the intensive lifestyle intervention (*n* = 2,570) or to receive diabetes support and education (*n* = 2,575). The mean age was 58.7 years and the mean BMI was 36. The median duration of diabetes was 5 years and 14% of the subjects reported a history of CVD. The primary endpoint was the first occurrence of a composite CV outcome. Initially, the composite outcome included death from CV causes, nonfatal MI, and nonfatal stroke. Since, in the first 2 years of the trial, the primary event rate in the control group was lower than expected, hospitalization for angina was added to the primary outcome and the follow-up was increased to a maximum of 13.5 years. On September 14, 2012, the intervention was terminated based on the futility analysis and recommendation from the Data Safety Monitoring Board (DSMB). There was no difference in the composite primary outcome with 403 events occurring in the intervention group and 418 in the control group (1.83 and 1.92 events per 100 person-years, respectively; HR in the intervention group, 0.95; 95% CI 0.83–1.09; *P* = 0.51). There were no statistically significant differences in the secondary outcomes between the two groups. Trial investigators submit several plausible reasons for the trial results. Sustained weight loss greater than what was achieved in the intervention group may be required to reduce the risk of CVD and the provision of education sessions; in addition, the increased use of statins in the control group may have lessened the difference between the two groups.

The CV safety and efficacy of many current agents used in the treatment of T2D, including the dipeptidyl peptidase-4 (DPP-4) inhibitor class of drugs, is not known. The Saxagliptin Assessment of Vascular Outcomes Recorded in Patients with Diabetes (SAVOR-TIMI 53) trial assessed the effect of saxagliptin on CV outcomes.[38] In the trial, 16,492 patients with T2D who either had history of, or were at risk for, CV events were assigned randomly to receive either saxagliptin or placebo and were followed for a median of 2.1 years. The primary endpoint was a composite of CV death, MI, or ischemic stroke, which was experienced by 613 patients in the saxagliptin group and 609 patients in the placebo group (7.3 and 7.2%, respectively; HR with saxagliptin 1.00; 95% CI 0.89–1.12; $P = 0.99$ for superiority; $P < 0.001$ for noninferiority). "On-treatment" analysis revealed similar results (HR = 1.03; 95% CI 0.91–1.17). More patients in the saxagliptin group, however, were hospitalized for HF as compared with the placebo group (3.5 vs. 2.8%; HR = 1.27; 95% CI 1.07–1.51; $P = 0.007$). Rate of acute (0.3% in the saxagliptin group and 0.2% in the placebo group) and chronic pancreatitis (<0.1% in the saxagliptin group and 0.1% in the placebo group) were similar in the two groups.

The Cardiovascular Outcomes Study of Alogliptin in Subjects with Type 2 Diabetes and Acute Coronary Syndrome (EXAMINE)[39] was a double-blind, noninferiority trial conducted with patients with T2D who had either an acute MI or unstable angina requiring hospitalization within the previous 15–90 days. In the trial, 5,380 patients were randomized to either alogliptin or placebo in addition to their existing antihyperglycemic and CV drug therapy and were followed for a median of 18 months. The primary endpoint was a composite of death from CV causes, nonfatal MI, or nonfatal stroke, which was experienced in 305 patients (11%) in the alogliptin group and 316 patients (11.8%) in the placebo group. These differences were not statistically significant (HR = 0.96; upper boundary of the one-sided repeated CI was 1.16; $P < 0.001$ for noninferiority). A1C was significantly lower with alogliptin than with placebo (mean difference –0.36%; $P < 0.001$). Incidences of hypoglycemia, cancer, and pancreatitis were similar with alogliptin and placebo. Although EXAMINE was conducted in very-high-risk CV patients with T2D with recent events, patients in SAVOR-TIMI 53 either had a history of a CV event or were at risk for CV events.

ONGOING TRIALS

Several trials are ongoing to assess CV outcomes in patients with T2D. The Sitagliptin Cardiovascular Outcome Study (0431-082 AM1; TECOS)[40] is designed to assess the CV outcome of long-term treatment with sitagliptin or placebo added to usual care in patients with T2D with a history of CVD. The Cardiovascular Outcome Study of Linagliptin Versus Glimepiride in Patients With Type 2 Diabetes (CAROLINA) trial[41] is assessing the long-term effects of another DPP-4 inhibitor, linagliptin, on CV morbidity and mortality and is investigating the glycemic parameters in patients with T2D who are at increased CV risk and receiving usual care with the comparator, glimepiride. The aim of Liraglutide Effect and Action in Diabetes: Evaluation of Cardiovascular Outcome Results—A Long Term Evaluation (LEADER)[42] is to determine the long-term effect of liraglutide on CV events in subjects with T2D. Another study, A Trial Comparing Cardiovascular Safety of Insulin Degludec Versus Insulin Glargine in Subjects With Type 2 Diabetes at High Risk of Cardiovascular Events (DEVOTE), is evaluating CV safety of insulin degludec as compared with insulin glargine in subjects with T2D who are at high risk of CV events.[42]

META-ANALYSES EXAMINING EFFECTS OF INTENSIVE GLYCEMIC CONTROL

Given the early termination of ACCORD and lower-than-anticipated event rates in ADVANCE and VADT, there was concern about these studies being underpowered to truly assess the effects of intensive glycemic control on CVD risk. As a result, four separate meta-analyses have been conducted since 2009 to explore the relationship between glycemic control and CVD events in subjects with T2D. The first one, conducted by Horwich et al.,[43] included 33,040 participants from UKPDS, ACCORD, ADVANCE, VADT, and PROactive. Results of this meta-analysis indicate that, overall, non-fatal MI was decreased by 17% and CHD events were reduced by 15% with no significant difference of intensive glycemic control on stroke and all-cause mortality.[8] A second meta-analysis by Kelley et al.[9] included 27,000 participants from UKPDS, ACCORD, ADVANCE, and VADT and revealed that intensive glycemic control was associated with a significant 10% relative reduction in CV events, mainly due to an 11% reduction in CHD events. Intensive glycemic control did not have a significant effect on rates of stroke, CV mortality, congestive HF, or all-cause mortality. When the combined results of ACCORD, ADVANCE, and VADT trials were analyzed, there was only a 10% nonsignificant relative reduction in CHD events (odds ratio [OR] 0.9; 95% CI 0.83–1.01). The overall analysis was indicative of the fact that the benefits of intensive glycemic control were at the cost of an increased risk for severe hypoglycemia (OR 2.3; CI 1.46–2.81). A third meta-analysis, conducted by Mannucci et al.,[44] indicated that intensive glycemic control was associated with a significant 11% relative reduction in CV events that was attributed to a decrease in MI rates by 14%. There was no effect of intensive glycemic control on rates of stroke, CV mortality, or all-cause mortality. Intensive glycemic control also was associated with significantly higher rates of hypoglycemic events as compared with standard control (OR 3.01; 95% CI 1.47–4.60).[10] Lastly, Turnbull et al.[35] reported a reduction in major in CV events by 9% (HR 0.91; 95% CI 0.84–0.99) with glycemic control, predominantly due to a significant 15% reduction in the rate of MI. There was no significant reduction in CV and total mortality with intensive glycemic control. Intensive glycemic control was associated with a two-fold higher risk of severe hypoglycemia. The ideal approach used to institute intensive glycemic control, and the rapidity and degree of A1C reduction that balances the benefit versus risk ratio for patients with T2D, remains unclear.

TREATMENT OF DYSLIPIDEMIA AND CARDIOVASCULAR DISEASE IN DIABETES

There is an increased prevalence of lipid abnormalities in patients with T2D, and this contributes to the risk of CVD in T2D. Subanalyses of diabetes subgroups of larger trials[45,46] and trials specifically in subjects with diabetes[47,48] have shown significant primary and secondary prevention of CVD events in patients with and without CHD. The Heart Protection Study (HPS)[49] enrolled 20,536 adults in the U.K. with coronary disease, other occlusive arterial disease, or diabetes and randomized the subjects to either 40 mg of simvastatin or placebo with a follow-up period of 5 years. Results showed a significant reduction in all-cause mortality (12.9% in the simvastatin group vs. 14.7% in the placebo group; $P = 0.0003$) due to a significant proportional reduction in coronary death rate (5.7 vs. 6.9%, respectively; $P = 0.0005$). Results of the extended post-trial follow-up of the HPS participants[51] showed that the significant reduction in vascular mortality and morbidity due to the average 5-year reduction in LDL cholesterol with simvastatin persisted in the subsequent 6 years. The Atorvastatin Study for Prevention of Cardiovascular End Points in Subjects With Type 2 Diabetes (ASPEN) trial[47] assessed the effect of 10 mg of atorvastatin versus placebo on CVD prevention specifically in T2D patients. The mean LDL cholesterol reduction in the atorvastatin group over 4 years was 29% versus placebo ($P <0.0001$). There was no significant difference in the composite endpoint (CV death, nonfatal MI, nonfatal stroke, recanalization, coronary artery bypass surgery, resuscitated cardiac arrest, and worsening or unstable angina requiring hospitalization) with the rates being 13.7% for the atorvastatin group and 15% in the placebo group (HR 0.90; 95% CI 0.73–1.12). During the course of the ASPEN trial, there was a change in the lipid treatment guidelines with recommendations for lower LDL cholesterol target levels. The DSMB thus recommended that the study medication be discontinued for all primary and secondary prevention subjects with an adjudicated endpoint and that usual care be provided. Thus, only 67% of the subjects in the atorvastatin group and 58% in the placebo group completed the double-blind phase receiving study medication. The results of this study may be related to these changes during the course of the trial. A meta-analysis by Kearney et al.,[50] which included data on >18,000 patients with diabetes from 14 randomized controlled trials (RCTs) of statin therapy with a mean follow-up of 4.3 years, demonstrated that each millimoles per liter reduction in LDL cholesterol resulted in 9% proportional reduction in all-cause mortality and 13% reduction in vascular mortality.

Although the LDL cholesterol target has been the focus of several trials, a low plasma level of high-density lipoprotein cholesterol (HDL-C) is a major risk factor for CHD. The Veterans Affairs High-Density Lipoprotein Intervention Trial (VA-HIT)[52] was undertaken to test the hypothesis that drug therapy to increase low HDL-C would decrease the incidence of major CHD events in men with CAD, HDL-C <40 mg/dl, and LDL-C ≤140 mg/dl. Patients were randomized to either 1,200 mg of gemfibrozil or placebo. The primary outcome was nonfatal MI or death from coronary causes with a median follow-up of 5.1 years. The overall reduction in the risk of an event was 4.4%. There was a reduction in relative risk of 22% (95% CI 7–35%; $P = 0.006$). There was a 24% reduction in the combined outcome of death from CHD, nonfatal MI, and stroke ($P <0.001$). The beneficial effect of gemfibrozil did not become apparent until 2 years after randomization. The Fenofibrate Intervention and Event Lowering in Diabetes (FIELD) study[53] was designed to assess the effects of long-term treatment with fenofibrate to raise HDL-C and lower triglyceride levels on coronary morbidity and mortality in patients with T2D between the ages of 50 and 75 years not taking statin therapy at study entry. Patients were randomized to micronized fenofibrate 200 mg or placebo. At 5 years follow-up, 5.9% of patients in the placebo arm and 5.2% in the fenofibrate arm had a coronary event (relative reduction of 11%; HR 0.89; 95% CI 0.75–1.05; P = 0.16). There was a significant relative reduction of 24% in non-fatal MI (HR 0.76; 95% CI 0.62–0.94; P = 0.01) and a nonsignificant increase in CHD mortality (HR 1.19; 95% CI 0.90–1.57; P = 0.22). Fenofibrate was associated with less albuminuria progression (P = 0.002) and less retinopathy laser treatment (5.2 vs. 3.6%, P = 0.0003). Another trial to focus on the HDL-C was the Atherosclerosis Intervention in Metabolic Syndrome with Low HDL/High Triglycerides: Impact on Global Health Outcomes (AIM-HIGH),[54] which tested whether extended-release (ER) niacin added to simvastatin to raise low levels of HDL-C was superior to simvastatin alone in reducing the risk due to low HLD-C in patients with established CVD. Patients were assigned to either ER niacin 1,500–2,000 mg/day or placebo. All patients received ezetimibe 10 mg in addition to simvastatin 40–80 mg/day. The primary endpoint was the first event of the composite of death from CHD, nonfatal MI, ischemic stroke, hospitalization for an acute coronary syndrome, or symptom-driven coronary or cerebral revascularization. After a mean follow-up period of 3 years, the trial was stopped due to lack of efficacy. At 2 years, niacin therapy had significantly increased the median HDL-C from 35 to 42 mg/dl and lowered the triglyceride level from 164 to 122 mg/dl. The primary endpoint occurred in 16.4% of patients in the niacin group and 16.2% in the placebo group (HR 1.02; 95% CI 0.87–1.21; P = 0.79). Thus, there was no clinical benefit from the addition of niacin to statin therapy in patients with LDL-C <70 mg/dl.

The ACCORD Lipid Trial[55] investigated whether combination therapy with statin and fibrate as compared to statin alone would reduce the risk of CVD in T2D patients at high risk for CVD. The primary outcome was the first occurrence of nonfatal MI, nonfatal stroke, or death from CV causes. There was no difference between the placebo and the fenofibrate group with regard to the percentage of patients with previous CVD or statin use. With a mean follow-up of 4.7 years, there was no significant difference in the rate of the primary outcome (HR in the fenofibrate group 0.92; 95% CI 0.79–1.08; P = 0.32) or the secondary outcomes.

There is an increased risk for incident diabetes with statin use.[50,56] A meta-analysis of >170,000 person's data from 27 randomized trials showed that individuals at low risk of vascular disease, including those who are using statins for primary prevention, benefited from statin use. There were reductions in major vascular events and vascular death without increase in death from other causes.[46] Thus, the risk-benefit ratio should be considered for the patient with regard to statin use.

BLOOD PRESSURE CONTROL AND CARDIOVASCULAR DISEASE IN DIABETES

Hypertension is a major risk factor for both CVD and microvascular complications. Epidemiological analyses show that BP >115/75 mmHg is associated with increased CV event rates[57–59] and that systolic BP >120 mmHg predicts long-term end-stage renal disease (ESRD). RCTs have demonstrated benefit by reduction of CHD events, stroke, and nephropathy when the systolic BP is lowered to <140 mmHg and the diastolic BP is lowered to <80 mmHg in patients with diabetes.[57,60–62] Trials studying the benefits of specific systolic and diastolic BP targets on CVD have been conducted as well.

In the Hypertension Optimal Treatment (HOT) trial,[61] 18,790 patients with hypertension and diastolic BP between 100 mmHg and 115 mmHg were assigned randomly to a target diastolic BP of ≤90, ≤85, or ≤80 mmHg. In each group, 8% of the subjects had diabetes and the mean systolic BP in all the groups was 169 ± 14 mmHg. The principal aims of this study were to assess the association of the target diastolic BPs and major CV events during antihypertensive treatment and the association between the major CV events and the diastolic BP achieved during treatment. At the end of the study, the average diastolic BP was reduced was by 20.3, 22.3, and 24.3 mmHg and the systolic BP was reduced by 26.2, 28.0, and 29.9 mmHg in the target groups ≤90, ≤85, and ≤80 mmHg, respectively. The lowest incidence of major CV events occurred at a mean achieved diastolic BP of 82.6 mmHg and at a mean achieved systolic BP of 138.5 mmHg. In patients with diabetes, there was a 51% reduction in major CV events in the ≤80 diastolic BP target group as compared with ≤90 mmHg (*P* = 0.05). The evidence for benefits from <140 mmHg systolic BP targets, however, are limited.

The ACCORD BP trial[63] investigated whether therapy targeting a normal systolic BP of <120 mmHg reduces major CV events in 4,733 subjects with T2D at high risk for CV events. Participants were randomized to either intensive therapy (target systolic BP <120 mmHg) or standard therapy (target BP <140 mmHg). The primary composite outcome was nonfatal MI, nonfatal stroke, or death from CV causes with a mean follow-up of 4.7 years. After 1 year, the mean systolic BP was 133.5 mmHg in the standard therapy group and 119.3 mmHg in the intensive therapy group. The annual rate of the primary outcome was 2.09% in the standard therapy group and 1.87% in the intensive therapy group (HR with intensive therapy was 0.88; 95% CI 0.97–1.06; *P* = 0.20). The annual rates of death from any cause were 1.19% in the standard therapy group and 1.28% in the intensive therapy group (HR 1.07; 95% CI 0.85–1.35; *P* = 0.55). The annual rate of stroke, a prespecified secondary outcome, was 0.53% in the standard therapy group and 0.32% in the intensive therapy group (HR 0.59; 95% CI 0.39–0.89; *P* = 0.01). Rate of macroalbuminuria was reduced (8.7% in the standard therapy group vs. 6.6% in the intensive therapy group; *P* = 0.009) although there was no difference in the frequency of ESRD or the need for dialysis between the two groups.

A meta-analysis by McBrien et al.[64] on RCTs of adults with T2D comparing prespecified BP targets found no significant reduction in mortality or nonfatal MI. There was a statistically significant reduction in stroke by 35% but the absolute risk reduction was only 1%. Indicators of microvascular complications were not examined. Another meta-analysis[65] included trials that compared BP goals and trials that compared treatment strategies. Results showed that a systolic BP goal of 130–135 mmHg was acceptable. When the systolic BP was <130 mmHg, there were reductions in stroke, a 10% reduction in mortality, and reduced onset and progression of albuminuria. There was no reduction of other CVD events, retinopathy, or neuropathy. Patients with a longer life expectancy, however, in whom renal benefits are expected from long-term, more stringent BP control or in whom the risk for stroke is a concern, lowering systolic BP to <130 mmHg may be appropriate, if this is achieved with few drugs and without side effects.[66]

Recently, the Eighth Joint National Committee (JNC 8) guidelines[67] have advocated a higher systolic and diastolic BP goals for the management of hypertension. In patients with hypertension ≥60 years, the recommendations are to treat the BP to <150/90 mmHg. For those between the ages of 30 and 59, the JNC has recommended that there is evidence to treat to a diastolic BP of <90 mmHg, but also suggested that evidence for setting a goal for systolic BP control in those between the ages of 30 and 59 was insufficient. For those <30 years old, the JNC again felt that evidence was insufficient to set a goal for diastolic BP, and thus the goal was set at BP of <140/90 mmHg based on expert opinion. Furthermore, the goals for BP control are the same for those hypertensive patients with diabetes and chronic kidney disease as for the general hypertensive population <60 years of age.

The 2014 American Diabetes Association position statement[68] maintains that patients with diabetes and hypertension should be treated to a systolic BP goal of <140 mmHg and diastolic BP of <80 mmHg. Furthermore, for younger patients, lower systolic BP target of <130 mmHg may be appropriate if the goal can be achieved without undue treatment burden.

CONCLUSION

Taking into consideration the evidence thus far, it is important to approach glucose lowering in the context of managing overall CV risk. Generally, A1C of <7% is thought to be appropriate for patients. Glycemic goals, however, should be individualized based on duration of diabetes, preexisting CVD and other comorbidities, age, and life expectancy. For example, more stringent goals are appropriate for a relatively young patient with no underlying CVD who has been recently diagnosed with diabetes. On the other hand, less intensive goals should be recommended for elderly patients with long-standing diabetes who may have established macrovascular disease in whom the risks associated with hypoglycemia could be significant. Intensive glycemic control consistently has been shown to produce a substantial benefit for preventing microvascular complications in both T1D and T2D. The entire effect of intensive glycemic control on macrovascular complications is yet to be clearly understood. In addition, goals for BP and lipid management should be individualized for the patient in the context of the existing comorbidities and the risk-benefit ratio. Although macrovascular disease is a major cause of death in patients with diabetes, microvascular complications cause substantial morbidity.

REFERENCES

1. Centers for Disease Control and Prevention. *Diabetes Public Health Resource*, Centers for Disease Control and Prevention, 2012. Available at www.cdc. gov/diabetes/projects/cda2.htm. Accessed 17 July 2013.

2. Gaede P, Vedel P, Parving HH, Pedersen O. Intensified multifactorial intervention in patients with type 2 diabetes mellitus and microalbuminuria: the Steno type 2 randomised study. *Lancet* 1999;353(9153):617–622.

3. Diabetes Control and Complications Trial Research Group 1. The effect of intensive treatment of diabetes on the development and progression of long-term complications in insulin-dependent diabetes mellitus. *N Engl J Med* 1993;329(14):977–986.

4. U.K. Prospective Diabetes Study Group 1. Intensive blood-glucose control with sulphonylureas or insulin compared with conventional treatment and risk of complications in patients with type 2 diabetes (UKPDS 33). *Lancet* 1998;352(9131):837–853.

5. Patel A, MacMahon S, Chalmers J, Neal B, Billot L, Woodward M, Marre M, Cooper M, Glasziou P, Grobbee D, Hamet P, Harrap S, Heller S, Liu L, Mancia G, Mogensen CE, Pan C, Poulter N, Rodgers A, Williams B, Bompoint S, de Galan BE, Joshi R, Travert F; ADVANCE Collaborative Group. Intensive blood glucose control and vascular outcomes in patients with type 2 diabetes. *N Engl J Med* 200;358(24):2560–2572.

6. Duckworth W, Abraira C, Moritz T, Reda D, Emanuele N, Reaven PD, Zieve FJ, Marks J, Davis SN, Hayward R, Warren SR, Goldman S, McCarren M, Vitek ME, Henderson WG, Huang GD; VADT Investigators. Glucose control and vascular complications in veterans with type 2 diabetes. *N Engl J Med* 2009;360(2):129–139.

7. Gerstein HC, Miller ME, Byington RP, Goff DC, Bigger JT, Buse JB, Cushman WC, Genuth S, Ismail-Beigi F, Grimm RH, Probstfield JL, Simons-Morton DG, Friedewald WT; Action to Control Cardiovascular Risk in Diabetes Study Group. Effects of intensive glucose lowering in type 2 diabetes. *N Engl J Med* 2008;358(24):2545–2559.

8. Macisaac RJ, Jerums G. Intensive glucose control and cardiovascular outcomes in type 2 diabetes. *Heart Lung Circ* 2011;20(10):647–654.

9. Kelly TN, Bazzano LA, Fonseca VA, Thethi TK, Reynolds K, He J. Systematic review: glucose control and cardiovascular disease in type 2 diabetes. *Ann Intern Med* 2009;151(6):394–403.

10. Ray KK, Seshasai SR, Wijesuriya S, Sivakumaran R, Nethercott S, Preiss D, Erqou S, Sattar N. Effect of intensive control of glucose on cardiovascular outcomes and death in patients with diabetes mellitus: a meta-analysis of randomised controlled trials. *Lancet* 2009;373(9677):1765–1772.

11. Desouza C, Raghavan VA, Fonseca VA. The enigma of glucose and cardiovascular disease. *Heart* 2010;96 (9):649–651.

12. Huxley R, Barzi F, Woodward M. Excess risk of fatal coronary heart disease associated with diabetes in men and women: meta-analysis of 37 prospective cohort studies. *BMJ* 2006;332(7533):73–78.

13. Myint PK, Sinha S, Wareham NJ, Bingham SA, Luben RN, Welch AA, Khaw KT. Glycated hemoglobin and risk of stroke in people without known diabetes in the European Prospective Investigation into Cancer (EPIC)-Norfolk prospective population study: a threshold relationship? *Stroke* 2007;38(2):271–275.

14. Fonseca VA. Ongoing clinical trials evaluating the cardiovascular safety and efficacy of therapeutic approaches to diabetes mellitus. *Am J Cardiol* 2011;108(Suppl 3):52B–8B.

15. Stratton IM, Adler AI, Neil HA, Matthews DR, Manley SE, Cull CA, Hadden D, Turner RC, Holman RR. Association of glycaemia with macrovascular and microvascular complications of type 2 diabetes (UKPDS 35): prospective observational study. *BMJ* 2000;321(7258):405–412.

16. Nathan DM, Cleary PA, Backlund JY, Genuth SM, Lachin JM, Orchard TJ, Raskin P, Zinman B; Diabetes Control and Complications Trial/Epidemiology of Diabetes Interventions and Complications (DCCT/EDIC) Study Research Group. Intensive diabetes treatment and cardiovascular disease in patients with type 1 diabetes. *N Engl J Med* 2005;353(25):2643–2653.

17. Gubitosi-Klug RA; DCCT/EDIC Research Group. The Diabetes Control and Complications Trial/Epidemiology of Diabetes Interventions and Complications study at 30 years: summary and future directions. *Diabetes Care* 2014;37(1):44–49.

18. Del Prato S. Megatrials in type 2 diabetes. From excitement to frustration? *Diabetologia* 2009;52(7):1219–1226.

19. Riddle MC, Ambrosius WT, Brillon DJ, Buse JB, Byington RP, Cohen RM, Goff DC, Malozowski S, Margolis KL, Probstfield JL, Schnall A, Seaquist ER; Action to Control Cardiovascular Risk in Diabetes Investigators. Epidemiologic relationships between A1C and all-cause mortality during a median 3.4-year follow-up of glycemic treatment in the ACCORD trial. *Diabetes Care* 2010;33(5):983–990.

20. Bonds DE, Miller ME, Bergenstal RM, Buse JB, Byington RP, Cutler JA, Dudl RJ, Ismail-Beigi F, Kimel AR, Hoogwerf B, Horowitz KR, Savage PJ, Seaquist ER, Simmons DL, Sivitz WI, Speril-Hillen JM, Sweeney ME. The association between symptomatic, severe hypoglycaemia and mortality in type 2 diabetes: retrospective epidemiological analysis of the ACCORD study. *BMJ* 2010;340:b4909.

21. Adler GK, Bonyhay I, Failing H, Waring E, Dotson S, Freeman R. Antecedent hypoglycemia impairs autonomic cardiovascular function: implications for rigorous glycemic control. *Diabetes* 2009;58(2):360–366.

22. Zhao Y, Campbell CR, Fonseca V, Shi L. Impact of hypoglycemia associated with antihyperglycemic medications on vascular risks in veterans with type 2 diabetes. *Diabetes Care* 2012;35(5):1126–1132.

23. Raz I, Wilson PW, Strojek K, Kowalska I, Bozikov V, Gitt AK, Jermendy G, Campaigne BN, Kerr L, Milicevic Z, Jacober SJ. Effects of prandial versus

fasting glycemia on cardiovascular outcomes in type 2 diabetes: the HEART2D trial. *Diabetes Care* 2009;32(3):381–386.

24. Kilpatrick ES, Rigby AS, Atkin SL. The effect of glucose variability on the risk of microvascular complications in type 1 diabetes. *Diabetes Care* 2006;29(7):1486–1490.

25. Frye RL, August P, Brooks MM, Hardison RM, Kelsey SF, MacGregor JM, Orchard TJ, Chaitman BR, Genuth SM, Goldberg SH, Hlatky MA, Jones TL, Molitch ME, Nesto RW, Sako EY, Sobel BE; BARI 2D Study Group. A randomized trial of therapies for type 2 diabetes and coronary artery disease. *N Engl J Med* 2009;360(24):2503–2515.

26. Dormandy JA, Charbonnel B, Eckland DJ, Erdmann E, Massi-Benedetti M, Moules IK, Skene AM, Tan MH, Lefèbvre PJ, Murray GD, Standl E, Wilcox RG, Wilhelmsen L, Betteridge J, Birkeland K, Golay A, Heine RJ, Korányi L, Laakso M, Mokán M, Norkus A, Pirags V, Podar T, Scheen A, Scherbaum W, Schernthaner G, Schmitz O, Skrha J, Smith U, Taton J; PROactive Investigators. Secondary prevention of macrovascular events in patients with type 2 diabetes in the PROactive Study (PROspective pioglitAzone Clinical Trial In macroVascular Events): a randomised controlled trial. *Lancet* 2005;366(9493):1279–1289.

27. Erdmann E, Charbonnel B, Wilcox RG, Skene AM, Massi-Benedetti M, Yates J, Tan M, Spanheimer R, Standl E, Dormandy JA; PROactive Investigators. Pioglitazone use and heart failure in patients with type 2 diabetes and preexisting cardiovascular disease: data from the PROactive study (PROactive 08). *Diabetes Care* 2007;30(11):2773–2778.

28. Gerstein HC, Bosch J, Dagenais GR, Díaz R, Jung H, Maggioni AP, Pogue J, Probstfield J, Ramachandran A, Riddle MC, Rydén LE, Yusuf S; ORIGIN Trial Investigators. Basal insulin and cardiovascular and other outcomes in dysglycemia. *N Engl J Med* 2012;367(4):319–328.

29. Sarwar N, Gao P, Seshasai SR, Gobin R, Kaptoge S, Di Angelantonio E, Ingelsson E, Lawlor DA, Selvin E, Stampfer M, Stehouwer CD, Lewington S, Pennells L, Thompson A, Sattar N, White IR, Ray KK, Danesh J; Emerging Risk Factors Collaboration. Diabetes mellitus, fasting blood glucose concentration, and risk of vascular disease: a collaborative meta-analysis of 102 prospective studies. *Lancet* 2010;375(9733):2215–2222.

30. Selvin E, Steffes MW, Zhu H, Matsushita K, Wagenknecht L, Pankow J, Coresh J, Brancati FL. Glycated hemoglobin, diabetes, and cardiovascular risk in nondiabetic adults. *N Engl J Med* 2010;362(9):800–811.

31. Gerstein HC, Santaguida P, Raina P, Morrison KM, Balion C, Hunt D, Yazdi H, Booker L. Annual incidence and relative risk of diabetes in people with various categories of dysglycemia: a systematic overview and meta-analysis of prospective studies. *Diabetes Res Clin Pract* 2007;78(3):305–312.

32. Anand SS, Dagenais GR, Mohan V, Diaz R, Probstfield J, Freeman R, Shaw J, Lanas F, Avezum A, Budaj A, Jung H, Desai D, Bosch J, Yusuf S, Gerstein

HC; EpiDREAM Investigators. Glucose levels are associated with cardiovascular disease and death in an international cohort of normal glycaemic and dysglycaemic men and women: the EpiDREAM cohort study. *Eur J Prev Cardiol* 2012;19(4):755–764.

33. Gerstein HC, Islam S, Anand S, Almahmeed W, Damasceno A, Dans A, Lang CC, Luna MA, McQueen M, Rangarajan S, Rosengren A, Wang X, Yusuf S. Dysglycaemia and the risk of acute myocardial infarction in multiple ethnic groups: an analysis of 15,780 patients from the INTERHEART study. *Diabetologia* 2010;53(12):2509–2517.

34. Seshasai SR, Kaptoge S, Thompson A, Di Angelantonio E, Gao P, Sarwar N, Whincup PH, Mukamal KJ, Gillum RF, Holme I, Njølstad I, Fletcher A, Nilsson P, Lewington S, Collins R, Gudnason V, Thompson SG, Sattar N, Selvin E, Hu FB, Danesh J; Emerging Risk Factors Collaboration. Diabetes mellitus, fasting glucose, and risk of cause-specific death. *N Engl J Med* 2011;364(9):829–841.

35. Turnbull FM, Abraira C, Anderson RJ, Byington RP, Chalmers JP, Duckworth WC, Evans GW, Gerstein HC, Holman RR, Moritz TE, Neal BC, Ninomiya T, Patel AA, Paul SK, Travert F, Woodward M; Control Group. Intensive glucose control and macrovascular outcomes in type 2 diabetes. *Diabetologia* 2009;52(11):2288–2298.

36. ORIGIN Trial Investigators. Characteristics associated with maintenance of mean A1C <6.5% in people with dysglycemia in the ORIGIN Trial. *Diabetes Care* 2013;36:2915–2922.

37. Wing RR, Bolin P, Brancati FL, Bray GA, Clark JM, Coday M, Crow RS, Curtis JM, Egan CM, Espeland MA, Evans M, Foreyt JP, Ghazarian S, Gregg EW, Harrison B, Hazuda HP, Hill JO, Horton ES, Hubbard VS, Jakicic JM, Jeffery RW, Johnson KC, Kahn SE, Kitabchi AE, Knowler WC, Lewis CE, Maschak-Carey BJ, Montez MG, Murillo A, Nathan DM, Patricio J, Peters A, Pi-Sunyer X, Pownall H, Reboussin D, Regensteiner JC, Rickman AD, Ryan DH, Safford M, Wadden TA, Wagenknecht LE, West DS, Williamson DF, Yanovski SZ; Look AHEAD Research Group. Cardiovascular effects of intensive lifestyle intervention in type 2 diabetes. *N Engl J Med* 2013;369(2):145–154.

38. Scirica BM, Bhatt DL, Braunwald E, Steg PG, Davidson J, Hirshberg B, Ohman P, Frederich R, Wiviott SD, Hoffman EB, Cavender MA, Udell JA, Desai NR, Mosenzon O, McGuire DK, Ray KK, Leiter LA, Raz I; SAVOR-TIMI 53 Steering Committee and Investigators. Saxagliptin and cardiovascular outcomes in patients with type 2 diabetes mellitus. *N Engl J Med* 2013;369(14):1317–1326.

39. White WB, Cannon CP, Heller SR, Nissen SE, Bergenstal RM, Bakris GL, Perez AT, Fleck PR, Mehta CR, Kupfer S, Wilson C, Cushman WC, Zannad F; EXAMINE Investigators. Alogliptin after acute coronary syndrome in patients with type 2 diabetes. *N Engl J Med* 2013;369(14):1327–1335.

40. Merck. *Sitagliptin Cardiovascular Outcome Study (0431-082 AM1) (TECOS)*. U.S. National Library of Medicine, 2012. Available at www.clinicaltrials.gov/ct2/show/NCT00790205?term=.+Sitagliptin+Cardiovascular+Outcome+Study+%280431-082+AM1%29+%28TECOS%29&rank=1. Accessed 10 January 2014.

41. Boehringer Ingelheim Pharmaceuticals. *CAROLINA: Cardiovascular Outcome Study of Linagliptin versus Glimepiride in Patients with Type 2 Diabetes*. U.S. National Library of Medicine, 2013. Available at www.clinicaltrials.gov/ct2/show/NCT01243424?term=CAROLINA+trial&rank=12. Accessed 10 January 2014.

42. Novo Nordisk. *Liraglutide Effect and Action in Diabetes: Evaluation of Cardiovascular Outcome Results—a Long Term Evaluation (LEADER)*. U.S. National Library of Medicine, 2013. Available at www.clinicaltrials.gov/ct2/show/NCT01179048?term=Liraglutide+Effect+and+Action+in+Diabetes%3A+Evaluation+of+Cardiovascular+Outcome+Results+-+A+Long+Term+Evaluation+%28LEADER%29&rank=1. Accessed 10 January 2014.

43. Horwich TB, Fonarow GC. Glucose, obesity, metabolic syndrome, and diabetes relevance to incidence of heart failure. *J Am Coll Cardiol* 2010;55(4):283–293.

44. Mannucci E, Monami M, Lamanna C, Gori F, Marchionni N. Prevention of cardiovascular disease through glycemic control in type 2 diabetes: a meta-analysis of randomized clinical trials. *Nutr Metab Cardiovasc Dis* 2009; 19(9):604–612.

45. Baigent C, Keech A, Kearney PM, Blackwell L, Buck G, Pollicino C, Kirby A, Sourjina T, Peto R, Collins R, Simes R; Cholesterol Treatment Trialists' (CTT) Collaborators. Efficacy and safety of cholesterol-lowering treatment: prospective meta-analysis of data from 90,056 participants in 14 randomised trials of statins. *Lancet* 2005;366(9493):1267–1278.

46. Mihaylova B, Emberson J, Blackwell L, Keech A, Simes J, Barnes EH, Voysey M, Gray A, Collins R, Baigent C; Cholesterol Treatment Trialists' (CTT) Collaborators. The effects of lowering LDL cholesterol with statin therapy in people at low risk of vascular disease: meta-analysis of individual data from 27 randomised trials. *Lancet* 2012;380(9841):581–590.

47. Knopp RH, d'Emden M, Smilde JG, Pocock SJ. Efficacy and safety of atorvastatin in the prevention of cardiovascular end points in subjects with type 2 diabetes: the Atorvastatin Study for Prevention of Coronary Heart Disease Endpoints in non-insulin-dependent diabetes mellitus (ASPEN). *Diabetes Care* 2006;29(7):1478–1485.

48. Colhoun HM, Betteridge DJ, Durrington PN, Hitman GA, Neil HA, Livingstone SJ, Thomason MJ, Mackness MI, Charlton-Menys V, Fuller JH; CARDS Investigators. Primary prevention of cardiovascular disease with atorvastatin in type 2 diabetes in the Collaborative Atorvastatin Diabetes Study (CARDS): Multicentre randomised placebo-controlled trial. *Lancet* 2004;364(9435):685–696.

49. Heart Protection Study Collaborative Group. MRC/BHF Heart Protection Study of cholesterol lowering with simvastatin in 20,536 high-risk individuals: a randomised placebo-controlled trial. *Lancet* 2002;360(9326):7–22.

50. Kearney PM, Blackwell L, Collins R, Keech A, Simes J, Peto R, Armitage J, Baigent C; Cholesterol Treatment Trialists' (CTT) Collaborators. Efficacy of cholesterol-lowering therapy in 18,686 people with diabetes in 14 randomised trials of statins: a meta-analysis. *Lancet* 2008;371(9607):117–125.

51. Bulbulia R, Bowman L, Wallendszus K, Parish S, Armitage J, Peto R, Collins R; Heart Protection Study Collaborative Group. Effects on 11-year mortality and morbidity of lowering LDL cholesterol with simvastatin for about 5 years in 20,536 high-risk individuals: a randomised controlled trial. *Lancet* 2011;378(9808):2013–2020.

52. Rubins HB, Robins SJ, Collins D, Fye CL, Anderson JW, Elam MB, Faas FH, Linares E, Schaefer EJ, Schectman G, Wilt TJ, Wittes J. Gemfibrozil for the secondary prevention of coronary heart disease in men with low levels of high-density lipoprotein cholesterol. Veterans Affairs High-Density Lipoprotein Cholesterol Intervention Trial Study Group. *N Engl J Med* 1999;341(6):410–418.

53. Keech A, Simes RJ, Barter P, Best J, Scott R, Taskinen MR, Forder P, Pillai A, Davis T, Glasziou P, Drury P, Kesäniemi YA, Sullivan D, Hunt D, Colman P, d'Emden M, Whiting M, Ehnholm C, Laakso M; FIELD Study Investigators. Effects of long-term fenofibrate therapy on cardiovascular events in 9795 people with type 2 diabetes mellitus (the FIELD study): randomised controlled trial. *Lancet* 2005;366(9500):1849–1861.

54. Boden WE, Probstfield JL, Anderson T, Chaitman BR, Desvignes-Nickens P, Koprowicz K, McBride R, Teo K, Weintraub W; AIM-HIGH Investigators. Niacin in patients with low HDL cholesterol levels receiving intensive statin therapy. *N Engl J Med* 2011;365(24):2255–2267.

55. Ginsberg HN, Elam MB, Lovato LC, Crouse JR, Leiter LA, Linz P, Friedewald WT, Buse JB, Gerstein HC, Probstfield J, Grimm RH, Ismail-Beigi F, Bigger JT, Goff DC, Cushman WC, Simons-Morton DG, Byington RP; ACCORD Study Group. Effects of combination lipid therapy in type 2 diabetes mellitus. *N Engl J Med* 2010;362(17):1563–1574.

56. Sattar N, Preiss D, Murray HM, Welsh P, Buckley BM, de Craen AJ, Seshasai SR, McMurray JJ, Freeman DJ, Jukema JW, Macfarlane PW, Packard CJ, Stott DJ, Westendorp RG, Shepherd J, Davis BR, Pressel SL, Marchioli R, Marfisi RM, Maggioni AP, Tavazzi L, Tognoni G, Kjekshus J, Pedersen TR, Cook TJ, Gotto AM, Clearfield MB, Downs JR, Nakamura H, Ohashi Y, Mizuno K, Ray KK, Ford I. Statins and risk of incident diabetes: a collaborative meta-analysis of randomised statin trials. *Lancet* 2010;375(9716):735–742.

57. Chobanian AV, Bakris GL, Black HR, Cushman WC, Green LA, Izzo JL, Jones DW, Materson BJ, Oparil S, Wright JT, Roccella EJ; Lung National Heart, and Blood Institute Joint National Committee on Prevention, Detec-

tion, Evaluation, and Treatment of High Blood Pressure, and National High Blood Pressure Education Program Coordinating Committee. The seventh report of the Joint National Committee on Prevention, Detection, Evaluation, and Treatment of High Blood Pressure: the JNC 7 report. *JAMA* 2003;289(19):2560–2572.

58. Lewington S, Clarke R, Qizilbash N, Peto R, Collins R; Prospective Studies Collaboration. Age-specific relevance of usual blood pressure to vascular mortality: a meta-analysis of individual data for one million adults in 61 prospective studies. *Lancet* 2002;360(9349):1903–1913.

59. Stamler J, Vaccaro O, Neaton JD, Wentworth D. Diabetes, other risk factors, and 12-yr cardiovascular mortality for men screened in the Multiple Risk Factor Intervention Trial. *Diabetes Care* 1993;16(2):434–444.

60. U.K. Prospective Diabetes Study Group. Tight blood pressure control and risk of macrovascular and microvascular complications in type 2 diabetes: UKPDS 38. *BMJ* 1998;317(7160):703–713.

61. Hansson L, Zanchetti A, Carruthers SG, Dahlöf B, Elmfeldt D, Julius S, Ménard J, Rahn KH, Wedel H, Westerling S. Effects of intensive blood-pressure lowering and low-dose aspirin in patients with hypertension: principal results of the Hypertension Optimal Treatment (HOT) randomised trial. HOT Study Group. *Lancet* 1998;351(9118):1755–1762.

62. Adler AI, Stratton IM, Neil HA, Yudkin JS, Matthews DR, Cull CA, Wright AD, Turner RC, Holman RR. Association of systolic blood pressure with macrovascular and microvascular complications of type 2 diabetes (UKPDS 36): prospective observational study. *BMJ* 2000;321(7258):412–419.

63. Cushman WC, Evans GW, Byington RP, Goff DC, Grimm RH, Cutler JA, Simons-Morton DG, Basile JN, Corson MA, Probstfield JL, Katz L, Peterson KA, Friedewald WT, Buse JB, Bigger JT, Gerstein HC, Ismail-Beigi F; ACCORD Study Group. Effects of intensive blood-pressure control in type 2 diabetes mellitus. *N Engl J Med* 2010;362(17):1575–1585.

64. McBrien K, Rabi DM, Campbell N, Barnieh L, Clement F, Hemmelgarn BR, Tonelli M, Leiter LA, Klarenbach SW, Manns BJ. Intensive and standard blood pressure targets in patients with type 2 diabetes mellitus: systematic review and meta-analysis. *Arch Intern Med* 2012;172(17):1296–1303.

65. Bangalore S, Kumar S, Lobach I, Messerli FH. Blood pressure targets in subjects with type 2 diabetes mellitus/impaired fasting glucose: observations from traditional and Bayesian random-effects meta-analyses of randomized trials. *Circulation* 2011;123(24):2799–2810.

66. American Diabetes Association. Standards of medical care in diabetes—2013. *Diabetes Care* 2013;36(Suppl 1):S11–S66.

67. James PA, Oparil S, Carter BL, Cushman WC, Dennison-Himmelfarb C, Handler J, Lackland DT, Lefevre ML, Mackenzie TD, Ogedegbe O, Smith SC, Svetkey LP, Taler SJ, Townsend RR, Wright JT, Narva AS, Ortiz E. 2014 evidence-based guideline for the management of high blood pressure in

adults: Report from the panel members appointed to the Eighth Joint National Committee (JNC 8). *JAMA* 2013;290(21):2805–2816.

68. American Diabetes Association. Standards of medical care in diabetes—2014. *Diabetes Care* 2014;37(Suppl 1):S14–S80.

Chapter 48
Peripheral Arterial Disease: Diagnosis and Management

Enrico Cagliero, MD

EPIDEMIOLOGY

Peripheral arterial disease (PAD) is a manifestation of atherosclerosis in the arterial tree of the lower extremities and is a marker for atherosclerotic disease in other vascular beds, specifically the coronary and cerebrovascular circulature. Together with peripheral neuropathy, PAD is a major risk factor for nontraumatic lower-extremities amputation (LEA), and diabetes contributes to >60% of LEA in the U.S. The most common symptom of PAD is intermittent claudication, defined as frank pain, cramping in the legs or fatigue that is present, reproducibly with walking, and quick relief with rest. More severe presentations include pain at rest, nonhealing foot ulcers, and tissue loss or gangrene, which frequently can lead to limb loss and is termed critical limb ischemia (CLI). Most patients with PAD are asymptomatic, however, thus making it difficult to determine the true prevalence of PAD in patients with diabetes.

Diabetes is a significant risk factor for the development of PAD, with the prevalence of PAD being approximately twice in patients with diabetes as compared with the overall population. Other major risk factors for PAD include increasing age, systolic blood pressure, total serum cholesterol, and smoking (or prior history of smoking). Diabetes duration, poor glycemic control, as assessed by A1C, and the presence of diabetic neuropathy are associated with an increased risk of PAD. African Americans and Hispanics have a higher prevalence of PAD than non-Hispanic Whites. In a large study, the prevalence of PAD, as assessed by the ankle-brachial index (ABI), was 9.5% in U.S. adults with diabetes, >40 years of age with 78% of cases of PAD being asymptomatic. In the U.K. Prospective Diabetes Study (UKPDS), the prevalence of PAD at diagnosis of type 2 diabetes (T2D) was 1%, but at 18 years' follow-up, the prevalence increased to 18%. The prevalence of the most severe consequence of PAD (i.e., nontraumatic LEA) is ~3–4%, with more recent data showing a significant 60% reduction in amputation rate, over the past 20 years. PAD is associated significantly with a twofold increase in risk of cardiac mortality.

PAD is more severe in patients with diabetes than in those without diabetes. Patients with diabetes tend to have worse arterial disease in the distal vessels below the knee versus in the aorta or iliac arteries. PAD in patients with diabetes frequently is associated with vascular calcifications in the intimal plaques and in the media (Monckeberg's sclerosis), and the disease is more diffuse with poor collateral circulation. Moreover, patients with diabetes have more foot ulcers and gangrene than patients without diabetes with lower incidence of rest pain. They

DOI: 10.2337/9781580405096.48

also tend to fare worse, with amputations rates as much as five times higher than PAD patients without diabetes and overall double mortality rates.

PATHOGENESIS

Diabetes is a disease characterized by abnormalities in the small and large vessels, and PAD is thought to be caused by the atherogenic processes that are observed in the entire arterial vasculature, especially the coronary and cerebrovascular arteries. Although the diabetic metabolic milieu is associated with numerous abnormalities that have been postulated to be pathogenetic to atherosclerosis, no clear mechanisms have been identified as causative to vascular disease in human diabetes. In experimental diabetes as well as in patients with diabetes, multiple factors that could play a pathogenetic role have been observed, including increased inflammation, endothelial cell dysfunction, vascular smooth muscle abnormalities, and prothrombotic changes.

CLINICAL MANIFESTATIONS

The clinical manifestation of PAD can vary from completely asymptomatic to the most common manifestation of intermittent claudication, defined as the inability to walk a given distance without the development of reproducible pain, cramps, or aches in the calves, thighs, or buttocks (depending on the anatomical location of the stenosed vessel), which is relieved rapidly by rest. The pain also can be described as "discomfort, heaviness, tightness" and therefore a detailed history is essential. Claudication usually comes after a period of walking pain-free and is worse when walking fast or uphill when oxygen requirements increase. The concomitant development of peripheral neuropathy in patients with diabetes leads to a decreased rate of symptoms compared with patients without diabetes who have similar degrees of PAD. Moreover, other diseases, such as spinal stenosis or nerve root compression, also can cause pain while walking. In those cases, however, the walking distance before the development of pain can vary from day to day, the pain is not quickly relieved by rest (can take >15–30 minutes), and frequently a change in body position, such as sitting or bending, is needed to get symptomatic relief.

As the disease progresses, pain, usually described as a deep ache, also will occur at rest, especially at night, and eventually the presence of nonhealing wounds, gangrene, and ischemic foot can occur. In cases of severe peripheral neuropathy, patients with diabetes who have CLI frequently present not with pain at rest but rather with foot ulcers, infection, and ultimately gangrene, leading to amputation if perfusion is not restored.

DIAGNOSIS

The evaluation of a patient with PAD relies on meticulous history, physical exam, noninvasive testing, and imaging studies. The physical exam will include visual inspection of both the feet and legs and palpation of peripheral pulses. Vascular insufficiency can be suggested by dependent rubor, pallor on elevation, absence of hair growth, cool dry skin, and dystrophic nails. The interdigital spaces should be examined for the presence of fissures, ulcerations, and infections. Neurological exam (reflexes, sensory, vibratory, and position testing) should be done and any foot deformity also noted. Palpation of bilateral femoral, popliteal, dorsalis pedis, and posterior tibial arteries is mandatory. Pulse assessment has been shown to have a high interobserver variability. In 10% of healthy individuals, the dorsalis pedis pulse can be absent, and in 2%, the posterior tibial is absent.

Although history and physical examination can help establish the diagnosis of PAD, noninvasive evaluation of lower-extremities circulation provides an accurate and reproducible measurement for the detection of PAD and the determination of its severity. The ABI determination is the most commonly performed test and has been suggested by the American Diabetes Association (ADA) as a screening test to be performed in all patients >50 years old with diabetes and patients <50 years old who have other PAD risk factors (smoking, hypertension, hyperlipidemia, or duration of diabetes >10 years). The test has a good reproducibility and small interobserver variability. The ABI is defined as the ratio of the systolic blood pressure in the ankle divided by the systolic blood pressure at the arm. It is measured in supine patients by using manual blood pressure cuffs and a handheld continuous wave Doppler ultrasound device. The higher of the two ankle pressures is divided by the higher brachial artery pressure. In subjects without PAD, the pressure at the ankle usually is 10–15 mmHg higher than the pressure at the arm, resulting in an ABI >1.10. As PAD develops, the ankle pressure decreases and the ABI also decreases. Although cutoff levels are somewhat arbitrary, ABI <0.90 is diagnostic of PAD, with ABI <0.6 usually indicating inadequate perfusion to heal a foot ulcer and ABI <0.4 likely associated with rest pain, gangrene, or ischemic ulcers. In patients with calcified and noncompressible arteries, the ABI might not be accurate, and the values could be elevated falsely; ABI >1.3 or 1.4 are indicative of poorly compressible arteries and should lead to alternative measurements of lower-extremity perfusion. The digital vessels are less prone to calcifications, and in patients with calcifications, the toe-brachial index is more accurate. Toe pressures are obtained by placing cuffs around each toe with a digital flow sensor beyond the cuff; a toe-to-brachial index >0.75 usually is considered normal.

After initial diagnosis of PAD is made with ABI, other noninvasive tests performed in a vascular laboratory would include the segmental pressure and pulse volume recording. The segmental pressure measurements, by placing three or four cuffs at various locations on the leg, help to identify the location of PAD (a drop in pressure >20 mmHg suggests the presence of an obstructive lesion between the two measured segments), while the analysis of the pressure waves (characterized by rapid systolic peak followed by rapid down stroke with a dicrotic notch) can help identify the location where PAD occurs. In patients with exertional pain, a stress test with ABI measurements at rest and after exercise can help identify whether the pain is caused by vascular disease or by nonvascular causes (while normal individuals show no fall in ankle pressure after 5 minutes' walk, patients with PAD experience a fall in ankle pressure with exercise). Measurements of tissue perfusion, such as the transcutaneous oxygen tension ($tcPO_2$), performed by placing probes on the foot and leg and using the chest as a reference site, can be useful to predict the presence of PAD. Such measurements are used most commonly to determine whether revascularization is needed in a limb with

CLI or chronic ulcer. Normal tcPO$_2$ levels are ~60 mmHg; levels <20 mmHg are indicative of severe PAD and need for revascularization to achieve healing.

When it is essential to determine the exact anatomical localization and characterization of the stenosis, for example in patients in whom revascularization is considered, several anatomical studies can be used. Duplex ultrasonography (DUS) is a technique that allows for direct visualization of the artery by using real-time B-mode imaging and color pulsed-wave Doppler ultrasonography. B-mode imaging permits visualization of the arterial wall layers and characterization of atherosclerotic plaques, whereas the pulsed-wave imaging measures flow velocity and detects turbulence in the blood flow. DUS results have been shown to correlate well with angiographic data; it is less accurate in aortoiliac segments because of obesity and bowel gas; and it has limited utility in providing details for the assessment of the more distal and smallest vessels. The gold standard for vascular imaging has long been the intra-arterial digital subtraction angiography (DSA), because of its superior ability to visualize distal small-caliber vessels. Improved technical advances in angiographic equipment and computer processing power have rendered this technique even more accurate, and it also has the unique advantage of permitting the use of catheter-based interventions for the treatment of lower-extremities ischemia at the same time of the imaging study. The disadvantage of this technique is the need for intra-arterial access (risk of bleeding, infections, atheroembolism, vascular access complications) and the infusion of contrast agents with the attendant risk of nephrotoxicity, which especially is of concern in patients with diabetes and underlying renal insufficiency. Two other imaging techniques that have emerged over the past few years are computed tomographic angiography (CTA) and magnetic resonance angiography (MRA). CTA is noninvasive with good spatial resolution, defines the anatomy and presence of stenosis, and provides additional diagnostic information about soft tissue abnormalities such as aneurysms. Moreover, it can be used in the presence of metal clips, stents, and prostheses. The major issues are the requirement for iodinated contrast and the significant amount of ionizing radiation. Contrast-enhanced MRA has the advantage over CTA that images are not obscured by calcium, and it does not require ionizing radiation; however, disadvantages include long acquisition time, inability to be used in patients with contraindications to magnetic resonance imaging, and recently—with the identification of a rare condition known as nephrogenic systemic fibrosis (NSF)—the need to have an estimated glomerular filtration rate >30 ml/minute/1.73 m^2. In current practice, when catheter-based interventions commonly are used, DSA could be the first anatomical study, thus allowing for endovascular treatment at the same time. For patients in whom surgery is the planned therapy, MRA or CTA provide excellent alternatives to DSA. The decision regarding which modality to use first frequently depends on physician preference and local availability and expertise with the given technique.

TREATMENT

Strategies addressing the risk factors for cardiovascular disease (CVD) are an essential component in the treatment of PAD. Smoking is the most significant risk factor for PAD, and smoking cessation should be an important component of the treatment for all patients with PAD. In the UKPDS, treatment of blood pressure was shown to decrease the risk of developing PAD in patients with T2D, and the role of lipid control in the prevention and treatment of CVD is well established. The role of glycemic control in macrovascular disease is more complex, and to date, no randomized trial has demonstrated a reduction in PAD with tight glucose control, although no studies have focused on PAD and the available trials were not powered to detect a difference in PAD. A comprehensive risk reduction approach (combined management of hypertension, hyperlipidemia, and hyperglycemia), such as the one used in the Steno trial, showed a significant reduction in overall cardiovascular events as well as PAD (amputation and lower-extremities revascularization).

The benefits of antiplatelet therapy in patients with PAD have been somewhat controversial. Old recommendations based on a subset analysis of the Antithrombotic Trialists' Collaboration showing a significant benefit of aspirin treatment in patients with PAD have been somewhat tempered by more recent data. The Prevention of Progression of Arterial Disease and Diabetes (POPADAD) trial showed that there was no benefit of aspirin therapy in patients with diabetes on both cardiac disease and PAD, and the Aspirin for Asymptomatic Atherosclerosis (AAA) trial also failed to show any beneficial effect of aspirin in patients with low ABI. Although there are many possible explanations for these two negative studies, the frequent association of PAD with more generalized atherosclerosis makes the use of aspirin in this patient population recommended for most patients. In fact the 2013 ADA clinical guidelines recommend the use of low-dose (75–162 mg) aspirin for primary prevention in patients with diabetes and an increased cardiovascular risk (men >50 and women >60 years old who have at least one additional risk factor, such as hypertension, hyperlipidemia, smoking, albuminuria, or a family history of CVD). Clopidogrel has been shown to reduce the risk of ischemic events in high-risk cardiovascular patients, and in the Clopidogrel versus Aspirin in Patients at Risk of Ischemic Events (CAPRIE) trial, clopidogrel was shown to have an additional benefit as compared with aspirin in such patients. Combination treatment of aspirin plus clopidogrel has not been shown to be superior to either of these agents alone in any randomized trials. On the basis of this evidence, the 2011 guidelines of the American College of Cardiology and American Heart Association recommended the use of antiplatelet therapy (aspirin or clopidogrel) in patients with symptomatic PAD as well as in asymptomatic patients with PAD and an ABI of <0.90 (even though the level of evidence for this latter group is less compelling). The use of anticoagulation therapy with warfarin has not been shown to have any benefit to prevent cardiovascular ischemic events and is potentially harmful secondary to the increased risk of major bleeding episodes.

In patients with symptomatic PAD (intermittent claudication but no CLI), medical therapy is recommended with supervised exercise as the cornerstone and possibly the use of pharmacological agents. Although the precise mechanism of action of exercise regimens remains unclear (no changes in ABI usually are observed after exercise), several clinical trials have demonstrated significant clinical benefits, including an average 150% increase in maximal walking time, pain-free walking, and maximal walking distance, in PAD patients undergoing supervised exercise regimens as compared with usual care. Supervised exercise regimens have been shown to be more effective than available medical therapy for PAD in the few clinical trials available and the recent Claudication: Exercise Versus Endoluminal Revascularization (CLEVER) study showed superior results in terms of treadmill walking performance in patients randomized to an exercise program versus patients randomized to stent revascularization. On the basis of these studies, supervised exercise training has been included in the guidelines of the American College of Cardiology and American Heart Association for the treatment of claudication patients with PAD. Another study also has extended these recommendations for patients with PAD who do not have symptoms: the treadmill exercise group showed significant improvement in exercise performance, whereas the control group showed a decline in a 6-minute walk distance test. The role of unsupervised training is less clear, with the data showing that supervised training is superior, yielding a 150-meter greater improvement in walking distance, possibly related to an improved patient adherence to the exercise regimen in a supervised setting.

Two drugs, both platelet aggregation inhibitors, are currently approved by the U.S. Food and Drug Administration for the medical therapy of intermittent claudication: pentoxifylline and cilostazol. Pentoxifylline is the less efficacious agent, and in a single head-to-head trial, it was no more effective than the placebo arm, whereas the cilostazol patients showed a significant 30% increase in maximal walking distance. Therefore, the use of pentoxifylline is limited to patients who cannot take cilostazol. Of note, the effects of supervised exercise regimens were of a greater magnitude than the effects of cilostazol. Cilostazol is taken 100 mg twice daily and in reduced doses (50 mg twice daily) in patients taking inhibitors of cytochrome P450 isoenzymes CYP2C19 or CYP3A4. This drug is contraindicated (black box warning) in patients with history of congestive heart failure of left-ventricular ejection fraction <40%. Cilostazol appears to be safe, but in a long-term study, >60% of patients stopped taking the medications by 3 years of follow-up, perhaps linked to its modest clinical efficacy. Recently, the results of a randomized clinical trial of the angiotensin-converting enzyme inhibitor ramipril in patients with PAD and intermittent claudication showed 77 and 123% increases in pain-free and maximum walking time as compared with placebo as well as an improvement in clinical symptoms as assessed by a PAD-specific questionnaire. The mechanisms of potential action of ramipril are not completely understood but potentially could include increased peripheral blood flow secondary to vasodilatation induced by reductions in angiotensin II. These changes, if confirmed in other studies, could be of a larger magnitude than those observed after therapy with cilostazol.

Revascularization is indicated in patients with PAD for two major reasons: *1*) intermittent claudication that is not responding to an adequate trial of supervised exercise and pharmacological therapy and that is disabling and *2*) CLI (i.e., pain at rest, nonhealing ulcer, or gangrene). Some patients with isolated iliac artery stenosis can undergo revascularization as a first-line treatment because the success rates for this lesion are great and the incidence of restenosis is low, but usually endovascular or surgical approaches to intermittent claudication are a second line of therapy. Moreover, after revascularization procedures, patients should follow strict cardiovascular risk factor modification and optimal medical therapy to lower the rates of cardiovascular events. For patients with CLI, the goal of revascularization procedures is to restore blood flow to the foot in at least one vessel and therefore permit healing of the lesions and avoid amputation. Two major approaches are available for revascularization in patients with CLI: bypass surgery and endovascular repair with balloon angioplasty, stenting with bare metal or drug-eluting stents. Although in the past bypass surgery was the cornerstone of revascularization and endovascular repair as a first-line therapy only for high-risk elderly patients or for patients who did not have an acceptable venous conduit, in recent years the approach has shifted with more endovascular procedures performed as initial revascularization therapy. The improvements in bypass surgical techniques have allowed low perioperative mortality (~3%) and good limb salvage rates (usually >80% at 5 years' follow-up), with vein graft to tibial or pedal arteries functioning for >5 years in 50–70% of patients. There is, however, significant postoperative morbidity (~20%) and wound complications, leading to prolonged hospitalizations, additional procedures, and discomfort for patients. Most studies have shown the importance of good-quality venous grafts, because the outcomes with prosthetic grafts are inferior. De novo stenosis of the vein conduit can occur in up to 30–40% of patients within the first 2 years after surgery, and therefore close monitoring of these patients is warranted. Data from multiple studies have shown that diabetes is not a risk factor for vein graft failure, but patients with diabetes are at increased risk for long-term mortality and limb loss. Careful attention to patient management perioperatively, including the use of statins and tight glycemic control, has been suggested to decrease perioperative events and complications and possibly to decrease the risk of graft failure and restenosis.

Recent advances in percutaneous revascularization techniques have made these procedures become first-line therapy for several patients with CLI. The reasons include the lower procedural risks as compared with surgery, recent data showing limb salvage rates comparable to the ones obtained with surgery, and the advances in techniques and equipment that have allowed more complex and long-segment occlusions to be treated successfully. Results from several single-center studies have shown that while limb salvage rates are comparable to surgical interventions, restenosis and reinterventions are quite common, with most of these series having been performed in less severe cases than in comparable surgical studies. Moreover, diabetes has been found to predict poorer outcomes after vascular procedures, and the technical success of the procedure does not necessarily correspond to clinical success for the patient. The Bypass versus Angioplasty in Severe Ischaemia of the Leg (BASIL) trial was designed to compare the outcome of bypass surgery versus angioplasty in patients with PAD. The initial short-term report showed that both strategies led to similar short-term outcomes with surgery being more expensive and with a higher morbidity rate. The long-term follow-up (minimum of 3 and maximum of 7 years) showed no differences between the two techniques in terms of overall survival or amputation-free survival; however, for patients who survived at least 2 years after randomization, the surgical approach was associated with a significant increase in overall survival and a trend for improved amputation-free survival. In addition, there was a significant crossover to bypass surgery, and patients who underwent bypass after initial endovascular procedure fared worse than patients who had surgery as the initial option. Therefore, the authors of the BASIL study concluded that bypass surgery with vein conduit offered the best initial approach for patients expected to survive ≥2 years and that angioplasty might be preferred in patients lacking venous conduit. A recent single-center prospective study of surgery versus revascularization showed that the choice of initial revascularization modality did not seem to affect outcomes but that patients with diabetes had worse clinical success and multiple revascularization procedures were needed in several of these patients. The role of new technical advances, such as drug-eluting stents, is not completely clear; recently, three randomized trials of drug-eluting versus bare-metal stents all showed significant higher 1-year patency rates in patients treated with drug-eluting stents.

Therefore, surgical interventions continue to remain the best primary treatment choice for patients with CLI especially in patients with acceptable surgical risk and longer life expectancy; they also frequently are required after failed endovascular interventions.

A multidisciplinary approach, including patients and their primary care physicians, has been demonstrated to help bring down the rates of LEAs in patients with diabetes. Higher screening rates with careful history and physical exams and ABI, aggressive risk reduction management plus supervised physical activity, and careful medical management also will help reduce the risk of CLI. All patients with CLI need a dedicated multidisciplinary team with technical experience taking care of these complex patients. As technological advances become available, more data will be needed to assess their cost-effective implementation in improving limb salvage rates.

BIBLIOGRAPHY

Adler AI, Stevens RJ, Neil A, Stratton IM, Boulton AJM, Holman RR, U.K. Prospective Diabetes Study Group. UKPDS 59: Hyperglycemia and other potentially modifiable risk factors for peripheral vascular disease in type 2 diabetes. *Diabetes Care* 2002;25:894–899.

Ahimastos AA, Walker PJ, Askew C, Leicht A, Pappas E, Blombery P, Reid CM, Golledge J, Kingwell BA. Effect of ramipril on walking times and quality of life among patients with peripheral arterial disease and intermittent claudication. A randomized controlled trial. *JAMA* 2013;309:453–460.

Andersen CA. Noninvasive assessment of lower extremity hemodynamics in individuals with diabetes mellitus. *J Vasc Surg* 2010;52:76S–80S.

American Diabetes Association. Peripheral arterial disease in people with diabetes. *Diabetes Care* 2003;26:3333–3341.

BASIL Trial Participants. Bypass versus Angioplasty in Severe Ischemia of the Leg (BASIL): multicentre, randomized controlled trial. *Lancet* 2005;366:1925–1934.

Belch J, MacCuish A, Campbell I, et al. The prevention of progression of arterial disease and diabetes (POPADAD) trial: factorial randomized placebo controlled trial of aspirin and antioxidants in patients with diabetes and asymptomatic peripheral arterial disease. *BMJ* 2008;337:a1840.

Bradbury AW, Adam DJ, Bell J, Forbes JF, Fowkes GR, Gillespie I, Vaughan Ruckley C, Raan GM. Bypass versus Angioplasty in Severe Ischemia of the Leg (BASIL) trial: an intention to treat analysis of amputation-free and overall survival in patients randomized to a bypass surgery–first or a balloon angioplasty-first revascularization strategy. *J Vasc Surg* 2010;51:5S–17S.

Conte MS. Challenges of distal bypass surgery in patients with diabetes: patient selection, techniques and outcomes. *J Vasc Surg* 2010;52:96S–103S.

Dawson DL, Cutler BS, Hiatt WR, Hobson II RW, Martin JD, Bortey EB, Forbes WP, Strandness DE. A comparison of cilostazol and pentoxifylline for treating intermittent claudication. *Am J Med* 2000;109:523–530.

Dick F, Diehm N, Galimanis A, Husmann M, Schmidli J, Baumgartner I. Surgical or endovascular revascularization in patients with critical limb ischemia: influence of diabetes mellitus on clinical outcome. *J Vasc Surg* 2007;45:751–761.

Fowkes FGR, Price JF, Stewart MCW, Butcher I, Leng GC, Pell ACH, Sandercock PAG, Fox KAA, Lowe, GDO, Murray GD; Aspirin for Asymptomatic Atherosclerosis Trialists. Aspirin for prevention of cardiovascular events in a general population screened for a low ankle brachial index. A randomized controlled trial. *JAMA* 2010;303:841–848.

Gaede P, Lund-Andersen H, Parving HH, Pedersen O. Effect of a multifactorial intervention on mortality in type 2 diabetes. *N Engl J Med* 2008;358:580–591.

Gregg EW, Sorlie P, Paulose-Ram R, Gu Q, Eberhardt MS, Woltz M, Burt L, Curtin L, Engelgau M, Geiss L. Prevalence of lower-extremity disease in the US adult population >40 years of age with and without diabetes. 1999-2000 National Health and Nutrition Examination Survey. *Diabetes Care* 2004;27:1591–1597.

Hamburg NM, Balady GJ. Exercise rehabilitation in peripheral artery disease. Functional impact and mechanisms of benefits. *Circulation* 123:87–97.

Jude EB, Oyibo SO, Chalmers N, Boulton AJM. Peripheral arterial disease in diabetic and nondiabetic patients. A comparison of severity and outcome. *Diabetes Care* 2001;24:1433–1437.

Lau JF, Weinbrg MD, Olin JW. Peripheral artery disease. Part 1: Clinical evaluation and noninvasive diagnosis. *Nat Rev Cardiol* 2011;8:405–418.

Li Y, Rios Burrows N, Gregg EW, Albright A, Geiss LS. Declining rates of hospitalization for nontraumatic lower-extremity amputation in the diabetic population aged 40 years or older: US, 1988-2008. *Diabetes Care* 2012;35:273–277.

Moss SE, Klein R, Klein BEK. The prevalence and incidence of lower extremities amputation in a diabetic population. *Arch Intern Med* 1992;152:610–616.

Murphy TP, Cutlip DE, Regensteiner JG, et al.; for the CLEVER Study Investigators. Supervised exercise versus primary stenting for claudication resulting from aortoiliac peripheral artery disease. Six-month outcome from the Claudication: Exercise Versus Endoluminal Revascularization (CLEVER) Study. *Circulation* 2012;125:130–139.

Rastan A, Tepe G, Krankeberg H, Zahorsky R, Beschorner U, Noory E, Sixt S, Schwarz T, Brechtel K, Bohme C, Neumann FJ, Zeller T. Sirolimus-eluting stents vs. bare-metal stents for treatment of focal lesions in infrapopliteal arteries: a double blind, multi-centre, randomized clinical trial. *Eur Heart J* 2011;32:2274–2281.

2011 Writing Group Members, 2005 Writing Group Members, ACCF/AHA Task Force Members. 2011 ACCF/AHA focused update of the guideline for the management of patients with peripheral artery disease (updating the 2005 guideline). A report of the American College of Cardiology Foundation/American Heart Association task force on practice guidelines. *Circulation* 2011;124:2020–2045.

Chapter 49
Dyslipidemia in Diabetes: Epidemiology, Complications, and Management

CRAIG WILLIAMS, PharmD, FNLA, BCPS
STEVEN HAFFNER, MD

INTRODUCTION

Diabetes is associated with a two- to tenfold increased risk of cardiovascular disease. In addition, patients with diabetes have increased rates of morbidity and mortality after a myocardial infarction (MI). In the general population, the incidences of MI and stroke are similar among older people with diabetes with poor risk factor control and people with preexisting coronary heart disease (CHD). Nevertheless, there is heterogeneity of risk for CHD among people with diabetes. Traditional risk factors such as smoking and hypertension remain important modifiers of CHD risk in this population. The initiation and progression of atherosclerosis in patients with diabetes, however, is driven by lipoprotein retention in the artery wall and the inflammatory response to that retention. Alterations in lipoprotein production and metabolism in patients with diabetes results in dyslipidemia and accelerates the process of atherosclerosis. In the U.K. Prospective Diabetes Study (UKPDS) 23,[1] the baseline predictors of cardiovascular disease in order of entry into a Cox proportional hazards model were as follows: 1) low-density lipoprotein (LDL) cholesterol, 2) high-density lipoprotein (HDL) cholesterol, 3) A1C, 4) systolic blood pressure, and 5) cigarette smoking.

The increased atherogenicity of lipoproteins in patients with diabetes explains the substantial benefit seen in clinical trials of lipid-lowering therapies. Although residual risk for CHD remains in patients with diabetes, an aggressive approach to controlling cholesterol will substantially lower the risk of MI and stroke.

PATHOPHYSIOLOGY AND PRESENTATION

Dyslipidemia refers to changes in multiple lipoproteins that may result from insulin resistance. In the normal hepatocyte, insulin stimulates the production of free fatty acids (FFA) and the degradation of apolipoprotein B100 (apoB). The primary protein constituent of very-low-density lipoprotein (VLDL), intermediate-density lipoprotein, and LDL is apoB. As insulin resistance develops and circulating concentrations of insulin rise, the pathway for FFA production remains insulin sensitive. The increased circulating concentrations of insulin therefore lead to increased hepatic production of FFAs. This occurs simultaneously with an increase in apoB secretion due to the loss of insulin-stimulated intracellular degradation of apoB. These changes, along with the increased secretion of fatty acids from adipo-

 DOI: 10.2337/9781580405096.49

cytes, substantially contribute to the alterations in the lipid profile that are seen in patients with type 2 diabetes (T2D).

Compared with people without diabetes, patients with diabetes or metabolic syndrome present with higher triglyceride (TG) levels, lower HDL cholesterol (HDL-C), and higher apoB but a relatively "normal" LDL cholesterol (LDL-C). On the basis of the observation of relatively normal LDL-C levels but higher TG and lower HDL-C, the focus in the past had been on fibrate and niacin therapy for diabetic dyslipidemia. Indeed, gemfibrozil has been shown to reduce CHD in people with diabetes in the Helsinki Heart Study and the Veterans Affairs High-Density Lipoprotein Cholesterol Intervention Trial, and fenofibrate reduced CHD in the newer Fenofibrate Intervention and Event Lowering in Diabetes (FIELD) trial.[2] Niacin reduced CHD in patients with elevated fasting blood glucose in the 3,908-patient Coronary Drug Project trial. The transition from the view of fibric acid or niacin as initial therapy to the current approach of statin-based LDL lowering as the initial therapy came from analyses of newer trials coupled with an increased understanding of the role of the different lipoproteins in the pathogenesis of diabetic vascular disease.

IMPLICATIONS FOR THERAPY

The lipoprotein changes described previously result in a larger number of smaller, denser LDL particles in the patient with diabetic dyslipidemia. Although TG is elevated and HDL-C is reduced, it is unclear what etiologic role these changes play in the macrovascular disease characterized by T2D. Indeed, patients with type 1 diabetes (T1D) rarely have alterations in TG or HDL-C but still experience accelerated atherosclerosis. Because dyslipidemia is uncommon in T1D, this increased macrovascular risk is thought to derive primarily from increased susceptibility of the diabetic arterial wall to circulating lipoproteins. The observation that macrovascular disease is accelerated in patients with diabetes but without dyslipidemia raised early questions regarding TG and HDL-C as clinical targets. Follow-up trials have supported this skepticism. In the 15,067-patient ILLUMI-NATE trial, which tested raising HDL-C with an inhibitor of the cholesteryl ester transfer protein, an increase was seen in the combined endpoint of nonfatal MI and cardiovascular death by 20%. In that trial, 45% of participants had diabetes at baseline. More recent work with HDL has highlighted that the functioning of this lipoprotein is more important than just the concentration of cholesterol carried by these particles (i.e., HDL-C). Thus, some individual patients with relatively low HDL-C values but high particle function may be relatively protected from atherosclerosis compared with other individuals with higher HDL-C values but poorer particle function. Tests for HDL particle function currently are available only in a research setting and future commercial use of such testing will depend on the development of effective HDL therapies.

Conversely, analyses of LDL-C–lowering trials have revealed a disproportionately greater benefit from LDL-C lowering in patients with diabetes (Table 49.1). Additionally, high-risk patients with diabetes (e.g., longer duration of diabetes, preexisting cardiovascular disease, older age) and patients with more severe dyslipidemia (higher TG and lower HDL-C) have greater benefit from an LDL-C lowering compared with low-risk patients with diabetes (Table 49.1).

Table 49.1 Reduction in 10-Year Risk of Major Cardiovascular Disease Endpoints (CHD Death/Nonfatal Myocardial Infarction) in Major Statin Trials, or Substudies of Major Trials, in Patients with Diabetes (*n* = 16,032)

Study	CVD prevention	Statin dose and comparator	Risk reduction (%)	Relative risk reduction (%)	Absolute risk reduction (%)	LDL-C reduction
4S-DM	2°	Simvastatin 20–40 mg vs. placebo	85.7 to 43.2	50	42.5	186 to 119 mg/dl (36%)
ASPEN 2	2°	Atorvastatin 10 mg vs. placebo	39.5 to 24.5	34	12.7	112 to 79 mg/dl (29%)
HPS-DM	2°	Simvastatin 40 mg vs. placebo	43.8 to 36.3	17	7.5	123 to 84 mg/dl (31%)
CARE-DM	2°	Pravastatin 40 mg vs. placebo	40.8 to 35.4	13	5.4	136 to 99 mg/dl (27%)
TNT-DM	2°	Atorvastatin 80 mg vs. 10 mg	26.3 to 21.6	18	4.7	99 to 77 mg/dl (22%)
HPS-DM	1°	Simvastatin 40 mg vs. placebo	17.5 to 11.5	34	6.0	124 to 86 mg/dl (31%)
CARDS	1°	Atorvastatin 10 mg vs. placebo	11.5 to 7.5	35	4	118 to 71 mg/dl (40%)
ASPEN	1°	Atorvastatin 10 mg vs. placebo	9.8 to 7.9	19	1.9	114 to 80 mg/dl (30%)
ASCOT-DM	1°	Atorvastatin 10 mg vs. placebo	11.1 to 10.2	8	0.9	125 to 82 mg/dl (34%)

Note: 1°, primary prevention; 2°, secondary prevention. Studies were of differing lengths (3.3–5.4 years) and used somewhat different endpoints, but all reported similar outcomes (rates of cardiovascular disease death and nonfatal MI). In this tabulation, results of the statin on 10-year risk of major cardiovascular disease outcomes (CHD death/nonfatal MI) are listed for comparison among studies. Correlation between 10-year cardiovascular disease risk of the control group and the absolute risk reduction with statin therapy is highly significant (*P* = 0.0007).

Trials not defined in text: ASPEN (Atorvastatin Study for Prevention of Coronary Heart Disease Endpoints in Non-insulin Dependent Diabetes Mellitus); CARE (Cholesterol And Reduction of Events trial); CARDS (Collaborative Atorvastatin Diabetes Study); ASCOT (Anglo-Scandinavian Cardiac Outcomes Trial).

Source: Analyses provided by Craig Williams, PharmD, Oregon Health & Science University, 2007. From American Diabetes Association. Standards of medical care in diabetes—2014. *Diabetes Care* 2014;37(Suppl 1):S14–S80.

In further support of a clinical approach that favors lowering LDL-C first was the finding in the FIELD trial of a substantially greater benefit of statins as compared with fenofibrate to reduce CHD endpoints in patients with diabetes.[2] FIELD was designed as a placebo-controlled study of fenofibrate in 9,795 patients with diabetes. Because the trial design allowed for use of nonstudy lipid-lowering therapy, there was a relatively high rate of statin drop-in (nearly 40% of placebo patients by study completion). Because fenofibrate modestly lowers LDL-C (12% in trial), there was a lower drop-in rate of statin usage in the patients randomized to fenofibrate (~20%). Although this difference in the use of statins complicated the analysis of the trial, it allowed the authors to analyze outcomes for patients receiving statin therapy compared with fenofibrate. It subsequently was reported that fenofibrate lowered CHD events by 19% compared with a 49% reduction for statins.

This finding from FIELD,[2] along with the LDL-C–lowering trials, complements the understanding of atherosclerosis as a disease of apoB lipoprotein retention and inflammation in the vascular wall. Although TG-rich VLDL remnant lipoproteins are elevated in diabetes and do contribute to atherosclerosis, the increased LDL particle count and mildly elevated LDL-C in diabetic dyslipidemia remains the proven target of pharmacological therapy. Whether additional LDL-C lowering with nonstatin agents will be helpful is being tested with ezetimibe in the ongoing IMPROVE-IT (IMproved Reduction of Outcomes: Vytorin Efficacy International Trial).

MANAGEMENT

CURRENT AMERICAN DIABETES ASSOCIATION AND NATIONAL CHOLESTEROL EDUCATION PROGRAM GUIDELINES WITH THE AMERICAN COLLEGE OF CARDIOLOGY AND THE AMERICAN HEART ASSOCIATION UPDATE

New guidelines for cholesterol management were released in late 2013 by the American College of Cardiology and the American Heart Association (ACC/AHA).[3] These guidelines were coauthored by many of the individuals involved with the National Cholesterol Education Program (NCEP) III guidelines, and they replace what would have been the NCEP IV guidelines.[4] These new guidelines are strictly evidence based and rely heavily on updated meta-analyses of the randomized clinical trials. Similar to the older NCEP guidelines as well as the current American Diabetes Association (ADA) guidelines,[5] the new ACC/AHA guidelines[3] give both primary and secondary goals for therapy in patients with diabetes.

Along with the ADA guidelines,[5] the ACC/AHA guidelines[3] focus primarily on statin therapy for patients with diabetes. There are notable differences, however, in the use of LDL-C as a therapeutic target (Table 49.2). Although the ADA guidelines retain LDL-C goals for patients, the new ACC/AHA guidelines[3] do not.

In the NCEP III guidelines,[4] LDL-C targets are emphasized, and although statins are the preferred agents for LDL-C lowering, combination therapy remains an option. Both the ADA guidelines[5] and ACC/AHA guidelines[3] emphasize that combination therapy remains largely untested. But an LDL-C–guided approach that

Table 49.2 Primary Goal and Priorities of Treatment from NCEP and ADA Guidelines

ADA

Primary goal (dyslipidemia/lipid management): Lifestyle modification focusing on the reduction of saturated fat, trans fat, and cholesterol intake; and increased physical activity for all patients with diabetes and prediabetes. Statin-based therapy should be added to lifestyle therapy for *1)* all patients with diabetes and with CVD or *2)* those with diabetes age >40 years with one additional cardiac risk factor.*

First priority: Statins for all high-risk patients with diabetes with an absolute LDL-C goal <100 mg/dl in patients without CVD and <70 mg/dl in patients with diabetes who have CVD.

Second priority: Relative LDL-C reduction ~40% if absolute LDL-C goals cannot be achieved due to high baseline LDL-C or poor response to therapy. Note that combination therapy to target HDL-C or TG is actively discouraged.

NCEP III

Primary goal: Lifestyle modification for all patients with diabetes and metabolic syndrome. LDL-C–lowering therapy, with statin-based regimen for all patients with diabetes aged >20 years.

First priority: Achieve absolute LDL-C <100 mg/dl in all patients with diabetes and <70 mg/dl in patients with diabetes who have CVD.

Second priority: After LDL-C goal is reached, consider intensification of pharmacotherapy† in patients with TG >200 mg/dl to reach a non-HDL-C goal (total cholesterol minus HDL-C), which is 30 mg/dl above the LDL-C goal (e.g., if LDL-C goal is <70 mg/dl, then non-HDL-C goal is <100 mg/dl).

ACC/AHA

Primary goal: Statin therapy for all patients with diabetes >40 years old.

First priority: Moderate-intensity statin to lower LDL-C by at least 30% from baseline.

Second priority: High-intensity statin to lower LDL-C by 50% from baseline for patients with diabetes and an estimated 10-year risk of atherosclerotic vascular events of >7.5%.

Note: CVD = cardiovascular disease; HDL = high-density lipoprotein; LDL = low-density lipoprotein.

*Risks include *1)* cigarette smoking, *2)* hypertension (blood pressure ≥140/90 mmHg), *3)* family history of premature cardiovascular disease (primary cardiac event in first-degree male relative <55 years of age or first-degree female relative <65 years of age), and *4)* age (men age ≥45 years, women age ≥55 years).

†Intensification of pharmacotherapy can include fibrate or niacin therapy or greater LDL-C lowering to reach non-HDL-C goal.

Sources: Data from Grundy SM, Cleeman JI, Merz CN, Brewer HB Jr, Clark LT, Hunninghake DB, Pasternak RC, Smith SC Jr, Stone NJ; National Heart, Lung, and Blood Institute; American College of Cardiology Foundation; American Heart Association. Implications of recent clinical trials for the National Cholesterol Education Program Adult Treatment Panel III Guidelines. *Circulation* 2004;110:227–239; American Diabetes Association. Standards of medical care in diabetes—2014. *Diabetes Care* 2004;37(Suppl 1):S14–S80.

NCEP has long endorsed remains a favored strategy by many clinicians when treating patients with diabetes. Understanding both the historic approach of an LDL-C–guided strategy as well as the reason for the changes in the new guidelines is imperative for the clinician who manages patients with diabetes.

The use of LDL-C as a surrogate goal in diabetes initially was based on observational data from the UKPDS[1] and now generally is supported by the newer trial data that have been discussed. The data for clinical outcomes, however, are derived largely from fixed-dose studies of statins with post hoc analyses that extrapolated the effects of different achieved LDL-C goals.

The choice to not target specific LDL-C levels in the ACC/AHA guidelines[3] is due to the fact that there have not been adequate studies that used a strategy of titrating to an LDL-C goal to justify any particular clinical target. Therefore, the ACC/AHA committee felt that an evidence-based recommendation could not be given for LDL-C goal-targeted therapy in patients with or without diabetes. The decision to remove LDL-C targets, however, remains controversial.

Despite this significant change in the ACC/AHA guidelines,[3] all three guidelines remain similar in many ways. They all focus on statin therapy and LDL-C, and this remains an appropriate approach in the patient with diabetes. Although the older NCEP guidelines[4] are less prescriptive regarding the agent or combination of agents used to achieve that goal, this generally is due to the fact that these guidelines predate much of the newer trial evidence that examined combination therapy.

A reasonable approach to incorporating all three current guidelines into clinical practice is to recognize that each one has both secondary as well as primary goals. To meet both goals for patients with diabetes means using a similar treatment strategy.

The secondary goals of the older NCEP guidelines[4] focus on subjects with an elevated TG level >200 mg/dl after meeting their LDL-C goals. These guidelines use non-HDL-C (total cholesterol minus HDL-C) as the secondary target. The non-HDL-C goal is always 30 mg/dl above the LDL-C goal. Although non-HDL-C can be lowered by either lowering LDL-C further or by raising HDL-C, the more evidence-based approach is to further lower LDL-C. The most evidence-based way to further lower LDL-C in patients with diabetes is to use higher doses of more potent statins. Thus, optimizing the use of statins is the best way to meet the goals of both the older NCEP guidelines and the newer ACC/AHA guidelines.[3,4]

The secondary goals of the ADA guidelines[5] also align well with the newer ACC/AHA recommendations in patients with diabetes. The ADA guidelines state that although TG <150 mg/dl and HDL-C >40 mg/dl (>50 mg/dl in women) is desirable, the only lipoprotein target for pharmacological therapy is LDL. Rather than focus on establishing a secondary lipoprotein goal, the ADA guidelines discuss reducing LDL-C ~40% if the absolute goals cannot be achieved. They actively discourage the use of niacin or fibrates to target HDL-C or TG. This approach results in first optimizing the statin therapy in clinical practice and therefore is similar to the new ACC/AHA guideline.[3]

The secondary goal of the new ACC/AHA guidelines is different.[3] It calls for use of high-intensity statin therapy to achieve an LDL-C reduction of at least 50% in diabetes patients who are higher risk (10-year risk of a major vascular event of >7.5%). The data for this secondary goal are extrapolated from data in patients without diabetes, however, and the therapies that are recommended as high intensity (atorvastatin 40 and 80 mg and rosuvastatin 20 and 40 mg) have little randomized trial data to support their use in patients with diabetes.

Considering the recommendations of all three guidelines and the evidence base for those recommendations, it is reasonable in patients with diabetes to follow the ADA-recommended approach of using a statin to lower LDL-C by ~40% from the pretreated baseline value. It also is reasonable based on the design of the trials and the meta-analysis conducted by the ACC/AHA to adopt the monitoring approach that is recommended by that guideline. In essence, because there are limited data to suggest what absolute value of LDL-C should be achieved in patients with diabetes, providers should focus instead on using a statin regimen that is well tolerated by the patient and that lowers LDL-C by ~40%. All reasonable effort should be made to ensure compliance with this regimen. Although many different statins and doses can be used to achieve this degree of LDL-C lowering, several agents are given in doses that do not routinely achieve this degree of lowering and should be avoided. Among these are simvastatin 10 mg, pravastatin 10 and 20 mg, lovastatin 20 mg, and all doses of fluvastatin except 80 mg. Patients taking any of these doses of the respective statin should be titrated to higher doses or onto a more potent statin unless those regimens are not tolerated. Multiple statins should be tried before alternative LDL-C–lowering agents are used.

Although the new ACC/AHA guidelines[3] have moved away from recommending absolute LDL-C targets for individual patients, it should be noted that the ADA guidelines[5] have retained LDL-C targets. Specifically, the ADA still endorses the approach of NCEP in recommending that most patients with diabetes should have an LDL-C <100 mg/dl and patients with diabetes and CHD should have an LDL-C <70 mg/dl if possible. Patients who have diabetes and established CVD experience particularly high rates of recurrent CVD events. In the subanalysis of patients with diabetes in the Scandinavian Simvastatin Survival Study (4S; a study with high baseline LDL-C), the patients who received placebo had a projected 10-year Framingham CHD event rate of nearly 90% (Table 49.1).

Statin therapy in patients with diabetes and CHD should be initiated irrespective of baseline LDL-C, with a goal of lowering LDL-C by ~40% from pretreatment values. A secondary goal of an LDL-C <70 mg/dl remains reasonable. There is a broader range of options for patients with diabetes but without CHD if baseline LDL-C is not elevated. In the NCEP guidelines,[4] if LDL-C in these patients is already <100 mg/dl, then additional lowering is optional. This is now outdated. The ADA guidelines[5] on this topic are similar to the new ACC/AHA guidelines[3] and are more aggressive. This position was informed greatly by the findings of the Heart Protection Study (HPS) from 2002.[6]

In the HPS,[6] the 5,963 patients with diabetes benefited from LDL-C lowering with 40 mg simvastatin regardless of baseline LDL-C. Patients with baseline LDL-C <100 mg/dl (and even <80 mg/dl) experienced similar relative reductions in CHD events as patients with elevated baseline LDL-C. A degree of caution is warranted in applying these findings to primary prevention in patients with diabetes because 50% of the patients with diabetes in HPS had CHD at study entry. On post hoc analysis, however, the patients with diabetes and without baseline CHD experienced a similar absolute risk reduction in CHD events compared with the patients with diabetes and with baseline CHD. This finding underlies the recommendation from both the ADA and the new ACC/AHA guidelines[3] that statin-based LDL-C lowering should be added to lifestyle therapy for any patient with diabetes >40 years old irrespective of baseline LDL-C. An updated meta-analysis from the Cholesterol Treatment Trialists[7] included 32,210 subjects with diabetes and supports this recommendation. The analysis, which included 26 clinical trials with statin-based therapy, found that more intensive lowering of LDL-C was associated with more CHD benefit compared with less intensive LDL-C lowering. The relative risk reduction was 25% for patients with T1D and 18% for patients with T2D, both of which were highly significant.

COMBINATION THERAPY

The definitive finding that more statin-based LDL-C lowering reduced CHD events in patients with diabetes compared with less-intense LDL-C lowering raised new questions about the role of combination lipid therapies in patients with diabetes. Combination therapy can be targeted to either further lower LDL-C with agents like ezetimibe or bile acid sequestrants or to raise HDL-C and lower TG with agents like niacin and fibrates. In 2005, an analysis of the FIELD trial[2] suggested that fibrate therapy likely offers little additional benefit in patients with diabetes who already are taking a statin. In 2009, the recommendations of the ADA moved further away from HDL-C and TG as therapeutic targets in favor of a greater focus on more intensive LDL-C goals. This was due to a lack of clinical trial support for combination therapy and the increased recognition that small, dense LDL is the primary atherosclerotic lipoprotein in patients with diabetes. In 2013, the recommendations changed again to actively discourage the use of combination therapy primarily because of two clinical trials.

In 2010, the Action to Control Cardiovascular Risk in Diabetes (ACCORD) trial[8] found no additional CHD benefit of adding fenofibrate to simvastatin in patients with T2D, and in 2011 the AIM-HIGH[9] (Atherothrombosis Intervention in Metabolic Syndrome with Low HDL/High Triglyceride: Impact on Global Health Outcomes) trial found no additional CHD benefit from adding niacin to an LDL-C–lowering regimen composed of simvastatin and ezetimibe. The findings of both trials were unexpected. Of note, in ACCORD, LDL-C was lowered an additional 10% by fenofibrate, but this result was similar to the 10% reduction in LDL-C seen in the placebo group that continued on their statin therapy. Compared with the placebo (statin-only) group, fenofibrate raised HDL-C by 2% and lowered TG by 15%.

Traditionally, providers have been concerned about the use of combination therapy because of the increased risk of myositis and rhabdomyolysis. The risk, however, of rhabdomyolysis with nicotinic acid in combination with statins is very low. The risk with the fibrates is higher and was highlighted by the increased mortality seen in subjects on gemfibrozil and cervistatin (Baycol) before cerivastatin was removed from the worldwide market. Because of differences in metabolism, the risk of combination therapy is higher when gemfibrozil is added to a statin compared with other fibrates. A component of the risk of statin plus fibrate is pharmacodynamic, however, and is unrelated to kinetics and metabolism. Therefore, any fibrate added to any statin carries a greater risk of rhabdomyolysis compared with statin monotherapy. Of note, fibrate monotherapy causes rhabdomyolysis about six times as commonly as statin monotherapy. Other clinical factors that increase risk and should be considered before this combination is used include renal dysfunction and hypothyroidism. Additional concerns with nicotinic acid relate to its possible effect on insulin resistance and increasing glucose intolerance. Older studies have suggested marked rises in A1C in subjects treated with 4 g/day nicotinic acid. More recent studies with smaller doses of nicotinic acid and careful attention to monitoring glycemic control have shown much smaller effects on A1C. Additionally, a reanalysis of the original Lipid Research Clinics study found that the benefit of niacin actually was greater in patients with an elevated fasting glucose at baseline. Therefore, it is likely that patients with diabetes or impaired fasting glucose derive disproportionately greater CHD benefit from niacin, despite a small worsening of glycemic control in some individuals.

APPROACH TO PATIENTS WITH PREDIABETES

The term "prediabetes" refers to abnormalities in glucose handling which result in glycemic values that are between normal and overt diabetes. Most prediabetes is due to peripheral insulin resistance, and many of these patients will exhibit other metabolic characteristics as a result of that insulin resistance. The co-occurrence of several of these characteristics has been termed "metabolic syndrome." According to the National Health and Nutrition Examination Survey data set, there are ~60% more patients in the U.S. with metabolic syndrome than with diabetes. Although there has been some controversy surrounding the term "metabolic syndrome," it remains a useful way to describe the clustering of cardiovascular risk factors (hypertension, glucose intolerance, and dyslipidemia) that often accompany obesity. Many patients who are medically obese (BMI >30 kg/m^2), however, do not have the metabolic syndrome. This individual discordance, despite the strong population association, underlies the ongoing controversy regarding the appropriate clinical use of the term. Notably, in 2007, the World Health Organization declined to recognize the metabolic syndrome as a distinct clinical entity in their 10th revision of the *International Classification of Diseases* manual, despite offering criteria for its definition in 1999. Despite this, and despite the controversy, the term "metabolic syndrome" does provide a meaningful context for both the clinician and the patient regarding the global cardiometabolic risk that often is found in people who are obese both with or without diabetes.

The NCEP Adult Treatment Panel (ATP)[10] defines the metabolic syndrome as the presence of three of five risk factors, including waist circumference, high TG, low HDL-C, hypertension, and a fasting glucose ≥110 mg/dl (Table 49.3). The prevalence of the metabolic syndrome in patients with T2D has been examined in several populations and appears to be ~80%. Although it is possible that the remaining patients with diabetes and without the metabolic syndrome are at lower risk of CHD, this aspect requires further study, and the substantial risk of CHD in T1D is a reminder that obesity does not have to be present for diabetes to pose a substantial CHD risk. The CHD risk of T1D was recently and nicely reviewed by Retnakaran et al.[11]

The NCEP nicely discusses that the primary therapy for metabolic syndrome is behavioral (i.e., weight loss and increased physical activity). As shown by Jensen

Table 49.3 CEP ATP III: The Metabolic Syndrome

Risk factor*	Defining level
Abdominal obesity (waist circumference)	
Men	>102 cm (>40 inches)
Women	>88 cm (>35 inches)
Triglycerides	≥150 mg/dl
HDL cholesterol	
Men	<40 mg/dl
Women	<50 mg/dl
Blood pressure	≥130/85 mmHg
Fasting glucose	≥110 mg/dl

Note: *Diagnosis of the metabolic syndrome is established when three or more of these risk factors are present.

Source: From the Expert Panel on Detection, Evaluation, and Treatment of High Blood Cholesterol in Adults. Executive summary of the third report of the National Cholesterol Education Program (NCEP) Expert Panel on Detection, Evaluation and Treatment of High Blood Cholesterol in Adults (Adult Treatment Panel III). *JAMA* 2001;285:2486–2497. Reprinted with permission from the publisher.

et al.,[12] obesity carries increased CHD risk independent of other lifestyle factors, including poor diet and smoking. Although aggressive targeting of lipids in obese patients without the metabolic syndrome currently is not advocated, the risk of CHD clearly is elevated in people without diabetes but with metabolic syndrome. Although the ADA *Standards of Medical Care*[5] has recommendations for the treatment of impaired glucose tolerance (IGT) to prevent diabetes, it does not use the term "metabolic syndrome" or discuss pharmacological interventions for CHD risk reduction in patients with IGT. In 2007 the ADA, in association with the American College of Cardiology (ACC),[13] convened a consensus development conference to address lipoprotein management in patients with insulin resistance and multiple cardiometabolic risk factors (hyperglycemia, dyslipidemia, and hypertension). Although the term "metabolic syndrome" is not used in the document, the population being discussed is the same. The resulting consensus statement, published in 2008, appropriately reiterates LDL as the primary lipoprotein driving the development of atherosclerosis in this insulin-resistant population. The treatment targets are less clear-cut.

Consistent with the NCEP update from 2004,[10] the statement calls for a goal LDL-C <70 mg/dl in patients with diabetes who have CHD. In those patients with cardiometabolic risk factors but without diabetes, however, they call for an LDL-C goal of <100 mg/dl as long as two out of the three following risk factors are present: smoking, hypertension, or early family history of CHD (Table 49.4). This approach to high-risk patients with the metabolic syndrome remains reasonable and is expected to be addressed in the next update of the NCEP guidelines.[10]

Table 49.4 Suggested Treatment Goals in Patients with Cardiometabolic Risk Factors and Lipoprotein Abnormalities

	LDL-C (mg/dl)	Goals Non-HDL-C (mg/dl)	apoB (mg/dl)
Highest-risk patients, including those with 1) known CVD or 2) diabetes plus one or more additional major CVD risk factor	<70	<100	<80
High-risk patients, including those with 1) no diabetes or known clinical CVD but two or more additional major CVD risk factors or 2) diabetes but no other major CVD risk factors	<100	<130	<90

Note: Other major risk factors (beyond dyslipoproteinemia) include smoking, hypertension, and family history of premature CHD.

ALTERNATIVE LIPOPROTEIN TARGETS

Although TG and HDL-C are inappropriate targets for pharmacotherapy, debate continues in regard to apoB. The 2008 ADA consensus statement on cardiometabolic risk identified apoB as a therapeutic target along with LDL-C and non-HDL-C (Table 49.4). Although apoB makes sense as a potential goal of therapy in patients with diabetes or the metabolic syndrome, it has yet to be used as a primary treatment target in a large outcomes trial. When the available outcomes studies with LDL-C–lowering therapy are examined post hoc, the results for the predictability of apoB compared with LDL-C and non-HD-C are mixed. The largest of those analyses, by Kastelein et al.,[14] analyzed the Incremental Decrease in End Points through Aggressive Lipid Lowering (IDEAL) and Treat to New Targets (TNT) trials together for a total of 18,889 patients and concluded that non-HDL-C and apoB were similarly predictive for CHD event reduction. Approximately 15% of the patients in those trials had diabetes, with an unknown but certainly higher percentage having the metabolic syndrome.

The larger issue with using apoB as a secondary target is the question of what to do with the patient who is at their LDL-C goal but not at their apoB goal. Although an elevated apoB could offer the opportunity to reinforce lifestyle counseling, the questions surrounding the role of combination lipid therapy that were discussed leave open the question of what therapeutic approach to take to lower apoB when LDL-C is already appropriately at goal. It is not clear how often apoB would be found to be elevated if patients with diabetes are strictly complying with the newer LDL-C goals of <70 and <100 mg/dl. Unpublished data suggest that number to be ~1 in 20 in patients with an LDL-C goal of <70 mg/dl.

Because of these unanswered questions about apoB and the established role of LDL-C in patients with metabolic syndrome and diabetes, the goals outlined in the ADA/ACC consensus statement[13] for LDL-C and non-HDL-C should be followed while we await further outcomes for combination therapy before adopting apoB as a routine secondary target in general practice.

CONCLUSION

People with T2D have a marked increase in CHD. For establishing cholesterol treatment goals, both the ADA and the new ACC/AHA guidelines[3] focus on the use of statin therapy. Although the ADA retains LDL-C treatment goals similar to the older NCEP ATP III guidelines,[10] it emphasizes that clinical trial data to support combination therapy is lacking. In this way, the ADA guidelines are similar to the newer ACC/AHA guidelines in primarily recommending statin therapy with a minimum reduction of LDL-C of ~40%. Although both the NCEP III[10] and ADA still recommend a goal LDL-C of <100 mg/dl, with a goal of <70 mg/dl in patients with diabetes who have CHD, this should now be considered a secondary goal and the emphasis in practice should be on the use of appropriate doses of statins to lower LDL-C by 30–50%. Secondary goal targeting in the NCEP guidelines also recommends lowering non-HDL-C in subjects who have a TG level >200 mg/dl to a goal that is 30 mg/dl above the LDL goal. Although the addition of LDL-C–lowering agents to statin therapy is still acceptable when necessary, it has yet to be proven in clinical trials. The combination of niacin or fibrates to target TG or HDL-C should be avoided in patients who are at LDL-C targets on a statin-based therapy. These differences are relatively minor, and the clear message from both organizations is for aggressive LDL-C lowering in patients with diabetes. Recent attention on the metabolic syndrome is appropriate, given the worldwide epidemic of obesity and CHD. Although the focus of therapy remains behavior and lifestyle intervention, pharmacological therapy should be used achieve the target values of specific risk factors. Because these patients have multiple risk factors for CHD by definition, an LDL-C goal of <100 mg/dl is appropriate in these patients as well.

REFERENCES

1. Turner RC, Millns H, Neil HA, Stratton IM, Manley SE, Matthews DR, Holman RR. Risk factors for coronary artery disease in non-insulin-dependent diabetes mellitus (UKPDS 23). *BMJ* 1998;316:823–828.

2. Keech A, Simes RJ, Barter P, Best J, Scott R, Taskinen MR, Forder P, Pillai A, Davis T, Glasziou P, Drury P, Kesäniemi YA, Sullivan D, Hunt D, Colman P, d'Emden M, Whiting M, Ehnholm C, Laakso M; FIELD study investigators. Effects of long-term fenofibrate therapy on cardiovascular events in 9795 people with type 2 diabetes mellitus (the FIELD study): randomized controlled trial. *Lancet* 2005;366:1849–1861.

3. ACC/AHA Guideline on the Treatment of Blood Cholesterol to Reduce Atherosclerotic Cardiovascular Risk in Adults. A report of the American Col-

lege of Cardiology/American Heart Association Task Force on practice guidelines. Published online ahead of print, 12 November 2013.

4. Expert Panel on Detection, Evaluation and Treatment of High Blood Cholesterol in Adults. Executive summary of the third report of the National Cholesterol Education Program (NCEP) Expert Panel on Detection, Evaluation and Treatment of High Blood Cholesterol in Adults (Adult Treatment Panel III). *JAMA* 2001;285:2486–2497.

5. American Diabetes Association. Standards of medical care in diabetes—2014. *Diabetes Care* 2014;37(Suppl 1):S14–S80.

6. Heart Protection Study Collaborative Group (HPS). MRC/BHF Heart Protection Study of cholesterol-lowering with simvastatin in 5963 people with diabetes: a randomized placebo-controlled trial. *Lancet* 2003;361:2005–2016.

7. Cholesterol Treatment Trialists' (CTT) Collaboration. Efficacy and safety of more intensive lowering of LDLc: a meta-analysis of data from 170,000 participants in 26 randomized trials. *Lancet* 2010;376:1670–1681.

8. Action to Control Cardiovascular Risk in Diabetes (ACCORD) Study Group. Effects of combination lipid therapy in type 2 diabetes mellitus. *N Engl J Med* 2010;362:1563–1574.

9. AIM-HIGH Investigators. Niacin in patients with low HDL cholesterol levels receiving intensive statin therapy. *N Engl J Med* 2011;365:2255–2267.

10. Grundy SM, Cleeman JI, Merz CN, Brewer HB Jr, Clark LT, Hunninghake DB, Pasternak RC, Smith SC Jr, Stone NJ; National Heart, Lung, and Blood Institute; American College of Cardiology Foundation; American Heart Association. Implications of recent clinical trials for the National Cholesterol Education Program Adult Treatment Panel III Guidelines. *Circulation* 2004;110:227–239.

11. Retnakaran R, Zinman B. Type 1 diabetes, hyperglycemia and the heart. *Lancet* 2008;371:1790–1799.

12. Jensen MK, Chiuve SE, Rimm EB, Dethlesfsen C, Tjonneland A, Joensen AM, Overvad K. Obesity, behavioral lifestyle factors, and risk of acute coronary events. *Circulation* 2008;117:3062–3069.

13. American Diabetes Association/American College of Cardiology. Foundation Consensus Statement: lipoprotein management in patients with cardiometabolic risk. *Diabetes Care* 2008;31:811–822.

14. Kastelein JJ, van der Steeg WA, Holme I, Gaffney M, Cater NB, Barter P, Deedwania P, Olsson AG, Boekholdt SM, Demicco DA, Szarek M, LaRosa JC, Pedersen TR, Grundy SM; TNT Study Group; IDEAL Study Group. Lipids, apolipoproteins, and their ratios in relation to cardiovascular events with statin treatment. *Circulation* 2008;117:3002–3009.

Chapter 50
Hypertension in Diabetes

Jorge Calles-Escandón, MD
Thomas A. Murphy, MD
Georges Saab, MD
Tariq Khan, MD

INTRODUCTION AND BACKGROUND

Hypertension, independent of any other risk factors,[1,2] is causative of both macro- and microvascular disease and is one of the main etiologies of renal failure and cardiovascular events (acute myocardial infarction, stroke, peripheral vascular disease, congestive heart failure). Treatment of hypertension is effective in decreasing these outcomes,[3] independent of specific medications and irrespective of renal disease.[4,5] Control of hypertension is particularly important in patients with diabetes, both to prevent cardiovascular disease and to minimize progression of renal and eye complications.[6] Moreover, a wide array of medications are now available that allow physicians and patients to attain blood pressure (BP) targets. It is therefore imperative that physicians treating patients with diabetes become familiar with the diagnosis and treatment of hypertension in their patients.

DEFINITION OF HYPERTENSION

This chapter uses the definitions suggested by the Eighth Report of the Joint National Committee (JNC 8) based on the average of properly measured BP at two or more visits (Table 50.1).[7]

Isolated systolic hypertension is considered to be present when BP is ≥140/<90 mmHg and isolated diastolic hypertension is considered to be present when BP is <140/≥90 mmHg.

These definitions apply to adults who are not taking antihypertensive medications and who are not acutely ill. If there is a disparity in category between the systolic and diastolic pressures, the higher value determines the severity of the

Table 50.1 Blood Pressure Targets

Category	Systolic BP (mmHg, Sys)	Diastolic BP (mmHg, Dias)
Normal	<120	<80
Prehypertension	129–130	80–89
Hypertension stage 1	140–159	90–99
Hypertension stage 2	≥160	≥100

DOI: 10.2337/9781580405096.50

hypertension. Similar but not identical definitions were suggested in the 2007 European Societies of Hypertension and Cardiology guidelines for the management of arterial hypertension.[8]

We want to emphasize the importance of properly measuring BP in the office setting. Unfortunately, current trends in medical practice have imposed serious limitations to the time available for measurement of BP. Physicians, however, must strive to create systems to properly accommodate this simple measurement, which has profound implications for the prevention of vascular outcomes in patients with diabetes. Patients should ideally rest for 5 minutes before measuring BP; subsequently, the arm should be positioned so that the cuff is at the level of the right atrium, the legs should not be crossed, and the measuring cuff should be in direct contact with the skin.

CLINICAL EPIDEMIOLOGY

The most comprehensive report examining the clinical epidemiology of hypertension in diabetes is the National Health and Nutrition Examination Survey (NHANES). Using the NHANES surveys from the periods 1988–1994, 1999–2004, and 2005–2008, the prevalent hypertension, defined as proposed by the JNC 7[9] or by self-reported hypertension treatment, increased from 51 to 66% ($P < 0.001$). The rates in patients with diabetes are higher than those observed in the general population of ~29%. The already increased cardiovascular risk of the patient with diabetes is increased further by the presence of hypertension.[10] The recently recognized twin epidemics of obesity and type 2 diabetes (T2D) in adults,[11] which also are affecting adolescents and children, more likely will have a negative impact on the prevalence of hypertension in future decades, and it heralds an increase in cardiovascular morbidity and mortality.[12]

Although hypertension is a common problem in patients with type 1 diabetes (T1D) and T2D, there are some differences between the two types of diabetes. The prevalence of hypertension in T1D is low at the time of initial diagnosis but demonstrates an increase to 33% 20 years after diagnosis and to 70% at 40 years of diabetes.[13] The rate of increase parallels the rate of progression of kidney disease. In contrast, the prevalence of hypertension in patients with newly diagnosed T2D is high (40%), and in many of these patients, it was documented without any evidence of kidney disease.[14] When diagnosed, patients with T2D are older and have had "silent" diabetes, both of which may increase the prevalence of hypertension individually, for many more years than those with T1D. Besides the effects of aging and increased glucose exposure, the hypertension of patients with T2D is associated with obesity and dyslipidemia (the so-called metabolic syndrome),[15,16] which may be related to insulin resistance and compensatory hyperinsulinemia, which has been shown to increase renal sodium retention.[10,17] Both obesity and diabetes are associated with endothelial dysfunction,[18] which promotes vasoconstriction and increased peripheral resistance. The RIACE study[19] in Italy found that high BMI, family history, albuminuria, and vascular disease (macro and micro) were quantitatively the most important phenotypic characteristics of patients with T2D and hypertension.

TREATMENT OF HYPERTENSION IN PATIENTS WITH DIABETES

Treatment of hypertension in diabetes has been found to prevent vascular complications, both macro- and microvascular. Evidence comes from well-conducted clinical trials, including U.K. Prospective Diabetes Study (UKPDS), Hypertension Optimal Treatment (HOT), and Action in Diabetes and Vascular Disease (ADVANCE) (see Table 50.2).

In the UKPDS trial,[20] close to 1,200 patients with T2D and hypertension (average at baseline = 160/94 mmHg) were randomly assigned to two treatments arms with different treatment targets in BP: *1*) BP <150/85 or *2*) BP <180/105 mmHg. The initial therapies selected were an angiotensin-converting enzyme (ACE) inhibitor (Captopril) or a β-blocker (atenolol). The UKPDS trial found that the more intensively treated arm achieved a BP of 144/82 mmHg, and the participants in this group had a reduction of diabetes-related endpoints (24%), including deaths, as well as reductions in incident rates of strokes (44%) and in deterioration in retinopathy and visual acuity in comparison with the group of patients in the less intensively treated arm. A follow-up study of UKPDS has found that these benefits are lost in the more intensively treated group if the BP is not maintained at similar levels than those achieved during the active trial.[20a] It should be noted, however, that the intensively treated group had a higher A1C (8.3 vs. 7.5%) at the start of the post-trial observational period, which may have offset the benefits of intense BP control.

Three thousand patients with diabetes participated in the HOT trial.[21] The relative risk of a cardiovascular event was reduced significantly in the group of T2D patients assigned to a treatment arm with a target for diastolic BP ≤80 mmHg compared with the group that had a diastolic target BP of ≤90 mmHg (relative risk [RR] = 0.49; 95% confidence interval [CI] 0.29–0.81). The HOT trial did not find a reduction in cardiovascular events when also including those without T2D. Furthermore, those with T2D only made up 8% of the entire study

Table 50.2 Summary of Major Trials of Hypertension Management in Patients with Type 2 Diabetes

Trial	Macrovascular events (AMI, stroke, CV death)	Microvascular complications (retinopathy, nephropathy)	Overall death
U.K. Prospective Diabetes Study (UKPDS)	↓↓	↓	↓
Hypertension Optimal Treatment (HOT)	↓		↓
Action in Diabetes and Vascular Disease (ADVANCE)	↓↓	↓↓	↓

population and the achieved BP was not reported for this subgroup. These findings might limit the conclusion of this study in T2D. Given the results of the other studies reported here, however, the results of the HOT trial provide further evidence that lowering BP in T2D is beneficial.

The ADVANCE trial[22] evaluated the effect of intensive BP and intensive glycemic control on cardiovascular events in patients with T2D with high cardiovascular risk and was designed as a placebo-controlled randomized trial. All 11,000 patients in the ADVANCE trial had T2D. The initial treatment in ADVANCE was a combination of an ACE inhibitor and a thiazide diuretic (treated group). Modifications in therapy (including additions of other medications) were left to the discretion of the treating MDs. At the end of the trial, the patients in the treated group had an average BP of 135/74 mmHg, lower than the BP observed in the placebo group (140/76 mmHg). Over a mean follow-up of 4.3 years, randomization to drug therapy was associated with a 9% lower risk of combined micro- and macrovascular events and a 14% lower risk of death as compared with placebo. The results were similar among those with and without hypertension at baseline and were not modified by baseline systolic BP.

These three major trials provide evidence that the treatment of hypertension is successful in decreasing the incident rates of cardiovascular events and microvascular complications in patients with T2D as well as in decreasing cardiovascular and overall mortality.

THE TARGET OF HYPERTENSION TREATMENT IN PATIENTS WITH DIABETES

The previously discussed trials do not allow us to define the optimal level of control of hypertension in which maximum benefit is achieved. Although the HOT trial randomized patients to various targets, the difference in achieved BP reduction in each arm was less than expected, limiting any determination of an optimal target. Statistical analysis of the UKPDS BP data suggests that there is a linear relation between the systolic pressure and outcomes.[23] Thus, a suggestion may be made that normalization of the BP should be the target of treatment of hypertension in patients with diabetes, and thus a universal target of BP may be recommended. The following paragraphs examine data from several trials examining whether this strategy in diabetes improves outcomes.

The Action to Control Cardiovascular Risk in Diabetes (ACCORD) trial[24] enrolled >10,000 patients with T2D in a 2 × 2 factorial design to test the hypothesis that intensive control of glucose would improve cardiovascular outcomes versus current standard of care control. Two other trials were embedded in ACCORD, the lipid trial, and the BP trial. The ACCORD BP trial randomly assigned 4,733 patients with T2D who had cardiovascular disease or at least two additional risk factors for cardiovascular disease to either intensive therapy (target systolic BP <120 mmHg) or standard therapy trial (target systolic BP <140 mmHg).[24] The targets were successfully reached in the two groups (intensive [INT] = 119 mmHg; and standard [STD] 133 mmHg) and sustained for >5 years (Figure 50.1). Patients treated in the INT group required a significantly larger number of BP-reducing

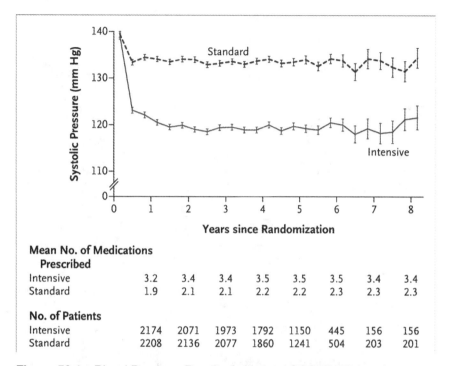

Figure 50.1—Blood Pressure Results from the ACCORD Trial and Average Number of Medications Needed to Attain Targets in Both Arms of Therapy. Reprinted with permission from the publisher.[24]

medications than the STD group (INT = 3.4 vs. STD = 2.1) and experienced a threefold higher incidence of serious side events (hypotension, hypokalemia) attributable to the use of medications (episodes of hypotension, syncope).

The ACCORD investigators reported that in spite of BP normalization, the INT group had *no* significant difference in the incident rate of the primary outcome (nonfatal myocardial infarction, nonfatal stroke, or death from cardiovascular causes) versus the STD group (1.87 vs. 2.09%; hazard ratio [HR] = 0.88). Moreover, ACCORD results showed a slight difference in the all-cause mortality rate (INT = 1.28 vs. STD = 1.19%) or in cardiovascular death (INT = 0.52 vs. STD = 0.49%). In contrast, INT treatment produced reductions in rates of total and nonfatal stroke (0.32 vs. 0.53% total stroke and 0.30 vs. 0.47% nonfatal stroke). The SANDS trial (Effect of Lower Targets for Blood Pressure and LDL Cholesterol on Atherosclerosis in Diabetes: the SANDS randomized trial)[25] enrolled 499 American Indian men and women who were randomized to aggressive (*n* = 252) versus standard (*n* = 247) treatment groups. Final BP levels were 117 (aggressive) and 129 (standard) mmHg. Both adverse events (38.5 and 26.7%; *P* = 0.005) and serious adverse events (*n* = 4 vs. 1; *P* = 0.18) secondary to

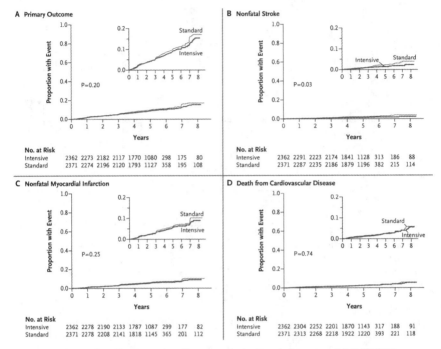

Figure 50.2—Cardiovascular Outcomes in Participants of ACCORD BP Trial.

Note: The insert in the panel indicates the rate of deaths attributable to cardiovascular disease. Panel B shows the only outcome that was different statistically between the two treatment arms. Reprinted with permission from the publisher.[24]

medications were higher in the aggressively treated group. In spite of much better lowering of BP, cardiovascular outcomes (1.6/100 and 1.5/100 person-years; $P = 0.87$) did not differ between groups.

Further support comes from a post hoc analysis of the ACCOMPLISH trial (described in the following section) in which 60% of the participants had diabetes. This analysis also found a reduction in the risk of stroke with an achieved systolic BP <120 mmHg but was offset by a higher risk of coronary events.[26] The analysis also found that cardiovascular events were similar for those who achieved a systolic BP 120 to <130 mmHg as compared to those with systolic BP 130 to <140 mmHg but significantly lower than those with systolic BP ≥140 mmHg. Conversely, those achieving a systolic BP 120 to <130 mmHg had a higher rate of worsening renal function compared with those achieving systolic BP 130 to <139 mmHg. This risk was even higher for those achieving systolic

BP <120 mmHg. Thus, these findings suggest that a reduction in systolic BP <140 mmHg is associated with a reduction in cardiovascular events, but reductions in systolic BP <130 mmHg were not associated with increased cardiovascular benefit (except for stroke) but were associated with a higher rate of adverse events.

The finding that normalization of BP can prevent strokes is intriguing. Some caveats, however, need to be considered:

1. A high number of patients ($n = 89$) have to be treated to prevent one stroke.
2. To achieve normalization of BP, the pharmacological treatment is complex; three or more classes of medications are needed and are associated with a threefold increase in side effects from the medications used.
3. As of now, we cannot define characteristics (genetic or phenotypes) of those patients who are candidates for normalization of BP for stroke prevention, a topic that deserves further research.

The BP target for patients with T2D and hypertension needs to be redefined, prompted primarily by the findings of ACCORD. For BP targeting, one size does not fit all, and targets should be personalized. In light of these trials, the overall target for patients with T2D and hypertension should be ≤140/80 mmHg. The latter target is particularly clear for patients with clinical characteristics similar to those of ACCORD participants. Contrary to a widely held belief, the participants of ACCORD are representative of a large segment of the patient population of patients with T2D, but needless to say, not all patients fit this profile. Special consideration is for those patients who have diabetes and established nephropathy with high levels of albuminuria, in whom the target may be a more stringent ≤130/80 mmHg. In a post hoc analysis of the Irbesartan Diabetic Nephropathy Trial,[27] a progressive reduction in cardiovascular and renal events was seen with lower achieved systolic BP up to 120 mmHg among participants with diabetic nephropathy. As stated previously, however, such post hoc analyses not unusually have failed to be confirmed by subsequent randomized trials (e.g., post hoc UKPDS vs. ACCORD), and thus future studies are required to strengthen this recommendation. Younger patients with T2D, without high risk of cardiovascular events, may be candidates for a lower target BP, an important consideration as age did not modify the results of ACCORD.

Data from ACCORD, SANDS, ABCD, and ACCOMPLISH do not support normalization of BP in patients with hypertension and T2D and clinical characteristics similar to the participants in these trials (high risk of cardiovascular events). The 2014 guidelines from the American Diabetes Association (ADA) for the BP target in patients with diabetes and hypertension now endorse a target BP ≤140/80 mmHg.

APPROACH TO TREATMENT OF HYPERTENSION IN PATIENTS WITH DIABETES

The treatment of hypertension in our patients with diabetes needs to be comprehensive and include strategies that fall into two categories: non-pharmacological and pharmacological. The scope of this chapter precludes it from examining both categories in detail. Instead, this chapter briefly discusses lifestyle modification, which is better provided by registered dietitians (RDs), certified diabetes educators (CDEs), and exercise physiologists, and dedicates more space to the discussion of use of medications.

LIFESTYLE MODIFICATION

Overall, the goals of lifestyle modification for BP management include the following:

- Reduction in sodium intake
- Body-weight loss (in obese patients)
- Tobacco cessation
- Exercise
- Moderation in alcohol intake

Numerous "diets" and exercise regimens have been advocated, most of which have little or no validation. An example of a successful and validated dietary approach to control of BP by changes in diet behavior is the Dietary Approaches to Stop Hypertension (DASH),[28-31] available online at the National Institutes of Health website.[32] We encourage physicians to establish close links with RDs, CDEs, and exercise physiologists, as these professionals are fully dedicated to non-pharmacological approaches, and hence they can provide in-depth counseling to our patients.

MEDICATIONS

The medication approach to the treatment of hypertension represents one of the most successful areas of pharmacological treatments in medicine. There is a large and ever-increasing array of medications for control of BP. The most important classes of drugs for treatment of hypertension in patients with diabetes are listed in Table 50.3 and are discussed in the next paragraphs, subsequent to which we delineate an approach for selection.

ACE Inhibitors

The class of ACE inhibitors has distinctive advantages when used in patients with hypertension and diabetes. First, and foremost, ACE inhibitors protect against the progression of increased albuminuria or even reverse it, even in cases with severely increased albuminuria.[33,34] The positive outcomes in albuminuria are seen in both T1D and T2D and are the basis for considering the ACE inhibitors in the primary prevention of diabetic nephropathy. Added to the renoprotective effects, ACE inhibitors have been shown to slow the progression of retinopathy. ACE inhibitors have no effects on serum lipids but may increase insulin sensitivity; in a small trial, ACE inhibitors reduced A1C from 8.6 to 6.5% with no changes in insulin dose, dietary intake, or body weight.[35,36] The side effects include cough, hyperkalemia, and increased serum creatinine, more so in patients with renal insufficiency. Clinically, the power of ACE inhibitors to lower BP is limited, so it is common to use them in in combination with

Table 50.3 Medications for Hypertension in Patients with Diabetes

Medication class	Positive effects besides ↓ BP	Negative side effects	Selection tier
Angiotensin-converting enzyme (ACE) inhibitors	↓ Albuminuria ↑ Insulin sensitivity	Cough ↓ Renal function ↑ Serum potassium	First tier
Angiotensin receptor blockers (ARB)	↓ Albuminuria ↑ Insulin sensitivity	↓ Renal function ↑ Serum potassium	First tier
Diuretics—thiazide type		↓ Serum potassium ↑ Glucose, lipids, uric acid	First tier (in combination) or second tier
β-Blockers	↓ CV events, CHF	↑ Asthma Masks hypoglycemia	Second tier
Calcium channel blockers	Neutral in glucose/lipids	↑ CHF	Second tier
α-Blockers		Orthostatic ↓BP	Third tier

Note: BP = blood pressure; CHF = coronary heart failure; CV = cardiovascular.

other agents, especially low-dose thiazide. Although it has been speculated that ACE inhibitors may provide a cardiovascular benefit,[37-44] the latter is more likely related to the decrease in BP rather than an intrinsic property of the ACE inhibitors.

Angiotensin II Receptor Blockers

Antgiotensin II receptor blockers (ARBs) have the same renoprotection benefits as ACE inhibitors.[45-48] The ARBs are also cardioprotective,[48] as evidenced by larger reductions in the primary composite cardiovascular endpoint and in cardiovascular and total mortality compared with a β-blocker. The ONTARGET trial[49] did not find a difference in the composite primary outcome between an ARB with an ACE inhibitor or the combination of both in 6,391 patients with diabetes.

ACE Inhibitors Plus ARBs

If both ACE inhibitors and ARBs have renoprotective effects as well as positive cardiovascular effects, then it is tempting to speculate that the combination of both classes of medications may have additive or even synergistic effects. This thought found some support in the randomized controlled trial of dual blockade of renin-angiotensin system in patients with hypertension, albuminuria, and non–insulin-dependent diabetes: the Candesartan and Lisinopril Microalbuminuria (CALM) trial, which showed that a combination of an ACE inhibitor and ARB had more power in reducing BP than either agent alone.[50,51] The ARB alone had less power in reducing albuminuria than the ACE inhibitor or the combination. The ONTARGET trial[49] tested an ARB versus an ACE inhibitor versus the combination of an ARB and an ACE inhibitor on renal outcomes (composite of dialysis plus doubling of serum creatinine plus death). The number of events for the composite primary outcome was similar for ARBs ($n = 1,147$ [13.4%]) and ACE inhibitors ($n = 1,150$ [13.5%]; HR = 1.00; 95% CI 0.92–1.09), but was increased with an ARB plus ACE inhibitor combination ($n = 1,233$ [14.5%]; HR = 1.09; CI 1.01–1.18; $P = 0.037$). The investigators of this trial found that an ARB is similar to an ACE inhibitor, but the ARB plus ACE inhibitor combination, in spite of reducing proteinuria to a greater extent than monotherapy, worsens major renal outcomes. Further evidence was provided in a recently published study,[52] which found similar results with combination therapy. Thus, based on the available evidence from published clinical trials, the combination of an ARB with an ACE inhibitor is not recommended.

It has been hypothesized that the reason for the negative results with combination ACE inhibitor and ARB therapy may be due to subsequent elevation of renin levels. If such a hypothesis were true, then the addition of a direct renin inhibitor (DRI) to an ACE inhibitor or ARB might offer a different approach to reduce cardiac and renal endpoints. The ALTITUDE trial, however, also found no difference in combined cardiac and renal endpoints and an increased risk of adverse events with the addition of the DRI aliskirin to an ACE inhibitor or an ARB.[53] Whether mineralocorticoid blockers added to ACE inhibitor or ARB therapy would have similar results warrants further study.

Thiazide Diuretics

Thiazide and thiazide-like diuretics are effective in lowering BP in patients with diabetes and hypertension by decreasing plasma volume.[54] The latter permits more effectiveness of the BP effect of an ACE inhibitor.[55] On the other hand, ACE inhibitors minimize hypokalemia (by lowering aldosterone release) and other side effects seen with thiazides. As a matter of fact, the currently used low doses of thiazides (12.5–25 mg/day) have minimal side effects as shown in the ALLHAT trial[39] as opposed to the previous experience with larger doses of these medications.

The ALLHAT trial[39] assessed the safety and efficacy of four different classes of medications as initial monotherapy: *1)* a thiazide-like diuretic (chorthalidone at small doses of 12.5 to 25 mg/day), *2)* a calcium channel blocker (CCB), *3)* an ACE inhibitor, or *4)* an α-blocker. Among the 33,000 participants, almost 40% had T2D. The α-blocker arm was stopped due to higher incidence of coronary heart failure (CHF).

Chlorthalidone was superior in the prevention of cardiovascular disease and stroke as compared with an ACE inhibitor. These differences were also true for the subgroup of patients with diabetes. The diuretic, however, induced a mild rise in the plasma glucose and increased incident rates of diabetes compared with the ACE inhibitor and the CCB.

The combination of thiazide diuretics to an ACE inhibitor or ARB offers several theoretical advantages. First, volume depletion induced by the thiazide diuretics and subsequent activation of the renin-angiotensin-aldosterone system can be mitigated by cotreatment with an ACE inhibitor or ARB. Second, given the diverging effects on potassium excretion, the combination may serve to help prevent hypo- or hyperkalemia.[39,55]

Calcium Channel Blockers

CCBs have good efficacy and few adverse effects on serum lipids or blood glucose, especially the nondihydropyridine CCBs. Some concerns regarding adverse increased cardiovascular morbidity and mortality[56] were not supported by large clinical trials.[21,57] Moreover, a CCB was associated with similar rates of coronary events as thiazides and ACE inhibitors,[39] but a higher rate of CHF was observed with the CCB compared with the diuretic (RR 1.42; 95% CI 1.23–1.64). When used in combination with an ACE inhibitor as initial therapy, a CCB was superior to an ACE inhibitor plus thiazide diuretic with fewer cardiovascular outcomes (8.8 vs. 11%).[58,59] In a head-to-head comparison, the ACCOMPLISH trial[60] found a CCB was superior to a thiazide diuretic when used as primary therapy in all participants treated with an ACE inhibitor, including the subgroup with T2D. The thiazide diuretic used in the ACCOMPLISH trial (hydrochlorothiazide) differed from that used in the ALLHAT trial (chlorthalidone). Whether this played a role in the outcome of ACCOMPLISH requires further study.

β-Blockers

In spite of masking hypoglycemia-related symptoms, β-blockers are used frequently for the treatment of high BP in patients with diabetes; the UKPDS showed that a β-blocker was as effective as an ACE inhibitor in lowering BP and in the prevention of vascular disease.[20,61]

A special class of β-blockers includes those with α-1-adrenergic–α-antagonism. In pretreated patients with an ACE inhibitor or an ARB, the addition of a β-blocker–α-1-blocker did not increase the blood levels of A1C in contrast to a β-blocker that was associated with worsening glycemia and an increase in A1C of 0.15%.[62] Besides the latter, the β-blocker–α-agent retards the progression to increased albuminuria (6.6% rate of progression) versus β-blocker (11.1% rate of progression). Whether the addition of a β-blocker with an α-antagonism had an impact on hard renal and cardiovascular endpoints is not known, and the recommendation to use these agents over other β-blockers will require further study.

α-Blockers

α-Blocker agents (α-agents) are associated commonly with orthostatic hypotension and are as effective in lowering BP as ACE inhibitors and CCBs. The ALLHAT trial[39] included a treatment arm with an α-agent that was stopped earlier than anticipated because of higher rates of new-onset CHF than in other treatment arms. In consequence, α-agents are not recommended as primary therapy but may be useful as a tertiary line of add-on therapy.

APPROACH FOR SELECTION OF MEDICATIONS

The main purposes of the treatment of hypertension in patients with diabetes are to prevent cardiovascular events and to prevent or slow progression of microvascular complications (in particular kidney and eye diseases).

On the basis of the overall evidence of the trials discussed in this chapter, an ACE inhibitor or an ARB is the preferred treatment choice as the initial therapy in any hypertensive patient with diabetes, and more so in those who have any degree of increased albuminuria.[6–8,63] As a matter of fact, most experts in the field of hypertension begin with an ACE inhibitor or an ARB in hypertensive patients with diabetes and with or without proteinuria. Although monotherapy can attain the goal BP in a good percent of patients with diabetes and stage I hypertension, stage II hypertension usually requires combination therapy as the initial treatment. Starting those patients on a combination therapy based on an ACE inhibitor (or an ARB) and a low dose of a thiazide is very common practice due to the large arrays of fixed combinations available in the market and ease of use; however, a CCB has been shown to be a superior choice.

If the BP does not achieve the target desired, add a CCB, a thiazide, or a β-blocker. Further escalation of treatment should be considered if target BP is not achieved with dual- or triple-agent combination by adding a third or fourth agent as indicated in Figure 50.2. The immense majority of patients will attain BP target (either <140 or <130 mmHg for special patients) with two or three agents. For those patients in whom the treatment still does not achieve a proper control of BP, however, then a vasodilator may be considered (e.g., hydralazine) or other agents considered depending upon clinical context (e.g., loop diuretics in patients with CHF or chronic renal failure). Mineralocorticoid receptor blockers also may be considered, but they require further studies with hard outcomes before definitive recommendations can be made.

A suggested approach for the initial selection of medications and subsequent additions is presented in Figure 50.3. A flow diagram for monitoring and ongoing adjustments is depicted in Figure 50.4. Consult an expert on hypertension if the control of BP is not achieved after three steps of medication additions.

CONCLUSION

Hypertension is a common finding in patients with diabetes. There is a whole body of evidence that supports the benefits of treating hypertension in patients with diabetes, most notably an improvement in macro- and microvascular outcomes. Modifications to lifestyle must be recommended to all patients with diabetes and blood pressure elevation. Use of medications is usually needed, and physicians should not shy away from using them to achieve the current target endorsed by the American Diabetes Association (<140/80 mmHg is the general recommendation, but in some cases <130/80 mmHg).

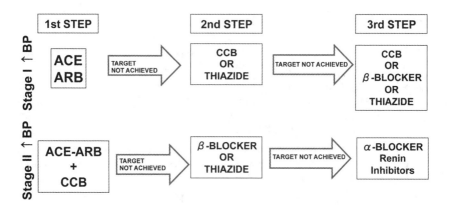

Figure 50.3—Overview of Medication Selection.

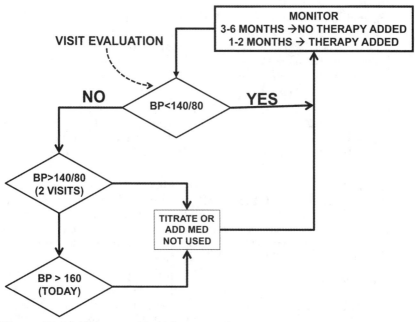

Figure 50.4—Treatment Flowchart.

REFERENCES

1. Kannel WB. Hypertensive risk assessment: Cardiovascular risk factors and hypertension. *J Clin Hypertens* 2004;6:393–399.

2. Feinleib M, Garrison RJ, Fabsitz R, Christian JC, Hrubec Z, Borhani NO, Kannel WB, Rosenman R, Schwartz JT, Wagner JO. The NHLBI twin study of cardiovascular disease risk factors: methodology and summary of results. *Am J Epidemiol* 1977;106:284–285.

3. Shea S, Cook EF, Kannel WB, Goldman L. Treatment of hypertension and its effect on cardiovascular risk factors: data from the Framingham Heart Study. *Circulation* 1985;71:22–30.

4. Ninomiya T, Perkovic V, Turnbull F, Neal B, Barzi F, Cass A, Baigent C, Chalmers J, Li N, Woodward M, MacMahon S. Blood pressure lowering and major cardiovascular events in people with and without chronic kidney disease: meta-analysis of randomised controlled trials. *BMJ* 2013;347:f5680–f5692.

5. Turnbull F, Neal B, Ninomiya T, Algert C, Arima H, Barzi F, Bulpitt C, Chalmers J, Fagard R, Gleason A, Heritier S, Li N, Perkovic V, Woodward M, MacMahon S. Effects of different regimens to lower blood pressure on major cardiovascular events in older and younger adults: meta-analysis of randomised trials. *BMJ* 2008;336:1121–1123.

6. Buse JB, Ginsberg HN, Bakris GL, Clark NG, Costa F, Eckel R, Fonseca V, Gerstein HC, Grundy S, Nesto RW, Pignone MP, Plutzky J, Porte D, Redberg R, Stitzel KF, Stone NJ. Primary prevention of cardiovascular diseases in people with diabetes mellitus: a scientific statement from the American Heart Association and the American Diabetes Association. *Diabetes Care* 2007;30:162–172.

7. James PA, Oparil S, Carter BL, Cushman WC, Dennison-Himmelfarb C, Handler J, Lackland DT, Lefevre ML, Mackenzie TD, Ogedegbe O, Smith SC Jr, Svetkey LP, Taler SJ, Townsend RR, Wright JT Jr, Narva AS, Ortiz E. 2014 evidence-based guideline for the management of high blood pressure in adults: report from the panel members appointed to the Eighth Joint National Committee (JNC 8). *JAMA* 2013;311:507–520.

8. Mancia G, Fagard R, Narkiewicz K, et al. 2013 ESH/ESC guidelines for the management of arterial hypertension: the Task Force for the Management of Arterial Hypertension of the European Society of Hypertension (ESH) and of the European Society of Cardiology (ESC). *J Hypertension* 2013;31:1281.

9. Chobanian AV, Bakris GL, Black HR, Cushman WC, Green LA, Izzo JL Jr, Jones DW, Materson BJ, Oparil S, Wright JT Jr, Roccella EJ. The Seventh Report of the Joint National Committee on Prevention, Detection, Evaluation, and Treatment of High Blood Pressure: the JNC 7 report. *JAMA* 2003;289:2560–2572.

10. Ferrannini E, Cushman WC. Diabetes and hypertension: the bad companions. *Lancet* 2012;380:601–610.

11. Colosia AD, Palencia R, Khan S. Prevalence of hypertension and obesity in patients with type 2 diabetes mellitus in observational studies: a systematic literature review. *Diabetes Metab Syndr Obes* 2013;6:327–338.

12. Rosner B, Cook NR, Daniels S, Falkner B. Childhood blood pressure trends and risk factors for high blood pressure: the NHANES experience 1988–2008. *Hypertension* 2013;62(2):247–254.

13. Parving HH, Hommel E, Mathiesen E, Skott P, Edsberg B, Bahnsen M, Lauritzen M, Hougaard P, Lauritzen E. Prevalence of microalbuminuria, arterial hypertension, retinopathy and neuropathy in patients with insulin dependent diabetes. *Br Med J (Clin Res Ed)* 1988;296:156–160.

14. Hypertension in Diabetes Study (HDS). I. Prevalence of hypertension in newly presenting type 2 diabetic patients and the association with risk factors for cardiovascular and diabetic complications. *J Hypertens* 1993;11:309–317.

15. Zimmet P, Alberti G. The metabolic syndrome: progress towards one definition for an epidemic of our time. *Nat Clin Pract Endocrinol Metab* 2008;4:239–246.

16. Alberti KG, Zimmet P, Shaw J. Metabolic syndrome—a new world-wide definition. A consensus statement from the International Diabetes Federation. *Diabet Med* 2006;23:469–480.

17. Nosadini R, Sambataro M, Thomaseth K, Pacini G, Cipollina MR, Brocco E, Solini A, Carraro A, Velussi M, Frigato F. Role of hyperglycemia and insulin resistance in determining sodium retention in non-insulin-dependent diabetes. *Kidney Int* 1993;44:139–146.

18. Calles-Escandon J, Cipolla M. Diabetes and endothelial dysfunction: a clinical perspective. *Endocr Rev* 2001;22:36–52.

19. Solini A, Penno G, Bonora E, Fondelli C, Orsi E, Arosio M, Trevisan R, Vedovato M, Cignarelli M, Andreozzi F, Nicolucci A, Pugliese G. Diverging association of reduced glomerular filtration rate and albuminuria with coronary and noncoronary events in patients with type 2 diabetes: the Renal Insufficiency and Cardiovascular Events (RIACE) Italian multicenter study. *Diabetes Care* 2012;35:143–149.

20. U.K. Prospective Diabetes Study Group. Tight blood pressure control and risk of macrovascular and microvascular complications in type 2 diabetes: UKPDS 38. *BMJ* 1998;317:703–713.

20a. Holman RR, Paul SK, Bethel MA, Neil HA, Matthews DR. Long-term follow-up after tight control of blood pressure in type 2 diabetes. *N Engl J Med* 2008;359.1565–1576.

21. Hansson L, Zanchetti A, Carruthers SG, Dahlof B, Elmfeldt D, Julius S, Menard J, Rahn KH, Wedel H, Westerling S. Effects of intensive blood-pressure lowering and low-dose aspirin in patients with hypertension: prin-

cipal results of the Hypertension Optimal Treatment (HOT) randomised trial. HOT Study Group. *Lancet* 1998;351:1755–1762.

22. Patel A, MacMahon S, Chalmers J, Neal B, Woodward M, Billot L, Harrap S, Poulter N, Marre M, Cooper M, Glasziou P, Grobbee DE, Hamet P, Heller S, Liu LS, Mancia G, Mogensen CE, Pan CY, Rodgers A, Williams B. Effects of a fixed combination of perindopril and indapamide on macrovascular and microvascular outcomes in patients with type 2 diabetes mellitus (the ADVANCE trial): a randomised controlled trial. *Lancet* 2007;370:829–840.

23. Adler AI, Stratton IM, Neil HA, Yudkin JS, Matthews DR, Cull CA, Wright AD, Turner RC, Holman RR. Association of systolic blood pressure with macrovascular and microvascular complications of type 2 diabetes (UKPDS 36): prospective observational study. *BMJ* 321:412–419.

24. Cushman WC, Evans GW, Byington RP, Goff DC Jr, Grimm RH Jr, Cutler JA, Simons-Morton DG, Basile JN, Corson MA, Probstfield JL, Katz L, Peterson KA, Friedewald WT, Buse JB, Bigger JT, Gerstein HC, Ismail-Beigi F. Effects of intensive blood-pressure control in type 2 diabetes mellitus. *N Engl J Med* 2010;362:1575–1585.

25. Howard BV, Roman MJ, Devereux RB, Fleg JL, Galloway JM, Henderson JA, Howard WJ, Lee ET, Mete M, Poolaw B, Ratner RE, Russell M, Silverman A, Stylianou M, Umans JG, Wang W, Weir MR, Weissman NJ, Wilson C, Yeh F, Zhu J. Effect of lower targets for blood pressure and LDL cholesterol on atherosclerosis in diabetes: the SANDS randomized trial. *JAMA* 2008;299:1678–1689.

26. Weber MA, Bakris GL, Hester A, Weir MR, Hua TA, Zappe D, Dahlof B, Velazquez EJ, Pitt B, Jamerson K. Systolic blood pressure and cardiovascular outcomes during treatment of hypertension. *Am J Med* 2013;126:501–508.

27. Evans M, Bain SC, Hogan S, Bilous RW. Irbesartan delays progression of nephropathy as measured by estimated glomerular filtration rate: post hoc analysis of the Irbesartan Diabetic Nephropathy Trial. *Nephrol Dial Transplant* 2012;27:2255–2263.

28. Appel LJ, Moore TJ, Obarzanek E, Vollmer WM, Svetkey LP, Sacks FM, Bray GA, Vogt TM, Cutler JA, Windhauser MM, Lin PH, Karanja N. A clinical trial of the effects of dietary patterns on blood pressure. DASH Collaborative Research Group. *N Engl J Med* 1997;336:1117–1124.

29. Conlin PR, Erlinger TP, Bohannon A, Miller ER III, Appel LJ, Svetkey LP, Moore TJ. The DASH diet enhances the blood pressure response to losartan in hypertensive patients. *Am J Hypertens* 2003;16:337–342.

30. Getchell WS, Svetkey LP, Appel LJ, Moore TJ, Bray GA, Obarzanek E. Summary of the Dietary Approaches to Stop Hypertension (DASH) randomized clinical trial. *Curr Treat Options Cardiovasc Med* 1999;1:295–300.

31. Hikmat F, Appel LJ. Effects of the DASH diet on blood pressure in patients with and without metabolic syndrome: results from the DASH trial. *J Hum Hypertens* 2013;28:170–175.

32. National Heart, Lung, and Blood Institute. Your guide to lowering your blood pressure with DASH. Available from www.nhlbi.nih.gov/health/public/heart/hbp/dash. Accessed 23 March 2014.

33. Bakris GL, Williams M, Dworkin L, Elliott WJ, Epstein M, Toto R, Tuttle K, Douglas J, Hsueh W, Sowers J. Preserving renal function in adults with hypertension and diabetes: a consensus approach. National Kidney Foundation Hypertension and Diabetes Executive Committees Working Group. *Am J Kidney Dis* 2000;36:646–661.

34. Barnett AH, Bain SC, Bouter P, Karlberg B, Madsbad S, Jervell J, Mustonen J. Angiotensin-receptor blockade versus converting-enzyme inhibition in type 2 diabetes and nephropathy. *N Engl J Med* 2004;351:1952–1961.

35. Alkharouf J, Nalinikumari K, Corry D, Tuck M. Long-term effects of the angiotensin converting enzyme inhibitor captopril on metabolic control in non-insulin-dependent diabetes mellitus. *Am J Hypertens* 1993;6:337–343.

36. Morris AD, Boyle DI, McMahon AD, Pearce H, Evans JM, Newton RW, Jung RT, MacDonald TM. ACE inhibitor use is associated with hospitalization for severe hypoglycemia in patients with diabetes. DARTS/MEMO Collaboration. Diabetes Audit and Research in Tayside, Scotland. Medicines Monitoring Unit. *Diabetes Care* 1997;20:1363–1367.

37. U.K. Prospective Diabetes Study Group. Efficacy of atenolol and captopril in reducing risk of macrovascular and microvascular complications in type 2 diabetes: UKPDS 39. *BMJ* 1998;317:713–720.

38. Heart Outcomes Prevention Evaluation Study Investigators. Effects of ramipril on cardiovascular and microvascular outcomes in people with diabetes mellitus: results of the HOPE study and MICRO-HOPE substudy. *Lancet* 2000;355:253–259.

39. Major outcomes in high-risk hypertensive patients randomized to angiotensin-converting enzyme inhibitor or calcium channel blocker vs diuretic: the Antihypertensive and Lipid-Lowering Treatment to Prevent Heart Attack Trial (ALLHAT). *JAMA* 2002;288:2981–2997.

40. Braunwald E, Domanski MJ, Fowler SE, Geller NL, Gersh BJ, Hsia J, Pfeffer MA, Rice MM, Rosenberg YD, Rouleau JL. Angiotensin-converting-enzyme inhibition in stable coronary artery disease. *N Engl J Med* 2004;351:2058–2068.

41. Fox KM. Efficacy of perindopril in reduction of cardiovascular events among patients with stable coronary artery disease: randomised, double blind, placebo-controlled, multicentre trial (the EUROPA study). *Lancet* 2003;362:782–788.

42. Fox KM, Bertrand ME, Remme WJ, Ferrari R, Simoons ML, Deckers JW. Efficacy of perindopril in reducing risk of cardiac events in patients with revascularized coronary artery disease. *Am Heart J* 2007;153:629–635.

43. Yusuf S, Sleight P, Pogue J, Bosch J, Davies R, Dagenais G. Effects of an angiotensin-converting-enzyme inhibitor, ramipril, on cardiovascular events in high-risk patients. The Heart Outcomes Prevention Evaluation Study Investigators. *N Engl J Med* 2000;342:145–153.

44. Braunwald E, Domanski MJ, Fowler SE, Geller NL, Gersh BJ, Hsia J, Pfeffer MA, Rice MM, Rosenberg YD, Rouleau JL. Angiotensin-converting-enzyme inhibition in stable coronary artery disease. *N Engl J Med* 2004;351:2058–2068.

45. Brenner BM, Cooper ME, de Zeeuw D, Keane WF, Mitch WE, Parving HH, Remuzzi G, Snapinn SM, Zhang Z, Shahinfar S. Effects of losartan on renal and cardiovascular outcomes in patients with type 2 diabetes and nephropathy. *N Engl J Med* 2001;345:861–869.

46. Lewis EJ, Hunsicker LG, Clarke WR, Berl T, Pohl MA, Lewis JB, Ritz E, Atkins RC, Rohde R, Raz I. Renoprotective effect of the angiotensin-receptor antagonist irbesartan in patients with nephropathy due to type 2 diabetes. *N Engl J Med* 2001;345:851–860.

47. Parving HH, Brenner BM, Cooper ME, de Zeeuw D, Keane WF, Mitch WE, Remuzzi G, Snapinn SM, Zhang Z, Shahinfar S. [Effect of losartan on renal and cardiovascular complications of patients with type 2 diabetes and nephropathy]. *Ugeskr Laeger* 2001;163:5514–5519.

48. Dahlof B, Devereux RB, Kjeldsen SE, Julius S, Beevers G, de Faire U, Fyhrquist F, Ibsen H, Kristiansson K, Lederballe-Pedersen O, Lindholm LH, Nieminen MS, Omvik P, Oparil S, Wedel H. Cardiovascular morbidity and mortality in the Losartan Intervention For Endpoint reduction in hypertension study (LIFE): a randomised trial against atenolol. *Lancet* 2002;359:995–1003.

49. Mann JF, Schmieder RE, McQueen M, Dyal L, Schumacher H, Pogue J, Wang X, Maggioni A, Budaj A, Chaithiraphan S, Dickstein K, Keltai M, Metsarinne K, Oto A, Parkhomenko A, Piegas LS, Svendsen TL, Teo KK, Yusuf S. Renal outcomes with telmisartan, ramipril, or both, in people at high vascular risk (the ONTARGET study): a multicentre, randomised, double-blind, controlled trial. *Lancet* 2008;372:547–553.

50. Andersen NH, Poulsen PL, Knudsen ST, Poulsen SH, Eiskjaer H, Hansen KW, Helleberg K, Mogensen CE. Long-term dual blockade with candesartan and lisinopril in hypertensive patients with diabetes: the CALM II study. *Diabetes Care* 2005;28:273–277.

51. Mogensen CE, Neldam S, Tikkanen I, Oren S, Viskoper R, Watts RW, Cooper ME. Randomised controlled trial of dual blockade of renin-angiotensin system in patients with hypertension, microalbuminuria, and non-insulin

dependent diabetes: the candesartan and lisinopril microalbuminuria (CALM) study. *BMJ* 2000;321:1440–1444.

52. Fried LF, Emanuele N, Zhang JH, Brophy M, Conner TA, Duckworth W, Leehey DJ, McCullough PA, O'Connor T, Palevsky PM, Reilly RF, Seliger SL, Warren SR, Watnick S, Peduzzi P, Guarino P. Combined angiotensin inhibition for the treatment of diabetic nephropathy. *N Engl J Med* 2013;369:1892–1903.

53. Parving HH, Brenner BM, McMurray JJ, de ZD, Haffner SM, Solomon SD, Chaturvedi N, Persson F, Desai AS, Nicolaides M, Richard A, Xiang Z, Brunel P, Pfeffer MA. Cardiorenal end points in a trial of aliskiren for type 2 diabetes. *N Engl J Med* 2012;367:2204–2213.

54. Passmore AP, Whitehead EM, Crawford V, McVeigh GE, Johnston GD. The antihypertensive and metabolic effects of low and conventional dose cyclopenthiazide in type II diabetics with hypertension. *Q J Med* 1991;81:919–928.

55. Weinberger MH. Influence of an angiotensin converting-enzyme inhibitor on diuretic-induced metabolic effects in hypertension. *Hypertension* 1983;5:III132–III138.

56. Estacio RO, Jeffers BW, Hiatt WR, Biggerstaff SL, Gifford N, Schrier RW. The effect of nisoldipine as compared with enalapril on cardiovascular outcomes in patients with non-insulin-dependent diabetes and hypertension. *N Engl J Med* 1998;338:645–652.

57. Tuomilehto J, Rastenyte D, Birkenhager WH, Thijs L, Antikainen R, Bulpitt CJ, Fletcher AE, Forette F, Goldhaber A, Palatini P, Sarti C, Fagard R. Effects of calcium-channel blockade in older patients with diabetes and systolic hypertension. Systolic Hypertension in Europe Trial Investigators. *N Engl J Med* 1999;340:677–684.

58. Bakris G, Briasoulis A, Dahlof B, Jamerson K, Weber MA, Kelly RY, Hester A, Hua T, Zappe D, Pitt B. Comparison of benazepril plus amlodipine or hydrochlorothiazide in high-risk patients with hypertension and coronary artery disease. *Am J Cardiol* 2013;112:255–259.

59. Jamerson K, Weber MA, Bakris GL, Dahlof B, Pitt B, Shi V, Hester A, Gupte J, Gatlin M, Velazquez EJ. Benazepril plus amlodipine or hydrochlorothiazide for hypertension in high-risk patients. *N Engl J Med* 2008;359:2417–2428.

60. Bakris G, Hester A, Weber M, Dahlof B, Pitt B, Velasquez E, Staikos-Byrne L, Shi V, Jamerson K. The diabetes subgroup baseline characteristics of the Avoiding Cardiovascular Events Through Combination Therapy in Patients Living With Systolic Hypertension (ACCOMPLISH) trial. *J Cardiometab Syndr* 2000;3:229–233.

61. U.K. Prospective Diabetes Study Group. Efficacy of atenolol and captopril in reducing risk of macrovascular and microvascular complications in type 2 diabetes: UKPDS 39. *BMJ* 1998;317:713–720.

62. Bakris GL, Fonseca V, Katholi RE, McGill JB, Messerli FH, Phillips RA, Raskin P, Wright JT Jr, Oakes R, Lukas MA, Anderson KM, Bell DS. Metabolic effects of carvedilol vs metoprolol in patients with type 2 diabetes mellitus and hypertension: a randomized controlled trial. *JAMA* 2004; 292:2227–2236.

63. American Diabetes Association. Executive summary: standards of medical care in diabetes—2014. *Diabetes Care* 2014;37(Suppl 1):S5–S13.

Chapter 51

Infections and Diabetes

Rajeev Sharma, MBBS, MD
Michael Augenbraun, MD, FACP, FIDSA
Mary Ann Banerji, MD, FACP

Host immune defenses are altered in patients with diabetes. Hyperglycemia and acidosis alter the functions of phagocytic cells and result in changing their movement toward the site of an infection and impairing their microbicidal activity. Subtle alterations in cell-mediated immunity predispose the patient to tuberculosis, coccidioidomycosis, and cryptococcosis. The host's metabolic state in diabetes also favors the specific nutritional requirements of some microbes. High glucose concentrations in blood and body fluids promote the overgrowth of certain fungal pathogens—particularly *Candida* species and *Zygomycetes*. *Zygomycetes* also grow more rapidly in an acidotic environment. Finally, mechanical factors largely contribute to the increased susceptibility of patients with diabetes to infections (Table 51.1). Treatment of infection in a patient with diabetes involves both antibiotic therapy and maintenance of good glycemic control. Table 51.2 provides an empiric antimicrobial treatment scheme for the management of the more common infections affecting diabetic patients. More specific details are described in subsequent sections.[1,2]

Evidence indicates that hyperglycemia is associated with increased infections, morbidity, and mortality. What is less clear is whether lowering the blood glucose to near-normal levels, especially in the setting of serious illness, improves infectious outcomes. A single randomized controlled trial (RCT) of mostly surgical cases in an intensive-care setting showed a clear benefit of maintaining blood glucoses between 80 and 110 mg/dl (4.4–6.1 mmol) in decreasing mortality and sepsis when compared with conventional glycemic control. Subsequently, many studies, including a large multicenter study of mixed surgical and medical patients

Table 51.1 Mechanical Factors Contributing to Infections in Patients with Diabetes

Physiological Change	Disease Process	Result
Ischemic changes	Chronic diabetic vascular disease	Mixed bacterial foot infections
Depressed cough reflex	Cerebrovascular insults	Pneumonia
Impaired bladder emptying	Autonomic neuropathy	Urinary tract infections
Fecal incontinence	Autonomic neuropathy	Cutaneous maceration
Impaired mobility	Various abnormalities	Pressure sores

DOI: 10.2337/9781580405096.51

Table 51.2 Empiric Antimicrobial Treatment

Organ system	Usual organism	Primary therapy	Alternate therapy
Urinary Tract			
Bacteriuria			
Asymptomatic male or female		No treatment	
Pregnancy	Aerobic Gram-negative bacilli and staph hemolyticus	amoxicillin, trimethoprim-sulfamethoxazole	
Acute uncomplicated cystitis/urethritis	*E. coli, Staph saphrophyticus*	trimethoprim-sulfamethoxazole or nitrofurantoin with pyridium	ciprofloxacin or levofloxacin or moxifloxacin or fosfomycin plus pyridium
Acute pyelonephritis	*E. coli* Enterococci		
Hospitalized		fluoroquinolones third-generation cephalosporin ampicillin + gentamicin piperacillin/tazobactam	ticarcillin/clavulanate or piperacillin/tazobactam vancomycin ampicillin/sulbactam
Perinephric abscess (drainage as required)			
With pyelonephritis	*E. coli*	Treat as for acute pyelonephritis as above	
With *S. aureus* bacteremia	*S. aureus*	naficillin or oxacillin	cephazolin vancomycin
Gall Bladder			
Cholecystitis	Enterobacteriaceae Enterococci, Bacteroides	piperacillin/ tazobactam ampicillin/sulbactam ticarcillin/clavulanate	ceftazidime plus metronidazole aztreonam plus clindamycin ampicillin plus gentamicin with or without metronidazole
If life threatening		imipenem/cilastatin or meropenem	
Emphysematous	Polymicrobial including Clostridium species	imipenem/cilastatin or meropenem	
Ear, Nose, and Throat			
Rhinocerebral mucormycosis	Mucor and Rhizopus species	Lipo Amphotericin B	
Invasive otitis externa	Pseudomonas aeruginosa	ciprofloxacin ceftazidime	imipenem/cilastatin meropenem piperacillin

Organ system	Usual organism	Primary therapy	Alternate therapy
Foot			
Non–limb threatening			
Mild, previously untreated*	S. aureus, strepto-cocci	clindamycin, cephalosporin amoxacillin/clavula-nate	
Chronic	Polymicrobial; S. aureus, strep, E. coli, Proteus, Klebsiella, Anaer-obes (e.g., B. fragilis)	ampicillin/sulbactam piperacillin/ tazobactam ticarcillin/clavulanate clindamycin plus cef-triaxone or cefotaxime	
Limb and life threatening	Polymicrobial: as above (see chronic infections)	imipenem/cilastatin or meropenem plus van-comycin	
Soft Tissue			
Necrotizing fasciitis	Group A streptococ-cus, Clostridia spe-cies, Polymicrobial	penicillin G plus clindamycin imipenem/cilastatin meropenem	

Note: *Shallow and no ischemia, abscess, or osteomyelitis. All antimicrobial use and dosing should take into account renal and hepatic function, clinical circumstance, contraindications, and drug toxicity. These are examples of regimens likely to be effective. Other regimens also may be effective in specific circumstances. Examples of third-generation cephalosporins are ceftriaxone and cefotaxime.

(Normoglycemia in Intensive Care Evaluation-Survival Using Glucose Algorithm Regulation [NICE-SUGAR]), showed no decrease in morbidity or mortality from sepsis. There is, however, clear evidence of increased hypoglycemia in all studies with intensive glycemic control. Thus, although patients may benefit from good glycemic control in terms of decreasing the intensity and severity of infections, in the intensive-care setting, there is no clear benefit beyond moderate glucose control, and intensive glucose control is likely to be associated with poorer overall outcomes. Moderate glucose control is recommended between 140 and 180 mg/dl (7.7 and 10 mmol/l) unless lower levels can be achieved safely.[3]

SUPERFICIAL TISSUE INFECTIONS

Minor trauma to tissues affected by vascular insufficiency often initiates superficial tissue infection. In addition, peripheral sensory neuropathy leads to the occurrence of an insensibility to minor injuries, which delays care. Infection may take the form of a cellulitis, soft tissue necrosis, draining sinus, or osteomyelitis. Although the feet are most commonly involved in these infections, a similar process can occur in the skin beneath pressure points. In both situations, tissue undermining can be extensive.

FOOT ULCERS AND DIABETES

Diabetic foot infections with ulcers are common and can be broadly divided into two categories: non–limb-threatening and limb-threatening infections. There are other more complex classifications.[4]

Non–Limb-Threatening Infections

Non–limb-threatening infections are associated with shallow ulcers, minimal cellulitis, minimal or no tissue necrosis, and no systemic symptoms. Treatment involves wound care and oral antibiotics. Gram-positive bacteria such as group A streptococci, *Staphylococcus aureus*, and possibly coagulase-negative staphylococci usually are involved. Oral antibiotics are acceptable to use depending on the severity of the infection and include dicloxacillin, cephalexin, amoxicillin/clavulanate, or clindamycin. A culture of the exudate would be useful if methicillin-resistant *S. aureus* (MRSA) is prevalent locally. Oral agents for MRSA include trimethoprim/sulfamethoxazole and doxycycline, and these two antibiotics generally have poor activity against β-hemolytic streptococci. Familiarity with local susceptibility patterns is helpful. Maintaining good control of glucose levels is very important. Frequent observation is necessary to ensure that healing occurs. Antibiotics should be given for at least 1–2 weeks' duration and potentially longer, depending on the clinical situation.

Limb-Threatening Infections

Limb-threatening infections are associated with ulcers that usually are deep; the infection extends to the subcutaneous tissue or deeper with significant tissue necrosis and systemic symptoms. Patients must be hospitalized, and surgical evaluation (and often intervention) is essential. The bacteriology of these infections includes Gram-positive bacteria, Gram-negative bacteria (e.g., *Escherichia coli* and *Pseudomonas aeruginosa*), and anaerobic bacteria (e.g., *Bacteroides fragilis* and *Peptostreptococcus species*). Deep-wound cultures and Gram stains (preferably scrapings or curettage of tissue) should be done to determine therapy. In addition to determining the bacteriology, antimicrobial susceptibility must be determined in view of the increasing antimicrobial resistance of Gram-negative and Gram-positive bacteria (i.e., MRSA). Empiric intravenous antibiotic therapy is directed at the presumed organisms previously mentioned. Examples of such regimens include piperacillin/tazobactam, ampicillin/sulbactam, ertrapenem, imipenem/cilastatin, or meropenem and there are many other potentially effective regimens.[4] The clinically recommended duration of therapy is around 2–4 weeks considering the clinical response. Any regimen used should take into account such features as local antimicrobial susceptibility data (i.e., the prevalence of MRSA), drug toxicity, and contraindications.

Patients with diabetes are more susceptible to developing severe necrotizing or gangrenous infections. These may be monomicrobial (i.e., caused by *Streptococcus* species, primarily β-hemolytic streptococcus such as group A) or polymicrobial. Immediate surgical intervention is warranted. Broad-spectrum antibiotic therapy is indicated for polymicrobial infection. In group A streptococcal necrotizing fasciitis (which may result in streptococcal toxic shock syndrome [TSS]), both high-dose penicillin and clindamycin should be used. Anecdotal data suggest that intravenous immune globulin may be beneficial in treating streptococcal TSS. The use of hyperbaric oxygen has shown mixed results and may be used as an adjunctive therapy in a select group of patients with diabetic foot ulcers that are difficult to heal.[5]

Osteomyelitis is a complication of deep tissue infection or a large foot ulcer. The diagnosis may be difficult to establish clinically and may require magnetic resonance imaging. Bone culture and histology are definitive diagnostic modalities and are used in cases of diagnostic uncertainty or poor therapeutic response to empiric treatment. Surgical removal of infected bone is one treatment option accompanied by a short course of antibiotic treatment. The medical treatment of persistent bone infection includes prolonged duration of antibiotics, usually >4 weeks.

MALIGNANT OTITIS EXTERNA

Malignant otitis externa is an infection usually caused by *P. aeruginosa* that occurs almost exclusively in patients with diabetes. It is a chronic erosive process that initially involves the soft tissue and cartilage around the external auditory canal. There is pain and drainage of purulent material and progressive destruction as the process progresses into the temporal and petrous bones and mastoids. The infection progresses regardless of tissue planes and ultimately reaches cranial nerves, the meninges, or the sigmoid sinus. Paralysis of nerves 7, 9, 10, 11, and possibly 12 may occur. A computed tomography (CT) scan of the head should be performed to identify the extent of bony involvement, intracranial extension, or presence of an abscess. CT changes are late findings, however. Therefore, early in the right clinical context, a nonspecific, but highly sensitive Technetium Tc 99m methylene diphosphate bone scan may be performed to increase the diagnostic probability. Treatment consists of local debridement of necrotic tissue and prolonged therapy with antipseudomonal antibiotics like ceftazidime or fluroquinolones, especially ciprofloxacin, along with good glucose control. Because osteomyelitis usually is present, the course of therapy should be at least 6–8 weeks.[6] Useful antimicrobial agents are listed in Table 51.2.

URINARY TRACT INFECTIONS

Patients with diabetes are at increased risk of urinary tract infections (UTI) and the risk increases with poor control and longer duration of diabetes. Women with diabetes have a two- to fourfold higher incidence of bacteriuria than women without diabetes and men with diabetes. *E. coli* and other Gram-negative bacteria cause most UTIs. UTI as a result of hematogenous infection most commonly is caused by *S. aureus*; it warrants serious consideration of line sepsis or endocarditis and further investigation. Although asymptomatic bacteriuria precedes symptomatic bacteriuria, there is no evidence that therapy for asymptomatic bacteriuria is beneficial because relapse rates are high and therapy does not prevent the development of symptomatic UTIs. Screening for asymptomatic bacteriuria in women with diabetes therefore is not recommended.[7]

Acute pyelonephritis is significantly more common in females than males. The clinical presentation and the response to therapy in patients with diabetes compared with those without diabetes are similar. A failure to respond to appropriate therapy raises the possibility of complications, including perinephric abscess, renal papillary necrosis, emphysematous cystitis, or emphysematous pyelonephritis. These complications need to be rapidly diagnosed and aggressively treated. When upper UTI is suspected, patients should be hospitalized and treated with intravenous antibiotics (usually broad spectrum and then tailored to culture results) and hydration. If there is poor response after 3–4 days of therapy, these complications should be explored using radiological investigations. The usual duration of therapy in uncomplicated infection with intravenous and subsequent oral antibiotics is 14 days.[8]

Candida UTIs usually are associated with indwelling bladder catheters or anatomic abnormalities. Less commonly, hematogenous spread occurs. *Candida* UTIs rarely occur otherwise. The presentation of *Candida* UTIs is similar to that of bacterial cystitis. Parenchymal involvement may result in pyelonephritis, abscess formation, or the development of fungus balls (which also may cause obstruction). Treatment consists of removal of the urinary catheters or the correction of anatomic abnormality. Most symptomatic infections are caused by *Candida albicans* and are treated with fluconazole. Resistance to fluconazole is rare. There is no clear benefit to treating asymptomatic infection unless there is a plan for instrumentation.

ABDOMINAL INFECTIONS

Cholecystitis incidence may be no more common in patients with diabetes compared with the general population, but emphysematous cholecystitis occurs with an increased frequency in these patients. Approximately 35% of the cases occur in patients with diabetes, and emphysematous cholecystitis is associated with increased mortality in 15% of patients with diabetes compared with <4% of individuals without diabetes. The presentation is similar to that of uncomplicated cholecystitis. The presence of crepitations, clinical deterioration, or failure to improve with conservative therapy should lead to radiological evaluation. Surgical intervention, in addition to broad-spectrum antimicrobial therapy, may be lifesaving.

PULMONARY INFECTIONS

It is not clear whether diabetes is associated with an increased incidence of pneumonia. However, the spectrum of pneumonia is different in patients with diabetes.[9] There is an increased frequency of infections with Gram-negative bacteria (e.g., *Klebsiella* and *E. coli*); *S. aureus*; *Mycobacterium tuberculosis*; and certain fungi, such as *Aspergillus, Mucor, Cryptococcus*, and *Coccidiodes*. Other infections caused by *Streptococcus pneumoniae* (especially bacteremia), the influenza virus, and *Legionella* may be associated with increased morbidity and mortality. This spectrum of pulmonary infections needs to be considered with regard to diagnosis, (empiric) treatment, and clinical follow-up to ensure that the infection is resolving appropriately.[10] Table 51.3 outlines an empiric approach to antimicrobial treatment for pulmonary infections.

Table 51.3 Empirical Selection of Antimicrobial Agents for Treating Patients with Community-Acquired Pneumonia

Outpatients

Generally preferred agents are (not in any particular order) as follows: doxycycline, a macrolide, or a respiratory fluoroquinolone. Selection considerations:
- These agents have activity against the most likely pathogens in this setting, which include *Streptococcus pneumoniae, Mycoplasma pneumoniae,* and *Chlamydia pneumoniae.*
- Selection should be influenced by regional antibiotic susceptibility patterns for *S. pneumoniae* and the presence of other risk factors for drug-resistant *S. pneumoniae.*
- Penicillin-resistant pneumococci may be resistant to macrolides and/or doxycycline. Consider use of respiratory fluroquinolones or β-lactam plus macrolide.
- For older patients or those with underlying comorbidities like diabetes, chronic lung, liver, or kidney disease, immunosuppression with a fluoroquinolone or a β-lactam plus macrolide may be a preferred choice; some authorities prefer to reserve fluoroquinolones for such patients.

Hospitalized patients

General medical ward and non-intensive-care-unit patients
Generally preferred agents are as follows: an extended-spectrum cephalosporin combined with a macrolide or a β-lactam/β-lactamase inhibitor combined with a macrolide or a fluoroquinolone (alone).

Intensive care unit
Generally preferred agents are as follows: an extended spectrum cephalosporin* or β-lactam/β-lactamase inhibitor† plus either fluoroquinolone‡ or macrolide§. Alternatives or modifying factors are as follows:
- Structural lung disease: antipseudomonal agents (piperacillin, piperacillin/tazobactam, carbapenem, or cefepime) plus a fluoroquinolone (including high-dose ciprofloxacin)
- β-lactam allergy: fluoroquinolone plus Aztreonam or β-lactam plus macrolide and aminoglycoside

Note: There is no recent update from the Infectious Diseases Society of America, but there is no change for community-acquired pneumonia.

*Extended-spectrum cephalosporin: cefotaxime or ceftriaxone.

†β-lactam/β-lactamase inhibitor: ampicillin/sulbactam or pipercillin/tazobactam.

‡Fluoroquinolone: gemifloxacin, levofloxacin, moxifloxacin, or other fluoroquinolone with enhanced activity against *pneumoniae* (for aspiration pneumonia, some fluoroquinolones show in vitro activity against anaerobic pulmonary pathogens, although there are no clinical studies to verify activity in vivo).

§Macrolide: azithromycin, clarithromycin, or erythromycin.

Source: Adapted from Mandell LA, Wunderink RG, Anzueto A, Bartlett JG, Campbell GD, Dean NC, Dowell SF, File TM Jr, Musher DM, Niederman MO, Torres A, Whitney OQ; Infectious Diseases Society of America; American Thoracic Society. Infectious Diseases Society of America/American Thoracic Society consensus guidelines on the management of community-acquired pneumonia in adults. *Clin Infect Dis* 2007;44(Suppl 2):S27–S72.

Reprinted with permission from the publisher.[10]

A large retrospective U.K. report with 7-year follow-up showed that of the community-acquired infections among elderly patients with diabetes, lower respiratory tract infections were the most common, followed by UTIs (155 and 99.6 per 1,000 patient-years, respectively) and sepsis. Within 28 days of diagnosis of pneumonia (10.6 per patient-year), 80% were hospitalized and 32% had died. These data should inform future preventive actions.[11]

Prevention of pneumonia should be addressed in all patients with diabetes. The Advisory Committee on Immunization Practices recommends that all patients with diabetes be vaccinated once with the pneumococcal vaccine and annually with the influenza vaccine. The evidence for the efficacy of pneumococcal vaccines for preventing pneumonia in the elderly with or without diabetes is not conclusive.

SPECIFIC ORGANISM-RELATED INFECTIONS

FUNGAL INFECTIONS AND MUCORMYCOSIS

Much less common but much more devastating is infection caused by the agents of mucormycosis (primarily the *Zygomycetes*). The syndrome most often seen in patients with diabetes is rhinocerebral mucormycosis. This is an invasive process caused by the mycelia of the genera *Mucor, Absidia, Rhizopus, Cunninghamella*, and others. The conidia of the organisms are unable to regenerate if ingested by normal macrophages, and the organisms are essentially nonpathogenic in the normal host. The growth of *Rhizopus* is inhibited by normal human serum. These fungi, however, can grow rapidly in the presence of high concentrations of glucose and in an acid environment. Both conditions prevail in the patient with ketoacidosis. In such patients, these organisms are able to germinate at the site of infections (usually the nares and the sinuses) and to begin a rapid necrotizing process that characterizes rhinocerebral mucormycosis. Within a few days, the process may extend from a small eschar on the nasal septum to involve the paranasal sinuses and orbit. The infection proceeds without regard for tissue planes. It can track into the brain within a few days, and the result often is lethal if not diagnosed and treated at an early stage.

Diagnosis is by prompt aggressive surgical biopsy, including tissues deep to the area of necrosis. *Zygomycetes* are different from other fungi in that they stain better with hematoxylin and eosin than with methenamine silver. Identification of irregular pleomorphic nonseptate branching hyphae is pathognomonic. *Zygomycetes* must be differentiated from *Aspergillus*, which is the most similar in appearance.

The hyphae of *Aspergillus* do not stain well with hematoxylin and eosin. Treatment of zygomycosis infection includes correction of ketoacidosis, vigorous and repeated surgical debridement, and antifungal therapy with amphotericin B. Azole antifungal drugs are not effective against *Zygomycetes*, although posaconazole, an orally administered triazole, has shown promise as a salvage therapy and an option for oral step-down therapy. Posaconazole is not approved by the U.S. Food and Drug Administration for the treatment of zygomycosis and is available for unlabeled use. Other fungal infections with increased incidence in diabetes are candidiasis, coccidioidomycosis, and aspergillosis.

HUMAN IMMUNODEFICIENCY INFECTION

According to World Health Organization statistics, AIDS, caused by HIV, affects nearly 35 million people in the world. Diabetes is common in these patients because of an increasing life span due to the availability of antiretroviral drug therapy, as well as due to a direct increased risk associated with both HIV infection and antiretroviral drug therapy. It is postulated that HIV proteins, like Tat and Vpr, cause increased tumor necrosis factor-α and inhibit peroxisome proliferator-activated receptor-γ activity, respectively, resulting in increased inflammation that may lead to insulin resistance. The antiretrovirals, including nucleoside reverse-transcriptase inhibitors (NRTIs) and protease inhibitors, also contribute to insulin resistance and diabetes.[12] More recently, NRTIs have been associated with less frequent diabetes. Management of HIV infection in diabetes is the same as in patients without diabetes. The interaction and adverse effect profile of different medications used for treatment of these diseases, however, can cause increased morbidity and mortality (e.g., lactic acidosis with metformin and NRTIs such as stavudine).

TUBERCULOSIS

Both type 1 and type 2 diabetes increase the risk for active and more severe tuberculosis. Among patients with diabetes, higher A1C levels are associated with a greater hazard of active tuberculosis. Thus, there is increased overlap of the population at risk for both diabetes and tuberculosis and the combination of the two represents a worldwide threat. All patients with diabetes should undergo tuberculin skin testing to diagnose latent tuberculosis infection. The risk of a patient with diabetes with a positive skin test developing active tuberculosis is two- to fourfold greater than that for a patient without diabetes with the same positive test. Patients with diabetes with a positive tuberculin skin test >10 mm should be considered strongly for preventive chemotherapy once active tuberculosis is excluded.[13] Diabetes increases tuberculosis risk because of hyperglycemia and impaired macrophage and lymphocyte function, leading to diminished ability to contain the organism. Conversely, an infection like tuberculosis worsens glycemic control in patients with diabetes. Pulmonary tuberculosis in patients with diabetes may present with an atypical radiographic pattern and distribution with lower lung involvement, multilobar and cavitary disease. The treatment of tuberculosis in diabetes is the same as in nondiabetic patients. Some studies have shown increased risk of treatment failure in diabetic patients. The glycemic control may worsen with antitubercular therapy, especially with rifampicin. The serum concentration of glyburide, glipizide, and pioglitazone are decreased when given concurrently with rifampicin. Finally, some patients on insulin therapy might have increased requirements when taking rifampicin.[14]

CONCLUSION

Infection in diabetes presents as a challenge due to altered host immune response, hyperglycemia, and delayed wound healing. Both humoral and cell-mediated immunity dysfunction result in infections being more common and/or severe in patients with diabetes, particularly those with poorly controlled glucose. The diagnostic techniques remain the same as for individuals without diabetes. The consensus is that glycemic targets during treatment for infections should be moderate (140–180 mg/dl). The response to treatment is probably less effective and prolonged in nature because of the noted risk factors.

REFERENCES

1. Joshi N, Caputo GM, Weitekamp MR, Karchmer AW. Infections in patients with diabetes mellitus. *N Engl J Med* 1999;341:1906–1912.

2. Calvert HM, Yoshikawa T. Infections in diabetes. *Infect Dis Clin North Am* 2001;15:407–421.

3. NICE-SUGAR Study Investigators; Finfer S Chittock DR, Su SY, Blair D, Foster D, Dhingra V, et al. Intensive versus conventional glucose control in critically ill patients. *N Engl J Med* 2009;360(13):1283–1297.

4. Lipsky BA, Berendt AR, Cornia PB, Pile JC, Peters EJ, Armstrong DG, Deery HG, Embil JM, Joseph WS, Karchmer AW, Pinzur MS, Senneville E; Infectious Diseases Society of America. 2012 Infectious Diseases Society of America clinical practice guideline for the diagnosis and treatment of diabetic foot infections. *Clin Infect Dis* 2012 ;54(12):e132–173.

5. Londahl M. Hyperbaric oxygen therapy as adjunctive treatment of diabetic foot ulcers. *Med Clin North Am* 2013;97(5):957–980.

6. Carfrae MJ, Kesser BW. Malignant otitis externa. *Otolaryngol Clin North Am* 2008;41(3):537–549.

7. Harding GKM, Zhanel GG, Nicolle LE, Cheang M; Manitoba Diabetes Urinary Tract Infection Study Group. Antimicrobial treatment in diabetic women with asymptomatic bacteriuria. *N Engl J Med* 2002;347:1576–1583.

8. Nicolle LE, Bradley S, Colgan R, Rice JC, Schaeffer A, Hooton TM; Infectious Diseases Society of America; American Society of Nephrology; American Geriatric Society. Infectious Diseases Society of America guidelines for the diagnosis and treatment of asymptomatic bacteriuria in adults. *Clin Infect Dis* 2005;40:643–654.

9. Fisher-Hoch SP, Mathews CE, McCormick JB. Obesity, diabetes and pneumonia: the menacing interface of non-communicable and infectious diseases. *Trop Med Int Health* 2013;18(12):1510–1519.

10. Mandell LA, Wunderink RG, Anzueto A, Bartlett JG, Campbell GD, Dean NC, Dowell SF, File TM Jr, Musher DM, Niederman MS, Torres A, Whitney CG; Infectious Diseases Society of America; American Thoracic Society. Infectious Diseases Society of America/American Thoracic Society consensus guidelines on the management of community-acquired pneumonia in adults. *Clin Infect Dis* 2007;44(Suppl 2):S27–S72.

11. McDonald HI, Nitsch D, Millett ERC, Sinclair A, Thomas SL. New estimates of the burden of acute community-acquired infections among older people with diabetes mellitus: a retrospective cohort study using linked electronic health records. *Diabet Med* 2013 Dec 16. Available at http://www.ncbi.nlm.nih.gov/pubmed/24341529. Accessed 31 March 2014.

12. Paik IJ, Kotler DP. The prevalence and pathogenesis of diabetes mellitus in treated HIV-infection. *Best Pract Res Clin Endocrinol Metab* 2011;25(3):469–478.

13. Dooley KE, Chaisson RE. Tuberculosis and diabetes mellitus: convergence of two epidemics. *Lancet Infect Dis* 2009;9(12):737–746.

14. Blumberg HM, Burman WJ, Chaisson RE, Daley CL, Etkind SC, Friedman LN, Fujiwara P, Grzemska M, Hopewell PC, Iseman MD, Jasmer RM, Koppaka V, Menzies RI, O'Brien RJ, Reves RR, Reichman LB, Simone PM, Starke JR, Vernon AA. American Thoracic Society/Centers for Disease Control and Prevention/Infectious Disease Society of America: treatment of tuberculosis. *Am J Respir Crit Care Med* 2003;167:603–663.

Chapter 52
Skin and Subcutaneous Tissues

Jean L. Bolognia, MD
Irwin M. Braverman, MD

T his chapter discusses several cutaneous disorders, including diabetic cheiro-arthropathy (waxy skin and stiff joints), scleredema, diabetic dermopathy, necrobiosis lipoidica (NL; diabeticorum), disseminated granuloma annulare, eruptive xanthomas, lipodystrophy, acanthosis nigricans, diabetic bullae, necrolytic migratory erythema (NME; glucagonoma syndrome), and reactions to oral hypoglycemic drugs and insulin. Patients who have diabetes as a component of the autoimmune polyendocrine syndrome have an increased prevalence of vitiligo, while individuals with diabetic nephropathy requiring dialysis can develop the keratotic papules of acquired perforating dermatosis. Cutaneous infections (e.g., candidiasis, pyoderma, and mucormycosis) and lower extremity ulcerations are covered in other chapters in this book.

PATHOPHYSIOLOGY

The underlying pathophysiology is theoretical in most of the cutaneous disorders associated with diabetes. The skin lesions of NL and diabetic dermopathy have histological evidence of microangiopathy, and this presumably plays a role in the formation of lesions. In diabetic cheiroarthropathy, the thickened dermis may be the result of an increase in glycosylated insoluble collagen. The epidermal hyperplasia seen in lesions of acanthosis nigricans is thought to result from the action of circulating insulin on insulin-like growth factor receptors on keratinocytes and fibroblasts, whereas the epidermal necrosis seen in NME may be a reflection of glucagon-induced hypoaminoacidemia. Hypertriglyceridemia and eruptive xanthomas in the setting of diabetes are presumably due to the effects of hypoinsulinemia on lipid metabolism in that they quickly resolve after insulin administration.

DIABETIC CHEIROARTHROPATHY

Up to 30% of young patients (ages 1–28 years) with type 1 diabetes (T1D) have painless limited mobility of the small and large joints, and in individuals with diabetes for >5 years, the severity of joint disease is correlated with microvascular complications. Although involvement of the small joints of the hands can be demonstrated by the failure of the palmar surfaces of the interphalangeal joints to approximate ("prayer sign") (Figure 52.1) or the inability to place the palms flat

 DOI: 10.2337/9781580405096.52

on a tabletop ("tabletop sign"), clinical detection may require passive extension of the digits. Approximately a third of patients with limited joint mobility have tight, thick, waxy skin of the dorsal aspect of the hands that is difficult to tent (i.e., is less extensible). This increased thickness can be confirmed by high-resolution ultrasonography, whereas thickening and enhancement of the flexor tendon sheaths may be seen by magnetic resonance imaging. Of note, thickened skin has been observed primarily in individuals with moderate to severe joint disease. These skin findings may reverse with improved control of diabetes, including pancreatic transplant; otherwise, there is no well-established treatment.

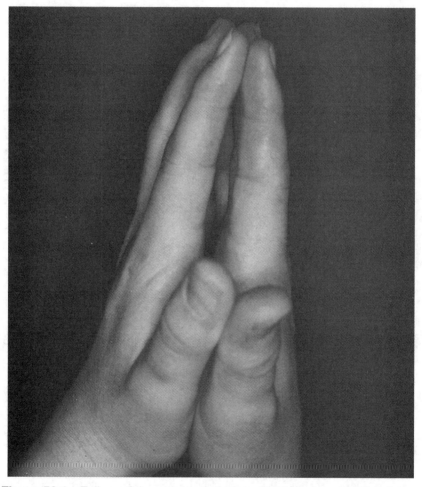

Figure 52.1—Failure of the palmar surfaces of interphalangeal joints to approximate in a patient with cheiroarthropathy, also referred to as stiff joints and waxy skin. This clinical finding is known as the "prayer sign."

SCLEREDEMA

In scleredema, there is a thickening of the skin due to the deposition of glycosaminoglycans (in particular, hyaluronic acid) within the dermis. Areas of involvement may not be visually apparent, although they can develop a *peau d'orange* (orange peel) appearance as a result of prominent and depressed follicular openings (Figure 52.2). The extent of involvement is best appreciated by palpation of the induration. Because scleredema is found most commonly on the upper back and posterior neck, the patient may be unaware of its presence. On physical examination, however, there is often decreased range of motion of the neck, especially dorsal extension. Less common sites of involvement include the face, upper arms, chest, lower back, and tongue. Rarely, there is cardiac, muscular, or esophageal involvement.

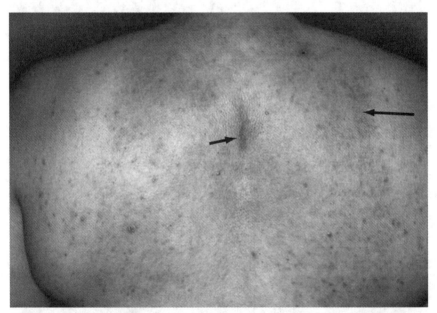

Figure 52.2—Scleredema of the upper back with overlying erythema (*large arrow*) and development of *peau d'orange* appearance centrally (*small arrow*).

Scleredema has been associated with a monoclonal gammopathy or preceding streptococcal and viral infections as well as T1D and type 2 diabetes (T2D; usually long-standing T2D). In the form seen in patients with diabetes, the induration may be accompanied by erythema (Figure 52.2), which might be misdiagnosed as treatment-resistant cellulitis.

There is no consistently effective treatment for scleredema, although sometimes, especially in patients without diabetes, spontaneous resolution may occur.

In symptomatic patients, a 12-week course of PUVA [psoralens (8-methoxypso-ralen, 0.4–0.6 mg/kg) plus ultraviolet A (UVA)] or UVA1 (340–400 nm) can be considered. In a small series of patients with T1D, intraperitoneal insulin delivery led to improvement after several months. For severe disease, there are case reports of the use of electron beam therapy.

DIABETIC DERMOPATHY

Diabetic dermopathy is characterized by multiple hyperpigmented macules on the extensor surface of the distal lower extremities (Figure 52.3). The individual lesions range in size from 0.5 to 2 cm, are oval or circular, and may have associated atrophy and scale. These skin changes also have been referred to as "shin spots" or "pigmented pretibial patches" and are thought to represent an abnormal response to trauma. In one series of 393 patients with T2D, 12.5% had evidence of diabetic dermopathy, whereas in a second series of 173 patients (with both T1D and T2D), 40% had such lesions, in particular, individuals >50 years of age. These skin lesions also may be seen in individuals without evidence of glucose intolerance, albeit less often. In general, the dermopathy is asymptomatic except for its appearance, and no effective treatment has been described. A higher prevalence of neuropathy, retinopathy, nephropathy, and large-vessel disease, however, has been reported in patients with diabetic dermopathy as compared with individuals without such skin lesions.

NECROBIOSIS LIPOIDICA

Skin lesions of NL (diabeticorum) are so named because of *1)* the presence of necrobiosis or degeneration of collagen in the dermis, *2)* the yellow color of most well-developed lesions due to carotene and lipid, and *3)* the association with diabetes. The disorder is characterized by red-brown to violet plaques that enlarge and frequently become yellow centrally (Figure 52.4). In addition, there is atrophy of the epidermis, which leads to shiny transparent skin and visualization of underlying dermal and subcutaneous vessels. The most common location for NL is the shin (seen in 90% of patients), but lesions also can occur on the scalp, face, and arms. Plaques may ulcerate, especially those on the distal lower extremities.

NL is uncommon, occurring in 0.1–0.3% of the population with diabetes, usually during the third or fourth decade of life. There is some disagreement, however, as to the proportion of patients with NL who actually have frank diabetes. The range that usually is cited is 40–65%, based primarily on clinical series from the 1950s and 1960s. In a more recent retrospective study of consecutive patients seen over a period of 25 years, only 7 (11%) of 65 patients with classic biopsy-proven NL had diabetes at presentation.

There is no well-established treatment for NL, but in small series, some success has been reported with topical corticosteroids (with or without occlusion), pentoxifylline (400 mg three times per day), nicotinamide (500 mg three times per day), clofazimine (200 mg/day), and dipyridamole (50–75 mg three to four times

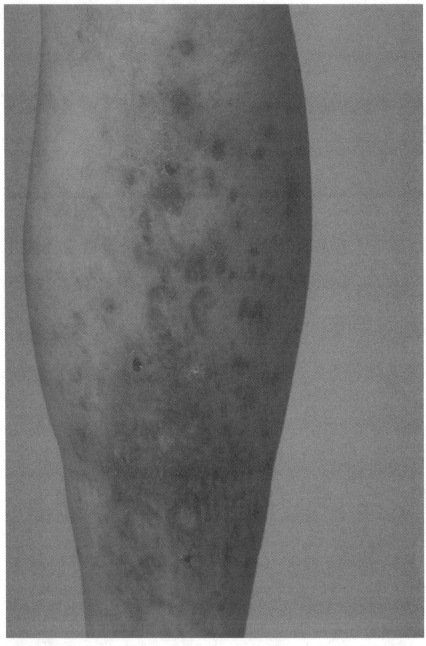

Figure 52.3—Hyperpigmented macules on the shin of a patient with diabetic dermopathy.

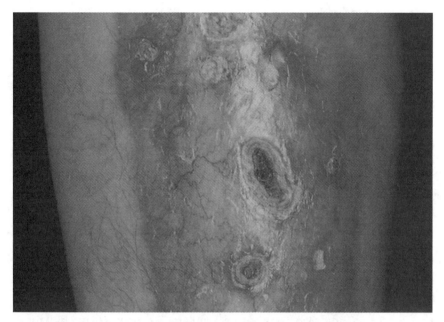

Figure 52.4—Necrobiosis lipoidica of the anterior lower extremity.

per day) plus low-dose aspirin (325 mg/day). A double-blind, placebo-controlled trial of a combination of the latter two medications, however, showed no significant benefit. Intralesional injections of corticosteroids (5 mg/ml triamcinolone acetonide) can be used to treat the active borders of the lesions. If ulceration occurs, the injections should be discontinued.

DISSEMINATED GRANULOMA ANNULARE

Granuloma annulare is characterized by annular or arciform plaques that form from the coalescence of skin-colored, pink, or red-brown papules (Figure 52.5). The skin in the center of the lesion may be normal or slightly erythematous in appearance. Most commonly, granuloma annulare has a localized acral distribution, but the lesions can be more numerous, papular, and located on the trunk as well as the extremities. The term generalized or disseminated granuloma annulare is used to describe the latter patients. The clinical diagnosis can be confirmed by performing a skin biopsy. A patient with generalized granuloma annulare should be screened for glucose intolerance because in one series of 100 patients with generalized granuloma annulare, 21% were shown to have diabetes. The etiology of granuloma annulare is unknown, and the treatment is empiric and includes topical and intralesional corticosteroids (5 mg/ml triamcinolone acetonide), topical calcineurin inhibitors (twice daily), oral niacinamide (500 mg three times per

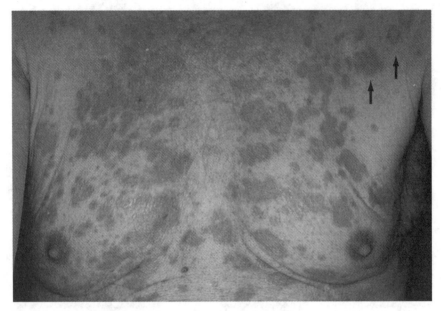

Figure 52.5—Generalized granuloma annulare. The annular shape of the lesions is best seen on the left shoulder (arrows).

day), and, in severe cases, PUVA two to three times per week or oral hydroxychloroquine (200–400 mg/day). There are also case reports of the use of tumor necrosis factor-α for extensive disease.

ERUPTIVE XANTHOMAS

There are several types of cutaneous xanthomas, including eruptive, tendinous, tuberous, and planar, which are reflections of hypercholesterolemia or hypertriglyceridemia. Eruptive xanthomas can appear suddenly, and the lesions are usually 4–6 mm in diameter, firm, and yellow with a red base; the elbows, knees, buttocks, and sites of trauma are favored sites (Figure 52.6). Biopsy findings are diagnostic and demonstrate collections of lipids within the dermis. The most common scenario for the appearance of eruptive xanthomas is hypertriglyceridemia in the setting of poorly controlled diabetes. Administration of insulin results in a decrease in the circulating levels of triglycerides, and the xanthomas resolve relatively quickly. Xanthelasma (plane xanthoma of the eyelids) is the least specific marker of hyperlipidemia because 50% of the patients have normal lipid levels. In addition, there is no clear-cut association between diabetes and xanthelasma.

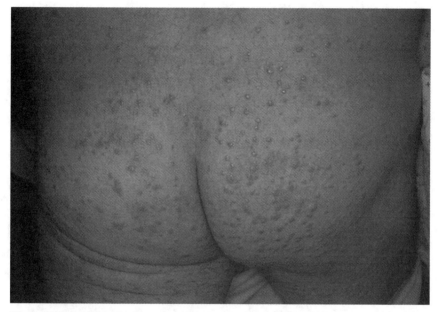

Figure 52.6—Eruptive xanthomas on the buttocks of a patient with poorly controlled diabetes.

LIPODYSTROPHY

Although the diseases outlined in this section are referred to as lipodystrophies, the patients have primarily lipoatrophy, and the lipoatrophy is divided into two major forms: total (generalized) and partial. In the generalized form, the entire body is involved. The onset is congenital (at birth or during infancy) in the familial (autosomal recessive) form of the disease and during the first to third decades of life in the sporadic form. In contrast, partial lipoatrophy usually involves the extremities or the upper portion of the body (face to hips), is sporadic or less often familial, and has its onset during childhood or at puberty. In biopsy specimens of areas of subcutaneous fat loss, the fat cells are present, but the cytoplasmic fat is absent.

Three forms of lipoatrophy are associated with insulin-resistant diabetes—familial generalized, familial partial, and acquired generalized. Patients with the inherited form of generalized lipoatrophy also have increased muscle mass, whereas individuals with all three forms have hypertriglyceridemia and fatty infiltration of the liver. In addition, those with familial (congenital) total lipoatrophy can have hyperpigmentation, acanthosis nigricans, and generalized hypertrichosis. The inherited forms of lipodystrophy are the result of mutations in genes that encode proteins involved in adipocyte differentiation, lipid droplet formation, and formation of the nuclear lamina.

ACANTHOSIS NIGRICANS

In acanthosis nigricans, velvety tan to dark-brown plaques are seen on the sides of the neck, axillae, and groin (Figure 52.7). Additional sites of involvement include the extensor surface of the small joints of the hand, the elbows, and the knees. Acanthosis nigricans can be a reflection of an underlying malignancy, usually adenocarcinoma of the gastrointestinal tract, but it is associated more commonly with insulin resistance and obesity.

The clinical spectrum in obese patients can range from euglycemia with mild hyperinsulinemia and tissue resistance to insulin-requiring diabetes. Acanthosis nigricans is also a cutaneous manifestation of the insulin-resistant syndromes (types A and B) and lipodystrophy (generalized and partial), as well as women with the HAIR-AN (hyperandrogenism, insulin resistance, acanthosis nigricans) syndrome. In obese patients, weight loss and improvement of tissue resistance to insulin has improved their acanthosis nigricans. Otherwise, treatment is limited to topical agents, such as tretinoin (0.05–0.1%), urea (10–25%), and α-hydroxy acids (lactic and glycolic), which can improve the cosmetic appearance.

DIABETIC BULLAE

The spontaneous formation of diabetic bullae (bullosis diabeticorum) in a primarily acral location (feet and distal lower extremities more than forearms and hands)

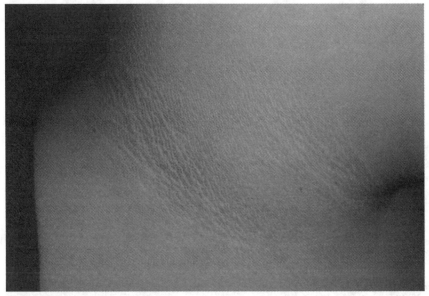

Figure 52.7—Velvety dark-brown plaques on the lateral neck of a patient with acanthosis nigricans.

is an uncommon manifestation of diabetes. The lesions arise from normal noninflamed skin and range in size from a few millimeters to several centimeters (Figure 52.8). The blisters are usually tense and contain clear viscous fluid that is sterile. There is no history of antecedent trauma, and the lesions may recur. Two major forms exist and are distinguished by the site of blister formation: *1*) the blister is intraepidermal and heals without scarring, or *2*) it is subepidermal and may heal with atrophy and mild scarring. Both types are found predominantly in middle-aged to elderly patients with long-standing diabetes who often have evidence of peripheral neuropathy. Other than local care—for example, drainage via placement of a small window in the roof of the most dependent portion of the bulla while leaving the remainder of the blister roof intact and topical antibiotics to prevent secondary infection—there is no specific recommended treatment.

NECROLYTIC MIGRATORY ERYTHEMA

Patients with NME have bright erythematous patches that most frequently are seen in the girdle area (lower abdomen, groin, buttocks, and thighs), perioral region, and extremities (Figure 52.9). The cutaneous finding that distinguishes NME from other migratory eruptions is the presence of superficial bullae at the active borders. Because the bullae rapidly break, only denuded areas and crusts may be observed clinically. These areas then heal with superficial desquamation as the erythema advances.

Histologically, swollen and necrotic keratinocytes are seen in the superficial layers of the epidermis, findings similar to those seen in acrodermatitis enteropathica. In addition to the cutaneous eruption, the patients frequently have glossitis, anemia, weight loss, and diarrhea, as well as diabetes.

Most patients with classic NME have an α-cell tumor of the pancreas and markedly elevated serum glucagon levels (a variant termed "necrolytic acral erythema" is a cutaneous marker of liver disease, usually due to hepatitis C virus). Removal of the pancreatic tumor can result in prompt resolution of the cutaneous eruption. In inoperable cases, the following treatments can lead to improvement: intermittent peripheral infusions of amino acids, zinc, and fatty acids; subcutaneous injections of the long-acting somatostatin analog octreotide acetate; somatostatin receptor-targeted radiotherapy; or transcatheter arterial embolization of hepatic metastases.

DRUG REACTIONS TO ORAL HYPOGLYCEMIC AGENTS AND INSULIN

Administration of oral hypoglycemic agents can lead to commonly recognized drug reactions, such as pruritus, urticaria, morbilliform eruptions, and Stevens–Johnson syndrome. Phototoxic (dose-related exaggerated sunburn) and photoallergic (idiosyncratic eczematous dermatitis in a photodistribution) eruptions are additional potential cutaneous side effects and are related to the sulfur moiety found in sulfonylureas. A unique reaction is the chlorpropamide alcohol flush, which is similar to the disulfiram alcohol flush; the latter is seen less often as the

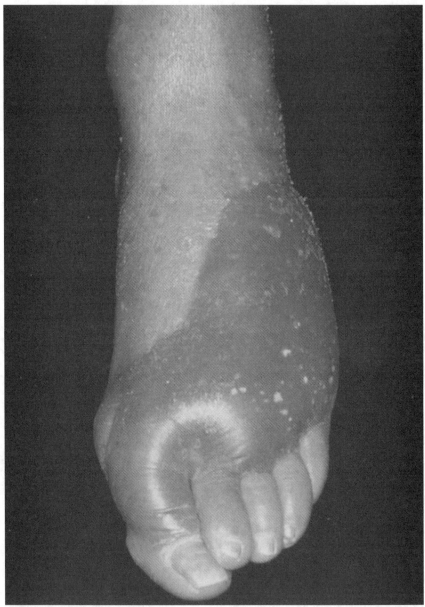

Figure 52.8—Tense large bulla on the dorsum of the foot that is characteristic of bullosis diabeticorum.

Source: Braverman IM. *Skin Signs of Systemic Disease.* 3rd ed. Philadelphia, Saunders, 1998. Reprinted with permission from the publisher.

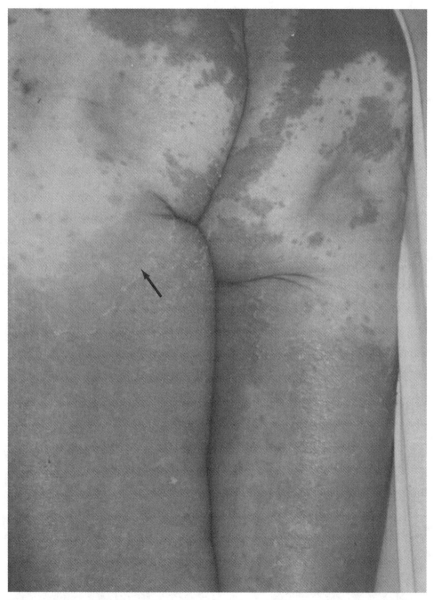

Figure 52.9—Angular erythematous patches on the buttocks and thighs of a patient with a gluoagonoma of the panoicas, aiiUw, peiipiieial des-quamation.

Source: Braverman IM. *Skin Signs of Systemic Disease.* 3rd ed. Philadelphia, Saunders, 1998. Reprinted with permission from the publisher.

use of second- and third-generation sulfonylureas increases. Lastly, rosiglitazone can lead to facial and peripheral edema.

The cutaneous reactions to insulin can be divided into localized reactions, generalized reactions, and lipoatrophy or lipohypertrophy. The localized reactions include pruritus, burning, erythema, induration, and, occasionally, ulceration at the insulin injection site. Allergic local reactions vary from the immediate formation of an urticarial lesion at the injection site to the appearance of a pruritic papule or nodule 24–48 hours after the injection. The latter lesions represent a delayed hypersensitivity reaction and, as such, heal slowly over a week or more and often leave residual hyperpigmentation. They frequently cease to form after several weeks or months. The primary treatment for persistent localized reactions is a switch to purer forms of insulin; if this is unsuccessful, the possibility of an allergy to the zinc, protamine, or preservative, such as paraben or meta-cresol, in the preparation should be considered as well as small quantities of natural latex rubber antigens from the insulin injection materials.

Generalized systemic reactions are uncommon and are characterized by pruritus, urticaria or angioedema, and serum sickness–like illnesses. The risk of a systemic reaction to insulin is related to the source and purification of the insulin, with bovine insulin having the highest incidence and human insulin the lowest. Diagnosis of immunoglobulin E (IgE)–mediated insulin allergy is based on measurement of specific IgE antibodies against insulin and protamine in addition to skin-prick or intracutaneous tests to insulin preparations and insulin additives. Treatment options for individuals already receiving human insulin include induction of tolerance via continuous subcutaneous insulin infusion, induction of tolerance via desensitization, and use of rapid-acting insulin analogs (e.g., insulin lispro).

Lipoatrophy at injection sites is seen with subcutaneous administration and is much less common with monocomponent or recombinant human insulin. Improvement in the areas of subcutaneous fat loss has been reported after injection of human insulin into the edge of the lipoatrophy. In patients already receiving human insulin, the use of a jet injector may prove beneficial. Lipohypertrophy (i.e., an increase in the amount of subcutaneous fat) can also be seen at the site of insulin injection. Treatment consists of rotation of injection sites and perhaps liposuction and the use of insulin lispro. Given the risk of malabsorption of insulin, injections should not be performed at sites of lipohypertrophy.

BIBLIOGRAPHY

Bolognia JL, Braverman IM. Cutaneous complications of type 1 diabetes. In *Type 1 Diabetes: Etiology and Treatment.* Sperling MA, Ed. Totowa, NJ, Humana Press, 2003, p. 485–499.

Braverman IM. *Skin Signs of Systemic Disease.* 3rd ed. Philadelphia, Saunders, 1998.

Heinzerling L, Raile K, Rochlitz H, Zuberbier T, Worm M. Insulin allergy: clinical manifestations and management strategies. *Allergy* 2008;63:148–155.

Jelenick JE. *The Skin in Diabetes.* Philadelphia, Lea & Febiger, 1986.

Krause WKH, Stutz N. *Cutaneous Manifestations of Endocrine Diseases.* Berlin, Springer, 2010.

Morgan AJ, Schwartz RA. Diabetic dermopathy: a subtle sign with grave implications. *J Am Acad Dermatol* 2008;58:447–451.

Perez MI, Kohn SR. Cutaneous manifestations of diabetes mellitus. *J Am Acad Dermatol* 1994;30:519–531.

Radermecker RP, Scheen AJ. Allergic reactions to insulin: effects of continuous subcutaneous insulin infusion and insulin analogues. *Diabetes Metab Res Rev* 2007;23:348–355.

Rosenbloom AL, Silverstein JH, Lezotte DC, Richardson K, McCallum M. Limited joint mobility in childhood diabetes mellitus indicates increased risk for microvascular disease. *N Engl J Med* 1981;305:191–194.

Tuchinda C, Kerr HA, Taylor CR, Jacobe H, Bergamo BM, Elmets C, Rivard J, Lim HW. UVA1 phototherapy for cutaneous diseases: an experience of 92 cases in the United States. *Photodermatol Photoimmunol Photomed* 2006;22:247–253.

Chapter 53

Hypogonadotropic Hypogonadism in Type 2 Diabetes

Paresh Dandona, MBBS, DPhil, FRCP, FACP, FACC, FACE
Ajay Chaudhuri, MBBS, MRCP (UK)
Sandeep Dhindsa, MBBS

Sidebar 53.1—Clinical Case

A 54-year-old man with type 2 diabetes (T2D) of 5 years' duration presents to a physician for consultation. He also has hypertension, hyperlipidemia, and erectile dysfunction. His BMI is 32 kg/m², and his blood pressure and pulse rate are 130/72 mmHg and 76 beats/minute, respectively. His medications are metformin 750 mg twice a day, glipizide XL 5 mg/day, aspirin 81 mg/day, atorvastatin 40 mg/day, ramipril 10 mg/day, and carvedilol 6.25 mg twice a day. He has tried sildenafil in the past but discontinued it due to lack of efficacy. On further questioning, he denies decrease in libido or energy. He is not depressed and has never had a fracture. Review of laboratory data show that his A1C is 6.5%, low-density lipoprotein (LDL) cholesterol is 80 mg/dl, high-density lipoprotein (HDL) cholesterol is 34 mg/dl, and triglycerides are 210 mg/dl. Urine albumin/creatinine ratio is 22 mg/gram. Complete blood count and metabolic panel are normal.
Question: Should testosterone concentration be measured in this patient?

Studies over the past few years have established clearly that at least 25% of men with type 2 diabetes (T2D) have subnormal free testosterone (FT) concentrations in association with inappropriately low luteinizing hormone (LH) and follicle-stimulating hormone (FSH) concentrations. These patients thus suffer from hypogonadotrophic hypogonadism (HH). Another 4% have subnormal testosterone concentrations with elevated LH and FSH concentrations.[1] Obesity and metabolic syndrome (MetS) also are associated with HH. This chapter reviews the information on this association, the clinical consequences of HH in these men, and the results of replacement with testosterone.

ASSOCIATION OF T2D WITH LOW TESTOSTERONE

It has been known for two decades that males with T2D frequently have low total testosterone concentrations.[2,3] It also has been shown in epidemiological studies that low testosterone concentrations predict the occurrence of T2D. Because testosterone is largely bound to sex hormone–binding globulin (SHBG, 44%) and albumin (54%), total testosterone does not reflect the bioavailability of testosterone at the cellular level.[4] Since SHBG concentrations also are low in obesity and

DOI: 10.2337/9781580405096.53

T2D, it was not clear whether FT concentrations were low in these patients and whether these patients were truly hypogonadal. Reliable assays for FT were not widely available until recently.

Assays based on equilibrium dialysis are the gold standard for measuring FT. FT measured by this technique represents 1.5 to 4% of total testosterone.[5] Equilibrium dialysis is a tedious, expensive, and time-consuming technique and therefore may not be suitable for population-based or large-size studies. FT measured by radioimmunoassay (an assay that still is used commonly) is unreliable because it represents a variable fraction (20–60%) of the FT measured by equilibrium dialysis.[6-8] FT also can be calculated from SHBG and testosterone using the method of Vermeulen et al.[7] This calculated FT has been shown to correlate very well with FT measured by equilibrium dialysis[6] and is well suited for epidemiological and clinical studies.

Subnormal FT concentrations in association with inappropriately low LH and FSH concentrations in men with T2D were first described in 2004.[1,9] These abnormalities were independent of the duration and severity of hyperglycemia (A1C). Magnetic resonance imaging (MRI) in these hypogonadal patients showed no abnormality in brain or the pituitary.[9] The response of LH and FSH to gonadotropin-releasing hormone agonist (GnRH) injection was normal. It now has been shown that kisspeptin injection also leads to an increase in gonadotropin and testosterone concentrations in men with T2D (discussed later in more detail).[10]

This association of HH with T2D now has been confirmed in several studies and is present in 25–40% of these men.[1,11-14] In this context, it is important that the Endocrine Society now includes T2D in the list of conditions known to have a high prevalence of hypogonadism and suggests screening men with T2D for hypogonadism.[15] These observations recently were extended to younger patients with T2D between the ages of 18 and 35 years who had HH at a rate of 33% when the usual normal range for middle age was employed, whereas the rate was 58% when the age-specific normal range for FT for the young was employed.[16] With the advent of more specific liquid chromatography tandem mass spectrometry (LC-MS/MS) assay for measuring total testosterone, the reference ranges for total testosterone and FT recently have been revised downward. Utilizing this methodology, in our most recent study, we found that 29% of men with T2D have subnormal FT concentrations, as measured by equilibrium dialysis.[17] Some 25% had HH, whereas 4% had hypergonadotropic hypogonadism.

Men with T2D who have low testosterone levels also have been found to have a high prevalence of symptoms suggestive of hypogonadism, such as fatigability and erectile dysfunction.[11] In all of these studies, total testosterone and FT concentrations were related inversely to BMI and age. The presence of low testosterone concentration, however, was not entirely dependent upon obesity since 25% of nonobese patients (31% of lean and 21% of overweight) also had HH.[9] HH is relatively rare in T1D and, therefore, is not a function of diabetes or hyperglycemia per se.[18] Thus, in view of the inverse relationship between BMI and testosterone concentrations in both T1D and T2D, HH probably is related to insulin resistance.[9,13,18] Previous studies have shown that hypogonadism is associated with upper-abdominal adiposity, insulin resistance, and MetS.[19,20] Treatment of systemic insulin resistance by rosiglitazone leads to a modest increase in testosterone concentrations in men with T2D,[21] without the restoration of testosterone concentrations to normal.

ASSOCIATION OF OBESITY AND METABOLIC SYNDROME WITH LOW TESTOSTERONE

Many studies have shown FT concentrations to be also low in the obese, especially in those with BMI ≥40kg/m²,[22,23] Giagulli et al. studied two groups of obese men (BMI <35 or ≥40 kg/m²) and compared them with nonobese subjects.[22] They found that 10 out of the 22 men with BMI ≥40 kg/m² had low FT, whereas none of the subjects with BMI <35 kg/m² were hypogonadal. Zumoff et al.[24] studied 48 healthy men (mean age 33.2 years) with BMI ranging from 21 to 95 kg/m² and collected blood samples every 20 minutes for a period of 24 hours. They found that the 24-hour mean FT and non–SHBG-bound testosterone correlated inversely with BMI. Vermeulen et al.[23] compared 35 obese men (mean BMI 41.1 kg/m²) with 54 lean men. The FT concentrations were 26% lower in the obese. The FT concentrations correlated inversely with BMI. The authors also compared LH pulsatility over 12 hours in eight obese and lean men and found that the mean integrated LH levels over 12 hours were significantly lower in obese men. FT concentrations correlated positively with the sum of LH pulse amplitudes in each individual.[23] These studies established that obesity is associated with HH. These studies, however, involved a small number of men. Some recent studies have examined the prevalence of hypogonadism in obesity in a much larger number of men. A study from the Netherlands in 160 obese men (mean age 58 years) found a 35.6% prevalence of HH.[25] Men with diabetes, however, were included in the obese population. Nielsen et al.[26] examined testosterone concentrations of 615 nonobese and 70 obese young Danish men (20–29 years of age) in association with subcutaneous and visceral fat mass, measured by DEXA and MRI. The purpose of this study was to investigate the impact of obesity on reference intervals for testosterone in young men. On the basis of study results, the reference interval of plasma FT in nonobese men was 0.29–0.78 nmol/l and in obese men it was 0.23–0.67 nmol/l. Total and bioavailable testosterone concentrations were related negatively to all measures of fat mass: 23% of obese young men had subnormal total testosterone concentrations, while 10% had subnormal total and bioavailable testosterone concentrations. The largest study in this regard compared the prevalence of low testosterone concentrations in obese men and men with T2D (mean age 60 years; range 45–96 years)[27]: 44% of men with diabetes and 33% of age-matched men without diabetes had subnormal FT concentrations, respectively. Forty percent of obese men and 50% of obese men with diabetes had subnormal FT concentrations. Thus, obesity is associated with a high prevalence of hypogonadism and the presence of diabetes adds to that risk.[1] This study, however, was restricted to a relative elderly population (age >45 years). Furthermore, these studies did not utilize LC-MS/MS methodology. Therefore, the actual prevalence of hypogonadism in obesity may be lower.

We recently studied the impact of obesity on testosterone concentrations in boys at the completion of puberty.[28] We compared the testosterone, LH, and FSH concentrations of 25 lean and 25 obese boys in Tanner stage 4 and 5. The FT concentrations (measured by equilibrium dialysis followed by LC-MS/MS) of obese boys were 40% lower than those of lean boys. The gonadotropin concentrations of lean and obese boys were similar. The testosterone concentrations were related inversely related to BMI, homeostatic model assessment insulin resistance (HOMA-IR), and C-reactive protein (CRP) concentrations.

Similar to the negative impact of obesity on testosterone concentrations in men, studies have highlighted the association of MetS with hypogonadism.[29] Kaplan et al. studied 864 men (mean age 52 years) and demonstrated that aging men with obesity and MetS have a significantly decreased total testosterone (150 and 300 mg/dl less in obese and severely obese respectively) compared with aging, metabolically healthy men.[30] FT concentrations decrease proportionally with increasing number of components of MetS.[31] In a population-based study of 1,896 middle-age Finnish males (345 of whom had MetS), Laaksonen et al. showed that FT and SHBG were 11 and 18% lower in MetS than in normal subjects, respectively.[20] Men with FT in the lowest third tertile were 1.7 times (after adjustment for age and BMI) more likely to have MetS. Low testosterone and low SHBG concentrations were associated with MetS, and its components, independent of BMI. Total testosterone, FT, and SHBG were associated inversely with concentrations of insulin, glucose, triglycerides, and CRP and were associated positively with HDL. Obesity might be the most important contributor to the presence of hypogonadism in MetS, and the linear inverse relationship of testosterone with BMI is preserved in the presence of MetS.[8,10] Thus, from the preceding discussion, it appears that insulin resistance in men is associated with HH.[32]

POSSIBLE PATHOPHYSIOLOGICAL MECHANISMS UNDERLYING HH IN T2D AND OBESITY

ROLE OF ESTRADIOL

Because testosterone and androstenedione in the male can be converted to estradiol and estrone, respectively, through the action of aromatase in the mesenchymal cells and preadipocytes of adipose tissue, it has been suggested that excessive estrogen secretion due to aromatase activity in the obese potentially may suppress the hypothalamic secretion of GnRH.[1,33] Therefore, it follows that the estradiol concentrations in men with HH and T2D or obesity should be elevated to account for the suppression of gonadotropin secretion. We have shown, however, that this widely believed presumption is not true.[34] We measured the estradiol concentrations in 240 men with T2D both with and without HH. Total estradiol concentrations were measured by immunoassay and free estradiol concentrations were calculated using SHBG. Total and free estradiol concentrations in men with HH were significantly lower than in those without HH.[34] To confirm these findings, total estradiol concentrations were measured in a subset of 102 men by the LC-MS/MS assay and free estradiol concentrations were measured by equilibrium dialysis (Figure 53.1).[34] Estradiol concentrations were 25% lower in men with HH. Free estradiol concentrations were related directly to FT concentrations, irrespective of age or BMI.[1] As mentioned, our recent data on young

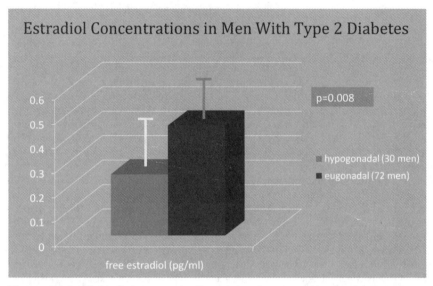

Figure 53.1—Estradiol concentrations were measured by liquid chromatography tandem mass spectrometry followed by equilibrium dialysis. Normal range 0.04–0.45 pg/ml. To convert from pg/ml to ng/dl, divide by 10. Mean ± SD estradiol concentrations were 0.38 ± 0.39 and 0.48 ± 0.27 pg/ml in hypogonadal and eugonadal men respectively. Median (25, 75 percentile) estradiol concentrations were 0.25 (0.12, 0.47) and 0.45 (0.28, 0.71) in hypogonadal and eugonadal men respectively. Figure adapted from published data.[32]

pubertal and postpubertal males (14–20 years of age) have shown that FT concentrations are ~40% lower in obese adolescents as compared with lean adolescents.[28] Similar to our study in middle-aged men with T2D, we found that estradiol concentrations also were significantly lower in adolescents with lower FT as compared to those with normal testosterone. The estradiol concentrations related directly to testosterone concentrations but not to BMI. Population-based studies such as the European Male Aging Study also showed that estradiol concentrations are lower in hypogonadal men as compared with eugonadal men, regardless of whether the hypogonadism is primary or secondary.[35] In fact, no study has shown increased concentrations of estradiol in hypogonadal men as compared with eugonadal men with obesity or T2D. The direct relationship between plasma estradiol and testosterone concentrations is consistent with the concept that estradiol concentrations are dependent on testosterone, the substrate for estradiol synthesis. Clomiphene (estrogen antagonist) and aromatase inhibitors (which decrease estradiol concentrations) have been shown to increase testosterone concentrations in obese men with low testosterone.[36] This, however, cannot be taken as evidence of estradiol as the cause of low testosterone in those men, because eugonadal men also respond to aromatase inhibition by an increase in testosterone concentrations. This occurs because estradiol has an inhibitory effect on gonadotropin secretion even in a normal physiological setting. A decrease in estradiol action or concentration would lower its inhibitory effect on gonadotropins, and eugonadal men may achieve even supranormal LH, FSH, and testosterone concentrations.[37] Elevated gonadotropin concentrations also are seen in men with congenital aromatase deficiency or the absence of estrogen receptor-α.[38,39] Clearly, the suppression of LH, FSH, and testosterone in T2D and obesity is not induced by circulating estradiol concentrations.[34]

ROLE OF INSULIN RESISTANCE

The selective deletion of the insulin receptor from neurons leads to a reduction in LH concentrations by 60–90% and low testosterone concentrations.[40] These animals respond to GnRH challenge by normal or supranormal release of LH. In addition, these animals had atrophic seminiferous tubules with markedly impaired or absent spermatogenesis. In addition, it is known that the incubation of hypothalamic neurons with insulin results in the facilitation of secretion of GnRH.[41,42] Thus, insulin action and insulin responsiveness in the brain are necessary for the maintenance of the functional integrity of the hypothalamo-hypophyseal-gonadal axis.

ROLE OF INFLAMMATORY MEDIATORS

Tumor necrosis factor-α (TNF-α) and interleukin-1β (IL-1β) have been shown to suppress hypothalamic GnRH and LH secretion in experimental animals and in vitro.[43,44] It therefore is relevant that CRP concentrations are increased markedly in hypogonadal men with T2D as compared with men with T2D and normal testosterone (6.5 mg/l versus 3.2 mg/l).[45] These data were confirmed by another study from Australia in which the median CRP concentration in patients with T2D with low total testosterone was 7.7 mg/l as compared with 4.5 mg/l in men with normal testosterone.[13] FT concentrations were related inversely to CRP concentrations. It thus is possible that inflammatory mediators may contribute to the suppression of the hypothalamo-hypophyseal axis and the syndrome of HH in T2D. The presence of inflammation also may contribute to insulin resistance since several inflammation-related mediators, such as suppressor of cytokine signaling-3 (SOCS-3), IκB kinase β (IKKβ), and c-Jun N-terminal kinase-1 (JNK-1) interfere with insulin signal transduction[46,47] and contribute to insulin resistance. These mediators also are known to be increased in obesity.[1,48]

ROLE OF LEPTIN

Leptin is known to play a permissive role in the regulation of reproductive axis. Leptin appears to serve as a signal of energy reserves to regulate the hypothalamo-pituitary-gonadal axis in relation to nutritional status.[49] Men and women with anorexia nervosa have low levels of leptin and hypogonadotropism. Absence of leptin gene or leptin signaling in humans results in HH.[50] Although there are extremely uncommon forms of human obesity because of a lack of the leptin gene, almost all obesity in humans is associated with leptin resistance and high leptin concentrations. It is possible that leptin resistance in hypothalamus or in some other neurons is responsible for the hypogonadotropism seen in obesity. Direct evidence in humans supporting or disproving this reasoning, however, is lacking.

ROLE OF KISSPEPTIN

It is now known that kisspeptin, a hypothalamic neuropeptide encoded by the KISS1 gene, and the presence of kisspeptin receptors on the GnRH neurons (G protein-coupled receptor 54), are obligate for the release of GnRH.[51,52] Humans with the absence of either kisspeptin gene or its receptor (GPR54) have HH.[52,53] Data from animal studies show that factors associated with decreased GnRH secretion, such as inflammation and estrogen, decrease KISS1 gene expression in the hypothalamus.[54,55] Intravenous injection of kisspeptin increases LH and testosterone concentrations in men with T2D and HH,[10] suggesting that the hypothalamic-pituitary-gonadal axis is intact per se in men with HH andT2D. However, the presumably metabolic insult in insulin resistance that results in hypogonadotropism is yet to be defined.

In summary, it is likely that there are several interlinked causative mechanisms underlying HH in men with T2D. It should be noted that human chorionic gonadotropin-induced testosterone secretion by Leydig cells is related inversely to insulin sensitivity (as measured by hyperinsulinemic euglycemic clamp) among men with varying degrees of glucose tolerance.[56] Thus, the lesion resulting in hypogonadism in obesity and T2D may occur at several levels of hypothalamic-pituitary-gonadal axis. The absence, however, of an increase in gonadotropin concentrations indicates that the primary defect in T2D and obesity is at the hypothalamo-hypophyseal level.[1]

WHAT COMES FIRST: HYPOGONADISM OR OBESITY OR T2D?

Since even young men with T2D and patients with newly discovered T2D have a high prevalence of HH, and obesity is associated with HH, it is possible that HH precedes diabetes. Several epidemiological studies have shown that low testosterone at baseline approximately doubles the odds of development of T2D.[1,57–59] Longitudinal data from the Boston Area Community Health Survey (BACH) cohort, however, show that testosterone in physiological concentrations does not have a significant impact on body composition parameters over a 5-year period.[60]

It generally is assumed that the association of low testosterone and obesity is bidirectional. Low testosterone predisposes to obesity and vice versa. Indeed, there are definite lines of evidence for both "directions" of this association in different clinical settings. Men who are rendered hypogonadal by GnRH agonist therapy for advanced prostate cancer increase their subcutaneous and visceral fat mass by 15–20%.[61] Consistent with this, they develop insulin resistance and their risk of incident T2D increases by 30%.[62] In the other "direction," boys who are obese prepubertally do not achieve normal testosterone concentrations at completion of puberty. Obese boys have 40% lower FT concentrations than lean boys.[28,63]

Hypogonadism also has been linked with future development of MetS. In an 11-year follow-up study, Laakonsen et al. showed that testosterone and SHBG predict MetS and T2D in middle-aged men.[59] The data, however, are more consistent with total testosterone than with FT.[64,65] It is possible that low SHBG concentrations may mediate a portion of this association. SHBG polymorphisms that lead to lower SHBG concentrations are strongly predictive of development of T2D, while those that lead to higher SHBG concentrations are protective.[66,67]

DOES HYPOGONADISM MATTER?
POSSIBLE CONSEQUENCES OF HYPOGONADISM

It is well accepted that low testosterone concentrations are associated with symptoms such as fatigue, lack of libido, and erectile dysfunction. Recent studies have described pathophysiological effects of subnormal testosterone concentrations beyond those related to sexual health, as will be discussed.

Symptoms of Sexual Dysfunction

Cross-sectional studies have found a high prevalence of low libido (64%), erectile dysfunction (74%), and fatigue (63%) in hypogonadal men with T2D.[11] The presence of these symptoms, however, was similarly high in eugonadal men with T2D (48, 65, and 57%, respectively). The treatment of erectile dysfunction with phosphodiesterase-5 inhibitors such as sildenafil in men with T2D is known to be not as effective as that in subjects without diabetes.[68]

Cardiovascular Disease

Recent evidence from longitudinal observational studies shows that low testosterone concentration is prospectively associated with an increase in the incidence of cardiovascular events.[1] Laughlin et al. prospectively followed 794 elderly men (mean age 71 years) for 20 years in a community setting.[69] The hazard ratio for men in the lowest quartile of bioavailable testosterone was 1.44 for all-cause mortality and 1.36 for cardiovascular mortality. Another prospective study (Osteoporotic Fracture in Men [MrOS] Swedish cohort)[70] that included 3,014 men (mean age 75 years, mean follow-up 4.5 years) showed a 65% increased risk of mortality in men with low FT (<6.1 ng/dl). Subnormal FT concentrations are associated with a 69% increased risk of stroke or transient ischemic attack.[71] A study in 930 men with coronary artery disease reported that a low testosterone at baseline was associated with increased mortality after 7 years of follow-up (21% vs. 12%).[72] Many cross-sectional, retrospective, case-control, and smaller studies also have demonstrated an association of low testosterone with increased mortality.[73–75] The relationship between cardiovascular mortality and low testosterone, however, was not seen in two longitudinal studies. These studies were done in relatively younger populations (mean ages 52 and 55 years) and had much lower mortality rates, which possibly can explain the lack of an association.[76,77] A recent meta-analysis of 11 trials (16,184 subjects, 9.7 years of follow-up) concluded that low total testosterone appeared to be associated with 35 and 25% higher risk of all-cause and cardiovascular mortality.[78] Substantial between-study heterogeneity, however, limited the ability to provide valid summary estimates. Relative risks for all-cause mortality were higher in studies that included older (>60 years) rather than younger men and in studies that had men with lower testosterone concentrations (<487 mg/dl). Most studies measured total testosterone, but not FT.

Two studies have looked at the association between subnormal testosterone concentrations and cardiovascular mortality specifically in men with T2D.[79] In 153 men with T2D and known coronary artery disease, subnormal FT concentration at baseline increased cardiovascular mortality by three times over 2 years.[1] In a more recent and larger study, 581 men with T2D in a diabetes clinic were followed for 5.8 years.[80] Low total testosterone concentrations (<300 mg/dl) were associated with a doubling of total mortality. After adjustment for age and SHBG, however, this significance in mortality was lost but approached significance ($P = 0.06$). Consistent with this, men with low FT (<6.5 ng/dl) did not have higher mortality than those with normal FT concentrations. Men, however, with markedly low total (<240 ng/dl) or bioavailable testosterone concentrations (<75 ng/dl) had 2.5 times higher all-cause and cardiovascular mortality.

In summary, evidence shows that testosterone concentrations are inversely associated with all-cause and cardiovascular mortality in men and that these associations are most evident when testosterone concentrations are much lower than the cut-offs used clinically to diagnose hypogonadism.

INSULIN SENSITIVITY

HH in men with T2D is associated with a higher BMI (3–4 kg/m^2), 12% more subcutaneous fat mass (measured by DEXA), and higher waist-to-hip ratio as compared with eugonadal men with T2D.[9,11,81] In one study involving men with T2D from the U.K., 74% of hypogonadal men were obese as compared with 54% of eugonadal men.[11] As yet, no study has measured visceral, intramuscular, or hepatic fat content in men with T2D both with and without HH. Many studies have documented that hypogonadism is associated with insulin resistance.[32,82] Preliminary data from a study comparing the insulin resistance in men with T2D with subnormal or normal testosterone concentrations recently were presented at the annual meetings of the ADA, the Endocrine Society, and the American Association of Clinical Endocrinologists.[1,83] Eighty-nine men with T2D had their insulin sensitivities measured by hyperinsulinemic euglycemic clamps. Thirty-nine men had HH and 42 were eugonadal. Men with HH had greater BMI (39 vs. 34 kg/m^2, $P = 0.002$) and fat mass (46 vs. 34 kg, $P < 0.001$) but similar age (54 vs. 52 years, $P = 0.4$) and A1C (7.1 vs. 7.2%, $P = 0.5$) as compared with eugonadal men. The glucose infusion rate was 30% lower in men with HH as compared with eugonadal men, even after adjustment for the difference in fat mass between the two groups ($P = 0.02$).

HEMATOCRIT

Hypogonadal men with T2D have a lower hematocrit than those with normal testosterone concentrations.[45] The prevalence of normocytic normochromic anemia in such patients is 38% as compared with 3% in those with normal testosterone concentrations. A large study (464 men) also found a direct correlation between FT concentrations and hemoglobin in men with T2D and renal insufficiency.[84] Testosterone regulates erythropoiesis.[85] It has not, however, yet been determined whether the association of anemia with hypogonadism in men with T2D is causal or is secondary to other confounding factors, such as inflammation. In these men, hemoglobin is related positively to testosterone but is related negative to CRP concentrations.[1,45]

BONE DENSITY

Hypogonadism is associated with a decrease in bone mineral density (BMD) and an increase in fracture rate.[86,87] Furthermore, trabecular bone architecture (measured by high-resolution MRI) deteriorates much more in hypogonadal men as compared with eugonadal men.[88] Hypogonadal men usually have lower estradiol concentrations as compared with eugonadal men because testosterone is the substrate for estradiol formation by aromatization.[35] In epidemiological studies, estradiol concentrations correlate more robustly with BMD than testosterone concentrations in men.[89] This is especially true of trabecular bone. Testosterone, however, appears to be an independent predictor of cortical bone density.[90,91] One study in men with T2D has shown that FT concentrations are associated positively with BMD in arms and ribs, but not with hip, spine, or total-body BMD values.[81] Another study has shown a positive relation of lumbar spine BMD with FT concentrations in men with T2D.[92] No study has evaluated the relation between BMD and free estradiol concentrations in men with T2D.[1] Neither are data available on the fracture rates of hypogonadal men with T2D. This group may be especially vulnerable to fractures since T2D in both men and women is associated with a higher fracture rate and poor bone quality, in spite of the fact that bone density in T2D is 5–10% higher than people without diabetes.[93]

PROSTATE-SPECIFIC ANTIGEN

Men with T2D have 20% lower prostate-specific antigen (PSA) concentrations than men without diabetes.[1,94] PSA concentrations are lower in hypogonadal than in eugonadal men with T2D (0.89 vs. 1.1 ng/ml).[95] It is interesting that the incidence of prostatic carcinoma is lower in men with diabetes. This is in contrast to the increased incidence of cancer in people with diabetes in various organs, including the colon, the kidney, the breast, the endometrium, and the pancreas.[96] The diminished incidence of prostate cancer in men with diabetes may receive a contribution from the high prevalence of HH and low testosterone concentrations. Epidemiological studies, however, do not support a causative role of testosterone in prostate cancer or a protection among men with hypogonadism from getting prostate cancer.[97] Similar to T2D, obesity also is associated with

10–30% lower PSA concentrations and lower prostate cancer incidence.[98] Obese men are half as likely to have PSA concentrations >4 mg/l.[99,100] The lower PSA concentrations may not be a result of lower testosterone concentrations in obesity and T2D, but rather they may due to the larger plasma volumes and hence hemodilution.[101] Prostate cancer progression and mortality, however, are increased in obese men, possibly related to later detection because of lower PSA concentrations.[102,103]

OBESITY, T2D, AND SPERMATOGENESIS

Some (but not all) studies have shown that BMI is related inversely to sperm counts, sperm morphology, and sperm motility.[104–109] Data are most consistent about the impact of morbid obesity on spermatogenesis. In a meta-analysis of 21 studies, BMI >40 kg/m² was associated with a doubling of risk of oligospermia (<40 million spermatozoa per ejaculate) or azoospermia.[110] Similar abnormalities have been found in diabetes (both T1D and T2D) and MetS.[111,112] The high prevalence of HH in obesity and T2D, especially in young men, may partially explain the high prevalence of infertility or oligospermia in these men. Studies comparing sperm parameters of obese men or men with diabetes both with and without HH have not been conducted. In one study, however, BMI was related negatively to semen quality even after adjustment for total testosterone concentrations.[113] This suggests that obesity-related factors other than testosterone may contribute to this association.

SHOULD TESTOSTERONE BE MEASURED IN EVERY MAN WITH T2D?

Because the frequency of subnormal FT concentrations in T2D is at least 25%, we believe that FT concentration should be measured in every patient with T2D. This is consistent with the Endocrine Society (U.S.) guidelines. The prevalence of hypothyroidism is between 5 and 8% in this population and yet we screen everyone for this condition. An Androgen Deficiency in Aging Male (ADAM) questionnaire should be administered in every patient with a low testosterone so that the presence of clinical hypogonadism can be established. If the case for the replacement of testosterone in patients with HH is not proven, as will be discussed, is there a case for measuring its concentrations in every patient with T2D? We believe that there is, because, like hypothyroidism, patients may slide gradually into this clinical state without any overt symptoms that may be revealed through direct questioning. "Asymptomatic" men may realize that they had been symptomatic only after a trial with testosterone. Such patients potentially may benefit from testosterone replacement therapy, as will be discussed.[1]

In contrast, it is not yet recommended that all obese men should be screened for hypogonadism. More studies need to be done to accurately define the prevalence of subnormal testosterone concentrations in obesity. Obese men should have their testosterone concentrations measured if they have signs or symptoms suggestive of hypogonadism.

Sidebar 53.2—Clinical Case Continued

The physician orders a serum FT concentration to be measured (by equilibrium dialysis) in the patient. If this methodology is not available, serum total testosterone and SHBG concentration should be measured and FT calculated.[7,9,17] LH and FSH concentrations also should be measured. If FT concentration is subnormal and LH and FSH are not high, prolactin concentration should be measured. Subnormal testosterone result should be repeated because an acute illness can lower serum testosterone concentrations transiently.

The patient's laboratory results now show a total testosterone of 205 ng/dl (250–1,100 ng/dl), SHBG 22 nmol/l (13–71 nmol/l), FT 2.9 ng/dl (3.5–15.5 ng/dl). His calculated FT concentration (http://www.issam.ch/freetesto.htm) is 4.9 ng/dl (6.5–25 ng/dl). LH, FSH, and prolactin were 3.4 international units (IU)/l, 4.9 IU/l, and 7 mg/l, respectively. His repeat FT concentration was also subnormal.

- Should an MRI of pituitary be done?
- Should he be screened for low bone mass with DEXA?
- Should he receive testosterone replacement therapy?

The patient has HH associated with T2D and obesity. Other causes of HH, such as hemochromatosis and pituitary adenoma, should be considered. MRI should be done if there is a deficiency of other pituitary hormones, headaches, or visual field defects. In one study of men with HH, pituitary macroadenomas were confined to men with total testosterone concentration <104 ng/dl. Thus, it would be prudent to do an MRI and screen for other pituitary hormone abnormalities if the total of FT is less than half the lower limit of normal. In the patient in this clinical case, an MRI was not done.

Hypogonadism is an indication to screen for osteopenia or osteoporosis. Hence, we believe, DEXA should be done. However, many physicians restrict DEXA to patients with testosterone concentrations less than half the lower limit of normal.

SHOULD MEN WITH T2D OR OBESITY AND LOW TESTOSTERONE BE REPLACED WITH TESTOSTERONE?

Issues To Be Considered in View of the Previous Data

The Endocrine Society recommends that men with low testosterone and symptoms of androgen deficiency be considered for therapy with testosterone.[15] The guidelines do not recommend treatment of asymptomatic men with low testosterone. The Institute of Medicine recommends that more short-term studies in selected populations should investigate the benefits and risks of testosterone therapy. Trials in men with T2D and obesity are important in this regard because both are associated commonly with hypogonadism. A few studies on testosterone replacement in men with T2D with low testosterone have emerged and are described in the following paragraphs.[1] Some studies of testosterone replacement in men with MetS or obesity also are discussed.

Insulin Resistance

Almost two decades ago, Marin et al. demonstrated an improvement in insulin sensitivity (as measured by euglycemic clamp) with oral and transdermal testosterone treatment in obese men without diabetes.[114-116] Four recent studies have shown a decrease in insulin resistance after testosterone therapy in hypogonadal men with T2D. Kapoor et al. studied the effects of treatment with intramuscular testosterone for 3 months in 24 hypogonadal men with T2D in a placebo-controlled double-blind crossover trial.[117] Homeostasis Model Assessment (HOMA)-IR decreased by 1.73 after testosterone therapy as compared with placebo. In another trial, 32 men with MetS and newly diagnosed T2D with total testosterone concentration of <350 ng/dl (12 nmol/l) were prescribed diet and exercise.[118] Half of them also were given transdermal testosterone for 1 year. Testosterone therapy resulted in greater improvements in insulin sensitivity (measured by HOMA-IR; –0.9) as compared with diet and exercise alone. A prospective, randomized double-blind multicenter trial of transdermal testosterone (3-g metered dose 2% gel for 1 year) therapy in 220 hypogonadal men with T2D or MetS recently was published (TIMES2 study; Testosterone replacement In hypogonadal men with either Metabolic Syndrome or T2D).[119] The primary endpoint of the study was change in insulin sensitivity, as measured by HOMA-IR. Patients were evaluated every 3 months; 136 men in the study had T2D, 176 men had MetS, and 92 men had both. Testosterone therapy resulted in a 15% ($P = 0.01$) decrease in HOMA-IR at 6-month and 1-year time-points in men with T2D as well as in those with MetS. One study in lean hypogonadal men with T2D with mean BMI of 24 kg/m^2 did not show any change in insulin sensitivity following treatment with low-dose intramuscular testosterone (100 mg every 3 weeks) for 3 months.[120] This dose is inadequate and may account for the lack of effect.[1] A small study in 22 Indian men with T2D did not show a change in HOMA-IR after intramuscular testosterone for 3 months.[121] A study in elderly nonobese (BMI 29 kg/m^2) men on replacement with testosterone patch (5 mg/day) for 2 years did not result in any change in insulin sensitivity and secretion measured by intravenous glucose tolerance test and mixed meal ingestion.[122] The study participants were not overtly hypogonadal but had low normal testosterone concentrations. The treatment resulted in small but significant increase in testosterone concentrations (371–483 ng/dl). It is, however, possible that the change in insulin sensitivity because of testosterone therapy occurs only in obese and presumably insulin-resistant men. Thus, it appears that insulin resistance improves with testosterone therapy in obese men with T2D. These studies have calculated HOMA-IR to measure insulin resistance. HOMA-IR has to be interpreted with caution in people with diabetes because of deficient insulin secretion. Therefore, the effect of testosterone on insulin sensitivity needed to be confirmed by use of hyperinsulinemic-euglycemic clamp methodology. It is not clear whether the effect is due to a change in body composition or is independent of this composition.[1]

We are conducting a randomized placebo-controlled trial of testosterone replacement for 6 months in men with HH and T2D. Preliminary results of patients who have completed the trial so far were presented at national endocrine meetings earlier this year.[83] Twenty-nine patients have been studied; 15 patients received intramuscular testosterone every 2 weeks, and 14 patients received intramuscular saline injections. Dose of testosterone was adjusted to keep the serum FT concentrations in the mid-normal range for healthy young men. Insulin sensitivity (measured by hyperinsulinemic-euglycemic clamps) increased by 25% in the testosterone group ($P = 0.01$) and did not change in the placebo group ($P = 0.75$). DEXA scans showed a gain of 2 kg of lean body mass ($P = 0.004$) and a loss of 2 kg of fat mass ($P = 0.02$) at 6 months. Unexpectedly, the change in insulin sensitivity after testosterone replacement was not related to the change in fat mass or lean mass.

Glycemic Control

In three of the previously mentioned studies, glycemic control also was evaluated by measuring A1C and fasting glucose. The small study by Kapoor et al. showed a decrease in fasting glucose (28 mg/dl) and A1C (0.37%) as compared with placebo with 3 months of testosterone replacement.[117] The trial in men with new-onset T2D with transdermal testosterone did show a decrease in A1C from 7.5 to 6.3% over a period of 1 year.[118] This was in conjunction with diet and exercise, but no hypoglycemic medications. The comparison group in this study was diet and exercise group. There was a decrease in A1C from 7.5 to 7.1% in this group. The mean fasting glucose decreased by 34 and 29 mg/dl in the testosterone and diet or exercise groups, respectively ($P = 0.06$ for comparison among groups). The larger trial (TIMES2), however, did not show a clear effect of testosterone replacement on A1C.[119] Medication changes were not allowed for the first 6 months of the study. Patients with T2D showed a trend toward an improvement in A1C at 1 year (–0.4%, $P = 0.057$) but not at 6 months ($P = 0.6$). Although no changes were made in patients' medications for the first 6 months, the study protocol allowed medication changes between 6 and 12 months; therefore, no clear conclusions can be made regarding the effect of testosterone therapy on glycemic control from this trial. There were no changes in fasting glucose or insulin. We did not find any change in A1C after testosterone treatment in men with T2D (as compared with the placebo group) in the previously mentioned National Institutes of Health (NIH) trial.[83] Thus, there appears to be a mild decrease in A1C with testosterone therapy in men with T2D, but the data are inconsistent and currently testosterone replacement cannot be recommended for glycemic control.[1]

Symptoms and Sexual Dysfunction

In the TIMES2 trial, there was an improvement in the International Index of Erectile Function (IIEF) score in the testosterone replacement group, mainly because of an increase in sexual desire, but other symptoms did not change. The smaller trial of intramuscular testosterone by Kapoor et al. in hypogonadal men with T2D showed an improvement in symptoms as measured by the ADAM questionnaire.[117] Although there are no specific studies assessing the effect of testosterone replacement on the effectiveness of phosphodiesterase IV inhibitors like sidenafil, studies in hypogonadal men without diabetes do show this benefit.[123] Sexual desire and satisfaction with erection improved after testosterone treatment in the NIH funded trial currently underway.[97]

Body Composition and Abdominal Adiposity

Heufelder et al. showed a decrease in waist circumference of 14 cm in men with new-onset T2D treated for 1 year with transdermal testosterone, diet, and exercise.[118] The control group, which was prescribed only diet and exercise, lost 5 cm. Kapoor et al. showed a decrease by 1.63 cm in waist circumference after intramuscular testosterone treatment.[117] In the TIMES2 trial, there was a small but statistically significant decrease in waist circumference (0.8 cm) in men with T2D who were treated with testosterone. Significantly, BMI did not change in any of the studies in spite of the decrease in abdominal girth.[1] According to Marin et al., a decrease in visceral obesity (measured by computed tomography scan) after testosterone therapy has been shown to occur in obese men without diabetes.[114,115] A large study on the effects of testosterone replacement on body composition in men with MetS recently was published.[124] This randomized double-blind trial included 184 men. As compared with the placebo arm, men treated with intramuscular testosterone for 30 weeks had a reduction of 4 kg of weight and 4.6 cm of waist circumference. HOMA-IR did not change. As mentioned previously, testosterone treatment resulted in a 2 kg gain in lean mass and 2 kg loss of fat mass after 6 months in men with T2D who were treated with intramuscular testosterone for 6 months.[83] There also were increases in arm and leg lean mass (1 kg each), while subcutaneous trunk fat mass decreased by 1.5 kg. There was no change in placebo group. Hepatic and visceral fat mass are being measured by MRI in this trial. Those results are not yet available.

Cardiovascular Outcomes

A recent meta-analysis of testosterone therapy trials ranging from 3 month to 3 years did not show any change in the rates of death, myocardial infarctions, revascularization procedures, or cardiac arrhythmias as compared with the placebo-nonintervention groups.[125] None of these trials, however, was powered to show a difference. Surprisingly, a recent trial of testosterone replacement therapy designed to study the effects of testosterone replacement for 6 months on muscle mass and strength in elderly men (>65 years) with limited mobility had to be discontinued prematurely because of a higher incidence (22% vs. 5%) of cardiovascular-related adverse events in the testosterone treatment arm as compared with the placebo arm.[126] This trial was not included in the previously mentioned meta-analysis. The study population had a high prevalence of chronic conditions, and it is possible that the results could have been due to chance alone. Other studies, however, in elderly population have not shown an increase in cardiac events after testosterone replacement.[127-129] The TIMES2 trial[119] reported that cardiovascular events occurred less commonly with testosterone than with placebo (4.6 vs. 10.7%; $P = 0.095$); however, this effect was short of significance. A recently published study (prospective cohort study in an endocrine clinic) investigated the effect of testosterone replacement therapy in 238 hypogonadal men with T2D on all-cause mortality.[80] Sixty-four hypogonadal men received testosterone (mean duration 42 ± 20 months), and 174 men were not treated. The mortality rate in untreated hypogonadal men was 20%, while hypogonadal men treated with testosterone had a mortality rate of 9.4% ($P = 0.002$). After multivariate adjustment, the hazard ratio for decreased survival in the untreated group was 2.3 (1.3–3.9, $P = 0.004$). By comparison, the mortality rate in a cohort of 340 men with normal testosterone concentrations was 9.1%. Testosterone replacement in the setting of heart failure also has been reported to have beneficial effects on exercise capacity, muscle strength, and HOMA-IR.[130]

One study showed a decrease of 15 mg/dl in total cholesterol but no change in LDL cholesterol, HDL cholesterol, or triglycerides after testosterone therapy for 3 months.[117] In the TIMES2 trial, men with MetS had a 15% decline in lipoprotein(a) and 7% decline in total and LDL concentrations. Men with T2D had similar trends, but the results were not significant. There was, however, a 6% decline in HDL concentrations in both the MetS and T2D groups.[119] No changes were seen in triglycerides, LDL, or HDL cholesterol concentrations in men with MetS.[124] No changes have been seen in blood pressure following testosterone treatment.[117,119]

Heufelder et al. showed a decrease in CRP concentrations (–0.5 mg/dl) and an increase in adiponectin (0.9 µg/ml) after testosterone therapy.[118] The study in men with MetS showed a decrease in CRP, TNF-α, and IL-1 after testosterone therapy.[124] CRP, IL-6, resistin, and TNF-α concentrations, however, did not change after intramuscular testosterone replacement for 3 months in a trial by Kapoor et al.[131] There also was a decrease in adiponectin after testosterone therapy. The reasons for the discrepancies between studies are not clear but could be related to the differences in study design, route of testosterone administration, and duration of therapy.[1]

Effect of Testosterone on Mediators of Inflammation and Insulin Resistance

It is now well accepted that inflammation can induce insulin resistance at a cellular level. IKKβ and SOCS-3 cause serine phosphorylation of insulin receptor substrate 1 (IRS-1). Free fatty acids, probably the best-accepted mediator of insulin resistance, are also proinflammatory. In the previously mentioned NIH-funded trial that we are doing, we found a 40% decline in free fatty acids after 6 months of testosterone replacement in men with HH and T2D.[132] Leptin, TNF-α, and CRP concentrations declined by 15–25%. IKKβ and SOCS-3 expression in mononuclear cells declined by 25%. JNK-1, another cellular inhibitor of insulin signaling, did not change. We currently are conducting analysis of adipose tissue and muscle tissue in these men to evaluate the expression and protein content of insulin signaling and inflammatory mediators to understand the molecular mechanisms underlying the improvement in insulin sensitivity by testosterone.

Safety Issues of Testosterone Replacement

The TIMES2 trial[119] did not show an increase in age-adjusted PSA values. PSA concentrations exceeded normal limits in four subjects at 12 months (three in testosterone treatment arm and one in placebo). Mean PSA concentrations also did not change after 1 year of therapy in the study by Heufelder et al.[118] In this context, it is important that the replacement of testosterone in hypogonadal patients in general does not lead to an increased risk of prostatic carcinoma, although the trials have been too limited in duration and number of patients.[125] Studies of testosterone replacement in men with MetS or obesity also have not shown any changes in PSA.[116,124]

CONCLUSION

HH is found in 25% of men with T2D. An additional 4% have HH. HH is common in obesity and MetS. Low testosterone concentrations in men with T2D are associated with an increased prevalence of symptoms of hypogonadism, obesity, very high CRP concentrations, mild anemia, insulin resistance, and decreased BMD. In addition, these men demonstrated an elevated risk (two to three times) of cardiovascular events and death in two small studies. Short-term studies of testosterone therapy have demonstrated an increase in libido. In addition, there is an increase in insulin sensitivity. Some, but not all studies, have shown an improvement in glycemia, body composition, and cardiovascular risk factors, such as cholesterol and CRP concentrations. Trials of a longer duration clearly are required to definitively establish the benefits and risks of testosterone replacement in patients with T2D or obesity and HH.[1]

REFERENCES

1. Dandona P, Dhindsa S. Update: Hypogonadotropic hypogonadism in type 2 diabetes and obesity. *J Clin Endocrinol Metab* 2011;96:2643–2651.

2. Barrett-Connor E, Khaw KT, Yen SS. Endogenous sex hormone levels in older adult men with diabetes mellitus. *Am J Epidemiol* 1990;132:895–901.

3. Andersson B, Marin P, Lissner L, Vermeulen A, Bjorntorp P. Testosterone concentrations in women and men with NIDDM. *Diabetes Care* 1994;17:405–411.

4. Dunn JF, Nisula BC, Rodbard D. Transport of steroid hormones: binding of 21 endogenous steroids to both testosterone-binding globulin and corticosteroid-binding globulin in human plasma. *J Clin Endocrinol Metab* 1981;53:58–68.

5. Winters SJ, Kelley DE, Goodpaster B. The analog free testosterone assay: are the results in men clinically useful? *Clin Chem* 1998;44:2178–2182.

6. Morley JE, Patrick P, Perry HM, 3rd. Evaluation of assays available to measure free testosterone. *Metabolism* 2002;51:554–559.

7. Vermeulen A, Verdonck L, Kaufman JM. A critical evaluation of simple methods for the estimation of free testosterone in serum. *J Clin Endocrinol Metab* 1999;84:3666–3672.

8. Rosner W. An extraordinarily inaccurate assay for free testosterone is still with us. *J Clin Endocrinol Metab* 2001;86:2903.

9. Dhindsa S, Prabhakar S, Sethi M, Bandyopadhyay A, Chaudhuri A, Dandona P. Frequent occurrence of hypogonadotropic hypogonadism in type 2 diabetes. *J Clin Endocrinol Metab* 2004;89:5462–5468.

10. George JT, Veldhuis JD, Tena-Sempere M, Millar RP, Anderson RA. Exploring the pathophysiology of hypogonadism in men with type 2 diabetes: kisspeptin-10 stimulates serum testosterone and LH secretion in men with type 2 diabetes and mild biochemical hypogonadism. *Clin Endocrinol (Oxf)* 2013;79:100–104.

11. Kapoor D, Aldred H, Clark S, Channer KS, Jones TH. Clinical and biochemical assessment of hypogonadism in men with type 2 diabetes: correlations with bioavailable testosterone and visceral adiposity. *Diabetes Care* 2007;30:911–917.

12. Rhoden EL, Ribeiro EP, Teloken C, Souto CA. Diabetes mellitus is associated with subnormal serum levels of free testosterone in men. *Br J U Int* 2005;96:867–870.

13. Grossmann M, Thomas MC, Panagiotopoulos S, Sharpe K, Macisaac RJ, Clarke S, Zajac JD, Jerums G. Low testosterone levels are common and associated with insulin resistance in men with diabetes. *J Clin Endocrinol Metab* 2008;93:1834–1840.

14. Corona G, Mannucci E, Petrone L, Ricca V, Balercia G, Mansani R, Chiarini V, Giommi R, Forti G, Maggi M. Association of hypogonadism and type II diabetes in men attending an outpatient erectile dysfunction clinic. *Int J Impot Res* 2006;18:190–197.

15. Bhasin S, Cunningham GR, Hayes FJ, Matsumoto AM, Snyder PJ, Swerdloff RS, Montori VM. Testosterone therapy in adult men with androgen deficiency syndromes: an Endocrine Society clinical practice guideline. *J Clin Endocrinol Metab* 2006;91:1995–2010.

16. Chandel A, Dhindsa S, Topiwala S, Chaudhuri A, Dandona P. Testosterone concentration in young patients with diabetes. *Diabetes Care* 2008;31:2013–2017.

17. Dhindsa S, Furlanetto R, Vora M, Chaudhuri A, Ghanim H, Dandona P. Low estradiol concentrations in males with subnormal testosterone concentrations and type 2 diabetes. *Diabetes Care* 2011;34:1–6.

18. Tomar R, Dhindsa S, Chaudhuri A, Mohanty P, Garg R, Dandona P. Contrasting testosterone concentrations in type 1 and type 2 diabetes. *Diabetes Care* 2006;29:1120–1122.

19. Haffner SM. Sex hormones, obesity, fat distribution, type 2 diabetes and insulin resistance: epidemiological and clinical correlation. *Int J Obes Relat Metab Disord* 2000;24(Suppl 2):S56–S58.

20. Laaksonen DE, Niskanen L, Punnonen K, Nyyssonen K, Tuomainen TP, Salonen R, Rauramaa R, Salonen JT. Sex hormones, inflammation and the metabolic syndrome: a population-based study. *Eur J Endocrinol* 2003;149:601–608.

21. Kapoor D, Channer KS, Jones TH. Rosiglitazone increases bioactive testosterone and reduces waist circumference in hypogonadal men with type 2 diabetes. *Diab Vasc Dis Res* 2008;5:135–137.

22. Giagulli VA, Kaufman JM, Vermeulen A. Pathogenesis of the decreased androgen levels in obese men. *J Clin Endocrinol Metab* 1994;79:997–1000.

23. Vermeulen A, Kaufman JM, Deslypere JP, Thomas G. Attenuated luteinizing hormone (LH) pulse amplitude but normal LH pulse frequency, and its rela-

tion to plasma androgens in hypogonadism of obese men. *J Clin Endocrinol Metab* 1993;76:1140–1146.

24. Zumoff B, Strain GW, Miller LK, Rosner W, Senie R, Seres DS, Rosenfeld RS. Plasma free and non-sex-hormone-binding-globulin-bound testosterone are decreased in obese men in proportion to their degree of obesity. *J Clin Endocrinol Metab* 1990;71:929–931.

25. Hofstra J, Loves S, van Wageningen B, Ruinemans-Koerts J, Jansen I, de Boer H. High prevalence of hypogonadotropic hypogonadism in men referred for obesity treatment. *Neth J Med* 2008;66:103–109.

26. Nielsen TL, Hagen C, Wraae K, Brixen K, Petersen PH, Haug E, Larsen R, Andersen M. Visceral and subcutaneous adipose tissue assessed by magnetic resonance imaging in relation to circulating androgens, sex hormone-binding globulin, and luteinizing hormone in young men. *J Clin Endocrinol Metab* 2007;92:2696–2705.

27. Dhindsa S, Miller MG, McWhirter CL, Mager DE, Ghanim H, Chaudhuri A, Dandona P. Testosterone concentrations in diabetic and nondiabetic obese men. *Diabetes Care* 2010;33:1186–1192.

28. Mogri M, Dhindsa S, Quattrin T, Ghanim H, Dandona P. Testosterone concentrations in young pubertal and post-pubertal obese males. *Clin Endocrinol (Oxf)* 2013;78:593–599.

29. Lunenfeld B. Testosterone deficiency and the metabolic syndrome. *Aging Male* 2007;10:53–56.

30. Kaplan SA, Meehan AG, Shah A. The age related decrease in testosterone is significantly exacerbated in obese men with the metabolic syndrome. What are the implications for the relatively high incidence of erectile dysfunction observed in these men? *J Urol* 2006;176:1524–1527; discussion 1527–1528.

31. Corona G, Mannucci E, Schulman C, Petrone L, Mansani R, Cilotti A, Balercia G, Chiarini V, Forti G, Maggi M. Psychobiologic correlates of the metabolic syndrome and associated sexual dysfunction. *Eur Urol* 2006;50:595–604; discussion 604.

32. Dandona P, Dhindsa S, Chaudhuri A, Bhatia V, Topiwala S, Mohanty P. Hypogonadotrophic hypogonadism in type 2 diabetes, obesity and the metabolic syndrome. *Curr Mol Med* 2008;8:816–828.

33. Pitteloud N, Dwyer AA, Decruz S, Lee H, Boepple PA, Crowley WF Jr, Hayes FJ. The relative role of gonadal sex steroids and gonadotropin-releasing hormone pulse frequency in the regulation of follicle-stimulating hormone secretion in men. *J Clin Endocrinol Metab* 2008;93:2686–2692.

34. Dhindsa S, Furlanetto R, Vora M, Ghanim H, Chaudhuri A, Dandona P. Low estradiol concentrations in men with subnormal testosterone concentrations and type 2 diabetes. *Diabetes Care* 2011;34:1854–1859.

35. Tajar A, Forti G, O'Neill TW, Lee DM, Silman AJ, Finn JD, Bartfai G, Boonen S, Casanueva FF, Giwercman A, et al. Characteristics of secondary,

primary, and compensated hypogonadism in aging men: evidence from the European Male Ageing Study. *J Clin Endocrinol Metab* 2010;95:1810–1818.

36. Loves S, Ruinemans-Koerts J, de Boer H. Letrozole once a week normalizes serum testosterone in obesity-related male hypogonadism. *Eur J Endocrinol* 2008;158:741–747.

37. T'Sjoen GG, Giagulli VA, Delva H, Crabbe P, De Bacquer D, Kaufman JM. Comparative assessment in young and elderly men of the gonadotropin response to aromatase inhibition. *J Clin Endocrinol Metab* 2005;90:5717–5722.

38. Smith EP, Boyd J, Frank GR, Takahashi H, Cohen RM, Specker B, Williams TC, Lubahn DB, Korach KS. Estrogen resistance caused by a mutation in the estrogen-receptor gene in a man. *N Engl J Med* 1994;331:1056–1061.

39. Carani C, Qin K, Simoni M, Faustini-Fustini M, Serpente S, Boyd J, Korach KS, Simpson ER. Effect of testosterone and estradiol in a man with aromatase deficiency. *N Engl J Med* 1997;337:91–95.

40. Bruning JC, Gautam D, Burks DJ, Gillette J, Schubert M, Orban PC, Klein R, Krone W, Muller-Wieland D, Kahn CR. Role of brain insulin receptor in control of body weight and reproduction. *Science* 2000;289:2122–2125.

41. Salvi R, Castillo E, Voirol MJ, Glauser M, Rey JP, Gaillard RC, Vollenweider P, Pralong FP. Gonadotropin-releasing hormone-expressing neurons immortalized conditionally are activated by insulin: implication of the mitogen-activated protein kinase pathway. *Endocrinology* 2006;147:816–826.

42. Gamba M, Pralong FP. Control of GnRH neuronal activity by metabolic factors: the role of leptin and insulin. *Mol Cell Endocrinol* 2006;254–255:133–139.

43. Watanobe H, Hayakawa Y. Hypothalamic interleukin-1 beta and tumor necrosis factor-alpha, but not interleukin-6, mediate the endotoxin-induced suppression of the reproductive axis in rats. *Endocrinology* 2003;144:4868–4875.

44. Russell SH, Small CJ, Stanley SA, Franks S, Ghatei MA, Bloom SR. The in vitro role of tumour necrosis factor-alpha and interleukin-6 in the hypothalamic-pituitary gonadal axis. *J Neuroendocrinol* 2001;13:296–301.

45. Bhatia V, Chaudhuri A, Tomar R, Dhindsa S, Ghanim H, Dandona P. Low testosterone and high C-reactive protein concentrations predict low hematocrit in type 2 diabetes. *Diabetes Care* 2006;29:2289–2294.

46. Vallerie SN, Furuhashi M, Fucho R, Hotamisligil GS. A predominant role for parenchymal c-Jun amino terminal kinase (JNK) in the regulation of systemic insulin sensitivity. *PLoS One* 2008;3:e3151.

47. Dandona P, Aljada A, Bandyopadhyay A. Inflammation: the link between insulin resistance, obesity and diabetes. *Trends Immunol* 2004;25:4–7.

48. Ghanim H, Aljada A, Daoud N, Deopurkar R, Chaudhuri A, Dandona P. Role of inflammatory mediators in the suppression of insulin receptor phosphorylation in circulating mononuclear cells of obese subjects. *Diabetologia* 2007;50:278–285.

49. Seth A, Stanley S, Jethwa P, Gardiner J, Ghatei M, Bloom S. Galanin-like peptide stimulates the release of gonadotropin-releasing hormone in vitro and may mediate the effects of leptin on the hypothalamo-pituitary-gonadal axis. *Endocrinology* 2004;145:743–750.

50. Farooqi IS, Matarese G, Lord GM, Keogh JM, Lawrence E, Agwu C, Sanna V, Jebb SA, Perna F, Fontana S, et al. Beneficial effects of leptin on obesity, T cell hyporesponsiveness, and neuroendocrine/metabolic dysfunction of human congenital leptin deficiency. *J Clin Invest* 2002;110:1093–1103.

51. Seminara SB, Messager S, Chatzidaki EE, Thresher RR, Acierno JS Jr, Shagoury JK, Bo-Abbas Y, Kuohung W, Schwinof KM, Hendrick AG, et al. The GPR54 gene as a regulator of puberty. *N Engl J Med* 2003;349:1614–1627.

52. de Roux N, Genin E, Carel JC, Matsuda F, Chaussain JL, Milgrom E. Hypogonadotropic hypogonadism due to loss of function of the KiSS1-derived peptide receptor GPR54. *Proc Natl Acad Sci USA* 2003;100:10972–10976.

53. Silveira LG, Noel SD, Silveira-Neto AP, Abreu AP, Brito VN, Santos MG, Bianco SD, Kuohung W, Xu S, Gryngarten M, et al. Mutations of the KISS1 gene in disorders of puberty. *J Clin Endocrinol Metab* 2010;95:2276–2280.

54. Iwasa T, Matsuzaki T, Murakami M, Shimizu F, Kuwahara A, Yasui T, Irahara M. Decreased expression of kisspeptin mediates acute immune/inflammatory stress-induced suppression of gonadotropin secretion in female rat. *J Endocrinol Invest* 2008;31:656–659.

55. Navarro VM, Castellano JM, Fernandez-Fernandez R, Barreiro ML, Roa J, Sanchez-Criado JE, Aguilar E, Dieguez C, Pinilla L, Tena-Sempere M. Developmental and hormonally regulated messenger ribonucleic acid expression of KiSS-1 and its putative receptor, GPR54, in rat hypothalamus and potent luteinizing hormone-releasing activity of KiSS-1 peptide. *Endocrinology* 2004;145:4565–4574.

56. Pitteloud N, Hardin M, Dwyer AA, Valassi E, Yialamas M, Elahi D, Hayes FJ. Increasing insulin resistance is associated with a decrease in Leydig cell testosterone secretion in men. *J Clin Endocrinol Metab* 2005;90:2636–2641.

57. Oh JY, Barrett-Connor E, Wedick NM, Wingard DL. Endogenous sex hormones and the development of type 2 diabetes in older men and women: the Rancho Bernardo study. *Diabetes Care* 2002;25:55–60.

58. Haffner SM, Shaten J, Stern MP, Smith GD, Kuller L. Low levels of sex hormone-binding globulin and testosterone predict the development of non-insulin-dependent diabetes mellitus in men. MRFIT Research Group. Multiple Risk Factor Intervention Trial. *Am J Epidemiol* 1996;143:889–897.

59. Laaksonen DE, Niskanen L, Punnonen K, Nyyssonen K, Tuomainen TP, Valkonen VP, Salonen R, Salonen JT. Testosterone and sex hormone-binding globulin predict the metabolic syndrome and diabetes in middle-aged men. *Diabetes Care* 2004;27:1036–1041.

60. Gates MA, Mekary RA, Chiu GR, Ding EL, Wittert GA, Araujo AB. Sex steroid hormone levels and body composition in men. *J Clin Endocrinol Metab* 2013;98:2442–2450.

61. Hamilton EJ, Gianatti E, Strauss BJ, Wentworth J, Lim-Joon D, Bolton D, Zajac JD, Grossmann M. Increase in visceral and subcutaneous abdominal fat in men with prostate cancer treated with androgen deprivation therapy. *Clin Endocrinol* 2011;74:377–383.

62. Grossmann M, Cheung AS, Zajac JD. Androgens and prostate cancer; pathogenesis and deprivation therapy. *Best Pract Res Clin Endocrinol Metab* 2013;27:603–616.

63. Moriarty-Kelsey M, Harwood JE, Travers SH, Zeitler PS, Nadeau KJ. Testosterone, obesity and insulin resistance in young males: evidence for an association between gonadal dysfunction and insulin resistance during puberty. *J Pediatr Endocrinol Metab* 2010;23:1281–1287.

64. Lakshman KM, Bhasin S, Araujo AB. Sex hormone-binding globulin as an independent predictor of incident type 2 diabetes mellitus in men. *J Gerontol A Biol Sci Med Sci* 2010;65:503–509.

65. Bhasin S, Jasjua GK, Pencina M, D'Agostino R Sr, Coviello AD, Vasan RS, Travison TG. Sex hormone-binding globulin, but not testosterone, is associated prospectively and independently with incident metabolic syndrome in men: the Framingham Heart study. *Diabetes Care* 2011;34:2464–2470.

66. Ding EL, Song Y, Manson JE, Hunter DJ, Lee CC, Rifai N, Buring JE, Gaziano JM, Liu S. Sex hormone-binding globulin and risk of type 2 diabetes in women and men. *N Engl J Med* 2009;361:1152–1163.

67. Perry JR, Weedon MN, Langenberg C, Jackson AU, Lyssenko V, Sparso T, Thorleifsson G, Grallert H, Ferrucci L, Maggio M, et al. Genetic evidence that raised sex hormone binding globulin (SHBG) levels reduce the risk of type 2 diabetes. *Hum Mol Genet* 2010;19:535–544.

68. Behrend L, Vibe-Petersen J, Perrild H. Sildenafil in the treatment of erectile dysfunction in men with diabetes: demand, efficacy and patient satisfaction. *Int J Impot Res* 2005;17:264–269.

69. Laughlin GA, Barrett-Connor E, Bergstrom J. Low serum testosterone and mortality in older men. *J Clin Endocrinol Metab* 2008;93:68–75.

70. Tivesten A, Vandenput L, Labrie F, Karlsson MK, Ljunggren O, Mellstrom D, Ohlsson C. Low serum testosterone and estradiol predict mortality in elderly men. *J Clin Endocrinol Metab* 2009;94:2482–2488.

71. Yeap BB, Hyde Z, Almeida OP, Norman PE, Chubb SA, Jamrozik K, Flicker L, Hankey GJ. Lower testosterone levels predict incident stroke and tran-

sient ischemic attack in older men. *J Clin Endocrinol Metab* 2009 Jul;94(7):2353–2359.

72. Malkin CJ, Pugh PJ, Morris PD, Asif S, Jones TH, Channer KS. Low serum testosterone and increased mortality in men with coronary heart disease. *Heart* 2010;96:1821–1825.

73. Khaw KT, Dowsett M, Folkerd E, Bingham S, Wareham N, Luben R, Welch A, Day N. Endogenous testosterone and mortality due to all causes, cardiovascular disease, and cancer in men: European Prospective Investigation into Cancer in Norfolk (EPIC-Norfolk) Prospective Population study. *Circulation* 2007;116:2694–2701.

74. Vikan T, Johnsen SH, Schirmer H, Njolstad I, Svartberg J. Endogenous testosterone and the prospective association with carotid atherosclerosis in men: the Tromso study. *Eur J Epidemiol* 2009;24:289–295.

75. Shores MM, Matsumoto AM, Sloan KL, Kivlahan DR. Low serum testosterone and mortality in male veterans. *Arch Intern Med* 2006;166:1660–1665.

76. Araujo AB, Kupelian V, Page ST, Handelsman DJ, Bremner WJ, McKinlay JB. Sex steroids and all-cause and cause-specific mortality in men. *Arch Intern Med* 2007;167:1252–1260.

77. Smith GD, Ben-Shlomo Y, Beswick A, Yarnell J, Lightman S, Elwood P. Cortisol, testosterone, and coronary heart disease: prospective evidence from the Caerphilly study. *Circulation* 2005;112:332–340.

78. Araujo AB, Dixon JM, Suarez EA, Murad MH, Guey LT, Wittert GA. Clinical review: Endogenous testosterone and mortality in men: a systematic review and meta-analysis. *J Clin Endocrinol Metab* 2011;96:3007–3019.

79. Ponikowska B, Jankowska EA, Maj J, Wegrzynowska-Teodorczyk K, Biel B, Reczuch K, Borodulin-Nadzieja L, Banasiak W, Ponikowski P. Gonadal and adrenal androgen deficiencies as independent predictors of increased cardiovascular mortality in men with type II diabetes mellitus and stable coronary artery disease. *Int J Cardiol* 2010 Sep 3;143(3):343–348.

80. Muraleedharan V, Marsh H, Kapoor D, Channer KS, Jones TH. Testosterone deficiency is associated with increased risk of mortality and testosterone replacement improves survival in men with type 2 diabetes. *Eur J Endocrinol* 2013 Oct 21;169(6):725–733.

81. Dhindsa S, Bhatia V, Dhindsa G, Chaudhuri A, Gollapudi GM, Dandona P. The effects of hypogonadism on body composition and bone mineral density in type 2 diabetic patients. *Diabetes Care* 2007;30:1860–1861.

82. Traish AM, Saad F, Feeley RJ, Guay A. The dark side of testosterone deficiency: III. Cardiovascular disease. *J Androl* 2009;30:477–494.

83. Dhindsa S, Batra M, Kuhadiya N, Sandhu S, Chaudhuri A, Ghanim H, Dandona P. Testosterone replacement decreases insulin resistance in hypogonadal men with type 2 diabetes. *The Endocrine Society (OR22-1), American Diabetes Association (1994-P), and AACE* (abstract #280) 2013.

84. Grossmann M, Panagiotopolous S, Sharpe K, MacIsaac RJ, Clarke S, Zajac JD, Jerums G, Thomas MC. Low testosterone and anaemia in men with type 2 diabetes. *Clin Endocrinol* 2009;70:547–553.

85. Shahidi NT. Androgens and erythropoiesis. *N Engl J Med* 1973;289:72–80.

86. Orwoll ES, Klein RF. Osteoporosis in men. *Endocr Rev* 1995;16:87–116.

87. Jackson JA, Riggs MW, Spiekerman AM. Testosterone deficiency as a risk factor for hip fractures in men: a case-control study. *Am J Med Sci* 1992;304:4–8.

88. Benito M, Gomberg B, Wehrli FW, Weening RH, Zemel B, Wright AC, Song HK, Cucchiara A, Snyder PJ. Deterioration of trabecular architecture in hypogonadal men. *J Clin Endocrinol Metab* 2003;88:1497–1502.

89. Khosla S, Melton LJ 3rd, Atkinson EJ, O'Fallon WM, Klee GG, Riggs BL. Relationship of serum sex steroid levels and bone turnover markers with bone mineral density in men and women: a key role for bioavailable estrogen. *J Clin Endocrinol Metab* 1998;83:2266–2274.

90. Mellstrom D, Johnell O, Ljunggren O, Eriksson AL, Lorentzon M, Mallmin H, Holmberg A, Redlund-Johnell I, Orwoll E, Ohlsson C. Free testosterone is an independent predictor of BMD and prevalent fractures in elderly men: MrOS Sweden. *J Bone Miner Res* 2006;21:529–535.

91. Lorentzon M, Swanson C, Andersson N, Mellstrom D, Ohlsson C. Free testosterone is a positive, whereas free estradiol is a negative, predictor of cortical bone size in young Swedish men: The GOOD study. *J Bone Miner Res* 2005;20:1334–1341.

92. Vasilkova O, Mokhort T, Sanec I, Sharshakova T, Hayashida N, Takamura N. Testosterone is an independent determinant of bone mineral density in men with type 2 diabetes mellitus. *Clin Chem Lab Med* 2011;49:99–103.

93. Schwartz AV, Vittinghoff E, Bauer DC, Hillier TA, Strotmeyer ES, Ensrud KE, Donaldson MG, Cauley JA, Harris TB, Koster A, et al. Association of BMD and FRAX score with risk of fracture in older adults with type 2 diabetes. *JAMA* 2011;305:2184–2192.

94. Werny DM, Saraiya M, Gregg EW. Prostate-specific antigen values in diabetic and nondiabetic US men, 2001-2002. *Am J Epidemiol* 2006;164:978–983.

95. Dhindsa S, Upadhyay M, Viswanathan P, Howard S, Chaudhuri A, Dandona P. Relationship of prostate-specific antigen to age and testosterone in men with type 2 diabetes mellitus. *Endocr Pract* 2008;14:1000–1005.

96. Inoue M, Iwasaki M, Otani T, Sasazuki S, Noda M, Tsugane S. Diabetes mellitus and the risk of cancer: results from a large scale population based cohort study in Japan. *Arch Intern Med* 2006;166:1871–1877.

97. Heikkila R, Aho K, Heliovaara M, Hakama M, Marniemi J, Reunanen A, Knekt P. Serum testosterone and sex hormone-binding globulin concentra-

tions and the risk of prostate carcinoma: a longitudinal study. *Cancer* 1999;86:312–315.

98. Werny DM, Thompson T, Saraiya M, Freedman D, Kottiri BJ, German RR, Wener M. Obesity is negatively associated with prostate-specific antigen in U.S. men, 2001-2004. *Cancer Epidemiol Biomarkers Prev* 2007;16:70–76.

99. Parekh N, Lin Y, Dipaola RS, Marcella S, Lu-Yao G. Obesity and prostate cancer detection: insights from three national surveys. *Am J Med* 2010;123:829–835.

100. Culp S, Porter M. The effect of obesity and lower serum prostate-specific antigen levels on prostate-cancer screening results in American men. *BJU Int* 2009;104:1457–1461.

101. Banez LL, Hamilton RJ, Partin AW, Vollmer RT, Sun L, Rodriguez C, Wang Y, Terris MK, Aronson WJ, Presti JC Jr, et al. Obesity-related plasma hemodilution and PSA concentration among men with prostate cancer. *JAMA* 2007;298:2275–2280.

102. Calle EE, Rodriguez C, Walker-Thurmond K, Thun MJ. Overweight, obesity, and mortality from cancer in a prospectively studied cohort of U.S. adults. *N Engl J Med* 2003;348:1625–1638.

103. Wright ME, Chang SC, Schatzkin A, Albanes D, Kipnis V, Mouw T, Hurwitz P, Hollenbeck A, Leitzmann MF. Prospective study of adiposity and weight change in relation to prostate cancer incidence and mortality. *Cancer* 2007;109:675–684.

104. Kort HI, Massey JB, Elsner CW, Mitchell-Leef D, Shapiro DB, Witt MA, Roudebush WE. Impact of body mass index values on sperm quantity and quality. *J Androl* 2006;27:450–452.

105. Pauli EM, Legro RS, Demers LM, Kunselman AR, Dodson WC, Lee PA. Diminished paternity and gonadal function with increasing obesity in men. *Fertil Steril* 2008;90:346–351.

106. Du Plessis SS, Cabler S, McAlister DA, Sabanegh E, Agarwal A. The effect of obesity on sperm disorders and male infertility. *Nat Rev Urol* 2010;7:153–161.

107. Jensen TK, Andersson AM, Jorgensen N, Andersen AG, Carlsen E, Petersen JH, Skakkebaek NE. Body mass index in relation to semen quality and reproductive hormones among 1,558 Danish men. *Fertil Steril* 2004;82:863–870.

108. Chavarro JE, Toth TL, Wright DL, Meeker JD, Hauser R. Body mass index in relation to semen quality, sperm DNA integrity, and serum reproductive hormone levels among men attending an infertility clinic. *Fertil Steril* 2010;93:2222–2231.

109. Aggerholm AS, Thulstrup AM, Toft G, Ramlau-Hansen CH, Bonde JP. Is overweight a risk factor for reduced semen quality and altered serum sex hormone profile? *Fertil Steril* 2008;90:619–626.

110. Sermondade N, Faure C, Fezeu L, Shayeb AG, Bonde JP, Jensen TK, Van Wely M, Cao J, Martini AC, Eskandar M, et al. BMI in relation to sperm count: an updated systematic review and collaborative meta-analysis. *Hum Reprod Update* 2013;19:221–231.

111. Shrivastav P, Swann J, Jeremy JY, Thompson C, Shaw RW, Dandona P. Sperm function and structure and seminal plasma prostanoid concentrations in men with IDDM. *Diabetes Care* 1989;12:742–744.

112. Kasturi SS, Tannir J, Brannigan RE. The metabolic syndrome and male infertility. *J Androl* 2008;29:251–259.

113. Qin DD, Yuan W, Zhou WJ, Cui YQ, Wu JQ, Gao ES. Do reproductive hormones explain the association between body mass index and semen quality? *Asian J Androl* 2007;9:827–834.

114. Marin P, Krotkiewski M, Bjorntorp P. Androgen treatment of middle-aged, obese men: effects on metabolism, muscle and adipose tissues. *Eur J Med* 1992;1:329–336.

115. Marin P, Holmang S, Jonsson L, Sjostrom L, Kvist H, Holm G, Lindstedt G, Bjorntorp P. The effects of testosterone treatment on body composition and metabolism in middle-aged obese men. *Int J Obes Relat Metab Disord* 1992;16:991–997.

116. Marin P, Holmang S, Gustafsson C, Jonsson L, Kvist H, Elander A, Eldh J, Sjostrom L, Holm G, Bjorntorp P. Androgen treatment of abdominally obese men. *Obes Res* 1993;1:245–251.

117. Kapoor D, Goodwin E, Channer KS, Jones TH. Testosterone replacement therapy improves insulin resistance, glycaemic control, visceral adiposity and hypercholesterolaemia in hypogonadal men with type 2 diabetes. *Eur J Endocrinol* 2006;154:899–906.

118. Heufelder AE, Saad F, Bunck MC, Gooren L. Fifty-two-week treatment with diet and exercise plus transdermal testosterone reverses the metabolic syndrome and improves glycemic control in men with newly diagnosed type 2 diabetes and subnormal plasma testosterone. *J Androl* 2009;30:726–733.

119. Jones TH, Arver S, Behre HM, Buvat J, Meuleman E, Moncada I, Morales AM, Volterrani M, Yellowlees A, Howell JD, et al. Testosterone replacement in hypogonadal men with type 2 diabetes and/or metabolic syndrome (the TIMES2 study). *Diabetes Care* 2011;34:828–837.

120. Lee CH, Kuo SW, Hung YJ, Hsieh CH, He CT, Yang TC, Lian WC, Chyi-Fan S, Pei D. The effect of testosterone supplement on insulin sensitivity, glucose effectiveness, and acute insulin response after glucose load in male type 2 diabetics. *Endocr Res* 2005;31:139–148.

121. Gopal RA, Bothra N, Acharya SV, Ganesh HK, Bandgar TR, Menon PS, Shah NS. Treatment of hypogonadism with testosterone in patients with type 2 diabetes mellitus. *Endocr Pract* 2010;16:570–576.

122. Basu R, Dalla Man C, Campioni M, Basu A, Nair KS, Jensen MD, Khosla S, Klee G, Toffolo G, Cobelli C, et al. Effect of 2 years of testosterone replacement on insulin secretion, insulin action, glucose effectiveness, hepatic insulin clearance, and postprandial glucose turnover in elderly men. *Diabetes Care* 2007;30:1972–1978.

123. Buvat J, Montorsi F, Maggi M, Porst H, Kaipia A, Colson MH, Cuzin B, Moncada I, Martin-Morales A, Yassin A, et al. Hypogonadal men nonresponders to the PDE5 inhibitor tadalafil benefit from normalization of testosterone levels with a 1% hydroalcoholic testosterone gel in the treatment of erectile dysfunction (TADTEST study). *J Sex Med* 2011;8:284–293.

124. Kalinchenko SY, Tishova YA, Mskhalaya GJ, Gooren LJ, Giltay EJ, Saad F. Effects of testosterone supplementation on markers of the metabolic syndrome and inflammation in hypogonadal men with the metabolic syndrome: the double-blinded placebo-controlled Moscow study. *Clin Endocrinol* 2010;73:602–612.

125. Fernandez-Balsells MM, Murad MH, Lane M, Lampropulos JF, Albuquerque F, Mullan RJ, Agrwal N, Elamin MB, Gallegos-Orozco JF, Wang AT, et al. Clinical review 1: adverse effects of testosterone therapy in adult men: a systematic review and meta-analysis. *J Clin Endocrinol Metab* 2010;95:2560–2575.

126. Basaria S, Coviello AD, Travison TG, Storer TW, Farwell WR, Jette AM, Eder R, Tennstedt S, Ulloor J, Zhang A, et al. Adverse events associated with testosterone administration. *N Engl J Med* 2010;363:109–122.

127. Srinivas-Shankar U, Roberts SA, Connolly MJ, O'Connell MD, Adams JE, Oldham JA, Wu FC. Effects of testosterone on muscle strength, physical function, body composition, and quality of life in intermediate-frail and frail elderly men: a randomized, double-blind, placebo-controlled study. *J Clin Endocrinol Metab* 2010;95:639–650.

128. Page ST, Amory JK, Bowman FD, Anawalt BD, Matsumoto AM, Bremner WJ, Tenover JL. Exogenous testosterone (T) alone or with finasteride increases physical performance, grip strength, and lean body mass in older men with low serum T. *J Clin Endocrinol Metab* 2005;90:1502–1510.

129. Nair KS, Rizza RA, O'Brien P, Dhatariya K, Short KR, Nehra A, Vittone JL, Klee GG, Basu A, Basu R, et al. DHEA in elderly women and DHEA or testosterone in elderly men. *N Engl J Med* 2006;355:1647–1659.

130. Caminiti G, Volterrani M, Iellamo F, Marazzi G, Massaro R, Miceli M, Mammi C, Piepoli M, Fini M, Rosano GM. Effect of long-acting testosterone treatment on functional exercise capacity, skeletal muscle performance, insulin resistance, and baroreflex sensitivity in elderly patients with chronic heart failure: a double-blind, placebo-controlled, randomized study. *J Am Coll Cardiol* 2009;54:919–927.

131. Kapoor D, Clarke S, Stanworth R, Channer KS, Jones TH. The effect of testosterone replacement therapy on adipocytokines and C-reactive protein

in hypogonadal men with type 2 diabetes. *Eur J Endocrinol* 2007;156:595–602.

132. Dhindsa S, Ghanim H, Green K, Batra M, Kuhadiya N, Sandhu S, Makdissi M, Chaudhuri A, Dandona P. Testosterone restores insulin sensitivity in males with hypogonadotropic hypogonadism (HH) through its novel anti-inflammatory actions and the suppression of free fatty acids (FFA), tumor necrosis factor (TNF) α, suppressor of cytokine signaling (SOCS)-3 and IκB kinase (IKK) β independently of weight loss. *American Diabetes Association 166-LB* (abstract) 2013.

Chapter 54

Clinical Implications of Nonalcoholic Fatty Liver Disease in Type 2 Diabetes

MARYANN MAXIMOS, DO
FERNANDO BRIL, MD
KENNETH CUSI, MD, FACP, FACE

INTRODUCTION

Nonalcoholic fatty liver disease (NAFLD) is a chronic condition in individuals without significant alcohol consumption and in whom other causes of liver disease, such as medications or other disease processes, have been excluded.[1] The hallmarks of the disease are insulin resistance and liver steatosis evidenced on imaging or liver biopsy. NAFLD can range from simple steatosis to severe nonalcoholic steatohepatitis (NASH) and ultimately can result in cirrhosis and hepatocellular carcinoma (HCC).[2,3]

The prevalence of obesity has been increasing worldwide and has many implications for the overall health of people. With obesity comes a deluge of medical problems, including type 2 diabetes (T2D), atherogenic dyslipidemia (elevated triglycerides [TGs], low high-density lipoprotein cholesterol [HDL-C], and small and dense low-density lipoprotein [LDL] particles), cardiovascular disease (CVD), obstructive sleep apnea, polycystic ovarian syndrome (PCOS), and NAFLD.[4] NAFLD may be present in nonobese individuals without the typical phenotype of the metabolic syndrome (more in younger patients) but closely associated with insulin resistance, particularly in adipose tissue as well as at the level of muscle and liver. Although the diagnosis and management of these medical conditions have been overall well standardized, this is not the case for NAFLD. In this condition, not only is it difficult to make the diagnosis, but its natural history and clinical implications are poorly understood, and pharmacologic interventions are not yet clearly established.[5] New data are emerging to help answer these important questions, with novel diagnostic tests and treatments, such as pioglitazone, which are likely to change patient management in the near future.

NAFLD is now a frequent problem for health care providers taking care of patients with T2D, in whom the disease is more prevalent and follows a more progressive course. This chapter will discuss the prevalence, natural history, and metabolic consequences of NAFLD. In addition, it reviews the best steps to establish the diagnosis and select treatment for this condition.

PREVALENCE

Worldwide estimates of NAFLD prevalence range between ~10 and ~35% in the general population (with the U.S. having one of the highest rates).[6] Among those with NAFLD, at least 30% have NASH.[7] Yet, the prevalence of NAFLD depends

DOI: 10.2337/9781580405096.54

on the method used to diagnose the disease. When solely using elevated liver aminotransferases, only between 7 and 11% of the population is believed to have NAFLD.[6] This is likely a gross misrepresentation of the actual prevalence of the disease, however, as most patients with NAFLD have normal aminotransferase levels.[8,9] When using ultrasound as a diagnostic measure, the prevalence of NAFLD is estimated to be between 17 and 46%[6] depending on the patient population being assessed. For example, in the Dionysos Nutrition and Liver Study,[10] the prevalence of NAFLD was 20% in 496 middle-age Italian patients not suspected of having liver disease. In a predominantly overweight or obese population, Williams et al.[7] found a 46% prevalence of NAFLD. Using the gold-standard technique of magnetic resonance and spectroscopy (MRS), in a large multiethnic population, the Dallas Heart Study reported an overall prevalence of ~34% in the U.S.[11] Of note, the prevalence in obese patients was much higher in this study. In fact, the prevalence of NAFLD exceeds 90% in morbidly obese patients undergoing bariatric surgery.[12,13] Those with dyslipidemia were found to have a prevalence of ~50%,[4,14] and patients who are obese or have T2D have the highest risk of developing NAFLD. Later in this chapter, we will review the advantages and disadvantages of these different imaging modalities. Finally, when using a liver biopsy to make the diagnosis of NAFLD, the prevalence has ranged from 20 to 50%,[15,16] similar to that found using varying imaging modalities.

In patients with T2D, the prevalence of NAFLD and NASH are much greater. Leite et al.[17] reported a 69% prevalence of NAFLD using ultrasound in patients with T2D, similar to the percentage found in an Italian[18] and Scottish population.[19] In our experience, >80% of obese patients with T2D screened by MRS have NAFLD. Indeed, nearly 80% of those with abnormal aminotransferases and 53% of those with normal aminotransferases have biopsy-proven NASH.[20] The prevalence of NAFLD has been less well studied in patients with type 1 diabetes (T1D). Targher et al.[21] studied >200 patients with T1D using ultrasound and liver aminotransferase levels and found a prevalence of nearly 55%. The patients with NAFLD had a higher BMI and were more insulin resistant than controls, thus posing the question of whether hyperglycemia *per se* or a combination of obesity and insulin resistance are the driving factors in the promotion of NAFLD.

It also has been suggested that there are ethnic variations in NAFLD, with Hispanics having the highest prevalence, followed by Caucasians, and finally African Americans.[7,9,22,23] In most studies, however, ethnicities were not well matched for risk factors for NAFLD. When controlling for obesity, Lomonaco et al.[24] found no significant increase in hepatic steatosis or NASH severity in Hispanics compared with Caucasians. In addition, contrary to common belief, Hispanics had similar severity of insulin resistance to Caucasians. They did show, however, that Hispanics with diabetes had slightly more fibrosis on liver biopsy than Caucasians. Other groups have attained similar findings.[25] In regard to the African American population, they are believed to have the lowest prevalence of NAFLD when compared with Hispanics and Caucasians. Guerrero et al.[26] conducted a reanalysis of the Dallas Heart Study, which found that the lower prevalence of steatosis among African Americans was associated closely with lower total body fat. It remains to be elucidated whether African Americans are truly less susceptible to the development of NAFLD, or if it is due to their leaner body habitus and better metabolic profiles in most studies. Still, African American patients with NAFLD may be at risk of NASH as reported in several studies,[7,27] and even at a higher risk of cirrhosis and HCC.[28] More work needs to be done in establishing the role of ethnicity in NAFLD and NASH, particularly in the African American population, which has been underrepresented in prior studies.

Although most of the published literature suggests an increasing prevalence of NAFLD in the adult population, the same is true in the pediatric population, largely because of the increasing incidence of obesity. Welsh et al.[29] demonstrated a threefold increase in prevalence of pediatric NAFLD from 1988 to 2010, when using BMI and abnormal aminotransferases as markers of disease. Given the adult data, we can extrapolate that this is likely an underrepresentation of the true prevalence of disease in the pediatric population. In regard to gender, men have a significantly higher prevalence of NAFLD and NASH when compared with females.[7,9,30] There has been, however, an increased prevalence in postmenopausal women, thus suggesting that sex hormone metabolism may have an effect on NAFLD.[31]

NATURAL HISTORY

Given the increasing rate of worldwide obesity, there will likely be a surge in patients with NAFLD and its related complications over the upcoming years. Proof of this is the nine-fold increase seen in the need for liver transplantation resulting from NASH from 2001 to 2009.[32] It is believed that if this rate of increase continues, NASH soon will surpass all other liver diseases as the number-one indication for liver transplantation.

The exact mechanisms and progression over time from simple steatosis to steatohepatitis are not fully elucidated. Nor is it clear which patients will advance from steatohepatitis to cirrhosis or HCC. Several studies[33–35] have looked at long-term outcomes in patients with NAFLD and NASH and have found that overall mortality in patients with NAFLD is increased when compared with healthy controls. When looking at the causes of death, the most common cause in patients with NAFLD and NASH is CVD, followed by liver disease and, in some studies, nonhepatic malignancies. Liver-related complications (end-stage liver disease and HCC) occur mainly in those with NASH.

As summarized in Figure 54.1, when followed over 2–6 years, about a third of patients with NASH have evidence of disease progression. Those at highest risk include older patients, those with obesity, and presence or family history of T2D. Patients with a fatty liver are at increased risk of developing T2D, even in the absence of obesity.[36,37] Prediabetes is also more common in patients with NAFLD compared with well-matched controls without liver disease.[38] A study by Loomba et al.[39] showed that the presence of T2D, and to a lesser degree a family history of diabetes, were both associated with a higher prevalence of fibrosis after adjustment for other confounding factors, confirming a prior landmark longitudinal study by Adams et al.[40] Also, after a mean follow-up of 3.7 years, Pais et al.[41] reported the development of NASH in two-thirds of patients with simple steatosis and progression to severe fibrosis in 40%, with the most important risk factor for progression being T2D. In addition, ~7% of those with NASH cirrhosis will

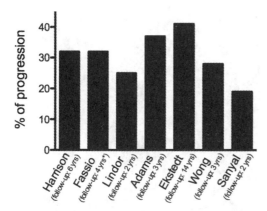

Figure 54.1—NASH and disease progression. Reprinted with permission from the publisher.[114]

develop HCC during 6.5 years of follow-up.[42,43] Again, patients with T2D and NASH are at the highest risk of developing HCC.[28]

T2D is associated with a much higher risk of developing steatohepatitis and cirrhosis, as well as HCC. The greatest challenge for physicians is to predict which patients will progress from NAFLD to NASH, and which will progress to fibrosis or HCC. Unfortunately, aside from unfavorable baseline clinical characteristics (such as obesity and diabetes) and severity of liver histology, there are no validated plasma biomarkers or imaging techniques that predict future disease at this time.

ROLE OF OBESITY AND METABOLIC ASSOCIATIONS

Although the exact mechanism behind the development of fatty liver disease is not fully understood, obesity plays a major role in the pathogenesis of NAFLD and NASH.[44] A schematic representation (Figure 54.2) illustrates that excessive intra-hepatic TG accumulation is the consequence of dysfunctional, insulin-resistant adipose tissue. In this setting (typical of obesity and T2D) diminished adipocyte insulin sensitivity (genetic, or acquired as in obesity) causes excessive rates of lipolysis and oversecretion of free fatty acids (FFA). Increased flux of FFA to the liver in turn, leads to stimulation of *de novo* lipogenesis, TG accumulation, and development of NAFLD. It is also hypothesized that this increased FFA flux through the mitochondria causes mitochondrial dysfunction, release of reactive oxygen species, activation of intrahepatocyte inflammatory pathways, and lipo-apoptosis.[7] This chronic "lipotoxicity" translates into necroinflammation and fibrosis, with eventual disease progression to cirrhosis or HCC. Increased liver FFA flux and altered mitochondrial fatty acid oxidation recently have been demonstrated in patients with NAFLD.[45] The resultant metabolic consequences are chronic hyperinsulinemia from hepatic insulin resistance and decreased insulin

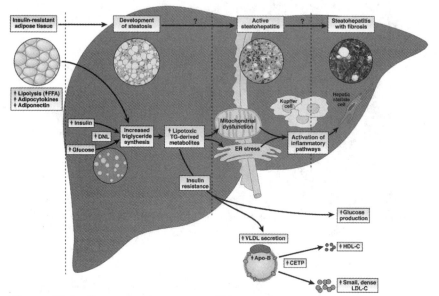

Figure 54.2—Excessive intrahepatic TG accumulation is the consequence of insulin-resistant adipose tissue. Reprinted with permission from the publisher.[5]

clearance,[46] dyslipidemia, and subclinical inflammation, all potentially contributing to premature CVD and diabetes.[4]

Although clinical evidence of the association between NAFLD and incident T2D comes from both retrospective[47] and prospective[48] studies, the link between CVD and NAFLD is supported mainly by cross-sectional studies that have relied on surrogate markers of CVD (carotid intimal-medial thickness, calcium score, endothelial dysfunction).[49] Also, in most of these studies, the diagnosis of NAFLD was made using liver aminotransferases or ultrasound rather than gold-standard techniques (MRS or histology). Although large, prospective studies assessing CV events in patients with NAFLD are lacking, those evaluating mortality consistently have reported an increase in deaths due to CVD in patients with a fatty liver. A frequently overlooked problem of these studies is that patients with NAFLD usually have a worse metabolic profile (higher BMI, more T2D, and worse dyslipidemia) than those without a fatty liver, something that cannot be completely corrected by statistical analysis. Therefore, data are insufficient at present to conclude that NAFLD is independently associated with CVD.

Many other conditions commonly seen in NAFLD may explain the increased CV risk of these patients. Very-low-density lipoproteins (VLDL) are not appropriately suppressed by insulin in these patients and the hepatic oversecretion of VLDL (which correlates with intrahepatic TG accumulation) translates into the typical dyslipidemic profile of patients with NAFLD, with high TGs, low HDL-C, and small and dense LDL particles.[50,51] In a study by Fabbrini et al.[52] hepatic steatosis, but not visceral fat, was associated with higher insulin resistance and worse dyslipidemia. Increased insulin resistance in patients with NAFLD in turn may translate into worse T2D control, requiring increased dosages of medication to achieve glycemic control.[53] Myocardial steatosis, impaired left ventricular energy metabolism, and diastolic dysfunction also have been correlated with hepatic steatosis, and can contribute to CVD.[49,54,55] NAFLD and CVD are linked closely, but the question remains whether this link is independent of all the other classic CV risk factors.

Other less well-supported associations have been described for a variety of comorbidities, including obstructive sleep apnea (OSA), vitamin D deficiency, colonic adenomas, hypothyroidism, and PCOS.[4]

A recent meta-analysis by Musso et al.[56] illustrated that there is an association with OSA in patients with NAFLD, linking it to an increased prevalence of NASH and fibrosis. It has been postulated that chronic intermittent hypoxia may promote hepatic TG accumulation, necroinflammation, and fibrosis through activation of several cellular pathways.[56] No adjustments in the previous meta-analysis, however, were made for insulin resistance or T2D. Therefore, overlapping risk factors between OSA and NAFLD may explain these results. Therefore, it may be prudent at present to screen patients with OSA for NAFLD and vice versa.

Targher et al.[57] reported an association between vitamin D deficiency and NAFLD when comparing 60 patients with NAFLD to 60 healthy controls, along with correlations in histologic severity. It has been hypothesized that vitamin D deficiency may play a role in insulin resistance, impaired insulin secretion, and upregulation of hepatic inflammatory and oxidative stress genes.[57] In our hands[58] and those of others,[59] however, no associations between vitamin D deficiency and severity of liver disease or insulin resistance at the levels of the skeletal muscle, adipose tissue, or liver were found. Needless to say, more work needs to be done in regard to vitamin D and its effects in NAFLD.

Colonic adenomas, and more important, colorectal neoplasm also have been associated with NAFLD and NASH. In a provocative cross-sectional study by Wong et al.[61] using liver MRS or biopsy, patients with NASH, but not those with simple steatosis, were found to have an increase in colorectal advanced neoplasm. Stadlmayr et al.[60] arrived at similar conclusions in 1,211 patients, but using liver ultrasound for the diagnosis of NAFLD. Yet, the debate remains as some studies have arrived at opposite conclusions.[62]

Hypothyroidism is another commonly encountered disease, which has been suggested to be associated with NAFLD. In a large cross-sectional study from China in ~4,000 patients, there was a significant association between NAFLD and hypothyroidism.[63] In addition, there was a steady increase in the prevalence of NAFLD and abnormal aminotransferase levels with worsening hypothyroidism. Although we also reported an association between hypothyroidism and NAFLD in a middle-age, obese population,[64] we found no evidence that hypothyroidism worsened liver disease in patients with NASH. This suggests that the association of these two entities may be linked more closely to obesity and its associated metabolic abnormalities than to the severity of liver disease itself.

NAFLD also may be evident in women with PCOS, because both conditions are associated with obesity and insulin resistance. A recent small cross-sectional study[65] comparing women with PCOS to healthy controls, well-matched for age and weight, showed that women with PCOS had a statistically higher prevalence of hepatic steatosis, metabolic syndrome, and elevated aminotransaminases. Similar results were reported in a smaller cross-sectional study using liver MRS for the diagnosis of NAFLD in women with hyperandrogenic PCOS.[66] Although both studies were relatively small and await confirmation, their results suggest that PCOS is associated with hepatic steatosis. Therefore, physicians should consider liver disease in all women with PCOS, regardless of their age.

As reviewed, NAFLD has been associated with several unrelated comorbidities. As studies have been rather small, retrospective, or included controls not well matched for age, BMI, or prevalence of T2D, it remains unclear whether these associations are real, or whether they are just the result of confounding factors affecting the analyses. Therefore, large, prospective, and well-controlled studies are much needed.

DIAGNOSIS

According to the American Association for the Study of Liver Diseases (AASLD) Practice Guidelines[1] for the diagnosis and management of NAFLD, the following criteria for the diagnosis are required: *1*) hepatic steatosis by imaging or histology; and *2*) no coexisting causes for chronic liver disease, such as significant alcohol consumption, medications, or other competing etiologies for hepatic steatosis.

The first step in the evaluation of any patient is performing a comprehensive history and physical exam. Many patients with NAFLD may have no physical exam findings, except for elevated BMI (although not always the case), and may be completely asymptomatic. Some patients, however, may exhibit generalized right upper-quadrant pain, hepatomegaly, or evidence of insulin resistance, such as acanthosis nigricans.[5,22] Oftentimes, elevations in liver aminotransferases, particularly alanine aminotransferase (ALT), will be present and should prompt additional evaluation. As was previously discussed, however, normal ALT levels are common in NAFLD,[8,67] and physicians therefore must have a high index of suspicion to diagnose NAFLD and NASH.

In the event that patients have elevated plasma aminotransferases, they must be evaluated for causative factors. One of the first things to evaluate is alcohol consumption, which should not be significant to make the diagnosis of NAFLD, although the definition is arbitrary. The AASLD Guidelines[1] recommend that ongoing or recent alcohol consumption not be higher than 21 drinks per week for men and 14 drinks per week for women, or otherwise would constitute significant alcohol consumption. Beyond alcohol, commonly used medications such as corticosteroids, diltiazem, amiodarone, valproic acid, and methotrexate can cause steatosis or elevations in liver aminotransferases, to name a few. Certain disease processes, such as hepatitis B and C, autoimmune hepatitis, primary biliary cirrhosis, α-1 antitrypsin deficiency, and Wilson's disease, also must be excluded in the evaluation of patients with hepatic steatosis.[4,43]

Once these considerations have been explored and found to be noncontributory, NAFLD must be considered. Although liver ultrasound is widely available, inexpensive, and has no radiation exposure, it is operator dependent and not as accurate in patients who are morbidly obese or who have <30% liver fat present.[68] Thus, using this tool, many patients are left undiagnosed. Another ultrasound-based technique is transient elastography (TE), which has been used throughout Europe, Asia, and Canada. It uses low-amplitude shear waves that propagate through the liver parenchyma and the velocity with which the wave moves is directly correlated with liver stiffness. Studies have shown that the TE was accurate when diagnosing cirrhosis and advanced fibrosis;[69] however, >20% of the studies performed were unable to be interpreted secondary to patient body habitus.[70]

Computed tomography provides better images when compared with ultrasound; however, it exposes patients to large amounts of radiation. It is able to detect moderate to severe degrees of steatosis, but it is unable to quantify the amount of fat present, and it cannot be used to follow disease progression or response to treatment.[68] Therefore, MRS is the gold-standard technique for diagnosis of NAFLD because of its high sensitivity and specificity for steatosis.[43] It has been shown to have a very good correlation with the amount of liver fat estimated by liver biopsy, and the technique has been extensively validated in the Dallas Heart Study.[11] Although MRS is an excellent tool to utilize in the diagnosis of NAFLD, it is not approved by the U.S. Food and Drug Administration and is available only in academic institutions for use in the research setting.[43] Recent work examining the role of magnetic resonance elastography in patients with NAFLD has been promising.[71]

Although noninvasive radiologic tools are helpful to make the diagnosis of NAFLD, they cannot accurately identify patients with NASH. At present, a liver biopsy is the only reliable means of diagnosing NASH.[1] Although it is a fairly well-tolerated procedure, it is also more invasive and carries the risk of bleeding, infection, and injury to adjacent organs. By obtaining liver tissue, it is possible to grade the severity of steatohepatitis and establish fibrosis stages. This allows confirmation of the diagnosis, determines disease severity and prognosis, and verifies need for treatment. The patients who are best suited for undergoing a liver biopsy are those with high-risk clinical factors, such as obesity and T2D, and with chronically elevated liver aminotransferases greater than two to three times the upper limit of normal, when other causes of liver disease have been excluded or when treatment options depend on biopsy results.[1,4,5] With better treatments for NASH becoming available to clinicians, and the fact that patients with T2D are at greater risk of NASH and cirrhosis, a liver biopsy may be considered more often in selected patients.

Over the past several years, there have been significant efforts to identify serologic indicators of NASH and fibrosis. Combined clinical (age, BMI, presence of diabetes, other) and laboratory (aminotransferase levels, platelet count, albumin, other) screening scores have been developed, such as the aspartate aminotransferase (AST)/ALT ratio, BARD (BMI ≥28=1 point, AST to ALT Ratio of ≥0.8=2 points, Diabetes=1 point), FIB-4 (Fibrosis-4 Score), Fatty Liver Index, NAFLD Fibrosis Score, and others, with easily obtainable clinical information. These scores have been tested by several different groups,[67,72] and although the FIB-4 and NAFLD Fibrosis Score show some promise, they have not been found to have ample accuracy or validity at this time and are useful largely to identify advanced, but not intermediate, stages of the disease.[4] Thus, more work needs to be done in identifying a noninvasive scoring system, which will accurately and consistently predict those with NASH without requiring patients to undergo a liver biopsy.

Another potential noninvasive biomarker, which recently has been examined widely, is caspase-cleaved cytokeratin-18 (CK-18),[4] a biomarker of hepatocyte apoptosis. Because hepatocyte apoptosis plays a critical role in the pathogenesis of NASH, CK-18 is believed to be increased in patients with NASH when compared with controls with steatosis alone.[5,73] A recent study, however, found a low sensitivity and specificity for CK-18 as a predictor of NAFLD, NASH, or fibrosis and found a weak correlation with steatosis, lobular inflammation, and fibrosis in a large cross-sectional study.[74] Thus, we believe that plasma CK-18 is an inadequate biomarker for the diagnosis or monitoring of NASH, but its value may increase in combination with other tests.

Although these modalities are used to diagnose NAFLD, the genetics behind this disease remain unclear.[75] Genetic variants described have involved molecules regulating insulin signaling, lipid metabolism, oxidative stress, or fibrogenesis. Research suggests that the strongest genetic signal for the presence of NAFLD is a single-nucleotide polymorphism, rs738409 (G allele), encoding isoleucine substitution for methionine (I148M) in a gene called patatin-like phospholipase A3 (PNPLA3). Located in adipose tissue and the liver, its main function is as a minor hydrolase to regulate lipolysis. Its true physiological relevance in NAFLD remains to be determined.[49] No genetic testing currently is recommended, however, for the diagnosis of NAFLD.[1]

See Table 54.1 for a summary of different tools used to make the diagnosis of NAFLD and Figure 54.3 for an algorithm to use in the diagnosis of NAFLD and NASH.

TREATMENT

LIFESTYLE MODIFICATIONS

Management of patients with NAFLD should be focused on lifestyle modifications, such as diet and exercise, as these currently are the standard of care. Multiple studies suggest that by implementing lifestyle modifications, specifically weight reduction, aminotransferase levels and hepatic steatosis improve when measured by ultrasound or MRS.[1] The information regarding the effect on liver histology is sparse, however.[76] Not only does weight reduction improve NAFLD, but evidence suggests that macronutrient composition and type of exercise (aerobic activity versus resistance activity) also may influence hepatic TG accumulation,[4] as these have both been shown to affect disease as well. In a 2009 study by Kirk et al.,[77] patients who were divided into low-carbohydrate versus high-carbohydrate caloric-restricted diets took similar amounts of time to lose 7% of body weight, and changes in the amount of liver fat as measured by MRS (38 vs. 45%, $P <0.001$ when compared to baseline) also were similar. A larger study conducted by Haufe et al.[78] in 2011, randomized 102 people to low-fat versus low-carbohydrate diets over a 24-week period. Patients in the low-fat group lost 6.5% body fat, whereas those in the low-carbohydrate group lost 7.5% ($P <0.001$). Both groups had a similar, statistically significant, change in liver fat when measured by

Table 54.1 Profile of Currently Available Diagnostic Tests for Nonalcoholic Fatty Liver Disease (NAFLD)

Diagnostic tool	Current cost	Current availability	Sensitivity	Specificity	Test limitations
Plasma AST/ALT	Low	High	+	+	Fluctuate over time; poor reflection of histology
Clinical scoring systems*	Low	High	++	++	Poor performance when intermediate disease severity
Plasma CK-18 levels	Intermediate	Low	++	++	Poor performance when intermediate disease severity
Ultrasound**	Low	High	+++	+++	Operator dependent
Computed tomography**	Intermediate	High	+++	+++	Involves radiation
MRI and spectroscopy (MRS)	High	Low	++++	++++	Only in research settings; contraindicated with noncompatible metal devices
Transient elastography†	Intermediate	Low	+++	+++	Operator dependent, obesity hampers testing
Liver biopsy	High	High	++++	++++	Invasive procedure

Note: AST = aspartate aminotransferase; ALT = alanine transaminase; CK-18 = cytokeratin-18.

*Clinical scoring systems such as FIB-4, BARD, Fatty Liver Index, NAFLD Fibrosis Score, and AST/ALT ratio.

†Used for the diagnosis of fibrosis.

**Sensitivity decreases in patients with liver fat <30%.

MRS (42 vs. 47%, *P* = NS between groups but *P* <0.001 when compared to baseline for both groups).

As summarized elsewhere,[43] several studies looking at exercise alone have indicated that although exercise may reduce liver fat content as measured by MRS, results were not as dramatic as with dietary interventions or integrated lifestyle modification programs. When combining exercise with diet modification, studies have shown a reduction in hemoglobin A1C and hepatic steatosis as measured by MRS.[79] Patients who lose >7% of body weight with a moderate-intensity hypoca-

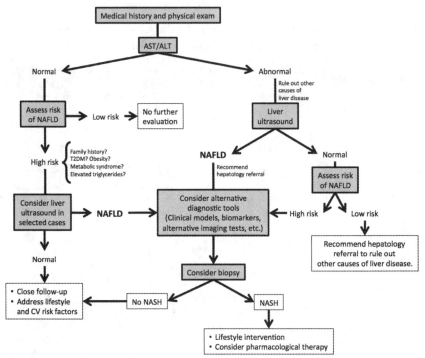

Figure 54.3—Diagnostic algorithm for NAFLD and NASH. From Bril and Cusi.[49]

loric diet plus exercise,[76] or with the addition of a weight-loss agent,[80] have a significant improvement in steatohepatitis but not in fibrosis.

BARIATRIC SURGERY

Given that lifestyle modification is often difficult, there has been a large amount of effort looking at the effects of bariatric surgery on those with obesity and NAFLD or NASH. Procedures such as laparoscopic adjustable banding, sleeve gastrectomy, and the Roux-en-Y gastric bypass have been the most studied procedures to date.[81] Surgeons should take advantage of these procedures and establish the diagnosis of NAFLD with a liver biopsy as the majority of these patients have NASH and many have advanced fibrosis. In the Longitudinal Assessment of Bariatric Surgery (LABS) Consortium, funded by the National Institutes of Health, only ~10% of patients undergoing bariatric surgery had a liver biopsy taken at the time of the procedure. It was estimated by the authors that >85% of those with NASH or advanced fibrosis did not undergo biopsy and went undiagnosed.[49] Bariatric surgery has been shown to have sustainable effects on weight loss, steatohepatitis, and often, but not always, on fibrosis when histology was reviewed. There are no prospective randomized controlled trials (RCTs), however, which led a Cochrane review to conclude that data are insufficient to make NASH a clear indication for the procedure.[82] In one of the few large, long-term prospective trials, there was not a marked effect on fibrosis.[83] It remains to be established whether histological improvement is just the result of weight reduction alone or whether there is an intrinsic metabolic effect on the liver from bariatric surgery. The AASLD Guidelines[1] do not believe bariatric surgery is contraindicated in an otherwise-eligible obese individual with NAFLD or NASH, but at present cannot recommend it specifically to treat NASH.

GLUCOSE-LOWERING AGENTS

Aside from lifestyle modifications and bariatric surgery, significant effort has been placed into studying and developing pharmaceutical options for the treatment of NAFLD and NASH. Because NAFLD has been shown to be associated with insulin resistance and diabetes, insulin sensitizers and other diabetic medications have been explored. Metformin was associated with a reduction in aminotransferases and insulin resistance in early studies, but in recent RCTs, it was found not to improve histolology.[4,49] Therefore, it is not recommended as a specific treatment for liver disease in adults with NASH.[1]

Many studies have looked at the effects of thiazolidinediones (TZDs) on patients with NAFLD and NASH. TZDs act as peroxisome proliferator-activated receptor-γ (PPAR-γ) agonists to improve insulin resistance in skeletal muscle, in adipose tissue, and at the level of the liver. The AASLD[1] recommends pioglitazone to treat steatohepatitis in patients with biopsy-proven NASH, particularly in patients with T2D. TZDs improve insulin sensitivity, plasma aminotransferases and histology (steatosis, inflammation, and ballooning) in patients with[84] and without[85,86] T2D. The **P**ioglitazone, **V**itamin **E**, or Placebo for **N**onalcoholic **S**teatohepatitis (PIVENS) study,[85] a large multicenter RCT, compared three interventions: pioglitazone versus vitamin E versus placebo. Although both pioglitazone and vitamin E were found to have statistically significant improvements in histology versus placebo, only the pioglitazone group had a statistically significant higher number of patients in whom there was resolution of NASH compared with placebo. In a recent RCT by Cusi,[87] 18 months of pioglitazone treatment (vs. placebo) in patients with prediabetes or T2D and NASH, led to a significant improvement in steatohepatitis. Moreover, it was shown to have a modest, but significant effect on fibrosis when compared with placebo. The TZD was well tolerated with no significant adverse events aside from a 2-kilogram weight gain on average. As reviewed elsewhere,[88] potential side effects of pioglitazone include weight gain (2–4 kilograms depending on dosing and duration of treatment), bladder cancer (males), potential bone loss (females), and mixed effects on the cardiovascular system (reduced risk of CV events but a slight increase in congestive heart failure[89]). Much work is needed to fully understand the long-term safety and efficacy of this medication.

There has been much interest in incretin mimetics, such as exenatide and liraglutide, because they promote weight loss and activation of hepatic glucagon-like peptide-1 (GLP-1) signaling causing reductions in hepatic steatosis in rodents.[90] These findings are thought to result from a direct effect on liver signaling pathways, such as GLP-1 receptors present in hepatocytes,[91] or indirectly via weight loss, which reverses lipotoxicity and reduces hyperglycemia. In a pilot study using twice-daily exenatide in patients with well-controlled T2D, the incretin-mimetic led to a ~20% reduction in hepatic steatosis as measured by MRS,[43] but it has not been shown to have a significant role in the reversal of NASH.[92] Results from ongoing RCTs are awaited to examine the potential of incretin-mimetics in patients with NAFLD or NASH.[49]

VITAMIN E

Another class of medications studied in detail is antioxidants, specifically vitamin E. It has been postulated that vitamin E has the potential to reduce the generation of hepatocyte reactive oxygen species and inhibit inflammatory cytokines. An extensive amount of research has been conducted in regard to vitamin E and its effects on NAFLD and NASH. In the PIVENS[85] trial, vitamin E was found to be beneficial in adult patients with NASH when liver histology was used as the primary outcome. On the contrary, the Effect of Vitamin E or Metformin for Treatment of Nonalcoholic Fatty Liver Disease in Children and Adolescents trial (TONIC),[93] did not meet the primary endpoint of a sustainable reduction in liver aminotransferase levels. When looking specifically at histology, the vitamin E arm showed no significant change in steatosis, inflammation, or fibrosis. Changes were noted in ballooning, however, thus affecting the prevalence of patients with NASH after treatment. Therefore, treatment with vitamin E may be attempted in patients without diabetes with biopsy-proven NASH, but more evidence is needed in regard to its efficacy in patients with diabetes or cirrhosis and in patients who do not have histologic confirmation of NAFLD.[1]

PENTOXIFYLLINE

Although the majority of the previously discussed treatments had modest to no effect on fibrosis, pentoxifylline (PTX) has been tested as an antifibrotic agent with anti-inflammatory properties (i.e., inhibition of cytokines such as tumor necrosis factor-α with reduction of free radical production).[4,49] In a small pilot study, Zein et al.[94] reported that PTX significantly improved steatosis, lobular inflammation, and fibrosis when compared with placebo. Additional studies[95] have shown that it decreases plasma levels of oxidized fatty acids compared with placebo and lipid-derived oxidative stress. At the current time, however, it is not recommended for use in patients with NAFLD until stronger evidence is found.

LIPID-LOWERING MEDICATIONS

The use of lipid-lowering medications has been the subject of a recent in-depth review.[96] In brief, statins are useful in the treatment of dyslipidemia, which is a known risk for CVD, the number-one metabolic complication of NAFLD. Several studies have shown that statins are safe to use in patients with liver disease, and no evidence has shown that patients with chronic liver disease,[97,98] including NAFLD and NASH, have an increased risk of liver injury from statins over those without liver disease. Thus, it is the recommendation of the AASLD[1] that statins can be used to treat dyslipidemia. Several small studies[99,100] have suggested that statins may even improve liver biochemistries and histology in patients with NASH. In the only pilot RCT[101] (n = 16) to date, however, there was no effect on liver histology. As reviewed elsewhere,[102] statins have been shown to improve liver biochemistries and steatosis by ultrasound, but results in histology have been rather inconsistent and likely not significant from a therapeutic perspective. Statins should not be used to improve liver histology of patients with NAFLD or NASH but essentially to prevent CVD.

Other lipid-lowering medications, such as niacin and fibrates, have been examined as well. An RCT from Fabbrini et al.[103] examined 27 obese subjects with NAFLD when taking placebo versus niacin versus fenofibrate. Neither niacin nor fenofibrate were found to affect intrahepatic TG as measured by MRS. In addition, niaspan caused hepatic, adipose tissue, and muscle insulin resistance (P <0.05), whereas fenofibrate had no effect on insulin action, which is consistent with other reports.[104]

MISCELLANEOUS MEDICATIONS

Many other medications have been evaluated for the treatment of NAFLD.[49,105] Few, however, have been assessed in large RCTs using liver histology as the primary endpoint. In addition, there have been conflicting results among the studies. For instance, ursodeoxycholic acid (UDCA), has been suggested to have a modest effect on steatosis and fibrosis in NASH, but studies have been small, most studies have been poorly controlled, and results overall have been inconsistent.[106] Omega-3 polyunsaturated fatty acid (PUFA) supplementation has generated significant interest, but thus far, studies have reported a minimal impact on liver aminotransferases or hepatic steatosis, and effects on liver histology in NASH are unknown. RCTs are underway to examine this further.

In addition to UDCA and PUFAs, orlistat (Xenical, a pancreatic lipase inhibitor that prevents the absorption of fats and is used for weight reduction) was found to improve liver histology in patients with NASH, in particular if ≥7% of total body weight was lost. Both the control group and those on orlistat lost similar amounts of weight, however, and both groups had a similar change in histology.[80] Thus, it is likely that these findings are due to weight loss alone and not necessarily to an intrinsic property attributable to the drug.

Most recently, there has been interest in regard to the farnesoid X receptor (FXR) ligand obeticholic acid (OCA), a semisynthetic derivative of the primary human bile acid chenodeoxycholic acid and the natural agonist of FXR (a hormone receptor that regulates glucose and lipid metabolism in the liver). This drug has been reported to improve insulin sensitivity and reduce markers of liver inflammation and fibrosis in patients with T2D and NAFLD after 6 weeks of treatment.[107] Moreover, positive results in patients with biopsy-proven NASH were reported with OCA after 72 weeks in the Farnesoid X Receptor (FXR) Ligand Obeticholic Acid in NASH Treatment Trial (FLINT) (a multicenter RCT). In a planned interim analysis, there was a statistical improvement (P = 0.0024 on an intention-to-treat basis) in the primary liver histological endpoint of an NAFLD activity score decrease of at least two points, with no worsening of fibrosis, in approximately half of the participants on OCA treatment.[49] Thus, OCA appears to be a promising treatment option for patients with NASH.

As can be appreciated in Table 54.2, there are currently very few treatment options that have been shown to be effective in large, long-term RCTs. According to the available evidence at this time, the best treatment option for patients with T2D may be pioglitazone. Therefore, early initiation of this drug may be considered in this population. In nondiabetic patients, both vitamin E and pioglitazone have been found to be effective. While obeticholic acid and incretin mimetics offer significant promise for the treatment of NAFLD, more work needs to be done to determine their long-term safety and efficacy in the treatment of NAFLD and NASH, especially in patients with T2D.

FUTURE DIRECTIONS

Although great strides have been made in the study of NAFLD, many knowledge gaps still exist. One such area that needs further attention is the study of NAFLD in the pediatric population; placing more emphasis on this age-group will be critical to halt, or at least ameliorate, the progression of this disease and its CV consequences later in life. It can be said that the field is at a stage comparable to diabetic nephropathy before the establishment of albumin excretion rates as a

Table 54.2 Pharmacologic Agents Tested for the Treatment of NAFLD or NASH

Medication	Results*	Outcomes
Glucose-lowering agents		
Metformin	Ineffective	AST/ALT,[93] histology,[108]
Pioglitazone	Effective	AST/ALT, MRS, histology[84–87]
Exenatide[†]	Effective (NAFLD)	AST/ALT, MRS[109]
Liraglutide[†]	Effective (NAFLD)	AST/ALT, CT[110]
Lipid-lowering agents		
Statins	Ineffective	AST/ALT,[111] histology[101]
Niacin	Ineffective	AST/ALT, MRS[103]
Fibrates	Ineffective	AST/ALT, MRS[103]
PUFA[†]	Mixed results	AST/ALT, MRS[112]
Orlistat**	Ineffective	Histology[80]
Vitamin E	Mixed results	AST/ALT,[85] histology[93]
Ursodeoxycholic acid	Mixed results	AST/ALT, histology[106]
Pentoxifylline	Effective	Histology,[94] AST/ALT[113]
Obeticholic acid	Effective	Histology[107]

Note: AST = aspartate aminotransferase; ALT = alanine transaminase; CT = computed tomography; MRS = magnetic resonance and spectroscopy; PUFA = polyunsaturated fatty acid.
*Drug was effective or ineffective in at least one large RCT. Mixed results: both effective and ineffective RCTs have been published.
**Results may be attributed to weight loss and not intrinsic effect of medication.
[†]No significant data on liver histology.

standard of care or of osteoporosis before the routine use of dual X-ray absorptiometry. Both conditions now are diagnosed and treated early on in a cost-effective manner. We predict that development of better early, noninvasive diagnostic tests that predict those at the greatest risk of NASH will make routine screening and early treatment mandatory. We envision that such testing will be incorporated as a standard of care for all patients with diabetes. Until then, increased clinician awareness; early identification of high-risk patients based on their clinical profile and the available tools; and treatment with lifestyle intervention, pioglitazone, and other emerging agents likely will have a major impact as we move forward in understanding NAFLD.

REFERENCES

1. Chalasani N, Younossi Z, Lavine JE, et al. The diagnosis and management of non-alcoholic fatty liver disease: practice guideline by the American Association for the Study of Liver Diseases, American College of Gastroenterology, and the American Gastroenterological Association. *Hepatology* 2012;55:2005–2023.

2. Fabbrini E, Sullivan S, Klein S. Obesity and nonalcoholic fatty liver disease: Biochemical, metabolic, and clinical implications. *Hepatology* 2010;51:679–689.

3. Gaggini M, Morelli M, Buzzigoli E, DeFronzo RA, Bugianesi E, Gastaldelli A. Non-alcoholic fatty liver disease (NAFLD) and its connection with insulin resistance, dyslipidemia, atherosclerosis and coronary heart disease. *Nutrients* 2013;5:1544–1560.

4. Torres DM, Williams CD, Harrison SA. Features, diagnosis, and treatment of nonalcoholic fatty liver disease. *Clin Gastroenterol Hepatol* 2012;10:837–858.

5. Lomonaco R, Chen J, Cusi K. An endocrine perspective of nonalcoholic fatty liver disease (NAFLD). *Ther Adv Endocrinol Metab* 2011;2:211–225.

6. Vernon G, Baranova A, Younossi ZM. Systematic review: the epidemiology and natural history of non-alcoholic fatty liver disease and non-alcoholic steatohepatitis in adults. *Aliment Pharmacol Ther* 2011;34:274–285.

7. Williams CD, Stengel J, Asike MI, et al. Prevalence of nonalcoholic fatty liver disease and nonalcoholic steatohepatitis among a largely middle-aged population utilizing ultrasound and liver biopsy: a prospective study. *Gastroenterology* 2011;140:124–131.

8. Fracanzani AL, Valenti L, Bugianesi E, et al. Risk of severe liver disease in nonalcoholic fatty liver disease with normal aminotransferase levels: a role for insulin resistance and diabetes. *Hepatology* 2008;48:792–798.

9. Browning JD, Szczepaniak LS, Dobbins R, et al. Prevalence of hepatic steatosis in an urban population in the United States: impact of ethnicity. *Hepatology* 2004;40:1387–1395.

10. Bedogni G, Miglioli L, Masutti F, Tiribelli C, Marchesini G, Bellentani S. Prevalence of and risk factors for nonalcoholic fatty liver disease: the Dionysos Nutrition and Liver Study. *Hepatology* 2005;42:44–52.

11. Szczepaniak LS, Nurenberg P, Leonard D, et al. Magnetic resonance spectroscopy to measure hepatic triglyceride content: prevalence of hepatic steatosis in the general population. *Am J Physiol Endocrinol Metab* 2005;288:E462–E468.

12. Haentjens P, Massaad D, Reynaert H, et al. Identifying non-alcoholic fatty liver disease among asymptomatic overweight and obese individuals by clinical and biochemical characteristics. *Acta Clin Belg* 2009;64:483–493.

13. Machado M, Marques-Vidal P, Cortez-Pinto H. Hepatic histology in obese patients undergoing bariatric surgery. *J Hepatol* 2006;45:600–606.

14. Ahmed MH, Barakat S, Almobarak AO. Nonalcoholic fatty liver disease and cardiovascular disease: has the time come for cardiologists to be hepatologists? *J Obes* 2012;483135.

15. Marcos A, Fisher RA, Ham JM, et al. Selection and outcome of living donors for adult to adult right lobe transplantation. *Transplantation* 2000;69:2410–2415.

16. Lee JY, Kim KM, Lee SG, et al. Prevalence and risk factors of non-alcoholic fatty liver disease in potential living liver donors in Korea: a review of 589 consecutive liver biopsies in a single center. *J Hepatol* 2007;47:239–244.

17. Leite NC, Salles GF, Araujo AL, Villela-Nogueira CA, Cardoso CR. Prevalence and associated factors of non-alcoholic fatty liver disease in patients with type-2 diabetes mellitus. *Liver Int* 2009;29:113–119.

18. Targher G, Bertolini L, Padovani R, et al. Prevalence of nonalcoholic fatty liver disease and its association with cardiovascular disease among type 2 diabetic patients. *Diabetes Care* 2007;30:1212–1218.

19. Williamson RM, Price JF, Glancy S, et al. Prevalence of and risk factors for hepatic steatosis and nonalcoholic fatty liver disease in people with type 2 diabetes: the Edinburgh type 2 Diabetes Study. *Diabetes Care* 2011;34:1139–1144.

20. Maximos M, Bril F, Portillo Sanchez P, et al. High risk of nonalcoholic fatty liver disease (NAFLD) and steatohepatitis (NASH) in obese patients with type 2 diabetes mellitus (T2DM) and normal liver aminotransferases. 2014;[Submitted Abstract to ADA Scientific Sessions].

21. Targher G, Bertolini L, Padovani R, et al. Prevalence of non-alcoholic fatty liver disease and its association with cardiovascular disease in patients with type 1 diabetes. *J Hepatol* 2010;53:713–718.

22. Neuschwander-Tetri BA, Clark JM, Bass NM, et al. Clinical, laboratory and histological associations in adults with nonalcoholic fatty liver disease. *Hepatology* 2010;52:913–924.

23. Mohanty SR, Troy TN, Huo D, O'Brien BL, Jensen DM, Hart J. Influence of ethnicity on histological differences in non-alcoholic fatty liver disease. *J Hepatol* 2009;50:797–804.

24. Lomonaco R, Ortiz-Lopez C, Orsak B, et al. Role of ethnicity in overweight and obese patients with nonalcoholic steatohepatitis. *Hepatology* 2011;54:837–845.

25. Bambha K, Belt P, Abraham M, et al. Ethnicity and nonalcoholic fatty liver disease. *Hepatology* 2012;55:769–780.

26. Guerrero R, Vega GL, Grundy SM, Browning JD. Ethnic differences in hepatic steatosis: an insulin resistance paradox? *Hepatology* 2009;49:791–801.

27. Kallwitz ER, Guzman G, TenCate V, et al. The histologic spectrum of liver disease in African-American, non-Hispanic white, and Hispanic obesity surgery patients. *Am J Gastroenterol* 2009;104:64–69.

28. El-Serag HB, Tran T, Everhart JE. Diabetes increases the risk of chronic liver disease and hepatocellular carcinoma. *Gastroenterology* 2004;126:460–468.

29. Welsh JA, Karpen S, Vos MB. Increasing prevalence of nonalcoholic fatty liver disease among United States adolescents, 1988–1994 to 2007–2010. *J Pediatr* 2013;162:496–500 e1.

30. Caballeria L, Pera G, Auladell MA, et al. Prevalence and factors associated with the presence of nonalcoholic fatty liver disease in an adult population in Spain. *Eur J Gastroenterol Hepatol* 2010;22:24–32.

31. Yang JD, Abdelmalek MF, Pang H, et al. Gender and menopause impact severity of fibrosis among patients with nonalcoholic steatohepatitis. *Hepatology* 2013. doi: 10.1002/hep.26761.

32. Charlton MR, Burns JM, Pedersen RA, Watt KD, Heimbach JK, Dierkhising RA. Frequency and outcomes of liver transplantation for nonalcoholic steatohepatitis in the United States. *Gastroenterology* 2011;141:1249–1253.

33. Adams LA, Harmsen S, St Sauver JL, et al. Nonalcoholic fatty liver disease increases risk of death among patients with diabetes: a community-based cohort study. *Am J Gastroenterol* 2010;105:1567–1573.

34. Stepanova M, Rafiq N, Younossi ZM. Components of metabolic syndrome are independent predictors of mortality in patients with chronic liver disease: a population-based study. *Gut* 2010;59:1410–1415.

35. Soderberg C, Stal P, Askling J, et al. Decreased survival of subjects with elevated liver function tests during a 28-year follow-up. *Hepatology* 2010;51:595–602.

36. Fan JG, Li F, Cai XB, Peng YD, Ao QH, Gao Y. The importance of metabolic factors for the increasing prevalence of fatty liver in Shanghai factory workers. *J Gastroenterol Hepatol* 2007;22:663–668.

37. Kim HJ, Kim HJ, Lee KE, et al. Metabolic significance of nonalcoholic fatty liver disease in nonobese, nondiabetic adults. *Arch Intern Med* 2004;164:2169–2175.

38. Ortiz-Lopez C, Lomonaco R, Orsak B, et al. Prevalence of prediabetes and diabetes and metabolic profile of patients with nonalcoholic fatty liver disease (NAFLD). *Diabetes Care* 2012;35:873–878.

39. Loomba R, Abraham M, Unalp A, et al. Association between diabetes, family history of diabetes, and risk of nonalcoholic steatohepatitis and fibrosis. *Hepatology* 2012;56:943–951.

40. Adams LA, Sanderson S, Lindor KD, Angulo P. The histological course of nonalcoholic fatty liver disease: a longitudinal study of 103 patients with sequential liver biopsies. *J Hepatol* 2005;42:132–138.

41. Pais R, Charlotte F, Fedchuk L, et al. A systematic review of follow-up biopsies reveals disease progression in patients with non-alcoholic fatty liver. *J Hepatol* 2013;59:550–556.

42. Bhala N, Angulo P, van der Poorten D, et al. The natural history of nonalcoholic fatty liver disease with advanced fibrosis or cirrhosis: an international collaborative study. *Hepatology* 2011;54:1208–1216.

43. Lomonaco R, Sunny NE, Bril F, Cusi K. Nonalcoholic fatty liver disease: current issues and novel treatment approaches. *Drugs* 2013;73:1–14.

44. Lomonaco R, Cusi K. In *Evidence-Based Management of Diabetes.* Buse JB, Vora, J, Eds. Shrewsbury, U.K., TFM Publishing, 2012, p. 383–404.

45. Sunny NE, Parks EJ, Browning JD, Burgess SC. Excessive hepatic mitochondrial TCA cycle and gluconeogenesis in humans with nonalcoholic fatty liver disease. *Cell Metab* 2011;14:804–810.

46. Bril F, Lomonaco R, Orsak B, et al. Relationship between disease severity, hyperinsulinemia and impaired insulin clearance in patients with nonalcoholic steatohepatitis (NASH). *Hepatology* 2013. doi: 10.1002/hep.26988.

47. Bae JC, Rhee EJ, Lee WY, et al. Combined effect of nonalcoholic fatty liver disease and impaired fasting glucose on the development of type 2 diabetes: a 4-year retrospective longitudinal study. *Diabetes Care* 2011;34:727–729.

48. Park SK, Seo MH, Shin HC, Ryoo JH. Clinical availability of nonalcoholic fatty liver disease as an early predictor of type 2 diabetes mellitus in Korean men: 5-year prospective cohort study. *Hepatology* 2013;57:1378–1383.

49. Bril F, Cusi K. Nonalcoholic fatty liver disease (NAFLD) in type 2 diabetes mellitus (T2DM): current controversies and future directions. *Diabetes Care.* In press.

50. Fabbrini E, Mohammed BS, Magkos F, Korenblat KM, Patterson BW, Klein S. Alterations in adipose tissue and hepatic lipid kinetics in obese men and women with nonalcoholic fatty liver disease. *Gastroenterology* 2008;134:424–431.

51. Kotronen A, Seppala-Lindroos A, Bergholm R, Yki-Jarvinen H. Tissue specificity of insulin resistance in humans: fat in the liver rather than muscle is associated with features of the metabolic syndrome. *Diabetologia* 2008;51:130–138.

52. Fabbrini E, Magkos F, Mohammed BS, et al. Intrahepatic fat, not visceral fat, is linked with metabolic complications of obesity. *Proc Natl Acad Sci U S A* 2009;106:15430–15435.

53. Juurinen L, Tiikkainen M, Hakkinen AM, Hakkarainen A, Yki-Jarvinen H. Effects of insulin therapy on liver fat content and hepatic insulin sensitivity in patients with type 2 diabetes. *Am J Physiol Endocrinol Metab* 2007;292:E829–E835.

54. Rijzewijk LJ, Jonker JT, van der Meer RW, et al. Effects of hepatic triglyceride content on myocardial metabolism in type 2 diabetes. *J Am Coll Cardiol* 2010;56:225–233.

55. Bonapace S, Perseghin G, Molon G, et al. Nonalcoholic fatty liver disease is associated with left ventricular diastolic dysfunction in patients with type 2 diabetes. *Diabetes Care* 2012;35:389–395.

56. Musso G, Cassader M, Olivetti C, Rosina F, Carbone G, Gambino R. Association of obstructive sleep apnea with the presence and severity of nonalcoholic fatty liver disease. A systematic review and meta-analysis. *Obes Rev* 2013;14:417–431.

57. Targher G, Bertolini L, Scala L, et al. Associations between serum 25-hydroxyvitamin D3 concentrations and liver histology in patients with non-alcoholic fatty liver disease. *Nutr Metab Cardiovasc Dis* 2007;17:517–524.

58. Bril F, Maximos M, Subbarayan S, Biernacki D, Cusi K. Plasma vitamin D deficiency and development of non-alcoholic fatty liver disease (NAFLD) and nonalcoholic steatohepatitis (NASH). Unpublished 2013.

59. de las Heras J, Rajakumar K, Lee S, Bacha F, Holick MF, Arslanian SA. 25-Hydroxyvitamin D in obese youth across the spectrum of glucose tolerance from normal to prediabetes to type 2 diabetes. *Diabetes Care* 2013;36:2048–2053.

60. Stadlmayr A, Aigner E, Steger B, et al. Nonalcoholic fatty liver disease: an independent risk factor for colorectal neoplasia. *J Intern Med* 2011;270:41–49.

61. Wong VW, Wong GL, Tsang SW, et al. High prevalence of colorectal neoplasm in patients with non-alcoholic steatohepatitis. *Gut* 2011;60:829–836.

62. Touzin NT, Bush KN, Williams CD, Harrison SA. Prevalence of colonic adenomas in patients with nonalcoholic fatty liver disease. *Ther Adv Gastroenterol* 2011;4:169–176.

63. Chung GE, Kim D, Kim W, et al. Non-alcoholic fatty liver disease across the spectrum of hypothyroidism. *J Hepatol* 2012;57:150–156.

64. Bril F, Lomonaco R, Orsak B, et al. Is there a link between hypothyroidism and nonalcoholic fatty liver disease? (Abstract.) *Hepatology* 2013;58:521A.

65. Karoli R, Fatima J, Chandra A, Gupta U, Islam FU, Singh G. Prevalence of hepatic steatosis in women with polycystic ovary syndrome. *J Hum Reprod Sci* 2013;6:9–14.

66. Jones H, Sprung VS, Pugh CJ, et al. Polycystic ovary syndrome with hyperandrogenism is characterized by an increased risk of hepatic steatosis compared to nonhyperandrogenic PCOS phenotypes and healthy controls, independent of obesity and insulin resistance. *J Clin Endocrinol Metab* 2012;97:3709–3716.

67. McPherson S, Anstee QM, Henderson E, Day CP, Burt AD. Are simple non-invasive scoring systems for fibrosis reliable in patients with NAFLD and normal ALT levels? *Eur J Gastroenterol Hepatol* 2013;25:652–658.

68. Ali R, Cusi K. New diagnostic and treatment approaches in non-alcoholic fatty liver disease (NAFLD). *Ann Med* 2009;41:265–278.

69. Nobili V, Vizzutti F, Arena U, et al. Accuracy and reproducibility of transient elastography for the diagnosis of fibrosis in pediatric nonalcoholic steatohepatitis. *Hepatology* 2008;48:442–448.

70. Wong VW, Vergniol J, Wong GL, et al. Diagnosis of fibrosis and cirrhosis using liver stiffness measurement in nonalcoholic fatty liver disease. *Hepatology* 2010;51:454–462.

71. Xanthakos SA, Podberesky DJ, Serai SD, et al. Use of magnetic resonance elastography to assess hepatic fibrosis in children with chronic liver disease. *J Pediatr* 2014;164:186–188.

72. Yoneda M, Imajo K, Eguchi Y, et al. Noninvasive scoring systems in patients with nonalcoholic fatty liver disease with normal alanine aminotransferase levels. *J Gastroenterol* 2013;48:1051–1060.

73. Feldstein AE, Wieckowska A, Lopez AR, Liu YC, Zein NN, McCullough AJ. Cytokeratin-18 fragment levels as noninvasive biomarkers for nonalcoholic steatohepatitis: a multicenter validation study. *Hepatology* 2009;50:1072–1078.

74. Cusi K, Chang Z, Harrison S, et al. Limited value of plasma cytokeratin-18 as a biomarker for NASH and fibrosis in patients with nonalcoholic fatty liver disease (NAFLD). *J Hepatol* 2014;60:167–174.

75. Anstee QM, Day CP. The genetics of NAFLD. *Nat Rev Gastroenterol Hepatol* 2013;10:645–655.

76. Promrat K, Kleiner DE, Niemeier HM, et al. Randomized controlled trial testing the effects of weight loss on nonalcoholic steatohepatitis. *Hepatology* 2010;51:121–129.

77. Kirk E, Reeds DN, Finck BN, Mayurranjan SM, Patterson BW, Klein S. Dietary fat and carbohydrates differentially alter insulin sensitivity during caloric restriction. *Gastroenterology* 2009;136:1552–1560.

78. Haufe S, Engeli S, Kast P, et al. Randomized comparison of reduced fat and reduced carbohydrate hypocaloric diets on intrahepatic fat in overweight and obese human subjects. *Hepatology* 2011;53:1504–1514.

79. Lazo M, Solga SF, Horska A, et al. Effect of a 12-month intensive lifestyle intervention on hepatic steatosis in adults with type 2 diabetes. *Diabetes Care* 2010;33:2156–2163.

80. Harrison SA, Fecht W, Brunt EM, Neuschwander-Tetri BA. Orlistat for overweight subjects with nonalcoholic steatohepatitis: a randomized, prospective trial. *Hepatology* 2009;49:80–86.

81. Mummadi RR, Kasturi KS, Chennareddygari S, Sood GK. Effect of bariatric surgery on nonalcoholic fatty liver disease: systematic review and meta-analysis. *Clin Gastroenterol Hepatol* 2008;6(12):1396–1402.

82. Chavez-Tapia NC, Tellez-Avila FI, Barrientos-Gutierrez T, Mendez-Sanchez N, Lizardi-Cervera J, Uribe M. Bariatric surgery for non-alcoholic steatohepatitis in obese patients. *Cochrane Database Syst Rev* 2010;CD007340.

83. Mathurin P, Hollebecque A, Arnalsteen L, et al. Prospective study of the long-term effects of bariatric surgery on liver injury in patients without advanced disease. *Gastroenterology* 2009;137:532–540.

84. Belfort R, Harrison SA, Brown K, et al. A placebo-controlled trial of pioglitazone in subjects with nonalcoholic steatohepatitis. *N Engl J Med* 2006;355:2297–2307.

85. Sanyal AJ, Chalasani N, Kowdley KV, et al. Pioglitazone, vitamin E, or placebo for nonalcoholic steatohepatitis. *N Engl J Med* 2010;362:1675–1685.

86. Aithal GP, Thomas J, Kaye P, et al. A randomized, double blind, placebo controlled trial of one year of pioglitazone in nondiabetic subjects with NASH. (Abstract.) *Hepatology* 2007;46(Suppl):295 (abstract 132).

87. Cusi K. Extended treatment with pioglitazone improves liver histology in patients with prediabetes or type 2 diabetes mellitus and NASH. *Hepatology* 2013;60:167–174

88. Yau H, Rivera K, Lomonaco R, Cusi K. The future of thiazolidinedione therapy in the management of type 2 diabetes mellitus. *Curr Diab Rep* 2013;13:329–341.

89. Lincoff AM, Wolski K, Nicholls SJ, Nissen SE. Pioglitazone and risk of cardiovascular events in patients with type 2 diabetes mellitus: a meta-analysis of randomized trials. *JAMA* 2007;298:1180–1188.

90. Ding X, Saxena NK, Lin S, Gupta NA, Anania FA. Exendin-4, a glucagon-like protein-1 (GLP-1) receptor agonist, reverses hepatic steatosis in ob/ob mice. *Hepatology* 2006;43:173–181.

91. Gupta NA, Mells J, Dunham RM, et al. Glucagon-like peptide-1 receptor is present on human hepatocytes and has a direct role in decreasing hepatic steatosis in vitro by modulating elements of the insulin signaling pathway. *Hepatology* 2010;51:1584–1592.

92. Kenny PR, Brady DE, Torres DM, Ragozzino L, Chalasani N, Harrison SA. Exenatide in the treatment of diabetic patients with non-alcoholic steatohepatitis: a case series. *Am J Gastroenterol* 2010;105:2707–2709.

93. Lavine JE, Schwimmer JB, Van Natta ML, et al. Effect of vitamin E or metformin for treatment of nonalcoholic fatty liver disease in children and adolescents: the TONIC randomized controlled trial. *JAMA* 2011;305:1659–1668.

94. Zein CO, Yerian LM, Gogate P, et al. Pentoxifylline improves nonalcoholic steatohepatitis: a randomized placebo-controlled trial. *Hepatology* 2011;54:1610–1619.

95. Zein CO, Lopez R, Fu X, et al. Pentoxifylline decreases oxidized lipid products in nonalcoholic steatohepatitis: new evidence on the potential therapeutic mechanism. *Hepatology* 2012;56:1291–1299.

96. Bril F, Lomonaco R, Cusi K. The challenge of managing dyslipidemia in patients with nonalcoholic fatty liver disease. *Clinical Lipidology* 2012;7:471–481.

97. Chalasani N, Aljadhey H, Kesterson J, Murray MD, Hall SD. Patients with elevated liver enzymes are not at higher risk for statin hepatotoxicity. *Gastroenterology* 2004;126:1287–1292.

98. Chalasani N. Statins and hepatotoxicity: focus on patients with fatty liver. *Hepatology* 2005;41:690–695.

99. Browning JD. Statins and hepatic steatosis: perspectives from the Dallas Heart Study. *Hepatology* 2006;44:466–471.

100. Athyros VG, Tziomalos K, Gossios TD, et al. Safety and efficacy of long-term statin treatment for cardiovascular events in patients with coronary heart disease and abnormal liver tests in the Greek Atorvastatin and Coronary Heart Disease Evaluation (GREACE) Study: a post-hoc analysis. *Lancet* 2010;376:1916–1922.

101. Nelson A, Torres DM, Morgan AE, Fincke C, Harrison SA. A pilot study using simvastatin in the treatment of nonalcoholic steatohepatitis: a randomized placebo-controlled trial. *J Clin Gastroenterol* 2009;43:990–994.

102. Bril F, Cusi K. Treatment of NAFLD/NASH. In *International Book of Diabetes*. DeFronzo R, Ferrannini E, Alberti KG, Zimmet P, Eds. In press.

103. Fabbrini E, Mohammed BS, Korenblat KM, et al. Effect of fenofibrate and niacin on intrahepatic triglyceride content, very low-density lipoprotein kinetics, and insulin action in obese subjects with nonalcoholic fatty liver disease. *J Clin Endocrinol Metab* 2010;95:2727–2735.

104. Belfort R, Berria R, Cornell J, Cusi K. Fenofibrate reduces systemic inflammation markers independent of its effects on lipid and glucose metabolism in patients with the metabolic syndrome. *J Clin Endocrinol Metab* 2010;95:829–836.

105. Musso G, Gambino R, Cassader M, Pagano G. A novel approach to control hyperglycemia in type 2 diabetes: sodium glucose co-transport (SGLT) inhibitors: systematic review and meta-analysis of randomized trials. *Ann Med* 2012;44:375–393.

106. Ratziu V. Treatment of NASH with ursodeoxycholic acid: pro. *Clin Res Hepatol Gastroenterol* 2012;36(Suppl 1):S41–S45.

107. Mudaliar S, Henry RR, Sanyal AJ, et al. Efficacy and safety of the farnesoid X receptor agonist obeticholic acid in patients with type 2 diabetes and nonalcoholic fatty liver disease. *Gastroenterology* 2013;145:574–582.

108. Haukeland JW, Konopski Z, Eggesbo HB, et al. Metformin in patients with non-alcoholic fatty liver disease: a randomized, controlled trial. *Scand J Gastroenterol* 2009;44:853–860.

109. Sathyanarayana P, Jogi M, Muthupillai R, Krishnamurthy R, Samson SL, Bajaj M. Effects of combined exenatide and pioglitazone therapy on hepatic fat content in type 2 diabetes. *Obesity* 2011;19:2310–2315.

110. Jendle J, Nauck MA, Matthews DR, et al. Weight loss with liraglutide, a once-daily human glucagon-like peptide-1 analogue for type 2 diabetes treatment as monotherapy or added to metformin, is primarily as a result of a reduction in fat tissue. *Diabetes Obes Metab* 2009;11:1163–1172.

111. Lewis JH, Mortensen ME, Zweig S, Fusco MJ, Medoff JR, Belder R. Efficacy and safety of high-dose pravastatin in hypercholesterolemic patients with well-compensated chronic liver disease: results of a prospective, randomized, double-blind, placebo-controlled, multicenter trial. *Hepatology* 2007;46:1453–1463.

112. Cussons AJ, Watts GF, Mori TA, Stuckey BG. Omega-3 fatty acid supplementation decreases liver fat content in polycystic ovary syndrome: a randomized controlled trial employing proton magnetic resonance spectroscopy. *J Clin Endocrinol Metab* 2009;94:3842–3848.

113. Lee YM, Sutedja DS, Wai CT, et al. A randomized controlled pilot study of pentoxifylline in patients with non-alcoholic steatohepatitis (NASH). *Hepatol Int* 2008;2:196–201.

114. Sunny NE, Bril F, Cusi K. Nonalcoholic fatty liver disease: current issues and novel treatment approaches. *Drugs* 2013;73:1–14.

Chapter 55

Diabetes and Cancer

Daniel J. Rubin, MD, MSc
Ajay D. Rao, MD, MMSc

INTRODUCTION

I
t is now well established that diabetes is associated with an increased lifetime risk of developing many forms of cancer.[1] The evidence is most compelling for type 2 diabetes (T2D), whereas far less data are available regarding an association between type 1 diabetes (T1D) and cancer. Insulin, both exogenous and endogenous, has been proposed as the primary mediator of this increased risk, mostly through its role as a growth promoter. In addition to insulin therapy, evidence is emerging for associations of noninsulin antidiabetic medications with cancer. Some agents, such as metformin, may decrease the risk of developing cancer, whereas others, such as sulfonylureas (SUs), may increase the risk. There is considerable uncertainty about these associations with antidiabetic medications, however, due to limitations in the data.

EPIDEMIOLOGY

Diabetes and cancer continue to be highly prevalent disease entities worldwide. What is more concerning is the rapid increase in the incidence rates of both. The concept of these two diseases coexisting is not new, as close to 60 years ago Elliot Joslin commented on the importance of studying the association of diabetes and cancer.[2] Early studies yielded conflicting results about a potential association. More recently, studies have shown that the risk for many hematological and solid malignancies is elevated in diabetic individuals, especially liver, pancreatic, and endometrial cancers (Table 55.1).

PRIMARY LIVER CANCER

Primary liver cancer represents the sixth most frequently occurring cancer in the world and the second most common cause of cancer mortality. Hepatocellular carcinoma (HCC) is the most common histological type.[3] Although there are clearly well-established factors that lead to HCC such as chronic alcoholism, hepatitis B or C virus, and rare autoimmune disorders, there is increasing evidence that T2D may make a significant contribution to HCC risk.[4] In a retrospective study utilizing the Surveillance, Epidemiology, and End Results (SEER)-Medicare databases, patients with HCC tended to have a higher prevalence of diabetes or impaired fasting glucose than compared to healthy controls (54.7% vs. 26.9%,

 DOI: 10.2337/9781580405096.55

Table 55.1 Relative Risks of Cancer in Different Organs of Diabetic Patients

Cancer		RR (95% CI)
Liver (El-Serag et al. 2006)	13 case-control studies 7 cohort studies	2.50 (1.8–3.5) 2.51 (1.9–3.2)
Pancreas (Huxley et al. 2005)	17 case-control studies 19 cohort studies	1.94 (1.53–2.46) 1.73 (1.59–1.88)
Kidney[a] (Lindblad et al. 1999, Washio et al. 2007)	1 cohort study 1 cohort study	1.50 (1.30–1.70) 2.22 (1.04–4.70)
Endometrium (Friberg et al. 2007)	13 case-control studies 3 cohort studies	2.22 (1.80–2.74) 1.62 (1.21–2.16)
Colon-rectum (Larsson et al. 2005)	6 case-control studies 9 cohort studies	1.36 (1.23–1.50) 1.29 (1.16–1.43)
Bladder (Larsson et al. 2006)	7 case-control studies 3 cohort studies	1.37 (1.04–1.80) 1.43 (1.18–1.74)
Non-Hodgkin's lymphoma (Mitri et al. 2008)	5 cohort studies 11 case-control studies	1.41 (1.07–1.88) 1.12 (0.95–1.31)
Breast (Larsson et al. 2007)	5 case-control studies 15 cohort studies	1.18 (1.05–1.32) 1.20 (1.11–1.30)
Prostate (Kasper & Giovannucci 2006)	9 case-control studies 10 cohort studies	0.89 (0.72–1.11) 0.81 (0.71–0.92)

[a] Data on kidney cancer were not obtained from meta-analysis.

Source: Vigneri P, Frasca F, Sciacca L, Pandini G, Vigneri R. Diabetes and cancer. *Endocr Relat Cancer* 2009;16(4):1103–1123. Reprinted with permission from the publisher.

$P < 0.0001$).[4] Furthermore, nonalcoholic fatty liver disease (NAFLD) and the metabolic syndrome are associated with prevalence of HCC.[5] In one retrospective study, patients with both NAFLD and HCC exhibited more features of the metabolic syndrome than non-NAFLD patients, and the prevalence of diabetes was nearly twofold higher in NAFLD patients (64%, $P < 0.05$).[5] Because diabetes represents a common component to these two entities, it is not surprising that although chronic hepatitis C infection confers the highest risk of HCC in an individual (odds ratio [OR] 39.89; 95% confidence interval [CI] 36.29–43.84), >60% of patients with HCC have a history of diabetes or obesity and the presence of diabetes or obesity is associated with an increased risk of HCC (OR 2.47; 95% CI 2.34–2.61).[6]

PANCREATIC CANCER

Pancreatic cancer is the fourth leading cause of cancer-related mortality in the United States. Approximately 80% of patients with pancreatic cancer have diabetes or glucose intolerance.[7] Because new-onset diabetes may be a clinical sign of

difference between OR and RR ?
developing

pancreatic cancer, it has been difficult to conclude that diabetes is a risk factor for pancreatic cancer.[8,9] For example, one study showed that 56% of patients with pancreatic cancer were diagnosed with diabetes within 2 years before the diagnosis of cancer, but when controlled for the duration of diabetes, there was no longer a significant association.[10] A meta-analysis in 1995 showed that individuals with diabetes for >5 years had a twofold greater risk of developing pancreatic cancer than individuals without diabetes.[8] In 2005, this study was updated with increased follow-up and unexpectedly showed that individuals with a shorter duration of diabetes (<4 years) had a higher risk of pancreatic cancer than those with a longer duration of diabetes (relative risk [RR] 2.1 vs. 1.5; $P = 0.005$).[11] Although it is clear that pancreatic cancer and diabetes are interrelated, it is still unclear which is the inciting incident.[12]

ENDOMETRIAL CANCER

Endometrial cancer is the fourth leading incident cancer in the U.S.[13] Epidemiological data have revealed both positive and negative associations between diabetes and endometrial cancer, with the majority of evidence supporting positive associations. When cohort studies were adjusted for BMI and other risk factors, however, the association between diabetes and endometrial cancer was attenuated.[14] Hence, shared factors, such as physical inactivity and obesity, may partially explain the observed higher risk of endometrial cancer in individuals with diabetes.[15] Interestingly, the presence of preexisting diabetes confers an increased overall mortality (hazard rate ratio [HRR] 1.7; 95% CI 1.1–2.5) in patients diagnosed with endometrial cancer, although not endometrial cancer–specific mortality.[16]

PATHOPHYSIOLOGY

The leading hypotheses by which diabetes is thought to affect the development or progression of cancer include hyperinsulinemia (endogenous or exogenous), hyperglycemia, and chronic inflammation.[1]

INSULIN AND INSULIN GROWTH FACTORS

Receptors for insulin and insulin-like growth factor (IGF) have been found on cancer cells. Activation of the IGF-1 receptor (IGR) can trigger insulin-mediated mitogenesis[17] and downstream signaling may stimulate not only cancer cells but also normal cells involved in cancer progression (Figure 55.1).[18,19] In addition, the presence of hyperglycemia may allow IGF-1 to stimulate vascular smooth muscle cell proliferation and migration.[20] Hyperinsulinemia also indirectly increases circulating free, bioactive IGF-1 levels by reducing the hepatic production of IGF-binding protein (IGFBP)-1 and possibly IGFBP-2.[21]

The role of insulin receptors in tumorigenesis is less clear than that of IGRs. Activation of the insulin receptor may lead to a prolonged mitogenic stimulus.[22] Inactivation of the tumor suppressor gene, p53, may lead to upregulation of the

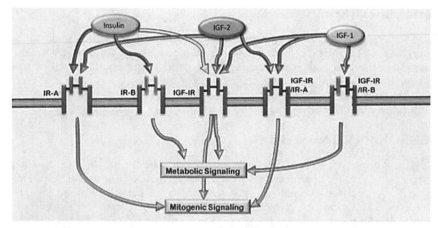

Figure 55.1—Insulin receptors and mitogenic signaling. Insulin signals primarily through insulin receptor-A (IR-A) and insulin receptor-B (IR-B) with lower affinity for insulin-like growth factor 1 receptor (IGF-1R). Binding of insulin and insulin-like growth factor 2 (IGF-2) to the IR-A by insulin predominantly results in mitogenic signaling.

Source: Adapted from Gallagher EJ, LeRoith D. Diabetes, cancer, and metformin: connections of metabolism and cell proliferation. *Ann N Y Acad Sci* 2011;1243:54–68. Reprinted with permission from the publisher.

insulin receptor.[23] Interestingly, functional insulin receptors emerge during the differentiation of embryonal cancer cells and may facilitate neoplastic growth.[22,24,25] In breast tumor cells, there may be an abnormal downregulation of insulin receptors characterized by an enhanced downstream effect (tyrosine kinase activity) that may offer a metabolic advantage to growing neoplastic cells.[26] Studies relating insulin receptor levels with breast cancer prognosis are conflicting, with some showing higher levels associated with a more favorable prognosis,[27,28] and others showing an association with a worse prognosis.[29] These differences may be related to the relationship between serum levels of insulin and regulation of insulin receptors.

Finally, there may be an indirect effect of hyperinsulinemia on other hormones crucial to the regulation of cancer biology. For example, increased circulating insulin may be associated with decreased levels of sex-hormone binding globulin. This in turn may result in increased levels of testosterone, interestingly in women, but not in men.[30] Androgens may promote the development of neoplastic lesions through growth factors and direct stimulation of cancer cells.[24] In addition, there may be increases in free estrogen levels that may play a role in inducing neoplasia of the breast, endometrium, and ovary.[31,32]

HYPERGLYCEMIA

Hyperglycemia is the fundamental derangement in diabetes and should not be overlooked as a potential mediator of tumorigenesis. Many cancers rely on glucose stores for energy. It is unclear whether hyperglycemia per se is a facilitator of neoplastic growth or just a surrogate for hyperinsulinemia. It is possible that there is a subset of tumors for which hyperglycemia confers a growth advantage and appropriate antihyperglycemic therapy may limit tumor growth.[1]

CHRONIC INFLAMMATION

In addition to the direct effects of insulin, both obesity and diabetes also may induce inflammatory pathways associated with malignant progression. Dysfunctional adipose tissue has been shown to secrete factors that attract monocytes and macrophages into adipose tissue. These obesity-associated disturbances can result in the development of insulin resistance, T2D, and obesity-related cardiovascular disease. Furthermore, obesity-induced inflammation is thought to be an important link between obesity and cancer. Several proinflammatory factors associated with obesity, such as tumor necrosis factor-α (TNF-α), interleukin (IL)-6, and matrix metalloproteinases may contribute to carcinogenesis.[33,34] Finally, oxidative stress also may create an environment that is favorable to tumor development in both obesity and diabetes.[35]

ASSOCIATIONS WITH OBESITY AND CANCER

Obesity is a risk factor for a number of cancers, including colorectal, breast (in postmenopausal women), ovarian, endometrial, renal, esophageal, pancreatic, gallbladder, and liver.[30,36,37]

The underlying link between obesity, the metabolic syndrome, and T2D is most likely insulin resistance and hyperinsulinemia. Chronic hyperinsulinemia has been associated with colon, breast, pancreatic, and endometrial cancer. The tumorigenic effects of insulin may be mediated by insulin receptors or changes in endogenous hormone metabolism secondary to the chronic hyperinsulinemia. Whether hyperinsulinemia is a cause or an effect remains unclear. Elevated IGF-1 levels also may mediate the increased risk of cancer among obese and diabetic individuals.[38]

COLON CANCER

Prospective cohort studies have shown increased risks of cancers of the colon or rectum among individuals with elevated blood levels of C-peptide.[39-41] In addition, numerous studies have suggested an association between obesity and colon carcinoma.[36,42-44] In one prospective cohort study, each kilogram of weight gained annually from age 20 to 50 years was associated with a 60% higher risk of colon cancer (95% CI 1.20–2.09).[44] The connection appears to be insulin resistance and hyperinsulinemia. For example, in animal models of colon cancer, a high-fat diet and high-glycemic food enhanced tumor promotion, as did the direct infusion of insulin.[45-48] Finally, there is evidence that there may be a link between insulin levels and colon cancer mortality. In the Risk Factors and Life Expectancy Project, those with hyperglycemia or metabolic syndrome experienced a threefold increase in colon cancer mortality.[49] In an adjuvant chemotherapy trial for colon cancer, those with diabetes had a significantly reduced survival (6 vs. 11.3 years) and a 21% increase in cancer recurrence, even after adjustment for prognostic factors and treatment-related side effects.[50]

BREAST CANCER

Obesity is a well-established risk factor for postmenopausal breast cancer incidence and mortality.[51] In a large cancer prevention study sponsored by the American Cancer Society, the adjustable risk attributable to overweight corresponded to ~30–50% of postmenopausal breast cancer death.[52] Obesity also has been associated with adverse features of breast cancer at diagnosis, including but not limited to, larger tumor size, advanced grade, and increased nodal involvement.[53-55]

The causal pathway linking diabetes, obesity, and breast cancer again involves hyperinsulinemia. In breast cancer cells, insulin receptors, IGRs, and the hybrid insulin-IGR are highly expressed.[18,56,57] There also may be significant interactions between the insulin–IGF system and other pathways, including the estrogen receptor (ER) pathway. Furthermore, there is also cross-talk between the ER and the IGR. One promising avenue of research to clarify the relationship between obesity and breast cancer has been in patients receiving adjuvant chemotherapy and hormonal therapy, where weight gain related to treatment is common. Several ongoing studies now are investigating the role of insulin resistance and treatment-related weight gain, and whether these factors mediate some of the adverse outcomes in patients already on treatment for breast cancer.

DIABETES THERAPIES ASSOCIATED WITH CANCER

Potential associations of diabetes therapies with cancer incidence and mortality are summarized in Table 55.2.

INSULIN

Insulin has been known to induce tumor growth since the 1960s, primarily through weak direct and indirect mitogenic properties.[58,59] The mitogenic potency of insulin analogs has been a theoretical concern. Similar to the pathophysiology of chronic hyperinsulinemia and its relation to malignancy, different affinities to the IGR have been implicated as a reason for potential growth-promoting and mitogenic properties of insulin analogs. Specifically, insulin glargine has high affinity to the IGR and mitogenicity in vitro.[60] Indeed, in 2009, one observational study in Germany reported a significantly increased risk of malignancy associated with insulin glargine in a dose-adjusted analysis.[61] The combined epidemiological and in vitro evidence at the time sparked considerable controversy.

Fortunately, more recent studies have provided strong evidence that insulin glargine does not, in fact, increase the risk of cancer. First, the analysis of the Ger-

Table 55.2 Associations of Diabetes Therapies with Cancer Incidence and Mortality

Antidiabetic medication	Overall CA	Bladder	Breast	Colorectal	Gastric	Liver	Lung	Pancreatic	Prostate	Renal	Thyroid	Mortality
α-Glucosidase inhibitors	None?	None?	--	--	↓↓?	--	--	--	--	--	None?	--
Glinides	↑?	--	--	↑?	↑?	↑?	↑?	↑?	--	--	--	--
Incretins	--	--	--	--	--	--	--	↑?	--	--	--	--
DPP-4 inhibitors	--	--	--	--	--	--	--	↑?	--	--	None	--
GLP-1 agonists	--	--	--	--	--	--	--	↑?	--	--	↑?	--
Insulin	↑?	↑?	--	↑?	--	↑?	↑?	↑?	--	--	--	↑?
Glargine	None	--	--	--	--	--	--	--	--	--	--	--
Metformin	↓?	None	None?	↓	None	↓	↓	↓	None?	--	None	↓
SGLT-2 inhibitors	--	--	--	--	--	--	--	--	--	--	--	--
Dapagliflozin	--	↑?	↑?	--	--	--	--	--	--	--	--	--
Canagliflozin	None	None	None	--	--	--	--	--	--	None	--	--
Sulfonylureas	↑?	None	None	None	None	--	None	↑↑	None	--	↑↑?	--
Thiazolidinediones	None	↑?	↓?	↓	None	↓	↓?	None	None	--	None	--
Pioglitazone	None?	↑	--	--	--	--	--	None	--	--	--	--
Rosiglitazone	--	None?	--	--	--	--	--	--	--	--	--	--

CA = cancer.

Note: No data for colesevelam, bromocriptine, insulin lispro, aspart, or glulisine.

↑/↓ = Up to 50% increase (↑) or decrease (↓) in risk; ↑↑/↓↓ = More than 50% increase (↑↑) or decrease (↓↓) in risk; ? = conflicting or limited data; -- = insufficient data man study had flaws, making the conclusions unsupportable.[62] Second, several other observational studies and combined data from 31 randomized controlled trials (RCTs), including 12,537 people in the Outcome Reduction with an Initial Glargine Intervention (ORIGIN) trial, have found no association of insulin glargine with cancer.[62–66] Third, 70% of insulin glargine is converted within 30 minutes of incubation to metabolites (M1 and M2), which have substantially less IGR affinity and mitogenic potential than human insulin.[67] Fourth, malignancy rates associated with insulin glargine are not significantly different than those associated with neutral protamine Hagedorn (NPH) or insulin detemir.[68] Thus, it has been suggested that the case of insulin glargine as a potential independent risk factor for cancer should be closed.

METFORMIN

In contrast to insulin therapy, a number of observational studies have suggested that metformin may be associated with a lower risk of developing cancer and longer survival with cancer. Estimates from systematic reviews and meta-analyses are a 20–39% decreased cancer risk associated with metformin use compared with nonuse.[69–72] Among diabetic patients with cancer exposed to metformin, mortality rates are reduced by 15–34% for all cancers combined,[69,73] by 45% among patients with pancreatic cancer (HR 0.55; 95% CI 0.32–0.96),[74] and by 48% among patients with breast cancer (HR 0.52; 95% CI 0.28–0.97).[75]

Meta-analyses of RCTs, however, fail to show any significant association of metformin exposure with either cancer incidence or mortality.[72,76] The discordance between the observational studies and the RCTs suggests that the apparent anticancer effect of metformin may be accounted for by residual confounding or bias.[69,77] Indeed, most of the observational studies reporting a decreased risk of incident cancer with metformin exposure may have failed to account for time-related biases.[77] Furthermore, the three studies that avoided these biases did not find an effect of metformin on cancer risk.[78–80]

Despite the conflicting clinical data, evidence from animal and in vitro studies supports a benefit of metformin in preventing and treating cancer. Metformin treatment inhibits proliferation of human lung, gastric, endometrial, hepatocellular, medullary thyroid, head and neck squamous, breast, and epithelial cancer cell lines.[81–83] Likewise, mouse studies show metformin inhibits the growth of gastric, hepatocellular, ovarian, and pancreatic cancer.[83,84] Metformin also has been demonstrated to improve the efficacy of several chemotherapeutic agents in multiple cancer models.[82,83]

A number of mechanisms may explain the potential anticarcinogenic effect of metformin (Figure 55.2).[83] First, metformin activates adenosine 5'-mono-phosphate-activated protein kinase (AMPK) through liver kinase B-1 (LKB-1), a tumor suppressor. AMPK inhibits protein synthesis and gluconeogenesis during cellular stress and inhibits mammalian target of rapamycin (mTOR). A downstream effector of growth signaling, mTOR is important in carcinogenesis. Second, metformin inhibits mTOR independent of AMPK by decreasing IGF-1 levels. Third, metformin induces cell-cycle arrest independent of AMPK by decreasing cyclin D1.[85] Additional mechanisms by which metformin may inhibit

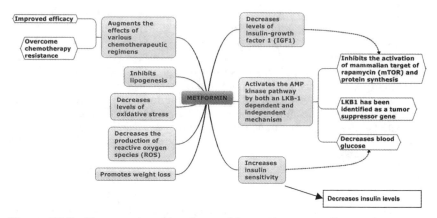

Figure 55.2—Proposed mechanisms of the anti-cancer effects of metformin.

Note: AMP = adenosine 5'-mono-phosphate-activated protein; LKB-1 = liver kinase B-1.

Source: Adapted from Rizos CV, Elisaf MS: Metformin and cancer. *Eur J Pharmacology* 2013;705(1–3):96–108. Reprinted with permission from the publisher.

cancer development and growth include promoting apoptosis, decreasing production of reactive oxygen species, modifying lipogenesis, and reducing growth factor signaling. Lastly, an indirect anticancer effect may be mediated by counteracting hyperinsulinemia, hyperglycemia, and weight gain.

THIAZOLIDINEDIONES

The cancer that has received the most attention as potentially linked with thiazolidinedione (TZD) therapy, especially pioglitazone, is bladder cancer. The Prospective Piogliazone Clinical Trial in Macrovascular Events (PROactive) study was the first clinical trial to raise concerns about a possible association between pioglitazone and bladder cancer.[86] This study of >5,000 patients designed to determine whether pioglitazone reduces cardiovascular events among high-risk patients with T2D reported a nonsignificant increased risk of bladder cancer among pioglitazone users relative to controls. In response, countries either removed pioglitazone from the market or warned against its use in patients with active or prior bladder cancer. Subsequent review of these cases, however, suggested that the incidence of bladder cancer was lower than initially reported and not different between groups.[87]

Nonetheless, the suggestion of a link between pioglitazone use and bladder cancer prompted many studies. Several systematic reviews and meta-analyses of mostly observational studies report a 17–23% increased risk of bladder cancer with pioglitazone use compared with nonuse.[88–91] The association tends to be stronger with higher cumulative dose and increasing duration of exposure. Despite the apparent increased risk of bladder cancer with pioglitazone therapy, the number needed to harm (NNH) is quite large at about 5 per 100,000 patient-years. This translates to one new case of bladder cancer for every 20,903 patients with T2D taking pioglitazone.[90]

Although one large, retrospective case-control study found an association between rosiglitazone use and increased bladder cancer incidence,[92] the predominance of evidence indicates there is no such association based on meta-analyses of multiple RCTs, case-control, and cohort studies.[88,89]

Conflicting data aside, the observational evidence linking TZD use with bladder cancer should be met with skepticism. As with most observational data, the modest association could be due to bias or residual confounding. Furthermore, the biological mechanism relating TZD use to bladder cancer is unknown, especially given that other peroxisome proliferator–activated receptor-γ (PPAR-γ) agonists have anticarcinogenic effects (see the following section).[93] Although studies in rats suggest that PPAR-γ agonists, including pioglitazone, may increase the risk of bladder cancer in a dose-dependent fashion, the applicability of rat studies to humans may be limited.[94] The association of PPAR-γ stimulation and bladder cancer is not observed in primates or mice. Additionally, male rats are more likely to develop bladder cancer than female rats, but this sex-specificity has not been found in other species, including humans. After reviewing the preclinical data on PPAR-γ agonists and carcinogenesis, the U.S. Food and Drug Administration (FDA) concluded that a credible mechanism to explain cancer formation does not exist.[93]

Potential Anticarcinogenic Effects of TZD Therapy

As mentioned previously, there is evidence to suggest that TZD therapy may provide an anticarcinogenic benefit. PPAR-γ receptors are expressed in many human cancers, including lung, prostate, bladder, colon, breast, and thyroid.[93] PPAR-γ ligands inhibit cellular proliferation, promote differentiation, induce apoptosis, and inhibit angiogenesis (Figure 55.3).[93,95] Some of these anticancer effects may be independent of the PPAR-γ system.[96] In addition, as with metformin, the indirect anticancer effects of TZDs may be mediated by a reduction in circulating insulin levels and hyperglycemia.

Despite the preclinical evidence suggesting a potential protective effect of TZDs, most studies have not found any association of TZD use with the incidence of cancer overall or specific tumors other than bladder cancer. Two systematic reviews and meta-analyses found no association of TZD therapy with overall cancer risk.[89,97] Studies also have found no association of TZD use with lung,[89] breast,[89] pancreatic,[89,98] prostate,[89] gastric,[99] or thyroid cancer.[100] In contrast, one meta-analysis limited to observational studies reported a 7–11% decreased incidence of colorectal, lung, and breast cancer associated with TZD therapy, which was of marginal statistical significance.[97]

INCRETIN-BASED THERAPIES

Glucagon-like peptide-1 receptor (GLP-1R) agonists and depeptidyl peptidase-4 (DPP-4) inhibitors potentiate incretin receptor signaling.[101] Most of the available data related to cancer are based on studies of exenatide and sitagliptin,

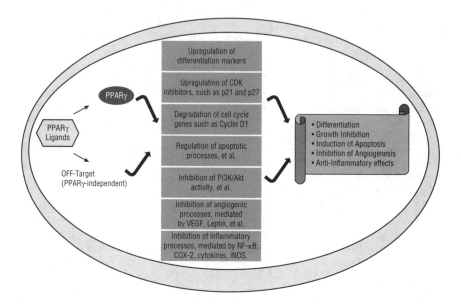

Figure 55.3—Proposed mechanisms of the anti-cancer effects of PPAR-γ agonists.

Source: Adapted from Mansure JJ, Nassim R, Kassouf W. Peroxisome proliferator-activated receptor gamma in bladder cancer: a promising therapeutic target. *Cancer Biol Ther* 2009;8(7):6–15. Reprinted with permission from the publisher.

the first approved GLP-1R agonist and DPP-4 inhibitor. The two cancers proposed to have a potential association with incretin-based therapies are pancreatic cancer and medullary thyroid carcinoma (MTC); however, these associations are controversial.

Pancreatic Cancer

The concern about incretin-based therapy and pancreatic cancer is based on several pieces of circumstantial evidence. First, these medications are associated with pancreatitis, and chronic pancreatitis is an established risk factor for pancreatic cancer.[102,103] Second, the transition from chronic pancreatitis to pancreatic cancer is characterized by intraepithelial neoplasia, intraductal papillary mucinous neoplasms, and pancreatic duct glands. Exenatide accelerates formation and growth of pancreatic intraepithelial neoplasia in rat and mouse models of chronic pancreatitis.[104] Treatment with sitagliptin of human islet amyloid polypeptide transgenic rats is associated with increased pancreatic ductal proliferation and ductal metaplasia.[105] Third, an analysis of the FDA Adverse Event Reporting System (FAERS) found an increased risk of pancreatic cancer associated with the use of incretin-based medications.[106] This non–FDA-sponsored analysis, however, is deeply flawed and likely yielded unreliable results, as will be discussed.

There is considerable evidence to cast doubt on a causal link between incretin-promoting therapy and pancreatic cancer. In contrast to the in vitro data associating GLP-1R stimulation with preneoplastic pancreatic lesions, the growth or survival of pancreatic cancer cells is not affected by exenatide.[107] Whether or not GLP-1R is expressed by pancreatic cancer cells is uncertain, as studies have generated conflicting results.[108,109] Furthermore, treatment with liraglutide, another GLP-1R agonist, for 87 weeks at plasma levels up to 60 times higher than those achieved with the maximum dose in humans was not associated with preneoplastic proliferative lesions or cancer in Cynomolgus monkeys.[110] Perhaps most convincingly, there have been no case reports of pancreatic cancer developing after initiation of a GLP-1R agonist or DPP-4 inhibitor in patients with a previously documented normal pancreas.[111] Lastly, there are critical limitations of the FAERS database, including disproportionate reporting, failure to validate specific diagnoses, and lack of information about confounders.[112] The FDA website therefore states that "FAERS data cannot be used to calculate the incidence of an adverse event of medication error in the U.S. population."[113] Europe's counterpart to the FDA, the European Medicines Agency, recently concluded little evidence supports an association of incretin-based therapy with pancreatic cancer.[114]

Medullary Thyroid Carcinoma

In vitro and animal studies raise some concern that incretin-based therapies may promote the development of MTC, a rare neuroendocrine tumor of thyroid C-cells.[101] GLP-1R stimulation of rat thyroid C-cell lines and thyroid tissues causes secretion of calcitonin,[115] a well-established biomarker for MTC.[116] Liraglutide treatment of rats at twofold greater doses than the maximum human dose increased the incidence of C-cell hyperplasia, whereas treatment at 10-fold the maximum human dose increased the incidence of C-cell tumors.[117] Development of tumors, however, did not affect survival. Additional support for a potential association of incretin-based therapies with MTC is that GLP-1R expression has been found in C-cells of 33% of normal human thyroid tissue (5 of 15 samples), 91% of MTC (11 of 12 samples), and 100% of C-cell hyperplasia (9 of 9 samples), whereas normal thyroid follicles did not express GLP-1R.[108] Lastly, an analysis of the FAERS found an increased odds of thyroid cancer, including MTC, associated with exenatide or liraglutide therapy.[106] As discussed, however, the FAERS analysis is flawed and likely yielded unreliable results.

Although these data suggest a potential link between incretin-promoting therapies and MTC, more compelling evidence raises substantial doubt about such an association. As with the rat models of bladder cancer, rat models of MTC are limited in their applicability to human MTC because of significant differences in incidence rates, histology, and GLP-1R expression.[101] Furthermore, it is unclear whether C-cell hyperplasia precedes sporadic cases of MTC, and the distinction between neoplastic and non-neoplastic C-cell hyperplasia is controversial.[118] In addition, the evidence for GLP-1R expression in thyroid tissue is controversial, with some studies finding that 0 or 27% of human MTCs express GLP-1R.[109,119]

The human data against an association between incretin-based treatment and MTC are perhaps most convincing. As with pancreatic cancer, there have been no case reports definitively linking GLP-1R agonist or DPP-4 inhibitor therapy with MTC.[111] Analysis of nine clinical trials including >5,000 patients revealed no consistent dose or time-dependent relationship between calcitonin levels and liraglutide treatment up 104 weeks.[120] Furthermore, the association reported in the FAERS is subject to bias and confounding, and DPP-4 inhibitors have not been linked with MTC.[111] Because MTC was reported only at incretin doses many times higher than those approved for use in humans and development of tumors did not affect survival, the FDA has concluded that the risk of MTC with incretin-based treatment is low.[121] Even if there is an increased risk of MTC with incretin-promoting therapy, because MTC is quite rare, the number of patients who would need to be treated for 1 year to yield one additional case of MTC would be very high (NNH 35,000–55,000 if the risk is doubled).[101] Given the uncertainty on this issue, the FDA mandated long-term studies to monitor the incidence of MTC.

SULFONYLUREAS

The evidence linking SU therapy with the risk of cancer is mixed, with some studies suggesting an increased risk, others no association, and some even a decreased risk of cancer. The most definitive data come from a systematic review and meta-analysis of 18 studies (2 RCTs, 6 cohort, and 10 case-control) involving 315,517 participants that found SU use is associated with a 55% increased overall risk of cancer in the cohort studies (RR 1.55; 95% CI 1.48–1.63).[72] In contrast, data from the RCTs and case-control studies failed to demonstrate a significant effect. Furthermore, there is evidence for publication bias and heterogeneity among the studies. It is possible, if not likely, that the association found in the cohort studies reflects residual confounding or bias.

Data examining potential associations between SU therapy and the risk of specific cancers are also mixed. A systematic review and meta-analysis of eight observational studies found a 70% increased risk of pancreatic cancer associated with SU use (OR 1.70; 95% CI 1.27–2.28).[98] There was, however, heterogeneity among the studies not explained by study design, setting, or comparator drug. A retrospective cohort of almost 1 million people drawn from the National Health Insurance database in Taiwan found that SU users were at 88% increased risk for thyroid cancer compared with nonusers (OR 1.88; 95% CI 1.20–2.95).[100] In contrast, studies have not found any association of SU therapy with colorectal, lung, prostate, pancreas, gastric, or bladder cancer.[99,122,123] Other studies have not found an increased risk of cancer in general or breast cancer specifically among SU users compared with metformin users.[124,125]

A small body of evidence suggests that gliclazide, a second-generation SU, may be protective against cancer. Observational studies have found a 33–60% reduction in overall cancer risk with gliclazide use compared with nonuse.[126,127] Another observational study found that gliclazide users had lower odds of mortality compared with glibenclamide users.[128] In vitro studies suggest an antioxidant effect of gliclazide, as treatment with the drug significantly reduced DNA damage induced by free radicals of human lymphocytes and mouse insulinoma cells.[129]

A few observational studies have found that SU exposure may increase the risk of mortality among individuals with cancer. One population-based retrospective cohort study of >10,000 new users of metformin or SUs drawn from administrative databases in Canada reported a 30% increased risk of cancer-related mortality among SU users compared with metformin users (HR 1.30; 95% CI 1.10–1.60).[130] Similarly, a retrospective cohort study of >8,000 patients with T2D in primary care practices in the United Kingdom found a 48% increased risk of mortality after a diagnosis of cancer among SU users relative to users of metformin (HR 1.48; 95% CI 1.29–1.71).[73] There are major limitations to these studies, however, as they are subject to time-related biases.[77] Furthermore, the increased risk associated with SU exposure may be due to a deleterious effect of SUs, a protective effect of metformin, or unmeasured confounders.

GLINIDES

Very few data have examined a potential association between glinide (i.e., repaglinide or nateglinide) therapy and cancer. A prospective case-control study based on the National Health Insurance database in Taiwan of nearly 109,000 newly diagnosed individuals with T2D reported a statistically significant 16% increased risk of cancer among glinide users compared with nonusers (OR 1.16; 95% CI 1.06–1.28).[122] Patients exposed to glinides in this study were at higher risk of colorectal, gastric, liver, lung, and pancreatic cancer. There was, however, no increase in the risk of cancer with increasing dose or duration of therapy, calling into question whether this association is real or a matter of bias or confounding. Another prospective case-control study, in which 195 diabetic participants with cancer were matched for multiple factors with 195 diabetic controls without cancer, failed to identify any link between repaglinide therapy and incident cancer.[127] This study included only 16 controls and 18 cases on repaglinide therapy, raising the issue that we simply do not have enough data on these medications to draw firm conclusions on their potential association with cancer.

α-GLUCOSIDASE INHIBITORS

Another class of medications for which data regarding associations with cancer are lacking is the α-glucosidase inhibitors (AGIs, e.g., acarbose and miglitol). The largest study to investigate an association between AGIs and overall cancer risk was conducted with the National Health Insurance database in Taiwan.[122] This prospective case-control study included 3,278 patients with T2D exposed to AGIs and found no association with incident cancer. Other observational studies using the same national database also found no association of AGI therapy with thyroid cancer or bladder cancer.[100,123] One study, however, did report a 62% decreased risk of gastric cancer that was statistically significant (HR 0.38; 95% CI 0.15–0.96).[131]

SGLT-2 INHIBITORS

Yet a third class of medications about which we have limited data on associations with cancer is the sodium-glucose cotransporter-2 (SGLT-2) inhibitors. Approved in the U.S. in 2013, canagliflozin, the first available agent, has not been associated with increased cancer risk in preapproval studies.[132,133] Concerns were raised, however, with dapagliflozin over a potential increase in bladder and breast cancer that ultimately contributed to the FDA's decision to initially reject the drug.[134] A recent systematic review and meta-analysis analyzed a pool of 5,501 patients treated with dapagliflozin and 3,184 patients who received placebo.[133] Among the patients treated with dapagliflozin, there were nine cases of bladder cancer, whereas there was only one case among placebo patients. Although these trials were not powered to distinguish statistical differences in bladder cancer rates, the observed incidence rate of nine cases exceeds the expected rate of two cases in an age-matched male population of patients with diabetes.[133] Similarly, nine women treated with dapagliflozin were reported to have breast cancer compared with one woman in the control group. Whether or not dapagliflozin truly increases the risk of cancer remains uncertain given that half of the bladder cancer cases and all of the breast cancer cases were detected within 12 months of starting therapy, and animal studies have not suggested an increased risk of cancer.[133,135] More experience with these agents is necessary to better estimate potential cancer risks.

CONCLUSION

Diabetes and cancer individually represent tremendous health burdens on society. It is now clear that diabetes increases the risk of certain cancers. Although some antidiabetic medications may increase the risk of cancer and others may decrease the risk of cancer, such conclusions are tenuous at best. Currently, available evidence is limited by a lack of RCTs and dedicated prospective studies, as well as insufficient follow-up time, particularly for newer agents.

REFERENCES

1. Giovannucci E, Harlan DM, Archer MC, Bergenstal RM, Gapstur SM, Habel LA, Pollak M, Regensteiner JG, Yee D. Diabetes and cancer: a consensus report. *Diabetes Care* 2010;33(7):1674–1685.

2. Joslin EP, Lombard HL, Burrows RE, Manning MD. Diabetes and cancer. *N Engl J Med* 1959;260(10):486–488.

3. Altekruse SF, McGlynn KA, Reichman ME. Hepatocellular carcinoma incidence, mortality, and survival trends in the United States from 1975 to 2005. *J Clin Oncol* 2009;27(9):1485–1491.

4. Welzel TM, Graubard BI, Zeuzem S, El-Serag HB, Davila JA, McGlynn KA. Metabolic syndrome increases the risk of primary liver cancer in the United States: a study in the SEER-Medicare database. *Hepatology* 2011;54(2):463–471.

5. Ertle J, Dechene A, Sowa JP, Penndorf V, Herzer K, Kaiser G, Schlaak JF, Gerken G, Syn WK, Canbay A. Non-alcoholic fatty liver disease progresses

to hepatocellular carcinoma in the absence of apparent cirrhosis. *Int J Cancer* 2011;128(10):2436–2443.

6. Welzel TM, Graubard BI, Quraishi S, Zeuzem S, Davila JA, El-Serag HB, McGlynn KA. Population-attributable fractions of risk factors for hepatocellular carcinoma in the United States. *Am J Gastroenterol* 2013;108(8):1314–1321.

7. Permert J, Ihse I, Jorfeldt L, von Schenck H, Arnqvist HJ, Larsson J. Pancreatic cancer is associated with impaired glucose metabolism. *Eur J Surg* 1993;159(2):101–107.

8. Everhart J, Wright D. Diabetes mellitus as a risk factor for pancreatic cancer: a meta-analysis. *JAMA* 1995;273(20):1605–1609.

9. Pannala R, Basu A, Petersen GM, Chari ST. New-onset diabetes: a potential clue to the early diagnosis of pancreatic cancer. *Lancet Oncology* 2009;10(1):88–95.

10. Gullo L, Pezzilli R, Morselli-Labate AM. Diabetes and the risk of pancreatic cancer. *N Engl J Med* 1994;331(2):81–84.

11. Huxley R, Ansary-Moghaddam A, Berrington de Gonzalez A, Barzi F, Woodward M. Type-II diabetes and pancreatic cancer: a meta-analysis of 36 studies. *Br J Cancer* 2005;92(11):2076–2083.

12. Magruder JT, Elahi D, Andersen DK. Diabetes and pancreatic cancer: chicken or egg? *Pancreas* 2011;40(3):339–351.

13. Landis SH, Murray T, Bolden S, Wingo PA. Cancer statistics, 1998. *Cancer J Clin* 1998;48(1):6–29.

14. Anderson KE, Anderson E, Mink PJ, Hong CP, Kushi LH, Sellers TA, Lazovich D, Folsom AR. Diabetes and endometrial cancer in the Iowa Women's Health Study. *Cancer Epidemiol Biomark Prev* 2011;10(6):611–616.

15. Zanders MMJ, Boll D, van Steenbergen LN, van de Poll-Franse LV, Haak HR. Effect of diabetes on endometrial cancer recurrence and survival. *Maturitas* 2013;74(1):37–43.

16. Chia VM, Newcomb PA, Trentham-Dietz A, Hampton JM. Obesity, diabetes, and other factors in relation to survival after endometrial cancer diagnosis. *Int Gynecol Cancer* 2007;17(2):441–446.

17. Denley A, Carroll JM, Brierley GV, Cosgrove L, Wallace J, Forbes B, Roberts CT Jr. Differential activation of insulin receptor substrates 1 and 2 by insulin-like growth factor-activated insulin receptors. *Mol Cell Bio* 2007;27(10):3569–3577.

18. Papa V, Pezzino V, Costantino A, Belfiore A, Giuffrida D, Frittitta L, Vannelli GB, Brand R, Goldfine ID, Vigneri R. Elevated insulin receptor content in human breast cancer. *J Clin Inest* 1990;86(5):1503–1510.

19. Novosyadlyy R, Lann DE, Vijayakumar A, Rowzee A, Lazzarino DA, Fierz Y, Carboni JM, Gottardis MM, Pennisi PA, Molinolo AA, Kurshan N, Mejia W,

Santopietro S, Yakar S, Wood TL, LeRoith D. Insulin-mediated acceleration of breast cancer development and progression in a nonobese model of type 2 diabetes. *Cancer Res* 2010;70(2):741–751.

20. Clemmons DR, Maile LA, Ling Y, Yarber J, Busby WH. Role of the integrin alpha-beta3 in mediating increased smooth muscle cell responsiveness to IGF-I in response to hyperglycemic stress. *Growth Hormone IGF Res* 2007;17(4):265–270.

21. Renehan AG, Frystyk J, Flyvbjerg A. Obesity and cancer risk: the role of the insulin-IGF axis. *Trends Endorinol Metab* 2006;17(8):328–336.

22. Nagarajan L, Anderson WB. Insulin promotes the growth of F9 embryonal carcinoma cells apparently by acting through its own receptor. *Biochem Biophys Research Comm* 1982;106(3):974–980.

23. Webster NJ, Resnik JL, Reichart DB, Strauss B, Haas M, Seely BL. Repression of the insulin receptor promoter by the tumor suppressor gene product p53: a possible mechanism for receptor overexpression in breast cancer. *Cancer Res* 1996;56(12):2781–2788.

24. Gupta K, Krishnaswamy G, Karnad A, Peiris AN. Insulin: a novel factor in carcinogenesis. *Am J Med Sci* 2002;323(3):140–145.

25. Heath J, Bell S, Rees AR. Appearance of functional insulin receptors during the differentiation of embryonal carcinoma cells. *J Cell Biol* 1981;91(1):293–297.

26. Frittitta L, Vigneri R, Papa V, Goldfine ID, Grasso G, Trischitta V. Structural and functional studies of insulin receptors in human breast cancer. *Breast Cancer Res Treat* 1993;25(1):73–82.

27. Mulligan AM, O'Malley FP, Ennis M, Fantus IG, Goodwin PJ. Insulin receptor is an independent predictor of a favorable outcome in early stage breast cancer. *Breast Cancer Res Treat* 2007;106(1):39–47.

28. Mathieu MC, Clark GM, Allred DC, Goldfine ID, Vigneri R. Insulin receptor expression and clinical outcome in node-negative breast cancer. *Proc Assoc Am Physicians* 1997;109(6):565–571.

29. Law JH, Habibi G, Hu K, Masoudi H, Wang MY, Stratford AL, Park E, Gee JM, Finlay P, Jones HE, Nicholson RI, Carboni J, Gottardis M, Pollak M, Dunn SE. Phosphorylated insulin-like growth factor-i/insulin receptor is present in all breast cancer subtypes and is related to poor survival. *Cancer Res* 2008;68(24):10238–10246.

30. Calle EE, Kaaks R. Overweight, obesity and cancer: epidemiological evidence and proposed mechanisms. *Nat Rev Cancer* 2004;4(8):579–591.

31. Adlercreutz H. Western diet and Western diseases: some hormonal and biochemical mechanisms and associations. *Scand J Clin Lab Invest* 1990;201:3–23.

32. Moseson M, Koenig KL, Shore RE, Pasternack BS. The influence of medical conditions associated with hormones on the risk of breast cancer. *Inter J Epidemiol* 1993;22(6):1000–1009.

33. Cozen W, Gebregziabher M, Conti DV, Van Den Berg DJ, Coetzee GA, Wang SS, Rothman N, Bernstein L, Hartge P, Morhbacher A, Coetzee SG, Salam MT, Wang W, Zadnick J, Ingles SA. Interleukin-6-related genotypes, body mass index, and risk of multiple myeloma and plasmacytoma. *Cancer Epidemiol Biomark Preven* 2006;15(11):2285–2291.

34. Egeblad M, Werb Z. New functions for the matrix metalloproteinases in cancer progression. *Nat Rev Cancer* 2002;2(3):161–174.

35. Katiyar SK, Meeran SM. Obesity increases the risk of UV radiation-induced oxidative stress and activation of MAPK and NF-kappaB signaling. *Free Radic Biol Med* 2007;42(2):299–310.

36. Calle EE, Rodriguez C, Walker-Thurmond K, Thun MJ. Overweight, obesity, and mortality from cancer in a prospectively studied cohort of U.S. adults. *N Engl J Med* 2003;348(17):1625–1638.

37. Reeves GK, Pirie K, Beral V, Green J, Spencer E, Bull D. Cancer incidence and mortality in relation to body mass index in the Million Women Study: Cohort study. *BMJ* 2007;335(7630):1134.

38. Cohen DH, LeRoith D. Obesity, type 2 diabetes, and cancer: the insulin and IGF connection. *Endocr Relat Cancer* 2012;19(5):F27–45.

39. Jenab M, Riboli E, Cleveland RJ, Norat T, Rinaldi S, Nieters A, Biessy C, Tjonneland A, Olsen A, Overvad K, Gronbaek H, Clavel-Chapelon F, Boutron-Ruault MC, Linseisen J, Boeing H, Pischon T, Trichopoulos D, Oikonomou E, Trichopoulou A, Panico S, Vineis P, Berrino F, Tumino R, Masala G, Peters PH, van Gils CH, Bueno-de-Mesquita HB, Ocke MC, Lund E, Mendez MA, Tormo MJ, Barricarte A, Martinez-Garcia C, Dorronsoro M, Quiros JR, Hallmans G, Palmqvist R, Berglund G, Manjer J, Key T, Allen NE, Bingham S, Khaw KT, Cust A, Kaaks R. Serum C-peptide, IGFBP-1 and IGFBP-2 and risk of colon and rectal cancers in the European Prospective Investigation into Cancer and Nutrition. *Int J Cancer* 2007;121(2):368–376.

40. Otani T, Iwasaki M, Sasazuki S, Inoue M, Tsugane S. Plasma C-peptide, insulin-like growth factor-I, insulin-like growth factor binding proteins and risk of colorectal cancer in a nested case-control study: the Japan Public Health Center-Based Prospective Study. *Int J Cancer* 2007;120(9):2007–2012.

41. Wei EK, Ma J, Pollak MN, Rifai N, Fuchs CS, Hankinson SE, Giovannucci E. A prospective study of C-peptide, insulin-like growth factor-I, insulin-like growth factor binding protein-1, and the risk of colorectal cancer in women. *Cancer Epidemiol Biomarkers Prev* 2005;14(4):850–855.

42. Murphy TK, Calle EE, Rodriguez C, Kahn HS, Thun MJ. Body mass index and colon cancer mortality in a large prospective study. *Am J Epidemiol* 2000;152(9):847–854.

43. Platz EA, Willett WC, Colditz GA, Rimm EB, Spiegelman D, Giovannucci E. Proportion of colon cancer risk that might be preventable in a cohort of middle-aged US men. *Cancer Causes Control* 2000;11(7):579–588.

44. Aleksandrova K, Pischon T, Buijsse B, May AM, Peeters PH, Bueno-de-Mesquita HB, Jenab M, Fedirko V, Dahm CC, Siersema PD, Freisling H, Ferrari P, Overvad K, Tjonneland A, Trichopoulou A, Lagiou P, Naska A, Pala V, Mattiello A, Ohlsson B, Jirstrom K, Key TJ, Khaw KT, Riboli E, Boeing H. Adult weight change and risk of colorectal cancer in the European Prospective Investigation into Cancer and Nutrition. *Eur J Cancer* 2013;49(16):3526–3536.

45. Corpet DE, Jacquinet C, Peiffer G, Tache S. Insulin injections promote the growth of aberrant crypt foci in the colon of rats. *Nutr Cancer* 1997;27(3):316–320.

46. Corpet DE, Peiffer G, Tache S. Glycemic index, nutrient density, and promotion of aberrant crypt foci in rat colon. *Nutr Cancer* 32(1):29-36,1998

47. Koohestani N, Tran TT, Lee W, Wolever TM, Bruce WR. Insulin resistance and promotion of aberrant crypt foci in the colons of rats on a high-fat diet. *Nutr Cancer* 1997;29(1):69–76.

48. Koohestani N, Chia MC, Pham NA, Tran TT, Minkin S, Wolever TM, Bruce WR. Aberrant crypt focus promotion and glucose intolerance: correlation in the rat across diets differing in fat, n-3 fatty acids and energy. *Carcinogenesis* 1998;19(9):1679–1684.

49. Trevisan M, Liu J, Muti P, Misciagna G, Menotti A, Fucci F. Markers of insulin resistance and colorectal cancer mortality. *Cancer Epidemiol Biomarkers Prev* 2001;10(9):937–941.

50. Meyerhardt JA, Catalano PJ, Haller DG, Mayer RJ, Macdonald JS, Benson AB 3rd, Fuchs CS. Impact of diabetes mellitus on outcomes in patients with colon cancer. *J Clin Oncol* 2003;21(3):433–440.

51. Stoll BA. Obesity and breast cancer. *Inter J Obes Metabolic Disord* 1996;20(5):389–392.

52. Petrelli JM, Calle EE, Rodriguez C, Thun MJ. Body mass index, height, and postmenopausal breast cancer mortality in a prospective cohort of US women. *Cancer Causes Control* 2002;13(4):325–332.

53. Cui Y, Whiteman MK, Flaws JA, Langenberg P, Tkaczuk KH, Bush TL. Body mass and stage of breast cancer at diagnosis. *Int J Cancer* 2002;98(2):279–283.

54. Maehle BO, Tretli S, Skjaerven R, Thorsen T. Premorbid body weight and its relations to primary tumour diameter in breast cancer patients: its dependence on estrogen and progesteron receptor status. *Breast Cancer Res Treat* 2001;68(2):159–169.

55. Daling JR, Malone KE, Doody DR, Johnson LG, Gralow JR, Porter PL. Relation of body mass index to tumor markers and survival among young women with invasive ductal breast carcinoma. *Cancer* 2001;92(4):720–729.

56. Pandini G, Vigneri R, Costantino A, Frasca F, Ippolito A, Fujita-Yamaguchi Y, Siddle K, Goldfine ID, Belfiore A. Insulin and insulin-like growth factor-I (IGF-I) receptor overexpression in breast cancers leads to insulin/IGF-I hybrid receptor overexpression: evidence for a second mechanism of IGF-I signaling. *Clin Cancer Res* 1999;5(7):1935–1944.

57. Belfiore A, Frittitta L, Costantino A, Frasca F, Pandini G, Sciacca L, Goldfine ID, Vigneri R. Insulin receptors in breast cancer. *Ann N Y Acad Sci* 1996;784:173–188.

58. Sandhu MS, Dunger DB, Giovannucci EL. Insulin, insulin-like growth factor-I (IGF-I), IGF binding proteins, their biologic interactions, and colorectal cancer. *J Natl Cancer Inst* 2002;94(13):972–980.

59. Tran TT, Medline A, Bruce WR. Insulin promotion of colon tumors in rats. *Cancer Epidemiol Biomarkers Prev* 1996;5(12):1013–1015.

60. Kurtzhals P, Schäffer L, Sørensen A, Kristensen C, Jonassen I, Schmid C, Trüb T. Correlations of receptor binding and metabolic and mitogenic potencies of insulin analogs designed for clinical use. *Diabetes* 2000;49(6):999–1005.

61. Hemkens LG, Grouven U, Bender R, Gunster C, Gutschmidt S, Selke GW, Sawicki PT. Risk of malignancies in patients with diabetes treated with human insulin or insulin analogues: a cohort study. *Diabetologia* 2009;52(9):1732–1744.

62. Pocock SJ, Smeeth L. Insulin glargine and malignancy: an unwarranted alarm. *Lancet* 2009;374(9689):511–513.

63. Home PD, Lagarenne P. Combined randomised controlled trial experience of malignancies in studies using insulin glargine. *Diabetologia* 2009;52(12):2499–2506.

64. Currie CJ, Poole CD, Gale EA. The influence of glucose-lowering therapies on cancer risk in type 2 diabetes. *Diabetologia* 2009;52(9):1766–1777.

65. Jonasson JM, Ljung R, Talback M, Haglund B, Gudbjornsdottir S, Steineck G. Insulin glargine use and short-term incidence of malignancies: a population-based follow-up study in Sweden. *Diabetologia* 2009;52(9):1745–1754.

66. Gerstein HC, Bosch J, Dagenais GR, Diaz R, Jung H, Maggioni AP, Pogue J, Probstfield J, Ramachandran A, Riddle MC, Ryden LE, Yusuf S. Basal insulin and cardiovascular and other outcomes in dysglycemia. *N Engl J Med* 2012;367(4):319–328.

67. Owens DR. Glargine and cancer: can we now suggest closure? *Diabetes Care* 2012;35(12):2426–2428.

68. Dejgaard A, Lynggaard H, Rastam J, Krogsgaard Thomsen M. No evidence of increased risk of malignancies in patients with diabetes treated with insulin detemir: a meta-analysis. *Diabetologia* 2009;52(12):2507–2512.

69. Noto II, Goto A, Tsujimoto T, Noda M. Cancer risk in diabetic patients treated with metformin: a systematic review and meta-analysis. *PLoS One* 2012;7(3):e33411.

70. Soranna D, Scotti L, Zambon A, Bosetti C, Grassi G, Catapano A, La Vecchia C, Mancia G, Corrao G. Cancer risk associated with use of metformin and sulfonylurea in type 2 diabetes: a meta-analysis. *Oncologist* 2012;17(6):813–822.

71. Decensi A, Puntoni M, Goodwin P, Cazzaniga M, Gennari A, Bonanni B, Gandini S. Metformin and cancer risk in diabetic patients: a systematic review and meta-analysis. *Cancer Prev Res* 2010;3(11):1451–1461.

72. Thakkar B, Aronis KN, Vamvini MT, Shields K, Mantzoros CS. Metformin and sulfonylureas in relation to cancer risk in type ii diabetes patients: a meta-analysis using primary data of published studies. *Metabolism* 2013;62(7):922–934.

73. Currie CJ, Poole CD, Jenkins-Jones S, Gale EA, Johnson JA, Morgan CL. Mortality after incident cancer in people with and without type 2 diabetes: impact of metformin on survival. *Diabetes Care* 2012;35(2):299–304.

74. He XX, Tu SM, Lee MH, Yeung SC. Thiazolidinediones and metformin associated with improved survival of diabetic prostate cancer patients. *Ann Oncol* 2011;22(12):2640–2645.

75. He X, Esteva FJ, Ensor J, Hortobagyi GN, Lee MH, Yeung SC. Metformin and thiazolidinediones are associated with improved breast cancer-specific survival of diabetic women with HER2+ breast cancer. *Ann Oncol* 2012;23(7):1771–1780.

76. Stevens RJ, Ali R, Bankhead CR, Bethel MA, Cairns BJ, Camisasca RP, Crowe FL, Farmer AJ, Harrison S, Hirst JA, Home P, Kahn SE, McLellan JH, Perera R, Pluddemann A, Ramachandran A, Roberts NW, Rose PW, Schweizer A, Viberti G, Holman RR. Cancer outcomes and all-cause mortality in adults allocated to metformin: Systematic review and collaborative meta-analysis of randomised clinical trials. *Diabetologia* 2012;55(10):2593–2603.

77. Suissa S, Azoulay L. Metformin and the risk of cancer: time-related biases in observational studies. *Diabetes Care* 2012;35(12):2665–2673.

78. Azoulay L, Dell'Aniello S, Gagnon B, Pollak M, Suissa S. Metformin and the incidence of prostate cancer in patients with type 2 diabetes. *Cancer Epidemiol Biomarkers Prev* 2011;20(2):337–344.

79. Ferrara A, Lewis JD, Quesenberry CP, Jr., Peng T, Strom BL, Van Den Eeden SK, Ehrlich SF, Habel LA. Cohort study of pioglitazone and cancer incidence in patients with diabetes. *Diabetes Care* 2011;34(4):923–929.

80. Smiechowski BB, Azoulay L, Yin H, Pollak MN, Suissa S. The use of metformin and the incidence of lung cancer in patients with type 2 diabetes. *Diabetes Care* 2013;36(1):124–129.

81. Zakikhani M, Dowling R, Fantus IG, Sonenberg N, Pollak M. Metformin is an AMP kinase-dependent growth inhibitor for breast cancer cells. *Cancer Res* 2006;66(21):10269–10273.

82. Gotlieb WH, Saumet J, Beauchamp M-C, Gu J, Lau S, Pollak MN, Bruchim I. In vitro metformin anti-neoplastic activity in epithelial ovarian cancer. *Gyn Oncol* 2008;110(2):246–250.

83. Rizos CV, Elisaf MS: Metformin and cancer. *Eur J Pharmacol* 2013;705(1–3):96–108.

84. Kisfalvi K, Eibl G, Sinnett-Smith J, Rozengurt E. Metformin disrupts crosstalk between g protein–coupled receptor and insulin receptor signaling systems and inhibits pancreatic cancer growth. *Cancer Res* 2009;69(16):6539–6545.

85. Sahra IB, Laurent K, Loubat A, Giorgetti-Peraldi S, Colosetti P, Auberger P, Tanti JF, Le Marchand-Brustel Y, Bost F. The antidiabetic drug metformin exerts an antitumoral effect in vitro and in vivo through a decrease of cyclin D1 level. *Oncogene* 2008;27(25):3576–3586.

86. Dormandy JA, Charbonnel B, Eckland DJ, Erdmann E, Massi-Benedetti M, Moules IK, Skene AM, Tan MH, Lefebvre PJ, Murray GD, Standl E, Wilcox RG, Wilhelmsen L, Betteridge J, Birkeland K, Golay A, Heine RJ, Koranyi L, Laakso M, Mokan M, Norkus A, Pirags V, Podar T, Scheen A, Scherbaum W, Schernthaner G, Schmitz O, Skrha J, Smith U, Taton J. Secondary prevention of macrovascular events in patients with type 2 diabetes in the PROactive Study (PROspective pioglitAzone Clinical Trial In macroVascular Events): a randomised controlled trial. *Lancet* 2005;366(9493):1279–1289.

87. Dormandy J, Bhattacharya M, de Bruyn A-RvT. Safety and tolerability of pioglitazone in high-risk patients with type 2 diabetes. *Drug Safety* 2009;32(3):187–202.

88. Colmers IN, Bowker SL, Majumdar SR, Johnson JA. Use of thiazolidinediones and the risk of bladder cancer among people with type 2 diabetes: a meta-analysis. *CMAJ* 2012;184(12):E675–683.

89. Bosetti C, Rosato V, Buniato D, Zambon A, La Vecchia C, Corrao G. Cancer risk for patients using thiazolidinediones for type 2 diabetes: a meta-analysis. *Oncologist* 2013;18(2):148–156.

90. Ferwana M, Firwana B, Hasan R, Al-Mallah MH, Kim S, Montori VM, Murad MH. Pioglitazone and risk of bladder cancer: a meta-analysis of controlled studies. *Diabet Med* 2013;30:1026–1032.

91. Zhu Z, Shen Z, Lu Y, Zhong S, Xu C. Increased risk of bladder cancer with pioglitazone therapy in patients with diabetes: a meta-analysis. *Diabetes Res Clin Pract* 2012;98(1):159–163.

92. Hsiao FY, Hsieh PH, Huang WF, Tsai YW, Gau CS. Risk of bladder cancer in diabetic patients treated with rosiglitazone or pioglitazone: a nested case-control study. *Drug Saf* 2013;36:643–649.

93. Mansure JJ, Nassim R, Kassouf W. Peroxisome proliferator-activated receptor gamma in bladder cancer: a promising therapeutic target. *Cancer Biol Ther* 2009;8(7):6–15.

94. Tseng CH, Tseng FH. Peroxisome proliferator-activated receptor agonists and bladder cancer: lessons from animal studies. *J Environ Sci Health C Environ Carcinog Ecotoxicol Rev* 2012;30(4):368–402.

95. Yoshizumi T, Ohta T, Ninomiya I, Terada I, Fushida S, Fujimura T, Nishimura G, Shimizu K, Yi S, Miwa K. Thiazolidinedione, a peroxisome proliferator-activated receptor-gamma ligand, inhibits growth and metastasis of HT-29 human colon cancer cells through differentiation-promoting effects. *Int J Oncol* 2004;25(3):631–639.

96. Galli A, Ceni E, Mello T, Polvani S, Tarocchi M, Buccoliero F, Lisi F, Cioni L, Ottanelli B, Foresta V, Mastrobuoni G, Moneti G, Pieraccini G, Surrenti C, Milani S. Thiazolidinediones inhibit hepatocarcinogenesis in hepatitis B virus–transgenic mice by peroxisome proliferator-activated receptor γ–independent regulation of nucleophosmin. *Hepatology* 2010;52(2):493–505.

97. Colmers IN, Bowker SL, Johnson JA. Thiazolidinedione use and cancer incidence in type 2 diabetes: a systematic review and meta-analysis. *Diabetes Metab* 2012;38(6):475–484.

98. Singh S, Singh PP, Singh AG, Murad MH, McWilliams RR, Chari ST. Antidiabetic medications and risk of pancreatic cancer in patients with diabetes mellitus: a systematic review and meta-analysis. *Am J Gastroenterol* 2013;108(4):510–519; quiz 520.

99. Chen Y-L, Cheng K-C, Lai S-W, Tsai IJ, Lin C-C, Sung F-C, Lin C-C, Chen P-C. Diabetes and risk of subsequent gastric cancer: a population-based cohort study in Taiwan. *Gastric Cancer* 2013;16(3):389–396.

100. Tseng CH. Thyroid cancer risk is not increased in diabetic patients. *PLoS One* 2012;7(12):e53096.

101. Drucker DJ, Sherman SI, Gorelick FS, Bergenstal RM, Sherwin RS, Buse JB. Incretin-based therapies for the treatment of type 2 diabetes: evaluation of the risks and benefits. *Diabetes Care* 2010;33(2):428–433.

102. Nauck MA, Friedrich N. Do GLP-1–based therapies increase cancer risk? *Diabetes Care* 2013;36(Suppl 2):S245–S252.

103. Lowenfels AB, Maisonneuve P, Cavallini G, Ammann RW, Lankisch PG, Andersen JR, Dimagno EP, Andren-Sandberg A, Domellof L. Pancreatitis and the risk of pancreatic cancer. International Pancreatitis Study Group. *N Engl J Med* 1993;328(20):1433–1437.

104. Gier B, Matveyenko AV, Kirakossian D, Dawson D, Dry SM, Butler PC. Chronic GLP-1 receptor activation by exendin-4 induces expansion of pan-

creatic duct glands in rats and accelerates formation of dysplastic lesions and chronic pancreatitis in the Kras(G12D) mouse model. *Diabetes* 2012;61(5):1250–1262.

105. Matveyenko AV, Dry S, Cox HI, Moshtaghian A, Gurlo T, Galasso R, Butler AE, Butler PC. Beneficial endocrine but adverse exocrine effects of sitagliptin in the human islet amyloid polypeptide transgenic rat model of type 2 diabetes: interactions with metformin. *Diabetes* 2009;58(7):1604–1615.

106. Butler PC, Elashoff M, Elashoff R, Gale EAM. A critical analysis of the clinical use of incretin-based therapies: are the GLP-1 therapies safe? *Diabetes Care* 2013;36(7):2118–2125.

107. Koehler JA, Drucker DJ. Activation of glucagon-like peptide-1 receptor signaling does not modify the growth or apoptosis of human pancreatic cancer cells. *Diabetes* 2006;55(5):1369–1379.

108. Gier B, Butler PC, Lai CK, Kirakossian D, DeNicola MM, Yeh MW. Glucagon like peptide-1 receptor expression in the human thyroid gland. *J Clin Endocrinol Metab* 2012;97(1):121–131.

109. Körner M, Stöckli M, Waser B, Reubi JC. GLP-1 receptor expression in human tumors and human normal tissues: potential for in vivo targeting. *J Nucl Med* 2007;48(5):736–743.

110. Nyborg NCB, Mølck A-M, Madsen LW, Bjerre Knudsen L. The human GLP-1 analog liraglutide and the pancreas: evidence for the absence of structural pancreatic changes in three species. *Diabetes* 2012;61(5):1243–1249.

111. Nauck MA. A critical analysis of the clinical use of incretin-based therapies: the benefits by far outweigh the potential risks. *Diabetes Care* 2013;36(7):2126–2132.

112. Drucker DJ, Sherman SI, Bergenstal RM, Buse JB. The safety of incretin-based therapies: review of the scientific evidence. *J Clin Endocrinol Metab* 2011;96(7):2027–2031.

113. U.S. Food and Drug Administration. FDA Adverse Event Reporting System (FAERS), 2013. Available at www.fda.gov/Drugs/GuidanceComplianceRegulatoryInformation/Surveillance/AdverseDrugEffects/default.htm. Accessed July 2013.

114. European Medicines Agency. Assessment report for GLP-1 based therapies, 2013. Available at www.ema.europa.eu/docs/en_GB/document_library/Report/2013/08/WC500147026.pdf. Accessed 21 August 2013.

115. Chiu WY, Shih SR, Tseng CH. A review on the association between glucagon-like peptide-1 receptor agonists and thyroid cancer. *Exp Diabetes Res* 2012.924160.

116. Costante G, Meringolo D, Durante C, Bianchi D, Nocera M, Tumino S, Crocetti U, Attard M, Maranghi M, Torlontano M, Filetti S. Predictive value of serum calcitonin levels for preoperative diagnosis of medullary thyroid

carcinoma in a cohort of 5817 consecutive patients with thyroid nodules. *J Clin Endocrinol Metab* 2007;92(2):450–455.

117. Bjerre Knudsen L, Madsen LW, Andersen S, Almholt K, de Boer AS, Drucker DJ, Gotfredsen C, Egerod FL, Hegelund AC, Jacobsen H, Jacobsen SD, Moses AC, Molck AM, Nielsen HS, Nowak J, Solberg H, Thi TD, Zdravkovic M, Moerch U. Glucagon-like Peptide-1 receptor agonists activate rodent thyroid C-cells causing calcitonin release and C-cell proliferation. *Endocrinology* 2010;151(4):1473–1486.

118. Verga U, Ferrero S, Vicentini L, Brambilla T, Cirello V, Muzza M, Beck-Peccoz P, Fugazzola L. Histopathological and molecular studies in patients with goiter and hypercalcitoninemia: reactive or neoplastic C-cell hyperplasia? *Endocr Relat Cancer* 2007;14(2):393–403.

119. Waser B, Beetschen K, Pellegata NS, Reubi JC. Incretin receptors in non-neoplastic and neoplastic thyroid C cells in rodents and humans: relevance for incretin-based diabetes therapy. *Neuroendocrinology* 2011;94(4):291–301.

120. Hegedüs L, Moses AC, Zdravkovic M, Le Thi T, Daniels GH. GLP-1 and calcitonin concentration in humans: lack of evidence of calcitonin release from sequential screening in over 5000 subjects with type 2 diabetes or non-diabetic obese subjects treated with the human GLP-1 analog, liraglutide. *J Clin Endocrinol Metab* 2011;96(3):853–860.

121. Parks M, Rosebraugh C. Weighing risks and benefits of liraglutide—The FDA's review of a new antidiabetic therapy. *N Engl J Med* 2010;362(9):774–777.

122. Chang CH, Lin JW, Wu LC, Lai MS, Chuang LM. Oral insulin secretagogues, insulin, and cancer risk in type 2 diabetes mellitus. *J Clin Endocrinol Metab* 2012;97(7):E1170–1175.

123. Tseng CH. Diabetes and risk of bladder cancer: a study using the National Health Insurance database in Taiwan. *Diabetologia* 2011;54(8):2009–2015.

124. Qiu H, Rhoads GG, Berlin JA, Marcella SW, Demissie K. Initial metformin or sulphonylurea exposure and cancer occurrence among patients with type 2 diabetes mellitus. *Diabet Obes Metab* 2013;15(4):349–357.

125. Redaniel MT, Jeffreys M, May MT, Ben-Shlomo Y, Martin RM. Associations of type 2 diabetes and diabetes treatment with breast cancer risk and mortality: a population-based cohort study among British women. *Cancer Causes Control* 2012;23(11):1785–1795.

126. Yang X, So WY, Ma RCW, Yu LWY, Ko GTC, Kong APS, Ng VWS, Luk AOY, Ozaki R, Tong PCY, Chow C-C, Chan JCN. Use of sulphonylurea and cancer in type 2 diabetes—The Hong Kong Diabetes Registry. *Diabetes Res Clin Pract* 2010;90(3):343–351.

127. Monami M, Lamanna C, Balzi D, Marchionni N, Mannucci E. Sulphonylureas and cancer: a case-control study. *Acta Diabetol* 2009;46(4):279–284.

128. Monami M, Balzi D, Lamanna C, Barchielli A, Masotti G, Buiatti E, Marchionni N, Mannucci E. Are sulphonylureas all the same? A cohort study on cardiovascular and cancer-related mortality. *Diabetes Metab Res Rev* 2007;23(6):479–484.

129. Sliwinska A, Blasiak J, Drzewoski J. Effect of gliclazide on DNA damage in human peripheral blood lymphocytes and insulinoma mouse cells. *Chem Biol Interact* 2006;162(3):259–267.

130. Bowker SL, Majumdar SR, Veugelers P, Johnson JA. Increased cancer-related mortality for patients with type 2 diabetes who use sulfonylureas or insulin. *Diabetes Care* 2006;29(2):254–258.

131. Chen SW, Tsan YT, Chen JD, Hsieh HI, Lee CH, Lin HH, Wang JD, Chen PC. Use of thiazolidinediones and the risk of colorectal cancer in patients with diabetes: a nationwide, population-based, case-control study. *Diabetes Care* 2013;36(2):369–375.

132. Riser Taylor S, Harris KB. The clinical efficacy and safety of sodium glucose cotransporter-2 inhibitors in adults with type 2 diabetes mellitus. *Pharmacotherapy* 2013;33:984–999.

133. Vasilakou D, Karagiannis T, Athanasiadou E, Mainou M, Liakos A, Bekiari E, Sarigianni M, Matthews DR, Tsapas A. Sodium–glucose cotransporter 2 inhibitors for type 2 diabetes: a systematic review and meta-analysis. *Ann Inter Med* 2013;159(4):262–274.

134. Jones D. Diabetes field cautiously upbeat despite possible setback for leading SGLT2 inhibitor. *Nat Rev Drug Discov* 2011;10(9):645–646.

135. Ferrannini E, Solini A. SGLT2 inhibition in diabetes mellitus: rationale and clinical prospects. *Nat Rev Endocrinol* 2012;8(8):495–502.

136. Vigneri P, Frasca F, Sciacca L, Pandini G, Vigneri R. Diabetes and cancer. *Endocr Relat Cancer* 2009;16(4):1103-1123.

137. Gallagher EJ, LeRoith D. Diabetes, cancer, and metformin: connections of metabolism and cell proliferation. *Ann NY Acad Sci* 2011;1243:54–68.

Index

Note: Page numbers followed by an *f* refer to figures. Page numbers followed by a *t* refer to tables. Page numbers in **bold** indicate in-depth coverage of the topic.

A

A1C
acarbose, 418
ACCORD, 681, 881
Action in Diabetes and Vascular
 Disease (ADVANCE) study,
 675, 881
albuminuria, 272
alogliptin, 884
α-glucosidase inhibitors, 416, 423
birth defects, 168
canagliflozin, 449
carbamylated hemoglobin, 771
cardiovascular disease, 877, 908
childhood obesity, 264
chronic kidney disease, 771–773
closed-loop (CL) artificial
 pancreas, 130
combination therapy, 516–517
continuous glucose monitoring,
 37–40
continuous subcutaneous infusion
 (CSII) pumps, 128–129
Cycloset, 437–438, 439*f*
dapagliflozin, 452
DCCT/EDIC, 682
degludec, 489
Diabetes Control and
 Complications Trial (DCCT), 674
diabetes in nontransplant patients,
 607–608
diabetes predictors, 86
Diabetes Surgery Study, 529
diabetic ketoacidosis, 632, 646
dipeptidyl peptidase-4 inhibitors,
 388–389, 390*t*, 392*t*, 393
distal symmetric polyneuropathy,
 799–800
elderly patients, 550–551
Epidemiology of Diabetes
 Interventions and Complications
 (EDIC) study, 674
erythropoietin-stimulating agents,
 771
exenatide, 404
fetal condition, 206
follow-up assessment, 112–113
glargine, 485
GLP-1 receptor agonist, 402,
 405–406
Glucovance, 351–352
hospital admission, 560
intensive lifestyle intervention
 programs, 58
laboratory tests, 846
less-stringent target, 760
maternal hypoglycemia, 200
medical nutrition therapy, 51,
 52*t*–53*t*, 62
metformin therapy, 345–346, 348
microvascular complications, 772
nateglinide, 367
nephropathy, 678
non-ICU settings, 589
oral antidiabetic agents, 364
panretinal photocoagulation,
 749–750

prediabetes, 78, 81, 314–315
pregnancy, 197–198, 201
preoperative levels, 588
retinopathy, 677–678
screening test, 2–3, 4*t*, 5–8, 9*f*
self-monitoring blood glucose, 36
stress hyperglycemia, 592
sulfonylureas, 363, 365
sulfonylureas secondary failure,
 366
testosterone replacement therapy,
 979
thiazolidinediones, 381–382
transplant outpatient diabetes
 management, 611
U.K. Prospective Diabetes Study,
 674–675, 682
Veterans Affairs Diabetes Trial
 (VADT), 681
youth with T2D, 268, 276
abatacept, 118, 121
abdominal adiposity, 263–264, 274,
 286, 967, 979–980
abdominal pain, 513*t*, 624–625
abdominal visceral fat, 246–247
abnormal dark adaptation, 753
abscess formation, 946
absolute insulin deficiency, 264, 623*f*,
 643
abusive home situation, 655
acanthosis nigricans, 18, 266, 315, 645,
 952, 959–960, 1000
acarbose, 320*t*, 370, 416, 418–419,
 422, 509*t*, 511*t*, 514–515, 535, 553,
 612*t*
ACCORD Blood Pressure trial, 879,
 888, 924–925, 926*f*
ACCORD Lipid trial, 879, 887, 924
acetaminophen, 32, 33*t*, 37–38
acetoacetic acid, 644
acetone, 625
acetyl-carnitine, 810
acidemia, 629
acidosis, 642–644, 648, 651, 653, 766*t*,
 767, 776, 941
acquired abnormalities, 220
acquired generalized lipoatrophy, 959
acquired immune deficiency syndrome
 (AIDS), 949
acquired perforating dermatosis, 952
acrodermatitis enteropathica, 961
acromegaly, 441
Action for Health in Diabetes (Look
 AHEAD) study, 523
Action in Diabetes and Vascular
 Disease (ADVANCE), 550, 675,
 683*t*–684*t*, 696–697, 703, 876, 881,
 923–924
 intensive glycemic control (IC),
  885
 macrovascular complications, 681
Action in Diabetes and Vascular
 Disease: Preterax and Diamicron
 Modified Release Controlled
 Evaluation (ADVANCE) trial, 368
Action to Control Cardiovascular Risk
 in Diabetes (ACCORD)
 A1C, 681, 881

cardiovascular autonomic
 neuropathy, 835, 840
cardiovascular disease, 876,
 879–880
chronic diabetes complications,
 675–676
chronic kidney disease, 773
distal symmetric polyneuropathy
 (DSP), 799
dyslipidemia, 915
elderly patients, 550
hypertension, 924–927
hypoglycemia, 696–697, 703
intensive glycemic control, 885
peripheral neuropathy, 802
Action to Control Cardiovascular Risk
 in Diabetes (ACCORD) Eye Study,
 675, 753
activity diary, 39
Activity Guidelines for Americans, 70
Actoplus Met, 349*t*, 354–355
Actos Now for Prevention of Diabetes
 study (ACT NOW), 320*t*, 381
actovegin, 810
acupuncture, 813*t*, 814
acute cardiac ischemia, 702
acute heart failure, 347
acute kidney injury (AKI), 766*t*, 767,
 770, 782*t*
acute pancreatitis, 622, 626, 654
acute pyelonephritis, 942*t*, 945
acute renal failure, 406, 587, 654
acute respiratory distress syndrome
 (ARDS), 642, 654
adaptive immune response, 100
adenocarcinoma, 18, 960
adenosine 3′,5′-monophosphate
 regulated insulin secretion, 362
adenosine 5′-mono-phosphate-
 activated protein kinase (AMPK),
 342, 1025
adenosine triphosphate (ATP), 363
adherence, 146–148, 291–292
adipocyte, 219, 530, 909
adipocyte hypertrophy, 241
adipocyte insulin sensitivity, 997
adipocyte-derived cytokines, 523
adipocytokine, 172, 379–380, 546,
 808
adipogenesis, 377
adipokine, 218–219
adiponectin, 157, 219, 246, 379–380,
 546, 981
adipose tissue, 157, 240–241, 377–379,
 624, 629, 994, 1022
adipose tissue–derived inflammatory
 markers, 809
adiposity indexes, 837
adjustable gastric band, 527, 1004
adolescent, 40, 58, 65–66, 70, 75, 79,
 105, 110, 136*t*, 138–138
 adult-monitored self-management,
  303
 bariatric surgery, 535
 body image, 301
 body mass index, 263
 cognitive behavioral therapy, 143
 crisis at diagnosis, 135

depression, 302
developmental issues, 302
diabetic ketoacidosis, 633
disordered eating, 146
family conflict, 145
family-based treatment, 134, 294
glycemic control, 683
insulin administration by adult, 655
insulin pump therapy, 129
insulin resistance, 266
interpersonal therapy, 143
nonadherent behavior, 774
school environment, 303
T2D, special issues with, 300–303
adrenal function assessment, 113
adrenal insufficiency, 566, 704, 712*t*
adult, 59*t*, 77, 79, 80*f*, 83, 97, 110, **621–640**
adult-monitored self-management, 297
advanced glycation end products (AGEs), 672, 808
aerobic capacity reserve (Vo_2R), 70–71
Affordable Care Act, 296
African American population
   A1C, 6
   diabetes complications, 671
   diabetic nephropathy, 763–764
   elderly population, 545
   gestational diabetes, 158, 172
   glucose intolerance, 182
   glycemic targets, 682–683
   lifestyle modification, 245
   nonalcoholic fatty liver disease (NAFLD), 995–996
   obesity and T2D in children, 265
   peripheral arterial disease, 898
   prediabetes, 669
   psychosocial issues and T2D, 301
   T2D, 15–16, 106*t*, 212, 265
   thiazolidinediones, 379
African Caribbean population, 798
African population, 16, 83, 314
African sleeping sickness, 671
age/aging, 217, 712*t*
AIDS (acquired immune deficiency syndrome), 949
alanine aminotransferase (ALT), 1000, 1008*t*
Alaska Native population, 81
albiglutide, 407
albumin, 197–199, 966
albumin-to-creatinine ratio (ACR), 272, 762, 765, 780
albuminuria
   ACE inhibitor, 928, 932
   ARB, 932
   assessment, 268
   cardiovascular disease, 878–879
   chronic diabetes complications, 674, 676, 678
   chronic kidney disease, 761, 778, 840
   diabetic nephropathy, 272, 762, 764
   exercise, 69
   pregnancy, 198
   T2D in youth, 268
alcohol
   diabetes risk factors, 86
   hypertension, 928
   hypoglycemia, 708, 712*t*
   insulin secretagogue, 370
   metformin, 347
   nonalcoholic fatty liver disease, 1000
   obesity and T2D, 252
   pregnancy, 198
   psychosocial and family issues in children, 140, 144

psychosocial issues and T2D, 286–287
T2D, 218
alcohol abuse, 622
alcoholic ketoacidosis, 645
alcoholism, 1018
aldose reductase (polyol) pathway, 671
aldose-reductase inhibitors, 810
aldosterone, 776
aldosteronoma-induced hypokalemia, 19
alefacept, 118–119
alkaline phosphatase, 774, 807
ALLHAT trial, 930–932
allodynia, 815
allograft rejection, 609
allopurinol, 770, 775, 777*t*, 849
alogliptin, 349*t*, 355–356, 388, 390*t*, 391, 392*t*, 393, 395*t*, 509*t*, 884
α-1 antitrypsin deficiency, 1000
α-1-adrenergic–α-antagonism, 931
α-blocker, 929*t*, 930, 931–932, 933*f*
α-blocker agents (α-agents), 931–932
α-cell function, 131
α-cell secretion, 402
α-cell tumor of the pancreas, 961
α-glucosidase inhibitors (AGIs), **416–434**
   A1C, 416
   basal insulin with a GLP-1 receptor agonist, 518
   blood pressure, 420
   cancer, 1024*t*, 1031
   cardiovascular risk factors, 420
   clinical efficacy of, 417–419
   DPP-4 inhibitor, 418
   elderly patients, 421, 553
   fasting plasma glucose, 421
   hypoglycemic agents, 418
   insulin in patients with T2D, 418–419
   insulin resistance, 420
   macrovascular complications, 420
   mechanisms of action, 416–417
   metformin, 418
   obesity and T2D in children, 276
   other effects of, 420
   in patients with IGT, efficacy of, 419
   in patients with T1D, efficacy of, 419
   pharmacological characteristics, 417
   pioglitazone, 418
   vs. placebo, 418
   postprandial hyperglycemia, 416, 421
   postprandial triglyceride rise, 420
   prevention strategies for T2D, 322
   with sulfonylureas, 418
   therapy, indications for, 421
   thiazolidinediones in comparison to, 418
   tolerability, 421–422
α-hydroxy acids, 960
α-interferon, 19
α-lipoic acid, 810, 849
α-melanocyte stimulating hormone (MSH), 252
alternate site testing, 29
ambulatory surgical patients, 596
amenorrhea, 146
American Association for the Study of Liver Diseases (AASLD) Practice Guidelines, 1000, 1004, 1006
American Association of Clinical Endocrinologists (AACE), 35*t*, 382, 394, 404, 406, 588, 974
American Association of Diabetes Educators (AADE), 22, 23, 61*t*, 62

American College of Cardiology and the American Heart Association (ACC/AHA), 902–903, 911, 912*t*, 913–915, 919
American College of Obstetricians and Gynecologists (ACOG), 17, 159, 175*t*, 182
American Diabetes Association and American Association for Clinical Endocrinologists (ADA/AACE), 587*t*, 592, 596
American Indian population, 81, 84, 156, 245, 263, 265, 545, 798, 925
American Urological Association Symptom Index, 847
amino acids, 222, 462, 961
aminoglycoside, 770, 782*t*, 947*t*
aminotransferases, 995, 1000, 1005
amitriptyline, 812*t*, 813
amlodipine, 779
amoxicillin/clavulanate, 852*t*, 870, 944
amphotericin B, 948
amputation, 544, 668, 675, 676*f*, 679, 796, 802, 864, 866*t*, 898–899
amylin, 131, 222
amylin analogs, 276, 777
amyloid-induced β-cell destruction, 221
anaerobic bacteria, 944
anaerobic intestinal bacteria, 422
anastomotic leak, 534
anatomic abnormality, 946
androgen, 1021
androgen deficiency, 977
Androgen Deficiency in Aging Male (ADAM) questionnaire, 976, 979
androgen synthesis and production, 377
androstenedione, 969
anemia, 3, 348, 608, 766, 771, 779–780, 836, 838, 961
anesthesia, 585–586
angina, 391
angioedema, 964
angiogenesis, 673
angiotensin II, 763–764, 903
angiotensin II receptor blockers (ARBs), 270, 273, 323, 451, 753, 763, 903, 929–930, 932, 933*f*
angiotensin receptor inhibitors
   cardiovascular autonomic neuropathy, 849
   chronic kidney disease, 770, 772*t*, 774, 777*t*
   diabetic nephropathy, 778
   pregnancy, 199
angiotensin system blockade, 778
angiotensin-converting enzyme (ACE) inhibitors, 69, 270, 273, 323, 451, 613*t*, 734, 753
   blood pressure, 930–932, 933*f*
   cardiovascular autonomic neuropathy, 849
   chronic kidney disease, 765, 770, 772*t*
   diabetic nephropathy, 763, 777*t*, 778
   hypertension, 923–924, 928–930
   intensive blood pressure control, 774
   pregnancy, 199, 208*t*, 209
angle-closure glaucoma, 743
animal-insulin formulations, 472
anion gap, 630, 648–649, 652
anion gap acidosis, 645
ankle-brachial index (ABI), 871, 898, 900, 905
anorectal motor function, 846
anorectic hormones, 530
anorexia nervosa, 815, 971
anthropometric measurements, 241

antibacterial agents, 371
antibiotics, 646, 770
antibody testing, 14–15
anti-CD3 monoclonal antibodies, 117–118
anti-CD3 monoclonal antibody teplizumab, 121
anti-CD20 monoclonal antibody, 118
anti-CD25 (daclizumab), 119
anticoagulation therapy, 371, 902
anticonvulsant, 811*t*, 813
antidepressant medication, 143
antidiabetic agent, 242, 348, 382, 1024*t*
antifungal agent, 371
antihyperglycemic agent, 342, 348, 391, 508, 509*t*, 510
antihypertensive treatment, 198–200, 209, 774, 778
anti-inflammatory T-lymphocytes, 118
anti-insulin receptor antibodies, 19
antilymphocyte antibodies, 768
antimicrobial treatment, 942*t*–943*t*, 947*t*
antioxidant, 169
antiplatelet therapy, 902
antipseudomonal agent, 945, 947*t*
antipsychotic medication, 289, 622–623
antirejection protocol, 566
antiretroviral drug therapy, 949
antitubercular therapy, 949
anti–vascular endothelial growth factor (VEGF) medication, 730, 741
anxiety/anxiety disorder, 286, 289*t*, 291, 298, 801
apiriprazole, 622
apolipoprotein, 451
apolipoprotein B, 270, 908–909, 911, 918–919
apoptosis, 169, 383, 1026
apoptosis signal-regulating kinase 1 (ASK1), 809
appetite suppressant, 250
Archimedes model, 325
aromatase inhibitor, 970–971
arrhythmias, 68*t*, 586, 590, 629, 646, 703, 834, 844, 880
arterial stiffness, 273
arteriolar attenuation, 816
arterio-venous fistula (AVF), 767, 769
arterio-venous graft (AVG), 768
arthritis, 239
artificial electron acceptors, 29
artificial pancreas system, 28, 36–37, **128–133**, 130–132, 131*t*, 707
ascorbate, 32
Asian American population, 2*t*, 315, 545
Asian population, 15, 84, 106*t*, 156, 158, 172, 219, 263, 314, 316, 763
Asian-Pacific Islander population, 81
aspartate aminotransferase (AST)/ALT ratio, 1001
aspergillosis, 949
Aspergillus, 946, 948
aspiration pneumonia, 654
aspirin, 370, 613*t*, 734, 902, 957
asthma, 641
asymmetric quadriparesis, 814
asymptomatic bacteriuria, 945
asymptomatic hypoglycemia, 699–700
atherogenic dyslipidemia, 533, 994
atherogenic effect, 703
atheroinflammation, 668
atherosclerosis, 271, 344*t*, 670, 702, 775, 898, 908–909, 911
Atherosclerosis Intervention in Metabolic Syndrome with Low HDL/High Triglycerides: Impact on Global Health Outcomes (AIM-HIGH), 886–887

Atherosclerosis Risk in Communities (ARIC) Study, 840
atherosclerotic lipoprotein, 915
Atkins diet, 246
atorvastatin, 886, 910*t*, 914
Atorvastatin Study for Prevention of Cardiovascular End Points in Subjects With Type 2 Diabetes (ASPEN) trial, 886
at-risk states, 6–9
atrophy, 112
attention deficit–hyperactivity disorder (ADHD), 149
attenuated linear growth, 277
atypical antipsychotics, 19
atypical diabetes, 16
auricular mucormycosis, 654
Australian Aborigines, 218
Australian Diabetes Risk Assessment Tool (AusDrisk), 315
autoantibodies, 99–100, 113
autoimmune disorders, 1018
autoimmune hepatitis, 1000
autoimmune polyendocrine syndrome, 952
autoimmunity, 13–14, 19, 98–100, 546
Autoimmunity-Blocking Antibody for Tolerance in Recently Diagnosed Type 1 Diabetes (AbATE) trial, 117
autologous hematopoietic stem cell transplantation (AHSCT), 119
autonomic nerve fibers, 808
autonomic nervous system, 679
autonomic neural dysfunction, 837
autonomic neuropathy, 68*t*, 69, 584, 670*t*, 679, 712*t*, 866*t*, 941*t*
autonomous neuropathy, 206
autosympathectomy, 865
Avandamet, 349*t*, 353–354
Avoiding Cardiovascular Events Through Combination Therapy in Patients Living With Systolic Hypertension (ACCOMPLISH) trial, 926–927, 931
axon reflex testing, 847
azathioprine, 117
azole antifungal drugs, 948
azoospermia, 976
azotemia, 770

B

bacillus Calmette-Guérin (BCG), 117
bacteremia, 587
bacterial cystitis, 847
bacterial infection, 609
balance loss, 801
balanitis, 451
balloon angioplasty, 904
band erosion, 534
band prolapse, 534
barbiturates, 371
bare-metal stent, 905
bariatric surgery, 277, **522–543**
    dyslipidemia, 533–534
    glycemia, 526–527
    nonalcoholic fatty liver disease, 995, 1004–1005
    nutritional deficiency, 534
    perioperative hyperglycemia, 592–594
    postoperative blood glucose management, 593–594
    randomized controlled trials, 527–530
    risks of, 534–535
    T2D, 530–532, 535–536
    types of, 523–532
    weight loss, 526
barium meal, 845

baroreflex sensitivity (BRS), 842, 844, 880
basal hepatic glucose production (HGP), 379
basal hyperglycemia, 554
baseline evaluation, 300
β-blocker–α-agent, 931
β-blockers, 217, 371, 772*t*, 923, 929, 931–932, 933*f*
β-blocking agent, 734
β-cell, 1, 99–100, 213
    apoptosis, 222, 393
    autoantibodies, 98
    autoimmunity, 100–101
    childhood obesity, 263
    compensation system, 213, 224
    dedifferentiation, 213*f*, 221*f*, 223
    defective, 215–223
    destruction, 97
    drug- or chemical-induced diabetes, 19
    dysfunction, 212–214, 216, 221, 223, 377, 380, 461, 463, 530
    exhaustion, 219–220, 221*f*, 222
    failure, 213
    function, 6, 15, 84, 116–120, 215, 217–218, 220–221, 276, 348–350, 473, 566
    function in children, 264–265
    genetic defects, 18
    genetic predisposition, 216–217
    glucagon-like peptide-1 (GLP-1), 402
    inflammation, 223
    K_{ATP} channel, 18, 363
    Kir6.2 subunit, 18
    mass, 218, 221
    membrane, 360, 361*f*
    neogenesis, 393
    other mechanisms, 217
    pancreatic, 157–158
    replacement, 130
    reserve, 365
    responsiveness, 585
    rest strategies, 220
    secretion, 379
    SUR1/Kir6.2, 362
    susceptibility, molecular mechanisms of, 216–217
    susceptible, 215
    type 1 diabetes (T1D), 13–14
    type 2 diabetes (T2D), 16
β-cell (HOMA-B%), 381
β-cell–specific polypeptide, 222
Beers criteria, 370
behavior modification, 40, 148, 284, 316
behavior problems, 144
behavior therapy, 144
behavioral family therapy, 144–145
behavioral health specialist, 144
behavioral intervention, 245, 655
behavioral issues, 291–293, 622
behavioral monitoring, 291–292
behavioral nonadherence, 291–292
behavioral strategies, 51, 62
behavioral therapy, 242
behavior-change interventions, 21–22
benzphetamine, 250
β-blocker–α-1-blocker, 931
β-glucosidases, 417
β-hemolytic streptococci, 944
β-hydroxybutyrate (BOHB), 625–626, 645–646, 647, 649
β-oxidation, 644
bevacizumab, 750–752
bezafibrate, 321*t*, 323
bicarbonate, 630, 649, 651–653, 776
biguanides, 322–323, 341, 391, 418, 509*t*, 511*t*, 596*t*, 611*t*

bilateral femoral arteries, 900
bile acid, 401
bile acid sequestrant, 509*t*, 511*t*, 516, 915
biliopancreatic diversion (BPD), 524*t*, 525–527, 530, 533–534
biliopancreatic diversion with duodenal switch (BPD-DS), 525
binge-eating disorder (BED), 287
biomechanical complications, 57
biosensor system, 29
bipolar disorder, 289
birth defect, 168–169
birth injury, 197
birth trauma, 158, 161
birth weight, 86, 163, 171, 177–178, 180*t*
bladder cancer, 383, 453–454, 511*t*, 1005, 1019*t*, 1024*t*, 1026–1027, 1032
bladder catheterization, 646, 771, 782*t*, 946
bladder contractility, 834
bladder dysfunction, 836, 838*t*, 841, 847, 853, 853*t*
bleeding diathesis, 767
blister, 961
blood count, 646
blood gasses, 647
blood glucose
　concentrations, 1
　fungal pathogens, 941
　meter, 28–36
　staircase, 714*f*
　target, 559–560
blood glucose level, 53*t*, 73, 74*t*, 101, 111, 128–129, 632, 648
　closed-loop (CL) artificial pancreas, 130–131
　criteria for resolution of DKA and HHS, 630–631
　distal symmetric polyneuropathy, 799
　maternal hypoglycemia, 200
　pregnancy, 197
　puberty, 139
blood glucose meter, 32*t*, 563
blood glucose monitoring, 25*t*, 75*t*, 129, 161. *See also* continuous glucose-monitoring (CGM); self-monitoring blood glucose (SMBG)
blood lipid profile, 247
blood pressure (BP). *See also* hypertension
　α-glucosidase inhibitors, 420
　cardiovascular disease, 887–889, 908
　chronic kidney disease, 760
　circadian rhythm, 840
　combination therapy, 515
　control, 773–774, 778
　dapagliflozin, 453
　diabetes self-management education, 62
　diabetic ketoacidosis in infants, children and adolescents, 653
　diabetic retinopathy, 734
　distal symmetric polyneuropathy, 800
　elderly patients, 550
　endothelial dysfunction, 670
　exercise, 67*t*, 68–69
　GLP-1 receptor agonists, 403
　lifestyle intervention, 58
　lifestyle modification, 247
　medical nutrition therapy, 51, 52*t*
　pregnancy, 198, 200, 206
　regulation, 839
　sodium-glucose cotransporter 2, 447, 450

T1D, 112
T2D in youth, 268
　target, 921, 921*t*
blood transfusion, 766*t*, 780–781
blood urea nitrogen/creatinine ratio, 453
blood-borne pathogens, 31
blurry vision, 268
body composition, 979–980
body fat, 241
body image, 146, 301
body mass index (BMI), 2*t*, 55*t*, 57–58, 84, 88, 101, 112, 181
　acanthosis nigracans, 266
　adolescents, 263
　bariatric surgery, 529*f*, 535
　carpal tunnel syndrome, 818
　children, 263
　hypogonadotropic hypogonadism, 968–969
　intrauterine exposure, 266
　obesity, 239–240, 522
　overweight, 239
　physical activity, 316
　screening tests, 315
　spermatogenesis, 976
　susceptible β-cells, 215
　T2D, 218–219, 268*t*
bone
　culture, 945
　density, 975
　density screening, 535, 611
　fracture, 354, 383, 511*t*, 611
　loss, 611, 1005
　remodeling, 807
　resorption, 807
bone mineral density (BMD), 975
bovine insulin, 964
bovine pancreas, 482
bowel, 783
bowel motility, 834
bradycardia, 843–844
brain, 240, 702, 704*t*
brain development, 140
brain-derived neurotrophic factor, 288
breast cancer, 178, 453–454, 486, 1019*t*, 1023, 1024*t*, 1025
breast tumor cells, 1021
breast-feeding, 100, 121, 183, 205, 209, 712*t*
breath test, 846
broad-spectrum antibiotics, 849, 852*t*
bromocriptine, 411, 435–436, 436*f*, 440–441, 509*t*, 511*t*, 516
bronchiolitis, 641
buformin, 341
bulbocavernosus reflex, 846–847
bulimia nervosa, 146
bullying, 303
bupropion-naltrexone, 252
Bypass Angioplasty Revascularization Investigation 2 Diabetes (BARI 2D), 368, 797, 802, 882
bypass surgery, 904

C

caffeine, 218
calcineurin inhibitor, 608, 613*t*, 958
calcitonin, 1029–1030
calcium, 202, 646–647, 773–774
calcium channel blocker (CCB), 270, 613*t*, 772*t*, 779, 929*t*, 930–932, 933*f*
calcium phosphorus, 774
callus, 865–866, 868
calmodulin, 360, 361*f*
caloric intake, 157, 176, 201–202, 217, 317*t*
Cambridge Risk Score, 315

Canadian Diabetes Association (CDA), 175*t*, 587*t*, 588
Canadian Diabetes Risk Assessment Questionnaire (CANRISK), 315
Canadian First Nations' Children data, 270, 272
canagliflozin, 449–452, 509*t*, 511*t*, 516, 1024*t*, 1031
cancer, 239, 247, 383, 393, 486, 487*t*, 522, 975–976. *See also under specific type*
　α-glucosidase inhibitor, 1031
　associations of diabetes therapies with cancer incidence and mortality, 1024*t*
　bladder, 1019*t*, 1024*t*, 1026–1027, 1032
　breast, 1019*t*, 1023, 1024*t*, 1025
　chemotherapy, 740
　chronic inflammation, 1022
　colon, 1022–1023
　and diabetes, **1018–1043**
　diabetes therapies associated with, 1023–1032
　endometrial, 1019*t*, 1020
　epidemiology, 1018–1020
　glinides, 1031
　hyperglycemia, 1022
　incretin-based therapies, 1027–1030
　insulin, 1020–1021, 1023, 1025
　insulin growth factor, 1020–1021
　liver, 1018–1019, 1024*t*
　metformin, 1025–1026
　non-Hodgkin's lymphoma, 1019*t*
　obesity, 1022–1023
　pancreatic, 1019–1020, 1024*t*, 1025
　pathophysiology, 1020–1022
　prostate, 1019*t*, 1024*t*
　relative risks in different organs of diabetic patients, 1019*t*
　sodium-glucose cotransporter 2, 1031–1032
　sulfonylureas, 1030–1031
　thiazolidinediones, 1026–1027
Candesartan and Lisinopril Microalbuminuria (CALM) trial, 929–930
Candida, 941, 946
candidiasis, 949
capillary blood glucose concentration, 647
capillary nonperfusion, 749
capillary refill time, 646
capsaicin cream, 812*t*–813*t*, 814
captopril, 209, 778
carbohydrate
　α-glucosidase inhibitors, 416–417
　bariatric surgery, 535
　elderly patients, 553
　exercise, 73, 74*t*–75*t*
　intolerance, 377
　medical nutrition therapy, 52*f*, 53*t*–54*t*
　metabolism, 377
　nutrition intervention, 60, 176–177
　pregnancy, 202
　weight loss, 246
carbonic anhydrase, 251
cardiac
　arrhythmia, 650
　bypass surgery, 583
　ischemia, 702, 880
　outflow tract, 169
　surgery, 582
　sympathetic nerve populations, 844
　sympathetic tone, 838
　ventricular repolarization, 702

cardiometabolic disease, 57
cardiometabolic risk, 532
cardiomyocytes, 368
cardioselective β-blockers, 849
cardiothoracic procedure, 582, 584, 590–591
cardiovagal function, 843
cardiovascular
    autonomic function, 843
    complications, 508
    death, 391, 393
    drug therapy, 391
    events, 58, 343, 369, 407, 491, 679, 680*f*, 681–682, 740, 775, 921, 923–924, 927, 929*t*, 932, 973
    health, 65
    mortality, 567, 974
    outcomes, 980
    reflex testing, 839
    risk factors, 323, 368, 403, 449–450, 472, 485, 487*t*, 588, 880–881
    safety, 371, 391
    safety trials, 393
cardiovascular autonomic neuropathy (CAN)
    assessment of symptoms, 843–845
    bladder dysfunction, 853
    diabetic autonomic neuropathy, 838–839, 842–843
    diabetic diarrhea, 849
    disease-modifying therapies, 848–849
    erectile dysfunction, 853
    gastroparesis, 849
    glycemic control, 679, 848
    imaging techniques for, 844–845
    intensive insulin therapy, 836
    multiple risk factor intervention, 848–849
    orthostatic hypotension, 849
    pathogenetic pathways, other therapies targeting, 849
    silent ischemia, 839
    symptomatic treatment, 849–853
    T1D, 835–836
    T2D, 835–836
    treatment, 848–853
cardiovascular autonomic reflex tests (CARTs), 843
cardiovascular disease (CVD)
    ADA recommendations for screening asymptomatic individuals for diabetes, 2*t*
    adipocytokines, 379
    blood pressure, 887–889
    chlorthalidone, 930
    chronic kidney disease, 773
    dyslipidemia, 885–887
    glycemic control, 668, 680*f*, 876
    hypogonadotropic hypogonadism, 973
    insulin resistance, 7
    intensive glycemic control, 885
    intensive lifestyle intervention programs, 244
    kidney transplant, 609
    LDL cholesterol, 914
    lifestyle modification, 552
    medical nutrition therapy, 51
    metabolic syndrome, 242
    mortality, 82, 876
    nonalcoholic fatty liver disease, 994, 996, 998
    obesity, 239–240
    perioperative hyperglycemia, 584
    pioglitazone, 1005
    primary goal and priorities of treatment, 912*t*

resting tachycardia, 836, 838
risk factors, 66–67, 241, 246
screening for diabetes complications, 669*t*
studies evaluating, 881–884
sulfonylureas, 371
T1D, 113
T2D, 315
T2D youth, 269, 271
thiazolidinediones, 382–383
transplantation, 613*t*
treatment needs T1D vs. T2D, 106*t*
trials, 683*t*, 884–885, 910*t*
caretaker, 294–296, 302
carotid artery intima-media thickness (IMT), 420
carpal tunnel syndrome (CTS), 818
casein, 121
cataract, 740–741, 752
cataract extraction, 676, 676*f*, 741
catecholamines, 585–586, 590, 643*f*
catheter-based interventions, 901
cationic drug, 348
Caucasian population, 13–14, 79, 81–82, 84, 106*t*, 172, 522, 669, 683*t*, 995
ceftazidime, 942*t*, 945
celiac antibody testing, 113
celiac disease, 106*t*
cell-cycle arrest, 1025
cell-mediated immunity, 941, 950
cellular apoptosis, 808
cellulitis, 943–944, 954
center-involved DME, 739
Centers for Disease Control and Prevention (CDC), 182, 325, 522, 668
Centers for Medicare and Medicaid Services (CMS), 22, 62
central nervous system (CNS), 217–218, 435, 441
central venous pressure, 646
Centre for Epidemiologic Studies Depression Scale (CES-D), 289*t*
cephalopelvic disproportion, 207
cephalosporins, 870
cerebral edema, 148, 630, 632, 642, 647, 649, 652–654
cerebral ischemia, 702
cerebrovascular accidents, 780
cerebrovascular disease, 876
cerebrovascular event, 623
certified diabetes educator (CDE), 23, 719, 928
Cesarean section, 161, 179, 181, 197, 207–208
Charcot neuroarthropathy (CN), 806–807, 864, 871–872
chemical-induced diabetes, 19
chemotherapeutic agents, 1025
chemotherapeutic protocol, 566
chemotherapy, 949, 1023
children, 15, 18, 38*t*, 39–40, 57, 59*t*, 70, 97, 99–100. *See also* toddlers; youth
    adherence problems, 146–147
    α-glucosidase inhibitors, 422
    behavior problems, 144
    body mass index, 263
    breast-fed, 183
    canagliflozin, 452
    cerebral edema, 642
    cognitive behavioral therapy, 143
    cognitive dysfunction, 709
    crisis at diagnosis, 135
    dehydration, 645
    diabetes and development, 135, 137–141
    diabetic ketoacidosis, 630
    ethnicity and T2D, 265–266

family-based treatment, 134, 294
genetic susceptibility T2D, 265
glycemic control, 683
heart rate, 836
hyperglycemia, 643
hyperglycemic-hyperosmolar syndrome, 642
hypertension, 644
insulin pump therapy, 129
insulin resistance phenotype, 266
intrauterine exposure, 266
lifestyle and T2D, 266
lifestyle modification of nutrition and activity, 274–275
macrovascular complications, 273
malnutrition, 217
metformin therapy, 345, 346*t*
microvascular complications, 272–273
morbidity, 642
mortality, 642, 652
nephropathy, 272–273
neuropathy, 273
nonalcoholic fatty liver disease, 272
obesity, 179
obesity and T2D, **263–283**
retinopathy, 272
self-management, 148
    T1D, 105, 108, 110
    T2D, 264–267, 269, 300–303, 621
Children's Depression Inventory, 289*t*
Chinese American population, 84
Chinese patients, 220, 242–243
Chinese population, 82–83
chloride, 632, 644*t*
chlorpropamide, 360*t*, 362, 365, 369–370, 721
chlorpropamide alcohol flush, 961
chlorthalidone, 930–931
chocolate, 218
cholecystitis, 273, 942*t*, 946
cholesterol, 33*t*, 51, 52*t*–53*t*, 57, 246–249
cholesterol-lowering agents, 199, 200*t*
cholestyramine, 849, 852*t*
chromosomes, 14, 18, 99
chronic
    care model, 23
    complications, 269
    diabetes complications, **668–695**
    inflammation, 1022
    pain, 547*t*, 548, 550
chronic inflammatory demyelinating polyneuropathy (CIDP), 795*t*, 815–817
chronic kidney disease (CKD), 3, 369, 381, 565, 608, 760–792, 782*t*, 840.
    See also end-stage renal disease; kidney transplantation
    ACE inhibition plus ACE receptor blockage in diabetes, 779
    acidosis, 776
    anemia, 780–781
    angiotensin system blockade, 778
    blood pressure control, 773–774
    cardiovascular disease and, 773
    costs associated with, 763, 781
    and diabetes, target goals, 771–773
    diabetes related, 763
    diabetic nephropathy, 763–764
    dialysis therapy, 780
    dietary protein restriction, 775
    drugs for treatment of diabetes, 776–783
    dyslipidemia, 775
    epidemiology, 761–763
    erythropoiesis-stimulating agents, 780
    gadolinium-containing contrast agents, 771

glomerulonephritis, 763
hyperkalemia, 776
hypertension, 763
hyperuricemia and treatment, 775
iatrogenic injury, 769–771
kidney failure in diabetes, 780–783
metabolic bone disease, 774
metformin therapy, 776
potassium, 776
recombinant erythropoietin, 779
renal function in patients with
  diabetes, 769–776
renoprotective management, 760
risk factors in pathophysiology,
  764
stages, 764–765
stages as applied to diabetes,
  760–769
staging, 761, 762t
statin therapy, 775
target hemoglobin, 779
therapy for azotemia in diabetes,
  767–769
chronic liver disease, 1000
chronic obstructive pulmonary disease
  (COPD), 566
chronic sensorimotor neuropathy, 865
cimetidine, 348, 770
ciprofloxacin, 942t, 945, 947t
circadian plasma prolactin levels, 435
circulatory volume, 628
cirrhosis, 276, 422, 608, 994, 996–997,
  1001
c-Jun N-terminal kinase (JNK), 586
c-Jun-N-terminal-kinase (JNK)
  activation, 809
c-Jun N-terminal kinase-1 (JNK-1),
  971, 981
CKD–Epidemiology Collaboration
  Equation (CKD-EPI), 761–762
classification, 13–20
claudication, 899, 903
clindamycin, 870, 943t, 944–945
clinic visits, 206
clinical accuracy, glucose meters, 33
Clinical Laboratory Improvement
  Amendments, 30
Clinical Laboratory Standards Institute,
  31
clinical status, 611
clinically significant DME (CSME),
  739
clock drawing test, 549
closed-loop (CL) artificial pancreas,
  130
cloud-based platform, 30
clozapine, 622
coagulase-negative staphylococci, 944
Coccidiodes, 946
coccidioidomycosis, 941, 949
coffee, 86
cognitive behavioral therapy (CBT),
  143, 146
cognitive concerns screening
  questionnaire, 149t
cognitive dysfunction, 547t, 549, 551
cognitive function, 291, 708–709
cognitive impairment, 286, 548
colesevelam, 509t, 511t, 516
collaborative care model, 298
collagen synthesis, 673
colon, 783
colon cancer, 1022–1023
colonic adenomas, 999
colonic ulceration, 422
colorectal cancer, 1019t, 1022, 1024t
colorectal neoplasm, 999
coma, 622, 630, 644
combination therapy, 508, 510, 512–
  515, 517–518

communication, 145
community-based group lifestyle
  weight loss program, 326
community-based service, 295
complementary and alternative
  medicine (CAM), 249
complex carbohydrates, 176, 422
complications, ix, 6, 52t, 107t, 269,
  668–728. *See also* macrovascular
  complications; microvascular
  complications; *under specific type*
Comprehensive Diabetic Foot Exam
  (CDFE), 866, 871
computer-assisted sensory examination
  (CASEs), 805
computer-based protocols, 568
concomitant drug treatment, 371
congenital aromatase deficiency,
  971
congenital malformations, 168–169,
  197–198
congenital nephrotic syndrome of the
  Finnish type, 764
congestive heart failure, 347, 382–383,
  511t, 879
connective tissue inhibitor, 782
consciousness, 653
constipation, 511t, 838t
continuous end-total CO_2 monitoring,
  647
continuous glucose monitoring (CGM),
  28, 36–40, 66, 75t, 109t, 110, 129,
  137, 200, 702, 707
continuous intravenous insulin therapy,
  564–569, 570f–572f, 573t, 587–589
continuous snapshot glucose
  monitoring, 38
continuous subcutaneous infusion
  (CSII) pumps, 107t, 128–129, 137,
  203–204, 564, 566, 568, 570t–572t,
  591, 594, 596, 964
continuous-wave Doppler ultrasound
  device, 900
contraception, 183, 199, 270
contrast sensitivity, 753
Copenhagen Recommendations, 204t
coping skills, 148
cord-to-maternal plasma
  concentrations, 179
corneal abrasion, 740, 743–744
corneal confocal microscopy (CCM),
  802, 805
coronary artery bypass graft (CABG),
  583
coronary artery disease (CAD), 69,
  380, 773, 876–880, 973–974
coronary heart disease (CHD), 109t,
  200, 420, 877, 885–886, 908–909,
  911, 914–918
coronary heart failure (CHF), 929–932
coronary ischemia, 702
coronary revascularization, 391
cortical atrophy, 702t, 709
cortical bone density, 975
corticosteroids, 209, 217, 563,
  607–608, 611, 622–623, 816, 955,
  957–958, 1000
cortisol, 585t, 586, 643f, 702, 704t
counterregulatory function, 679
counterregulatory hormones, 585–586,
  623–624, 641, 643, 701–702, 713
cow's milk, 100, 121
C-peptide, 117–119, 810, 849, 1022
C-peptide/insulin molar ratio, 379
C-peptide levels, 162
C-peptide–related signaling pathways,
  808
C-peptide secretion, 97, 98f
cranial imaging, 654
cranial nerve, 740

cranial nerve posture, 653
cranial neuropathy, 795t, 817
C-reactive protein, 158, 246, 249,
  545, 969
C-reactive protein (CRP)
  concentrations, 971, 975, 981
creatinine, 33t, 276, 395t, 613t, 627f,
  646
Crede maneuver, 853t
critical care surgery patients, 584
critical limb ischemia (CLI), 898,
  900–901, 903–905
critically ill patients, 610t, 629
Cryptococcus, 946
CTLA4 (cytotoxic T-lymphocyte-
  associated protein 4), 99
cultural beliefs, 293, 295
cyclophosphamide, 770
Cycloset, **435–444**
  all-cause safety trial, 438, 440–441
  cardiovascular events, 440
  cardiovascular safety, 438–439
  dosing, 435–436
  drug-drug interactions, 441
  with ergot-related drugs, 441
  lactation, 441
  mechanisms of action, 436–437
  with metformin, 438
  with oral antidiabetic agents,
    437–438
  pediatric population, 441
  pharmacokinetics, 435
  phase 3 efficacy trials, 437–441
  pregnancy, 441
  with sulfonylureas, 437–438
  with thiazolidinediones, 438
  tolerability and safety, 438
  warnings, 441
cyclosporine, 116–117, 608
cyclosporine-induced nephrotoxicity,
  117
CYP2C9 pharmacogenomic studies,
  363
CYP3A4, 435
cystic fibrosis, 18
cystic-fibrosis–related diabetes
  (CFRD), 13, 18–19
cystic ovaries, 18
cystometry, 847
cytochrome-C, 29, 809
cytochrome P450 enzyme system
  3A4, 371
cytochrome P450 isoenzymes
  inhibitors, 903
cytochrome P450 system, 435
cytokines, 219, 223, 624, 641
cytoplasmic fat, 959
cytosol, 809
cytosolic glucose concentration, 671

D

Da Qing IGT and Diabetes Study,
  242–243, 316, 317t–321t, 324
Dallas Heart Study, 995, 1001
dapagliflozin, 448, 452–454, 509t,
  511t, 1024t, 1032
DASH Eating Plan, 248t
DASH-Sodium trial, 247
dawn phenomenon, 470, 474, 706–707
DCCT/EDIC, 836–837, 839, 848
de novo lipogenesis, 997
de novo stenosis, 904
dead-in-bed syndrome, 703
death, 158, 366, 680f, 702, 779, 923t,
  926f
decerebrate posture, 653
decorticate posture, 653
deep tissue infection, 679
deep-wound cultures, 944

dehydration
  chronic kidney disease, 776
  diabetic ketoacidosis and
    hyperglycemic hyperosmolar,
    621–622, 623*f*, 625, 627*f*, 628
  diabetic ketoacidosis in infants,
    children, and adolescents, 643*f*,
    644–646, 648
  elderly patients, 548, 584
  exercise, 68*t*, 69
delayed gastric emptying, 403–404,
    625, 840
dementia, 286, 709
depression
  diabetes complications, 668
  diabetes risk factors, 86
  distal symmetric polyneuropathy,
    801
  elderly patients, 547*t*, 548–549
  insulin omission, 655
  obesity and T2D, 252, 273
  psychosocial and family issues in
    children, 140, 142–144
  psychosocial issues related to
    T2D, 284–286, 289*t*, 291,
    298, 303
  self-management behaviors, 21
  self-monitoring blood glucose, 36
  youth, 302
"designer" fungus, 29
dextrose, 628, 631
diabetes. *See also under specific type*
  adults, age-adjusted county-level
    estimates among, 80*f*
  age group, prevalence by, 81*f*
  burnout, 142–143, 147
  camps, 139
  cancer and, **1018–1043**
  classification, 13–20
  complications, 52*t*, 109*t*, 669–673,
    678–682. *see also under specific
    type*
  costs associated with, ix, 239, 242,
    285, 544, 633, 668
  defined, 1
  determinants of prevalence, 81–82
  diagnosis, 1–12
  economic implications, 82–83
  education, 21–27, 60, 61*t*, 79*f*,
    105, 110, 112, 269, 284, 288,
    292, 296, 464, 592, 656, 709
  educator, 23–24, 25*t*, 61
  epidemic, 87–88
  geographic region, prevalence by,
    78–79, 100
  as a global problem, 82–87
  incidents, 81–82
  management, 140–141
  morbidity, 284
  mortality, 81–82
  number and percentage of U.S.
    population with diagnosed, 78*f*
  pathophysiology in, 705
  presentation, 705
  prevention, 57, 87, 277, 316–326,
    781
  race/ethnicity, 79*f*, 81*f*
  remission, 58, 532–534
  risk assessment, 314–315
  risk factors, 8, 83–85
  risk stratification, 87
  screening, 1–6, 9*f*, 315
  self-care behaviors/adherence,
    290*t*
  sex, 79*f*
  socioeconomic factors, 86
  U.S. adults, magnitude and trends
    of, 77–79, 80*f*, 81
Diabetes Bowel Symptom
  Questionnaire (DBSQ), 845

Diabetes Control and Complications
  Trial (DCCT), 3, 28, 107*t*, 128, 674,
  676, 698*f*, 734, 799–800, 877–878
  cardiovascular autonomic
    neuropathy, 835, 848
  chronic kidney disease (CKD),
    771
  dementia, 709
  diabetic nephropathy, 882
  diabetic retinopathy (DR), 744,
    882
  distal symmetric polyneuropathy
    (DSP), 796, 798
  hyperglycemia and diabetic
    neuropathy, 808
  hypoglycemia, 699
  microalbuminuria, 764
  ocular complications, 729
  retinopathy, 677
Diabetes Control and Complications
  Trial (DCCT)-Epidemiology
  of Diabetes Interventions and
  Complications (EDIC), 366–367,
  678–680, 683*t*–684*t*, 802
Diabetes Distress Scale (DDS17), 290*t*
Diabetes Eating Problem Survey–
  Revised (DEPS-R), 289*t*
Diabetes Empowerment Scale (DES),
  290*t*
Diabetes Knowledge Test (DKT), 290*t*
diabetes, **559–581**
Diabetes Outcome Progression Trial
  (ADOPT), 365–367, 369–370, 382
Diabetes Prevention Program (DPP), 8,
  57–58, 65, 243–245, 380–381, 528,
  669, 781, 837, 849
Diabetes Prevention Trial–Type 1
  (DPT-1) Study Group, 120
Diabetes Reduction Assessment
  with Ramipril and Rosiglitazone
  Medication (DREAM), 320*t*, 381
Diabetes Self-Care Profile (DSCP),
  290*t*
diabetes self-management, 21–22, 25*t*
Diabetes Self-Management Assessment
  Report Tool (D-SMART), 290*t*
diabetes self-management education
  (DSME), 21–24, 25*t*, 59*t*, 61–62,
  110
diabetes self-management support
  (DSMS), 21, 24, 25*t*, 59*t*
Diabetes Surgery Study, 529*f*, 533
Diabetes Treatment and Satiety Scale
  (DTSS-20), 289*t*
diabetes-focused physical examination,
  112
diabetes-related distress, 21
diabetes-related neovascularization,
  748
diabetes-specific social skills, 148
diabetic amyotrophy, 814–815
diabetic anorexia, 816
diabetic autonomic neuropathy,
  834–863
  clinical features and implications,
    838–842
  diagnosis, 842–848
  epidemiology and natural history,
    834–837
  incidence and prevalence,
    835–836
  natural history, 836
  other manifestations, 842
  pathogenesis, 837–842
  risk factors, 836–837
  symptomatic treatment of,
    850*t*–853*t*
  treatment, 848–853
diabetic bullae, 952, 960–961
diabetic cachexia, 816

diabetic cardiomyopathy, 839
diabetic cheiroarthropathy, 952–955
diabetic dermopathy, 952, 955, 956*f*
diabetic diarrhea, 838*t*, 840, 849, 852*t*
diabetic focal mononeuropathies,
  817–818
diabetic foot, 865, 867*t*, 870–871
diabetic foot ulceration (DFU),
  864–875
diabetic ketoacidosis (DKA), **621–640**
  acidosis, 651
  adolescents, **641–667**, 642
  behavioral intervention, 655
  bicarbonate, 630
  cerebral edema, 652–654
  children, **641–667**
  children, care management, 647
  children, risk factors, 641–642
  clinical and biochemical
    monitoring, 647–648
  clinical manifestations, 644–645
  complications of treatment,
    631–632, 652–654
  criteria for resolution, 630–631
  definition of, 642–643
  diagnostic criteria, 624–625, 626*t*
  differential diagnosis, 645
  disordered eating, 146
  emergency assessment, 645–646
  epidemiology, 621–622, 641–642
  exercise, 73
  fluid therapy, 628–629
  glycemic management in patients
    with T1D, 591
  hyperglycemic crisis, immediate
    follow-up care for, 631
  infants, **641–667**
  insulin, 629, 648–649
  insulin and T2D, 464
  intensive care units and non-ICU,
    561, 563
  laboratory findings, 625–626
  latent autoimmune diabetes of
    adults, 162
  management, 645–648
  neurocognitive difficulties, 148
  noncompliance, 622
  oral fluids and transition to SC
    insulin injections, 651–652
  pathophysiology, 643–644
  perioperative hyperglycemia,
    583
  phosphate, 630, 651
  potassium, 629–630, 650–651
  precipitating cause, 622–623
  pregnancy, 201, 204
  presentation, 645
  prevention, 632–633, 654–656
  programs to raise awareness,
    654–655
  psychological factors, 622
  psychosocial and family issues in
    children, 138, 141
  psychosocial issues, 641–642
  screening in high risk individuals,
    655–656
  secondary prevention in
    established patients, 655–656
  sick day management, 656
  supportive measures, 646
  symptoms and signs, 623–624
  T1D, 14, 108, 109*t*, 110
  T2D, 16
  T2D in youth, 268–269, 275
  treatment, 626, 628
  undiagnosed patients, 654–655
  volume expansion, 648
diabetic macular edema (DME), 729,
  731, 734, 741, 743, 748, 751–752
diabetic mononeuropathies, 794

diabetic nephropathy, 763, 782, 881, 927–928
  current thinking in pathophysiology of, 763–764
  genetic susceptibility, 764
diabetic peripheral neuropathy (DPN)
  atypical forms of, 794, 814–818
  classification of, 794
  current therapies, **793–833**
  definition of, 793
  distal symmetric polyneuropathy (DSP), 794, 814–818
  forms of, 794–814
diabetic radiculoplexus neuropathy (DRPN), 814–815
Diabetic Retinopathy Clinical Research Network (DRCR.net), 730, 734, 750–751
diabetic retinopathy (DR)
  ACE inhibitor, 928
  ACCORD-Eye, 675
  Action in Diabetes and Vascular Disease (ADVANCE) study, 675
  Airlie House classification, 737
  cataract extraction, 741
  chronic diabetes complications, 668, 673, 677–678
  clinical manifestations, 732t
  Diabetes Control and Complications Trial, 674, 676, 882
  diabetes screening test, 2
  emerging therapies for the treatment of, 753–755
  exercise, 68–69
  hemoglobin A1C, 677–678
  macrovascular complications, 878
  management of, **748–759**
  nonalcoholic fatty liver disease, 272
  ocular complications, 729–734
  prediabetes, 669
  pregnancy, 198–199, 200t, 206
  risk factors, 738
  T2D prevention strategies, 315
  treatment-induced diabetic SFN, 816
Diabetic Retinopathy Study (DRS), 729, 731, 749
Diabetic Retinopathy Vitrectomy Study, 734, 750
diabeticorum, 952
diabetogenic hormones, 157
diagnostic CGM, 38–39
diagnostic tests, 1009
Dialysis Outcomes and Practice Patterns Study (DOPPS), 765, 772
dialysis therapy, 761, 767, 781, 864
DiaPep277, 118–119
diarrhea, 511t, 513t, 961
diary, 39
diastolic dysfunction, 839, 999
diazoxide, 535
dicloxacillin, 944
diclofenac, 371, 422, 451–452, 770, 849
diet, 246–249, 317t–319t, 545, 547t, 552–553, 712t, 810, 1002
Dietary Approaches to Stop Hypertension (DASH), 247, 928
Dietary Guidelines for Americans, 56t
dietary interventions, 176–177, 242, 316
dietitians, 57, 60–61, 63, 201
digoxin, 371, 422, 451–452, 770, 849
dilated retinal exam, 112, 198–199, 268
dining out, 129
Dionysos Nutrition and Liver Study, 995
dipeptidyl peptidase-4 inhibitors (DPP-4), **387–400**, 596t, 612t, 777, 884, 1027

α-glucosidase inhibitors, 416, 418
antihyperglycemic agent, 509t
  with canagliflozin, 449
  cancer, 1024t, 1029–1030
  in clinical practice, 394
  combination therapy, 390t, 514–515
  to degludec, 489
  efficacy of, 388–389, 391, 393–394
  elderly patients, 553, 565
  GLP-1 receptor agonist, 401–402, 404
  GLP-1 receptor agonist and, 389
  hypoglycemia, 391, 451
  insulin and, 391
  with LX4211, 455
  mechanisms of action, 387–388
  metformin, 349, 355–357
  metformin therapy and, 389, 390t, 391, 394
  metformin therapy with, 516
  obesity and T2D, 276
  pharmacodynamic properties, 388
  pharmacokinetic properties, 388
  randomized controlled trials, 391
  sulfonylureas and, 389, 391
  thiazolidinediones and, 389, 391
  tolerability and safety, 391, 393
  triple oral combination therapy, 389, 392t
diplopia, 817
dipyridamole, 955
direct electron transfer technology, 29
direct renin inhibitor (DRI), 930
disaccharides, 416–417
disease management, 291–293
disease-modifying therapies, 809
disordered eating behavior (DEB), 140, 146, 287–288, 291, 302–303, 622, 655
disposition index (DI), 213, 214f, 264–265
disseminated granuloma annulare, 952, 957–958
distal hypothesis, 531
distal symmetric polyneuropathy (DSP), 670t, 794–814, 796t, 814–818
  age, 800
  α-lipoic acid, 810
  anticonvulsants, 813
  Charcot neuroarthropathy, 806–807
  clinical diagnosis of, 801–803
  confirmed, 802
  corneal confocal microscopy, 805
  C-peptide, 810
  diabetic foot ulcers, 806
  diagnosis of, 800
  diagnostic tests, 803–806
  disease-modifying therapies, 809–810
  epidemiology of, 795–800
  glycemic control, 809
  height, 800
  history, 801–803
  incidence and prevalence, 795–798
  intraepidermal nerve fiber density, 805
  late complications of, 806–807
  lifestyle intervention, 810
  multiple risk factor intervention, 810
  natural history of, 798–799
  nerve axon reflex and flare response, 805–806
  nerve conduction studies, 803–804
  other agents, 810

other treatment approaches, 813–814
pathogenesis, 807–809
quantitative sensory testing, 804–805
quantitative sudomotor axon reflex testing, 806
risk factors, 799–800
serotonin and norepinephrine reuptake inhibitor, 813
skin biopsy, 805
subclinical, 802
symptomatic therapies, 811
symptoms and signs, 801–803
treatment, 809–811, 813–814
tricyclic antidepressants, 813
distal tubular sodium, 776
disulfiram alcohol flush, 961, 964
diuretics, 270, 766t, 770, 772t, 776
dopamine receptor antagonists, 441, 509t, 511t
dopaminergic tone, 435
dorsal root ganglia, 808
dorsalis pedis arteries, 900
dot hemorrhages, 734
Down syndrome, 19
doxycycline, 944, 947t
D-phenylalanine, 359
DQ molecule, 99
DR haplotype DQB1*0602 gene, 14
DR haplotypes, 14
DR3/DR4 heterozygotes, 99
driving, 140, 200
Drug Enforcement Administration (DEA), 250–251
drug-eluting stents, 905
drug-induced diabetes, 19
drug-metabolizing enzymes, 363
drugs, 140, 144, 286–287, 645. See *also* drug use; medication therapy
drug-specific side effects, 369–370
dual-energy X-ray absorptiometry scan, 241, 968, 974, 979, 1009
ductal cells, 223, 393
dulaglutide, 407–408
duloxetine, 811t–812t, 813–814
duplex ultrasonography (DUS), 901
dysautonomia, 815–816
dysesthesias, 801, 815
dysfibrinolysis, 668
dysglycemia, 77, 367
dyslipidemia, 536, 752–753, 772t, 775, **908–920**
  alternative lipoprotein targets, 918–919
  American Diabetes Association and National Cholesterol Education program guidelines with the American College of Cardiology and the American Heart Association update, 911
  bariatric surgery, 524t, 533–534
  cardiometabolic risk factors and lipoprotein abnormalities, 918t
  cardiovascular disease, 885–887
  combination therapy, 915–916
  diabetic neuropathies, 808
  distal symmetric polyneuropathy, 801
  hypertension, 922
  implications for therapy, 909, 911
  lipid-lowering therapy, 1006
  macrovascular complications, 668
  management, 911, 913–915
  National Cholesterol Education Program (NCEP) Expert Panel on Detection, Evaluation and Treatment of High Blood Cholesterol in Adults (Adult Treatment Panel III), 917t

nonalcoholic fatty liver disease, 995, 999
obesity and T2D, 244–245, 269–271, 273
pathophysiology and presentation, 908–909
prediabetes, 916–917
primary goal and priorities of treatment from NCEP and ADA guidelines, 912t
T2D prevention strategies, 315
therapy, 675

E

early adult transition, 141
Early Treatment Diabetic Retinopathy Study (ETDRS), 675, 729, 731, 734, 738–739, 749, 751
eating behavior, 289t
Eating Disorder Examination-Questionnaire (EDE-Q), 289t
ectopic fat, 264
ectopic lipids, 241
edema, 383, 866t
Eighth Report of the Joint National Committee (JNC 8), 889, 921
elderly patients, 39, 69, 294–295, 297
  α-glucosidase inhibitors, 421
  chronic pain, 548, 550
  cognitive dysfunction, 548–549, 551
  community-acquired infections, 948
  dementia, 709
  depression, 547t, 548–549
  diabetes in the, **544–558**
  dialysis therapy, 769
  diet, 552–553
  dipeptidyl peptidase-4 inhibitors, 394
  environmental impact, 545
  exercise, 552
  falls, 549, 552
  functional decline, 548
  gastrointestinal disturbance, 394
  genetic predisposition, 545
  geriatric syndrome, 548–550
  glinide, 359
  Glucovance, 351
  glycemic control, 682
  goal setting, 547t, 550–551
  hearing impairment, 550
  hyperglycemia, 548
  hypoglycemia, 370–371, 547t, 550–551
  lifestyle modification, 552–553
  management strategy, 546, 547t
  metformin therapy, 345
  mortality, 622
  noninsulin hypoglycemic agents, 553–554
  oral agents, 553–554
  other commonly occurring medical conditions, 550
  other factors, 545–546
  overall approach and principles of care, 546–552
  pharmacological management of diabetes in, 553–554
  polypharmacy, 548–550
  scope of the problem, 544
  self-care barriers, 547t–548t
  socioeconomic factors, 544
  sulfonylureas and hypoglycemia, 565
  testosterone replacement therapy, 980
  treatment strategies, 547t, 552–554

urinary incontinence, 548, 550
vision impairment, 550
electrical stimulation therapies, 814
electrocardiogram (ECG), 843
electrocardiographic monitoring, 646, 650
electrolyte, 623f, 627f, 643f, 644, 646, 648
electrolyte imbalance, 628
electrophysiological testing, 753
ELEMENT trials, 493–494
embryo development, 198
embryonal cancer cells, 1021
empagliflozin, 454
emphysema, 654
emphysematous cholecystitis, 946
emphysematous cystitis, 946
emphysematous pyelonephritis, 946
employment, 294
enalapril, 209, 779
endocannabinoids, 288
endocarditis, 945
endocrinologist, 765–767
endogenous insulin secretion, 480
endometrial cancer, 1019t, 1020
endophthalmitis, 740
endoplasmic reticulum (ER) stress, 169, 213f, 221f, 222, 808–809
endothelial dysfunction, 584, 670–671, 922
endothelial function, 66, 67t, 249, 583–584, 848
endothelial nitric oxide synthase (eNOS), 441, 672f
endothelin antagonist, 782
end-stage liver disease, 996
end-stage renal disease (ESRD)
  chronic diabetes complications, 668, 676, 678
  chronic kidney disease, 760, 767–770, 776, 779, 781
  combination therapy, 511t
  diabetic foot, 866t, 887
  DPP-4 inhibitor, 395t
  elderly patients, 544
  GLP-1 receptor agonist, 407t
  obesity and T2D, 272
energy balance, 239
energy homeostasis, 218
enterovirus, 101
entrapment mononeuropathies, 818
enuresis, 655
environmental factors, 14, 86
environmental insult, 98
environmental toxins, 217
Epidemiology of Diabetes Interventions and Complications (EDIC) study, 673–674, 677, 796, 798–800, 835, 877
epidermis, 955
epidural analgesia, 586
epinephrine, 480, 585t, 702, 704t, 705–706
equilibrium dialysis, 967
erectile dysfunction, 834, 836, 841, 846, 853, 853t, 967, 973
eruptive xanthomas, 952, 958, 959f
erythema, 954, 964
erythrocytosis, 161
erythromycin, 371, 720, 852t
erythropoiesis, 975
erythropoiesis-stimulating agent (ESA), 766t, 771, 772t, 780–781
erythropoietin, 3, 779, 850t–851t
Escherichia coli, 482, 942t, 945
esophageal dysfunction, 838t, 840
estimated glomerular filtration rate (eGFR), 347, 451–451, 761, 762, 766, 769–771, 775–778, 780, 782t
estradiol, 969–971, 975

estrogen, 969
estrogen receptor-α, 971
estrone, 969
ethnicity
  diabetic foot, 866t
  distal symmetric polyneuropathy, 798
  elderly population, 545
  gestational diabetes, 182
  obesity and T2D, 245
  obesity and T2D in children, 263, 265–266, 268t
  psychosocial issues and T2D, 293, 295
  T1D, 106t
  T2D, 216, 219
  T2D prevention strategies, 315
  thiazolidinediones, 377, 379
euglycemic-hyperinsulinemic clamp studies, 343, 379
eugonadal men, 970–971, 973
EURODIAB IDDM Complications Study, 81, 621, 796–798, 800, 835–836, 840
European Male Aging Study, 970
European Medicines Agency (EMA), 393, 494–495, 851t–852t, 1029
European Nicotinamide Diabetes Intervention Trial (ENDIT), 120
European population, 314
evidence-based practice, 143
Examination of Cardiovascular Outcomes with Alogliptin versus Standard of Care (EXAMINE) trial, 391, 393
excessive fetal growth, 178, 197, 206, 209
excitatory glutamate receptors, 251
exenatide, 387, 402, 403t, 404, 405t, 404–407, 510t, 513t, 514, 517–518, 553, 777, 1005–1006
  cancer, 1028–1029
exendin-4, 387, 402
exercise, **65–76**, 1002. *See also* physical activity
  acute, effects of, 72
  aerobic, 66, 67t–68t, 70–71, 177, 247, 274, 810
  benefits, 66–67
  cardiovascular risk factors, 71–72
  compliance, 71–72
  continuous glucose monitoring, 66
  cooldown phase, 71
  diabetes prevention programs, 317t–319t
  distal symmetrical polyneuropathy, 810
  duration, 70–71
  elderly patients, 552
  exercise-related insulin adjustments, 66
  food, 73
  frequency, 70–71
  gestational diabetes, 162, 177–178
  guidelines, 69–72
  high-intensity, 70
  hyperglycemia, 66–68, 73, 75t
  hypertension, 928
  hypoglycemia, 66–67, 68t, 73–75, 75t, 702, 707–708, 711t–712t
  insulin, 73
  insulin pump, 66, 129
  intensity, 70–71
  intolerance, 838–839, 842f, 843
  lack of, 213
  moderate intensity, 70
  monitoring, 71–72
  motivation and participation, 72
  multiple-dose insulin regimens, 66
  muscle-strengthening, 70

nonalcoholic fatty liver disease, 1003
peripheral arterial disease, 902–903
pre-exercise checklist T1D, 74*t*
pregnancy, 157
progression, 71–72
resistance, 67*t*, 70–71, 274, 552, 810
risks, 67–69
screening, 69
selection of type, 69–70
self-monitoring blood glucose, 66
snack, 708
specific considerations in diabetes, 72
strength-training, 66
structure of sessions, 71
supervision, 71–72
T1D, 65–66, 73–75
T2D, 65–66, 68, 75
vigorous, 70
warm-up phase, 71
exercise physiologist, 928
exercise-related insulin adjustments, 66
exocrine cell proliferation, 393
exocrine pancreas, 18–19
extracellular fluid, 628
eye care, 745
eye complications, 921
eye exam, 613*t*, 670*t*, 743*t*
eye surgery, 582
ezetimibe, 775, 887, 911, 915

F

falls, 549, 801
familial clustering, 671
familial lipoatrophy, 959
family
  conflict, 144–146
  environment, 138
  issues, **134–155**, 294
  mythologies, 301
  physician, 765–767
  planning, 182–183
  therapy, 144
Family Environment Scale (FES), 289*t*
family-based behavioral lifestyle intervention, 273–274
family-based treatment, 134–135, 300–303
farnesoid X receptor (FXR), 1007
fasting hyperglycemia, 157
fasting lipid profile, 268, 613*t*
fasting plasma glucose (FPG)
  acarbose, 417–418
  α-glucosidase inhibitors, 421
  bariatric surgery, 529*f*
  cardiovascular autonomic neuropathy, 837
  cardiovascular events, 883
  Cycloset, 437
  degludec, 489
  detemir, 486
  diabetes after transplant, 608
  diabetes diagnosis, 1–3, 4*t*, 5–7, 9*f*
  diabetes epidemiology, 77–78, 81, 86
  empagliflozin, 454
  gestational diabetes, 173
  GLP-1 receptor agonists, 405
  Glucovance, 351
  laboratory tests, 846
  Metaglip, 350
  metformin therapy, 345–346, 348
  non-ICU settings, 589
  obesity and T2D in children, 267–268
  peripheral vascular disease, 670

rosiglitazone, 382
testosterone replacement therapy, 979
thiazolidinediones, 381
U.K. Prospective Diabetes Study, 674–675
fat, 54*t*, 85, 87, 177, 202, 213, 241, 248*t*, 317*t*
fat cell, 177, 377
fat oxidation, 240
fat stores, 218–219
fat-to-muscle ratio, 545
fatty acid chain, 486
fatty acids, 171, 202, 216, 218–219, 378, 462, 961
fatty acyl carnitine, 624
fatty acyl CoA, 624
fatty liver, 996
Fatty Liver Index, 1001
FDA Adverse Event Reporting System (FAERS), 393, 1028–1030
fecal incontinence, 841, 941*t*
feedback, 292
feet, 72, 111, 670*t*, 800
female sexual dysfunction, 838*t*, 841
fenfluramine, 251
fenofibrate, 675, 753, 886–887, 911, 915–916, 1007
Fenofibrate Intervention and Event Lowering in Diabetes (FIELD) study, 675, 886–887, 909, 911
fertility, 198, 344
fetal
  anomalies, 199
  cardiac structure, 206
  complications, 156
  condition, 206–207
  congenital malformations, 169
  death, 199
  demise, 181
  development, 198
  growth, 206–207
  growth restriction, 206
  hepatosplenomegaly, 161
  hyperglycemia, 158, 162, 170
  hyperinsulinemia, 158, 162, 209
  macrosomia, 176, 181, 207
  maternal ketoacidosis, 204
  organ development, 168
  overgrowth, 170–172
  risk, 161
  surveillance, 207
  well-being, 207
fetopathy, 158
fever, 625, 632
FIB-4 (Fibrosis-4 Score), 1001
fibrates, 675–676, 909, 913, 915, 1007, 1008*t*
fibric acid, 909
fibric acid medication, 271, 323
fibrinogen, 239
fibrinolysis, 673
fibroblasts, 952
fibrosis, 673, 996–997, 999, 1001, 1004–1005
fibrous tissue proliferation, 734, 737–738, 744
fibular nerve, 817
financial resources, 292, 296
Finnish Diabetes Prevention Study (DPS), 65, 87, 243, 315–316, 317*t*–321*t*, 322, 324, 837
Finnish Diabetes Risk Assessment (FINDRISK), 315, 324
Fistula First Initiative, 769
flavin adenine dinucleotide (FAD), 29
fluconazole, 946
fluid balance, 770

fluid intake, 632, 647, 653
fluid output, 647
fluid overload, 767
fluorescein angiography, 732*t*–733*t*, 734, 739, 751*f*
fluorescence, 37
fluoxetine, 277
fluroquinolones, 942*t*, 945
fluvastatin, 914
focal argon laser photocoagulation, 739, 748
focal laser, 732*t*–733*t*
focal neuropathies, 794, 795*t*
folate, 348
folic acid, 162, 169, 198, 200–202
follicle-stimulating hormone (FSH), 966–967, 971
food, 51, 52*f*, 52*t*, 58, 60, 73, 74*t*–75*t*, 248*t*
food additive, 217
Food and Drug Administration (FDA), 34
food diary, 39
food guide pyramid, 60
food intake, 287–288, 553, 712*t*
food record, 61
foot, 112–113, 796
  care education, 809
  deformities, 679, 866, 900
  examination, 613*t*
  infection, 941*t*, 943*t*
  ulceration, 668, 796, 802, 804–806, 866*t*, 898, 944–945
foregut hypothesis, 531–532
40/400 club, 706
fosfomycin, 942*t*
Fox M1 gene, 158
FoxO1, 223
Framingham Heart Study, 82, 84, 836, 914
frank infarction, 584
free fatty acids
  bariatric surgery, 523
  Cycloset, 436–437, 442
  diabetic ketoacidosis and hyperglycemic hyperosmolar, 623*f*, 624, 629
  diabetic ketoacidosis in infants, children and adolescents, 643*f*, 644
  dyslipidemia, 908–909
  gestational diabetes, 157
  nonalcoholic fatty liver disease, 997
  obesity and T2D, 241
  testosterone replacement therapy, 981
  thiazolidinediones, 379
free radical–mediated oxidative stress, 810
free testosterone (FT), 966–970, 973–974, 976
frequently sampled intravenous glucose tolerance test (FSIVGT), 379
fruits, 248*t*, 317*t*
functional decline, 548
fundus photography, 739, 742, 749*f*, 751*f*, 754*f*
fungal infection, 609, 948–949
fungus balls, 946
furosemide, 348, 770

G

gabapentin, 811*t*, 813
GAD-65, 162
GAD-alum vaccine, 121
gadolinium-containing contrast agents (GCCA), 771
Galega officinalis, 341

γ-aminobutyrate, 251
gangrene, 871, 898, 944
gastric
 bypass, 252–253
 restrictive procedure, 525, 532
 surgery, 58
gastric emptying studies, 845–846
gastroenterologist, 272
gastrointestinal
 disease, 239
 hormones, 532
 lipase inhibitor, 277
gastrointestinal autonomic neuropathy,
 838t, 840–841. *See* gastroparesis
gastrointestinal disturbance
 α-glucosidase inhibitors, 417,
 421–422
 combination therapy, 511t, 513t,
 517–518
 Cycloset, 438
 diabetic ketoacidosis and
 hyperglycemic hyperosmolar,
 625, 630
 DPP-4 inhibitor, 391, 394
 GLP-1 receptor agonist, 406
 insulin secretagogue, 365
 metformin, 347
 thiazolidinediones, 387
 transplant impact on other diabetes
 care, 613t
gastrointestinal rest, 586
gastrointestinal tract, 530, 960
gastroparesis, 513t, 712t, 720–721,
 835–836, 838t, 840, 851t
 cardiovascular autonomic
 neuropathy, 849
 gastric emptying studies, 845–846
 symptoms, 845
 T1D, 835–836
 T2D, 835–836
GDH pyrroloquinolinequinone (GDH-
 PQQ), 29, 32
gemfibrozil, 371, 909, 915
gene-probing technology, 216
generalized anxiety disorder, 286
Generalized Anxiety Disorder 7-Item
 Scale (GAD-7), 289t
generalized hypertrichosis, 959
gene(s). *See also under specific type*
 ABCC8, 363
 APOL1, 671
 DD polymorphism, 764
 DR haplotype DQB1*0602
 gene, 14
 Fox M1 gene, 158
 glucokinase gene, 18
 hepatic nuclear factor-1α gene, 363
 KCNJ11, 363
 KISS1 gene, 972
 NFATc4, 608
 non-HLA genes, 99
 patatin-like phospholipase A3
 (PNPLA3), 1002
 Pax3, 169
 proglucagon, 401
 transcription factor 7-like 2
 (TCF7L2), 217
 tumor suppressor p53, 1021
genetic-epigenetic insulin resistance,
 269
genetic(s)
 defects, 18
 predisposition, 216–217, 671
 susceptibility, 98–99, 101, 265,
 268t, 315, 672f
 syndromes, 19
 T2D risk factor, 221f
genital infection, 451
genito-urinary infection, 511t, 516
genotype score, 84

geriatric diabetes scale, 549
geriatric syndrome, 547t, 548–550
gestational diabetes (GDM), 1–2, 13,
 175t, 268t
 baby, 162–163
 classification, 16–17
 complications, 161
 congenital malformations,
 168–169
 costs associated with, 163
 diabetic retinopathy, 753
 diagnostic criteria, **156–167**
 diagnostic tests, alternative, 161
 differential diagnosis, 162
 epidemiology, **156–167**
 ethnicity, 172
 exercise, 177–178
 fetal overgrowth, 170–172
 glucose control, 173–181
 Hyperglycemia and Adverse
 Pregnancy Outcomes, 161
 intensive lifestyle intervention
 programs, 57
 long-term follow-up and
 prevention, 162
 management, **168–196**
 metformin therapy, 347
 mother, 162
 pathophysiology, 157–158
 population data, 156
 preeclampsia, 172
 pregnancy, treatment during,
 173–181
 prevalence, 156
 risk factors, 158
 screening tests, 158–160, 315
 still births, 169–170
 T2D risk factor, 17
 thiazolidinediones, 380
gestational hypertension, 174
ghrelin, 288, 531
Gila monster, 387, 402
Glasgow coma scale, 646
glaucoma, 740, 752
glaucoma surgery, 742
glibenclamide, 1030
gliclazide, 363, 368, 509t, 1030
glimepiride, 276, 360t, 365, 368, 389,
 392t, 449, 509t, 511t, 553, 776, 885
glinides, 323, **359–376**, 362, 369
 antidiabetic medications,
 comparison with other, 372
 cancer, 1024t, 1031
 cardiovascular outcomes, effects
 on, 368–369
 cost, 372
 pharmacologic properties and
 mechanisms of, 359–361
 safety, 371–372
 T2D, 371–372
 use and efficacy of, 367–368
glipizide, 276, 321f, 323, 349t,
 352–353, 360t, 362, 453, 509t, 511t,
 553, 776, 949
Global Partnership for Effective
 Diabetes Management, 394
glomerular filtration rate (GFR)
 anemia, 779
 chronic diabetes complications,
 669t, 678
 chronic kidney disease, 760–761,
 763–765, 767, 775
 diabetic ketoacidosis and
 hyperglycemic hyperosmolar,
 624
 hemoglobin levels, 780
 transplantation, diabetes treatment
 after, 612t, 644
glomerular hemodynamics, 840
glomerular hypertension, 763

glomerular hypertrophy, 763
glomerulosclerosis, 763
glomerulotubular imbalance, 446
glossitis, 961
GLP-1 receptor agonists, 35, 251, 276,
 612t, 721, 777
 adverse events and safety
 concerns, 406–407
 clinical trials, 404–406
 clinical use, 402–404
 diabetes and cancer, 1027, 1029
 DPP-4 inhibitor, 387, 389, 393
 elderly patients, 553
 future developments, 407–408
 glycemic control with the currently
 available, 405t
 mimetics, history of development
 and key characteristics of,
 401–402
 oral agents with, 516–517
 oral medications, 514–515
 pancreatitis, 406
 sodium-glucose cotransporter
 2, 449
 T1D, 408
 T2D, **401–415**
GLP-1 receptors (GLP-1R), 401
GLP-2, 217
glucagon, 212, 216, 342, 405, 585t,
 624, 643f, 702, 704t, 705
 failure, 701
 levels, 585–586
 secretion, 387–388
glucagon-containing α-cells, 223
glucagon-induced hypoaminoacidemia,
 952
glucagon-like peptide-1 (GLP-1)
 bariatric surgery, 526t, 531–532,
 535
 DPP-4 inhibitor, 387–388
 intensive care units and non-ICU,
 565
 metformin, 343, 356
 nonalcoholic fatty liver disease,
 1005
 sodium-glucose cotransporter 2,
 454–455
 T2D, 216–217, 401
 thiazolidinediones, 381
glucagonoma syndrome, 952
glucagon-secreting α-cells, 221
glucocorticoids, 19, 158, 591, 641, 712t
glucokinase gene, 18
glucolipotoxicity, 221f, 222–223
gluconeogenesis, 342, 585, 623, 623f,
 643–644, 1025
gluconeogenic enzymes, 623
glucoregulatory hormones, 212
glucose, 530, 626t, 627f, 647, 876–880.
 See also blood glucose levels
 control, 173–181, 175t, 610, 683t
 data, 30
 hypothesis, 673–674
 levels, 514, 799
 meter, 176
 monitoring, 28–36, **28–50**, 36–40,
 56t, 58–59, 174, 176
 oxidase, 29, 32
 oxidation, 169
 sensors, 37
 target, 173–174
 toxicity, 213f, 221f, 222, 463–464
 uptake, 343
glucose clamp studies, 485–486, 489,
 492–493
glucose dehydrogenase (GDH), 29
glucose disposal (M) value, 379
glucose homeostasis system, 217–218,
 363
glucose infusion rate (GIR), 492–493